a LANGE medical book

Basic and Clinical Endocrinology

Third Edition

Edited By

Francis S. Greenspan, MD
Clinical Professor of Medicine and Radiology
Department of Medicine, and Chief, Thyroid Clinic
University of California, San Francisco

APPLETON & LANGE
Norwalk, Connecticut/San Mateo, California

0-8385-0545-7

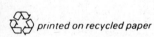 *printed on recycled paper*

 Copyright © 1991 by Appleton & Lange
A Publishing Division of Prentice Hall
Copyright © 1983 by Lange Medical Publications

92 93 94 95 / 10 9 8 7 6 5 4 3 2
Prentice Hall International (UK) Limited, *London*
Prentice Hall of Australia Pty. Limited, *Sydney*
Prentice Hall Canada, Inc., *Toronto*
Prentice Hall Hispanoamericana, S.A., *Mexico*
Prentice Hall of India Private Limited, *New Delhi*
Simon & Schuster Asia Pte. Ltd., *Singapore*
Editora Prentice Hall do Brasil Ltda., *Rio de Janeiro*
Prentice Hall, *Englewood Cliffs, New Jersey*

ISBN: 0-8385-0545-7
ISSN: 0891-2068

Production Editor: Laura K. Giesman
Designer: Steven M. Byrum

PRINTED IN THE UNITED STATES OF AMERICA

ISBN 0-8385-0545-7

90000

9 780838 505458

Table of Contents

The Authors

Claude D. Arnaud, MD
Professor of Medicine and Physiology, University of California, San Francisco, and Chief, Division of Gerontology and Geriatric Medicine, Director, Center for Biomedical Research on Aging, San Francisco.

David C. Aron, MD
Associate Professor, Case Western Reserve University School of Medicine, and Chief Endocrinology Section, Veterans Administration Medical Center, Cleveland, Ohio.

John D. Baxter, MD
Professor of Medicine and Biochemistry and Biophysics, Director of the Metabolic Research Unit, and Chief of the Division of Endocrinology, Moffitt Hospital and University of California, San Francisco.

Christopher C. Benz, MD
Associate Professor of Medicine, Cancer Research Institute, University of California, San Francisco.

Edward G. Biglieri, MD
Chief of Endocrinology, San Francisco General Hospital, and Professor of Medicine, University of California, San Francisco.

Glenn D. Braunstein, MD
Chairman, Department of Medicine, Cedars-Sinai Medical Center, Los Angeles, and Professor of Medicine, University of California, Los Angeles.

Bayard D. Catherwood, MD
Associate Professor of Medicine, Emory University, Atlanta, and Chief, Endocrinology and Metabolism Section, Veterans Administration Medical Center, Atlanta.

Felix A. Conte, MD
Professor of Pediatrics, University of California, San Francisco.

Haile T. Debas, MD
Professor and Chairman of the Department of Surgery, University of California, San Francisco.

Leonard J. Deftos, MD
Professor of Medicine, University of California, San Diego.

Clifford W. Deveney, MD
Associate Professor of Surgery, University of Pennsylvania, Philadelphia; Adjunct Associate Professor of Surgery, Medical College of Pennsylvania, Philadelphia; and Chief, Surgical Service Veterans Administration Medical Center, Philadelphia.

James W. Findling, MD
Associate Clinical Professor of Medicine, University of Wisconsin and Medical College of Wisconsin, Milwaukee.

Marie L. Foegh, MD, DSc
Associate Professor, Department of Surgery, Georgetown University, and Associate Director of Transplantation, Georgetown University, Hospital, Washington DC.

Peter H. Forsham, MD
Professor Emeritus of Medicine and Pediatrics, University of California, San Francisco.

William F. Ganong, MD
Lange Professor of Physiology, University of California, San Francisco.

Barry J. Gertz, MD, PhD
Clinical Assistant Professor of Medicine, Robert Wood Johnson Medical School, University of Medicine and Dentistry of New Jersey, and Director, Clinical Research, Merck Sharp and Dohme Research Laboratories, Rahway.

Alan Goldfien, MD
Professor Emeritus, Department of Medicine, Obstetrics, Gynecology, and Reproductive Sciences, University of California, San Francisco, and Senior Staff, Cardiovascular Research Institute, University of California, San Francisco.

Charles J. Grossman, PhD
Professor, Xavier University, Cincinnati; Associate Professor of Medicine, University of Cincinnati,

and Research Physiologist, Veterans Administration Medical Center, Cincinnati.

Francis S. Greenspan, MD
Clinical Professor of Medicine and Radiology, Department of Medicine, and Chief, Thyroid Clinic, University of California, San Francisco.

Susan L. Greenspan, MD
Instructor in Medicine, Harvard Medical School, and Associate in Medicine, Beth Israel Hospital, Boston.

Melvin M. Grumbach, MD
Edward B. Shaw Professor and Chairman, Department of Pediatrics, University of California, San Francisco.

Markus Hecker, PhD
Senior Scientist, The William Harvey Research Institute, St. Bartholomew's Hospital Medical College, Charterhouse Square, London.

Philip G. Hoffman, Jr., MD, PhD†
Associate Clinical Professor of Obstetrics, Gynecology, and Reproductive Sciences, University of California, San Francisco, and Associate Clinical Director, Reproductive Medicine, Syntex Research, Palo Alto.

John P. Kane, MD, PhD
Professor of Medicine and Biochemistry and Biophysics, University of California, San Francisco.

John H. Karam, MD
Professor of Medicine, Chief Clinical Endocrinology, University of California, San Francisco.

Claudio E. Kater, MD
Associate Professor of Medicine, and Director, Adrenal and Hypertension Unit, Division of Endocrinology, Escola Paulista de Medicina, Sao Paulo, Brazil.

John L. Kitzmiller, MD
Professor and Chief of Obstetrics, University of California, San Francisco.

Felix O. Kolb, MD
Clinical Professor of Medicine, University of California, San Francisco.

Brian J. Lewis, MD
Clinical Professor of Medicine, Cancer Research Institute, University of California, San Francisco.

Mary J. Malloy, MD
Clinical Professor of Pediatrics and Medicine, University of California, San Francisco.

Mary C. Martin, MD
Assistant Professor of Obstetrics, Gynecology, and Reproductive Sciences, University of California, San Francisco.

Scott E. Monroe, MD
Adjunct Associate Professor of Obstetrics, Gynecology, and Reproductive Sciences, University of California, San Francisco.

Sean J. Mulvihill, MD
Assistant Professor of Surgery, School of Medicine, University of California, San Francisco.

David J. Ramsay, DM, DPhil
Professor of Physiology, University of California, San Francisco.

Peter W. Ramwell, PhD
Professor of Physiology and Biophysics Georgetown University Medical Center Washington, D.C.

Basil Rapoport, MB, ChB
Professor of Medicine, University of California, San Francisco, and Staff Physician, Veterans Administration Medical Center, San Francisco.

Neil M. Resnick, MD
Assistant Professor of Medicine, Harvard Medical School, and Chief of Geriatrics, Brigham & Woman's Hospital, Boston.

Patricia R. Salber, MD, FACP, FACEP
Assistant Clinical Professor of Medicine, University of California, San Francisco.

E. Martin Spencer, MD, PhD
Director, Laboratory of Growth and Development, Children's Hospital, San Francisco.

Gordon J. Strewler, MD
Associate Professor of Medicine, University of California, and Chief, Endocrine Unit, Veteran's Administration Medical Center, San Francisco.

Dennis M. Styne, MD
Chair, Department of Pediatrics, University of California, Davis School of Medicine, Sacramento.

Robert N. Taylor, MD, PhD
Assistant Professor, Department of Obstetrics, Gynecology, and Reproductive Sciences, University of California, San Francisco.

---

†deceased

J. Blake Tyrrell, MD
Associate Clinical Professor of Medicine, Metabolic Research Unit, University of California, San Francisco.

Lawrence W. Way, MD
Professor of Surgery, University of California, San Francisco, and Chief of Surgical Service, Veterans Administration Medical Center, San Francisco.

John A. Williams, MD, PhD
Professor of Physiology and Internal Medicine, and Chair, Department of Physiology, University of Michigan, Ann Arbor.

Clinton W. Young, MD
Assistant Clinical Professor of Medicine, University of California, San Francisco.

Preface

The third edition of *Basic & Clinical Endocrinology* is a compact yet comprehensive and authoritative review of the rapidly expanding field of endocrinology, in which new concepts, new diagnostic techniques, and new therapeutic methods are continually being developed. For example, the recent advances in molecular biology have greatly enhanced our understanding of hormone secretion and action. The reader will not only be brought up-to-date on such advances and concepts but will also benefit from the extensive research and clinical experience of the authors, who place these advances in proper perspective and present them in a well written and easily understandable text.

Distinctive Features

This book provides comprehensive coverage of the endocrine system in its usual scope (Pituitary, Thyroid, Adrenal, Gonads, Parathyroid, Pancreas) as well as coverage of neuroendocrine, renal, gastrointestinal, and paracrine and autocrine hormones. In addition, specific areas of endocrinology such as growth, puberty, sexual differentiation, lipoprotein metabolism, obesity, metabolic bone disease, aging, and others are carefully reviewed with particular reference to clinical problems. Carefully chosen illustrations add clarity to the discussions, and decision matrix charts provide guidance in therapy. In every subject area, the clinical aspects of each endocrine problem are discussed by experienced clinicians with emphasis on the practical management of clinical problems. Current references for further reading are appended to each chapter.

Each chapter has been reviewed and updated to include the most recent concepts of pathophysiology and therapy. Several new chapters have been added and several others rewritten by new authors. These include:

- Immunoendocrinology: An analysis of the important interrelationships between the endocrine and immune systems.
- The Eicosanoids: A review of prostaglandins, thromboxanes, leukotrienes and related compounds.
- Hormones and Cancer: The current status of hormones in the diagnosis and treatment of malignancies.
- Humoral Manifestations of Malignancy: A discussion of hormones produced by tumors and how they may be used in the diagnosis and management of the neoplasm, as well as the potential physiologic significance of these substances.
- Geriatric Endocrinology: The changes in the endocrine system that occur with aging and how these changes modify the diagnosis and treatment of endocrine disorders in the elderly.
- The Appendix contains a very useful Table of Normal Hormone Test Results, in both American and International units.

Intended Audience

This book will serve the needs of first- and second-year medical students taking an initial endocrinology course, as well as those taking endocrinology electives during clinical years. It will also allow residents, fellows, family physicians, internists, and other subspecialists to remain fully current on the latest scientific and clinical information in endocrinology.

Francis S. Greenspan, MD

San Francisco, CA
June 1990

Mechanisms of Hormone Secretion & Action

1

John A. Williams, MD, PhD

Hormones are molecules that are synthesized and secreted by specialized cells, released into the blood, and exert biochemical effects on target cells at a distance from their site of origin. Some hormones such as thyroid-stimulating hormone act exclusively on one target tissue (in this case the thyroid gland); other hormones such as insulin and thyroid hormone act on many cell types, including (in this example) liver, brain, and skin. The specificity of hormone action is determined by the presence of specific hormone receptors on or in these target cells. The cellular response, however, is determined by the genetic programming of the particular cell. Thus, the same hormone may have different actions on different tissues. For example, adrenal glucocorticoids cause cytolysis of lymphocytes but induce enzymes necessary for the production of glucose in the liver.

Classes of Hormones
(Table 1–1)

Hormones have diverse molecular structures ranging from single modified amino acids (epinephrine) through lipids (estrogen, cortisol) to proteins (glucagon, insulin, growth hormone). In correlating properties of hormones with physiologic actions, it is generally useful to categorize them as (1) peptides and proteins, (2) steroids, and (3) amines or amino acid derivatives (Table 1–1). This listing is representative and not complete, since new molecules with hormonal activity are continually being discovered. For example, an area of investigation that is particularly active at present is the identification of new gastrointestinal hormones.

Hormones as Regulatory Molecules

Hormones make up one class of regulatory molecules; they act in ways similar to other regulatory molecules such as the neurotransmitters, paracrine agents, and metabolites. In general, the mechanism of intercellular regulation consists of perception of a stimulus by a cell by means of a specialized cell receptor, followed by the cellular response. In the case of hormone action, the stimulating hormone becomes bound to its

Acronyms Used in This Chapter	
ACTH	Adrenocorticotropic hormone
ADP	Adenosine diphosphate
AMP	Adenosine monophosphate
ATP	Adenosine triphosphate
AUG	Adenine-uridine-guanine
cAMP	Cyclic adenosine monophosphate
cGMP	Cyclic guanosine monophosphate
DAG	Diacylglycerol
DNA	Deoxyribonucleic acid
DOPA	Dihydroxyphenylalanine
FSH	Follicle-stimulating hormone
GDP	Guanosine diphosphate
GnRH	Gonadotropin-releasing hormone
GRE	Glucocorticoid regulatory element
GTP	Guanosine triphosphate
hCG	Human chorionic gonadotropin
HRE	Hormone-responsive element
IGF	Insulinlike growth factor
LH	Luteinizing hormone
mRNA	Messenger ribonucleic acid
MSH	Melanocyte-stimulating hormone
NAD	Nicotinamide adenine dinucleotide
PNMT	Phenylethanolamine-N-methyltransferase
RNA	Ribonucleic acid
SRP	Signal recognition particle
TRH	Thyrotropin-releasing hormone
TSH	Thyroid-stimulating hormone (thyrotropin)

specific receptor on or in the cell, and the result is a cascade of intracellular events including integration of several stimuli and amplification of the original bound stimulus, culminating in the cellular response. The stimulus may consist of only a few molecules of hormone per target cell. Intracellular amplification generally involves either intracellular messengers such as cAMP and Ca^{2+} or the synthesis of new RNA and protein. Cellular regulation by hormones, then, follows the same general pattern of **cell activation** observed in the control of other biologic processes; examples are the development of an egg following fertilization, the contraction of muscle following electrical excitation, and the activation, following ex-

Table 1–1. Classes of hormones based on structure.

Peptides and Proteins		Steroids	Amines
Glycoprotein	**Polypeptides**	**Steroids**	**Amines**
Follicle-stimulating hormone (FSH) Human chorionic gonadotropin (hCG) Luteinizing hormone (LH) Thyroid-stimulating hormone (TSH)	Adrenocorticotropic hormone (ACTH) Angiotensin Calcitonin Cholecystokinin Erythropoietin Gastrin Glucagon Growth hormone Insulin Insulinlike growth peptides (somatomedins) Melanocyte-stimulating hormone (MSH) Nerve growth factor Oxytocin Parathyroid hormone Prolactin Relaxin Secretin Somatostatin Vasopressin (ADH)	Aldosterone Cortisol Estradiol Progesterone Testosterone Vitamin D	Epinephrine Norepinephrine Thyroxine (T_4) Triiodothyronine (T_3)

posure to antigen, of a quiescent lymphocyte into one that actively synthesizes specific antibody.

Hormone Specificity Through Unique Receptors

Binding sites for peptide hormones and catecholamines are generally large glycoproteins on or in cellular membranes, including the plasma membrane, Golgi complex, and (in some cases) nuclear membrane. Hormones initially bind to receptors on the cell surface membrane (plasma membrane) that is exposed to the cell's environment. It is not clear whether binding sites in intracellular membranes, such as those on the Golgi complex, endoplasmic reticulum, and nuclear membrane, play a role in hormone action or are merely being transported to or from the plasma membrane as part of a general turnover of membrane proteins. In contrast to polypeptide hormones, the known receptors for steroids and thyroid hormones are located chiefly within the cell. Steroid receptors are located in the cytoplasm and nucleus; thyroid receptors are located in the plasma membrane, nucleus, and mitochondria. Steroid and thyroid hormones are small lipophilic molecules that are taken up through the cell membranes. Although the mechanism of cellular penetration is not fully understood, passive diffusion may operate in some situations and specific transport processes in others. Once inside the cell, these hormones interact with intracellular receptors. In some cases, the action of these hormones may be initiated by their initial interactions with cell membrane receptors.

While receptors (as distinct from binding proteins) must have the potential to be coupled to a biologic response, the receptor itself is a separate unit involved with recognition. In general, hormone-receptor interactions are noncovalent; they are reversible, involving hydrogen bonding, hydrophobic, and electrostatic forces. In the case of membrane receptors, which are normally coupled to an effector protein (adenylate cyclase, phospholipase C), addition of a new receptor by cell fusion or reimplantation of a solubilized receptor to a previously unresponsive cell possessing the effector system will allow that cell to respond to that hormone.

Abnormalities in or absences of specific receptors are now known to underlie some pathologic states, including insulin resistance, testicular feminization, and certain types of dwarfism, diabetes insipidus, and pseudohypoparathyroidism.

SYNTHESIS & SECRETION OF HORMONES

POLYPEPTIDE & AMINE HORMONES

The cells that secrete polypeptide hormones have many common structural features (Fig 1–1) related to the synthesis, packaging, and release of these molecules. Polypeptide hormones, along with other proteins destined for export from the cell, are synthesized on membrane-bound ribosomes and then sequestered in the cisternae of the endoplasmic reticulum. By contrast, proteins destined to remain in the cell are synthesized on free ribosomes.

Initially, the messenger RNA (mRNA) specific for the polypeptide hormone attaches to a free ribosome, and this is followed by initiation of translation at an adenine-uridine-guanine (AUG) initiation codon (Fig 1–2). Translation continues until a portion of the nas-

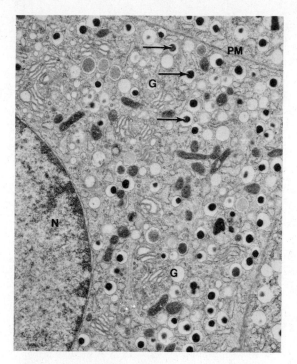

Figure 1–1. Electron micrograph of a portion of a pancreatic B cell, showing the features of cells secreting polypeptide hormones. N, nucleus; PM, plasma membrane; G, Golgi complex; arrows, granules. (Courtesy of EP Reaven.)

cent peptide called the "signal sequence" emerges from the ribosome. For polypeptide hormones, the signal sequence is located at the amino terminal of the nascent peptide. This sequence binds with high affinity to a ribonucleoprotein complex called the signal recognition particle (SRP). SRP is composed of 5 polypeptides and a 7S RNA that may base-pair with and so activate ribosomal RNA. After SRP selects and separates out nascent secretory protein-ribosome complexes, it then binds to an SRP receptor of "docking protein" in the endoplasmic reticulum membrane. The nascent polypeptide is then extruded, signal peptide first, through the membrane of the endoplasmic reticulum and into its lumen. While the signal sequence usually contains a number of hydrophobic amino acids, there is no common sequence between secretory proteins, and the mechanism of passage across the membrane remains largely unknown.

The complete molecule, including the signal peptide, is referred to as a **prehormone;** its lifetime is very short, however, as the signal peptide is rapidly cleaved off by a trypsinlike enzyme present in the endoplasmic reticulum.

In many cases, further modifications of the hormone occur before its secretion, such as the addition of sugars to the glycoprotein hormones hCG, TSH, LH, and FSH. If extra amino acids are still present following cleavage of the signal peptide, this form of the molecule is referred to as a **prohormone.** In the case of

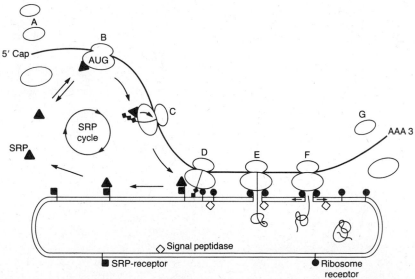

Figure 1–2. Synthesis and sequestration of polypeptide hormones. Synthesis begins at the left as ribosomal subunits aggregate (*A*) and begin to read the mRNA (*B*). The signal recognition particle (SRP) then binds to a "signal sequence" of the nascent polypeptide (*C*) and subsequently binds to an SRP receptor in the membrane of the endoplasmic reticulum (*D*). Ribosome receptors help to stabilize this interaction. The nascent polypeptide is then extruded into the lumen of the endoplasmic reticulum (*E*) and released (*F*). The amino terminal signal sequence is cleaved by a signal peptidase and the ribosome dissociates and is recycled (*G*). SRP is also recycled after the ribosome attaches to the endoplasmic reticulum. (Reproduced and modified, with permission, from Walter P, Lingappa VR: *Annu Rev Cell Biol* 1986;2:499.)

insulin, the prohormone proinsulin is a single chain, which allows folding and apposition of the 2 ends of the molecule so that interchain disulfide bonds can be correctly formed. When the middle sequence of proinsulin, the connecting (C) peptide, is removed, the mature 2-chain form of insulin remains.

In some cases, the prohormone may be the precursor for multiple peptides and is referred to as a **polyprotein.** The best-studied example is pro-opiomelanocortin, which in different portions of the pituitary and brain is cleaved to yield different peptides, including ACTH, MSH, and β-endorphin.

Following synthesis and sequestration within the lumen of the endoplasmic reticulum, the newly synthesized hormone moves to the Golgi region by vesicular transport and is there packaged into granules or vesicles (Fig 1–3). This intracellular transport is guided by microtubules and can be blocked by drugs such as colchicine that disrupt microtubules. It is in the Golgi region that terminal glycosylation occurs as well as conversion of prohormones to mature hormones. In some cases, substances such as proteins, amines (eg, dopamine), ATP, and Ca^{2+} are packaged along with the hormone into secretory granules. In this form the hormone is stored within the cell until its secretion is required. Storage pools allow the secretion of hormones at a rate much higher than the synthetic rate for brief periods. Since the prohormone molecules must be distinguished from proteins destined for immediate or "constitutive secretion," which follow a different cellular pathway, distinct sorting sequences or receptors are presumed to be involved in directing the prohormone to the secretory granule.

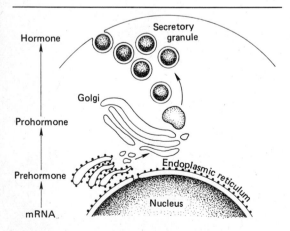

Figure 1–3. Intracellular transport of protein from the endoplasmic reticulum to the Golgi complex, packaging of newly synthesized polypeptide hormone into secretory granules, and release of hormone by exocytosis. At left are listed the molecular forms of the hormone (or information coding for the hormone) present in that portion of the cell.

Thyroid Hormones

The synthesis of thyroid hormones proceeds in part by the steps of synthesis and packaging discussed above in that thyroid hormones are first synthesized within the matrix of a large glycoprotein, thyroglobulin (Fig 1–4). Newly synthesized thyroglobulin is packaged in the Golgi region into vesicles and secreted into a specialized compartment, the follicular lumen. During this process of secretion, iodide that has been transported into the thyroid is oxidized by a peroxidase located on the apical plasma membrane. Oxidized iodine combines covalently with tyrosine residues of the protein to form mono- and diiodotyrosine. Two iodotyrosine residues then undergo a coupling reaction to form iodothyronine while still within the thyroglobulin matrix. The mature thyroglobulin in the follicular lumen thus can be considered a prohormone, since it contains a number of potential thyroid hormone molecules within its structure.

Conversion of the prohormone thyroglobulin to thyroid hormone requires phagocytosis or pinocytosis of colloid from the thyroid follicular lumen followed by lysosomal digestion. The released thyroid hormone then leaves the cell by an unknown avenue. The supply of thyroid hormone stored within follicular lumens may be sufficient to maintain normal secretory rates for several months. For more information on thyroid hormones, see Chapter 9.

Catecholamines

Cells that secrete the catecholamine hormones epinephrine and norepinephrine are similar to those that secrete polypeptide hormones in that they contain prominent secretory granules. The process of catecholamine synthesis and packaging is somewhat different, however (Fig 1–5). The endoplasmic reticulum and Golgi complex synthesize the secretory granule containing catecholamine transporters, the enzyme dopamine β-hydroxylase, and other proteins in a manner similar to the way they produce secretory granules for polypeptide hormones. The catecholamine hormones themselves, however, are synthesized directly from tyrosine by a series of enzymatic steps (see Chapter 13) and ultimately concentrated in the secretory granule. Tyrosine is converted to DOPA, which is then converted to dopamine in the cytoplasm. Dopamine is taken up by the catecholamine transporter in the granule membrane and converted in the granule to norepinephrine. Cells of the adrenal medulla, unlike most sympathetic neurons, also contain the enzyme phenylethanolamine-N-methyltransferase (PNMT) that catalyzes the conversion of norepinephrine to epinephrine. This enzyme is in the cytoplasm, so norepinephrine must leave the granule to be methylated. Because both norepinephrine and epinephrine can be taken up by isolated granules, an equilibrium must exist between the granules and the cytoplasm, though most of the catecholamine is stored in the granules

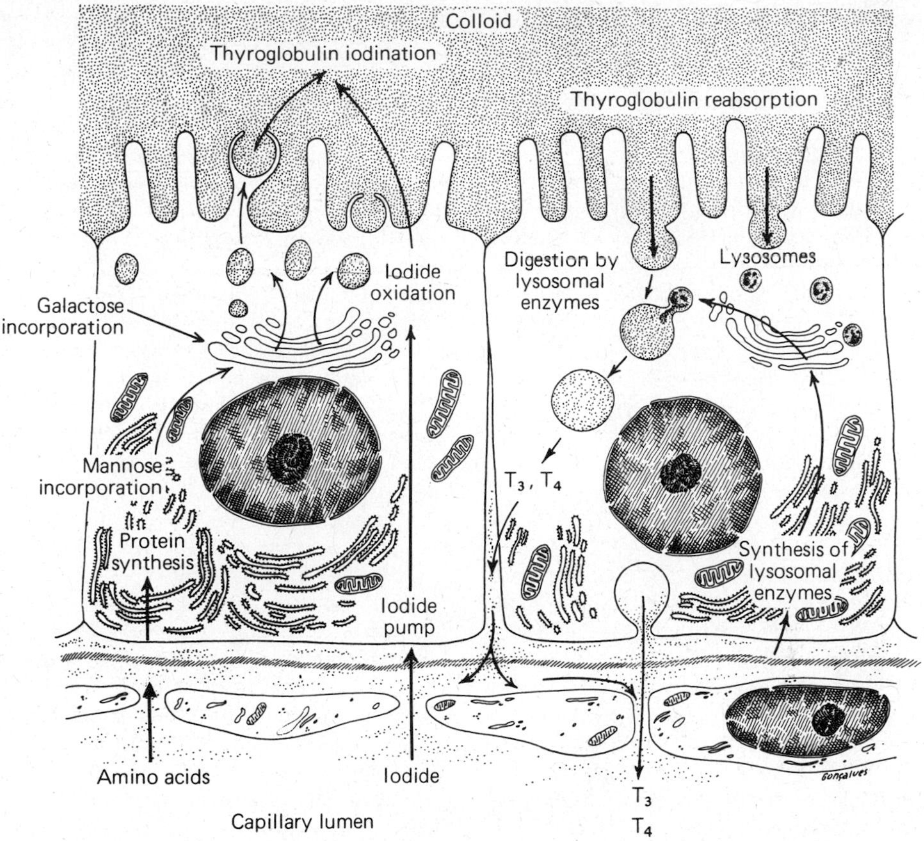

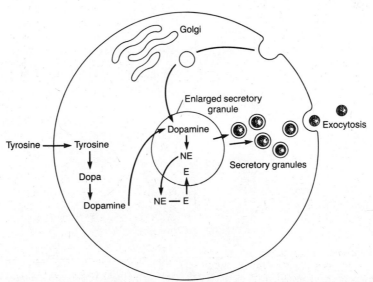

Figure 1–4. Processes of synthesis and iodination of thyroglobulin **(left)** and its reabsorption and digestion **(right)**. These events occur in the same cell. (Reproduced, with permission, from Junqueira LC, Carneiro J, Kelley R: *Basic Histology,* 6th ed. Appleton & Lange, 1989.)

Figure 1–5. Synthesis and packaging of norepinephrine (NE) and epinephrine (E). Tyrosine is converted in the cytoplasm to dopamine, which is concentrated within secretory granules and converted to NE and E. Following release of the granule contents, the empty vesicles or their membranes are recycled through the Golgi complex and then refilled.

complexed with ATP and proteins of poorly understood function called chromogranins. All of the granule contents are released together when the granule fuses with the plasma membrane.

Protein & Amine Hormones (Stimulus-Secretion Coupling)

Secretory granules store enough polypeptide and catecholamine hormones to maintain normal secretory rates for hours to days. Variations in the rate of hormone secretion into the blood are acutely caused by control of the rate at which secretory granule contents are released from the cell by exocytosis. In this process, the membrane surrounding the secretory granule fuses with the cell membrane, the intervening membrane breaks down, and the contents of the granule are released into the extracellular space. Calcium ions are necessary for fusion to occur; they play an important role in the control of secretion. The concentration of cytoplasmic Ca^{2+} is maintained at around 10^{-7} mol/L, which is much lower than the concentrations outside the cell and within certain intracellular organelles such as the endoplasmic reticulum and mitochondria. In the process of stimulus-secretion coupling, the agent inducing secretion acts on a receptor on the endocrine cell to open channels in the membrane selective for Ca^{2+}, which either allows Ca^{2+} to enter the cell (resulting in electrical changes or action potentials) or releases Ca^{2+} stored in intracellular organelles into the cytoplasm. The latter effect is initiated by the receptor activating a phospholipase C, which hydrolyzes phosphatidylinositides. One of the products of this cleavage, inositol trisphosphate, acts as an intracellular messenger to release stored Ca^{2+}. Another product, diacylglycerol (DAG), activates protein kinase C. This process is similar to the action of many hormones, which is discussed in the Intracellular Messengers section, below (see Fig 1–16). The increased concentrations of cytoplasmic Ca^{2+} and DAG then trigger fusion of the secretory granule and exocytosis of the hormone. Exocytosis also involves ATP, GTP, other cytoplasmic proteins, and probably a release site or receptor protein in the plasma membrane.

Endocrine cells are now known to contain contractile proteins such as actin and myosin. There is increasing evidence that these proteins may be important both in moving secretory granules to the plasma membrane and bringing about their subsequent fusion. Along with Ca^{2+} in some secretory cells, cAMP also plays an ancillary role in the control of hormone secretion. Specific Ca^{2+}- and cAMP-activated protein kinases are probably involved, as discussed later in the section on hormone action.

STEROID HORMONES

In contrast to polypeptide hormones, appreciable amounts of steroid hormones are not stored within the cells that produce them. Steroid hormones are able to pass through membranes and leave the cell rapidly after synthesis. As a result, the rate of secretion of most steroid hormones is controlled by the rate of synthesis. Steroid synthesis begins with cholesterol, and the various steps (primarily oxidative) in synthesis take place within the cytoplasm, smooth endoplasmic reticulum, and mitochondria. Cells secreting steroids generally contain an abundant supply of these organelles (Fig 1–6) plus prominent lipid droplets containing the cholesterol precursor.

Control of the rate of steroid synthesis (Fig 1–7) is

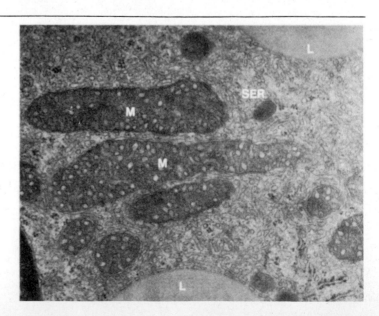

Figure 1–6. Electron micrograph of a portion of a cell from human adrenal cortex showing the common features of steroid-secreting cells. M, mitochondrion; L, lipid droplet; SER, smooth endoplasmic reticulum. (Courtesy of JA Long.)

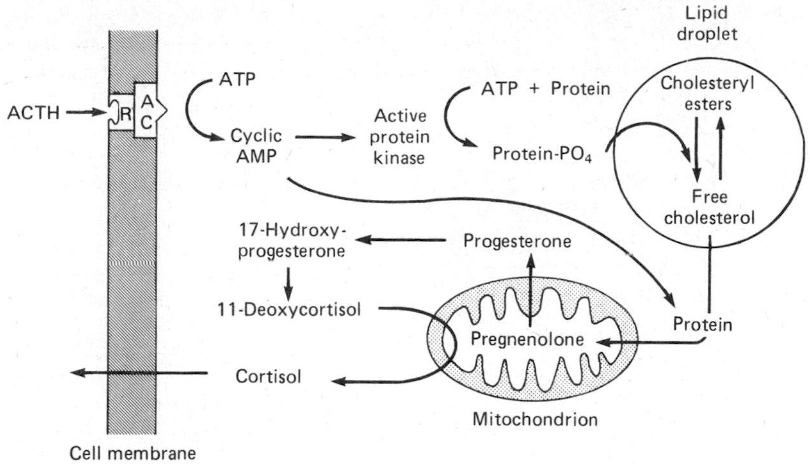

Figure 1–7. Synthesis and secretion of the steroid hormone cortisol from the adrenal cortex in response to stimulation by ACTH. ACTH binds to specific receptors on the cell membrane, activates adenylate cyclase, and increases the formation of cAMP. Cyclic AMP, by activating protein kinase, brings about increased synthesis of pregnenolone from cholesterol. Pregnenolone is subsequently converted through several intermediates to cortisol, leaves the cell, and enters the circulation.

by regulation of rate-limiting enzymes in the biosynthetic pathway—specifically, the initial hydroxylations and side-chain cleavage of cholesterol within the mitochondrion that result in the production of pregnenolone. In the case of adrenal and gonadal steroids, whose synthesis is controlled by tropic hormones, the stimulating hormone interacts with a specific receptor that leads to activation of adenylate cyclase and a rise in cAMP. Cyclic AMP then brings about a change in the activity of enzymes that are rate-limiting for steroid synthesis. This process also requires the synthesis of new protein that is rapidly turning over; the role of these proteins is as yet unknown.

Ca^{2+} also plays a role in the regulation of steroid synthesis. Ca^{2+} is necessary in the adrenal cortex both for ACTH to increase the level of cAMP and for the subsequent action of cAMP. In the mitochondria of kidney tubule cells, the level of Ca^{2+} appears to be an important regulator in the production of another steroid hormone, 1,25-dihydroxycholecalciferol, which is the active form of vitamin D.

HORMONE ACTION

HORMONE RECEPTORS

Hormone receptors on or in cells have 2 distinct roles: to distinguish a particular hormone from other hormones and regulatory molecules and to translate the hormonal signal into an appropriate cellular response. A receptor must have an affinity for its hormone that is high enough in relation to the concentration of the hormone in the blood so that the amount of hormone-receptor complex will increase or decrease in response to a change in the level of hormone present in the cell's environment. To ensure specificity, the affinity of the receptor for its hormone must be much higher than its affinity for other hormones. In general, the concentration of hormones in blood is 10^{-11} to 10^{-7} mol/L.

Kinetics of Hormone Binding

Biochemical studies of the properties of hormone receptors employ radiolabeled hormone and either intact target cells or a subcellular fraction prepared from the target cell that contains the receptor. Initially, hormone-receptor binding occurs as a bimolecular reaction:

$$[H] + [R] \underset{k_2}{\overset{k_1}{\rightleftharpoons}} [HR] \qquad \dots (1)$$

where [H] is the concentration of free hormone, [R] the concentration of free receptor, [HR] the concentration of the hormone-receptor complex, and k_1 and k_2 the rate constants for association and dissociation, respectively. When such a system is at equilibrium, the rates of the forward and backward reactions are equal, and

$$\frac{[H][R]}{[HR]} = \frac{k_2}{k_1} = K_d \qquad \dots (2)$$

where K_d is the equilibrium dissociation constant, a measure of the receptor's affinity for the hormone. Since the biologic response to the hormone is controlled by a signal generated in proportion to the number of hormone-receptor complexes, the equation can be rearranged as

$$\text{Biologic response} \propto [HR] = [H][R]\frac{1}{K_d} \quad \ldots \text{(3)}$$

In addition to the concentration of the free hormone, the concentration of receptors ([R]) and their affinity (K_d) influence the biologic response. It is thus important to be able to determine these parameters.

For any value of K_d and with the total number of receptors ([R_0]) remaining constant, the number of hormone-receptor complexes, usually referred to as "bound hormone," shows a predictable hyperbolic relationship with regard to the concentration of free hormone (Fig 1–8). At high concentrations of hormone, [HR] approaches a maximum equal to [R_0], since all of the receptor sites are filled; at half-maximal occupancy, when [R] = [HR], the free hormone concentration equals K_d. To make the data easier to interpret, various mathematic transformations are usually used, of which the most common is the Scatchard plot. Since [R_0] = [R] + [HR], we can substitute [R_0] − [HR] for [R] in equation (2) and rearrange to yield

$$\frac{[HR]}{[H]} = \frac{[R_0] - [HR]}{K_d} = \frac{[HR]}{K_d} + \frac{[R_0]}{K_d} \quad \ldots \text{(4)}$$

Since, in this equation, [R_0] and K_d are constants, the equation describes a straight line when bound/free hormone ([HR]/[H]) is plotted against bound hormone ([HR]) (Fig 1–8B). The slope of this line yields the K_d (slope = $-1/K_d$), whereas the line cuts the x axis at [R_0], the binding capacity.

In general, the binding of steroid and thyroid hormones (and some polypeptide hormones) to target cells or semipurified receptors results in linear Scatchard plots. The affinity (K_d) of most receptors is in the range of 10^{-10} to 10^{-8} mol/L, and the total number of receptors, [R_0] = 4000–100,000/cell.

In the case of certain polypeptide hormones, however, such as insulin, the binding data yield a curved rather than a linear Scatchard plot (Fig 1–8C). This curved plot may indicate 2 or more classes of specific receptors of differing binding affinity. The curvilinear Scatchard plot for hormone-receptor interaction could also result from negative cooperative interactions among a homogeneous class of receptors. It has been proposed that the binding of a hormone molecule to one receptor would decrease the affinity of the surrounding receptors for the same hormone. Evidence has been presented for negative cooperative interactions in the binding of insulin, although the issue is controversial.

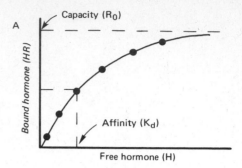

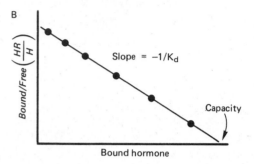

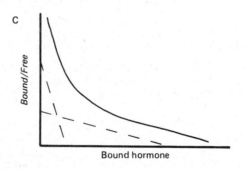

Figure 1–8. Binding of hormone to its specific receptor. **A:** Plot of bound versus free hormone over a range of free hormone concentrations. The dashed line indicates the asymptote; the value of free hormone at which half the receptors are saturated is the K_d or affinity constant. **B:** Scatchard transformation of the data in (A). The linear plot is indicative of a single binding site. **C:** Curvilinear Scatchard plot. The dashed lines indicate the contributions of 2 separate binding sites the sum of whose occupancy yields the curvilinear Scatchard plot.

Relation of Hormone-Receptor Occupancy to Biologic Response

The simplest relationship between receptor occupancy and the evoked biologic response is seen when there is a close correlation between the concentration of hormone required to occupy the receptor and for induction of the biologic response (Fig 1–9). For example, the fractional occupancy of glucocorticoid receptors in cultured hepatoma cells parallels induction of the enzyme tyrosine aminotransferase. In other

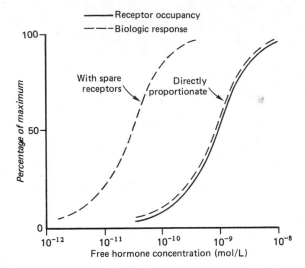

Figure 1–9. Relationship between receptor occupancy and induced biologic response as free hormone concentration is increased. Receptor occupancy is 50% of maximum when the free hormone concentration equals the K_d of the receptor.

cases, only a small percentage of the hormone receptors must be occupied to generate a maximal response (Fig 1–9). These additional receptors, which are occupied when hormone concentration reaches a level above that necessary to induce the maximal biologic response, are termed "spare" or reserve receptors. All the receptors are identical, potentially functional, and contribute to hormone sensitivity. An example is the stimulation of glucose transport in fat and muscle cells by insulin; in these cells, occupancy of only 2–10% of the insulin receptors leads to a maximal increase in the rate of glucose transport. This relationship increases the sensitivity of the system and in the case of the fat cell allows a receptor with a K_d of about 10^{-9} mol/L to respond to plasma concentrations of insulin that are approximately 100 times lower. Since "spare" receptors increase hormone sensitivity (equation [3]), a decrease in the number of spare receptors produced either by regulatory processes or by experimental manipulation leads to a decrease in hormone sensitivity (measured as the concentration of hormone necessary to elicit a half-maximal response). The maximal response of the tissue, however, is preserved if sufficient hormone is presented to the cell.

Regulation of Receptor Concentration

The number of receptors for polypeptide and catecholamine and, to a lesser extent, steroid hormones is extensively regulated by the homologous hormone and in some cases by other hormones. Most commonly, negative regulation of the number of hormone receptors occurs in response to changes in plasma hormone levels. In response to a high plasma concentration of the hormone, the number of receptors decreases— "down-regulation" or "densitization"—resulting in reduced sensitivity of the target cell. An example of this is seen in obesity, where high circulating levels of insulin are associated with a decreased number of functional insulin receptors. Regulation in the opposite direction ("up-regulation") is seen in the developing ovarian follicle, where increasing local concentrations of estrogen and FSH increase the number of receptors to luteinizing hormone (LH).

Regulation of the number of polypeptide receptors in the plasma membrane is believed to be due in part to the fact that receptors, like other membrane proteins, are not static but are being continually synthesized, inserted into the plasma membrane, removed, and degraded.

Removal of Receptors

The process of removing receptors from the cell surface plasma membrane is related in part to the phenomenon of cellular entry of polypeptide hormones. Since hormones have been isolated, characterized, and radioactively labeled to high specific activity, more is known about hormones than about their receptors. Convincing ultrastructural and biochemical evidence is now available that polypeptide hormones and growth factors such as insulin, prolactin, and nerve growth factor rapidly penetrate target cells, with all or part of the molecules remaining structurally intact. The best understood model for the receptor-mediated entry of hormones and other proteins is based on the entry of low-density lipoproteins and some polypeptide hormones into fibroblasts. The ligand binds to receptors located over specialized areas termed "coated pits," which are indentations in the membrane covered on the inside by a basketlike structure composed of the protein clathrin. The membrane containing the receptor and ligand is then endocytosed, forming a coated vesicle that rapidly loses its clathrin coat. The resulting smooth vesicle, termed an endosome or receptosome, is acidic; at this stage, the bound hormone may dissociate from the receptor. In different cells and for different ligands, the endosome may fuse with lysosomes, leading to degradation of both receptor and ligand; the receptor may remain intact and recycle back to the plasma membrane and be reutilized, or the hormone (ligand) may escape the vesicle to enter the cytoplasm.

Hormones, however, are also taken up into cells such as those of the liver and pancreas, where coated vesicles are not prominent. At present, it is not clear what biologic activities of hormones initially binding to plasma (cell surface) membrane receptors are mediated either by the internalized hormone or its receptor. Other internalized proteins, however, such as nerve growth factor and diphtheria toxin, are established as having intracellular sites of action.

Molecular Structure of Receptors

The primary molecular structure of many receptors is now known from molecular cloning experiments that allow the amino acid sequence of a receptor to be deduced from its coding nucleic acid sequence. The secondary structure, posttranslational modifications, and membrane-spanning domains of receptors can only be inferred from these data, but they have allowed us to define receptor families on the basis of some striking structural homologies (Fig 1–10).

For example, receptors for steroid and thyroid hormones are intracellular proteins that bind small hydrophobic ligands as well as DNA. They have a highly homologous central DNA-binding region, a carboxyl terminal hormone-binding region, and a variable amino terminal. The DNA-binding region, which is rich in cysteine residues, is believed to form loops or "fingers" coordinated by zinc ions that may interact with DNA. Since steroid and thyroid hormones are structurally dissimilar, the common receptor structure is presumably a reflection of the similar mechanisms they use to regulate gene expression. In addition, the thyroid hormone receptor appears to be the cellular counterpart of a viral oncogene, erb-A.

Two families of membrane receptors have been identified and studied. The first family includes the receptors for insulin, IGF-I, and EGF, which appear to be related because they all have a large external hormone-binding region, a short hydrophobic membrane-spanning domain, and a moderate-sized intracellular domain with tyrosine kinase activity. The EGF receptor is a single protein; the insulin receptor is a tetramer with alpha and beta subunits that arise from a common precursor and are connected by disul-

fide bonds. The alpha subunit, which is entirely external, includes the ligand-binding domain, while the beta subunit encompasses the transmembrane and intracellular domains. The low-density lipoprotein (LDL) receptor and the IGF-II or mannose 6-phosphate receptor are structurally similar to this family but they lack tyrosine kinase activity. Ligand internalization is a prominent feature of all of these receptors.

The second family of membrane receptors are those that interact with G proteins (see the next section). The alpha- and beta-adrenergic receptors and muscarinic cholinergic receptors appear to possess 7 hydrophobic membrane-spanning regions, 2 short and one moderate-sized cytoplasmic loops, and one cytoplasmic carboxyl terminal tail. These receptors are homologous to the visual pigment rhodopsin. The ligand-binding region of these receptors, which is still being defined, appears to involve the transmembrane segments and the outside loops, while the G protein-interacting region is intracellular. Individual receptors with this structure interact with all the known major classes of G proteins. Thus, other membrane receptors that interact with G proteins, such as those for glucagon, vasopressin, TRH, and CCK, will probably have similar structures. For both membrane and steroid receptors, hybrid or chimeric receptors have been engineered with recombinant DNA technology. Such studies are identifying the binding and information transfer portions of receptors as separate entities.

INTRACELLULAR MESSENGERS

Steroid and thyroid hormones are able either to interact with the plasma membrane or to penetrate intracellularly and combine with intracellular messengers that can directly mediate their actions. By contrast, polypeptide hormones and catecholamines that interact with receptors on the cell membrane generally act through intracellular messengers to alter processes within the cell. The 2 major classes of intracellular messengers are cyclic nucleotides, primarily cAMP and the Ca^{2+}-phospholipid system (Table 1–2). For many hormones, however, the primary intracellular messenger is unknown. In the case of insulin and epidermal growth factor, the receptor itself has been shown to possess protein kinase activity selectivity for tyrosine residues. Thus, receptor-mediated protein phosphorylation may be involved in intracellular signal transduction for these hormones.

Intracellular messengers ("second messengers") are generated by an effector protein such as adenylate cyclase or a Ca^{2+} channel protein that is an entity distinct from the hormone receptor itself. Both receptor and effector proteins are believed to be mobile within the plane of the membrane and are influenced by the state of fluidity of membrane lipids. In this

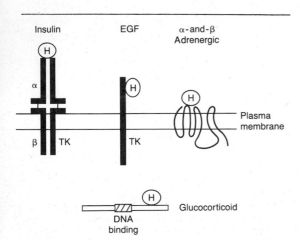

Figure 1–10. Proposed structures for different types of hormone receptors derived from molecular cloning experiments. H, hormone (grossly indicates the ligand-binding region); TK, tyrosine kinase.

Table 1–2. Division of polypeptide hormones and other regulators according to intracellular messenger system.

cAMP	Ca²⁺-DAG	Tyrosine Kinase
Increase cAMP		
ACTH	Acetylcholine	Epidermal growth
Beta-adrenergic	Alpha-adrenergic	factor
catecholamines	catecholamines	Insulin
Calcitonin	Angiotensin	Insulinlike growth
FSH	Cholecystokinin	peptide I
Glucagon	Gastrin	
LH	Oxytocin	
Parathyroid	Vasopressin	
hormone	TRH	
Secretin	GnRH	
TSH		
Vasopressin		
Decrease cAMP		
Acetylcholine		
Alpha-adrenergic		
catecholamines		
Dopamine		
Opiate Peptides		
Somatostatin		

"mobile receptor model," occupied receptors can move laterally within the membrane and make contact with and activate effectors (Fig 1–11). The phenomenon of spare receptors can be explained on the basis that there are more receptors than effectors. This model also explains the ability of multiple hormones, each acting on distinct receptors, to activate the same effector system. In fat cells, for example, at least 5 different hormones activate adenylate cyclase, whereas in liver 3 different hormones increase intracellular Ca²⁺. It is unlikely that a single protein could contain 5 different receptor sites, whereas there could easily be a number of receptors clustered around and able to make contact with and activate a single effector protein.

G Proteins as Receptor-Effector Couplers

Not only are receptors and effectors usually separate entities—they are now known to be coupled by a family of proteins called G proteins that bind and hy-

drolyze GTP. G proteins were originally identified as a component in the activation of adenylate cyclase; they also contribute to the inhibition of adenylate cyclase, the activation of phospholipases C and A₂, the regulation of K⁺ and Ca²⁺ channels, and the perception of light and odor. G proteins are heterotrimeric proteins with unique alpha subunits and common or extremely similar beta and gamma subunits. The alpha subunit binds guanine nucleotides, is NAD-ribosylated in response to cholera and pertussis toxins, and usually interacts with specific effectors. The beta-gamma dimer may anchor the complex to the membrane or in some cases directly activate an effector.

In the most generally accepted model of G protein function, receptor occupancy leads to the binding of GTP in place of GDP by the G protein's alpha subunit (Fig 1–12). The receptor-G protein complex rapidly dissociates, so that each receptor may activate multiple G proteins, and the G protein dissociates into the GTP-α subunit and the beta-gamma dimer. This dis-

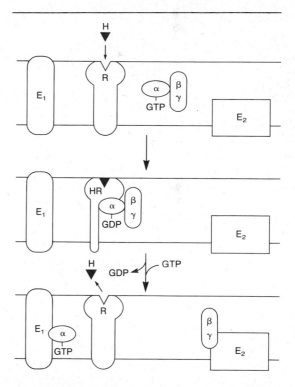

Figure 1–12. Possible mechanism by which a hormone receptor could activate 2 effectors, E₁ and E₂, via a single G protein. Activation by the beta-gamma subunit complex is currently controversial. Effectors include membrane enzymes (adenylate cyclase or phospholipase C) and ion channels. (Reproduced, with permission, from Dunlap K, et al. *Trend Neural Sci* 1987;**10**:241.) H, hormone; R, receptor; HR, hormone bound to receptor; GDP, guanosine diphosphate; GTP, guanosine triphosphate; α,β,γ, G protein subunits

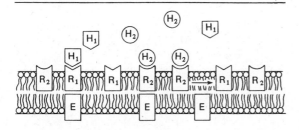

Figure 1–11. Highly schematic model of 2 types of hormone receptors, R₁ and R₂, which selectively bind hormones H₁ and H₂ and are able to diffuse laterally and interact with a single type of effector, E, in a fluid mosaic membrane.

sociation causes the receptor's affinity for the hormone to decrease, leading to dissociation of the hormone from the receptor. The GTP-α subunit activates the effector until an intrinsic GTPase hydrolyzes the GTP to GDP, after which the inactive GDP-α recombines with the beta-gamma dimer. This model explains the permanent activation of the effector by nonhydrolyzable GTP analogues and also provides an alternative inhibitory pathway by which excess beta-gamma subunits may recombine with and thereby inactivate free GTP-α subunits.

Cyclic AMP

The prototype intracellular messenger is cAMP; it was discovered by Sutherland and his colleagues, who showed that it was produced by the enzyme adenylate cyclase present in plasma membrane. After it is activated by the hormone-receptor complex, adenylate cyclase catalyzes the conversion of ATP to cAMP (Fig 1–13). Mg^{2+} is required for this reaction, as the substrate is Mg^{2+}-ATP complex. Adenylate cyclase is a distinct glycoprotein, with a molecular weight of 150,000, that can be solubilized with detergent and

activated directly by the diterpene Forskolin. Adenylate cyclase is also activated by cholera toxin and guanine nucleotides, particularly GTP and its nonhydrolyzable analogues. Biochemical and genetic evidence indicates that the latter agents act on a pair of homologous G proteins, as described in the previous section. One of these, G_s, mediates the stimulation of adenylate cyclase, while the other, G_i, inhibits the cyclase. Hormone receptors that increase cAMP interact with G_s, while those that decrease cAMP (Table 1–2) interact with G_i. The alpha subunits α_s and α_i contain the guanine nucleotide-binding site and a site that can be ADP-ribosylated. Alpha$_s$ can be ADP-ribosylated by cholera toxin, which causes the dissociation of the alpha subunit and permanently activates the cyclase. Alpha$_i$ can be ADP-ribosylated by pertussis toxin, which blocks the dissociation of the subunits and impairs the ability of the inhibitory peptides to inhibit the cyclase.

The activity of adenylate cyclase may also be modulated by other factors. Ca^{2+} inhibits adenylate cyclase in a number of tissues, whereas the Ca^{2+}-calmodulin complex (see next section) is known to activate certain

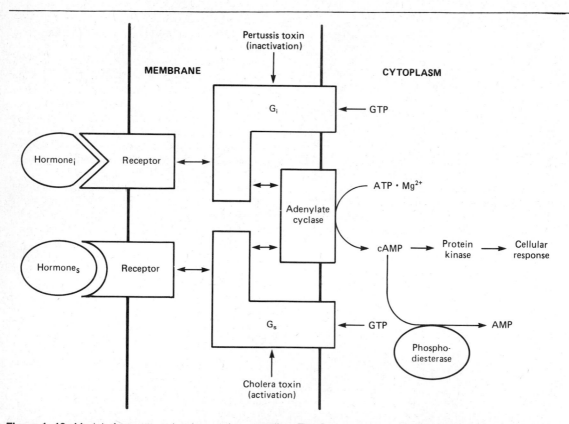

Figure 1–13. Model of receptor-adenylate cyclase coupling. The G_s (stimulating nucleotide) protein is shown coupling the hormone-receptor complex to its effector subunit (adenylate cyclase). The cAMP formed can either combine with protein kinase to initiate a cellular response or be metabolized (inactivated) by a specific phosphodiesterase. The G_i (inhibitory nucleotide) protein would inhibit adenylate cyclase. Hormone *i*, inhibitory hormone; hormone *s*, stimulating hormone; GTP, guanosine triphosphate; ATP, adenosine triphosphate; AMP, adenosine monophosphate.

cyclases. The activity of adenylate cyclase is also affected in various cells by prostaglandins and adenosine (see Chapter 4).

Cyclic AMP normally exists at very low levels (10^{-8} to 10^{-6} mol/L) in all cells. It is continually being degraded by a specific enzyme, cAMP phosphodiesterase, such that a rise in cellular cAMP induced by hormone activation of adenylate cyclase is rapidly reversed when removal of the hormone stops the production of cAMP. This phosphodiesterase is inhibited by methylxanthines such as caffeine and theophylline.

All of the presently known actions of cAMP in eukaryotes involve phosphorylation of proteins catalyzed by cAMP-activated protein kinases. The mechanism of this activation is shown in Fig 1–14. Normally, this protein kinase is inactivated by binding to a regulatory subunit. When cAMP is elevated, it binds to this regulatory subunit, causing it to release the active catalytic subunit. The active kinase then catalyzes the phosphorylation from ATP of serine and threonine residues of target proteins. This phosphorylation brings about changes in the activity of these proteins. Examples are the phosphorylation of phosphorylase kinase in liver and muscle to activate glycogenolysis and of hormone-sensitive lipase in adipose tissue to activate lypolysis. A great many other structural and enzymatic proteins are phosphorylated in response to various hormones, but in most instances the physiologic effects are not yet known.

Calcium (Ca²⁺)

Ionic calcium (Ca^{2+}) is a well-established intracellular messenger important in coupling excitation to contraction in muscle, excitation to transmitter release in nerves, and secretagogue action to secretion in various exocrine and endocrine glands. The importance of Ca^{2+} as an intracellular messenger in the action of a number of hormones is becoming increasingly apparent (Table 1–2).

The free cytoplasmic Ca^{2+} concentration is highly regulated to maintain a very low intracellular concentration. In various cell types, a Ca^{2+}-activated ATPase that directly uses ATP to transport Ca^{2+} out of the cell has been described. Ca^{2+} is also taken up

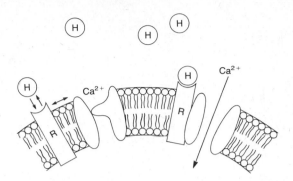

Figure 1–15. Hormone receptors (R) that bind hormone (H) and control the opening of selective Ca^{2+} channels in the cell membrane.

(buffered) by intracellular organelles, including mitochondria and endoplasmic reticulum. At rest, the cytoplasmic concentration of Ca^{2+} is maintained at 10^{-7} mol/L or less. A rise in cytoplasmic Ca^{2+} can then be brought about either by the opening of Ca^{2+} channels in the membrane (Fig 1–15) or by release of Ca^{2+} from intracellular organelles such as endoplasmic reticulum. Analogous to the activation of adenylate cyclase, multiple hormones and neurotransmitters may activate the same Ca^{2+} channels, suggesting separate receptor and Ca^{2+} channel subunits.

Probably most actions of Ca^{2+} as an intracellular messenger result from its binding to Ca^{2+}-binding proteins. The major Ca^{2+}-binding protein involved in the action of hormones is **calmodulin,** a small, highly acidic protein that binds 4 Ca^{2+} molecules per mole with an affinity (K_d) of about 10^{-6} mol/L. Calmodulin may exist as an integral subunit of an enzyme (Fig 1–16A) and confer Ca^{2+} sensitivity on the enzyme, as is the case with phosphorylase kinase. Alternatively, the Ca^{2+}-calmodulin complex may bind to other proteins and alter their activity (Fig 1–16B). An example is the activation of Ca^{2+}-regulated cyclic nucleotide phosphodiesterase by the Ca^{2+}-calmodulin complex in brain and other tissues. In the liver, where Ca^{2+} mediates the action of a number of hormones (ie, epinephrine, vasopressin, and angiotensin), a number of proteins (10–15) are phosphorylated following ex-

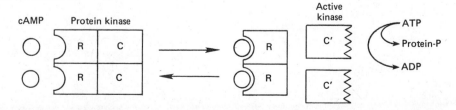

Figure 1–14. Activation of protein kinase by cAMP. R, regulatory subunit; C, repressed catalytic subunit; C′, active catalytic subunit.

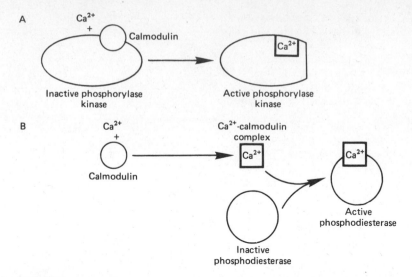

Figure 1–16. Mechanisms of enzyme activation by Ca^{2+} acting through binding to the Ca^{2+} receptor protein calmodulin. **A:** Ca^{2+} combines with calmodulin present as a subunit of phosphorylase kinase to activate the enzyme. **B:** Ca^{2+} combines with free calmodulin, and the Ca^{2+}-calmodulin complex then binds to and activates phosphodiesterase.

posure of hepatocytes to these hormones. It seems likely, therefore, that many of the actions of Ca^{2+} will be found to be mediated by Ca^{2+}-activated kinases.

Related to the above Ca^{2+} system is the newly described phospholipid-activated, Ca^{2+}-dependent kinase system, the "C" kinase. An accelerated turnover of membrane phosphatidylinositol and its phosphorylated derivatives usually accompanies cell activation by calcium-dependent hormones. This activation (Fig 1–17), which is calcium-independent, involves a unique but not yet isolated G protein called G_p that activates a phospholipase C to cleave polyphosphoinositides to yield diacylglycerol and inositol phosphate. This diglyceride is rich in arachidonic acid and serves as a prostaglandin precursor; but in the presence of another membrane phospholipid (phosphatidylserine) and calcium, it activates a specific protein kinase, the C kinase. Moreover, one of the water-soluble inositol metabolites, inositol triphosphate, appears to act as an intracellular messenger to release stored intracellular Ca^{2+}. The C kinase may then work in concert with Ca^{2+}-calmodulin-regulated protein kinases to mediate hormone action.

Cyclic GMP

Ca^{2+} is also related to another cyclic nucleotide, cyclic guanosine monophosphate (cGMP). The formation of cGMP is catalyzed by guanylate cyclase, an enzyme present in both the plasma membrane and the cytoplasm. The cytoplasmic form is activated by Ca^{2+}. As a result, in almost all cases where there is a rise in cytoplasmic Ca^{2+}, there is a parallel rise in cGMP. The membrane guanylate cyclase may be receptor activated. Increasing evidence suggests that

atrial natriuretic peptides may act through such a mechanism.

COMMON MECHANISMS OF HORMONE ACTION

Membrane Permeability & Transport

Hormones regulate the cellular entry and exit of a large number of ions, metabolites, and biosynthetic precursors. Ions and small organic molecules frequently move across membranes by means of channels or carriers composed of specialized proteins whose purpose is to increase the rate of movement across the membrane. A molecule moving across a membrane down its electrochemical gradient is said to be undergoing **passive transport.** Passive transport may show kinetic characteristics of diffusion or, if mediated by a carrier, saturation kinetics analogous to enzyme activity. When cellular energy is used (usually by means of an ATPase enzyme) to move the transported molecule against its electrochemical gradient, it is undergoing **active transport.** Hormones affect all of these types of transport processes. These actions are important both in regulating the biosynthetic and metabolic activities of individual cells and in regulating the movement of ions and other molecules across cells such as in the intestine, kidney tubules, and bone.

Hormones regulate the movement of molecules across membranes by at least 4 different mechanisms: (1) alteration of the affinity of the transport mechanism for the molecule being transported; (2) activation of previously inactive transport mechanisms present in

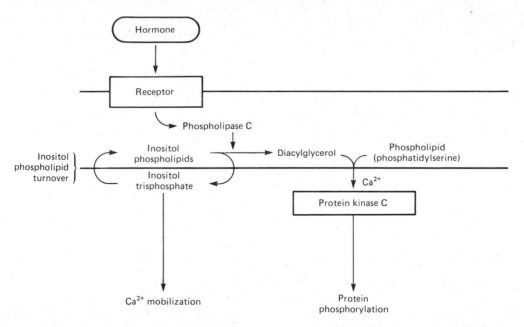

Figure 1–17. Schematic diagram of the mechanism by which a hormone or other signal acts via phospholipase C in the cell membrane to activate protein kinase C and increase inositol phospholipid turnover. One of the phosphorylated inositol derivatives, inositol trisphosphate, also acts to mobilize intracellular Ca^{2+}. (Modified and reproduced, with permission, from Nishizuka Y et al: Phospholipid turnover in hormone action. *Recent Prog Horm Res* 1984;**40:**301.)

the plasma membrane; (3) insertion into the plasma membrane of preexisting transport mechanisms present inside the cell; and (4) synthesis of new transport proteins.

A. Glucose and Amino Acid Transport: The cellular uptake of glucose and amino acids is stimulated by hormones in a large number of target tissues. The earliest and best-studied example is the stimulation of glucose entry into fat and muscle cells by insulin. Glucose crosses the plasma membrane by means of a transport protein, the glucose carrier, that facilitates glucose entry into cells. Because the number of carriers is limited, this "facilitated diffusion" shows saturation kinetics that can be characterized by a K_m (the concentration at which transport is half-maximal) and a J_{max} (the maximal rate of transport). Insulin increases the J_{max} by bringing about the insertion of new carriers from the cell interior into the plasma membrane. This action of insulin is rapid (seconds to minutes) and does not require new protein synthesis. Other hormones also increase glucose uptake by their target cells; examples include TSH acting on thyroid cells and cholecystokinin acting on pancreatic acinar cells.

The cellular uptake of amino acids also involves a number of transport proteins that mediate amino acid entry by facilitated diffusion. In some cases, the entry of amino acids is driven by Na^+, which also binds to the carrier and, by moving down its electrochemical gradient, serves to concentrate the amino acid inside the cell. Acceleration of amino acid transport is brought about by a variety of hormones, including in-

sulin, glucagon, growth hormone, and thyroid hormone. Thyroid hormone appears to act directly on the plasma membrane (Fig 1–21) independently of its effects on nuclear functions.

Other small molecules such as uridine and thymidine that are important as biosynthetic precursors enter cells by carrier-mediated facilitated diffusion. The transport of these molecules is stimulated by a number of polypeptide tropic hormones and by gonadal steroids acting on their respective target tissues.

B. Ion Transport: Cellular ionic balance is regulated to a great extent by the Na^+-K^+ ATPase that actively transports Na^+ out of and K^+ into cells. This active transport balances the passive entry of Na^+ and efflux of K^+ that occur by diffusion. Other ions either diffuse passively across the plasma membrane or their movements are coupled to Na^+ via carrier proteins. Two hormones that increase the activity of the Na^+-K^+ ATPase in a number of tissues are insulin and thyroid hormone. The effects of insulin are rapid and separate from its effects on glucose transport. The stimulation by thyroid hormone is slower, requiring the synthesis of new Na^+-K^+ ATPase molecules. The increased Na^+ transport induced by thyroid hormone is the basis for part of the action of thyroid hormones to stimulate oxygen consumption and heat production (calorigenesis). Another specialized form of ion transport is the uptake of iodide by the thyroid, which is increased by TSH.

C. Epithelial Transport: Epithelia are specialized sheets or tubules of cells whose function is to separate

2 compartments and regulate the transport of water and other molecules. For example, in the distal tubule of the kidney (Fig 1–18), aldosterone acts to increase the reabsorption of Na^+. Na^+ enters the cell from the lumen of the tubule down its electrochemical gradient by means of a specialized transport protein and then is actively transported out of the cell into capillaries by means of Na^+-K^+ ATPase located in the basolateral membrane of the tubular cell. Aldosterone induces the synthesis of new Na^+ channel protein (see section on nuclear regulation) that facilitates the entry of Na^+ into the cell. It also induces the production of other proteins that increase mitochondrial ATP synthesis for the transport of Na^+ out of the cell.

In an analogous manner, vitamin D, a steroidlike substance, increases the transepithelial absorption of Ca^{2+} and PO_4^{3-} of the small intestine. Growth hormone also increases Ca^{2+} and PO_4^{3-} absorption, while Ca^{2+} absorption is inhibited by adrenal glucocorticoids.

Other hormones regulating epithelial transport include parathyroid hormone in bone and kidney; gastrin, which increases the secretion of H^+-rich gastric juice by parietal cells of the stomach, and secretin, which increases the secretion of HCO_3^--rich pancreatic juice by the duct cells of the pancreas.

Enzyme Activation

Many effects of polypeptide and catecholamine hormones on intracellular enzymes involve alterations in the activity of preexisting enzymes rather than the synthesis or induction of new enzymes. These effects are generally slower than those regulating membrane transport, occurring in minutes to hours, but are also independent of the synthesis of new protein. Insulin, for example, has well-established effects on the activity of various enzymes involved in the metabolism of glucose, amino acids, fatty acids, and nucleotides.

Major mechanisms by which hormones affect enzyme activity are phosphorylation and dephosphorylation. The first and best-studied example of phosphorylation is the regulation of glycogen metabolism in liver and muscle (Fig 1–19). The activity of both glycogen synthetase and phosphorylase is regulated by phosphorylation; in the case of phosphorylase, addition of phosphate activates the enzyme, whereas in the case of glycogen synthetase, it inhibits the enzyme. Thus, hormones such as epinephrine and glucagon, by increasing the activity of several kinases (including phosphorylase kinase), bring about the net conversion of glycogen to glucose. Insulin, possibly by activating a phosphatase, increases the activity of glycogen synthetase and accelerates the formation of glycogen.

Many other enzymes responsive to insulin have

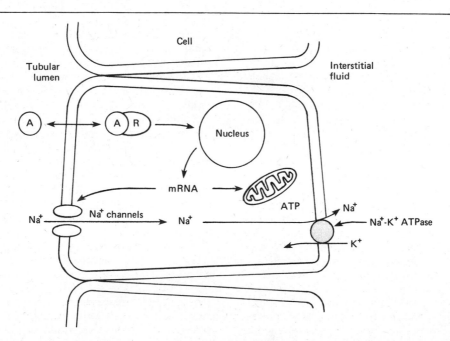

Figure 1–18. Mechanism by which aldosterone increases the resorption of Na^+ by cells of the distal nephron. Aldosterone (A) enters the cell and binds to a cytoplasmic receptor (R). The aldosterone-receptor complexes then enter the nucleus and induce the synthesis of proteins, including the Na^+ channel protein that mediates the entry of Na^+ from the lumen into the cell and mitochondrial proteins necessary to synthesize more ATP used by the Na^+-K^+ ATPase to pump Na^+ out of the cell and into the interstitial fluid.

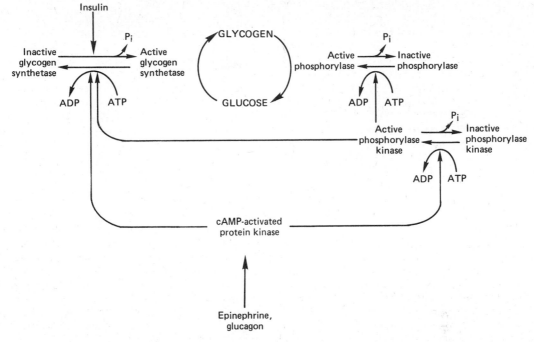

Figure 1–19. Simplified scheme of glycogen synthesis and breakdown.

been shown to be regulated by phosphorylation and dephosphorylation independently of the cAMP activated protein kinases. A well-studied example is the regulation of pyruvate dehydrogenase, a mitochondrial enzyme complex that produces acetyl-CoA necessary for lipid synthesis. Exposure of adipose tissue to insulin rapidly increases pyruvate dehydrogenase activity as a result of dephosphorylation. Insulin also activates pyruvate kinase and hydroxymethylglutaryl-CoA reductase and inhibits hormone-sensitive lipase—all by dephosphorylation processes. It is not known in any of these cases whether insulin activates phosphatases or inhibits kinases.

Both of the second messengers (cAMP and Ca^{2+}) can act by phosphorylation mechanisms. An example where the 2 intracellular messengers act together is the regulation of phosphorylase kinase, the enzyme that phosphorylates phosphorylase. Phosphorylase kinase is a multisubunit enzyme and can be activated independently by cAMP-activated protein kinase, which phosphorylates its alpha and beta subunits, or by Ca^{2+}, which binds to the delta subunit, calmodulin. The 2 intracellular regulators potentiate each other in that cAMP-induced phosphorylation increases the sensitivity of the enzyme to Ca^{2+}. Almost all hormones (including steroids) alter the state of phosphorylation of a small number of proteins in target cells. In most cases, however, the identity and functional role of the phosphorylated protein are unknown.

Besides phosphorylation, other enzymes can be directly activated by specialized binding proteins. Cal-

modulin, the protein that serves as the Ca^{2+} receptor for hormones utilizing Ca^{2+} as intracellular messenger, binds to and regulates a number of enzymes, including cyclic nucleotide phosphodiesterase, certain adenylate cyclases, and the Ca^{2+}-ATPase present in the cell membrane that acts to transport Ca^{2+} out of the cells.

Other ways in which enzyme activities can be regulated that may ultimately prove to be affected by hormones include aggregation of subunits, adenylation, methylation, and changes in the local concentration of ions or cofactors.

Nuclear Regulation

Certain actions of steroid, thyroid, and polypeptide hormones are brought about by increasing the number of a few specific types of mRNA. This effect is usually caused by altering the rate of transcription of the gene and so changing the amount of mRNA present. In some cases, hormones can affect the degradation of mRNA molecules. Hormone actions mediated by this mechanism are generally delayed in onset and blocked by inhibitors of RNA synthesis.

A. Steroid Hormones: Nuclear regulation has been studied most extensively for steroid hormones. Most of the known actions of steroids, as well as those of vitamins A and D, appear to follow this pathway (Fig 1–20). As previously mentioned, steroid hormones bind to receptors in the cytoplasm and nucleus. Specific receptor proteins have been found for all classes of steroids; they bind biologically active steroids with

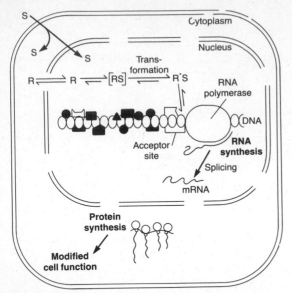

Figure 1–20. Current understanding of steroid hormone action. The steroids enter target cells through diffusion or a transport mechanism and bind to a receptor protein in the nucleus. The activated steroid-receptor complex can then bind to chromatin and act on specific DNA sequences termed glucocorticoid regulatory elements (GREs). RNA polymerase then binds to the GRE, new mRNA molecules are transcribed, and finally new protein is synthesized. S, steroid; R, receptor; RS, steroid-receptor complex. (Reproduced, with permission, from Walters MR: *Endocr Rev* 1985;6:512.)

higher affinity for the more active hormones. When the hormone binds to the receptor, a physical change occurs that activates the complex's ability to regulate transcription. Some steroid hormone antagonists bind to the receptor but do not activate it; other antagonists bind to the receptor but produce an activated complex that cannot stimulate transcription.

The receptors for glucocorticoids have recently been shown to be associated with a heat-stable protein. A model currently under investigation for all steroid hormones is that the activation step results in the dissociation of the heat-stable protein from the receptor. This exposes the DNA-binding site on the receptor, allowing the steroid-receptor complex to bind to the DNA.

Steroid hormone receptors bind to DNA sequences called **hormone-responsive elements (HREs).** These sequences act like the "enhancer" elements. They are distinct from the promoter where RNA polymerase initiates its actions and can be located upstream or downstream (in terms of the direction of transcription) from the promoter. Several HREs can exist for the same receptor. For example, progesterone and glucocorticoid receptors generally bind to the same HRE, whereas estrogen receptors bind to different HREs. The receptor-hormone complex bound to the HRE enhances (positive control) or diminishes

(negative control) the activity of the promoter. With positive control, the hormone-receptor-DNA complex may enhance the binding of other transcription factors, whereas with negative control, the complex may decrease the binding or activity of such factors. The differentiation of the cell plus the presence of the relevant receptor dictates whether the hormone will act on a specific regulated gene; thus, a particular gene may be regulated by the hormone in one tissue but not in another.

These effects on hormone-responsive elements ultimately modulate the concentration levels of pre-mRNAs, mRNAs, and their translational products. This allows the regulation of the amount of specific enzymes as well as enzyme activity, as described in the preceding sections. (See also Chapter 2, Fig 2–5.)

B. Thyroid Hormones: Thyroid hormones are now also known to regulate nuclear function (Fig 1–21). Thyroid hormones readily enter cells, but their uptake mechanism is unknown. They may either diffuse through the lipid bilayers of the cell membrane by virtue of their hydrophobicity or enter cells by means of a transport mechanism similar to that used by amino acids. After entry, thyroid hormones bind to cytoplasmic binding proteins that concentrate hormone intracellularly. It is the free thyroid hormone in the cell that

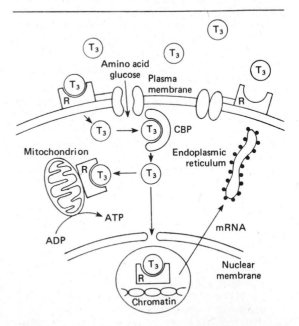

Figure 1–21. Proposed mechanism of thyroid hormone action. Thyroid hormone (in this case triiodothyronine, or T_3) binds to a receptor protein (R) on the cell surface and increases the uptake of glucose and amino acids. T_3 also enters the cell, where it reacts with cytoplasmic binding proteins (CBP) and receptors on chromatin and mitochondria. In the nucleus, the T_3-receptor complex leads to the synthesis of new protein.

binds directly to receptors on or in the nucleus. Other receptors are present in mitochondria and may mediate certain effects of thyroid hormone on oxygen consumption.

Nuclear receptors for thyroid hormones are acidic proteins that bind to DNA but are also influenced by the histone proteins present in chromatin. It is this interaction with histones that maintains the higher specificity for triiodothyronine (T_3) as compared to thyroxine (T_4) (see Chapter 9). The finding of thyroid hormone receptors associated with chromatin suggests that the hormone influences nuclear functions. Specific mRNAs known to be increased by thyroid hormones include those coding for growth hormone, liver $\alpha_{2\mu}$-globulin, and Na^+-K^+ ATPase. In general, these effects of thyroid hormones are slow, taking 1–2 days to reach a maximum.

C. Polypeptide Hormones: Several polypeptide hormones exert transcriptional and translational effects on nucleic acid and protein synthesis. Polypeptide hormones act on target cells via intracellular messengers such as cAMP and diacylglycerol to induce the binding of regulatory proteins to hormone-responsive elements. The resulting complexes then regulate the transcription of specific genes. Other hormones such as insulin, growth hormone, and prolactin, which do not have established intracellular mediators, also regulate gene transcription. For example, insulin has widespread effects on liver, pancreas, adipose tissue, and mammary gland. How the information is transmitted from these receptors to chromatin is not yet clear.

Other effects of polypeptide hormones on the ribosomal translation of preexisting mRNA are also known. In the muscle, fat, and liver of diabetic animals, there is decreased protein synthesis. Insulin increases the assembly of polysomes. Growth hormone administration in vivo also increases the rate of protein synthesis by subsequently isolated muscle ribosomes.

SUMMARY & CONCLUSIONS

The action of hormones is initiated by interaction with receptors specific for the hormone. In the case of polypeptide and amine hormones, these receptors are localized on the plasma membranes. Occupancy of these membrane receptors directly regulates membrane functions. Effects on intracellular functions are mediated by intracellular messengers such as cAMP and Ca^{2+}. Steroid and thyroid hormones interact chiefly with intracellular receptors. Receptors for steroid hormones are present in the cytoplasm and nucleus and, when occupied, regulate nuclear function. Some receptors for thyroid hormone are present in the nucleus and regulate nuclear function; others present in mitochondria and plasma membrane regulate the responsiveness of these organelles. Many actions of steroid and thyroid hormones require the synthesis of new proteins and are relatively slow compared to those actions of polypeptide and amine hormones that do not require synthetic events. Lastly, we must be careful not to take rigid positions on the ways in which different classes of hormones act, since mechanisms of action are still being discovered.

REFERENCES

Baxter JD, Funder JW: Hormone receptors. *N Engl J Med* 1979;**301:**1149.

Berridge, MJ: Inositol trisphosphate and diacylglycerol: Two interacting second messengers. *Annu Rev Biochem* 1987;**56:**159.

Czech MP: New perspectives on the mechanism of insulin action. *Recent Prog Horm Res* 1984;**40:**347.

DeLisle RC, Williams JA: Regulation of membrane fusion in secretory exocytosis. *Annu Rev Physiol* 1986;**48:** 225.

Evans RM: The steroid and thyroid hormone receptor superfamily. *Science* 1988;**240:**889.

Goldfine ID: The insulin receptor: Molecular biology and transmembrane signaling. *Endocr Rev* 1987;**8:**235.

Kelly RB: Pathways of protein secretion in eukaryotes. *Science* 1985;**230:**25.

King AC, Cuatrecasas P: Peptide hormone-induced receptor mobility, aggregation, and internalization. *N Engl J Med* 1981;**305:**77.

Neer EJ, Clapham DE: Roles of G protein subunits in transmembrane signaling. *Nature* 1988;**333:**129.

Nishizuka Y: The role of protein kinase C in cell surface signal transduction and tumor promotion. *Nature* 1984;**308:**693.

O'Malley BW: Steroid hormone action in eukaryotic cells. *J Clin Invest* 1984;**74:**307.

Pastan I, Willingham MC: Receptor-mediated endocytosis: Coated pits, receptosomes and the Golgi. *Trends Biochem Sci* 1983;**8:**250.

Rasmussen H: The Calcium messenger system: *N Engl J Med* 1986;**314:**1094,1164.

Walter P, Lingappa V: Mechanism of protein translocation across the endoplasmic reticulum membrane. *Annu Rev Cell Biol* 1986;**2:**499.

2 Gene Expression & Recombinant DNA in Endocrinology & Metabolism

John D. Baxter, MD, & Barry J. Gertz, MD, PhD

Over the past few decades, significant data have accumulated concerning the detailed structure and function of genes. This information is now being used to devise more sophisticated and direct means of diagnosing, preventing, and treating disease. The technology that has been developed, particularly the genetic engineering techniques of recombinant DNA, is also providing new approaches to understanding human physiology and the pathogenesis of disease.

Human insulin and growth hormone produced by recombinant DNA techniques are already available for clinical use, and numerous additional applications for recombinant DNA technology are forthcoming. Many new drugs will be developed, capabilities for predicting susceptibility to disease and for diagnosing disease will be greatly expanded, and new types of therapy (eg, gene transfer) may also become available. The physician will therefore require some understanding of this new technology in order to apply it to the management of endocrine and metabolic diseases and to assess its strengths and weaknesses. The rapid development of technology will also raise ethical issues whose consideration requires knowledge of gene function, gene regulation, and recombinant DNA techniques. The purpose of this chapter is to provide a conceptual framework for understanding gene expression and the role of recombinant DNA in endocrinology.

GENES & THEIR EXPRESSION

The modern era of molecular biology received its greatest impetus in 1953, when Watson and Crick reported the structure of deoxyribonucleic acid (DNA). This finding provided an understanding of how replication occurs (ie, through complementary base pairing) and thus how the genetic profile of an organism can be maintained from generation to generation. The

The material in this chapter is based on material written by the authors for a chapter entitled "Gene Expression and Recombinant DNA in Endocrinology and Metabolism" in: *Endocrinology and Metabolism,* 2nd ed. Felig P et al (editors). McGraw-Hill, 1987.

Acronyms Used in This Chapter

ACTH	Adrenocorticotropic hormone
cDNA	Complementary DNA
CGRP	Calcitonin gene-related peptide
DNA	Deoxyribonucleic acid
HMG-CoA	3-Hydroxy-3-methylglutaryl-coenzyme A
LDL	Low-density lipoprotein
GRE	Glucocorticoid regulatory element
NMR	Nuclear magnetic resonance
PCR	Polymerase chain reaction
mRNA	Messenger RNA
PTH	Parathyroid hormone
RFLP	Restriction fragment length polymorphism
RNA	Ribonucleic acid
rRNA	Ribosomal RNA
tRNA	Transfer RNA

discovery was followed by a series of breakthroughs revealing (1) the way in which the DNA of a cell evolves and replicates; (2) the means by which the DNA is expressed (ie, how it is transcribed into ribonucleic acid [RNA]) and how these transcripts are then either translated into protein (eg, for messenger RNA [mRNA]) or utilized in other ways (as with transfer RNA [tRNA], ribosomal RNA [rRNA], etc); and (3) the means by which gene expression is controlled. Knowledge in these areas continues to accumulate at an impressive rate.

Important aspects of the structure and function of DNA are briefly described below. For more detailed information, the reader is encouraged to consult the general references at the end of this chapter.

DNA Structure

The structure of DNA is shown in Figs 2–1 and 2–2. The backbone of DNA is composed of deoxyribose molecules linked by connecting phosphate groups. These bonds occur through the $3'$-hydroxyl moiety of the first sugar and the $5'$-hydroxyl moiety of the next sugar. Since the $5'$ moiety of the first sugar and the $3'$ moiety of the last sugar are free, the direction of the

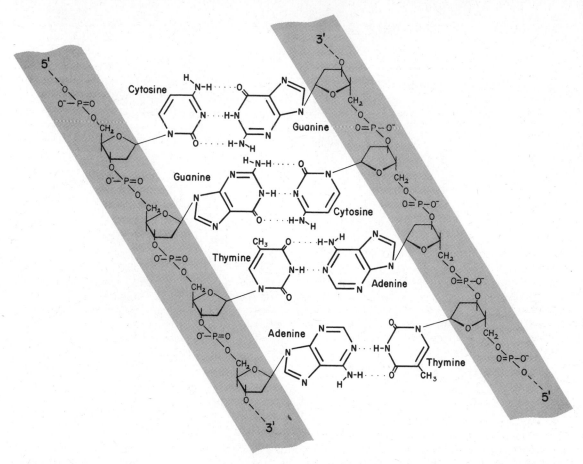

Figure 2–1. Structural features of a short segment of double-stranded DNA. Shaded areas show the sugar-phosphate backbones running antiparallel to one another (one running from 5′ to 3′ and the other from 3′ to 5′). The unshaded area shows the pyrimidines cytosine (C) and thymine (T), the purines guanine (G) and adenine (A), and the hydrogen bonding of C to G and A to T.

molecule is said to be from 5′ to 3′. These designations serve as a reference for orientation. Genes are described as being transcribed from 5′ to 3′, since the first sugar of the RNA product contains a 5′-triphosphate group. The 5′ end of a gene ordinarily refers to its transcriptional start site, or the "upstream" portion of the gene; the 3′ end designates the "downstream" portion of the gene, where transcription is terminated.

Connected to each sugar of the DNA backbone is one of 4 **bases:** adenine (A), guanine (G), cytosine (C), or thymine (T). Adenine and guanine are **purines,** whereas cytosine and thymine are **pyrimidines.** A base to which only a sugar is attached is called a **nucleoside;** a base to which both a sugar and a phosphate group are attached is called a **nucleotide.** For example, adenine (base) bound to ribose is termed adenosine (nucleoside); adenosine coupled to a phosphate group

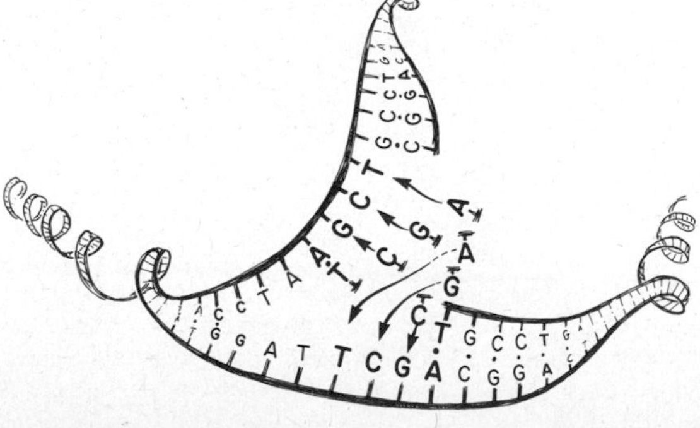

Figure 2–2. Highly simplified depiction of the essential features of DNA replication. The double helix unwinds, and 2 daughter strands of DNA are synthesized. Each of the resulting DNA molecules contains one strand of the original (parent) DNA molecule (semiconservative replication). Complementary base pairing directs the sequence of addition of nucleoside triphosphates by DNA polymerase (not shown). Each daughter strand of DNA is synthesized in the direction of 5′ to 3′, requiring one strand to be synthesized in a discontinuous fashion.

is designated adenylic acid (nucleotide). When nucleotides are linked together in a polymer, they generate a **nucleic acid.**

DNA is composed of 2 strands of nucleic acid that are antiparallel to each other (ie, running in opposite directions) such that the A moieties of one strand are hydrogen-bonded to the T moieties of the complementary strand and the C and G moieties are similarly bonded to each other. This **complementary base pairing** means that the order of the bases along one strand of DNA dictates the order along the other strand. This feature is the critical one in DNA replication and transcription for determining, respectively, the precise structures of DNA progeny and of RNA products of genes. The 2 strands are wound around each other in a configuration called a **double helix.** Within the nucleus of a cell, the DNA is packaged into chromatin, a highly ordered structure composed of DNA and proteins.

It is the order of bases along the DNA strand that can be construed as the "secret of life." This order, along with precise base pairing, permits "like to replicate like" and allows for information storage. It is in a sense the body's "computer program" for transmitting similar information to progeny, for directing cells of the developing embryo to differentiate properly into adult anatomic structures, and for directing all of the complex metabolic functions of the cell.

DNA Replication

When DNA replicates (Fig 2–2), the individual strands are separated and nucleoside triphosphates are aligned along the phosphodiester backbones by complementary base pairing. The sugar moieties are then connected enzymatically, resulting in complementary DNA strands. The many steps in this process are highly complex and outside the scope of this chapter, but the result is 2 daughter strands of DNA that are identical to the original DNA. Because one strand of each daughter DNA molecule is from the parent and the other is newly synthesized, the process is called **semiconservative replication.**

RNA Structure & Function

The first step in gene expression is the transcription of DNA into RNA (Fig 2–3). While the structures of RNA and DNA are similar in most respects, there are several differences: (1) The sugar moiety of RNA is ribose instead of deoxyribose. (2) In RNA, the base uracil (U) replaces T, and U therefore base-pairs with A. RNA in mammalian cells is ordinarily not double-stranded, although the RNA may fold in on itself ("secondary structure") and produce some double-stranded portions. Some of the RNA viruses, however, are double-stranded.

There are 3 major classes of RNA: mRNA, tRNA, and rRNA and several other minor RNA classes. **mRNA** contains sequences that are translated into protein (see below). **tRNA** is involved in transferring amino acids into protein. **rRNA,** along with proteins, forms **ribosomes,** structures that also are involved in protein synthesis. As described in Chapter 1 and illustrated in Fig 1–2, mRNA binds to the ribosome along with the tRNA molecules. Each type of tRNA in the series of tRNA molecules is specific for an amino acid that can bind to the tRNA covalently. Such "charged" tRNA molecules participate in the incorporation of amino acids into protein through the formation of peptide bonds. Of the minor RNA species, small nuclear RNAs participate in RNA processing (see below).

Gene Structure & Expression

In addition to the segments of DNA that are copied into RNA, there are some segments that are involved in receiving signals that either inhibit or facilitate gene transcription (**control sequences,** or **regulatory sequences**). Other regions determine where the enzymes involved in transcription (ie, the RNA polymerases) are to start and at what basal level a specific gene is to be expressed. These latter regions are called **promot-**

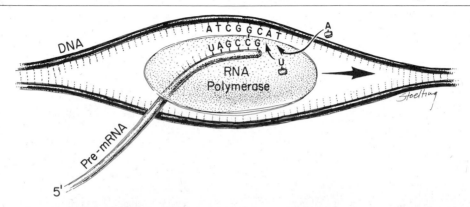

Figure 2–3. Synthesis of RNA. The DNA template is shown to open over the region where transcription of a precursor species (in this case depicted as pre-mRNA) is taking place. The enzyme RNA polymerase directs the addition of ribonucleoside triphosphates into the growing mRNA, with the actual sequence determined by complementary base pairing of purines and pyrimidines. In RNA, the pyrimidine uracil (U) base-pairs with adenine (A).

ers. In the case of RNA polymerase II, involved in transcription of genes that encode mRNA molecules, the promoter is located just upstream from the starting point of transcription. The 2 strands of DNA are separated during transcription, and RNA polymerase facilitates base pairing along one of the strands and subsequent polymerization from individual ribonucleoside triphosphates that serve as building blocks (Figs 2–2 and 2–3). At the end of the gene are poorly defined signals that terminate transcription.

The structure of a mammalian gene encoding an mRNA is shown in Fig 2–4. In the initial stage of expression of this gene, a precursor (**pre-mRNA**) is formed from transcription of the DNA that consists of **exons** (sequences whose transcripts occur in mature mRNA), **introns** (sequences that interrupt the exons) and 3'-flanking sequences (see below). Posttranscriptional processing leads to the formation of mature mRNA and results in the removal of the intron transcripts. This induces the formation of small nuclear ribonuclear protein particles or snRNPs, the participation of several small nuclear RNAs, and the involvement of the RNA itself in the processes of excisions of the introns and ligations of the exons. In most mRNA molecules, 2 other modifications occur: (1) The 3' end is cleaved, and a chain of A (adenosine) residues (**the poly [A] tail**) is added to the newly generated 3' end of

the mRNA. (2) A **cap,** consisting of a methylated nucleotide inserted in the reverse orientation, is added to the 5' end of the mRNA. The DNA upstream from the start of transcription is called the **5'-flanking DNA,** and that downstream from the completion of transcription is called the **3'-flanking DNA,** although the latter usually refers to the DNA following the poly(A) addition site.

Introns are present in most genes that code for mRNA, but their number varies; there may be as many as 50 in exceptional cases. They are not found in bacterial genes. In a few cases, DNA structures important for regulating the expression of the gene are found in introns. For example, a structure that binds the glucocorticoid receptor and contributes to responsiveness to this class of hormones is found in an intron of the human growth hormone gene.

The fact that genes are split into introns and exons has probably facilitated the process of evolution of genes. One critical mechanism for gene evolution probably involves the movement of DNA segments into existing genes, in which case the inserted segment could, for example, contain structures that (1) code for additional amino acids or (2) regulate the expression of the new gene in a different way. The advantage of introns for such rearrangements of DNA is that the genetic events can be somewhat imprecise. For exam-

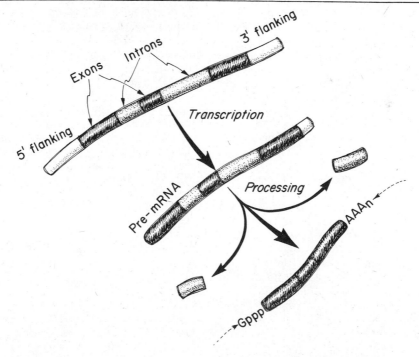

Figure 2–4. The initial steps in gene expression of a typical eukaryotic gene encoding a polypeptide. Exons (regions present in the mature transcript) and introns (regions destined to be excised from the primary transcript) are distinguished in the parent gene by shading. Both the exons and introns are transcribed into the primary gene product, or pre-mRNA. This precursor species then undergoes several processing steps, including splicing of the exons associated with removal of the introns, addition of a cap at the 5' end, and cleavage and polyadenylation at the 3' end. The mature transcript is then transported into the cytoplasm. These processing steps may occur sequentially.

ple, the insertion of a segment that consists of an exon flanked by 2 introns into an intron of an existing gene would result in an altered mRNA product of the gene, and the protein translated from the mRNA would have an additional segment of amino acids supplied by the added exon. For this evolutionary event to occur, all that is needed are breaks in the DNA in the middle of the intron in segments that do not contain critical control structures such as those which affect RNA processing; it introns and their removal by processing did not occur, such insertions would be more difficult to achieve without compromising the original gene.

After the mRNA is formed in the nucleus, it is transported to the cell cytoplasm, where it is translated into a protein whose amino acid sequence is determined by the codons of the mRNA according to the genetic code. Each **codon** consists of 3 nucleotides. The first codon of the mRNA that is translated is always AUG, which codes for methionine, and codons for other amino acids then follow. Individual amino acids are each covalently linked to a specific tRNA. These tRNA molecules bind to the mRNA through an **anticodon loop** containing 3 nucleotides that are complementary to the codons of the mRNA. For example, UAC on the anticodon loop pairs with AUG on the mRNA. Whereas each codon is unambiguous in terms of the amino acid specificity, the code is redundant in that more than one codon specifies a given amino acid (except for tryptophan and methionine). Thus, if the nucleic acid sequence of an mRNA is known, the amino acid sequence of its protein translation product will be known with certainty. Conversely, if the amino acid sequence of a protein is known, the nucleic acid sequence of the mRNA and the gene from which it is transcribed can only be partially known. At the end of each coding segment is a "stop" codon, which is UAA, UAG, or UGA; these do not recognize tRNA, and when the ribosome reaches them as it moves along the mRNA in the process of protein synthesis, translation ceases and the ribosome dissociates from the mRNA.

As discussed in Chapter 1, many proteins result from modification of the primary translation product, or precursor protein. For example, a signal peptide sequence that can target a protein for secretion may be removed from a preprotein during the entry of the protein into the secretory apparatus (as with the conversion of preproinsulin to proinsulin). Further proteolysis can follow, eg, the conversion of proinsulin to insulin, or the release of ACTH, a 39-amino-acid protein, from a much larger protein (pro-opiomelanocortin). In some cases, sugars or other chemical groups are added after translation.

REGULATION OF GENE EXPRESSION

During development of an organism, cells must differentiate in order to perform specialized functions. Furthermore, hormones, neurotransmitters, and other regulatory signals must be able to control the expression of DNA in various tissues in different ways. The molecular mechanisms involved in the regulation of gene expression are just beginning to be understood. Although many of the steps in the process of gene expression are regulated, the principal control appears to be at the level of transcription of the DNA into pre-mRNA.

In most cases, the structure of genes in the germ line cells is essentially identical to that in the various differentiated or somatic cells. However, in some cases, the bases of DNA are modified such that gene expression is altered. For example, cytosine residues can be methylated, and this can inhibit expression of the gene. The methylation patterns can also be inherited. Methylation appears to contribute to the inactivation of one of the X chromosomes in cells that contain two X chromosomes. The result is transcriptional activity of only one of each pair of X chromosomes in a given cell. In other cases, DNA undergoes rearrangement or mutation (or both). This occurs, for example, with cells of the immune system, in which both rearrangement and mutation of the immunoglobulin gene regions permit millions of different immunoglobulin genes to be formed from a relatively small number of genes present in the progenitor cells.

Details are beginning to emerge about the regulation of transcription. Promoter structures for different genes (discussed in a previous section) may vary in their capacity to initiate transcription, and these affect the total level of activity of the gene. Regulatory sequences also affect the efficiency of the promoter in initiating transcription. Two examples illustrate this point. The growth hormone gene contains 2 regulatory sequences located upstream from the promoter that are critical for efficient transcription initiation. These 2 sequences are homologous with a class of sequences first identified in *Drosophila* called **homeo box sequences** that regulate *Drosophila* development. The sequences regulate growth hormone gene expression by binding to a specific protein found in pituitary cells but not in other types of cells. This partly explains why the growth hormone promoter is active only in pituitary cells. Several other proteins (some that are not specific to pituitary cells and some that are receptors for hormones such as thyroid hormone) also bind near the growth hormone promoter. Interactions between these proteins appear to influence the initiation of transcription by RNA polymerase. A second example is the regulatory structure mediating glucocorticoid hormone action. As described in Chapter 1, glucocorticoids bind to intracellular receptors, and the steroid-receptor complex binds to DNA. The site on DNA where these receptors act is called the **glucocorticoid regulatory element** (GRE). The receptor complex binds to the GRE more tightly than to random DNA, and this binding enhances RNA polymerase action at the promoter located near the GRE (Fig 2–5). (See also Fig 1–20.) GREs found in glucocorticoid-responsive genes are usually located in the 5′-flanking DNA (less

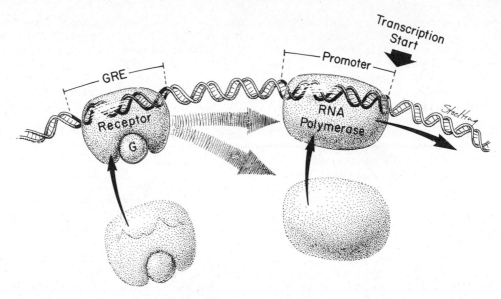

Figure 2–5. Regulatory structure mediating glucocorticoid (G) hormone action. The steroid-receptor complex binds to a specific DNA sequence called the glucocorticoid regulatory element (GRE). This binding event, in some unknown fashion, enhances (or in some cases inhibits) the interaction of RNA polymerase with the promoter of the glucocorticoid-regulated gene. The result is stimulation (or inhibition) of transcription of the gene.

commonly in introns) at a distance of a few to several thousand nucleotides away from the promoter. Similar mechanisms operate for the other classes of steroid hormones, vitamin D, thyroid hormone, and other nuclear-acting factors. Thus, these regulatory sequences can be thought of as "cassettes" of information inserted in the vicinity of a promoter that ordinarily bind regulatory proteins, some of which respond to regulatory ligands such as hormones that in turn affect promoter activity.

Gene expression can also be regulated at the level of RNA processing or mRNA turnover, although this is a less common mechanism than transcriptional control. For example, pre-mRNA from the calcitonin gene can be processed in 2 different ways that vary in the sequences removed. In brain and certain other tissues, the result is an mRNA that encodes calcitonin gene-related peptide (CGRP). In the parafollicular cells of the thyroid gland, calcitonin mRNA is primarily made. These 2 types of mRNA have in common the sequences at the 5' end that encode the amino-terminal portion of the precursor protein molecules. They differ in the 3' sequences that encode the carboxy-terminal portions of the molecules. Thus, this mechanism allows one gene to functionally serve as 2 genes. Variable RNA processing has been described for transcripts of the growth hormone and prolactin genes, although the differences in the resulting mRNA molecules are less striking. Hormones and other factors can regulate mRNA levels (and, consequently, protein levels) by affecting mRNA stability. Estrogens, for example, cause accumulation of ovalbumin mRNA in the chicken oviduct, owing in part to a steroid-mediated decrease in the rate of ovalbumin mRNA breakdown

with a consequent increase in the level of ovalbumin mRNA. The rates of degradation of particular mRNAs can be dictated by nucleotide sequences in either the 5'-untranslated, translated, or 3'-untranslated portions of the mRNA. How this is accomplished is as yet unknown.

There are several instances in which regulation of the efficiency of mRNA translation is observed, although these are unusual.

Finally, it should be emphasized that the activity of proteins is extensively controlled by hormones and other regulatory substances, as described in Chapter 1. Modification reactions such as phosphorylation control not only cytoplasmic events and the activity of cell surface receptors but also the activity of protein factors that affect transcription and other nuclear processes.

GENE EVOLUTION

Genes are generated during evolution through rearrangements, additions, or deletions of DNA segments; mutations of nucleotides; and duplications. The products of such duplication events can then evolve independently. This is the probable origin of the so-called **gene families,** which can comprise from a few to many genes. Related genes in these families can be identified through similarities in their overall organization and homologies (similarities) in their nucleotide sequences.

Examples of hormone gene families are (1) growth hormone, prolactin, and placental lactogen (chorionic somatomammotropin); (2) insulin and the somatomedins; and (3) the glycoprotein hormones (thyroid-stimulating hormone, chorionic gonadotropin, luteinizing hormone, and follicle-stimulating hormone). In this first example, the genes for growth hormone, prolactin, and placental lactogen all have a similar overall structure, with 5 exons separated by 4 introns. The sequences encoding the hormones have considerable homology, and when their exons are aligned to maximize this sequence similarity, the introns interrupt the coding sequences at similar locations. For the glycoprotein hormones, the same gene encodes the alpha subunit of the various hormones in the group, whereas the beta subunits of the hormones, although similar, are unique for each hormone. Another family of genes encodes the receptors for the steroid hormones, vitamin D, thyroid hormone, retinoic acid, and probably other ligands.

GENETIC DISEASE MECHANISMS

The precise molecular mechanisms for most of the genetic diseases encountered by endocrinologists are not known. Examples of diseases with a genetic basis are pseudohypoparathyroidism, vitamin D resistance, testicular feminization, congenital adrenal hyperplasia, some forms of dwarfism, type II diabetes mellitus, other rarer forms of diabetes mellitus, and disorders of lipid and lipoprotein metabolism. In other circumstances, the inherited defect is an increased susceptibility to developing a disease, eg, type I diabetes mellitus and the multiple endocrine neoplasia syndromes.

A number of molecular mechanisms can account for genetic disease. These have been examined in detail for many nonendocrine diseases such as the thalassemias; they have recently been established for many of the endocrine disorders. In some cases, mutations (such as those that alter a codon or generate a stop codon) change the amino acid sequence and result in a defective protein. For example, in vitamin D resistance, a mutation that changes one amino acid in the protein of the vitamin D receptor that binds to DNA results in defective receptor-DNA binding. Mutations sometimes result in an RNA product that does not accumulate in adequate quantities. Alternatively, deletion or insertion of genetic material can disrupt gene function or result in an abnormal RNA product. Mutations can also affect the processing of pre-mRNA into mRNA by occurring at sites on the gene required to specify proper processing. Finally, the entire gene can be deleted, as has been reported to occur in a rare form of growth hormone deficiency. For most genetic diseases, several independent mutations have resulted in the population of afflicted individuals. For example, over 10 different mutations have been found to produce familial hypercholesterolemia that results from defective or low levels of low-density lipoprotein (LDL) receptors. Several types of mutations also account for the 21-hydroxylase syndromes. Both of these conditions and many other genetic diseases are surprisingly prevalent; this suggests that these defects may have been selected for during evolution because they once provided an advantage to their carriers. This would be analogous to the protection conferred by sickle cell anemia and α-thalassemia against malaria.

RECOMBINANT DNA TECHNOLOGY

The essence of recombinant DNA technology is that isolated fragments of DNA can be cut and ligated together outside of living cells. This recombinant DNA can then be inserted back into a living cell of a prokaryote (nonnucleated cell such as a bacterium) or eukaryote (nucleated cell such as yeast or a mammalian cell) in which it can be replicated. In this way, starting from a single molecule, many new molecules can be obtained. These molecules can be used to study basic biologic processes such as how cells regulate gene expression. Alternatively, the technology can be put to practical uses such as the production of hormones that cannot be synthesized in adequate quantity or purity by other means. The methods available for producing recombinant DNA molecules have made it easier in many circumstances to work with DNA to yield novel protein products than to work with protein molecules themselves.

A major development that led to this new technology involved studies of the process of restriction and modification in bacteria whereby bacteria destroy foreign DNA yet protect their own genetic information by appropriate modifications. These studies led to the discovery of the **restriction enzymes** or **restriction endonucleases,** that bind to DNA at specific sequences and cleave it at these loci in a characteristic fashion. Fig 2–6 illustrates the action of the first restriction enzyme discovered, EcoRI, which was derived from *Escherichia coli.* (The name of each enzyme incorporates part of the name of the bacterium from which it was derived.) These enzymes allow scientists to cleave DNA at specific sites. Thus, a DNA fragment incubated with EcoRI will be cleaved at all sequences containing the structure shown in the figure. In this case, the cleavage will yield short single-stranded ends that are complementary to each other ("sticky ends"). If one of the resulting pieces is isolated and incubated with a DNA fragment from another source that has been cut with the same enzyme, the 2 complementary ends will base-pair. These hybrid DNA molecules can then be ligated together enzymatically to form a recombinant DNA molecule. Cleavage with some restriction enzymes yields fragments without sticky ends; these blunt-ended fragments can be ligated to other blunt-ended fragments, although this is somewhat less efficient.

Plasmids are frequently the starting material for such reconstructions; they serve as "vectors" for prop-

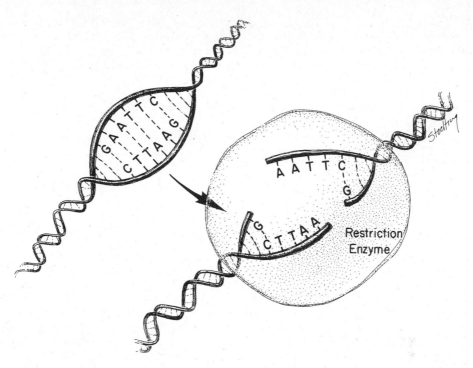

Figure 2–6. Endonucleolytic cleavage of DNA by the restriction enzyme EcoRI. The 6-base-pair sequence recognized by the restriction endonuclease is enlarged for purposes of illustration. The result of cleavage is 2 single-stranded "sticky ends," ie, ends overhanging 3 nucleotide complementary DNA segments.

agating recombinant DNA molecules. These are circular pieces of double-stranded DNA that replicate in bacterial "hosts" as episomes—ie, they replicate extrachromosomally. They frequently transmit antibiotic resistance; eg, they may contain a gene for β-lactamase that confers ampicillin resistance. A recombinant plasmid may be constructed as depicted in Fig 2–7 and inserted into a bacterium, usually *E coli,* by a process that makes the bacterium permeable and thus able to take up foreign DNA. The plasmid can subsequently replicate within the bacterial cell, and in this way the inserted DNA is replicated and transmitted along with the other genes carried on the plasmid. If a plasmid containing an antibiotic resistance gene is used, bacteria harboring the plasmid can be enriched by culturing them in the presence of the antibiotic. The population of cells derived from a single parent cell harboring a unique piece of foreign DNA is referred to as a **clone of cells,** and the DNA contained within them is said to be cloned (Fig 2–8). Once a clone is obtained, the bacteria can be grown in mass quantities, the plasmid DNA isolated and separated from other bacterial constituents, and the inserted DNA released from the plasmid by cleavage with the same restriction enzyme used for its initial isolation. This DNA can then be separated from the plasmid DNA by electrophoretic techniques and characterized.

Bacteriophages are viruses that infect bacteria. Variants of bacteriophage λ are used extensively as vectors for molecular cloning. This process involves inserting foreign DNA into the middle of the single chromosome in these variants. This recombinant DNA can then be incubated with the bacteriophage proteins ("packaged") to produce viable bacteriophages. These bacteriophages are then used to infect "lawns" of bacteria. During infection, a single phage particle attacks a bacterium, inserts its DNA into the bacterium, and then replicates within it. These bacteriophages mature and eventually lyse the bacterium. The released bacteriophages then infect the neighboring bacteria and repeat the process. Each starting virus finally produces a clear "plaque" of lysed bacteria containing a clone of that bacteriophage. Individual clones of bacteriophages can be propagated by letting them infect other bacteria cultures. Bacteriophages are particularly efficient for producing a large number of clones that each contain a single fragment from a starting mixture containing many DNAs, because the viral DNA gets into cells more efficiently than plasmid DNA does. Also, larger pieces of DNA can be inserted into bacteriophages than into plasmids. Three types of bacteriophage λ variants are used commonly: λgt10, λgt11, and cosmids. λgt10 is used for general cloning; λgt11 contains an inserted bacterial promoter and other structures that allow inserted DNA to be "expressed," ie, transcribed and the transcript translated into protein. Cosmids can accept particularly large pieces of DNA.

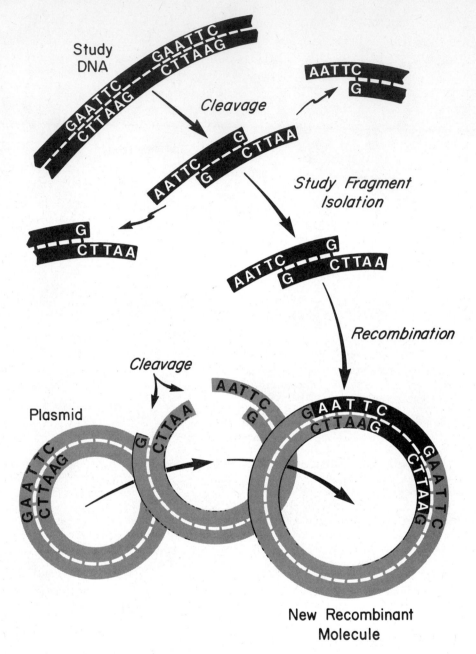

Figure 2–7. Generation of a recombinant DNA molecule. The study DNA is cleaved with a restriction enzyme (in this case, EcoRI), and the released fragment is purified (eg, separated from the parent DNA on the basis of size by agarose gel electrophoresis). A suitable plasmid containing a unique site for the same enzyme is prepared by cleavage with the enzyme and is then mixed with the purified fragment. The complementary overhanging ends anneal to one another and are then ligated together enzymatically (DNA ligase) to yield a new recombinant molecule.

HYBRIDIZATION

A fundamental property of single-stranded DNA or RNA is its propensity to anneal through base pairing (ie, hybridize) to a complementary strand of DNA or RNA. This is a very precise process based on the hy-drogen bonding of A to T or U and of C to G, which permits a single-stranded nucleic acid to find its complement among millions of noncomplementary competing molecules. Recombinant DNA technology makes extensive use of this property. For example, a homogeneous piece of DNA, after radiolabeling, can

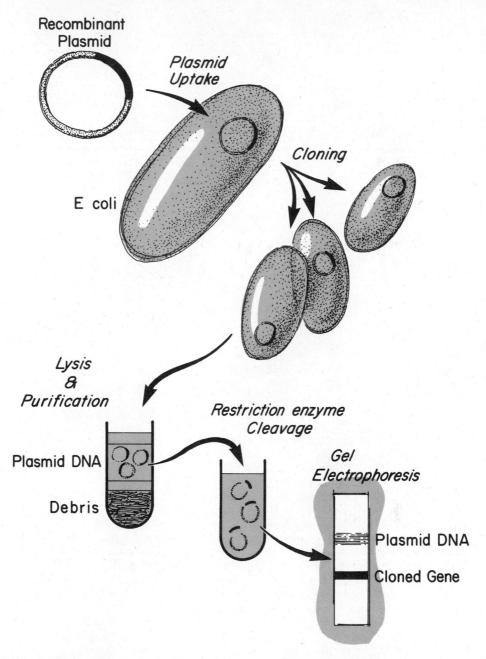

Figure 2–8. Cloning of DNA. Bacteria are treated to facilitate the uptake of recombinant plasmids containing the DNA insert of interest. Culturing in the presence of an antibiotic selects for those bacteria harboring a plasmid containing an appropriate antibiotic-resistance gene (resident on the same plasmid as the insert). Those bacteria that have failed to take up the plasmid will succumb to the antibiotic. Single colonies (a clone) of the now-resistant bacteria are selected for mass culture and are then lysed and the cloned plasmid DNA purified. Cleavage with the appropriate restriction enzyme will release the DNA insert, yielding quantities of homogeneous DNA suitable for further experimentation (eg, for sequencing or preparation of specific radiolabeled DNA probes).

be used as a **probe** (1) to identify a complementary piece of DNA or RNA that has been size-fractionated on a gel; (2) to localize a single colony of bacteria (from among thousands) that harbors a plasmid containing complementary sequences; or (3) to quantify levels of a specific mRNA. The latter process consists of: allowing the probe to hybridize to a mixture of mRNA molecules, either in solution or after the RNA has been transferred to filter paper; eliminating the nonhybridized probe; and then measuring the radioactivity in the hybrids, which reflects the amount of specific mRNA present.

DNA SEQUENCING

Another breakthrough that has facilitated the development of recombinant DNA technology was the design of methods to rapidly sequence DNA. Two methods are currently available.

The **chemical degradation technique** of Maxam and Gilbert relies on the systematic cleavage of homogeneous DNA fragments radiolabeled at one end. Reaction conditions cause the cleavage to occur only at one of the 4 nucleotides (A residues, for instance); only one of the susceptible positions in a DNA molecule is usually cleaved. The result is a series of DNA fragments extending from the radiolabeled end to each location of the given nucleotide (ie, at each A) in the original DNA fragment. These can be visualized after size fractionation of the DNA and radioautography; the size of each band corresponds to the position of the base in the starting DNA.

The **chain termination technique** of Sanger uses a homogeneous population of single-stranded DNA molecules as templates for complementary DNA synthesis. DNA synthesis is initiated at a particular site with the use of a small "primer" oligonucleotide that hybridizes to a specific sequence. DNA synthesis then proceeds in the presence of radiolabeled nucleoside triphosphate precursors. In addition, the reaction is performed in the presence of a nucleotide analog in which the 3′-OH group has been modified so that, after its incorporation, further elongation beyond the nucleotide cannot proceed. Four separate reactions are run, each reaction including a separate modified nucleotide (dideoxy ATP, for example) in addition to the 4 unmodified nucleotides. The chosen conditions cause the synthesis of the complementary DNA molecule to be terminated at low frequency at each site of a given base (A in this example). The resulting radiolabeled fragments, terminated at each nucleotide, are then size-fractionated on gels; the size of the band corresponds to the position of the complementary base in the original template DNA.

By use of these methods, even genes that are several thousand nucleotides in length can be sequenced in a reasonable period of time. Thus, once a gene is obtained in pure form, its primary structure, or nucleotide sequence, can be determined rapidly and accurately. These methods have been refined and automated to such an extent that the sequencing of the entire human genome is now a realistic possibility.

POLYMERASE CHAIN REACTION

The recently developed **polymerase chain reaction** (**PCR**) method is now being widely used to amplify DNA. This process involves incubating 2 DNA "primer" molecules and DNA polymerase with a given DNA or mixture of DNAs. The first primer hybridizes to complementary sequences at one end of the DNA to be amplified and primes the initiation of DNA replication at that site. The second primer is complementary to the opposite DNA strand at the other end of the DNA to be amplified. Thus, the polymerase first synthesizes DNA strands initiated from each of the primers. The polymerase is heat stable, and after each round of replication the DNA strands are denatured by heating and then the mixture is brought back to the reaction temperature and the next round of replication is allowed to proceed. DNA synthesized after the first 2 rounds of replication will be primed dominantly from the newly synthesized copies such that these copies will have termini corresponding to the location of the primers. With progressive cycles, the DNA sequences spanning the region between the 2 primers are enormously amplified. Thus, the starting DNA needs to contain a minute fraction (even one copy) of the DNA to be amplified. This PCR-amplified DNA can then be analyzed, by DNA sequencing or hybridization, for example, or used for molecular cloning. The PCR methodology is particularly suitable for analyzing genetic diseases. For example, any mutation in the amplified DNA will be revealed when it is sequenced. PCR will probably be used increasingly to diagnose genetic diseases, to detect foreign DNA such as viral or bacterial DNA in biologic specimens, and to perform molecular cloning.

SOURCES OF DNA FOR MOLECULAR CLONING

Three different sources of DNA are ordinarily used for molecular cloning: DNA produced by chemical synthesis, cellular mRNA transcribed into DNA by the process of reverse transcription, and chromosomal DNA.

DNA Synthesis

DNA molecules composed of as many as 70 nucleotides can now be synthesized rapidly by mechanical synthesizers. An entire gene can be constructed by combining several oligonucleotides synthesized in this fashion. This approach was used for the first recombinant DNA synthesis of human insulin. At the time this was done, the sequence of the insulin gene had not yet been determined, but the amino acid sequence of human insulin was known. Based on this knowledge, DNA fragments encoding the A and B chains of insulin were synthesized and each was used to program clones of bacteria to produce the respective chains. The resulting chains were then purified from the bacteria and joined chemically to yield insulin.

More commonly, smaller DNA segments are produced to facilitate recombinant DNA research. For example, small DNA segments containing restriction enzyme sites are added to the ends of DNA fragments to construct recombinant DNA molecules. Chemically synthesized fragments are used as probes to detect complementary DNA or RNA molecules. Synthetic DNA can be used to prepare hybrid genes that are combinations of different mammalian or bacterial genes. These may be used for protein production in the appropriate host cell.

Reverse Transcription of mRNA

Cellular mRNA encoding a particular protein can be isolated from cells that produce the specific protein product. DNA strands complementary to this mRNA (cDNA) can be produced from the mRNA template using deoxyribonucleoside triphosphates and the enzyme reverse transcriptase. This enzyme is isolated from retroviruses, RNA viruses that copy their RNA into DNA (reverse transcription). As discussed in a previous section, most mRNA molecules have a poly(A) tail, and this tail can be hybridized (annealed) to an oligomer of polydeoxythymidylate (oligo-dT) that serves as a required "primer" to initiate the reverse transcription. After the RNA is transcribed, it is destroyed, and the single-stranded cDNA formed through transcription is then copied into a double-stranded molecule. This latter step is facilitated either by the reverse transcriptase that can also copy DNA into DNA or by DNA polymerase.

One of several different methods can be used to insert the cDNA into a plasmid or bacteriophage vector. For example, chemically synthesized double-stranded DNA "linker" molecules containing an appropriate restriction site can be ligated to the ends of the fragment, and the entire fragment can then be inserted into the vector at the same restriction enzyme site (Fig 2–7).

Since any given cell contains thousands of different mRNA molecules, reverse transcription of total cellular mRNA will yield thousands of different cDNA molecules. To obtain a particular cDNA from this mixture, the investigator usually generates a large number of clones from the cDNA, thereby yielding a so-called cDNA library. After this library is inserted into a suitable vector and cloned into the appropriate host cell, up to millions of clones may exist, each harboring the same parent plasmid but a different cDNA insert. These must be screened to find the clone of bacteria containing plasmids or bacteriophages with the cDNA insert of interest. Screening of a cDNA library may be performed in several ways, 2 of which will be discussed.

First, if even a portion of the amino acid sequence of the protein encoded by the mRNA is known, this information can be used, through knowledge of the genetic code, to predict a partial DNA sequence for the cDNA. Small oligonucleotide DNA molecules that contain the nucleotide sequence complementary to the cDNA are then synthesized and radiolabeled. The DNA of the

clones comprising the cDNA library is transferred to filter papers and hybridized to the labeled oligonucleotides. The DNA from those clones with the correct cDNA—but not other cDNAs—will hybridize to the oligonucleotide probes. The clones can then be grown in large-scale culture for further analysis.

A second approach for screening a cDNA library is to insert the cDNA into a site in the vector that is somewhere in the middle of a bacterial gene, so that the codons of the cDNA will be expressed as part of a "fusion protein" containing bacterial and cDNA-encoded amino acid sequences. Screening this cDNA expression library with an antibody to the protein product of interest will permit identification of the clone producing the appropriate fusion protein and thus harboring the correct cDNA-containing vector.

To rigorously establish that the cDNA isolated by screening methods is in fact the correct one, the nucleotide sequence of the cDNA is determined. This is then compared with the amino acid sequence of the protein.

Chromosomal Genes

Using techniques analogous to those employed for cDNA cloning, the portions of a chromosome that contain the gene of interest can be cloned. Chromosomal DNA isolated from cell nuclei is cleaved into fragments with a restriction enzyme and the resultant fragments ligated into the appropriate bacteriophage DNA are cloned. A radiolabeled cDNA or chemically synthesized oligonucleotide may then be used to screen for the clone of bacteriophage with the chromosomal insert of interest. This is done by transferring the bacteriophage to a filter paper and then hybridizing the filter-bound phage DNA to the radioactive probe.

TRANSFER OF CLONED GENES INTO MAMMALIAN CELLS

DNA can be transferred, or "transfected," into mammalian cells in several ways to study gene function or produce proteins for scientific or commercial uses. For example, it can be microinjected into the cell nucleus. Alternatively, calcium phosphate precipitates of DNA can be prepared that will be phagocytosed by the cells. Bacteria that contain plasmids with inserted DNA can be stripped of their cell wall to form protoplasts that will fuse to mammalian cells. Direct electroporation of plasmid DNA into recipient cells is also sometimes used. In addition, viral vectors (eg, from retroviruses or bovine papillomavirus) have been designed to deliver the DNA of interest into target cells.

Most of the transfected DNA will not become integrated into the host chromosome and be stably expressed. However, some of this DNA may be transiently expressed, and its function can be studied for a short time (hours to days; transient expression assays). In other circumstances, it is desirable to isolate those few cells in which the transfected DNA has become integrated and therefore replicated along with the host DNA. This can be achieved, for example, by "co-transfecting" the DNA of interest with DNA containing a "selectable" gene, such as the gene encoding resistance to neomycin. In this case, when the cells are then cultured in the presence of an analogue of neomycin that ordinarily kills the cells, only the cells that both integrate and express the neomycin resistance gene will survive and propagate. These cells will usually have integrated the study gene as well.

Mammalian cells can amplify certain DNA sequences, including transfected DNA. Cells that harbor such amplified DNA can be selected for by applying pressure like that described above with neomycin resistance. This method is used extensively to select for mammalian cells that contain large numbers of a transfected gene and also (in many cases) to produce large quantities of its product.

Gene transfer into mammalian cells has been enormously useful for studying the mechanisms of gene expression and its regulation. A convenient way to study gene function after transfection is to link the promoter to be studied to the coding sequences of a "reporter" gene (such as that which encodes for chloramphenicol acetyltransferase [CAT] or lucidiferase) whose function is easily measured. For example, information about the glucocorticoid regulatory element shown in Fig 2–5 was derived chiefly from such gene transfer studies. Initially, these studies involved transferring a cloned glucocorticoid-responsive gene into a mammalian cell, which normally does not express that specific gene, and documenting that the transferred gene was glucocorticoid-responsive. This type of experiment demonstrates that elements responsive to the steroid reside somewhere on the cloned DNA that was transferred. Follow-up studies have included deleting the putative steroid regulatory sequences prior to gene transfer to demonstrate extinction of hormone responsiveness and splicing the putative control sequence to another gene that ordinarily is not steroid-regulated and demonstrating that the hybrid gene is glucocorticoid-responsive. Analogous methods are also used to study the mechanisms of hormone receptor function. For example, when a cell that is not ordinarily glucocorticoid-responsive is cotransfected with a glucocorticoid-responsive gene and one encoding the glucocorticoid receptor, the cell becomes responsive to the steroid. The function of individual domains of the receptor can be analyzed by constructing mutant receptor genes and transfecting them to assess their activities.

PRODUCTION OF MEDICALLY IMPORTANT PROTEINS BY RECOMBINANT DNA TECHNIQUES

A major use of recombinant DNA technology is to produce medically useful proteins. Employing genes to produce the proteins encoded by them is presently

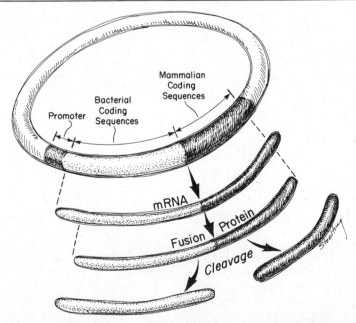

Figure 2–9. Expression of a mammalian protein as a fusion protein in bacteria. Sequences coding for a mammalian protein are linked to sequences coding for a bacterial protein. The linkage occurs in phase with respect to the genetic code. The hybrid protein gene is expressed under the control of the bacterial promoter. If engineered properly, the fusion protein can be cleaved (chemically or enzymatically) to release the mammalian protein, which can then be further purified.

the only means available for producing moderate-sized to large proteins in quantity. Although the methods for chemically synthesizing peptides have improved considerably in recent years, they have not progressed to the point where large proteins (eg, > 100 amino acids) can be made efficiently. Whereas some proteins, such as insulin, can be obtained by isolating them from animals, this approach (even for insulin) has its limitations and is impractical when large quantities of scarce proteins are needed, as is the case with interferon and erythropoietin.

As discussed earlier, genes must have regulatory sequences to be expressed. If mammalian DNA sequences are inserted randomly into bacteria, they will usually not be expressed efficiently. Therefore, sequences that encode the desired proteins must be inserted downstream from bacterial regulatory sequences that can direct the synthesis of the desired protein. These sequences would include a promoter; those encoding a ribosomal binding site; and an AUG codon, which codes for methionine and is necessary in mRNA to initiate translation. By this method of direct expression, the synthesized proteins can frequently be obtained in yields that represent several percent of the total bacterial proteins. These proteins are then purified from the bacteria. An alternative approach is the synthesis of a fusion (hybrid) protein from which the desired protein can be cleaved (Fig 2–9). To do this, the DNA sequences encoding the desired protein are inserted into the middle of the coding sequences of the bacterial gene. The bacterium synthesizes a hybrid protein containing sequences of bacterial and mammalian amino acids, with the sequences joined at a site that is susceptible to proteolytic or chemical cleavage. The mammalian protein can then be released from the fusion protein with the appropriate enzymes or chemical reagent. This approach was used for the first bacterial synthesis of human insulin and β-endorphin, and it offers particular advantages for the production of smaller proteins that alone are usually degraded rapidly in bacteria.

In some cases, proteins are produced more efficiently by yeasts than by bacteria. These organisms have plasmids similar to those of bacteria, and the approaches used for protein synthesis are similar to those described above. One useful feature of yeasts is that they can be programmed to secrete their expressed proteins into the medium, a feature that aids in purification.

Mammalian cells are being used increasingly for the production of recombinant DNA-derived proteins. This research has been stimulated by methods that increase the production yields and allow for the use of media that are devoid of expensive animal serum. An advantage of the use of mammalian cells is that these cells can add important carbohydrate groups to the proteins when this is necessary; this may not be done correctly by yeasts and is not performed at all by bacteria. Plasminogen activators now in clinical use and more complex proteins such as factor VIII are being produced by mammalian cells.

PRODUCTS OF RECOMBINANT DNA TECHNOLOGY

The human body produces thousands of different proteins, including those that function as hormones or enzymes, and deficiencies or excesses of many of these proteins can contribute to human disease. A large potential for clinical use of recombinant DNA products exists in this area. Technology is aimed at producing pure proteins, protein antagonists, and protein derivatives that possess a more limited and thus clinically more specific range of activities compared to the parent protein. The following is a brief review of progress in this area related to endocrinology.

Human insulin prepared by recombinant techniques is now available, and this ensures an unlimited supply of this hormone. **Growth hormone** has now replaced the cadaver-derived human growth hormone, which may in some cases be contaminated with Creutzfeldt-Jakob virus. **Erythropoietin** is useful for treating certain anemias and may decrease the need for transfusion and thereby reduce the risk of transfusion-associated complications, eg, in patients with renal failure. **Atrial natriuretic factor** is being tested in humans for the treatment of hypertension, heart failure, renal failure, and related states. Recombinant DNA-produced growth factors such as **epidermal growth factor** and fibroblast growth factor may promote wound repair. Relaxin may be useful in obstetric practice for relaxing the pelvis of a pregnant woman enough to permit the passage of a large fetus. **Pulmonary surfactant protein** may be useful in neonatology; this protein is deficient in patients with neonatal respiratory distress syndrome.

Products targeted principally at nonendocrinologic diseases may also become part of the armamentarium of endocrinologists. A number of agents being tested for anticancer activity, such as the **interferons, tumor necrosis factor,** and **interleukins,** may prove useful in treating endocrine neoplasia or ectopic hormone-producing cancers. Recombinant DNA technology is also being used to develop **vaccines** that potentially could prevent viral illnesses thought to be involved in the pathogenesis of diseases such as diabetes mellitus.

Not only can naturally occurring proteins be made, but variant proteins can be produced with specific advantages. The structures of genes can be altered so that they produce variants of the natural compounds. In addition, hybrid molecules can be produced by linking together parts of different genes to form a protein that has, for example, greater agonist activity than the natural compound or more specificity for a particular response. The activities of hybrid and variant immunoglobulin and tissue plasminogen molecules are currently being tested. Molecules with antagonist activity are also being produced. For example, **parathyroid hormone (PTH) antagonists,** produced by deleting amino acids from the amino terminus of PTH, might be useful in treating hypercalcemic states associated with excess PTH or PTH-like activity.

DRUG DELIVERY SYSTEMS

Most of the products of recombinant DNA technology are proteins that cannot be given orally for therapy. In general, they are unstable and poorly absorbed from the gastrointestinal tract. Thus, they must be given by injection, and this limits their use. A number of drug delivery systems are also being developed to overcome this problem. One approach involves the development of implantable devices that release medication at appropriate intervals during a prolonged period. Administration of peptides through the nose, rectum, and lungs is also being investigated. The nasal mucosa takes up some peptides, such as vasopressin and calcitonin, efficiently enough to be therapeutically effective. The nasal mucosa takes up larger proteins poorly when they are administered alone, but the inclusion of "enhancer" substances can promote their uptake. One such system involves mixing the protein with a bile salt analogue and spraying the mixture into the nose. This system has been shown to be effective over short periods for delivering insulin to diabetics. Because intranasally administered peptides are absorbed rapidly into the circulation, mimicking intravenous delivery, they may be particularly useful when pulsatile kinetics are desired, as when insulin is used for postprandial hyperglycemia. Liposomes may ultimately be useful for delivering parenterally administered drugs to particular sites. For example, drugs encapsulated by liposomes are preferentially taken up by reticuloendothelial cells, so this method could be used to deliver cytotoxic drugs to cancers involving these cells. Alternatively, ligands that bind to specific cell types could possibly be incorporated into liposomes to deliver them with encapsulated drugs to these cells.

RATIONAL DRUG DESIGN

Drug design has traditionally started with biologically active materials that occur in nature. Some of these materials have emerged as pharmaceuticals themselves (insulin and penicillin, for example). In other cases, naturally occurring compounds have been modified to improve the resulting drug's efficiency. Thus, the precursors to converting enzyme inhibitors came from snake venom, and those to hydroxymethylglutaryl-coenzyme A (HMG-CoA) reductase inhibitors (that block cholesterol biosynthesis) came from fungi. However, powerful new methods for rational drug design are now available—including recombinant DNA technology, more sophisticated means for determining protein structures such as x-ray diffraction and nuclear magnetic resonance (NMR), spectroscopy, and newer computer modeling techniques—that should accelerate the rate of pharmaceutical development. These methods can be applied to identified potential sites of action or targets for pharmaceuticals. In endocrinology, these targets are typically hormone receptors (eg, those for steroids, catecholamines, or peptides) or enzymes (eg, renin, converting enzyme, or HMG-CoA reductase), but they can also be specific viral protein or other regulatory molecules. Recombinant DNA techniques can now produce these targets in quantities sufficient to determine their 3-dimensional structures. Once the configuration of the binding site for a drug is known, drugs that stimulate or inhibit the site can be more rationally and more effectively designed.

DIAGNOSIS OF GENETIC DISEASE USING DNA

The DNA of a patient's cells obtained from blood, amniotic fluid, or biopsy material can be readily analyzed utilizing recombinant DNA technology. Tests based on DNA analysis are available for diagnosis of such classic genetic diseases as the thalassemias, sickle cell anemia, and phenylketonuria, and these tests have recently been applied to such endocrinologic conditions as multiple endocrine adenoma (MEA) type I. Genetic differences also contribute to many more common diseases in which the specific genetic defect has not yet been defined (eg, hypertension and type II diabetes mellitus), and the ability to analyze genes in detail may allow for the detection of DNA segments responsible for these diseases and thus provide a new means for diagnosis and study of these disorders.

Although a gene can be isolated from an individual and its primary structure determined, this procedure is cumbersome at present and not yet adaptable for general clinical use. However, when the locus of the proposed defect is strongly suspected, the PCR methodology, discussed in an earlier section, can be successfully employed.

Currently, the most prevalent technique for diagnosing genetic diseases is **restriction fragment length polymorphism** (RFLP) methodology. This approach generally involves isolating DNA from a patient and his or her relatives, cleaving it with restriction enzymes, running it on gels, transferring it to nitrocellulose filters, and hybridizing it with particular DNA probes. This method relies heavily on analysis of **genetic polymorphisms**—ie, differences in the primary structures of genes, such as differences between the 2 alleles of a given gene in the same individual or between the genes of different individuals. Such differences can occur in the gene sequences that are transcribed or in the 5'- or 3'-flanking DNA. Polymorphisms are generated in the process of replication of the DNA, when mutations occur at low frequency. Most of these are "silent" in that they have no effect on the function of the gene or on its products. Nevertheless, these mutations are inherited and can be used as **genetic markers.**

The following is an illustration of one use of polymorphism analysis. Assume, for instance, that a mutation in one base occurs in an individual and that this results in a genetic trait—eg, susceptibility to developing a disease such as diabetes mellitus. Somewhere in or around the affected gene, this individual is likely to have additional differences in comparison to other people. Occasionally, these differences result in the generation or loss of a restriction endonuclease cleavage site (Fig 2–10). In this case, cleavage of the affected individual's DNA with the restriction enzyme will result in DNA fragments that differ in size from those of other

people. Subjecting the fragments to size fractionation on a gel and performing hybridization to a radiolabeled probe from the gene as described above will allow identification of the aberrant fragment. Since the restriction site polymorphism will be inherited along with the mutation that results in disease susceptibility, this polymorphism can be used as a genetic marker for the disease. This type of analysis only requires an established linkage between a disease and a restriction fragment length polymorphism (RFLP) and an appropriate DNA probe; it is not necessary to know anything about the gene product.

In practice, the RFLP pattern is compared in afflicted and nonafflicted family members to establish the diagnosis; multiple mutations of independent origin commonly account for a given genetic disease, so a different RFLP pattern will exist for unrelated afflicted patients. For diseases such as sickle cell anemia, however, in which a single mutation accounts for all known cases, a change in a restriction enzyme site at the locus of the mutation can be used for general diagnosis.

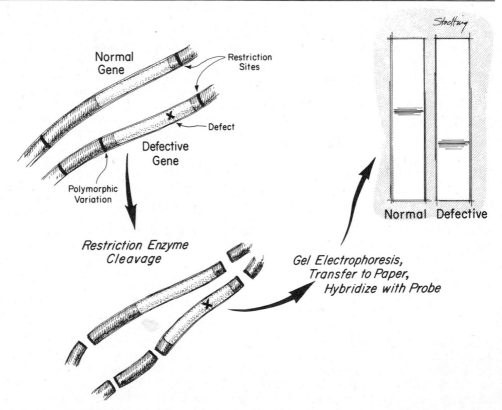

Figure 2–10. Use of restriction fragment length polymorphisms (RFLPs) as genetic markers of disease. In the case illustrated, a mutation resulting in a defective gene is associated with a polymorphic variation in the 5'-flanking DNA, and this results in the presence of a restriction site not present in unafflicted individuals. Cleavage with the appropriate restriction enzyme will yield a smaller fragment for the defective gene than for the normal gene. Subjecting the various fragments to size fractionation on a gel and to hybridization to a radiolabeled probe will allow identification of the aberrant fragment. This obviates the need for isolation and cloning of the genomic DNA to identify the mutation within the gene.

TRANSGENIC ANIMALS

Transgenic animals contain foreign DNA in their genomes. The availability of transgenic mice is greatly changing the study of gene function; when this technology is adapted to other animals, it is also likely to change animal husbandry techniques. Transgenic mice are prepared by microinjecting DNA into a fertilized mouse egg and then placing the egg into a pseudopregnant mouse. The recipient mouse then produces offspring containing the transfected DNA. Because the transfected DNA was placed in the egg, all of the cells of the resulting offspring will usually contain the transfected DNA. The progeny from such animals can then be used to produce more offspring containing the foreign DNA.

The use of transgenic mice has opened up many new and promising areas of study. For example, DNA containing the 5'-flanking DNA segment of the growth hormone gene can be linked to the coding sequences for another gene that is not ordinarily expressed in the pituitary. When this DNA is used to prepare transgenic mice, the foreign gene is expressed in pituitary cells but not in other types of cells. This experiment indicates that the DNA signals directing the pituitary-specific expression of this gene are contained in the transfected 5'-flanking DNA segment. In another example, a heterologous promoter such as that for the metallothionein gene can be linked to growth hormone coding sequences. The metallothionein promoter will be active in a large number of tissues that in turn will produce growth hormone. Thus, when this DNA is used for the microinjection, the offspring produced grow unusually large. This technique could be adapted to species such as fish to produce food more efficiently. A final example involves the 5'-flanking DNA segment of the alpha subunit of the glycoprotein gene being linked to a gene whose product stimulates cell replication (eg, the simian virus 40 T antigen gene). When this DNA is used for the microinjection, the resulting transgenic animals develop pituitary tumors that produce gonadotropin and contain gonadotropin-releasing hormone receptors. These tumors can be used to obtain and propagate cells that were previously unavailable for culture and study.

POTENTIAL FOR GENE THERAPY

Since genes can be transferred into mammalian cells and function after such transfer, it follows that genes might be inserted into the cells of patients where they could function, in effect, as therapeutic agents. For example, if the insulin gene could be appropriately transferred into a patient with type I diabetes mellitus, this gene could deliver insulin to the patient on a continuing basis, thereby obviating the need for insulin injections.

Similar considerations apply to other diseases such as the thalassemias, sickle cell anemia, and hypoparathyroidism and other hormonal deficiency states. Conversely, gene transfer therapy could also be used to treat states of pathologic excess, such as hypercholesterolemia or hypertension, by using genes that would lower cholesterol levels or blood pressure. However, the first applications of gene therapy will probably involve more severe conditions such as immunodeficiency states, cancer, and certain enzyme defects. Note that this type of therapy involves inserting foreign genes into somatic cells, which are not transmitted to offspring, whereas the preparation of transgenic animals involves inserting foreign genes into germ line cells, which are transmitted to offspring.

Most researchers now agree that gene therapy will ultimately be possible. However, a number of problems must be solved before it becomes generally applicable. In many cases, the gene must be delivered to the right tissue, eg, globin genes to erythroid cells and adenosine deaminase genes to bone marrow-derived cells. Similarly, for the LDL receptor gene to lower cholesterol levels, it has to function in the liver. Retroviruses have already been used to insert functional LDL receptor genes into hepatic cells, and transgenic mice overexpressing transfected LDL receptor genes have low serum cholesterol levels. In cases of hormone deficiency, however, such tissue-specific expression may not be necessary. In many cases, the gene must only function adequately, not excessively. For example, the insulin gene should not overfunction and produce hypoglycemia; ideally, expression of the transferred gene should respond to blood glucose levels. When genes are integrated into dividing cells, a mutation may occur at the site of integration that could lead to malignant transformation of the cell. One way to prevent this may involve removing target cells from the body, transferring the gene, documenting its proper function, demonstrating that the cells are not malignantly transformed, and then delivering them back to appropriate locations in the body. These cells might also be inserted in a capsule or a subcutaneous site so they could be removed if it became desirable to terminate treatment.

ETHICAL & BIOSAFETY CONSIDERATIONS

Recombinant DNA technology, like most other technologies, has the potential for misuse, either accidental or deliberate. When it first emerged in the 1970s, great concern was raised about its overall safety. It was feared, for example, that *E coli* harboring potentially toxic genes, if accidentally leaked into the environment, would propagate and cause great damage. Fortunately, most of these concerns have now been allayed; the strains of *E coli* used in the laboratory do not multiply well outside the laboratory or in the human intestine, and in general environmental pressure actually impairs the survival of organisms harboring cloned genes. Nevertheless, the potential does exist for inserting genes into organisms in ways that could produce harmful results. In addition, a general fear exists that gene therapy might be inherently immoral, or that it might be used to create individuals with undesirable traits, as popularized in the science fiction literature. For these and other reasons, most agree that there should be guidelines for conducting recombinant DNA research, as is now the case.

IMPACT OF MOLECULAR BIOLOGY ON MEDICINE

The basic information about genes and their function has been the greatest contribution of recombinant DNA technology, notwithstanding the numerous practical applications already achieved (as discussed earlier in this chapter). In addition, these applications themselves have provided means for increasing the body of knowledge. For example, the availability of substantial supplies, of proteins such as erythropoietin, other hematopoietic hormones, renin, and growth hormone provide a way to learn much more about their actions, biologic roles, and therapeutic uses.

Recent progress in cancer research is also illustrative. The study of retroviruses that can induce neoplastic transformation has generated information about potential mechanisms by which normal cells may become neoplastic. Many of these retroviruses carry a viral oncogene that can induce tumors. These oncogenes are similar to genes ("proto-oncogenes") in the normal cells from which the oncogenes were obtained. The products of the proto-oncogenes regulate cellular processes. Viral oncogenes are denoted by a

"v" preceding the name of the virus that harbors the gene; cellular genes are denoted by a preceding "c." These oncogenes may be related to growth factors (v-*sis* and a platelet-derived growth factor receptor subunit), growth factor receptors (v-*erb* B and the epidermal growth factor receptor; v-*fms* and the macrophage colony-stimulating factor receptor), protein-tyrosine kinase (v-*src*, v-*abl*), signal transduction-mediating guanyl nucleotide-binding proteins (v-*ras*), DNA-binding transcriptional regulatory proteins (v-*jun*, v-*fos*, v-*myc*) including the thyroid hormone receptor (v-*erb* A), and protein-serine kinase (v-*mos*). Other retroviruses stimulate the expression of cellular genes by inserting their RNA near these genes and then overriding their normal control elements. Sometimes the retroviruses also alter the structure of the gene products. In several human tumors, expression of certain proto-oncogenes is increased; in many cases, these genes are even amplified (c-*erb* B in epidermal cancer cells). Also, certain chromosomal translocations found in human tumors (c-*abl* gene in chronic myelogenous leukemia) occur at or near proto-oncogenes. In other tumors, proto-oncogene mutations have been found. Thus, the excessive or abnormal function of these genes appears to contribute to the malignant state. Other cellular genes appear to be "anti-oncogenes": The inactivation of their products by other viral products or by the mutation of the anti-oncogene (hereditary retinoblastoma) appears to participate in the development of cancer. Altogether, the evidence suggests that several steps are generally required to develop a tumor, that more than one gene may participate in the malignant state, and that heterogeneity and changes in oncogene expression can occur in a given tumor and can affect the course and progression of the malignancy. As more of these genes and their products are identified and their functions understood, better strategies can be devised to monitor and treat these disorders.

REFERENCES

General

Basic Biotechnology. Bu'luck J, Kristiansen B (editors). Academic Press, London 1987.

Biochemistry (3rd Ed). Stryer L (editor). WH Freeman & Company, New York 1988.

Current Protocols in Molecular Biology (Vols 1 and 2). Ausubel FM et al (editors). Green Publishing Assoc & Wiley Interscience, New York 1988.

Lewin B: *Genes II*. Wiley, 1985.

Molecular Cell Biology. Darnell J, Lodish H, Baltimore D (editors). Scientific American Book, New York 1986.

Watson JD et al: *Molecular Biology of the Gene*. Benjamin/Cummings Publishing Company, Inc, Menlo Park, CA 1987 pp 1163.

Regulation of Gene Expression & Gene Transfer

Akerblom IE et al: Negative regulation by glucocorticoids through interference with a c-AMP responsive enhancer. *Science* 1988;**241**:350.

Bentley DL, Groudine M: Sequence requirements for premature termination of transcription in the human c-myc gene. *Cell* 1988;**53**:245.

Bos TJ et al: v-*jun* encodes a nuclear protein with enhancer properties of AP-1. *Cell* 1988;**52**:705.

Botstein D, Fink GR: Yeast: An experimental organism for modern biology. *Science* 240;**1988**:1439.

Casey JL et al: Iron-responsive elements: Regulatory RNA sequences that control mRNA levels and translation. *Science* 1988;**240**:924.

Curran T, Franza BR Jr: Fos and Jun: The AP-1 connection. *Cell* 1988;**55**:395.

Dawid IB, Sargent TD: Xenopus laevis in developmental and molecular biology. *Science* 1988;**240**:1443.

Dorn A, Benoist C, Mathis D: New B-lymphocyte-specific enhancer-binding protein. *Mol Cell Biol* 1989;**9**:312.

Evans RM: The steroid and thyroid hormone receptor and superfamily. *Science* 1988;**240**:889.

Fromental C et al: Cooperativity and hierarchical levels of functional organization in the SV40 enhancer. *Cell* 1988;**54**:943.

Gartler SM, Riggs AD: Mammalian x-chromosome inactivation. *Annu Rev Genet* 1983;**17**:155.

Hyman SE et al: A common *trans*-acting factor is involved in transcriptional regulation of neurotransmitter genes by cyclic AMP. *Mol Cell Biol* 1988;**8**:4225.

Ingraham HA et al: A tissue-specific transcription factor containing a homeodomain specifies a pituitary phenotype. *Cell* 1988;**55**:519.

Jaenisch R: Transgenic animals. *Science* 1988;**240**:1468.

Kornberg A: DNA replication. *J Biol Chem* 1988;**263**:1.

Oro AE, Hollenberg SM, Evans RM: Transcriptional inhibition by a glucocorticoid receptor beta-galactosidase fusion protein. *Cell* 1988;**55**:1109.

Pelletier J, Sonenberg N: Internal initiation of translation of eukaryotic mRNA directed by a sequence derived from poliovirus RNA. *Nature* 1988;**334**:320.

Ptashne M: How gene activators work. *Sci Am* 1989;**260**:41.

Robertson M: The post-RNA world. *Nature* 1988;**335**:16.

Rosenfeld MG, Amara SG, Evans RM: Alternative RNA processing: Determining neuronal phenotype. *Science* 1984;**225**:1315.

Ross J: The turnover of messenger RNA. *Sci Am* 1989;**April**:48.

Scharp PA: RNA splicing and genes. *JAMA* 1988;**260**:3035.

Schleif R: DNA binding by proteins. *Science* 1988;**241**:1182.

Schuler GD, Cole MD: GM-CSF and oncogene mRNA stabilities are independently regulated in trans in a mouse monocyte tumor. *Cell* 1988;**55**:1115.

Schüle R et al: Many transcription factors interact synergistically with steroid receptors. *Science* 1988;**242**:1418.

Tsai SY et al: Molecular interactions of steroid hormone receptor with its enhancer element: Evidence for receptor dimer formation. *Cell* 1988;**55**:361.

Walden WE et al: Translational repression in eukaryotes: Partial purification and characterization of a repressor of ferritin mRNA translation. *Proc Natl Acad Sci USA* 1988;**85**:9503.

Wolffe AP, Brown DD: Developmental regulation of two 5S ribosomal RNA genes. *Science* 1988;**241**:1626.

Gene Evolution

Gilbert W: Genes in pieces revisited. *Science* 1985;**228**:823.

Howard JC: Molecular evolution: How old is a polymorphism? *Nature* 1988;**332**:588.

McConnell et al: The origin of MHC class II gene polymorphism within the genus *Mus*. *Nature* 1988;**332**:651.

Ohta T: Time for acquiring a new gene by duplication. *Proc Natl Acad Sci USA* 1988;**85**:3509.

Rotter JI, Diamond JM: What maintains the frequencing of human genetic diseases? *Nature* 1987;**329**:289.

Mechanisms & Diagnosis of Genetic Diseases

Aritonarakis SE: Diagnosis of genetic disorders at the DNA level. *N Engl J Med* 1989;**320**:153.

Brown MS, Goldstein JL: A receptor-mediated pathway for cholesterol homeostasis. *Science* 1986;**232**:34.

Donis-Keller H et al: A genetic linkage map of the human genome. *Cell* 1987;**51**:319.

Elias S, Annas GJ: Routine prenatal genetic screening. *N Engl J Med* 1987;**317**:1407.

Engleber NC, Eisenstein BI: The impact of new cloning techniques on the diagnosis and treatment of infectious disease. *N Engl J Med* 1984;**311**:892.

Genetic markers for neurofibromatosis. (Editorial) *Lancet* 1988;**September 24**:719.

Hobbs HH et al: Multiple crm mutations in familial hypercholesterolemia: Evidence for 13 alleles, including four deletions. *J Clin Invest* 1988;**81**:909.

Hughes MR et al: Point mutations in the human vitamin D receptor gene associated with hypocalcemic rickets. *Science* 1988;**242**:1702.

Kadowaki T et al: Two mutant alleles of the insulin receptor gene in a patient with extreme insulin resistance. *Science* 1988;**240**:787.

Li H et al: Amplification and analysis of DNA sequences in single human sperm and diploid cells. *Nature* 1988;**335**:414.

McKusick VA: The new genetics and clinical medicine: A summing up. *Hosp Prac* 1988;**July 15**:79.

Martin JB: Molecular genetics: Applications to the clinical neurosciences. *Science* 1987;**238**:765.

Miller WL: Molecular biology of steroid hormone synthesis. *Endocr Rev* 1988;**9**:295.

Moller DE, Flier JS: Detection of an alteration in the insulin-receptor gene in a patient with insulin resistance, acanthosis nigricans, and the polycystic ovary syndrome (type A insulin resistance). *N Engl J Med* 1988;**319**:1526.

Phillips JA: Genetic diagnosis: Differentiating growth disorders. *Hosp Pract* (April) 1985;**20**:85.

Rotter JI, Rimoin DL: The genetics of diabetes. *Hosp Pract* 1987;**May 15**:79.

Schimke RN: Multiple endocrine neoplasia: Search for the oncogenic trigger. *N Engl J Med* 1986;**314**:1315.

Saiki RK et al: Diagnosis of sickle cell anemia and beta-thalassemia with enzymatically amplified DNA and nonradioactive allele-specific oligonucleotide probes. *N Engl J Med* 1988;**319**:537.

Seizinger BR et al: Genetic linkage of von Recklinghausen neurofibromatosis to the nerve growth factor receptor gene. *Cell* 1987;**49**:589.

White R, Lalouel J-M: Chromosome mapping with DNA markers. *Sci Am* 1988;**258**:40.

White R, Caskey CT: The human as an experimental system in molecular genetics. *Science* 1988;**240**:1483.

Yoshimasa Y et al: Insulin-resistant diabetes due to a point mutation that prevents insulin proreceptor processing. *Science* 1988;**240**:784.

Cloning Methodology & DNA Sequencing

Caruthers MH: Gene synthesis machines: DNA chemistry and its uses. *Science* 1985;**230:**281.

Church GM, Kieffer-Higgins S: Multiplex DNA sequencing. *Science* 1988;**240:**185.

Roberts L: Who owns the human genome? *Science* 1987;**237:**258.

Polymerase Chain Reaction Technology

Loh EY et al: Polymerase chain reaction with single-sided specificity: Analysis of T cell receptor delta chain. *Science* 1989;**243:**217.

Saiki RK et al: Primer-directed enzymatic amplification of DNA with a thermostable DNA polymerase. *Science* 1988;**239:**487.

Stoflet ES et al: Genomic amplification with transcript sequencing. *Science* 1988;**239:**491.

Genetic Engineering

Erslev A: Erythropoietin coming of age. *N Engl J Med* 1987;**316:**101.

Haber E et al: Innovative approaches to plasminogen activator therapy. *Science* 1989;**243:**51.

Nienhuis AW: Hematopoietic growth factors: Biologic complexity and clinical promise. *N Engl J Med* 1988;**318:**916.

Rosenberg SA et al: A progress report on the treatment of 157 patients with advanced cancer using lymphokine-activated killer cells and interleukin-2 or high-dose interleukin-2 alone. *N Engl J Med* 1987;**316:**889.

Drug Delivery Systems

Gordon GS et al: Nasal absorption of insulin: Enhancement by hydrophobic bile salts. *Proc Natl Acad Sci USA* 1985;**82:**7419.

Kirsh R, Bugelski PJ, Poste G: Drug delivery to macrophages for the therapy of cancer and infectious diseases. *Ann NY Acad Sci* 1987;**507:**141.

Papahadjopoulos D, Gabizon A: Targeting of liposomes to tumor cells in vivo. *Ann NY Acad Sci* 1987;**507:**64.

Rational Drug Design

Bash PA et al: Calculation of the relative change in binding free energy of a protein-inhibitor complex. *Science* 1987;**235:**574.

Blundell TL, Sibanda BL, Sternberg MJE, Thornton JM: Knowledge-based prediction of protein structures and the design of novel molecules. *Nature* 1987;**326:**347.

DesJarlais RL et al: Docking flexible ligands to mac-romolecular receptors by molecular shape. *J Med Chem* 1986;**29:**2149.

Kuypeer LF et al: Receptor-based design of dihydrofolate reductase inhibitors: Comparison of crystallographically determined enzyme binding with enzyme affinity in a series of carboxy-substituted trimethoprim analogues. *J Med Chem* 1985;**28:**303.

Sielecki AR et al: Structure of human recombinant renin, a target for cardiovascular-active drugs, at 2.5 A resolution. *Science*

Wuthrich K: Protein structure determination in solution by nuclear magnetic resonance spectroscopy. *Science* 1989;**243:**45.

Gene Therapy

Hofmann SL et al: Overexpression of low density lipoprotein (LDL) receptor eliminates LDL from plasma in transgenic mice. *Science* 1988;**239:**1277.

Roberts L: Human gene therapy test. *Science* 1988;**July 22:**419.

Roberts L: New targets for human gene therapy. *Science* 1988;**241:**906.

Zwiebel JA, Freeman SM, Kantoff PW, Cornetta K, Ryan US, Anderson WF: High-level recombinant gene expression in rabbit endothelial cells transduced by retroviral vectors. *Science* 1989;**243:**220.

Oncogenes & Cancer

Arnold A, Staunton CE, Kim HG, Gaz RD, Kronenberg HM: Monoclonality and abnormal parathyroid hormone genes in parathyroid adenomas. *N Engl J Med* 1988;**318:**658.

Kolata G: Oncogenes give breast cancer prognosis. *Science* 1987;**235:**160.

Larsson C, Skogseid B, Oberg K, Nakamura Y, Nordenskjöld M: Multiple endocrine neoplasia type 1 gene maps to chromosome 11 and is lost in insulinoma. *Nature* 1988;**332:**85.

Nowell PC: Molecular events in tumor development. *N Engl J Med* 1988;**319:**575.

Simpson NE, Kidd KK, Goodfellow PJ, McDermid H, Myers S, Kidd JR, Jackson CE, Duncan AMV, Farrer LA, Brasch K, Castiglione C, Genel M, Gertner J, Greenberg CR, Gusella JF, Holden JJA, White BN. Assignment of multiple endocrine neoplasia type 2A to chromosome 10 by linkage. *Nature* 1987;**328:**528.

Tong L et al: Structural differences between a ras oncogene protein and the normal protein. *Nature* 1989;**337:**90.

Varmus H: Retroviruses. *Science* 1988;**240:**1427.

Weinberg RA: Finding the anti-oncogene. *Sci Am* 1988;**259:**44.

3

Immunoendocrinology

Charles J. Grossman, PhD

In 1898, an Italian investigator named Calzolari reported that castrated rabbits exhibited enlarged thymus glands. Because the thymus is an organ of the immune system, while the gonads are organs of the endocrine system, this technically made Calzolari the founder of the hybrid discipline **immunoendocrinology**. In 1940, Chiodi was able to repeat and extend these studies using the rat. The evidence that has accumulated since then suggests that the endocrine and immune systems interact extensively to regulate each other.

Many endocrine organs appear to be involved in some aspect of this regulatory process. These include (but probably are not limited to) the hypothalamus, pituitary, gonads, adrenals, pineal, thyroid, and thymus. Furthermore, many of these organs are themselves affected by immune function. The autonomic nervous system is also involved in this regulation; it affects the hypothalamus, pituitary, adrenal, thymus, gut-associated lymphatic tissue, lymph nodes, and bone marrow. While such direct neurologic control of the immune system is not discussed in this chapter, these additional pathways do undoubtedly play a role in regulation of the immune response.

ORGANIZATION & FUNCTION OF THE IMMUNE SYSTEM

The immune system is designed to identify foreign ("not of the body") substances and adaptively respond to this stimulus with various classes of immunologic cells and products. The final outcome, or **response,** is the removal of the offending cell or substance from the body. In this way the immune system functions much like any other sensory (stimulus-response) system in an organism.

The immune system must respond to the invader organism, or **antigen,** with great specificity. In humans, the immune system can be divided into the **innate (nonspecific)** and the **adaptive (specific, acquired) immune systems.** When an infectious particle (antigen) enters the body, it first encounters the barriers of the innate immune system. These barriers include chemicals (such as lysozyme), inflammation, phagocytosis, and the alternative complement sys-

Acronyms Used in This Chapter

ACTH	Adrenocorticotropic hormone
CRH	Corticotropin-releasing hormone
FSH	Follicle-stimulating hormone
GH	Growth Hormone (somatotropin)
GIF	Glucocorticoid-increasing factor
GnRH	Gonadotropin-releasing hormone
HBs Ag	Hepatitis B surface antigen
HLA	Human leukocyte antigen
HPAT	Hypothalamic-pituitary-adrenal-thymic axis
HPGT	Hypothalamic-pituitary-gonadal-thymic axis
HPT	Hypothalamic-pituitary-thyroid axis
IL-1	Interleukin-1
IL-2	Interleukin-2
IFN	Interferon
LH	Luteinizing hormone
MHC	Major histocompatibility complex
MLR	Mixed lymphocyte reaction
PHA	Phytohemagglutinin
PHP	Pineal-hypothalamic-pituitary axis
SLE	Systemic lupus erythematosis
Th	Helper/inducer T lymphocytes
Ts	Suppressor/cytotoxic T lymphocytes
T_3	Triiodothyronine
T_4	Thyroxine

tem. If these defenses are ineffective, specific immune responses are activated.

Specific immune responses include all reactions that are mediated by lymphocytes. When B and T lymphocytes initially identify an antigen, a **primary immune response** occurs. This response entails the production of both circulating and local antibodies as well as cytotoxic (or killer) T lymphocytes. After this primary immune response is completed, any subsequent challenge with the same antigen will generate a **secondary immune response** consisting of the production of antibodies specific to that antigen. This acquired response is possible because of the long-term memory retained by memory cells in this system (Fig 3–1).

During human development, the precursor lymphocytes migrate from the bone marrow into the thymus, where they mature into **thymus-derived** or **T lympho-**

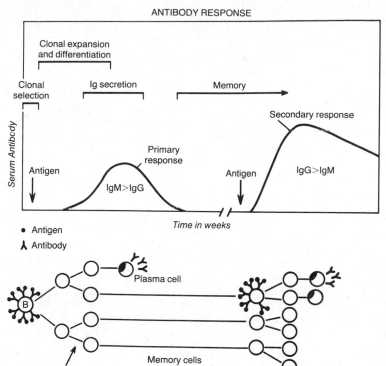

ANTIBODY RESPONSE

Figure 3–1. Antibody response in the serum against a conventional thymus-dependent antigen. The top panel depicts the serum levels of antibody after primary and secondary challenges. The bottom panel illustrates the cellular events in B, T, and plasma cells. Arrows indicate the interactions between helper T cells and B cells. Reproduced, with permission, from Unanue ER, Benacerraf B: *Textbook of Immunology*, 2nd ed. Williams & Wilkins, 1984.

cytes. They also develop in another location (probably the bone marrow but perhaps the lymphatic tissue of the gut), where they become **B lymphocytes.** The mature T and B lymphocytes then migrate to the lymph nodes and spleen, where they mediate the cellular and humoral responses of the specific immune system. The **cellular immune system** is mediated by T lymphocytes, whereas the **humoral immune system** is mediated by antibodies produced by B lymphocytes. Many T lymphocytes circulate between the blood and the lymphatic fluid. While a few B lymphocytes do circulate, most of them remain in the lymph nodes and spleen.

When T cells of the cellular immune system are stimulated by antigen, they form clones and produce various subclasses of effector T cells. These include **cytotoxic T lymphocytes (killer cells), helper T (Th) lymphocytes,** and **suppressor T (Ts) lymphocytes.** Killer cells can directly destroy target cells by producing cytotoxic **lymphokines.** Helper T cells help the B cell to produce antibodies (perhaps by producing lymphokines such as interleukin-2). Suppressor T cells inhibit the B cell from producing antibodies (also perhaps by producing lymphokines; Fig 3–2).

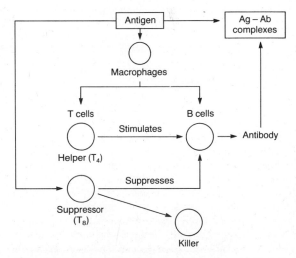

Figure 3–2. Simplified immune regulation scheme illustrating the relationships between macrophages, helper T cells, suppressor T cells, and B cells. Macrophages present degraded antigenic determinants to T and B cells as well as major histocompatibility complex (MHC) gene products.

When cells of the humoral immune system are stimulated by antigen, they form clones of plasma cells and produce **antibodies,** or **immunoglobulins.** These immunoglobulins (found in 5 structural classes: IgA, IgD, IgE, IgG, and IgM) have a variety of effects on the antigen-containing cells toward which they are structurally directed. Antibodies can precipitate and agglutinate the antigenic structures, opsonize the antigenic structures to make them easier for neutrophils and macrophages to phagocytose, and activate the classic pathway of the complement system.

Macrophages play an important role in the immune system. Macrophages can nonspecifically phagocytose foreign invaders, and they release various growth factors (including interleukin-1) that stimulate clonal formation of the B and T cells. To form these clones, the macrophages must present degraded pieces of the invader organism (**antigenic determinants**) to the precursor B and T cells (Fig 3–2). Macrophages and lymphocytes interact reciprocally, because the activated T lymphocytes eventually move to an infection site and release lymphokines that attract macrophages (and neutrophils) to the area. These lymphokines also activate the macrophages, increasing their phagocytic effectiveness. Various complement proteins generated during the activation of the complement system also attract and activate macrophages. Finally, both monokines and lymphokines, which mediate many steps in these immunologic responses, could probably be classified as hormones, because they are released by monocytes or lymphocytes and they affect target cells (other leukocytes). The effects of sex steroids on the production or action of monokines and lymphokines are currently unknown, but glucocorticoids do regulate the production of these leukocyte "hormones."

EFFECTS OF ENDOCRINE ABLATIONS & REPLACEMENTS ON THE IMMUNE RESPONSE

To study the effects of a hormone on the immune system, immunoendocrinologists often use the classic experimental method of ablating (removing) an endocrine organ and then replacing the hormone of interest. In fact, when a hormone or factor is still in the early stages of being purified, biologic assay is frequently the only way to measure it. For example, to study the effects of gonadal steroids on the immune system, both the direct effects on target lymphocytes and the possible effects on thymic hormone release must be measured. Because such thymic hormones are not adequately purified (although an RIA assay has been developed for one of the thymosin fractions), biologic assay remains the most effective way to measure the effects of steroids on immune function.

Using the ablation and replacement method, many investigators after Calzolari have reported increased thymic weight in experimental animals due to both castration and adrenalectomy. They have also shown that replacement of sex steroids or glucocorticoids reduces the degree of thymic hypertrophy and hyperplasia. This increase is only temporary, however; thymic weight is eventually reduced in animals that have been castrated for a long time. These observations partly explain the increased mass of thymic tissue reported in young children and the decreased mass reported in adolescents after the onset of puberty.

Other immunologic effects of castration in animals and humans include enlargement of the peripheral lymph nodes and spleen, increased incidence of graft-versus-host disease, decreased skin graft rejection time, and stimulation of in vitro T lymphocyte mitogen responsiveness mediated by circulating thymic serum factors. All these responses are mediated by the cellular immune system, suggesting that castration increases immune response.

The effects of gonadectomy on humoral immunity are still controversial. Some investigators report an increase in overall antibody production after gonadectomy, some report a decrease, and some report no changes. Other investigators have reported that gonadectomy alters the relative amounts of antibody classes produced. All seem to agree, however, that females have higher titers of various classes of circulating antibodies than do males and that estrogen treatment stimulates antibody production. Gonadectomy probably does not produce a single reproducible effect because of the complexity of the pathway that regulates B lymphocytes. This pathway involves interactions between macrophages, helper T lymphocytes, suppressor T lymphocytes, B lymphocytes, and the anti-idiotypic network.

SEXUALLY DIMORPHIC IMMUNE RESPONSE

Many clinical and experimental studies have shown that the immune response is **sexually dimorphic.** In other words, the cellular and humoral immune responses in nonpregnant, healthy adult females are generally more active than those in healthy adult males. This sexual dimorphism is frequently not seen until puberty, so it may partly result from the different ratios of gonadal steroids (estrogens:androgens) in males and females.

Circulating levels of the major immunoglobulin classes found in females far exceed those found in males of the same species, age, and physiologic condition. For example, many in vivo and in vitro studies in both humans and animals have found higher levels of

IgG, IgM, and IgA in females than in males. In addition, challenge with antigens (such as poliovirus) stimulates higher titers of antibodies in females than in males.

The cellular immune response is also greater in females than in males. Using skin graft rejection time to measure cellular immunity, females have been shown to reject skin allografts more consistently and more rapidly than do males. In addition, gonadectomy and steroid replacement alter this pattern.

EFFECTS OF PREGNANCY ON THE IMMUNE RESPONSE

Pregnancy significantly depresses the cellular immune response but does not greatly affect the humoral immune response. Because the cellular immune system mediates acute and early tissue rejection, this depression of the cellular immune response prevents maternal rejection of fetal antigens. The results of many studies support this conclusion. For example, some studies suggest that the cellular immune response in women who have had repeated early spontaneous abortions is not as depressed as it is in women who have carried their pregnancies to term. Other studies report that pregnant women do not reject foreign skin grafts as effectively as nonpregnant women, that their reactivity to PPD (tuberculin skin test) is decreased, and that their lymphocyte response (as measured in vitro by mitogen [phytohemagglutinin, PHA] or mixed lymphocyte reaction [MLR] assays) is depressed. Many studies with animals have demonstrated similar responses during pregnancy.

In humans, this immunosuppression is most apparent during the second and third trimesters of pregnancy. At that time, maternal lymphocytes proliferate less in response to soluble antigens and allogeneic lymphocytes. Decreased cell-mediated cytotoxicity (as measured by the killing of virally infected target cells) and reduced numbers of Th lymphocytes (helper/inducer) have also been reported during this period. This immunosuppression is clinically supported by the observed increase in the occurrence of smallpox, polio, viral hepatitis, varicella-zoster, influenza, rubella, cytomegalovirus infection, and pulmonary and systemic mycoses during pregnancy.

Furthermore, 3–6 months after the birth of a child, preexisting maternal autoimmune diseases such as Hashimoto's thyroiditis and Graves' disease may be exacerbated (see Chapter 10). This further supports the view that while the elevated levels of sex steroids during pregnancy depress the immune response, the postpartum reduction in sex steroid levels stimulates immune reactivity.

The thymus, which is a target organ for sex steroids and glucocorticoids, is also affected during pregnancy. Studies suggest that pregnancy causes the thymic lobules to significantly involute and atrophy, and that it reduces the number of cortical thymocytes but does not change the number of medullary thymocytes. Cortical thymocytes are glucocorticoid-sensitive, so their numbers are also increased by steroid withdrawal after castration; medullary thymocytes respond poorly in vitro to mitogens. Thus, during pregnancy, the number of reactive cortical thymocytes may be reduced to zero, while the original number of nonreactive medullary thymocytes is still present. This may partly explain the reduced immune response at this time. This hyporeactive immune response could also be due to the presence of regulatory (suppressor) Ts lymphocytes in the placenta as well as to the selective expression of histocompatibility antigens by various placental cells.

Altogether, the evidence strongly suggests that the immunosuppression associated with pregnancy is clinically significant and may be involved in the survival of the fetal allograft. The mechanism of this effect is still not entirely clear (see Mechanism of Sexually Dimorphic Immune Response, below), but elevated levels of sex steroids (estrogen and progesterone) appear to play a central role in this process.

HORMONAL REGULATION OF THE IMMUNE RESPONSE

This section details the known effects of steroid, thyroid, and pituitary hormones on the immune system. These effects are summarized in Table 3–1.

STEROID HORMONES

Estrogens

Estrogenic steroids can be both immunostimulating and immunoinhibiting agents. For example, estrogens can enhance the synthesis of antibodies by the humoral immune system. However, estrogens appear to act both directly and indirectly to strongly inhibit the cell-mediated immune response. They may act directly by affecting the target lymphocyte (which possesses estrogen receptors) and indirectly by releasing or inhibiting the release of hormones from the **thymic reticuloepithelial cells.**

Estrogen treatment inhibits or depresses cutaneous delayed hypersensitivity reactions, cancer immune surveillance, and graft rejection responses, all of which are mediated by effector T lymphocytes. Estrogen treatment also depresses the function of natural killer cells, produces lymphopenia, and inhibits the release of thymic hormones. In women taking oral contraceptives containing conjugated estrogen either

Table 3–1. Summary of effects of hormones on the immune system.

Hormone	Dose	Cellular Male	Cellular Female	Humoral Male	Humoral Female	Comment
Estrogen	Absent	↑	↑↑	↑±	↑±	Generally increases immune surveillance.
	Physiologic	↓	↑	↓	↑	Possible cause of sexual dimorphism.
	Pregnant	−	↓↓	−	↓±	May stimulate suppressor T cells.
Androgen	Absent	↑	↑	±	±	Functions with estrogen.
	Physiologic	±	↓±	±	↓±	Functions with estrogen.
	Pregnant	−	↓?	−	↓?	Requires further study.
Progesterone	Physiologic	±?	↓?	?	?	Requires prior estrogen priming. May play a role in immune regulation in female during luteal phase.
	Pregnant	−	↓↓	−	↓?	Probably functions with estrogen as potent immunosuppressive agent.
Glucocorticoid	Absent	↑↑↑	↑↑↑	↑↑	↑↑	Functions directly via lymphocyte receptors, but hypoglycemia may also depress lymphocyte function.
	Physiologic	↓↑	↓↑	↓↑	↓↑	Prevents overactivity of immune response. May function with monokines or lymphokines.
	Pharmacologic	↓↓↓	↓↓↓	↓↓↓	↓↓↓	Specific depressive effects depend on the concentration, type of glucocorticoid, length of treatment, and route of administration.
Growth hormone (GH)	Absent	↓	↓	↓	↓	Functions with prolactin.
	Physiologic	±	↑	±	↑	Possible cause of sexual dimorphism.
Prolactin	Absent	↓	↓	↓	↓	Functions with GH.
	Physiologic	±	↑	±	↑	Possible cause of sexual dimorphism.
Thyroid hormone	Absent	↓	↓	↓	↓	May function with GH. Interactions with other hormones that affect immune response are currently unknown.
	Physiologic	↓↑	↓↑	↓↑	↓↑	Maintains immune system. Elevated thyroid hormone may stimulate suppressor T cells.

alone or with medroxyprogesterone, the in vitro mitogenic response of peripheral lymphocytes may also be inhibited.

A similar depression in the cellular immune response has been reported for prostatic cancer patients being treated with estrogenic steroids (diethylstilbestrol). Thus, estrogen therapy may actually cause the immune depression frequently observed in these patients. Such therapy, while effective in the short run, could inhibit immune surveillance and increase the chance of metastases in such patients in the long run.

As mentioned previously, estrogen may also play a role in autoimmune disease because a variety of immunologic disorders are more prevalent in women than in men. The disorders most notable in humans are idiopathic thrombocytopenic purpura, rheumatoid arthritis, and systemic lupus erythematosus (SLE). In SLE, 16α-hydroxylation of estradiol is often increased, leading to the production of potent estrogenic metabolites. In response, the levels of circulating antinuclear antibodies rise, perhaps owing to the stimulation of the humoral immune system and the depression of suppressor T lymphocytes. This may result in exacerbation of the disease. Other possible estrogen-linked disease reports include more Asian influenza deaths in pregnant women than in nonpregnant women and more frequent coccidioidomycosis-related complications in women than in men (see Chapters 17 and 20).

Androgens

Androgens clearly modify the immune response, although they probably work with estrogens and the thymic reticuloepithelial cells. Both reticuloepithelial cells and certain classes of T lymphocytes reportedly possess androgen receptors. Sex differences have also been noted for patients infected with hepatitis B virus. Apparently the incidence of the postinfection carrier state (HBs Ag) is greater in males than in females, as is the prevalence of chronic liver damage due to the virus. Similarly, the incidence of diseases associated with hepatitis B infection (eg, Hodgkin's disease, lepromatous leprosy, primary hepatocellular carcinoma, chronic renal disease) is higher in males than in females. The virus may possess a surface antigen that cross-reacts with a male-associated antigen in humans. This would explain the impaired graft survival rate observed in patients who are chronic carriers of HBs Ag and in those who receive a donor male kidney.

Antibodies in these recipient carriers may bind to the antigens on the donor kidney and promote rejection.

Use of danazol (an androgenic steroid) has been reported to decrease attacks of hereditary angioedema. However, it is not clear if the steroid is affecting the immune response or increasing production of C1 esterase inhibitor via anabolic effects on the liver.

Progestins

Under certain circumstances, progesterone is a potent immunosuppressive agent. It is not immunosuppressive under all experimental conditions, because progesterone receptors must be generated in the target tissue to demonstrate this effect. Before such receptors can be generated, progestin-sensitive target tissues such as the uterus and thymic reticuloepithelial cells must be primed with estrogen.

The immunosuppressive effects of progesterone are similar to those reported for the estrogens and androgens. For example, progestins can strongly inhibit the cellular immune response. Some studies have found that progesterone depressed the rejection of skin grafts in experimental animals, including hamsters, mice, rats, and monkeys. In studies that used progesterone or 20α-dihydroprogesterone to inhibit the blastogenic response of lymphocytes, the levels of progestins employed closely matched those found in the human placenta during the latter months of pregnancy. This evidence supports the theory that progesterone helps to prevent the maternal system from rejecting the fetal graft.

Glucocorticoids

Glucocorticoids have long been known as potent immunosuppressive agents. Cortisol (or corticosterone in rats and mice) at both physiologic and pharmacologic levels effectively depresses both the cellular and humoral immune systems. However, under certain experimental conditions, low concentrations may be immunostimulatory. Organs of the immune system, including the thymic reticuloepithelial cells, perhaps spleen matrix cells, and various classes of both mature and developing effector lymphocytes, all possess glucocorticoid receptors. In addition, castration and adrenalectomy cause the same changes in thymic mass and structure.

Glucocorticoids produce widespread effects on the immune system (Fig 3–3). Glucocorticoids inhibit T lymphocyte activity, depress antibody production by B lymphocytes, reduce natural killer cell activity, and depress the inflammatory response capability of macrophages. They may also inhibit growth factor (IL-1, IL-2) production, block interferon production by activated T lymphocytes, and inhibit the interactions of the Th and B cells. In experimental animals, cortisone treatment also reduces the number of small lymphocytes in thymus-independent areas of the peripheral lymphatic tissue. It may do this by reducing the migration of the B lymphocytes from the bone marrow to the germinal centers in these peripheral lymphatic organs (spleen, lymph nodes) and by producing germinal center atrophy.

THYROID HORMONES

Proper humoral and cellular immune system function is absolutely dependent on the availability of triiodothyronine (T_3) and thyroxine (T_4) elaborated by the thyroid gland. For example, T_4 and somatotropin treatment will completely reconstitute both the cellular and humoral immune responses of the hypopituitary dwarf mouse. In addition, propylthiouracil blocks thyroid hormone release and depresses immune response. Animals treated with propylthiouracil demonstrate impaired primary immune responses; complete recovery is induced in these animals by T_4 treatment.

Pathologic conditions involving the thyroid and associated hormones have been well studied. For example, the hyperthyroidism of Graves' disease and the hypothroidism of Hashimoto's disease involve similar immunologic elements. Thyroid autoantibodies are present in both conditions, with associated lymphocyte infiltration of the thyroid. Both conditions also involve classes of T lymphocytes being sensitized to thyroid cell antigens. In Graves' disease, the levels of circulating suppressor T lymphocytes are reduced (perhaps as a result of higher T_4 levels) and the TSH thyroid cell receptor may act as an antigen. Thus, in the absence of Ts cells, increased antibody production by B cells (plasma cells) may produce a class of immunoglobulins (IgA, IgE, IgG, IgM) that bind to the TSH receptor to block or stimulate cAMP effects. Interestingly, Graves' disease may spontaneously evolve to Hashimoto's disease and vice versa (see Chapter 10).

PITUITARY HORMONES

Somatotropin

Recent studies have shown that somatotropin, or growth hormone (GH), can establish immunocompetence and enhance both the cytotoxic T lymphocyte and helper T lymphocyte functions of normal thymocytes but not of cortisol-resistant thymocytes. The thymic medulla contains such glucocorticoid-resistant thymocytes, so GH exerts its effects on the thymocytes in the cortex. Because the tightly packed cortex contains the relatively immature proliferating cells, while the medulla contains more mature cells, GH may contribute to the development of immature T cells into mature effector classes. These immature cells probably possess GH receptors.

The concentration of GH appears to affect the response of T lymphocytes in mitogen-driven blasto-

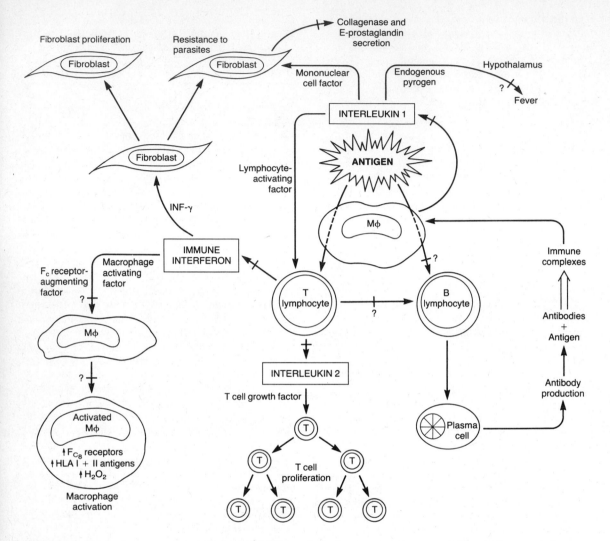

Figure 3–3. The immune system and glucocorticoid effects on the immune cytokine network. Bars indicate paths known or suspected (?) to be blocked by glucocorticoids. Reproduced, with permission, from Munck A, Guyre PM: *Steroid Hormone Resistance*. Chrousos GP, Loriaux DL, Lipsett MB (editors). Plenum Press, 1986.

genic assay. Low (≤ 10 ng/mL) or high (≥ 100 ng/mL) concentrations of GH are less immunostimulatory than are intermediate concentrations (25–50 ng/mL). How this in vitro observation relates to the in vivo effects of GH remains unclear. However, GH can reestablish immunocompetence in hypophysectomized rats and thymectomized, irradiated, lymphocyte-transplanted mice (Fig 3–4).

The immunostimulatory role of GH is further supported by studies of both runt and wasting diseases, immunologic deficiency disorders found in animals. Runt disease is due to a graft-versus-host reaction resulting from the infusion of mature donor lymphocytes into an immunocompromised recipient animal (or human); GH treatment exacerbates this disorder. Wast-

ing disease occurs when the T lymphocytes of an animal are unable to mature. This disease can be induced by neonatal thymectomy. In such thymectomized animals, immunocompetence can be reestablished by the infusion of replacement stem cells, especially if GH is administered at the same time. DiGeorge syndrome and Good's syndrome in humans may be similar to wasting disease in animals, but the effects of GH replacement on the course of these disorders is unknown.

Some clinical studies have suggested a relationship between GH effects and immunity in humans. For example, serum from acromegalic patients stimulated lymphocyte transformation more effectively than did serum from hypopituitary dwarfs. In addition, abnor-

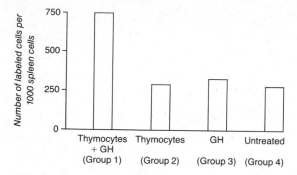

Figure 3–4. Growth hormone- or somatotropin-induced immunocompetence in thymocytes. Historadioautography of spleen cells of neonatally thymectomized CR-recipient mice. On day 1, groups 1 and 2 received 5×10^6 thymocytes of adult C_3H donors. Groups 1 and 3 received 100 µg GH daily. Group 4 was untreated. All mice were killed on day 4. [^3H]-thymidine, 0.8 µg/g body weight, was injected into all groups 1 hour before sacrifice. Results are expressed as the number of labeled cells per 1000 spleen cells counted. Reproduced, with permission, from Pierpaoli W, Fabris N, Sorkin E: *Hormones and Immune Response.* Wolstenholme GE, Knight J (editors). Churchill, 1970.

malities in circulating antibodies have been observed in children and adults with GH deficiencies; many of these abnormalities can be corrected by GH treatment. Other studies have shown that some children suffering from acute lymphoblastic leukemia have elevated GH and somatomedin levels that may be reduced after remission. Finally, hypophysectomy has suppressed the course of T cell leukemia in rats.

Prolactin

Prolactin is another pituitary hormone that can restore immune reactivity in hypophysectomized animals. This immunoenhancing effect, which has been reported for both the humoral and cellular immune systems, appears to be both dependent on dose and inhibited by bromocriptine (a prolactin antagonist). Prolactin may produce these effects by enhancing the development of immature thymocytes into mature effector cells. Prolactin treatment in animals can stimulate the expression of the theta antigen on fetal stem cells.

In nude mice, prolactin levels are significantly lowered, while luteotropic hormone levels are elevated. Implantation of thymic tissue in these animals lowered LH levels and raised prolactin levels into the normal range. This response is probably caused by hormones elaborated by the thymus that affect release of hormones from the pituitary. This evidence supports the model of reciprocal interaction between the thymus and pituitary.

EXTERNAL FACTORS IN THE HORMAL REGULATION OF THE IMMUNE RESPONSE

STRESS

Stress is bodily or mental tension produced by physical, chemical, or emotional stimuli. The strength and duration of this tension is variable and probably depends on the kind of stressor present; the duration of stress; and, in experiments, the species, sex, and physiologic condition of the animal. Stress appears to affect either directly or indirectly all of an animal's organ systems.

While stress factors can undoubtedly alter the immune response, the extent of these alterations is unclear. However, many stress conditions reportedly elevate circulating levels of glucocorticoid, although these levels may return to normal if the stress continues. These raised glucocorticoid levels are frequently accompanied by decreased estrogen and androgen levels. For example, in men, exercise, surgical, or psychologic stress that elevates cortisol levels may also lower circulating testosterone levels, while in women labor stress that elevates cortisol levels may also lower circulating estriol levels.

Because glucocorticoids and gonadal steroids have opposite effects on immune function, stress should initially produce both immunodepression (via increased glucocorticoid levels) and immunostimulation (via reduced gonadal steroid levels). Furthermore, the estrogen:androgen ratio is involved in the sexually dimorphic immune response, so stress may produce different immunologic effects in females than in males. In some experimental animals, stress does stimulate the immune response in females while inhibiting that response in males.

The key to the complex regulation of the immune response by the adrenal and gonadal axes appears to involve the effects of corticotropin-releasing hormone (CRH) on ACTH and LH release (Fig 3–5). Because CRH (which classically elevates ACTH levels) inhibits the release of LH but not FSH, stress inhibits gonadal function and stimulates adrenal function. Furthermore, estrogen stimulates the release of ACTH, so the adrenal response to castration is quite different in males and females. In females, prepubertal ovariectomy results in decreased pituitary secretion of ACTH caused by decreased pituitary sensitivity to CRH stimulation. In males, orchiectomy results in increased pituitary secretion of ACTH caused by pituitary hyperresponsiveness to CRH stimulation.

This information suggests several tentative conclusions. First, stress produces complex physiologic in-

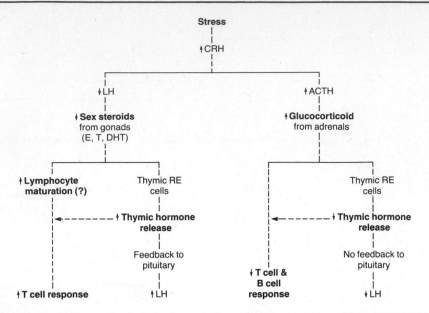

Figure 3–5. Proposed mechanism showing the endocrine interactions involved in the initial stress response. Reproduced, with permission, from Grossman CJ: Stress and the immune response: Interactions of peptides, gonadal steroids, and the immune system. In: *Frontiers of Stress Research.* Weiner H et al (editors). [In press.]

teractions that may alter immune response, frequently by reducing it. Second, under certain conditions (which require further clarification) stress may produce sexually dimorphic effects on immune response, possibly in response to differences in estrogen- or androgen-mediated secretion of ACTH. Third, during a stress response, the initial decrease in sex steroid levels and the increase in glucocorticoid levels may prevent excessive inhibition of the immune system, eventually bringing it back to equilibrium. Fourth and finally, regulation of the immune response by gonadal steroids and glucocorticoids is mediated by hormonal axes involving the hypothalamus, pituitary, adrenal cortex, gonads, and thymus. An axis involving the secretion of IL-1 from monocytes and glucocorticoid-increasing factor (GIF) from lymphocytes may also be involved in this system (see Immunoendocrine Interactions Involved in the Regulation of the Immune Response, below).

CIRCADIAN RHYTHM

Circadian (nyctohemeral) rhythm is the daily rhythmic repetition of certain physiologic phenomena in living organisms. This rhythm affects light-dark cyclic changes in metabolic activity (glycolysis, oxidative metabolism, and biliary function) and mitotic index (spontaneous or induced mitosis) in dividing cells. Because clonal formation during an immune response depends on cell division (blastogenic transformation), circadian rhythm could affect the development of precursor lymphocytes into mature effector cells.

Circadian rhythm seems to alter gonadal steroid,

thymic hormone, and glucocorticoid levels, which are clearly involved in regulating immune response. Melatonin, which is synthesized in the dark by the pineal, is central to this regulation because it inhibits the release of GnRH and CRH from the hypothalamus, which, in turn, reduces the release of LH, FSH, and ACTH from the pituitary. Thus, the levels of both sex steroids and glucocorticoids are lowered during the dark phase. Studies have demonstrated that maximal cellular and humoral immune reactivity in animals occurs during the dark phase (when glucocorticoid levels are lowered and thymic hormone levels are raised), while minimal immune reactivity occurs in the light phase (when glucocorticoid levels are elevated and thymic hormone levels are lowered). In humans, diurnal fluctuations in both thymic hormone and cortisol levels have also been reported. These results suggest the existence of a pineal-hypothalamic-pituitary axis that governs the other hormonal axes involving the hypothalamus and pituitary, resulting in changes in immune response. (See Regulation of the HPGT & HPAT Axes by the Pineal-Hypothalamic-Pituitary [PHP] Axis, below.)

IMMUNOENDOCRINE INTERACTIONS INVOLVED IN THE REGULATION OF THE IMMUNE RESPONSE

As mentioned previously, interactions between the endocrine and immune systems are not unidirectional.

Recent studies indicate that immune interactions can affect levels of circulating hormones. For example, the immune system may regulate the metabolism and circulating levels of both estrogen and progesterone, which significantly affect immune system function. This may explain the delayed vaginal opening and lowered levels of circulating gonadotropins, gonadal hormones, glucocorticoids, and GH in neonatally thymectomized female mice. The following axes are proposed feedback mechanisms that help to explain the known immunoendocrine interactions involved in regulation of the immune response.

HYPOTHALAMIC-PITUITARY-GONADAL-THYMIC (HPGT) AXIS

This system (Fig 3–6) consists of the following steps: (1) Increasing levels of the sex steroids (estradiol and testosterone) released by the gonads (2) decrease the amount of gonadotropin-releasing hormone (GnRH) released by the hypothalamus, which in turn (3) decreases the amount of gonadotropins (luteinizing hormone [LH] and follicle-stimulating hormone [FSH]) released by the anterior pituitary. This subsequently (4) decreases the amount of sex steroids secreted by the gonads, which (5) probably increases the amount of thymic hormone released. These thymic hormones then directly stimulate effector lymphocyte function. The elevated levels of one thymic hormone, thymosin β_4, (6) increase the amount of GnRH released by the hypothalamus and so (7) increase the amount of LH and FSH released by the anterior pituitary. This (1) increases the amount of sex steroids released by the gonads, beginning the self-regulating cycle again.

The sex steroids may also directly affect lympho-

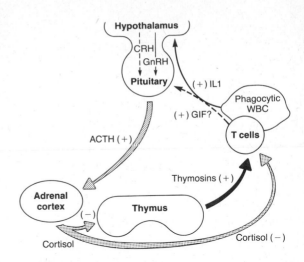

Figure 3–7. Proposed relationship between the HPAT axis, GIF, and IL-1. (−) = Inhibitory, (+) = stimulatory.

cytes through steroid receptors. While developing lymphocytes probably do not possess such receptors, evidence exists that lymphocytes undergoing blastogenic transformation do possess them. This suggests that sex steroids may affect the development of immature lymphoblasts into mature effector lymphocytes.

HYPOTHALAMIC-PITUITARY-ADRENAL-THYMIC (HPAT) AXIS

This system (Fig 3–7) consists of the following steps: (1) Increasing levels of glucocorticoids (cortisol and corticosterone) released by the adrenal cortex (2) decrease the amount of corticotropin-releasing hormone (CRH) released by the hypothalamus. This in turn (3) decreases the amount of adrenocorticotropic hormone (ACTH) released by the pituitary, which subsequently (4) decreases the amount of glucocorticoid released by the adrenal cortex. The lowered level of circulating glucocorticoid directly stimulates the activity of various classes of mature lymphocytes and may also speed the development of immature lymphoblasts into effector lymphocytes. The lowered levels of glucocorticoid also (5) increase the amount of thymic hormones released; these hormones also influence effector lymphocyte function and probably maturation. This elevated level of thymic hormone (1) may increase the amount of glucocorticoid released by the adrenal cortex through positive feedback on the hypothalamus and pituitary by substances called GIF and IL-1 that are released by effector lymphocytes and monocytes. A negative feedback on the hypothalamus and pituitary by thymic hormone has been postulated but has not been conclusively proved.

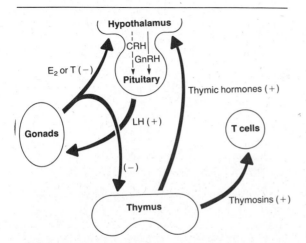

Figure 3–6. Endocrine interactions of the hypothalamic-pituitary-gonadal-thymic (HPGT) axis. (−) = Inhibitory, (+) = stimulatory.

Regulation of the HPAT Axis by GIF & IL-1

Glucocorticoid-increasing factor (GIF) is a lymphokinelike substance produced by lymphocytes in culture. When administered to animals in vivo, it reportedly increases the amount of ACTH released by the pituitary, which in turn increases the amount of glucocorticoid released by the adrenal cortex. Recently, the monokine interleukin-1 (IL-1) has also been reported to raise glucocorticoid levels by stimulating the release of ACTH from the pituitary. IL-1 may act directly on the pituitary or indirectly by increasing the amount of CRH released by the hypothalamus. The elevated levels of circulating glucocorticoid stimulated by GIF and IL-1 should theoretically depress, or downregulate, the ongoing immune response. GIF does function in experimental animals in vivo, but it is still unclear whether IL-1 is able to cross the blood-brain barrier to effect these changes. If IL-1 can cross this barrier and then act on the hypothalamus to increase the release of CRH, it would affect both the HPGT and HPAT axes and promote further regulatory effects on the immune response.

REGULATION OF THE HPGT & HPAT AXES BY THE PINEAL-HYPOTHALAMIC-PITUITARY (PHP) AXIS

The PHP axis (Fig 3–8) is the system hypothesized to account for the effects of circadian rhythm on immune response. It consists of the following steps: (1) Lengthening dark phases of the light-dark cycle (2) increase the amount of melatonin released by the pineal. The increase (3) inhibits the release of both CRH and GnRH from the hypothalamus. The reduction in CRH (4A) inhibits the HPAT axis and so lowers the circulating levels of ACTH and then glucocorticoids; the reduction in GnRH (4B) inhibits the HPGT axis and so lowers the circulating levels of LH, FSH, and then sex steroids. The lowered levels of glucocorticoids and sex steroids then (5) stimulate the immune response. They may also elevate the level of thymic hormones.

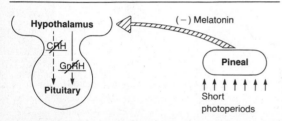

Figure 3–8. Endocrine interactions of the pineal-hypothalamic-pituitary (PHP) axis. (−) = Inhibitory.

INTERACTIONS BETWEEN THE HPGT & HPAT AXES

The release of CRH both stimulates the release of ACTH and inhibits the release of GnRH (Fig 3–5). Therefore, under conditions that stimulate adrenal function, such as stress, the immunosuppressive effect of elevated glucocorticoid levels might be countered by the immunostimulatory effect of lowered sex steroid levels. This may act as a self-regulating mechanism on both developing and mature lymphocytes to prevent excessive depression of the immune response and to increase the number of mature lymphocytes. The overall effect would be to protect the body from disease organisms while circulating glucocorticoid levels are elevated. Fig 3–9 presents an overview of the interactions between the axes hypothesized to regulate the immune response.

THE HYPOTHALAMIC-PITUITARY-THYROID (HPT) AXIS

This axis may play a role in regulation of the immune response, and thymic hormones may also be involved. Thyroid hormone does stimulate elements of the immune system, but the relationship between the HPT axis and immune system regulation is currently unknown.

MECHANISM OF THE SEXUALLY DIMORPHIC IMMUNE RESPONSE

It seems clear that the immune response is affected by hormones and that females possess a more active immune response than do males. This sexually dimorphic response is not apparent until puberty, so sex hormones appear to be responsible for this difference. Fig 3–10 presents a proposed mechanism to explain this dimorphism. This mechanism may change as new information becomes available.

According to this mechanism, the female estrogen:androgen ratio results in elevated levels of prolactin as well as basal GH secretion. The elevated levels of GH and prolactin stimulate both helper and cytotoxic T lymphocyte function. This stimulates the cellular immune response (causing increased tissue rejection, increased PPD response, etc) and also stimulates B lymphocytes (as mediated by activated helper T cells) to produce more antibodies. Increased estrogen secretion also reduces the release of thymic hormone, a hormone that is thought to stimulate suppressor T cells. Thus, the absence of this hormone would reduce suppressor T cell function and increase B cell production of antibodies. This would account for the prevalence of autoimmune diseases in females.

The male estrogen:androgen ratio, however, results

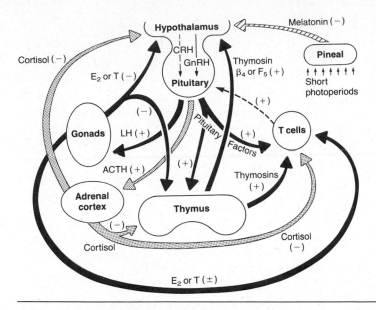

Figure 3–9. An overview of various hormonal axes involved in regulation of the immune system. (−) = Inhibitory, (+) = stimulatory, (±) = variable effects.

in little, if any, circulating prolactin and pulsatile GH secretion. Because the high levels of GH produced by pulsatile secretion are less stimulatory than lower levels, these GH peaks may depress lymphocyte blast transformation. Furthermore, testosterone can be metabolized in the male into either estradiol or dihydrotestosterone. While estrogens are either immunostimulatory or immunoinhibitory, the effect of dihydrotestosterone on the immune system is unclear, although thymic reticuloepithelial cells do have dihydrotestosterone receptors. The result is that the male possesses a less active immune response than does the female.

The more active immune response of the female serves a purpose that is currently unclear but that prob-ably involves the female's reproductive role. For example, the immune response is depressed during pregnancy to maintain the fetus and then reactivated after parturition. Furthermore, antibody transfer across the placenta and during nursing helps to protect the infant from disease until its own immune system is functional. This keeps both mother and baby infection-free during this sensitive period in the child's development. Such an increased humoral immune response might also be due to the development of a more active cellular immune system in the female, because one element of this system, the Th cell, assists in antibody production. The mechanism proposed here provides both new information and new questions to be investigated.

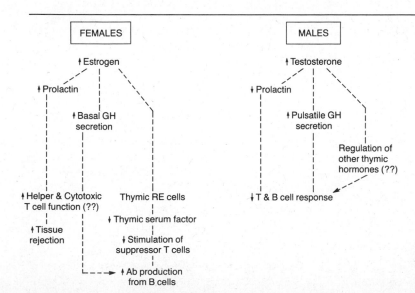

Figure 3–10. Proposed mechanism showing the endocrine interactions responsible for the dimorphic immune response. Both the cellular and humoral immune responses are generally more active in females than in males.

REFERENCES

Ablin RJ et al: Modulatory effects of oestrogen on immunological responsiveness. 2. Suppression of tumor-associated immunity in patients with prostatic cancer. *Clin Exp Immunol* 1979;**38**:83.

Berkenbosch F et al: Corticotropin-releasing factor-producing neurons in the rat activated by interleukin-1. *Science* 1987;**238**:524.

Burman KD, Baker JR Jr: Immune mechanisms in Graves' disease. *Endocr Rev* 1985;**6**:183.

Grossman CJ: Regulation of the immune system by sex steroids. *Endocr Rev* 1984;**5**:435.

Grossman CJ: Stress and the immune response: Interactions of peptides, gonadal steroids and the immune system. In: *Fourth Conference, International Symposium on Neuronal Control of Bodily Functions: New Frontiers of Stress Research;* Trier, Germany; September 1987. [In press.]

Grossman CJ, Roselle GA: The control of immune response by endocrine factors and the clinical significance of such regulation. *Prog Clin Biochem Med* 1986;**4**:9.

Kidd A et al: Immunologic aspects of Graves' and Hashimoto's diseases. *Metabolism* 1980;**29**:80.

Roitt IM, Brostoff J, Male D: *Immunology.* Mosby, 1985.

The Eicosanoids: Prostaglandins, Thromboxanes, Leukotrienes, & Related Compounds

4

Marie L Foegh, MD, Markus Hecker, PhD, & Peter W Ramwell, PhD

Prostaglandins and related fatty acid derivatives are among the most potent naturally occurring substances and are becoming increasingly recognized as important cell regulatory substances. This is reflected in the vast literature on eicosanoids, the large number of clinical pharmacologic studies, and the increasing number of compounds entering the market. However, their physiologic role is still not well defined, although their role in endocrinologic diseases is becoming clearer.

EICOSANOID SYNTHESIS

Several biologically active lipids are formed from the same precursor as the prostaglandins through interrelated enzymatic pathways. The general term **eicosanoids** is used to refer to these compounds, since they can all be derived from dietary polyunsaturated fatty acids with 18-, 20-, or 22-carbon skeletons. Among these fatty acids, **arachidonic acid** (all-*cis*-5,8,11,14-eicosatetraenoic acid; 20:4n-6) is the most important and abundant precursor for the biosynthesis of eicosanoids in humans. **Linoleic** (18:2n-6), **α-linoleic** (18:3n-3) and **arachidonic acids** are the only fatty acids known to be essential for the complete nutrition of many species of animals, including humans. Arachidonic acid is formed from linoleic acid in most mammals via desaturation and chain elongation to **dihomo-γ-linoleic acid** (20:3n-6) and subsequent desaturation. However, linoleic and linolenic acids are not synthesized in humans, so they must be supplied in the diet. For example, oils from cold water fish supply the highly unsaturated eicosapentaenoic (20:5n-3) and docosahexaenoic acids (22:6n-3).

Eicosanoids are not stored in the cell, so their biosynthesis is limited by the availability of free arachidonic acid. Arachidonic acid is released from membrane lipids and other lipid esters by phospholipases that are activated by various stimuli. In response to these stimuli—which vary from cell to cell—**phos**-

pholipase A$_2$ or a combination of **phospholipase C** and **diglyceride lipase** catalyzes the cleavage of the esterified arachidonic acid from the 2 position of specific glycerophospholipids that make up part of the lipid bilayer of the cell membrane (Fig 4–1). Once free, arachidonic acid is deesterified and oxidized by enzymes that are variably distributed among different cells. Not all cells make all products; for example, the endothelium synthesizes primarily PGE$_2$ and PGI$_2$, whereas platelets produce TXA$_2$ and 12-HETE.

Three pathways involve the oxidation of the polyunsaturated fatty acid precursors: the cyclooxygenase, cytochrome P-450, and lipoxygenase pathways.

The Cyclooxygenase Pathway

A. Prostaglandin Biosynthesis: In the 1930s, an unknown lipidlike substance was found in human seminal fluid that decreased blood pressure in rabbits. It was called prostaglandin because it was assumed to originate from the prostate gland; it is now known to originate from the seminal vesicles. In 1962, the first 2 prostaglandins were isolated and characterized—each

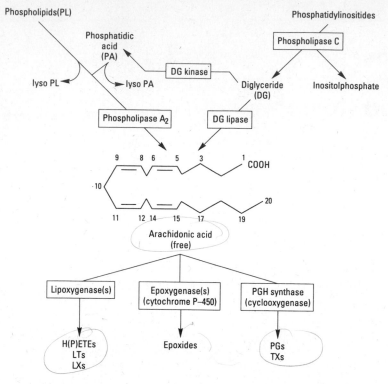

Figure 4–1. Pathways of arachidonic acid release and metabolism.

was found to contain a cyclopentane ring. They were named prostaglandins E and F (PGE and PGF) because of their respective solvent partitioning into ether and phosphate buffer (*fosfat* in Swedish). Today the nomenclature of prostaglandins describes 10 different rings, designated by the letters A through J, that are characterized by variations in the functional groups attached to carbons 9 and 11 of their common cyclopentane ring (Fig 4–2). Each of the 10 compounds may contain 1, 2, or 3 double bonds in the aliphatic side chains, depending upon the degree of unsaturation of the precursor polyenoic acid. For PGF, a subscript α or β refers to the spatial configuration of the carbon 9 hydroxyl group. The activity of these compounds depends on this configuration—only PGF_α compounds are biologically active.

The first step in prostaglandin biosynthesis is the uptake of 2 molecules of oxygen, which catalyzes the prostaglandin endoperoxide synthase or **cyclooxygenase.** The enzyme, which exists in most animals, is widely distributed throughout the body (but not in mature erythrocytes and lymphocytes). The synthesis of prostaglandins from arachidonic acid leads to an unstable endoperoxide, PGG_2. The C15-hydroperoxy group is rapidly reduced to a hydroxyl group, forming the endoperoxide PGH_2 (Fig 4–2). The cyclooxygenase reaction is inhibited by all **nonsteroidal antiinflammatory drugs (NSAIDs)** such as aspirin or indomethacin, which block the cyclooxygenase enzyme.

A variety of biologically active prostaglandins originate from the endoperoxides. Depending on the tissue, PGH_2 is converted to PGD_2 or PGE_2 by corresponding isomerases. PGE_2 can be transformed to PGF_2 by an enzyme named **prostaglandin E 9-ketoreductase.** In addition, 2 other compounds are formed, prostacyclin (PGI_2) and thromboxane A_2 (TXA_2).

B. Prostacyclin and Thromboxane Biosynthesis: Aggregating platelets (thrombocytes) release **thromboxane A_2 (TXA_2)** from the prostaglandin endoperoxides. It differs from these endoperoxides in that it contains an oxan:oxetane ring. The oxetane ring spontaneously hydrolyzes ($t_{1/2} = 30$ s at 37 °C and physiologic pH) to the biologically inactive TXB_2. In contrast to PGE compounds, TXA_2 contracts smooth muscle and induces platelet aggregation at low nanomolar concentrations. Its formation is catalyzed by **thromboxane synthase,** which is mainly present in platelets and macrophages. The enzyme also forms equimolar amounts of 12-hydroxy-5,8,10-heptadecatrienoic acid (HHT) and malondialdehyde, 2 products of as yet undefined biologic significance.

The endoperoxide is also transformed to PGI_2 by **prostacyclin synthase,** which is present in endothelial and smooth muscle cells, fibroblasts, and macro-

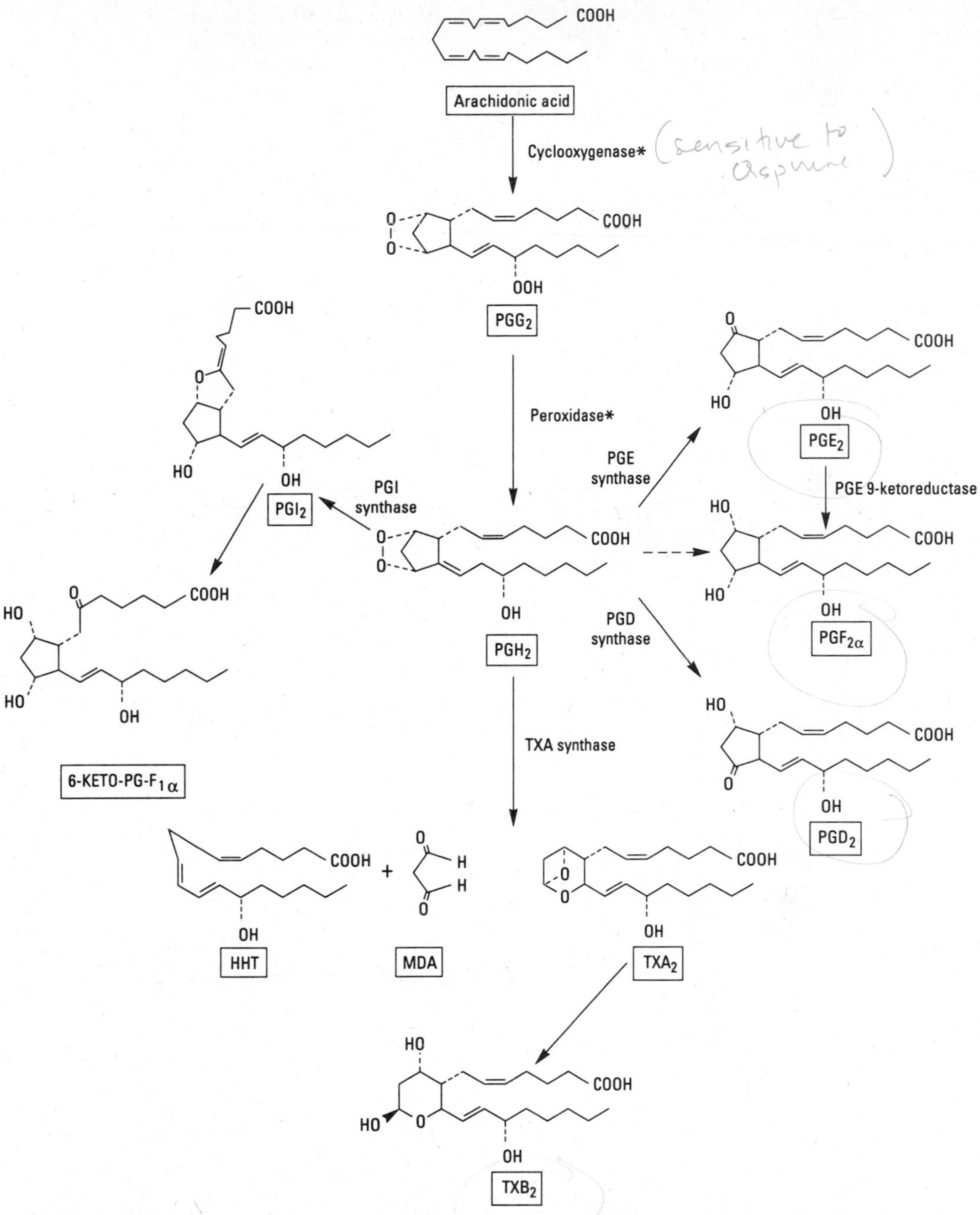

Figure 4–2. Prostaglandin and thromboxane biosynthesis. The asterisks indicate that both cyclooxygenase and peroxidase reactions are catalyzed by a single enzyme, prostaglandin endoperoxide (PGH) synthase.

phages. In contrast to TXA$_2$, PGI$_2$ strongly inhibits platelet aggregation and relaxes smooth muscle. Like TXA$_2$, PGI$_2$ hydrolyzes spontaneously ($t_{1/2}$ = 3 min at 37 °C and physiologic pH) to the biologically inactive 6-keto-PGF$_{1\alpha}$. Thus TXA$_2$ and PGI$_2$ are formed from the same precursor by 2 very similar types of enzymes, yet they have mutually antagonistic properties. Both

undergo rapid hydrolysis to inactive products that can be measured easily in the clinical laboratory.

The Cytochrome P-450 Pathway

In addition to being metabolized by the cyclooxygenase or lipoxygenase pathway, arachidonic acid can be also oxygenated by microsomal cytochrome

P-450 monooxygenases. This process yields various ω oxidation products as well as several epoxides and their corresponding diol derivatives. These and other closely related compounds are being investigated for their biologic activity on vascular smooth muscle and transporting epithelia.

The Lipoxygenase Pathway

The third pathway of arachidonic acid oxygenation is by lipoxygenases, which incorporate one oxygen molecule into the polyunsaturated precursor fatty acid (Fig 4–3). The regional specificity of these lipoxygenases is designated by the position of the carbon bearing the resulting hydroperoxy group in the product. Arachidonic acid is primarily converted into 5-HPETE, 12-HPETE, and 15-HPETE. In the cell, these unstable intermediates are metabolized by peroxidases to their corresponding hydroxy derivatives, HETEs. These derivatives either yield other biologically active substances or are directly biologically active.

The 5- and 12-lipoxygenases are widely distributed in mammalian tissues; in contrast to cyclooxygenase, lipoxygenases also occur in plants such as potato and soybean. This finding may indicate that the lipoxygenase pathway of polyenoic fatty acid oxygenation is phylogenetically older. Both 5- and 15-lipoxygenase contribute to the formation of leukotrienes and various trihydroxyeicosatetranoic acids, including the **lipoxins.**

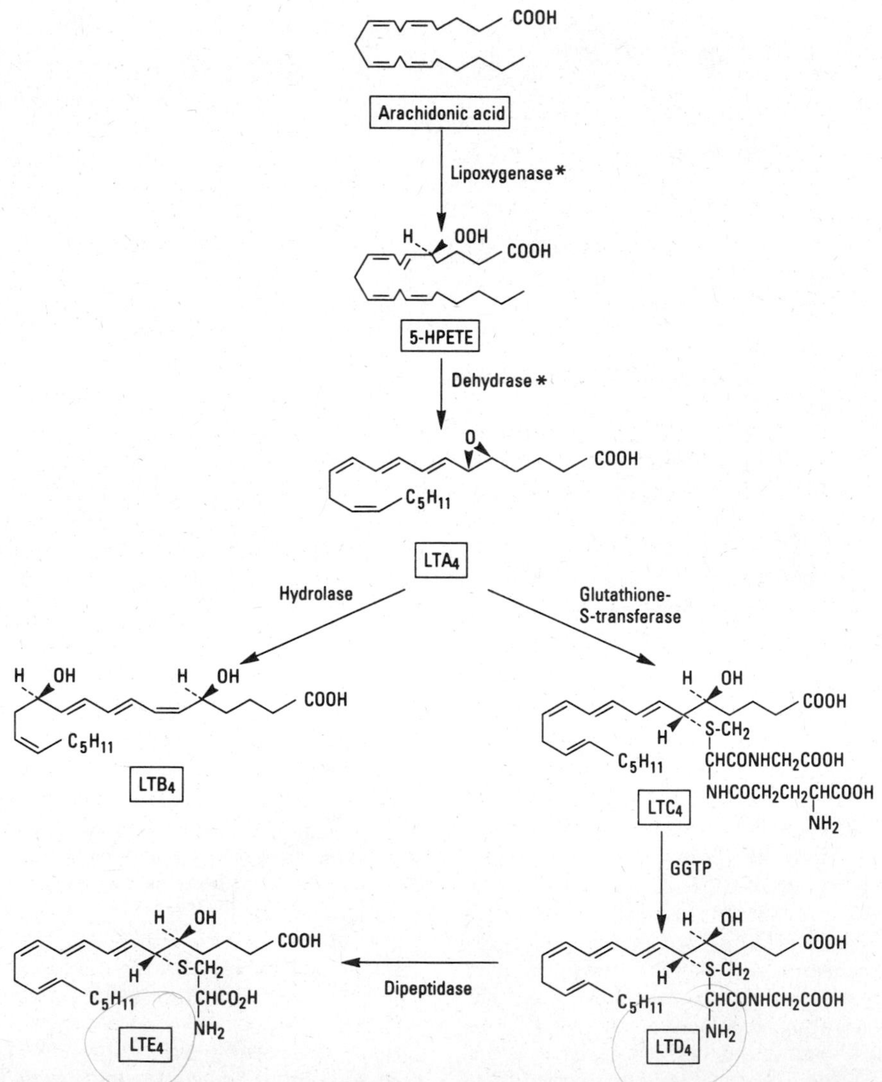

Figure 4–3. Leukotriene biosynthesis. The asterisks indicate that both the lipoxygenase and dehydrase reactions are driven by the enzyme 5-lipoxygenase. GGTP = γ-glutamyltranspeptidase. Compound names are shown in boxes.

Leukotrienes are potent biologically active compounds that are synthesized by the 5-lipoxygenase pathway in leukocytes and mast cells. Before their structures were known, they were recognized in perfusates of lung as the **slow-reacting substance(s) of anaphylaxis (SRS-A)** that are released following immunologic challenge. SRS-A is now known to be a mixture of the peptidoleukotrienes LTC_4, LTD_4, and LTE_4. The name leukotrienes reflects their discovery in leukocytes and their conjugated triene structure that produces their characteristic ultraviolet absorption spectrum. Again the subscript denotes the number of double bonds present. Leukotriene synthesis occurs only via the 5-lipoxygenase pathway (Fig 4–3), where the intermediate 5-HPETE is reduced by a dehydrase to LTA_4. This product is either hydrolyzed to LTB_4 by an epoxide hydrolase or converted into LTC_4 by the addition of the tripeptide glutathione through a specific **glutathione S-transferase.** Removal of the glutamic acid by **γ-glutamyltranspeptidase** leads to the formation of LTD_4. Further removal of the glycine residue by a dipeptidase yields LTE_4. The 5-lipoxygenase of human neutrophils stimulates calcium ions, which may translocate the enzyme from the cytosol to the membrane.

EICOSANOID METABOLISM

Prostaglandins are rapidly catabolized in the body. Thus, 97% of an intravenous dose of PGE_2 is eliminated from the plasma within 90 seconds. Prostaglandin degrading enzymes, which are widely distributed in the body, are most active in lung, kidney, spleen, adipose tissue, and intestine. The pulmonary vascular bed is particularly efficient at inactivating circulating prostaglandins. First, the C15-hydroxyl group, which is essential for the biologic activity of all prostaglandins, is oxidized to the corresponding ketone by a specific oxidoreductase, **prostaglandin 15-hydroxydehydrogenase (PGDH).** The resulting carbonyl compound is reduced to its 13,14-dihydro derivative by **prostaglandin Δ^{13}-reductase** (Fig 4–4). These first 2 reactions happen within a few minutes, whereas the second phase of prostaglandin catabolism entails the slower β and ω oxidation of the side chains. The second phase produces polar dicarboxylic acids that are freely excreted into the urine. Another pathway forms the corresponding 13,14-dihydro derivatives. The major metabolites of TXB_2 in plasma and urine are 11-dehydro-TXB_2 and 2,3-dinor-TXB, respectively. These compounds can be measured clinically.

Cytochrome P-450 monooxygenases from the kidney and liver catalyze β and ω-1 oxidation of most eicosanoids. By adding groups that block metabolism at the 13 and 15 positions or at the end of the aliphatic side chains many clinically effective long-acting analogues can be derived.

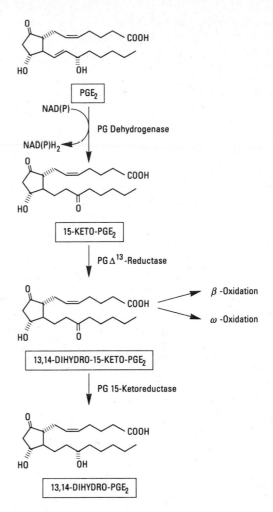

Figure 4–4. Catabolism of prostanoids. The figure illustrates the enzymatic degradation of PGE_2. PGD_2, $PGF_{2\alpha}$, 6-keto-$PGF_{1\alpha}$, and HHT are also metabolized this way, whereas TXB_2 is converted into its 2,3-dinor derivative by β oxidation.

INHIBITION OF EICOSANOID METABOLISM

Corticosteroids block all of the known pathways of eicosanoid metabolism by preventing the release of arachidonic acid. The steroids are thought to stimulate the synthesis of several Ca^{2+}-binding proteins collectively called **lipocortins.** Lipocortins inhibit phospholipase A_2 activity, probably by interfering with phospholipid binding, and thus prevent arachidonic acid release. NSAIDs (eg, aspirin, indomethacin, and ibuprofen) block both prostaglandin and thromboxane formation by inhibiting cyclooxygenase. Aspirin is a particularly long-lasting inhibitor of platelet cyclooxygenase and, therefore, TXA_2 biosynthesis, since it irreversibly acetylates the enzyme. Platelet cyclooxygenase cannot be restored via protein biosynthesis because platelets lack a nucleus. Selective thromboxane synthase inhibitors are being tested in pulmonary hypertension and preeclampsia.

Selective inhibitors of the lipoxygenase pathway are also being tested for a number of indications. With a few exceptions, NSAIDs do not inhibit lipoxygenase activity at concentrations that markedly inhibit cyclooxygenase activity.

EICOSANOID MECHANISM OF ACTION

The eicosanoids appear to produce a bewildering array of biologic effects. In essence, however, they increase either cytosolic Ca^{2+} or cyclic AMP in the cell. Most of the eicosanoids' effects on reproductive, vascular, airway, and gut smooth muscle are either contractile responses, which can be blocked with extra- or intracellular calcium antagonists, or relaxation (dilation) responses, which can be enhanced by cyclic AMP phosphodiesterase inhibitors or cyclic AMP analogues. These intracellular responses are species-, organ-, and receptor-specific.

Endocrine mechanisms that depend on the generation of intracellular cyclic AMP can also generally respond to the prostanoids, which generate cyclic AMP such as PGE, PGD, and PGI compounds. Thus, these prostaglandins can mimic the action of TSH on the thyroid as well as the action of LH (generating progesterone) on the corpus luteum.

In contrast, $PGF_{2\alpha}$, TXA_2, the endoperoxides, and the leukotrienes do not generate cyclic AMP but elicit Ca^{2+} fluxes. The increased intracellular Ca^{2+} levels then usually trigger smooth muscle contraction. This occurs in the oxytocic responses to both $PGF_{2\alpha}$ and PGE_2. However, PGE_2 also increases the level of intracellular cyclic AMP in the myometrium. This moderate increase is insufficient to promote relaxation in the presence of the huge Ca^{2+} level changes, so the contractile response does occur.

Eicosanoid receptors are membrane bound and several of them have been solubilized. Intracellular eicosanoid synthesis can up- and down-regulate the number of these receptors. The sex steroids and corticosteroids affect intracellular eicosanoid synthesis and so the response of the cells to eicosanoids. However, in some instances, PGE compounds can inhibit the effect of adenylate cyclase by acting on its regulatory elements.

PGE, PGI, and PGD compounds normally increase cyclic AMP levels. This action partly explains the apparently anomalous effect of these compounds on norepinephrine-induced lipolysis and the effect of antidiuretic hormone in some preparations of transporting epithelia.

Eicosanoids may elicit the release of arachidonic acid and so stimulate eicosanoid synthesis by a posi-

tive feedback mechanism. Thus, leukotrienes can generate thromboxane from peritoneal macrophages, an effect that is blocked by indomethacin. This phenomena may be clinically significant.

It may also be useful to determine how much the different pathways of arachidonate metabolism can be diverted by the different inhibitors. The sensitivity of some asthmatic patients to nonsteroidal anti-inflammatory drugs may be due to the diversion of arachidonate from the cyclooxygenase pathway, which would convert it to prostaglandins, to the 5-lipoxygenase pathway, which uses it to generate the bronchoconstrictor leukotrienes. The leukotrienes can also be generated by platelet-activating factor (PAF), which is inhibited by both 5-lipoxygenase inhibitors and specific PAF receptor antagonists. In the guinea pig asthma model, PAF can promote bronchoconstriction by releasing TXA_2, which is blocked by TXA_2 synthase inhibitors and receptor antagonists and indomethacin. Thus, pathologic agents such as PAF or endotoxin can act as a Ca^{2+} ionophore to release arachidonate, which is then metabolized to different eicosanoids, depending on cell type and species. Therefore, highly specific antagonists may not be the best therapeutic agents for asthma. The main reason to use a specific antagonist would be to spare the production of the PGE and PGI compounds, which in many situations may be cytoprotective.

The PGE compounds are thought to produce this gastric cytoprotection partly by elevating cytosolic cyclic AMP concentrations and partly by stabilizing platelets and protecting blood vessels from inflammatory agents. The cytoprotective effect may also be related to the action of the PGE compounds on monocytes, macrophages, PMNs, and eosinophils as well as platelets, since PGE treatment prevents the release of inflammatory mediators such as free radicals, thromboxane, leukotrienes, HETEs, and PAF as well as other types of inflammatory mediators such as cytokines. The hypothesis that PGE compounds were inflammatory was based on the assumption that PGE_2 produced edema. Instead, the leukotrienes are now known to dramatically increase tissue permeability and so cause edema. The NSAIDs exert their effect partly by blocking synthesis of PGG_2, which yields PGH_2 and an inflammatory oxygenated free radical.

EICOSANOID PHYSIOLOGY & PATHOPHYSIOLOGY

Nearly all cells of all animal species produce eicosanoids, since they form a system that preserves hemostasis. This system interacts with and modulates the many substances involved in injury and inflammation such as vasoactive amines, kallikreins and kinins, clotting factors, platelet-activating factor, and others. The effects of eicosanoids are summarized in Table 4–1.

Table 4–1. Effects of Eicosanoids.

PGI$_2$, PGE$_2$, PGD$_2$	TXA$_2$	LTB$_4$
Vasodilation ↑	Vasoconstriction ↑	Vascular permeability ↑
Cytoprotection ↑	Platelet aggregation ↑	Ca^{2+} flux ↑
Platelet aggregation ↓	Lymphocyte proliferation ↑	T cell proliferation ↑
Leukocyte aggregation ↓	Bronchoconstriction ↑	Leukocyte aggregation ↑
Cyclic AMP ↑	[1]Ca^{2+} flux ↑	INF-γ ↑
IL-1 and IL-2 ↓		IL-1 ↑
T cell proliferation ↓	**PGF$_{2\alpha}$**	IL-2 ↑
Lymphocyte migration ↓		Natural killer cell cytotoxicity ↑
DR antigen expression ↓	Vasoconstriction ↑	Chemoattractant ↑
	Bronchoconstriction ↑	
	Smooth muscle contraction ↑	**LTC$_4$, LTD$_4$**
		Bronchoconstriction ↑
		Vascular permeability ↑
		INF-γ ↑

PGI$_2$ = Prostacyclin, PGE$_2$ = Prostaglandin E$_2$, PGD$_2$ = Prostaglandin D$_2$, TXA$_2$ = Thromboxane A$_2$
LTB$_4$ = Leukotriene B$_4$, LTC$_4$ = Leukotriene C$_4$, LTD$_4$ = Leukotriene D$_4$
IL-1 = Interleukin-1, IL-2 = Interleukin-2
Cyclic AMP = Cyclic Adenomonophosphate, Ca^{2+} = Calcium, INF-γ = Interferon-γ
[1]Shown with TXA$_2$ mimics

Cardiovascular System

Several prostaglandins, including prostacyclin, promote vasodilation by activating adenylate cyclase. Prostacyclin—which is mainly synthesized by the endothelium—originally appeared to be a circulating hormone. However, little if any PGI$_2$ escapes immediate degradation. In the microcirculation, PGE$_2$ is also an important endothelial product. The potent vasodilator **endothelium-derived relaxing factor (EDRF)** is released from the endothelium along with PGE$_2$ and PGI$_2$; EDRF is not an eicosanoid. Both PGI$_2$ and EDRF have short half-lives. The action of EDRF is mediated by the soluble enzyme guanylate cyclase in vascular smooth muscle; unlike PGE$_2$ and PGI$_2$, its formation is not blocked by NSAIDs. Thus, the regulation of the microcirculation appears to depend on both prostanoate and nonprostanoate compounds synthesized by the endothelium.

The eicosanoids are involved in **thrombosis** mainly because TXA$_2$ promotes platelet aggregation and PGI$_2$ inhibits it. Prostacyclin inhibits platelet aggregation but does not inhibit platelet adhesion to the endothelium, platelet spreading, or granule release. However, evidence exists that PGI$_2$ and PGE$_2$ analogues can inhibit the development of atherosclerosis from studies that involved feeding animals with cholesterol.

Inhibition of platelet cyclooxygenase produces only a mild hemostatic defect. This result is supported by the modest hemostatic defects noted in patients with diseases involving deficiencies of platelet cyclooxygenase and thromboxane synthase, because those patients have no history of thrombosis. Blockage of either of these 2 enzymes inhibits secondary aggregation of platelets induced by ADP, by low concentrations of thrombin and collagen, or by epinephrine. Thus, these platelet enzymes are not necessary for platelet function but may amplify an aggregating stimulus. Clearly, the most important physiologic factors act through other pathways.

During the development of deep vein thrombosis, thromboxane and its metabolites are excreted in the urine, probably because the whole platelet pool is activated. This phenomenon occurs to a lesser extent in kidney transplant patients experiencing organ rejection. Elevated urinary excretion of thromboxane metabolites is also seen in patients before infarction and during unstable angina.

Respiratory System

PGE$_2$ is a powerful bronchodilator when given in aerosol form. Unfortunately, it also promotes coughing, and it has been difficult to obtain an analogue that possesses only the bronchodilator properties. Both PGF$_{2\alpha}$ and TXA$_2$ are strong bronchoconstrictors and may, with PAF, be mediators in asthma.

The identification of the leukotrienes (LTC$_4$, LTD$_4$, and LTE$_4$) with SRS-A expanded the known role of eicosanoids as mediators in asthma and other immune responses. The leukotrienes increase mucus secretion as well as promoting bronchoconstriction. In addition, leukotrienes and TXA$_2$ may be partly responsible for the adult respiratory distress syndrome. Other pathologic mediators such as PAF are not only direct bronchoconstrictors, but they can also release (depending on the species) PGF$_{2\alpha}$, thromboxane, and leukotrienes.

Renal System

Both the renal medulla and the cortex synthesize prostaglandins, but the synthetic capacity of the medulla is substantially greater than that of the cortex. These functional areas synthesize several hydroxyeicosatetraenoic acids, leukotrienes, cytochrome P-450 products, and epoxides that plan an important autoregulatory role in renal function. These compounds modify both renal hemodynamics and glomerular and tubular function. This regulatory role is particularly important in marginally functioning kidneys, as shown by the decline in kidney function associated with the use of cyclooxygenase inhibitors in elderly patients or patients with renal disease.

The major eicosanoid products of the renal cortex are PGE_2 and PGI_2. Both compounds increase renin release; however, renin release is normally under adrenergic control. The glomeruli contain mesangial cells that also synthesize small amounts of TXA_2. This very potent vasoconstrictor does not appear to be responsible for regulating glomerular function in healthy humans.

PGE_1, PGE_2 and PGI_2 increase glomerular filtration through their vasodilatory effects. These prostaglandins also increase water and sodium excretion. The increase in water clearance is probably caused by attenuating the action of antidiuretic hormone (ADH) on adenylate cyclase. This natriuretic effect may be caused by either the direct inhibition of sodium reabsorption in the distal tubule or by increased medullary blood flow. The loop diuretic furosemide exerts some of its effect by stimulating cyclooxygenase activity. In the normal kidney, this increases the synthesis of the vasodilator prostaglandins. Therefore, patient response to the loop diuretic will be diminished if a cyclooxygenase inhibitor is concurrently administered.

Like ADH, TXA_2 appears to increase water transport in the toad bladder. This finding led to the suggestion that ADH may exert part of its effect by increasing TXA_2 synthesis. The normal kidney synthesizes only small amounts of TXA_2. In renal conditions involving inflammatory cell infiltration of the interstitium (such as glomerulonephritis and renal transplant rejection), the inflammatory cells (monocyte-macrophages) release substantial amounts of TXA_2. This increased concentration of TXA_2 causes intrarenal vasoconstriction (and perhaps an ADH-like effect), leading to diminished renal function. Administration of TXA_2-synthase inhibitors or antagonists to these patients and to patients with preeclampsia may improve renal function.

Increased TXA_2 formation and decreased PGE_2 and PGI_2 synthesis have been observed in hypertensive animals. These changes may be either primary contributing factors or secondary responses. Increased TXA_2 formation is also seen in animals with cyclosporin-induced nephrotoxicity, but a causal relationship between the 2 has yet to be established.

PGE_2 may also be involved in renal phosphate excretion, because PGE_2 antagonizes the inhibition of phosphate reabsorption by parathyroid hormone (PTH) in the proximal tubule. However, the physiologic role of this eicosanoid may be limited, since the proximal tubule, the major site for phosphate transport, produces few prostaglandins.

The roles of leukotrienes and cytochrome P-450 products in the kidney are currently speculative. More information is needed to suggest any specific renal functions for these compounds.

Gastrointestinal System

The word cytoprotection was coined to describe the protective effect of the E prostaglandins against gastric ulcers in animals. These prostaglandins were independently discovered to inhibit gastric acid secretion in 1967. Since then, numerous experimental and clinical investigations have shown that PGE and its analogues protect against gastric ulcers produced by either steroids or NSAIDs.

Increased leukotriene formation in colonic mucosa has been demonstrated in patients with inflammatory bowel diseases. Whether these products play any pathophysiologic role has not yet been established.

Immune System

Monocyte-macrophages are the only cells of the immune system that can synthesize all the eicosanoids. T and B lymphocytes are interesting exceptions to the general rule that all nucleated cells produce eicosanoids. However, interaction between the lymphocytes and monocyte-macrophages may cause the lymphocytes to release arachidonic acid from their cell membranes. The arachidonic acid is then used by the monocyte-macrophage for eicosanoid synthesis (Table 4–2).

The eicosanoids modulate the effects of the immune system, as illustrated in the cellular immune response. As shown in Fig 4–5, PGE_2 and PGI_2 affect T cell proliferation like corticosteroids do. They inhibit T cell clonal expansion by inhibiting interleukin-1 and -2 and class II antigen expression on macrophages or other antigen-presenting cells. The leukotrienes, TXA_2, and PAF stimulate T cell clonal expansion. These compounds stimulate the formation of interleukin-1 and -2 as well as the expression of interleukin-2 receptors. The leukotrienes also promote interferon-γ release and can stimulate interferon-γ in place of interleukin-2. These in vitro effects of the eicosanoids and PAF agree with in vivo findings in animals of acute organ transplant rejection, as described below. The association between the use of the steroidal anti-inflammatory drugs and increased risk of

Table 4–2. Different Cell Types and Their Formation of Eicosanoids and PAF.

Cell Type	Eicosanoid
Macrophages	Leukotrienes, TXA_2, PGE_2, PAF, HETEs
Lymphocytes	Arachidonic acid
Platelets	TXA_2, HETEs
Endothelial cells	PGI_2, HETEs
Eosinophils	PGE_2, TXA_2, 15-HPETE, PAF, Leukotrienes
PMNs	Leukotrienes

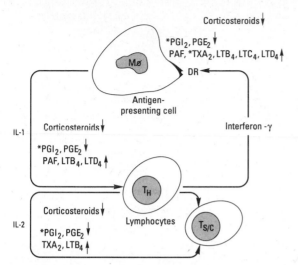

Figure 4–5. Modulation of macrophage and lymphocyte interactions by eicosanoids, platelet-activating factor (PAF), and corticosteroids. Corticosteroids, PGE$_2$, and possibly PGI$_2$ inhibit the effect of interleukin-1 (IL-1) on T cell lymphocytes. PAF, LTB$_4$, and LTD$_4$ stimulate IL-1 expression. These compounds exert similar inhibitory and stimulatory effects on the action of interferon-γ on the macrophage, and on the action of interleukin-2 (IL-2). Agents marked with an asterisk are suspected, but not yet proven, to have the indicated effects. DR = Class II MHC (major histocompatibility complex) 2 receptor, T = T lymphocytes. Mφ = macrophage, T$_H$ = Helper T cell, Ts/c = Suppressor/cytotoxic T cell (Modified and reproduced, with permission, from: Foegh ML, Ramwell PW: PAF and Transplant Immunology. In: Braquet P (editor): *The Role of Platelet Activating Factor in Immune Disorders.* Karger, 1988.)

infection is well established; however, the nonsteroidal anti-inflammatory drugs do not seem to alter patient responses to infections.

A. Inflammation: Edema is caused by leukotrienes LTC$_4$ and LTD$_4$ and is facilitated by the formation of the vasodilatory prostaglandins. The prostaglandins are not chemoattractants, but leukotrienes, especially LTB$_4$, and some of the HETEs (eg, 12-HETE) are strong chemoattractant agents. Thus, researchers are attempting to develop drugs that inhibit both the 5-lipoxygenase and the cyclooxygenase pathways.

B. Rheumatoid Arthritis: In this autoimmune disease, immune complexes are deposited in the affected joints, causing an inflammatory response that is amplified by eicosanoids and PAF. Lymphocytes and macrophages accumulate in the synovium, while polymorphonuclearleukocytes (PMNs) are located mainly in the synovial fluid. The major eicosanoids produced by PMNs are leukotrienes, which facilitate T cell proliferation and act as chemoattractants. Macrophages synthesize most eicosanoids and PAF. Human macrophages synthesize the cyclooxygenase

products PGE$_2$ and TXA$_2$, in addition to large amounts of leukotrienes.

PGE$_2$ has been proposed as an inflammatory mediator in arthritis. However, this theory does not incorporate the well-established inhibitory effect of PGE$_2$ on cellular immune responses. Therefore the hypothesis is now regarded as speculation. Another theory suggests that the undoubted benefits of NSAIDs on rheumatoid arthritis are caused by other mechanisms, ie, by reducing free radical formation. Corticosteroids are more potent than the NSAIDs in treating rheumatoid arthritis; this may be partly due to their inhibition of leukotriene formation, which is not an effect of the NSAIDs.

Female Reproductive System

A. Ovary: Prostaglandins are formed in the granulosa cells of the preovulatory follicle in response to gonadotropins. The highest levels of prostaglandins in the ovary are found at the time of ovulation.

PGF$_{2\alpha}$ is the endogenous luteolytic hormone in many species. In women, however, both PGF$_{2\alpha}$ and PGE analogues fail to elicit luteolysis. The physiologic significance of the PGF$_{2\alpha}$ produced in the human ovary is unknown.

B. Fallopian Tubes: The fallopian tubes synthesize both PGF$_{2\alpha}$ and PGE$_2$. The circular isthmus muscles contract in response to PGF$_{2\alpha}$ and relax in response to PGE$_2$. The longitudinal muscles are contracted by PGE$_2$. Thus, the prostaglandins may contribute to the regulation of ovum transport.

C. Blastocyst Implantation: Cyclooxygenase products have no proven role in human blastocyst implantation. Fertility in women is not affected by nonsteroidal anti-inflammatory drugs. In mice, however, PGE$_2$ promotes implantation and indomethacin inhibits its nidation.

D. Uterus: PGF$_{2\alpha}$ contracts the uterine muscle in vitro and in vivo. PGE$_2$ relaxes the uterine muscle in vitro. In vivo E prostaglandins contract the myometrium but the degree of contraction depends on the time of the menstrual cycle and on pregnancy.

The concentration of prostaglandins in the amniotic fluid increases over the course of pregnancy. This increase may be related to initiation of labor.

PGE$_2$ and prostacyclin play a role in decreasing vascular tone in pregnancy. Decreased prostacyclin production and the concomitant increase in TXA$_2$ synthesis may be responsible for the increased blood pressure in preeclampsia.

Male Reproductive System

The role of prostaglandins in semen is still conjectural. The major source of these prostaglandins is the seminal vesicle; the prostate and the testes synthesize only small amounts. Semen from fertile men contains about 400 μg/mL of PGE$_2$ and PGF$_{2\alpha}$ and their 19-hydroxy metabolites. There are about 20 times more PGE than PGF compounds in fertile semen, although this ratio varies greatly between individuals. However, within individuals this ratio remains fairly constant as long as the sperm characteristics are unchanged. The factors that regulate the concentration of prostaglandins in human seminal plasma are not known in detail, but testosterone does promote prostaglandin production. Thromboxane and leukotrienes have not been found in seminal plasma. Men with low seminal concentrations of prostaglandins are relatively infertile. It is known that large oral doses of aspirin reduce the prostaglandin content of seminal plasma.

Central & Peripheral Nervous Systems

Some of the eicosanoids affect the secretion of neurohormones in vitro. For example, PGE compounds inhibit growth hormone and prolactin release and, as mentioned earlier, LTC_4 stimulates LHRH secretion. These effects on neurohormones may not play any physiologic or pathophysiologic role, since they have not been reported in women receiving PGE compounds.

Prostaglandins are probably involved in fever, however. PGE_1 and PGE_2 increase body temperature, especially when administered into the cerebral ventricles. Recently pyrogens have been shown to release interleukin-1, which in turn promotes the synthesis and release of PGE_2. This synthesis is blocked by aspirin and other NSAIDs.

Intraventricular administration of PGD_2 produces other effects. This compound induces natural sleep (as determined by EEG analysis) in a number of species, including primates.

Recent data indicate that 12-HPETE may act as a neurotransmitter in *Aplysia* neurons. In addition, recent reports state that very high dilutions of LTC_4 specifically increase the release of LHRH from isolated rat anterior pituitary cells. Taken together, these data indicate that products of the lipoxygenase pathway can function as neurotransmitters.

PGE compounds inhibit the release of norepinephrine from sympathetic presynaptic nerve endings. Moreover, NSAIDs increase this release, suggesting that these prostaglandins play a physiologic role in this process. Thus, the vasoconstriction observed after treatment with cyclooxygenase inhibitors may be due to increased release of norepinephrine as well as inhibition of the endothelial synthesis of vasodilators (PGE_2 and PGI_2).

CLINICAL PHARMACOLOGY & THERAPEUTICS

Several approaches have been used in the clinical application of eicosanoids. First, stable long-acting analogues of PGE_1, PGE_2, and prostacyclin have been developed that increase intracellular cAMP. Therefore, these analogues can be regarded as cytoprotective. Second, enzyme inhibitors and receptor antagonists have been developed for interdiction and decreased expression of the "pathologic" eicosanoids, such as thromboxane and the leukotrienes. Third, knowledge of eicosanoid synthesis and metabolism has led to the development of new nonsteroidal anti-inflammatory drugs that inhibit cyclooxygenase with improved pharmacokinetic and pharmacodynamic effects. Finally, dietary manipulation—to change the polyunsaturated fatty acid precursors in the cell membrane phospholipids and so eicosanoid synthesis—is under active investigation.

THERAPEUTIC USES OF EICOSANOIDS

Gynecologic & Obstetric Uses

A. ABORTION: PGE_2 and $PGF_{2\alpha}$ are well known for their oxytocic actions. The ability of the E and F prostaglandins and their analogues to terminate pregnancy at any stage by promoting uterine contractions has been adapted to routine clinical use. The drugs are used for first- and second-trimester abortion and priming or ripening of the cervix before abortion. These prostaglandins appear to soften the cervix by increasing proteoglycan and changing the biophysical properties of collagen.

Early studies found that intravenously administered PGE_2 and $PGF_{2\alpha}$ produced abortion in about 80% of cases. The success rate was dependent on dose, duration of infusion, and parity of the woman. Dose-limiting side effects included vomiting, diarrhea, hyperthermia, and bronchoconstriction. Intra-amniotic administration of $PGF_{2\alpha}$ has close to a 100% success rate with fewer and less severe side effects than intravenous administration. The drug available for this route of administration is dinoprost tromethamine, a (tris [hydroxymethyl] aminomethane) salt of $PGF_{2\alpha}$, or Prostin F2 Alpha, with which it shares its pharmacologic actions. This drug is used to induce second-trimester abortions and is usually administered as a single 40-mg intra-amniotic injection. The abortion is normally completed within 20 hours.

The most serious side effect of intra-amniotic administration is cardiovascular collapse. Most of the reported cases have been diagnosed as anaphylactic shock, but others may have been due to the drug's escaping into the circulation and causing severe pulmonary hypertension. In pregnant anesthetized women, 300 μg $PGF_{2\alpha}$/min intravenously increases pulmonary resistance by 100% and increases the work of the right side of the heart 3-fold. Thus, only minimal amounts of the 40-mg intra-amniotic dose need to reach the circulation to cause cardiovascular effects. This problem may be avoided by instilling the drug under ultrasonic guidance.

Intramuscular injection can also be used to induce abortion. The drug used is carboprost tromethamine (15-methyl $PGF_{2\alpha}$, Prostin/15M); the carbon 15 methyl group prolongs the duration of action. Unlike the one-time intra-uterine instillation of dinoprost, carboprost is given repeatedly up to the total dose of 2.6 mg normally required to cause abortion.

The third route of administration used to induce abortion is the intravaginal route. Dinoprostone, a synthetic PGE_2 analogue, is administered as vaginal suppositories. It directly affects both the cervix and the uterus. The cervix is normally firm, with a small orificium, but PGE softens the collagenase of the cervix, leading to its easy dilation. PGE also stimulates contraction of the uterus, facilitating the expulsion of the fetus. The usual dose is 20 mg repeated at 3–5 hour intervals depending on the response of the uterus. Abortion is usually achieved within 90 hours, but nearly 25% of cases are incomplete and require additional intervention.

The use of PGE analogues for "menstrual regulation" or very early abortions—within 1–2 weeks after the last menstrual period—has been explored extensively. The major problems of this use were recently solved by combining the PGE analogues with an antiprogestin. (See Chapter 17.)

B. Induction of Labor: Numerous studies have shown that PGE_2, and $PGF_{2\alpha}$, and their analogues effectively initiate and stimulate labor. There appears to be no difference in the efficacy of the 2 drugs when administered intravenously, but $PGF_{2\alpha}$ is one-tenth as potent as PGE_2. These agents and oxytocin have similar success rates and comparable induction to delivery intervals. The side effects of the prostaglandins are moderate, with a slightly higher incidence of nausea, vomiting, and diarrhea than that produced by oxytocin. However, $PGF_{2\alpha}$ has more gastrointestinal side effects than PGE_2. Neither drug has an adverse effect on the maternal cardiovascular system in the recommended doses. In fact, PGE_2 has to be infused at a rate about 20 times that used for induction of labor to decrease blood pressure and increase heart rate. $PGF_{2\alpha}$ is a bronchoconstrictor and should be used with caution in asthmatics; however, neither asthmatic attacks nor bronchoconstriction have been observed during the induction of labor. Although both PGE_2 and $PGF_{2\alpha}$ pass the fetoplacental barrier (as does oxytocin), no fetal side effects are seen.

Theoretically, PGE_2 and $PGF_{2\alpha}$ should be superior to oxytocin for inducing labor in women with preeclampsia or with cardiac and renal diseases because, unlike oxytocin, they have no antidiuretic effect. In addition, PGE_2 has natriuretic effects. However, the clinical benefits of these advantages have not been documented. In cases of intrauterine fetal death, the prostaglandins alone or with oxytocin seem to effectively cause delivery. In some cases of postpartum bleeding, 15-methyl-$PGF_{2\alpha}$ will successfully control hemorrhage when oxytocin and methylergonovine fail to do so.

The effects of oral PGE_2 administration (0.5–1.5 mg/h) have been compared to those of intravenous oxytocin and oral demoxytocin, an oxytocin derivative, in the induction of labor. Oral PGE_2 is superior to the oral oxytocin derivative and in most studies is as efficient as intravenous oxytocin. However, the only currently available form of PGE_2 is dinoprostone (vaginal suppositories), although this route of administration is slightly less effective than intravenous oxytocin. Vaginal PGE_2 administration is also used to soften the cervix before inducing labor. Oral $PGF_{2\alpha}$ has too many gastrointestinal side effects to be useful for inducing labor. (See Chapter 20.)

Cardiovascular Uses

A. Patent of Ductus Arteriosus: Patency of the fetal ductus arteriosus is now generally believed to be dependent on PGE_2 and PGI_2 synthesis. In certain rare types of congenital heart diseases (transposition of the great arteries, pulmonary atresia, and pulmonary artery stenosis) it is important to maintain the patency of the ductus arteriosus before surgery. This is done with alprostadil, PGE_1, whose pharmacologic action resembles those of PGE_2 and PGI_2. Like PGE_2, PGE_1 is a vasodilator and an inhibitor of platelet aggregation, and it contracts uterine and intestinal smooth muscle. There are no absolute contraindications for the use of this drug, but in cases of respiratory distress syndrome it is not recommended. The most common side effects include apnea, bradycardia, hypotension, and hyperpyrexia. Because of rapid pulmonary clearance, the drug has to be continuously infused at an initial dose of 0.05–0.1 μg/kg/min, which may be increased to 0.4 μg/kg/min. Prolonged treatment has been associated with ductal fragility and rupture.

B. Systemic Hypertension: The vasodilator effects of PGE and PGA compounds have been studied extensively in hypertensive patients. These compounds also promote sodium diuresis. The first study involved the inadvertent conversion of PGE_2 to PGA_2 during the extraction of rabbit renal medulla. The powerful diuretic effect of these compounds was discovered almost incidentally after their hemodynamic effects. Prostacyclin lowers peripheral and coronary resistance. It has been used to treat both primary and secondary pulmonary hypertension (which sometimes occurs after mitral valve surgery). However, its pulmonary vasodilator effects are not specific enough, so the patient's blood pressure must also be supported with pressor drugs.

Several studies have investigated the use of PGE and PGI_2 compounds to treat Raynaud's disease and peripheral atherosclerosis. In the latter condition, prolonged infusions have been used to permit "remodeling" of the vessel wall and to enhance regression of atherosclerotic ulcers.

Immunologic Uses

Acute organ transplant rejection is caused by a cellular immune response. Administration of PGI_2 to renal transplant patients has reversed the rejection process in some cases. Experimental in vitro and in vivo data show that PGE_2 and PGI_2 can prevent T cell proliferation and organ graft rejection, whereas prevention of TXA_2 and leukotriene formation attenuates organ graft rejection. In kidney transplant patients excretion of TXB_2 in the urine increases during acute graft rejection. The eicosanoids have not yet been proved to cause organ transplant rejection; however, corticosteroids are still the primary treatment for acute transplant rejection.

THERAPEUTIC INHIBITION OF EICOSANOID GENERATION

Gynecologic & Obstetric Uses

A. Dysmenorrhea: Primary dysmenorrhea is attributed to increased endometrial synthesis of PGE_2 and $PGF_{2\alpha}$ during menstruation, with contractions of the uterus that lead to ischemic pain. NSAIDs successfully inhibit the formation of these prostaglandins and so relieve dysmenorrhea in 75–85% of cases. Some of these drugs are available over the counter. Aspirin is also effective for treatment of dysmenorrhea, but since it has low potency and is quickly hydrolyzed, large doses and frequent administration are necessary. These drugs are contraindicated for dysmenorrhea, as for other uses, by the presence of gastric or duodenal ulcer or decreased renal function. Treatment for dysmenorrhea is short term, continued only during the period of menstrual cramps.

B. Risk of Preeclampsia: Low dose aspirin (60 mg daily) has recently been used to successfully prevent preeclampsia and pregnancy-induced hypertension when administered from 12 and 28 weeks of pregnancy, respectively. This preventative effect may be due to a decrease in platelet TXA_2 formation. However, these benefits may also be due to effects of aspirin that are not related to prostaglandins. TXA_2 synthase inhibitors have been used to treat preeclampsia, but the results of this treatment are inconclusive.

C. Preterm Labor: Non-steroidal inflammatory drugs like indomethacin have been used to treat preterm labour. They seem to exert some beneficial effect, as expected from the known oxytocic action of the PGEs and $PGF_{2\alpha}$. However, this application may be contraindicated because it has been associated with an increased incidence of primary pulmonary hypertension in the newborn.

Cardiovascular Uses

A. Closure of Patent Ductus Arteriosus: In delayed closure of the ductus arteriosus, cyclooxygenase inhibitors can be used to inhibit synthesis of the vasodilators PGE_2 and PGI_2 and so close the ductus. Premature infants who develop respiratory distress due to failure of ductus closure can often be treated very successfully with indomethacin. This treatment precludes the need for surgical closure of the ductus.

B. Risk of Myocardial Infarction: Epidemiologic studies in the USA and UK indicate that low doses of aspirin reduce the risk of death due to myocardial infarction but perhaps increase overall mortality rates and produce a higher incidence of stroke. However, the beneficial effects of aspirin may relate to its other acetylating properties and not its acetylation of cyclooxygenase.

Other Uses

A. Asthma: Corticosteroids and cromolyn sodium are the major eicosanoid-related drugs used in asthma. Corticosteroids inhibit all eicosanoid synthesis and thus also inhibit eicosanoid mediator release. Cromolyn inhibits the release of eicosanoids and the other mediators such as histamine and PAF. PAF, leukotriene antagonists, and lipoxygenase inhibitors may become useful in treating acute asthmatic attacks and hypersensitivity reactions. Unfortunately, these approaches have not yet been very successful in the treatment of asthma.

B. Risk of Gastrointestinal Ulcers: Recently the synthetic analogue 16,16-methyl-PGE_1 was approved for prophylactic treatment against ulcers in patients receiving steroidal or nonsteroidal anti-inflammatory agents. This and other PGE analogues are cytoprotective at low doses and inhibit gastric acid secretion at higher doses. The side effects are abdominal discomfort and occasional diarrhea; both effects are dose related.

C. Arthritis: Aspirin has been used to treat arthritis for nearly a century, but its mechanism of action, namely, inhibition of cyclooxygenase activity, was not discovered until 1971. Aspirin and other anti-inflammatory agents that inhibit cyclooxygenase are diflunisal (a salicylic acid derivative), ibuprofen, indomethacin, fenoprofen, meclofenamate, naproxen, sulindac, and tolmetin. Corticosteroids may produce more beneficial effects because they inhibit leukotriene formation, which is not an effect of these cyclooxygenase inhibitors.

DIETARY MODULATION OF EICOSANOID GENERATION

It is difficult to define and employ a diet that consists of just one or 2 different long chain polyunsaturated fatty acids, so it is also difficult to interpret the effects of adding each of these polyenoic acids to the diet. Two approaches have been used. The first adds corn, safflower, and sunflower oils, which contain linoleic acid (C18:n-2) to the diet. The second approach adds oils containing C20- and C22-polyenoic acids. Both types of diets change the phospholipid composition of cell membranes by replacing arachidonic acid with the dietary fatty acids. It has been claimed that the synthesis of both TXA_2 and PGI_2 is reduced and that changes in platelet aggregation, vasomotor spasm, and cholesterol metabolism follow. However, none of these interventions have been convincingly shown to modify the natural history of the disease that they address. As indicated above, there are many documented and possible oxidation products of the different polyenoic acids. It is probably naive to ascribe the effects reported thus far to related metabolites. Carefully controlled clinical studies will be needed before these questions can be satisfactorily answered.

However, subjects on diets containing highly saturated fatty acids clearly show increased platelet aggregation when compared with other study groups. Such diets always reduce the composition of polyunsaturated fatty acids in phospholipids. These diets (eg, in Finland and the USA) are associated with higher rates of myocardial infarction than are more polyunsaturated diets (eg, in Italy).

REFERENCES

Foegh ML et al (editors): *Alexis Carrel Conference on Lipid Mediators in Organ Transplantation*. Vol 18, Suppl 4. Grune & Stratton, 1986.

Lands WEM (Editor): *Polyunsaturated Fatty Acids and Eicosanoids*. American Oil Chemists Society, 1987.

Samuelsson B, Paoletti R, Ramwell PW (editors): *Advances in Prostaglandin, Thromboxane and Leukotriene Research*. Vol 17. Raven Press, 1987.

Watkins WD et al (editors): *Prostaglandins in Clinical Practice*. Raven Press. [In press.]

5

Neuroendocrinology

William F. Ganong, MD

Research in the science of neuroendocrinology has demonstrated that the brain regulates the secretion of the endocrine glands and that hormones in turn act on the central nervous system to modify brain function. The brain-endocrine interactions are multiple, complex, and important, both in terms of normal physiology and in terms of the pathophysiology of disease. This chapter is a general review of neuroendocrine control mechanisms. Details of the neural regulation of individual hormones are presented in the chapters on those hormones.

Nerve cells and gland cells resemble each other in many ways. Both secrete chemical messengers that produce responses in target cells. Both have electrical activity, and this activity increases when the cells release their chemical messengers. Like gland cells, nerve cells secrete hormones that enter the circulation. In addition, nerve cells and gland cells often secrete the same substance, and the same peptide or amine can be secreted by neurons as a neurotransmitter, by neurons as a neural hormone, and by gland cells as a classic hormone. A partial list of substances known to perform these multiple functions is shown in Table 5–1.

Chemical messengers not only mediate cell-to-cell communication via synaptic junctions (neural communication) and via messengers in the circulating body fluids (endocrine communication), but some messengers may diffuse in the interstitial fluid to target cells without entering the bloodstream. This form of communication is called paracrine communication (Fig 5–1). **Paracrine communication** occurs when the messengers act on other cells; **autocrine communication** occurs when the messengers act on the cells that secreted them. Paracrine communication has been postulated to occur in the case of somatostatin in the pancreatic islets; in the case of catecholamines and serotonin, in the brain; and in the case of GnRH, in sympathetic ganglia. It may be an even more widespread phenomenon, but its existence is difficult to prove. Another form of communication involves transfer of substances between adjacent cells via gap junctions without extracellular release of chemical messengers.

Acronyms Used in This Chapter

ACTH	Adrenocorticotropic hormone
cAMP	Cyclic adenosine monophosphate
CCK	Cholecystokinin
CRH	Corticotropin-releasing hormone
DNA	Deoxyribonucleic acid
FSH	Follicle-stimulating hormone
GAP	GnRH-associated peptide
GH	Growth hormone (somatotropin)
GnRH	Gonadotropin-releasing hormone
GRH	Growth hormone-releasing hormone
LH	Luteinizing hormone
β-LPH	β-Lipotropin
mRNA	Messenger ribonucleic acid
PIH	Prolactin-inhibiting hormone
PRH	Prolactin-releasing hormone
RNA	Ribonucleic acid
SIF	Small intensely fluorescent (cells)
TRH	Thyrotropin-releasing hormone
TSH	Thyroid-stimulating hormone (thyrotropin)
VIP	Vasoactive intestinal polypeptide

BRAIN CONTROL OF ENDOCRINE FUNCTIONS

Neural regulation of endocrine function is achieved via input to neurons that secrete hypothalamic hormones, via the innervation of the intermediate lobe of the pituitary, and via the autonomic innervation of glands such as the pancreatic islets that are not directly controlled by tropic hormones from the pituitary gland. The posterior lobe of the pituitary gland is made up of the endings of neurons that secrete oxytocin and vasopressin into the general circulation, whereas the hormones of the anterior lobe of the pituitary are regulated by hypothalamic hypophyseotropic hormones reaching them in the portal hypophyseal vessels. These vessels provide a direct vascular path from the

Table 5–1. Neuroendocrine messengers: Substances that function as neurotransmitters, neural hormones, and classic hormones.

	Neuro-transmitter (Present in Nerve Endings)	Hormone Secreted by Neurons	Hormone Secreted by Endocrine Cells
Dopamine	+	+	+
Norepinephrine	+	+	+
Epinephrine	+		+
Somatostatin	+	+	+
Gonadotropin-releasing hormone (GnRH)	+	+	+
Thyrotropin-releasing hormone (TRH)	+	+	
Oxytocin	+	+	+
Vasopressin	+	+	+
Vasoactive intestinal polypeptide (VIP)	+	+	
Cholecystokinin (CCK)	+		+
Glucagon	+		+
Enkephalins	+		+
Pro-opiomelano-cortin derivatives	+		+
Other anterior pituitary hormones	+		+

brain to the anterior pituitary. Humans and several other species of mammals have no intermediate lobe, but in the species that do, its secretion is controlled in part by an inhibitory innervation from the hypothalamus. In addition, the secretion of the hormones of the adrenal medulla, pineal, kidney, parathyroid gland, and pancreatic islet cells is influenced by their autonomic innervation.

RELATION OF THE PITUITARY TO THE BRAIN

The main nuclei of the hypothalamus and the relationship of this part of the brain to the pituitary gland are shown in Fig 5–2. The posterior lobe of the pituitary arises embryologically as an evagination of the ventral hypothalamus, whereas the anterior and intermediate lobes of the pituitary are derived from Rathke's pouch, an evagination of the pharynx. The posterior lobe retains its neural character throughout life. In this lobe, the axons of neurons with their cell bodies in the supraoptic and paraventricular nuclei of the hypothalamus end on capillaries that drain via the posterior lobe veins and the cavernous sinuses to the general circulation. The anterior lobe receives no functionally important innervation from the hypothalamus, but its secretion is controlled by the hypothalamic hypophyseotropic hormones secreted into the portal hypophyseal vessels (Fig 5–3). This special system of blood vessels provides a short, direct connection between the ventral hypothalamus and the anterior lobe. It begins in a primary plexus of capillaries in the median eminence of the hypothalamus. Some of the capillaries lie on the ventral surface of the median eminence, and some form loops that penetrate the substance of the median eminence. The capillaries drain into the short sinusoidal portal hypophyseal vessels that pass down the pituitary stalk and break up into capillaries surrounding the cells of the adenohypophysis.

Dopamine-secreting neurons that have their cell bodies in the arcuate nuclei and neighboring areas (see below) send axons to the posterior lobe and, in those

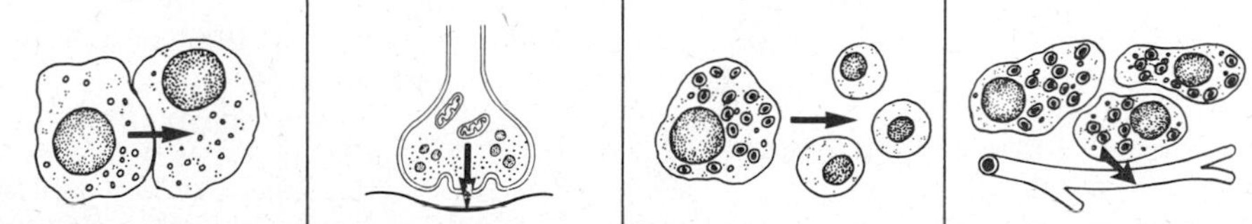

	GAP JUNCTIONS	SYNAPTIC	PARACRINE	ENDOCRINE
Message transmission	Directly from cell to cell	Across synaptic cleft	By diffusion in interstitial fluid	By circulating body fluids
Local or general	Local	Local	Locally diffuse	General
Specificity depends on	Anatomic location	Anatomic location and receptors	Receptors	Receptors

Figure 5–1. Intercellular communication by chemical mediators.

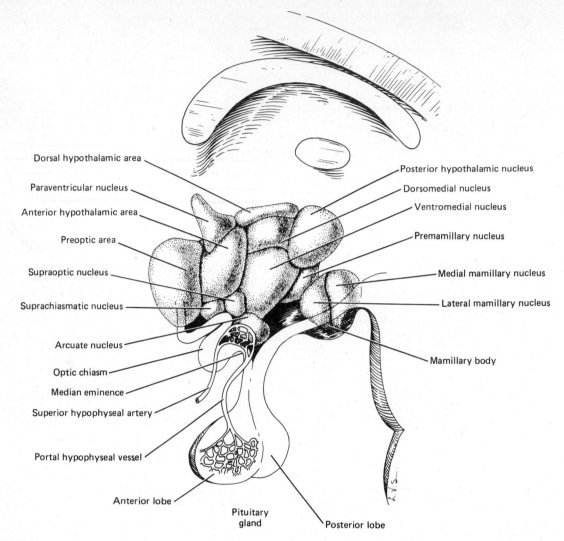

Figure 5–2. The human hypothalamus, with a superimposed diagrammatic representation of the portal hypophyseal vessels. (Reproduced, with permission, from Ganong WF: *Review of Medical Physiology,* 14th ed. Appleton & Lange, 1989.)

species that have one, the intermediate lobe as well. The function of this tuberohypophyseal innervation is unknown in the case of the posterior lobe; in the case of the intermediate lobe, it inhibits the secretion of intermediate lobe hormones.

HYPOTHALAMIC HORMONES

The exact number of hormones secreted by neurons in the hypothalamus is unclear, but 8 have been fully characterized and their structures determined (Table 5–2).

Posterior Pituitary Hormones

Oxytocin and arginine vasopressin are the 2 peptides known to be secreted from the posterior lobe of the pituitary in humans and most other mammals. Each peptide is synthesized in the hypothalamus as part of a preprohormone in the cell bodies of neurons in the supraoptic nuclei and the lateral and superior parts of the paraventricular nuclei (Fig 5–4). The preprohormone includes the peptide and an associated protein or **neurophysin** specific for the peptide. Neurons synthesize one peptide or the other—not both—and there are oxytocin-synthesizing and vasopressin-synthesizing neurons in both nuclei. Synthesis occurs in the ribosomes, and the preprohormone enters the rough endoplasmic reticulum, where the leader sequence is removed. The prohormone molecules are packaged into secretory granules in the Golgi apparatus, and the secretory granules migrate along the axons by axoplasmic flow to the endings in the posterior lobe. The

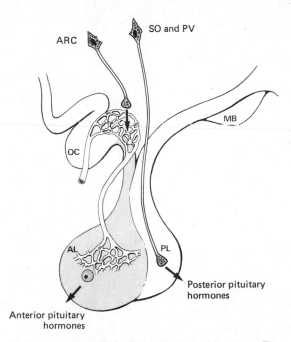

Figure 5–3. Secretion of hypothalamic hormones. The hormones of the posterior lobe (PL) are released into the general circulation from the endings of supraoptic and paraventricular neurons, whereas hypophyseotropic hormones are secreted into the portal hypophyseal circulation from the endings of arcuate and other hypothalamic neurons. AL, anterior lobe; MB, mamillary bodies; OC, optic chiasm.

packaged molecules undergo further processing as the granules move along the axons, and the bond between the peptide and its neurophysin is hydrolyzed before they are released from the endings. Secretion occurs by exocytosis, so that the octapeptides and neurophysins are released in equimolar amounts. Secretion is initiated by action potentials reaching the endings along the hormone-secreting neurons; thus, the neurons not only function as gland cells that synthesize and secrete the peptides, but they have propagated action potentials like other neurons. The action potentials increase the Ca^{2+} influx at the endings, and this triggers exocytosis. Physiologic control of the secretion of vasopressin and oxytocin and their functions are considered in detail in Chapter 9.

Hypophyseotropic Hormones

Most of the hypophyseotropic hormones stimulate the secretion of anterior pituitary hormones, but growth hormone and prolactin are also regulated by inhibitory hypophyseotropic hormones (Fig 5–5). There is also some overlap of function among the hypophyseotropic hormones.

TRH stimulates the secretion of TSH and prolactin. Its prolactin-stimulating activity is marked, but it probably does not have a major physiologic role as a prolactin-releasing hormone, because in most situations in which prolactin secretion is stimulated, there is no concomitant increase in TSH secretion. The cell bodies of the TRH-secreting neurons are located mostly in the medial portions of the paraventricular

Table 5–2. Hypothalamic hormones.

Hormone	Structure
Posterior pituitary hormones	
Arginine vasopressin	┌─ S ──────── S ─┐ Cys-Tyr-Phe-Gln-Asn-Cys-Pro-Arg-Gly-NH$_2$
Oxytocin	┌─ S ──────── S ─┐ Cys-Tyr-Ile-Gln-Asn-Cys-Pro-Leu-Gly-NH$_2$
Hypophyseotropic hormones	
Thyrotropin-releasing hormone (TRH)	(pyro)Glu-His-Pro-NH$_2$
Gonadotropin-releasing hormone (GnRH)	(pyro)Glu-His-Trp-Ser-Tyr-Gly-Leu-Arg-Pro-Gly-NH$_2$
Somatostatin[1]	┌─────── S ──────────── S ─────────┐ Ala-Gly-Cys-Lys-Asn-Phe-Phe-Trp-Lys-Thr-Phe-Thr-Ser-Cys
Growth hormone – releasing hormone (GRH)	Tyr-Ala-Asp-Ala-Ile-Phe-Thr-Asn-Ser-Tyr-Arg-Lys-Val-Leu-Gly-Gln-Leu-Ser-Ala-Arg-Lys-Leu-Leu-Gln-Asp-Ile-Met-Ser-Arg-Gln-Gln-Gly-Glu-Ser-Asn-Gln-Glu-Arg-Gly-Ala-Arg-Ala-Arg-Leu-NH$_2$
Prolactin-inhibiting hormone (PIH, dopamine)	HO⟍ HO⟋⟨benzene ring⟩— CH$_2$CH$_2$NH$_2$
Corticotropin-releasing hormone (CRH)	Ser-Gln-Glu-Pro-Pro-Ile-Ser-Leu-Asp-Leu-Thr-Phe-His-Leu-Leu-Arg-Glu-Val-Leu-Glu-Met-Thr-Lys-Ala-Asp-Gln-Leu-Ala-Gln-Gln-Ala-His-Ser-Asn-Arg-Lys-Leu-Leu-Asp-Ile-Ala-NH$_2$

[1] In addition to the tetradecapeptide shown here (somatostatin 14), an N-terminal extended molecule (somatostatin 28) and a 12-amino acid form (Somatostatin 28 [1-12]) are found in most tissues.

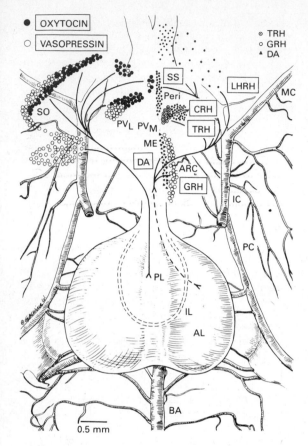

Figure 5–4. Location of cell bodies of hypophyseotropic hormone-secreting neurons projected on a ventral view of the hypothalamus and pituitary of the rat. AL, anterior lobe; ARC, arcuate nucleus; BA, basilar artery; IC, internal carotid; IL, intermediate lobe; MC, middle cerebral; ME, median eminence; PC, posterior cerebral; peri, periventricular nucleus; PL, posterior lobe; PV$_L$ and PV$_M$, lateral and medial portions of paraventricular nucleus; SO, supraoptic nucleus. The names of the hormones are enclosed in the boxes. (Courtesy of LW Swanson and ET Cunningham Jr.)

nuclei (Fig 5–4), and their axonal endings are mainly located in the medial portion of the external layer of the median eminence.

GnRH, which is also known as LHRH, stimulates the secretion of FSH as well as LH, and it has not been possible to separate its LH- and FSH-releasing activities by changing the structure of the molecule. Some hypothalamic extracts have been reported to produce selective stimulation of FSH secretion, but efforts to purify an FSH-releasing hormone (FRH) have failed. Consequently, there is a good possibility that there is only one gonadotropin-releasing hormone and that this hypophyseotropic hormone regulates the secretion of both gonadotropins. Evidence indicating that LH and FSH come from the same anterior pituitary cell makes this hypothesis even more attractive. However, it is difficult to prove that a separate FRH does not exist.

Most of the neurons that secrete GnRH have their cell bodies in the anterior hypothalamus, particularly in the preoptic area (Fig 5–4). Their axons converge on the median eminence and terminate primarily in the lateral portions of the external layer of the median eminence, especially near the pituitary stalk.

Somatostatin inhibits growth hormone (GH) secretion. It also inhibits TSH secretion, and administration of antisomatostatin antibodies causes a rise in circulating TSH. However, the physiologic role of somatostatin in the regulation of TSH secretion is unknown. The cells that secrete somatostatin into the portal hypophyseal blood have their cell bodies in the periventricular region immediately above the optic chiasm (Fig 5–4). Their axons terminate diffusely in all parts of the external layer of the median eminence.

GRH stimulates growth hormone secretion. The cell bodies of the GRH-secreting neurons are located in the arcuate nuclei (Fig 5–4), and the neuronal endings are in the external layer of the median eminence.

Dopamine is the principal and very possibly the only physiologically significant prolactin-inhibiting hormone (PIH). This catecholamine is secreted into

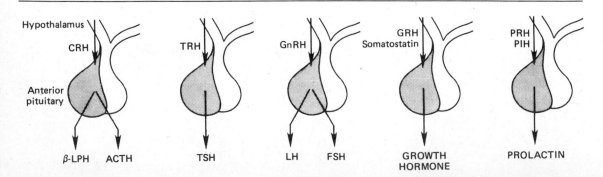

Figure 5–5. Effects of individual hypothalamic hypophyseotropic hormones on anterior pituitary secretion.

the portal hypophyseal vessels by neurons of the tuberoinfundibular dopaminergic system that have their cell bodies in the arcuate nuclei and their endings in the external layer of the median eminence (Fig 5–4). The bulk of the endings are located laterally in the same area as the GnRH endings, but some dopaminergic neurons also end in the medial part of the external layer.

There is considerable physiologic evidence for the existence of a prolactin-releasing hormone (PRH) in addition to PIH, but no single PRH has been identified. Instead, several different peptides with prolactin-releasing activity have been found in the hypothalamus, including oxytocin and vasoactive intestinal polypeptide (VIP). TRH also shows prolactin-releasing activity, as mentioned above. These peptides may act singly or together to stimulate prolactin secretion in various situations, or an additional major PRH may exist that has yet to be isolated and characterized.

CRH stimulates the secretion of β-lipotropin (β-LPH) as well as adrenocorticotropic hormone (ACTH). These pituitary hormones are formed in the same secretory granules from a large precursor molecule called **pro-opiomelanocortin** and are released in equimolar amounts by exocytosis (see Chapter 6). The CRH-secreting neurons are located in the anterior portion of the paraventricular nuclei just lateral to the TRH-secreting neurons (Fig 5–4), and their axons terminate in all parts of the external layer of the median eminence. Vasopressin has a moderate amount of CRH activity and may potentiate the activity of the CRH in the paraventricular neurons. In addition, angiotensin II and several other substances act directly on the pituitary to stimulate ACTH secretion, but their physiologic role in the regulation of ACTH secretion is unknown.

The genes for TRH, GnRH, somatostatin, GRH, and CRH have been cloned and the structures of their preprohormones have been determined. Prepro-TRH contains 5 copies of the TRH sequence. Prepro-GnRH consists of a signal sequence, the GnRH sequence, and then a 56-amino-acid polypeptide called GnRH-associated peptide (GAP). GAP, which appears to be secreted, exhibits prolactin-inhibiting activity in some preparations, but its physiologic role as a PIH is uncertain. The C-terminal end of preprosomatostatin is hydrolyzed to form the tetradecapeptide somatostatin 14, an N-terminal extended form of the hormone containing 28 amino acid residues (somatostatin 28), and a duodecapeptide from the N-terminal extension (somatostatin 28 [1–12]). Many tissues contain all 3 forms.

Hypophyseotropic Hormones Outside the Hypothalamus

All of the chemically identified hypothalamic hormones except GRH have also been found in other parts of the brain and in other organs of the body. Somatostatin is a neurotransmitter secreted in various parts of the brain, including primary afferent neurons conducting sensory impulses to the dorsal horn of the spinal cord. Somatostatin is also secreted by typical endocrine cells—the D cells—in the pancreatic islets and the gastrointestinal mucosa. From the latter location and possibly from the pancreas as well, somatostatin enters the general circulation and functions as a gastrointestinal hormone. TRH is also found in nerve endings in various parts of the brain and in the gastrointestinal tract. GnRH is found in neurons not only in the median eminence but also in other circumventricular organs (see below), and it or a very closely related peptide appear to be the neurotransmitter responsible for a slow excitatory response in sympathetic ganglia. CRH-containing fibers project from the paraventricular nuclei to the brain stem. Dopamine is found in many parts of the nervous system and in interneurons called small intensely fluorescent (SIF) cells in sympathetic ganglia. Oxytocin and vasopressin are found in neurons projecting from the hypothalamus to the brain stem and spinal cord. They are also found in the gonads. In addition, posterior lobe-like peptides and TRH are found in invertebrates. Thus, during the evolution of the pituitary, existing neurotransmitters and neurohormones were probably preempted to become the hypothalamic hormones secreted by or involved in the regulation of the pituitary gland.

Other Hormones Common to the Brain, Pituitary, & Gastrointestinal Tract

In addition to somatostatin and TRH, many gastrointestinal hormones are found in neurons in the brain as well as secretory cells or neurons in the gastric and intestinal mucosa. These hormones have no established function in the regulation of anterior pituitary secretion, although high concentrations of vasoactive intestinal polypeptide (VIP) have been found in portal hypophyseal blood, supporting its proposed role as a physiologic PRH (see above). In addition, ACTH, β-LPH, and the other derivatives of pro-opiomelanocortin are found not only in the anterior and intermediate lobes of the pituitary but also in neurons with their cell bodies in the arcuate nuclei of the hypothalamus. The function of these neurons is unknown. There is also evidence for the existence of prolactin, LH, and other anterior pituitary hormones in the brain.

NEUROTRANSMITTERS THAT AFFECT THE SECRETION OF HYPOTHALAMIC HORMONES

Afferent neural pathways converge from many different parts of the brain onto the neurons that secrete hypothalamic hormones. Not surprisingly, many different neurotransmitters are secreted by the neurons in these pathways, and drugs that modify the functions of neurotransmitters consequently affect the secretion of anterior and posterior pituitary hormones. Cholinergic discharge in the brain increases vasopressin secretion and may increase prolactin secretion. Discharge of gamma-aminobutyric acid-secreting neurons inhibits ACTH secretion, and histamine may be an excitatory mediator for ACTH. However, the transmitters that have received the most attention are the brain monoamines serotonin, dopamine, norepinephrine, and epinephrine. This is partly because the neurons secreting these substances can be identified by fluorescent or immunocytochemical techniques and partly because some diseases and various drugs used in the treatment of hypertension and psychiatric illness affect brain amine metabolism to the point that they alter pituitary function. Enkephalins and endorphins have also received considerable attention.

Most and possibly all of the hypophyseotropic hormones are secreted in a pulsatile rather than a tonic, steady fashion. For GnRH, this has important physiologic consequences and therapeutic implications. When GnRH is infused at a steady rate, it rapidly down-regulates its receptors on gonadotropes in the pituitary, resulting in the inhibition rather than the stimulation of LH secretion. Therefore, long-acting GnRH agonists can be used clinically to inhibit LH secretion, and pulsatile GnRH administration (at intervals of 1–2 hours) can be used to stimulate LH secretion in the treatment of infertility. This subject is discussed in more detail in Chapter 17.

Dopamine

The dopaminergic neurons in the brain are summarized in Fig 5–6. As noted above, the tuberoinfundibular dopaminergic system is the source of the dopamine that inhibits prolactin secretion. The other dopaminergic systems include the nigrostriatal system, which is concerned with the regulation of movement and is disrupted in Parkinson's disease; the mesocortical dopaminergic system, which is probably concerned with mental functions and may discharge abnormally in schizophrenia; and several small systems in and near the hypothalamus. There is some evidence that in addition to its inhibitory effect on prolactin, dopamine stimulates growth hormone secretion in humans, but there is little convincing evidence that dopamine plays a role in regulating the secretion of any other anterior pituitary hormones.

Norepinephrine

The noradrenergic neurons in the brain are summarized in Fig 5–7. They are divided into 2 systems, the locus ceruleus and the lateral tegmental. The locus ceruleus system consists of neurons with cell bodies in the locus ceruleus that project to all parts of the central nervous system. However, hypothalamic innervation from the locus ceruleus is limited to the supraoptic and paraventricular nuclei and parts of the dorsal hypothalamus, and there is little evidence that this system is involved in the regulation of endocrine function. The lateral tegmental system is made up of neurons with cell bodies in several nuclei in the pons and medulla that project to the spinal cord and to all parts of the hypothalamus. This system includes many noradrenergic neurons projecting from sites in or near the nucleus of the tractus solitarius where afferent fibers from the arterial baroreceptors end. In experimental animals, central release of norepinephrine increases the secretion of TSH, GH, LH, and FSH. It decreases the secretion of ACTH and apparently has a similar effect on oxytocin and vasopressin release, but it has no effect on prolactin secretion. Thus, norepinephrine plays

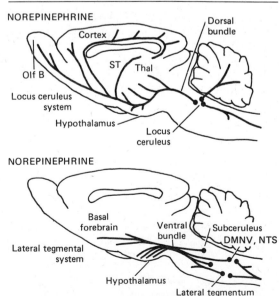

Figure 5–7. Noradrenergic neurons in the brain. Olf B, olfactory bulb; ST, stria terminalis; DMNV, dorsal motor nucleus of vagus; NTS, nucleus tractus solitarii. (Reproduced, with permission, from Ganong WF: *Review of Medical Physiology*, 14th ed. Appleton & Lange, 1989.)

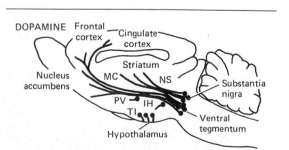

Figure 5–6. Dopaminergic neurons in the brain. The neurons are projected on a sagittal view of the rat brain. IH, incertohypothalamic system; MC, mesocortical system; NS, nigrostriatal system; PV, periventricular system; TI, tuberoinfundibular and tuberohypophyseal system. (Reproduced, with permission, from Ganong WF: *Review of Medical Physiology*, 14th ed. Appleton & Lange, 1989.)

an important role in regulating the secretion of hypophyseotropic hormones.

Epinephrine

Epinephrine-secreting neurons project from the medulla oblongata to the spinal cord and the hypothalamus (Fig 5–8). These neurons are involved in blood pressure regulation and are located so that they could exert effects on endocrine function. However, there is as yet little direct evidence that they play an important endocrine role.

Serotonin

Serotoninergic neurons have their cell bodies in the raphe nuclei in the midbrain, pons, and medulla and, like the dopaminergic and noradrenergic systems, project to the spinal cord and many different parts of the brain (Fig 5–9). Serotoninergic discharge increases prolactin secretion, probably by increasing the secretion of a PRH. Serotoninergic neurons also project to the suprachiasmatic nuclei, and lesions of these nuclei disrupt a variety of circadian rhythms, including the regular cycles in adrenocortical secretion and pineal secretion (see below). Drugs that decrease central secretion of serotonin abolish the circadian fluctuation in adrenocortical secretion, presumably via an effect on the suprachiasmatic nuclei.

Opioid Peptides

Many different opioid peptides have now been described. All are formed from 3 large precursor molecules (Table 5–3). All the precursors are found in the brain. They are also found outside the brain: **Preproenkephalin** is found in the adrenal medulla; **prepro-opiomelanocortin** is found in the anterior and intermediate lobes of the pituitary gland; and **preprodynorphin** and preproenkephalin are found in the gastrointestinal tract. The functions of these substances in peripheral tissues are considered in the chapters on the hormones of the adrenal medulla (Chapter 14), the anterior pituitary (Chapter 6), and the gastroin-

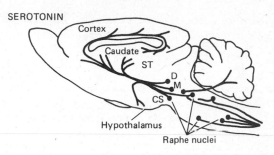

Figure 5–9. Serotoninergic neurons in the brain. CS, D, and M, central superior, dorsal, and medial raphe nuclei. ST, stria terminalis. (Reproduced, with permission, from Ganong WF: *Review of Medical Physiology,* 14th ed. Appleton & Lange, 1989.)

testinal tract (Chapter 21). In the brain, the opioid peptides produced from the precursors, particularly met-enkephalin and leu-enkephalin, are probably synaptic transmitters. There is considerable evidence that opioid peptides occur in the neural pathways involved in the regulation of anterior and posterior pituitary secretion. In humans, the effects of opioids on growth hormone and TSH secretion are unsettled, but it appears that opioids in the brain inhibit the secretion of ACTH, LH, and vasopressin, whereas they increase the secretion of prolactin. However, the nature of the opioids involved, the location of the opioid-secreting neurons, and the exact role of the pathways in the regulation of pituitary secretion are still unknown.

BRAIN REGULATION OF THE SECRETION OF OTHER HORMONES

Melatonin

The pineal gland secretes melatonin, an indole it produces by 5-methoxylation and N-acetylation of serotonin (Fig 5–10). There is some evidence that melatonin is also synthesized in the hypothalamus and in other parts of the body, but the melatonin in the circulation comes from the pineal. The pineal also appears to release melatonin into the cerebrospinal fluid, and cerebrospinal fluid levels are higher than those in plasma. The circulating melatonin level is markedly dependent on the incident light, with high levels in darkness (Fig 5–11). However, the function of melatonin is unknown. It has antigonadotropic activity in certain doses and under certain circumstances in experimental animals, but there is no good evidence for a physiologic antigonadotropic effect in humans.

The pineal is an excellent example of a gland that is under neural control. The light signals that regulate melatonin secretion are integrated in the suprachiasmatic nuclei, and disruption of these hypothalamic nuclei abolishes the light-dark fluctuations in circulating melatonin. From the suprachiasmatic nuclei, impulses

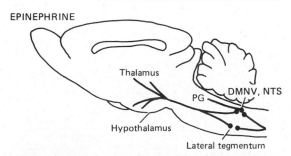

Figure 5–8. Epinephrine-secreting (adrenergic) neurons in the brain. PG, periaqueductal gray. (Reproduced, with permission, from Ganong WF: *Review of Medical Physiology,* 14th ed. Appleton & Lange, 1989.)

Table 5–3. Opioid peptides and their precursors.[1]

Precursor	Opioid Peptides	Structures
Preproenkephalin	Met-enkephalin Leu-enkephalin Octapeptide Heptapeptide	$Tyr\text{-}Gly\text{-}Gly\text{-}Phe\text{-}Met_5$ $Tyr\text{-}Gly\text{-}Gly\text{-}Phe\text{-}Leu_5$ $Tyr\text{-}Gly\text{-}Gly\text{-}Phe\text{-}Met\text{-}Arg\text{-}Gly\text{-}Leu_8$ $Tyr\text{-}Gly\text{-}Gly\text{-}Phe\text{-}Met\text{-}Arg\text{-}Phe_7$
Prepro-opiomelanocortin	β-Endorphin and other endorphins	See Chapter 6 and Fig 6–3.
Preprodynorphin	Dynorphin 1–8 Dynorphin 1–17 α-Neoendorphin β-Neoendorphin	$Tyr\text{-}Gly\text{-}Gly\text{-}Phe\text{-}Leu\text{-}Arg\text{-}Arg\text{-}Ile_8$ $Tyr\text{-}Gly\text{-}Gly\text{-}Phe\text{-}Leu\text{-}Arg\text{-}Arg\text{-}Ile\text{-}Arg\text{-}Pro\text{-}Lys\text{-}Leu\text{-}Lys\text{-}Trp\text{-}Asp\text{-}Asn\text{-}Gln_{17}$ $Tyr\text{-}Gly\text{-}Gly\text{-}Phe\text{-}Leu\text{-}Arg\text{-}Lys\text{-}Tyr\text{-}Pro\text{-}Lys_{10}$ $Tyr\text{-}Gly\text{-}Gly\text{-}Phe\text{-}Leu\text{-}Arg\text{-}Lys\text{-}Tyr\text{-}Pro_9$

[1]Reproduced, with permission, from Ganong WF: *Review of Medical Physiology,* 14th ed. Appleton & Lange, 1989.

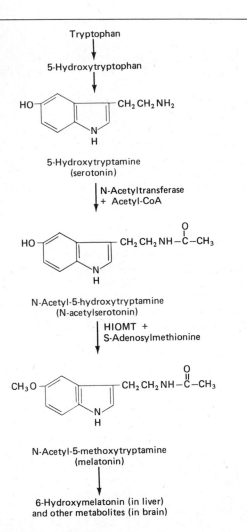

Figure 5–10. Formation and metabolism of melatonin. HIOMT, hydroxyindole-O-methyltransferase. (Reproduced, with permission, from Ganong WF: *Review of Medical Physiology,* 14th ed. Appleton & Lange, 1989.)

descend to the spinal cord and on each side pass via preganglionic sympathetic fibers in the thoracic region to the superior cervical ganglion. From the superior cervical ganglion, postganglionic neurons pass to the pineal gland via the nervi conarii. Norepinephrine released at these endings acts via beta-adrenergic receptors and cAMP to increase the synthesis of the enzyme N-acetyltransferase in the pineal and thus increase melatonin synthesis. The beta receptors show fluctuations in sensitivity with variations in the amount of norepinephrine reaching them; they are more sensitive after decreased exposure to norepinephrine and less sensitive after increased exposure. The receptors have been extensively studied, because they provide an excellent example of the role of receptors in the regulation of an endocrine gland.

Adrenal Medullary Hormones

The adrenal medulla is another endocrine gland under direct neural control. Its secretory cells are in effect postganglionic sympathetic neurons that have lost their axons and become endocrine cells. Consequently, they are innervated by preganglionic sympathetic neurons from the intermediolateral gray column of the spinal cord, and the transmitter that regulates adrenal medullary secretion is acetylcholine. The regulation of adrenal medullary secretion is discussed in detail in Chapter 14. Only a small part of the circulating norepinephrine comes from the adrenal medulla, however. The rest diffuses into the circulation from postganglionic noradrenergic endings in the viscera.

Renal, Parathyroid, & Pancreatic Hormones

Hormone secretion by the kidneys, the parathyroid glands, and the pancreatic islets is regulated in part by postganglionic sympathetic nerve fibers that secrete norepinephrine, and the islet cells also receive a parasympathetic cholinergic secretomotor innervation. In each of these instances, the neural components com-

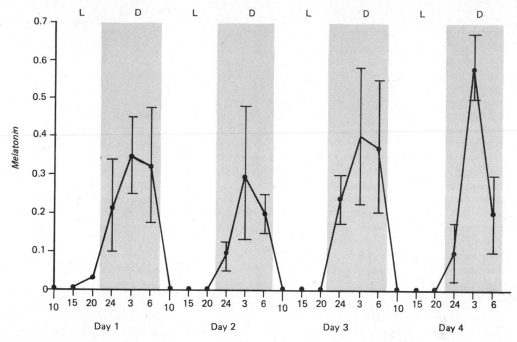

Figure 5–11. Plasma melatonin (in melatonin equivalents per 10 mL) in 5 normal adult men. Hours and days are represented on the horizontal scale, with light and dark phases indicated by L and D, respectively. (Reproduced, with permission, from Pelham RW et al: Twenty-four-hour cycle of a melatonin-like substance in the plasma of human males. *J Clin Endocrinol Metab* 1973;**37**:341.)

plement nonneural factors that play a major role in the regulation of secretion.

A. Renin: The secretion of renin from the juxtaglomerular cells in the kidney is a good example of autonomic regulation. Renin secretion is increased by increased discharge of the sympathetic nerves to the kidneys, but it is also increased by a reduction in intrarenal arterial pressure and a decrease in sodium and chloride crossing the macula densa at the start of each distal tubule. The latter 2 effects are direct and independent of renal innervation. The effect of sympathetic discharge is exerted via β_1-adrenergic receptors probably situated directly on the juxtaglomerular cells. The sympathetic pathway provides a direct mechanism by which psychologic and other stressful stimuli can increase renin secretion. Renin secretion is considered in detail in Chapter 15.

B. Erythropoietin: The secretion of the renal factor erythropoietin, which stimulates red blood cell maturation, is also increased by sympathetic discharge via beta-adrenergic receptors, although the secretion of this factor is primarily regulated by the amount of oxygen supplied to the tissues.

C. Parathyroid Hormone: Parathyroid hormone secretion is increased by increased sympathetic discharge via beta-adrenergic receptors, although the secretion of this hormone is primarily controlled by the amount of calcium ion (Ca^{2+}) in the blood perfusing the parathyroid glands. The regulation of parathyroid secretion is discussed in detail in Chapter 11.

D. Insulin: The secretion of insulin from the B cells and glucagon from the A cells of the pancreatic islets is increased by cholinergic mechanisms when the vagal nerve fibers innervating the pancreas are stimulated. Stimulation of the sympathetic innervation increases the secretion of insulin and glucagon via stimulation of beta-adrenergic receptors and inhibits the secretion of these hormones via alpha-adrenergic receptors. In the case of insulin, the alpha-inhibitory mechanism normally predominates, so that the net effect of sympathetic stimulation is inhibition of insulin secretion, whereas in the case of glucagon, the beta-excitatory mechanism predominates. There is evidence that the autonomic fibers also regulate the secretion of somatostatin and pancreatic polypeptide in the pancreatic islets. However, the secretion of insulin and glucagon is primarily regulated by glucose and other products of metabolism acting directly on the secretory cells. The regulation of islet cell secretion is considered in detail in Chapter 22.

EFFECTS OF HORMONES ON THE BRAIN

MECHANISMS OF HORMONE ACTION

Some of the multiple effects of hormones on the brain are indirect and are produced via hormone-induced changes in blood glucose, calcium, and the like. Others are direct and, in the case of hormones that penetrate the brain, may be due to direct actions of the hormone on neurons. In the case of hormones that do not penetrate the brain, the hormone-induced changes in brain function are mediated via the circumventricular organs, a unique group of brain structures that by their location outside the blood-brain barrier provide channels for chemical communication between the brain and the rest of the body.

Circumventricular Organs

The circumventricular organs are located in the midline portions of the brain that surround the third and fourth ventricles. Each has fenestrated capillaries, the type of highly permeable capillaries found in endocrine glands, the kidneys, and the intestinal epithelium. Each is readily penetrated by substances in the circulating blood, including peptides and other relatively large molecules. This is in marked contrast to the rest of the brain, where capillary endothelial junctions are tight and even small molecules have difficulty penetrating brain tissue. Thus, the circumventricular organs are outside the blood-brain barrier. However, they have intimate neural connections with the rest of the brain.

The established circumventricular organs (Fig 5–12) are the **area postrema,** located at the caudal end of the fourth ventricle; the **subfornical organ,** located in the dorsal part of the third ventricle between the columns of the fornix; the **organum vasculosum of the lamina terminalis,** located over the optic chiasm in the thin layer of tissue that forms the rostral boundary of the third ventricle; and the **neurohypophysis** and adjacent **median eminence** of the hypothalamus, located below the third ventricle. The pineal gland has fenestrated capillaries, like other endocrine organs, but—except for its sympathetic innervation (see above)—it lacks direct neural connections with the brain. The subcommissural organ does not have fenestrated capillaries, and although it has some of the histologic characteristics of a circumventricular organ, it probably has some other function.

The circumventricular organs are in a position to permit transport of large molecules from the brain to the circulation, and molecules in the blood that do not cross the blood-brain barrier can act on receptors in

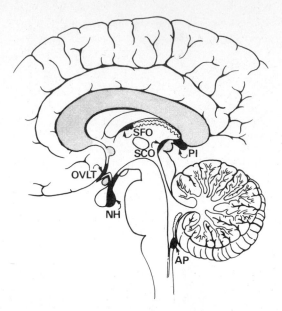

Figure 5–12. Circumventricular organs. The neurohypophysis (NH) and adjacent median eminence, the organum vasculosum of the lamina terminalis (OVLT), the subfornical organ (SFO), and the area postrema (AP) are shown projected on a sagittal section of the human brain. The pineal (PI) and the subcommissural organ (SCO) are also shown but probably do not function as circumventricular organs. (Reproduced, with permission, from Ganong WF: *Review of Medical Physiology,* 14th ed. Appleton & Lange, 1989.)

them. The neurohypophysis and median eminence function as **neurohemal organs,** sites where hypothalamic hormones secreted by neurons enter the general circulation (in the case of the posterior lobe hormones) and the portal hypophyseal circulation (in the case of the hypophyseotropic hormones). The circumventricular organs are also in an excellent position to function as **chemoreceptor trigger zones** where blood-borne chemicals can act on sensory cells to trigger changes in neural function without disruption of the blood-brain barrier. They carry out this function in particular for circulating peptides such as angiotensin II that affect brain function.

INDIRECT EFFECTS OF HORMONES ON THE BRAIN

Insulin produces changes in mental function, sweating, nervousness, convulsions, coma, and death by lowering blood glucose, the obligatory short-term substrate for brain metabolic processes. This is in contrast to the specific action of insulin on the glucoreceptor cells in the ventromedial nuclei of the hypothalamus to increase glucose utilization and thus produce satiety.

Hypocalcemia due to parathyroid hormone deficiency causes the changes in neural function that produce tetany, and hypercalcemia due to hyperparathyroidism produces changes in mental function that on occasion can be severe. Indeed, patients with chronic hypoglycemia and patients with hyperparathyroidism have been admitted to mental hospitals because of psychotic behavior, and their behavioral symptoms were subsequently relieved by treatment of the endocrine disease. Hypothyroidism can also cause mental symptoms, but the pathophysiologic basis of these symptoms is uncertain. Patients with hyperthyroidism are alert, nervous, and hyperphagic, but the first 2 effects are probably secondary to increased sympathetic activity, whereas hyperphagia is secondary to loss of calories as a consequence of hypermetabolism.

DIRECT EFFECTS OF HORMONES ON THE BRAIN

Hormones That Penetrate Brain Tissue

A. Effects of Steroids on Brain Function: Protein-bound steroids do not penetrate the brain, but free steroids enter with relative ease because of their high lipid solubility. Consequently, the brain level of active steroids is generally at least as high as the active, free fraction in plasma. The cells that take up the steroids have been identified as neurons by radioautography and are located throughout the central nervous system. Glucocorticoids, testosterone, estrogen, and progesterone all have effects on brain function.

Glucocorticoids increase the predominant frequency of the alpha rhythm of the EEG and produce mental symptoms that range from euphoria and bulimia to frank psychotic behavior. The mental symptoms associated with Cushing's syndrome are described in more detail in Chapter 12. Adrenal insufficiency is also associated with personality changes, although these are usually mild and subtle, and slowing of the basic frequency of the alpha rhythm is so characteristic that the EEG has been used as an aid in the diagnosis of Addison's disease. In rats, corticosterone binds to hippocampal neurons and stimulates DNA-dependent mRNA synthesis, but the physiologic significance of this action is unknown.

Progesterone in large doses stimulates sexual behavior in experimental animals, and smaller doses facilitate the effects of estrogens (see below). In addition, progesterone causes hyperthermia, probably by an action on the brain, and is believed to be responsible for the rise in basal body temperature at the time of ovulation in women.

Testosterone is responsible for male sexual behavior in many species of mammals, and sexual activity is reduced or abolished by castration. The site of this action of testosterone is the hypothalamus. In humans, male sex behavior is not dependent on testosterone and

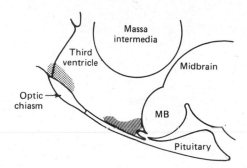

Figure 5–13. Loci where implantations of estrogens in the hypothalamus affect ovarian weight and sexual behavior in rats. The implants that stimulate sexual behavior are located anteriorly, above the optic chiasm (dotted area). They are separate from the posterior ventral sites (striped area), where implants inhibit LH secretion, causing ovarian atrophy. MB, mamillary body. (Reproduced, with permission, from Ganong WF: *Review of Medical Physiology,* 14th ed. Appleton & Lange, 1989.)

persists for long periods following castration. However, testosterone still acts on the brain to intensify sexual interest. Heterosexual drive in men is stimulated by estrogens as well as androgens, and increased libido with markedly decreased potency can be a problem in men being treated for prostatic cancer with large doses of estrogens.

Estrogens are responsible for the period of heat at the time of ovulation in females of species that have an estrous rather than a menstrual cycle. During heat, the female seeks out the male and engages in copulation, whereas during the rest of the cycle she rebuffs sexual advances. Evidence from lesion experiments and local implantation of steroids (Fig 5–13) indicates that estrogens produce heat by an action on the anterior hypothalamus. Androgens also intensify female sexual behavior in adult females. Primates have a menstrual rather than an estrous cycle without a clearly defined period of heat, but in monkeys and apes, the rise in circulating estrogens at the time of ovulation is associated with increased sexual activity. A few studies suggest that a midcycle increase in sexual activity also occurs in women. Ovariectomized and postmenopausal women have little or no loss of libido. However, they still have circulating androgens and estrogens of adrenal origin, and it has been claimed that if the adrenals as well as the ovaries are removed, sexual activity is markedly reduced.

B. Effects of Gonadal Steroids on Brain Development: In addition to its effects on adult sexual behavior, testosterone acts just after birth in rats to "masculinize" the brain. The transient rise in circulating testosterone at this time has no observable immediate effect on brain function, but it causes the animal to display the male pattern of sex behavior and the noncyclic male pattern of gonadotropin secretion when the animal becomes an adult. The same changes can be produced in female rats by a single injection of testosterone up to the fifth day of life. If male rats are castrated at birth, they develop the female pattern of sexual behavior and the female cyclic pattern of gonadotropin secretion in adulthood. The mechanism by which a brief exposure to testosterone produces lifelong changes in brain function is still unknown.

Changes similar to those occurring in rats can be produced in other laboratory animals, although in species in which the young are born more mature than they are in the rat, the animals must be treated before rather than after birth by administering androgens to the mother. In monkeys, early exposure to androgen does not change the pattern of gonadotropin secretion in adulthood, but it does produce masculinization of behavior. In women with congenital adrenal hyperplasia and the adrenogenital syndrome, the androgens also fail to alter the pattern of gonadotropin secretion; these women menstruate regularly when treated with glucocorticoids. However, it has been claimed that the behavior of these women is measurably masculinized.

There is some evidence that the androgens that masculinize the brain are actually converted to estrogens by **aromatization** before exerting their effects. Aromatization occurs in various parts of the brain. Proponents of the view that aromatization is necessary for masculinization argue that estrogens do not masculinize normal females, because young females have an avid estrogen-binding protein in their blood and tissues. However, aromatization has not yet been proved to be a necessary step for masculinization.

C. Thyroid Hormones on Brain Development: Thyroid hormones penetrate the brain and have marked effects on brain development in early life. If untreated, cretins with congenital hypothyroidism develop severe mental retardation. In animals that are hypothyroid from birth, neurons fail to develop to their normal size, there are fewer synaptic endings than normal, and dendritic trees are stunted. These morphologic changes are associated with abnormalities of brain enzyme concentrations and impaired RNA synthesis.

Hormones That Act Via Circumventricular Organs

Angiotensin II acts on the brain to produce several important effects. It increases water intake, blood pressure, and secretion of vasopressin. However, like most peptides, angiotensin II does not cross the blood-brain barrier; instead, it exerts its central effects by acting on the circumventricular organs. The increase in water intake is due primarily to the action of circulating angiotensin II on the subfornical organ, although the organum vasculosum of the lamina terminalis may have a secondary role in mediating this dipsogenic effect. In most but not all species studied, the blood pressure-raising effect is due to an action on the area postrema. The increase in vasopressin secretion appears to be due to an action on the subfornical organ. Angiotensin II also increases ACTH secretion, but it is uncertain how much, if any, of this effect is due to a direct action on the pituitary.

Insulin is also found in circumventricular organs in relatively large amounts, and there is evidence for retrograde transport of insulin to the cell bodies of the neurons innervating the circumventricular organs. However, the physiologic role of insulin at this site is unknown.

When administered systemically in small doses, posterior pituitary peptides have been reported to produce changes in the extinction of conditioned avoidance responses and other psychologic responses. It is difficult to see how these substances could penetrate the brain to produce the observed effects, but an effect mediated via the circumventricular organs is a possibility.

REFERENCES

Brownstein MH, Russell JT, Gainer H: Synthesis, transport and release of posterior pituitary hormones. *Science* 1980;**207**:373.

Cooper JR, Bloom FE, Roth RH: *The Biochemical Basis of Neuropharmacology,* 5th ed. Oxford Univ Press, 1986.

Delitala G, Mota M, Serio M: *Opioid Modulation of Endocrine Function.* Raven Press, 1984.

Fitzimons JT: *The Physiology of Thirst and Sodium Appetite.* Cambridge Univ Press, 1979.

Ganong WF: *Review of Medical Physiology,* 14th ed. Appleton & Lange, 1989.

Ganong WF: The role of catecholamines and acetylcholine in the regulation of endocrine function. *Life Sci* 1974; **15**:1401.

Guillemin R et al: Growth hormone-releasing factor: Chemistry and physiology. *Proc Soc Exp Biol Med* 1984; **175**:407.

Krieger DT, Liotta AS: Pituitary hormones in brain: Where, how and why? *Science* 1979;**205**:366.

Martin JB, Reichlin S: *Clinical Neuroendocrinology.* 2nd ed. Davis, 1987.

Martini L, Ganong WP (editors): *Frontiers in Neuroendocrinology.* Vol 10. Raven Press, 1988.

Mayo KE, Evans RM, Rosenfeld GM: Genes encoding mammalian neuroendocrine peptides: Strategies toward their identification and analysis. *Ann Rev Physiol* 1986;**48**:431.

Preslock JP: The pineal gland: Basic implications and clinical correlation. *Endocr Rev* 1984;**5**:282.

Weiner RI, Ganong WF: Role of brain monoamines and histamine in regulation of anterior pituitary secretion. *Physiol Rev* 1978;**58**:905.

Wood C, Porte DJR: Neural control of the endocrine pancreas. *Physiol Rev* 1974;**54**:596.

Anterior Pituitary Gland

6

James W. Findling, MD, & J. Blake Tyrrell, MD

Immunoassay techniques that measure the secretory products of the pituitary and advances in the neuroradiologic evaluation of the sella turcica have improved the diagnosis of pituitary disorders. Transsphenoidal microsurgery, bromocriptine, and somatostatin analogues such as octreotide acetate now allow earlier and more effective therapy. This chapter describes the clinical evaluation of the anterior pituitary (adenohypophysis), including its anatomy, embryology, and histology; the physiologic action and secretion of its major hormones; and disorders of the gland with respect to neuroradiologic findings and secretory hypo- and hyperfunction.

EMBRYOLOGY

The human fetal pituitary anlage is initially recognizable at 4–5 weeks of gestation, and rapid cytologic differentiation leads to a mature hypothalamic-pituitary unit at 20 weeks. The adenohypophysis originates from Rathke's pouch, an ectodermal evagination of the oropharynx, and migrates to join the neurohypophysis (an outpouching of the third ventricle). The portion of Rathke's pouch in contact with the neurohypophysis develops less extensively and forms the intermediate lobe. This lobe remains intact in some species, but in humans its cells become interspersed with those of the anterior lobe. These cells do, however, develop the capacity to synthesize and secrete pro-opiomelanocortin, adrenocorticotropic hormone (ACTH), and related peptide hormones.

Remnants of Rathke's pouch may persist at the boundary of the neurohypophysis, resulting in small colloid cysts. In addition, cells may persist in the lower portion of Rathke's pouch beneath the sphenoid bone, the pharyngeal pituitary. These cells have the potential to secrete hormones and have been reported to undergo adenomatous change.

ANATOMY
(Figs 6–1 and 6–2)

Gross Anatomy

The pituitary gland lies at the base of the skull in a portion of the sphenoid bone called the sella turcica

Acronyms Used in This Chapter

ACTH	Adrenocorticotropic hormone
AVP	Arginine vasopressin
cAMP	Cyclic adenosine monophosphate
CLIP	Corticotropinlike intermediate lobe peptide
CRH	Corticotropin-releasing hormone
FSH	Follicle-stimulating hormone
GABA	Gamma-aminobutyric acid
GH	Growth hormone
GnRH	Gonadotropin-releasing hormone
GRH	Growth hormone-releasing hormone
hCG	Human chorionic gonadotropin
hGH	Human growth hormone
hMG	Human menopausal gonadotropin
hPL	Human placental lactogen
LH	Luteinizing hormone
LPH	Lipotropin
MEN	Multiple endocrine neoplasia
MRI	Magnetic resonance imaging
MSH	Melanocyte-stimulating hormone
PRL	Prolactin
SHBG	Sex hormone-binding globulin
SIADH	Syndrome of inappropriate secretion of vasopressin (antidiuretic hormone)
TRH	Thyrotropin-releasing hormone
TSH	Thyroid-stimulating hormone (thyrotropin)
VER	Visual evoked response
VIP	Vasoactive intestinal polypeptide

("Turkish saddle"). The anterior portion, the tuberculum sellae, is flanked by posterior projections of the sphenoid wings, the anterior clinoid processes; the dorsum sellae form the posterior wall, and their upper corners project into the posterior clinoid processes. The gland is surrounded by dura, and the roof is formed by a reflection of the dura attached to the clinoid processes, the diaphragma sellae. In healthy individuals, the arachnoid membrane and, therefore, cerebrospinal fluid are prevented from entering the sella turcica by the diaphragma sellae. The pituitary stalk and its blood vessels pass through an opening in this diaphragm. The lateral walls of the gland are in direct apposition to the cavernous sinuses and separated from them by dural membranes. The optic chiasm lies 5–10 mm above the diaphragma sellae and anterior to the stalk (Fig 6–1).

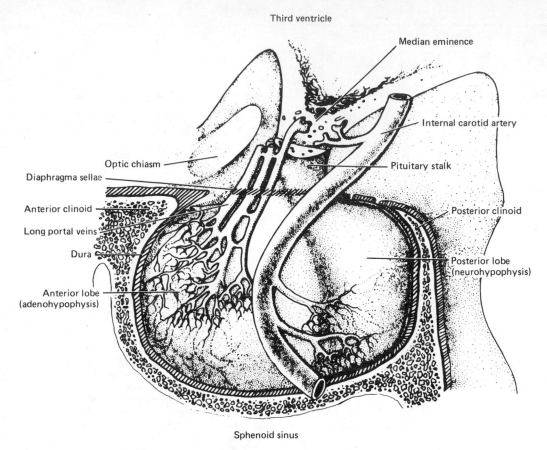

Third ventricle

Median eminence

Internal carotid artery

Optic chiasm

Pituitary stalk

Diaphragma sellae

Anterior clinoid

Posterior clinoid

Long portal veins

Dura

Posterior lobe
(neurohypophysis)

Anterior lobe
(adenohypophysis)

Sphenoid sinus

Figure 6–1. Anatomic relationships and blood supply of the pituitary gland. (Reproduced, with permission, from Frohman LA: Diseases of the anterior pituitary. Chap 7, pp 151–231, in: *Endocrinology and Metabolism*. Felig P et al [editors]. McGraw-Hill, 1981.)

The size of the pituitary gland, of which the anterior lobe constitutes two-thirds, varies considerably. It measures approximately $15 \times 10 \times 6$ mm and weighs 500–900 mg; it may double in size during pregnancy. Since the sella turcica tends to conform to the shape and size of the gland, there is considerable variability in the contour of this bony structure.

Blood Supply

The anterior pituitary is the most richly vascularized of all mammalian tissues, receiving 0.8 mL/g/min from a portal circulation connecting the median eminence of the hypothalamus and the anterior pituitary. This arterial blood is supplied by the internal carotid arteries via middle and inferior hypophyseal arteries. The arteries form a capillary network in the median eminence of the hypothalamus that recombines in long portal veins draining down the pituitary stalk to the anterior lobe, where they break up into another capillary network and re-form into venous channels. The posterior pituitary is supplied directly from branches of the middle and inferior hypophyseal arteries (Fig 6–1).

Venous drainage of the pituitary, the route through which anterior pituitary hormones reach the systemic circulation, is variable, but venous channels eventually drain via the cavernous sinus posteriorly into the superior and inferior petrosal sinuses to the jugular bulb and vein (Fig 6–2).

Recent evidence indicates that there is also retrograde blood flow between the pituitary and hypothalamus, providing a means of direct feedback between pituitary hormones and their neuroendocrine control.

Histology

The cells of the anterior pituitary were originally classified using techniques for staining intracellular granules as acidophils, basophils, and chromophobe cells. Immunocytochemical and electron microscopic techniques now permit classification of cells by their specific secretory products: somatotrophs (growth hormone [GH]–secreting cells), lactotrophs (prolactin [PRL]–secreting cells), thyrotrophs (cells secreting thyroid-stimulating hormone [thyrotropin; TSH]), cor-

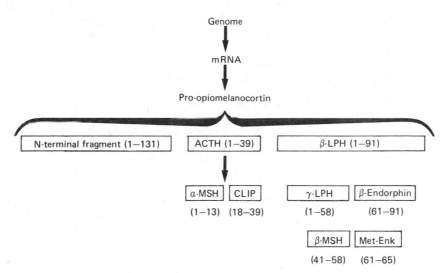

Figure 6–3. The processing of pro-opiomelanocortin (MW 28,500) into its biologically active peptide hormones. Abbreviations are expanded in the text.

(61–65) within β-LPH and β-endorphin, there is no evidence that it is secreted separately by the pituitary.

The N-terminal fragment (131 amino acids) of pro-opiomelanocortin has been isolated and sequenced. The first 76 amino acids of this N-terminal sequence appear to be the physiologically relevant form of this fragment. Plasma levels of this peptide increase in response to hypoglycemic stress. It may be an adrenal growth factor and may potentiate ACTH action on steroidogenesis.

Function

The primary effect of ACTH is to stimulate the secretion of glucocorticoids, mineralocorticoids, and androgenic steroids from the adrenal cortex (see Chapters 12 and 13). The amino-terminal end (residues 1–18) is responsible for this biologic activity. ACTH binds to receptors on the adrenal cortex and provokes steroidogenesis through the mediation of cyclic 3′,5′-adenosine monophosphate (cyclic AMP, cAMP).

The hyperpigmentation observed in states of ACTH hypersecretion (eg, Addison's disease, Nelson's syndrome) appears to be primarily due to ACTH. Because α- and β-MSH do not exist as separate hormones in humans, the exact cause of this increased pigmentation remains unclear.

The physiologic function of β-LPH and its family of peptide hormones, including β-endorphin, is not completely understood. However, it is known that both β-LPH and β-endorphin have the same secretory dynamics as ACTH; they increase in response to stress, hypoglycemia, and metyrapone and are suppressible with glucocorticoids. These hormones, including the N-terminal fragment, also parallel ACTH in disease states—eg, they are elevated in Addison's disease, Cushing's disease, and Nelson's syndrome and suppressed by glucocorticord excess.

Furthermore, there is evidence that β-endorphin acts as an "endogenous opiate," suggesting a role in pain appreciation. It may affect the endocrine regulation of other pituitary hormones and perhaps also the neural control of breathing. A hyperendorphin syndrome reported in a child with necrotizing encephalomyelopathy suggests that it may be a causative factor in disease states.

Measurement

It is more difficult to measure plasma ACTH by radioimmunoassay than the other anterior pituitary hormones. Its low concentration, instability in human plasma, and structural homology within its family of peptides create technical difficulties. However, the development of an immunoradiometric assay using monoclonal antibodies to ACTH has provided a sensitive and practical clinical assay for the evaluation of pituitary-adrenal disorders. The basal morning concentration ranges from 20 pg/mL to 100 pg/mL (4.4–22.2 pmol/L). Its short plasma half-life (7–12 minutes) and episodic secretion cause wide and rapid fluctuations both in its plasma concentration and in that of cortisol. Because ACTH adheres avidly to glass (a phenomenon that is utilized for extraction in some radioimmunoassay procedures), specimens should be collected in chilled, anticoagulated plastic tubes. Plasma should be separated and frozen immediately after collection to avoid destruction by plasma peptidases.

Although β-LPH has a longer half-life than ACTH and is more stable in plasma, its measurement has not been extensively utilized. Current data suggest that the normal concentration of β-LPH is 10–40 pg/mL (1–4 pmol/L).

Various levels of β-endorphin have been reported, but limitations exist because of cross-reactivity of antisera with β-LPH. Because chromatographic procedures are essential to determine plasma levels accurately, this hormone's measurement remains investigational.

The normal level of the N-terminal fragment in human plasma appears to be less than 100 pg/mL; measurements are not clinically available.

Secretion

The physiologic secretion of ACTH is mediated through neural influences by means of a complex of hormones, the most important of which is corticotropin-releasing hormone (CRH) (Fig 6–4). Although CRH was the first recognized hypothalamic hormone, it was not isolated until 1981, when Vale et al identified the 41-amino-acid peptide in ovine hypothalami. The structure of human CRH has also been identified and is identical to that of rat CRH. CRH has a long plasma half-life (approximately 60 minutes), and both arginine vasopressin (AVP) and angiotensin II potentiate the CRH-mediated secretion of ACTH. In contrast, oxytocin inhibits CRH-mediated ACTH secretion.

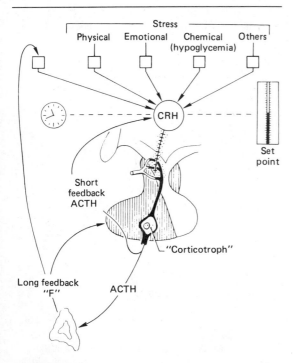

Figure 6–4. The hypothalamic-pituitary-adrenal axis, illustrating negative feedback by cortisol ("F") at the hypothalamic and pituitary levels. A short negative feedback loop of ACTH on the secretion of corticotropin-releasing hormone (CRH) also exists. (Reproduced, with permission, from Gwinup G, Johnson B: Clinical testing of the hypothalamic-pituitary-adrenocortical system in states of hypo- and hypercortisolism. *Metabolism* 1975;**24**:777.)

CRH is also secreted from human placenta; the level of this hormone increases significantly during late pregnancy and delivery. The role of CRH in the control of maternal hypothalamic-pituitary-adrenal function is uncertain.

CRH stimulates ACTH in a pulsatile manner, with diurnal rhythmicity causing a peak before awakening and a decline as the day progresses. The diurnal rhythm is a reflection of neural control and provokes concordant diurnal secretion of cortisol from the adrenal cortex (Fig 6–5). This episodic release of ACTH is independent of circulating cortisol levels—ie, the magnitude of an ACTH impulse is not related to preceding plasma cortisol levels. An example is the persistence of diurnal rhythm in patients with primary adrenal failure (Addison's disease). ACTH secretion also increases in response to feeding in both humans and animals.

Many types of stresses stimulate ACTH, often superseding the normal diurnal rhythmicity. Physical, emotional, and chemical stresses such as pain, trauma, hypoxia, acute hypoglycemia, cold exposure, surgery, depression, and pyrogen and vasopressin administration have all been shown to stimulate ACTH and cortisol secretion. The increase in ACTH levels during stress is mediated by vasopressin as well as CRH. Although physiologic cortisol levels do not blunt the ACTH response to stress, exogenous corticosteroids in high doses suppress it.

Negative feedback of cortisol and synthetic glucocorticoids on ACTH secretion occurs at both the hypothalamic and pituitary levels and appears to act by 2 mechanisms: "Fast feedback" is sensitive to the rate of change in cortisol levels, while "slow feedback" is sensitive to the absolute cortisol level. The first mechanism is probably nonnuclear; ie, this phenomenon occurs too rapidly to be explained by the influence of corticosteroids on nuclear transcription of the specific mRNA responsible for ACTH. "Slow feedback," occurring later, may be explained by a nuclear-mediated mechanism and a subsequent decrease in synthesis of ACTH. This latter form of negative feedback is the type probed by the clinical dexamethasone suppression test. In addition to the negative feedback of corticoids, ACTH also exerts a negative feedback effect on (ie, inhibits) its own secretion (short loop feedback).

GROWTH HORMONE

Biosynthesis

Growth hormone (GH; somatotropin) is a 191-amino-acid polypeptide hormone (MW 21,500) synthesized and secreted by the somatotrophs of the anterior pituitary. It is derived from a larger precursor peptide, preGH (MW 28,000), which is also secreted but which has no physiologic significance. GH, PRL, and human placental lactogen (hPL) probably evolved as a single

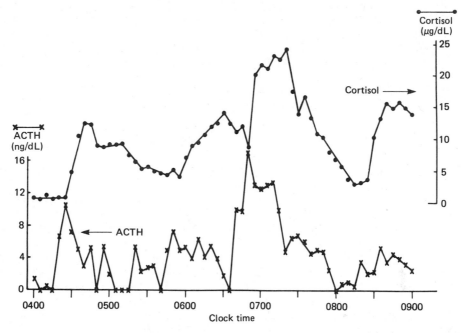

Figure 6–5. The episodic, pulsatile pattern of ACTH secretion and its concordance with cortisol secretion in a healthy human subject during the early morning. (Reproduced, with permission, from Gallagher TF et al: ACTH and cortisol secretory patterns in man. *J Clin Endocrinol Metab* 1973;**36**:1058.)

molecule; although they have subsequently diverged in both structure and functional importance, they continue to share intrinsic lactogenic and growth-promoting activity.

Function

As its name implies, the primary function of growth hormone (somatotropin) is promotion of linear growth. Its basic metabolic effects serve to achieve this result, but most of the growth-promoting effects are mediated by the somatomedins, a family of small peptides produced in the liver. These fascinating insulinlike growth factors are discussed in Chapter 7.

Growth hormone, via the somatomedins, increases protein synthesis by enhancing amino acid uptake and directly accelerating the transcription and translation of mRNA. In addition, GH tends to decrease protein catabolism by mobilizing fat as a more efficient fuel source: It directly causes the release of fatty acids from adipose tissue and enhances their conversion to acetyl-CoA, from which energy is derived. This protein-sparing effect may be the most important mechanism by which GH promotes growth and development.

GH also affects carbohydrate metabolism. In excess, it decreases carbohydrate utilization and impairs glucose uptake into cells. This GH-induced insulin resistance appears to be due to a postreceptor impairment in insulin action. These events result in glucose intolerance, which in turn stimulates insulin secretion.

Measurement

GH circulates unbound in plasma and has a half-life of 20–50 minutes. The healthy adult secretes approximately 400 μg/d (18.6 nmol/d); in contrast, young adolescents secrete about 700 μg/d (32.5 nmol/d). The availability of specific antisera to GH allows measurement of serum levels and reproducibility in different laboratories. Because the structure of GH is similar to that of hPL, GH antiserum will cross-react, and determinations during pregnancy are therefore unreliable.

The early morning GH concentration in fasting adults is less than 5 ng/mL (232 pmol/L) and usually less than 2 ng/mL (93 pmol/L). There are no significant sex differences.

Concentrations of somatomedins can now be determined by both radioreceptor assays and radioimmunoassays. Determining the levels of these mediators of GH action may result in more accurate assessment of the biologic activity of GH (see Chapter 7).

Secretion

The secretion of GH is mediated by 2 hypothalamic hormones: growth hormone–releasing hormone (GRH) and somatostatin (growth hormone–inhibiting hormone). These hypothalamic influences are tightly regulated by an integrated system of neural, metabolic, and hormonal factors. Because neither GRH nor somatostatin can be measured directly, the net result of any factor on GH secretion must be considered as the sum of its effects on these hypothalamic hormones. Table 6–2 summarizes the many factors that affect GH secretion in physiologic, pharmacologic, and pathologic states.

A. GRH: Two peptides (of 40 and 44 amino acids) with potent GH-releasing activity have been isolated from separate pancreatic tumors in patients with acromegaly. Full biologic activity of these releasing factors appears to reside in the 1–27 amino acid sequence of the N-terminal portion of the molecule. Human GRH is strikingly similar to many gastrointestinal peptides, including secretin, gastrin, vasoactive intestinal polypeptide (VIP), and gastric inhibitory peptide. Like CRH, GRH has a rather long half-life (50 minutes).

Table 6–2. Factors affecting growth hormone secretion.[1]

Increase	Decrease[2]
Physiologic	
Sleep	Postprandial hyperglycemia
Exercise	Elevated free fatty acids
Stress (physical or psychologic)	
Postprandial:	
Hyperaminoacidemia	
Hypoglycemia (relative)	
Pharmacologic	
Hypoglycemia:	Hormones:
Absolute: insulin or 2-deoxyglucose	Somatostatin
Relative: postglucagon	Growth hormone
Hormones:	Progesterone
GRH	Glucocorticoids
Peptide (ACTH, α-MSH, vasopressin)	Neurotransmitters, etc:
Estrogen	Alpha-adrenergic antagonists (phentolamine)
Neurotransmitters, etc:	Beta-adrenergic agonists (isoproterenol)
Alpha-adrenergic agonists (clonidine)	Serotonin antagonists (methysergide)
Beta-adrenergic antagonists (propranolol)	Dopamine antagonists (phenothiazines)
Serotonin precursors	
Dopamine agonists (levodopa, apomorphine, bromocriptine)	
GABA agonists (muscimol)	
Potassium infusion	
Pyrogens (*Pseudomonas* endotoxin)	
Pathologic	
Protein depletion and starvation	Obesity
Anorexia nervosa	Acromegaly: dopamine agonists
Ectopic production of GRH	Hypo- and hyperthyroidism
Chronic renal failure	
Acromegaly:	
TRH	
GnRH	

[1]Modified and reproduced, with permission, from Frohman LA: Diseases of the anterior pituitary. Chap 7, pp 151–231, in: *Endocrinology and Metabolism,* Felig P et al (editors). McGraw-Hill, 1981.
[2]Suppressive effects of some factors can be demonstrated only in the presence of a stimulus.

The administration of GRH to humans appears to be a useful means of assessing GH secretory reserves and characterizing states of GH deficiency. GRH may also be useful therapeutically for treatment of GH deficiency.

Other peptide hormones such as vasopressin, ACTH, and α-MSH may act as GH-releasing factors when present in pharmacologic amounts. Even thyrotropin- and gonadotropin-releasing hormones (TRH and GnRH) often cause GH secretion in patients with acromegaly; however, it is not certain whether any of these effects are mediated by the hypothalamus or represent direct effects on the somatotroph.

B. Somatostatin: Somatostatin was isolated and characterized in 1973 by Brazeau et al while searching for GRH. Since then, this tetradecapeptide molecule has been found not only in the hypothalamus but also in the D cells of the pancreatic islets and the gastrointestinal mucosa. In addition to its profound inhibitory effect on GH secretion in spite of all provocative stimuli, somatostatin also has important inhibitory influences on many other hormones, including TSH, insulin, glucagon, gastrin, secretin, and VIP. A long-acting analogue of somatostatin, octreotide acetate, has recently been developed and used therapeutically in the management of GH excess.

C. Neural Control: The neural control of basal GH secretion results in irregular and intermittent release associated with sleep and varying with age. Peak levels occur 1–4 hours after the onset of sleep (during stages 3 and 4) (Fig 6–6). These nocturnal sleep bursts, which account for nearly 70% of daily GH secretion, are greater in children and tend to decrease with age. Glucose infusion will not suppress this episodic release. Emotional, physical, and chemical stress, including surgery, trauma, exercise, electroshock therapy, and pyrogen administration, provoke GH release; and impairment of secretion, leading to growth failure, has been well documented in children with severe emotional deprivation.

D. Metabolic Control: The metabolic factors affecting GH secretion include all fuel substrates: carbohydrate, protein, and fat. Glucose administration, orally or intravenously, lowers GH in healthy subjects and provides a simple physiologic maneuver useful in the diagnosis of acromegaly (see below). In contrast, hypoglycemia stimulates GH release. This effect depends on intracellular glycopenia, since the administration of 2-deoxyglucose (a glucose analogue that causes intracellular glucose deficiency) also increases GH. This response to hypoglycemia depends on both the rate of change in blood glucose and the absolute level attained. GH increases have been noted during the recovery phase of a glucose tolerance test as blood glucose declines from the hyperglycemic to the euglycemic range.

A protein meal or intravenous infusion of amino acids (eg, arginine) causes GH release. Paradoxically, states of protein-calorie malnutrition also increase

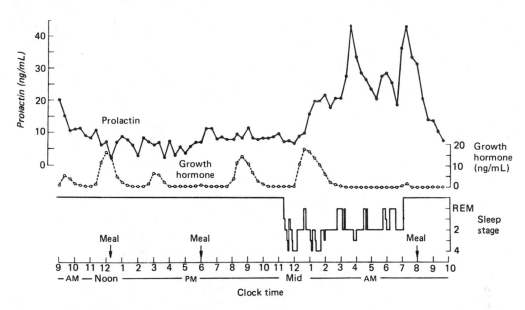

Figure 6–6. Sleep-associated changes in prolactin (PRL) and growth hormone (GH) secretion in humans. Peak levels of GH occur during sleep stages 3 or 4; the increase in PRL is observed 1–2 hours after sleep begins and is not associated with a specific sleep phase. (Reproduced, with permission, from Sassin JF et al: Human prolactin: 24-hour pattern with increased release during sleep. *Science* 1972;**177**:1205.)

GH, possibly as a result of decreased somatomedin production and lack of inhibitory feedback.

Fatty acids suppress GH responses to certain stimuli, including arginine and hypoglycemia. Fasting stimulates GH secretion, possibly as a means of mobilizing fat as an energy source and preventing protein loss.

E. Effects of Other Hormones: Many hormones also influence GH secretion: Responses to stimuli are blunted in states of cortisol excess and during hypo- and hyperthyroidism; although estrogen enhances GH secretion in response to stimulation, estradiol has been used to treat acromegaly because it decreases somatomedin production.

F. Effects of Neuropharmacologic Agents: Many neurotransmitters and neuropharmacologic agents affect GH secretion. Biogenic amine agonists and antagonists act at the hypothalamic level and alter GRH or somatostatin release. Dopaminergic, alpha-adrenergic, and serotoninergic agents all stimulate GH release.

Dopamine agonists such as levodopa, apomorphine, and bromocriptine increase GH secretion, whereas dopaminergic antagonists such as phenothiazines inhibit GH. The effect of levodopa, a precursor of both norepinephrine and dopamine, may be mediated by its conversion to norepinephrine, since its effect is blocked by the alpha-adrenergic antagonist phentolamine. Moreover, phentolamine suppresses GH release in response to other stimuli such as hypoglycemia, exercise, and arginine, emphasizing the

importance of alpha-adrenergic mechanisms in modulating GH secretion.

Beta-adrenergic agonists inhibit GH, and beta-adrenergic antagonists such as propranolol enhance secretion to provocative stimuli.

PROLACTIN

Biosynthesis

Prolactin (PRL) is a 198-amino-acid polypeptide hormone (MW 22,000) synthesized and secreted from the lactotrophs of the anterior pituitary. Despite evolution from an ancestral hormone common to GH and human placental lactogen (hPL), PRL shares only 16% of its residues with the former and 13% with hPL. A precursor molecule (MW 40,000–50,000) is also secreted and may constitute 8–20% of the PRL plasma immunoreactivity in healthy persons and in patients with PRL-secreting pituitary tumors.

Function

The primary effect of PRL is stimulation of lactation in the postpartum period (see Chapter 20). During pregnancy, PRL secretion increases and, in concert with many other hormones (estrogen, progesterone, hPL, insulin, and cortisol), promotes additional breast development in preparation for milk production. Despite its importance during pregnancy, PRL has not been demonstrated to play a role in the development of normal breast tissue in humans. During pregnancy, estrogen enhances breast development but blunts the effect of PRL on lactation; the decrease in both estrogen and progesterone after parturition allows initiation of lactation. Accordingly, galactorrhea may accompany the discontinuance of oral contraceptives or estrogen therapy. Although PRL secretion falls in the postpartum period, lactation is maintained by persistent breast suckling.

PRL levels are very high in the fetus and in newborn infants, declining during the first few months of life.

Although PRL does not appear to play a physiologic role in the regulation of gonadal function, hyperprolactinemia in humans leads to hypogonadism. In women, initially there is a shortening of the luteal phase; subsequently, anovulation, oligomenorrhea or amenorrhea, and infertility occur. In men, PRL excess leads to decreased testosterone synthesis and spermatogenesis, which clinically present as decreased libido, impotence, and infertility. The exact mechanisms of PRL inhibition of gonadal function are unclear, but the principal one appears to be alteration of hypothalamic-pituitary control of gonadotropin secretion. Basal LH and FSH levels are normal or subnormal; however, their pulsatile secretion is decreased and the midcycle LH surge is suppressed in women. Gonadotropin reserve, as assessed with GnRH, is usually normal or even exaggerated. PRL may also directly affect gonadal function by inhibiting the action of the gonadotropins on the ovary and testis, although the importance of this mechanism is less clear.

In addition, hyperprolactinemia in humans has been associated with glucose intolerance and hyperinsulinemia, and PRL may play a role as a diabetogenic factor during late pregnancy. Metabolic actions of PRL may occasionally mimic those of GH. Administration of ovine PRL to GH-deficient patients has resulted in positive nitrogen balance, lipolysis, and limited skeletal growth.

Prolactin also influences behavior patterns of numerous animal species. In humans, hyperprolactinemia has been associated with both anxiety and depression.

In several species, PRL is involved in the regulation of osmolality by influencing salt and water metabolism, although this effect has not been observed in humans. In salmon, it is critical for the adjustment from salt to fresh water.

Measurement

Reliable radioimmunoassay techniques for PRL are available; with specific antisera, there is no cross-reactivity with either GH or hPL.

The PRL secretory rate is approximately 400 μg/d (18.6 nmol/d). The hormone is cleared by the liver (75%) and the kidney (25%), and its half-time of disappearance from plasma is about 50 minutes.

Basal levels of PRL in adults vary considerably, with a mean of 13 ng/mL (590 pmol/L) in women and 5 ng/mL (227 pmol/L) in men. The upper range of normal in most laboratories is 15–25 ng/mL (681–1136 pmol/L).

Secretion

The hypothalamic control of PRL secretion, unlike that of the other pituitary hormones, is predominantly inhibitory. Thus, disruption of the hypothalamic-pituitary connection by stalk section, hypothalamic lesions, or pituitary autotransplantation increases PRL secretion. Presently, dopamine is thought to be the primary factor inhibiting PRL release; it has been found in the portal circulation and binds to dopamine receptors in rat lactotrophs. The administration of dopamine or its precursor levodopa, either in vitro or in vivo, inhibits PRL release; drugs that block dopamine receptors (eg, phenothiazines, metoclopramide) or cause hypothalamic dopamine depletion (reserpine, methyldopa) stimulate PRL release. The physiologic, pathologic, and pharmacologic factors influencing PRL secretion are listed in Table 6–3.

A. Prolactin-Releasing Factors: Hypothalamic extracts also contain fractions that stimulate release of PRL from the lactotroph. The best-studied of these PRL-releasing factors is TRH, which evokes release of PRL at a threshold dose similar to that which stimu-

Table 6–3. Factors affecting prolactin secretion.

Increase	Decrease
Physiologic	
Pregnancy	
Nursing	
Nipple stimulation	
Exercise	
Stress (hypoglycemia)	
Sleep	
Seizures	
Neonatal	
Pharmacologic	
TRH	Dopamine agonists (levo-
Estrogen	dopa, apomorphine, bro-
VIP	mocriptine, pergolide)
Dopamine antagonists (phe-	GABA
nothiazines, haloperidol,	
metoclopramide, reser-	
pine, methyldopa, amox-	
apine, opiates)	
Opioids	
Monoamine oxidase inhibi-	
tors	
Cimetidine (intravenous)	
Verapamil	
Licorice	
Pathologic	
Pituitary tumors	Pseudohypoparathyroidism
Hypothalamic/pituitary stalk	Pituitary destruction or re-
lesions	moval
Neuraxis irradiation	Lymphocytic hypophysitis
Chest wall lesions	
Spinal cord lesions	
Hypothyroidism	
Chronic renal failure	
Severe liver disease	

lates release of TSH. An exaggerated response of both TSH and PRL to TRH is observed in primary hypothyroidism, and their responses are blunted in hyperthyroidism. However, there are several discordant responses, suggesting that TRH is not the only PRL-releasing factor. The PRL increase associated with sleep, during stress, and after nipple stimulation or suckling is not accompanied by an increase in TSH.

Another hypothalamic peptide, VIP, stimulates PRL release in humans. Serotoninergic pathways may also stimulate PRL secretion, as demonstrated by the increased PRL secretion after the administration of serotonin precursors and by the reduction of secretion following treatment with serotonin antagonists. The neurotransmitter gamma-aminobutyric acid (GABA) and cholinergic pathways appear to inhibit PRL release.

B. Episodic and Sleep-Related Secretion: PRL secretion is episodic. An increase is observed 60–90 minutes after sleep begins but, in contrast to GH, is not associated with a specific sleep phase. Peak levels are usually attained between 4 and 7 AM (Fig 6–6). This sleep-associated augmentation of PRL release is not part of a circadian rhythm, like that of ACTH; it is related strictly to the sleeping period regardless of when it occurs during the day.

C. Other Stimuli: A variety of stresses, including surgery, exercise, hypoglycemia, and acute myocardial infarction, cause significant elevation of PRL levels. Nipple stimulation in nonpregnant women also increases PRL. This neurogenic reflex may also occur from chest wall injury such as mechanical trauma, burns, surgery, and herpes zoster of thoracic dermatomes. This reflex discharge of PRL is abolished by denervation of the nipple or by spinal cord or brain stem lesions. Several studies have also shown that seizures stimulate PRL secretion; the measurement of PRL levels 30–90 minutes after a seizure may distinguish true seizures from pseudoseizures.

D. Effects of Other Hormones: Many hormones influence PRL release. Estrogens increase the mitotic activity of lactotrophs, and their administration will augment basal and stimulated PRL secretion after 2–3 days of use (an effect that is of special clinical importance in patients with PRL-secreting pituitary adenomas); glucocorticoids tend to suppress TRH-induced PRL secretion; and thyroid hormone administration may blunt the PRL response to TRH.

E. Effects of Pharmacologic Agents: (Table 6–3.) Many pharmacologic agents alter PRL secretion. Dopamine agonists (eg, bromocriptine) decrease secretion, forming the basis for their use in states of PRL excess. Dopamine antagonists (eg, phenothiazines) augment PRL release and serve as provocative agents in assessing PRL secretory capacity. There is good correlation between the antipsychotic potency of these drugs and their hyperprolactinemic response, perhaps related to the extent of dopamine antagonism. Serotonin agonists will enhance PRL secretion; serotonin

receptor blockers suppress stress- and nursing-associated PRL release.

THYROTROPIN

Biosynthesis

Thyrotropin (thyroid-stimulating hormone, TSH) is a glycoprotein (MW 28,000) composed of 2 noncovalently linked subunits termed alpha and beta. The structure of the alpha subunit of TSH resembles that of the other glycoprotein molecules—FSH, LH, and human chorionic gonadotropin (hCG)—but the beta subunit differs in these glycoproteins and is responsible for their biologic and immunologic specificity. The peptides of these subunits appear to be synthesized separately and united before the carbohydrate groups are attached. The intact molecule is then secreted, as are small amounts of nonlinked subunits.

Function

The beta subunit of TSH attaches to high-affinity receptors in the thyroid, stimulating iodide uptake, hormonogenesis, and release of T_4 and T_3. This occurs through activation of adenylate cyclase and the generation of cAMP. TSH secretion also causes an increase in gland size and vascularity by promoting mRNA and protein synthesis. For a more detailed description of TSH action, see Chapter 10.

Measurement

TSH circulates unbound in the blood with a half-life of 50–60 minutes. The availability of monoclonal antibodies directed against different parts of the TSH molecule has allowed the development of ultrasensitive techniques (immunoradiometric assay) for measuring TSH concentration. The normal range is usually 0.4–4.8 µIU/mL (0.4–4.8 mIU/L). These new assays are helpful in the diagnosis of primary hypothyroidism and hyperthyroidism; however, TSH levels alone cannot be used to evaluate pituitary or hypothalamic hypothyroidism.

Radioimmunoassay techniques have also been developed for determination of the alpha subunit. The alpha subunit can be detected in about 80% of normals, with a range of 0.5–2 ng/mL. Plasma alpha subunit levels increase after administration of TRH in normal subjects, and basal levels are elevated in primary hypothyroidism and in patients with pure alpha subunit-secreting pituitary adenomas.

Secretion

The secretion of TSH is controlled by both stimulatory (TRH) and inhibitory (somatostatin) influences from the hypothalamus and in addition is modulated by the feedback inhibition of thyroid hormone on the hypothalamic-pituitary axis (Fig 6–7). Thyrotropin-releasing hormone (TRH), a tripeptide, is the major hypothalamic factor in TSH secretion. TRH

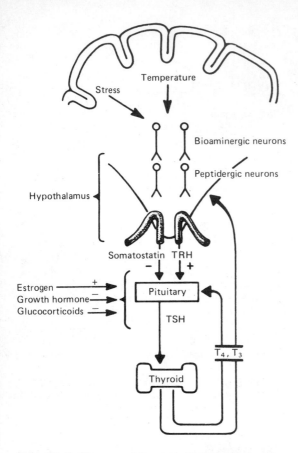

Figure 6–7. Diagram of the hypothalamic-pituitary-thyroid axis, illustrating the negative feedback of thyroid hormones (T_4, T_3) predominantly at the pituitary level. Hypothalamic factors may stimulate (TRH) or suppress (somatostatin) TSH secretion. Estrogen, GH, and glucocorticoids influence the effects of TRH on TSH secretion. (Reproduced, with permission, from Martin JB, Reichlin S, Brown GM: *Clinical Neuroendocrinology.* Davis, 1977.)

has been found in the hypothalamus as well as the portal blood; perfusion of pituitary stalk vessels with TRH evokes TSH release, and interruption of the hypothalamic-pituitary portal vessels decreases TSH secretion. The availability of synthetic TRH has led to many studies involving its relationship with TSH secretion.

A. TRH: The response of TSH to TRH is modulated by the circulating concentration of thyroid hormones. Small changes in serum levels (even within the physiologic range) cause substantial alterations in the TSH response to TRH. As shown in Fig 6–8, the administration of T_3 (15 μg) and T_4 (60 μg) to healthy persons for 3–4 weeks suppresses the TSH response to TRH despite only small increases in circulating T_3 and T_4 levels. Thus, the secretion of TSH is inversely proportionate to the concentration of thyroid hormone.

The set point (the level at which TSH secretion is maintained) is determined by TRH. Deviations from

this set point result in appropriate changes in TSH release. Administration of TRH increases TSH within 2 minutes, and this response is blocked by previous T_3 administration; however, larger doses of TRH may overcome this blockade—suggesting that both T_3 and TRH act at the pituitary level to influence TSH secretion. In addition, T_3 and T_4 inhibit mRNA for TRH synthesis in the hypothalamus, indicating that a negative feedback mechanism operates at this level also.

B. Somatostatin: This inhibitory hypothalamic peptide plays a role in the physiologic secretion of TSH by augmenting the direct inhibitory effect of thyroid hormone on the thyrotrophs. Infusion of somatostatin blunts the early morning TSH surge and will suppress high levels of TSH in primary hypothyroidism. Octreotide acetate, a long-acting somatostatin analogue, has been used successfully to inhibit TSH secretion in some patients with TSH-secreting pituitary tumors. Hypothyroidism occasionally follows the treatment of GH-deficient children, perhaps because GH therapy would stimulate somatostatin and subsequently decrease TSH.

C. Neural Control: In addition to these hypothalamic influences on TSH secretion, neurally mediated factors may be important. Dopamine physiologically inhibits TSH secretion. Intravenous dopamine administration will decrease TSH in both healthy and hypothyroid subjects as well as blunt the TSH response to TRH. Thus, as expected, dopaminergic agonists such as bromocriptine inhibit TSH secretion and dopaminergic antagonists such as metaclopramide increase TSH secretion in euthyroid subjects. Bromocriptine has also been effective in the management of some TSH-secreting pituitary tumors. Episodic or pulsatile TSH secretion has been demonstrated, with the highest levels during the early morning and lower levels in the late afternoon and early evening.

D. Temperature and Stress: Because thyroid hormone has such a critical role in the regulation of thermogenesis, the cold-induced increase of TSH in rats is not surprising. Nonetheless, neither acute nor chronic exposure to cold in adult humans has been shown to stimulate TSH release.

The effects of stress could affect TSH at various levels of the hypothalamic-pituitary-thyroid axis or by alteration of peripheral thyroid metabolism; however, except for insulin-induced hypoglycemia, stressful stimuli have not been demonstrated to have a direct influence on the secretion of TSH in humans.

E. Effects of Cortisol and Estrogens: Hormones such as cortisol and estrogens are also involved in TSH regulation. Glucocorticoid excess has been shown to impair the sensitivity of the pituitary to TRH and to be able to lower serum TSH to undetectable levels. However, estrogens increase the sensitivity of the thyrotroph to TRH; women have a greater TSH response to TRH than men do, and pretreatment of men with estradiol will increase their TRH-induced TSH response. (See also Chapter 10.)

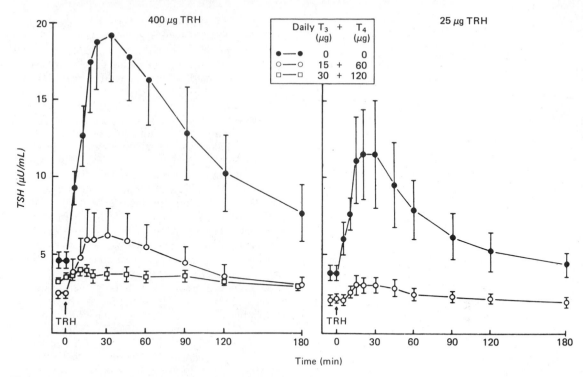

Figure 6–8. Administration of small doses of T_3 (15 µg) and T_4 (60 µg) healthy subjects inhibits the TSH response to 2 doses (400 µg, left; 25 µg, right) of TRH (protirelin). (Reproduced, with permission, from Snyder PJ, Utiger RD: Inhibition of thyrotropin-releasing hormone by small quantities of thyroid hormones. *J Clin Invest* 1972;**51**:2077.)

GONADOTROPINS: LUTEINIZING HORMONE, FOLLICLE-STIMULATING HORMONE

Biosynthesis

Luteinizing hormone (LH) and follicle-stimulating hormone (FSH) are glycoprotein gonadotropins composed of alpha and beta subunits and secreted by the same cell. The specific beta subunit confers on these hormones their unique biologic activity, as it does with TSH and hCG. The biologic activity of hCG, a placental glycoprotein, closely resembles that of LH. Human menopausal gonadotropin (hMG, menotropins)—an altered mixture of pituitary gonadotropins recovered from the urine of postmenopausal women—is a preparation with FSH-like activity. Menotropins and chorionic gonadotropin are used clinically for induction of spermatogenesis or ovulation (see Chapters 16 and 17).

Function

LH and FSH bind to receptors in the ovary and testis and regulate gonadal function by promoting sex steroid production and gametogenesis. These effects are mediated by the production of cyclic nucleotides.

In men, LH stimulates testosterone production from the interstitial cells of the testes (Leydig cells). For this reason, LH was formerly called interstitial cell-stimulating hormone (ICSH). Maturation of sper-

matozoa, however, requires both LH and FSH. FSH stimulates testicular growth and enhances the production of an androgen-binding protein by the Sertoli cells, which are a component of the testicular tubule necessary for sustaining the maturing sperm cell. This androgen-binding protein causes high local concentrations of testosterone near the sperm, an essential factor in the development of normal spermatogenesis (see Chapter 16).

In women, LH stimulates estrogen and progesterone production from the ovary. A surge of LH in the mid menstrual cycle is responsible for ovulation, and continued LH secretion subsequently stimulates the corpus luteum to produce progesterone by enhancing the conversion of cholesterol to pregnenolone. Development of the ovarian follicle is largely under FSH control, and the secretion of estrogen from this follicle is dependent on both FSH and LH.

Measurement

The development of immunoradiometric assays for LH and FSH in serum has provided sensitive and specific measurement of these hormones, and has made urinary gonadotropin excretion obsolete as an index of pituitary secretion. Presently, most laboratories utilize an International Reference Preparation (Second IRP/hMG) as a reference standard, and values for LH and FSH are expressed in mIU/mL.

Table 6–4. Normal gonadotropin responses (±SD) to GnRH (100 µg).

	Mean Maximum Δ LH (mIU/mL)(IU/L)	Mean Maximum Δ FSH (mIU/mL)(IU/L)
Women		
Folicular phase	17 (± 3)	3 (± 1)
Around LH peak	162 (± 49)	8 (± 3)
Luteal phase	49 (± 8)	3 (± 0.4)
Men		
Age 18–40	32 (± 6)	3 (± 1)
Age > 65	23 (± 4)	3 (± 1)

The normal levels of LH and FSH vary with the age of the subject. They are low before puberty and elevated in postmenopausal women. A nocturnal rise of LH in boys and the cyclic secretion of FSH and LH in girls usually herald the onset of puberty before clinical signs are apparent. In women, LH and FSH vary during the menstrual cycle; during the initial phase of the cycle (follicular), LH steadily increases, with a midcycle surge that initiates ovulation. FSH, on the other hand, initially rises and then decreases during the later follicular phase until the midcycle surge, which is concordant with LH. Both LH and FSH levels fall steadily after ovulation (Fig 6–9). (See Chapter 17.)

LH and FSH levels in men are similar to those in women during the follicular phase before the ovulatory increase. The alpha subunit, shared by all the pituitary glycoprotein hormones, can also be measured (see TSH) and will rise following GnRH administration. The normal levels of LH and FSH are shown in Table 6–4.

Secretion

The secretion of LH and FSH is controlled by a single stimulatory hypothalamic hormone, gonadotropin-releasing hormone (GnRH). GnRH, isolated by Schally et al in 1972, is a linear decapeptide that stimulates only LH and FSH; it has no effect on other pituitary hormones except in some patients with acromegaly and Cushing's disease, in whom it may augment GH and ACTH secretion, respectively. GnRH maintains basal gonadotropin secretion, generates the phasic release of gonadotropins for ovulation, and determines the onset of puberty.

A. Episodic Secretion: In both males and females, secretion of LH and FSH is episodic, with secretory bursts that occur each hour and are mediated by a concordant episodic release of GnRH. The amplitude of these secretory surges is greater in patients with primary hypogonadism. The pulsatile nature of GnRH release is critical for sustaining gonadotropin secretion. A continuous, prolonged infusion of GnRH in women evokes an initial increase in LH and FSH followed by prolonged suppression of gonadotropin se-

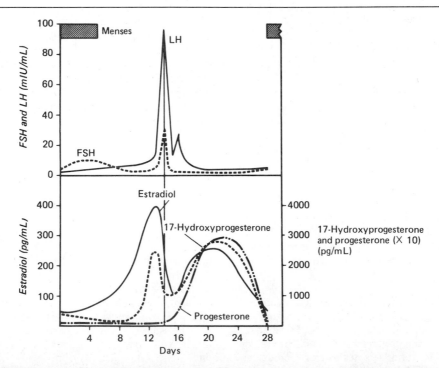

Figure 6–9. The secretory pattern of gonadotropins (LH, FSH) and sex steroids (estradiol, progesterone) during the normal female menstrual cycle. A midcycle surge of LH and FSH, stimulated by the rise in estradiol during the follicular phase, results in ovulation. After ovulation, the luteinized follicle secretes progesterone. (Reproduced, with permission, from Odell WD, Moyer DL: *Physiology of Reproduction*. Mosby, 1971.)

cretion. This phenomenon may be explained by down-regulation of GnRH receptors on the pituitary gonadotrophs. Consequently, long-acting synthetic analogs of GnRH may be used clinically to suppress LH and FSH secretion in conditions such as precocious puberty.

B. Positive Feedback: Circulating sex steroids affect GnRH secretion and thus LH and FSH secretion by both positive and negative (inhibitory) feedback mechanisms. During the menstrual cycle, estrogens provide a positive influence on GnRH effects on LH and FSH secretion, and the rise in estrogen during the follicular phase is the stimulus for the LH and FSH ovulatory surge. This phenomenon suggests that the secretion of estrogen is to some extent influenced by an intrinsic ovarian cycle. Progesterone amplifies the duration of the LH and FSH surge and augments the effect of estrogen. After this midcycle surge, the developed egg leaves the ovary. Ovulation occurs approximately 10–12 hours after the LH peak and 24–36 hours after the estradiol peak. The remaining follicular cells in the ovary are converted, under the influence of LH, to a progesterone-secreting structure, the corpus luteum. After about 12 days, the corpus luteum involutes, resulting in decreased estrogen and progesterone levels and then uterine bleeding. (See Chapter 17.)

C. Negative Feedback: Negative feedback effects of sex steroids on gonadotropin secretion also occur. In women, primary gonadal failure or menopause results in elevations of LH and FSH, which can be suppressed with long-term, high-dose estrogen therapy. However, a shorter duration of low-dose estrogen may enhance the LH response to GnRH. In men, primary gonadal failure with low circulating testosterone levels is also associated with elevated gonadotropins. However, testosterone is not the sole inhibitor of gonadotropin secretion in men, since selective destruction of the tubules (eg, by cyclophosphamide therapy) results in azoospermia and elevation of only FSH.

Inhibin, a polypeptide (MW 32,000) secreted by the Sertoli cells of the seminiferous tubules, is the major factor that inhibits FSH secretion by negative feedback. Inhibin, which has been purified and sequenced by analysis of its complementary DNA, consists of separate alpha and beta subunits connected by a disulfide bridge. Androgens stimulate inhibin production; this peptide may help to locally regulate spermatogenesis.

ENDOCRINOLOGIC EVALUATION OF THE HYPOTHALAMIC-PITUITARY AXIS

The precise assessment of the hypothalamic-pituitary axis has been made possible by radioimmunoassays of the major anterior pituitary hormones and by the introduction of 4 synthetic hypothalamic hormones: TRH (protirelin) and GnRH (gonadorelin), which are available commercially; and the newly synthesized ovine CRH and human GRH (GRH-40 and GRH-44). In addition, anterior pituitary function is also evaluated by measuring the specific target gland hormone secretion. Evaluation of the hypothalamic-pituitary axis should be performed carefully and the results interpreted critically, because the diagnosis of secretory abnormalities may indicate lifelong hormonal replacement in states of pituitary insufficiency or the necessity for surgical or radiation therapy in states of pituitary hypersecretion.

This section describes a practical approach to the evaluation of the hypothalamic-pituitary unit. The principles involved in testing each pituitary hormone are described, as well as special situations (eg, drugs, obesity) that may interfere with pituitary function or pituitary testing. Specific protocols for performing and interpreting diagnostic procedures are outlined at the end of this section. The clinical manifestations of either hypo- or hypersecretion of anterior pituitary hormones are discussed in subsequent sections.

EVALUATION OF ACTH

ACTH deficiency leads to adrenocortical insufficiency, characterized by decreased secretion of cortisol and the adrenal androgens; aldosterone secretion, controlled primarily by the renin-angiotensin axis, is usually maintained. Urine metabolites of adrenocorticosteroid secretion—17-hydroxycorticosteroids, 17-ketogenic steroids, and 17-ketosteroids—have long been used in the assessment of adrenal function; however, the development of specific plasma measurements of cortisol as well as other adrenal steroids has made these urine measurements obsolete (see Chapter 12).

Plasma ACTH Levels
Although ACTH can be directly determined in plasma, basal measurements are usually unreliable indicators of pituitary secretory reserve, since its short plasma half-life and episodic secretion result in wide fluctuations in plasma levels. Therefore, the interpretation of plasma ACTH levels requires the simultaneous assessment of cortisol secretion by the adrenal cortex. These measurements are of greatest utility in differentiating primary and secondary adrenocortical insufficiency and in establishing the etiology of Cushing's syndrome (see the later section on Cushing's disease and also Chapter 12).

Evaluation of ACTH Deficiency
In evaluating ACTH deficiency, measurement of basal cortisol levels is also unreliable. Although morning cortisol values are usually less than 10 μg/dL (0.28 μmol/L) in states of diminished pituitary ACTH

reserve, such low levels also occur in normal subjects because of the episodic nature of ACTH secretion. In addition, patients with ACTH deficiency following removal of ACTH-secreting pituitary adenomas or withdrawal of synthetic glucocorticoid therapy may have basal cortisol values exceeding 10 μg/dL (0.28 μmol/L) that fail to increase in response to a stressful stimulus. Consequently, the diagnosis of ACTH hyposecretion (secondary adrenal insufficiency) must be established by provocative testing of the reserve capacity of the hypothalamic-pituitary axis.

Adrenal Stimulation

Since adrenal atrophy develops as a consequence of prolonged ACTH deficiency, the initial and most convenient approach to evaluation of the hypothalamic-pituitary-adrenal axis is assessment of the plasma cortisol response to synthetic ACTH (cosyntropin; Cortrosyn). In normal individuals, injection of cosyntropin (250 μg) causes a rapid increase (within 30 minutes) of cortisol to at least 18 μg/dL (0.49 μmol/L), and this response usually correlates with the cortisol response to insulin-induced hypoglycemia and the 11-deoxycortisol rise after administration of metyrapone (discussed below). A subnormal cortisol response to ACTH confirms adrenocortical insufficiency. Although in most circumstances a normal ACTH stimulation test indicates adequate basal ACTH secretion, a normal response does not directly evaluate the ability of the hypothalamic-pituitary axis to respond to stress (see Chapter 12). Thus, patients withdrawn from long-term glucocorticoid therapy may have an adequate increase in cortisol following exogenous ACTH that precedes complete recovery of the hypothalamic-pituitary-adrenal axis. Therefore, such patients should receive glucocorticoids during periods of stress for at least 1 year after steroids are discontinued, unless the hypothalamic-pituitary axis is shown to be responsive to stress as described below.

Pituitary Stimulation

Direct evaluation of pituitary ACTH reserve can be performed by means of insulin-induced hypoglycemia, metyrapone administration, or CRH stimulation. These studies are unnecessary if the cortisol response to rapid ACTH stimulation is subnormal. The former 2 studies do not distinguish hypothalamic (CRH) from pituitary (ACTH) dysfunction; however, CRH stimulation may be useful for this purpose.

A. Insulin-Induced Hypoglycemia: The stimulus of neuroglycopenia associated with hypoglycemia (blood glucose < 40 mg/dL) evokes a stress-mediated activation of the hypothalamic-pituitary-adrenal axis. Subjects should experience adrenergic symptoms (diaphoresis, tachycardia, weakness, headache) associated with the fall in blood sugar. In normal persons, plasma cortisol increases to more than 18 μg/dL (0.49 μmol/L) following symptomatic hypoglycemia, indicating normal ACTH reserve. Although plasma ACTH

also rises, its determination has not proved to be as useful, since pulsatile secretion requires frequent sampling, and the normal response is not well standardized. Although insulin-induced hypoglycemia most reliably predicts ACTH secretory capacity in times of stress, this procedure requires a physician's presence and is contraindicated in elderly patients, patients with cerebrovascular or cardiovascular disease, and those with seizure disorders. It should be used with caution in patients in whom diminished adrenal reserve is suspected, since severe hypoglycemia may occur; in these patients, the test should always be preceded by the ACTH adrenal stimulation test.

B. Metyrapone Stimulation: Metyrapone administration is an alternative method for assessing ACTH secretory reserve. Metyrapone inhibits 11β-hydroxylase, the enzyme that catalyzes the final step in cortisol biosynthesis (see Chapter 12). The inhibition of cortisol secretion interrupts negative feedback on the hypothalamic-pituitary axis, resulting in a compensatory increase in ACTH. The increase in ACTH secretion stimulates increased steroid biosynthesis proximal to 11β-hydroxylase, and the increase can be detected as an increase in the precursor steroid (11-deoxycortisol) in plasma or by increases in urinary 17-hydroxycorticosteroids, which measure the urinary metabolite of 11-deoxycortisol. Two methods are available. The overnight test is preferred because of its simplicity; its is performed by administering 2–3 g of metyrapone orally at midnight. Plasma 11-deoxycortisol is determined the following morning and rises to greater than 7 μg/dL (0.19 μmol/L) in healthy individuals. Again, the test should be used cautiously in patients with suspected adrenal insufficiency and should be preceded by a rapid ACTH stimulation test (see above). Metyrapone may also be given in does of 750 mg every 4 hours for 24 hours, with collection of urine for 17-hydroxycorticosteroid determination before, during, and for 24 hours after metyrapone. The urinary 17-hydroxycorticosteroid concentration doubles in healthy individuals. The test is cumbersome because of the difficulty in collecting 24-hour urine samples, and there is a danger of provoking symptomatic adrenal insufficiency because of the large metyrapone doses.

C. CRH Stimulation: Ovine CRH has been administered intravenously as a means of assessing ACTH secretory dynamics. In healthy subjects, CRH (1 μg/kg) provokes a peak ACTH response within 15 minutes and a peak cortisol response within 30–60 minutes. This dose may be associated with mild flushing, occasional shortness of breath, tachycardia, and hypotension. Patients with primary adrenal insufficiency have elevated basal ACTH levels and exaggerated responses to CRH. Secondary adrenal insufficiency results in an absent ACTH response to CRH in patients with pituitary corticotroph destruction; however, hypothalamic dysfunction causes a prolonged and augmented ACTH response to CRH with a delayed peak. This test may also be useful in the differential diagnosis of ACTH-dependent Cushing's syndrome (see below).

ACTH Hypersecretion

ACTH hypersecretion is manifested by adrenocortical hyperfunction (Cushing's syndrome). The evaluation of ACTH excess relies upon dexamethasone suppression of plasma cortisol and urine steroids. Basal urine free cortisol and plasma ACTH determinations are also helpful. The diagnosis and differential diagnosis of ACTH hypersecrction are outlined in a later section on Cushing's disease and also in Chapter 12.

EVALUATION OF GROWTH HORMONE

The evaluation of GH secretory reserve is important in the assessment of children with short stature and in adults with suspected hypopituitarism. Because basal levels of GH are usually low and do not distinguish between normal and GH-deficient conditions, it is necessary to perform provocative tests.

Insulin-Induced Hypoglycemia

The most reliable stimulus of GH secretion is insulin-induced hypoglycemia. In normal individuals, GH levels will increase to more than 10 ng/mL (465 pmol/L) after adequate hypoglycemia is achieved. Since 10–20% of normal individuals fail to respond to hypoglycemia, other stimulatory tests may be necessary.

Tests with Levodopa, Arginine, & Other Stimuli

GH will also rise after oral administration of 500 mg of levodopa, a precursor of dopamine and norepinephrine that readily crosses the blood-brain barrier. About 80% of healthy subjects have a GH response greater than 6 ng/mL (279 pmol/L), and the mean maximal response is 28 ng/mL (1302 pmol/L). This test is safer than insulin-induced hypoglycemia in older patients. An infusion of arginine (0.5 g/kg to a maximum of 30 g) will raise GH in 70% of healthy individuals. Pretreatment with estrogen will enhance this response in many of the nonresponders, most of whom are men. Other stimuli, such as propranolol and glucagon, have also been utilized in considering GH secretory capacity.

GRH Test

Both forms of human pancreatic GRH (GRH-40 and GRH-44) have been used investigationally to evaluate GH secretory capacity. A dose of GRH (1 μg/kg) promptly stimulates GH; the mean peak is 10–15 ng/mL (465–697 pmol/L) at 30–60 minutes in healthy subjects. There is usually a small increase in somatomedin-C levels 24 hours after the administration of GRH. This test may be helpful in some patients in differentiating hypothalamic and pituitary causes of GH deficiency.

Exercise Test

In children with possible GH deficiency, an exercise test requiring 15 minutes of rapid stair-climbing is a convenient way to assess GH secretion. Hypogonadal or prepubertal children are usually pretreated for 3 days with estrogen, and an increment of greater than 5 ng/mL (232 pmol/L) constitutes a normal response.

GH Hypersecretion

The evaluation of GH hypersecretion is discussed in the section on acromegaly and is most conveniently assessed by suppression testing with oral glucose.

EVALUATION OF PROLACTIN

PRL secretion by the pituitary is the most resistant to local damage, and demonstration of decreased PRL secretory reserve indicates severe intrinsic pituitary disease. The evaluation of PRL secretion must also rely upon provocative testing, since basal PRL levels in healthy individuals may be at the lower limits of assay detectability.

Prolactin Reserve

The administration of TRH (500 μg intravenously) is the simplest and most reliable means of assessing PRL reserve. Although the response of PRL to TRH varies somewhat according to sex and age (Table 6–5), PRL levels usually increase 2-fold 15–30 minutes after TRH administration. In addition, insulin-induced hypoglycemia will evoke a stress-related increase in PRL.

Table 6–5. Normal responses to TSH and prolactin to TRH (500 μg)[1]

	TSH (μU/mL) (mU/L)	
Maximum Δ TSH		
Women and men age < 40	≥ 6	≥ 6
Men age 40–79	≥ 2	≥ 2
Time of maximum Δ TSH (min)	≤45	
	Prolactin (ng/mL) (pmol/L)	
Basal, men and women	<15 (<681)	
Maximum Δ prolactin		
Men age 20–39	15–40	(681–1818)
Men age 40–59	10–50	(454–2272)
Men age 60–79	5–90	(227–4090)
Women age 20–39	30–120	(1363–5454)
Women age 40–59	20–120	(909–5454)
Women age 60–79	10–100	(454–4545)

[1] Reproduced, with permission, from Snyder PJ et al: Diagnostic value of thyrotrophin-releasing hormone in pituitary and hypothalamic diseases: Assessment of thyrotrophin and prolactin secretion in 100 patients. *Ann Intern Med* 1974;**81**:751.

PRL Hypersecretion

PRL hypersecretion is a common endocrine problem, and differential diagnosis is often difficult. Clinical evaluation of hyperprolactinemia is discussed in the section on prolactinomas.

EVALUATION OF TSH

Basal Measurements

The laboratory evaluation of TSH secretory reserve begins with an assessment of target gland secretion; thyroid function tests (T_4RIA, T_3RIA, free thyroxine index [FT_4I]) should be performed. Normal thyroid function studies in a clinically euthyroid patient indicate adequate TSH secretion, and no further studies are warranted. Laboratory evidence of hypothyroidism requires a TSH level, and with primary thyroid gland failure, the TSH level will be elevated. Low or normal TSH suggests hypothalamic-pituitary dysfunction.

TRH Test

The introduction of synthetic TRH (protirelin) has made it possible to evaluate the complete hypothalamic-pituitary-thyroid axis. The TRH test was useful for the diagnosis of hyperthyroidism; however, the supersensitive TSH assay can distinguish hyperthyroidism from euthyroidism in most patients, so the TRH response test is now rarely indicated for this purpose (see Chapter 10). However, the TRH test may help to differentiate pituitary from hypothalamic disease. In healthy subjects, protirelin (500 μg intravenously) produces an increase of TSH of at least 6 μU/mL (6 mU/L) within 15–30 minutes (Table 6–5). In patients with primary hypothyroidism, an exaggerated TSH response to protirelin is observed; however, this test is helpful only in those few patients with primary hypothyroidism who have normal basal TSH levels. An impaired or absent TSH response in hypothyroid patients implicates hypothalamic-pituitary failure. Patients with hypothalamic disease often show a delayed TSH response (60–120 minutes) to TRH (see Fig 10–16) and, less commonly, an exaggerated TSH increase. Unlike gonadotropic function, prolonged TRH deficiency does not impair TSH responsiveness. An intrinsic pituitary disorder characteristically results in a subnormal or absent TSH response to TRH; however, many patients with hypothyroidism and pituitary disease have normal response to TRH, or responses that resemble hypothalamic dysfunction. Accordingly, the TRH test is not always a reliable way to differentiate pituitary from hypothalamic disease.

Responsiveness to TRH is often impaired in patients with hypothalamic pituitary disease (eg, acromegaly, Cushing's syndrome) who are euthyroid. Since GH or cortisol excess may decrease the TSH response to TRH, an absent response does not always indicate destruction of thyrotrophs. (See also Chapter 10.)

EVALUATION OF LH & FSH

Testosterone & Estrogen Levels

The evaluation of gonadotropin function also requires assessment of target gland secretory function, and measurement of gonadal steroids (testosterone in men, estradiol in women) is useful in the diagnosis of hypogonadism. In women, the presence of regular menstrual cycles is strong evidence that the hypothalamic-pituitary-gonadal axis is intact. Estradiol levels rarely fall below 50 pg/mL (184 pmol/L), even during the early follicular phase. A level of less than 30 pg/mL (110 pmol/L) in the presence of oligomenorrhea or amenorrhea is indicative of gonadal failure. In men, serum testosterone (normal range, 3–9 ng/mL) (10–31 nmol/L) is a sensitive index of gonadal function.

LH & FSH Levels

In the presence of gonadal insufficiency, high LH and FSH levels are a sign of primary gonadal disease; low or normal LH and FSH suggest hypothalamic-pituitary dysfunction (hypogonadotropic hypogonadism).

GnRH Test

LH and FSH secretory reserves may be assessed with the use of synthetic GnRH (gonadorelin, Factrel). Administration of GnRH (100 μg intravenously) causes a prompt increase in plasma LH and a lesser and slower increase in FSH (for normal responses, see Table 6–4). The LH response to GnRH is lowest during the follicular phase and greatest during the ovulatory surge. Normal subjects may have no FSH response to GnRH. On the other hand, in prepubertal children and in some patients with hyperprolactinemia, the FSH response is greater than that of LH.

A single GnRH test does not distinguish hypothalamic from pituitary disease in patients with hypogonadotropic hypogonadism. Patients with disturbances of the hypothalamus and pituitary may have an absent, normal, or exaggerated gonadotropin response to GnRH. Hypothalamic disease with long-standing GnRH deficiency results in an absent LH response to GnRH, but normal responsiveness may be restored with more prolonged and intermittent stimulation. Such a return of responsiveness provides evidence for intact pituitary gonadotrophs.

Clomiphene Test

The hypothalamic-pituitary-gonadal axis can also be assessed by administering clomiphene citrate, an antiestrogen that blocks estrogen receptors, causing a state of functional estrogen deficiency resulting in GnRH and gonadotropin release. The occurrence of a normal menstrual period approximately 12 days after administration of the drug or evidence of ovulation by basal body temperature constitutes a normal response. Failure of LH levels to increase after 5–10 days of clomiphene in a patient with a normal GnRH test suggests hypothalamic disease.

PROBLEMS IN EVALUATION OF THE HYPOTHALAMIC-PITUITARY AXIS

Several metabolic abnormalities must be taken into account when assessing the hypothalamic-pituitary axis. This section briefly outlines some of the disorders that may cause confusion and lead to misinterpretation of pituitary function tests. The effects of drugs are described in the next section.

Obesity

GH dynamics are impaired in many obese patients; all provocative stimuli, including insulin-induced hypoglycemia, arginine, levodopa, and glucagon plus propranolol, often fail to provoke GH secretion. The GH response to GRH is also impaired in obesity, but it significantly improves with weight loss. Obesity may increase urinary 17-hydroxycorticosteroid levels and the cortisol secretory rate, but plasma cortisol demonstrates normal diurnal variation and responds to hypoglycemia. The cortisol response to CRH is also blunted in obesity.

Diabetes Mellitus

Although glucose normally suppresses GH secretion, most type I diabetic individuals have normal or elevated GH levels that often do not rise in response to hypoglycemia or arginine. Levodopa will increase GH in some diabetic patients, and even a dopamine infusion (which produces no GH change in nondiabetic subjects, since it does not cross the blood-brain barrier) will stimulate GH in diabetic patients. Despite the increased GH secretion in patients with inadequately controlled diabetes, the GH response to GRH in insulin-dependent diabetic patients is similar to that of nondiabetic subjects.

Uremia

Basal levels of GH, PRL, LH, FSH, TSH, and free cortisol tend to be elevated, for the most part owing to prolongation of their plasma half-life. GH may paradoxically increase following glucose administration and is often hyperresponsive to a hypoglycemic stimulus. Although the administration of TRH (protirelin) has no effect on GH secretion in healthy subjects, the drug may increase GH in patients with chronic renal failure. The response of PRL to TRH is blunted and prolonged. Gonadotropin response to synthetic GnRH usually remains intact. Dexamethasone suppression of cortisol may be impaired.

Starvation/Anorexia Nervosa

GH secretion increases with fasting and malnutrition, and such conditions may cause a paradoxical increase in GH following glucose administration. Severe starvation, such as occurs in patients with anorexia

nervosa, may result in low levels of gonadal steroids. LH and FSH responses to GnRH may be intact despite a state of functional hypogonadotropic hypogonadism. Cortisol levels may be increased and fail to suppress adequately with dexamethasone. PRL and TSH dynamics are usually normal despite a marked decrease in circulating total thyroid hormones (see Chapter 10).

Depression

Depression may alter the ability of dexamethasone to suppress plasma cortisol and may elevate cortisol secretion; the response to insulin-induced hypoglycemia usually remains intact. The ACTH response to CRH is blunted in endogenous depression. Some depressed patients also have abnormal GH dynamics: TRH may increase GH, and hypoglycemia or levodopa may fail to increase GH. These patients may also show blunted TSH responses to TRH.

EFFECTS OF PHARMACOLOGIC AGENTS ON HYPOTHALAMIC-PITUITARY FUNCTION

Glucocorticoid excess impairs the GH response to hypoglycemia, the TSH response to TRH, and the LH response to GnRH. Estrogens tend to augment GH dynamics as well as the PRL and TSH response to TRH. Estrogens increase plasma cortisol secondary to a rise in corticosteroid-binding globulin and may result in inadequate suppression with dexamethasone. Estrogens may also produce a subnormal response to metyrapone testing by accelerating the metabolism of metyrapone.

Phenytoin enhances the metabolism of metyrapone and dexamethasone, making studies with these agents difficult to interpret. Phenothiazines may blunt the GH response to hypoglycemia and levodopa and frequently cause hyperprolactinemia. The many other pharmacologic agents that increase PRL secretion are listed in Table 6–3.

Narcotics, including heroin, morphine, and methadone, may all raise PRL levels and suppress GH and cortisol response to hypoglycemia.

In chronic alcoholics, alcohol excess or withdrawal may increase cortisol levels and cause inadequate dexamethasone suppression and an impaired cortisol increase after hypoglycemia.

Many drugs interfere with urine steroid collection (17-hydroxycorticosteroids and 17-ketosteroids), but since these measurements are no longer essential, such problems can be avoided.

ENDOCRINE TESTS OF HYPOTHALAMIC-PITUITARY FUNCTION

The methods for performing endocrine tests and the normal responses are described below. The indications for and the clinical utility of these procedures are described in the preceding section and will be mentioned again in the section on pituitary and hypothalamic disorders. Some of these procedures may be performed simultaneously; eg, the administration of insulin, TRH, and GnRH provides combined stimulation of the major anterior pituitary hormones. Alternatively, the rapid ACTH stimulation test may be combined with TRH and GnRH stimulation. When performed simultaneously, the methods, doses, sampling times, and interpretation of the various hormonal responses are identical with those described below for the individual procedures. The combined use of all the hypothalamic releasing factors (TRH, GnRH, CRH, and GRH) during a single test is a useful way to assess the integrity of anterior pituitary function.

Rapid ACTH Stimulation Test (Cortrosyn Test)

Method: Administer synthetic $ACTH_{1-24}$ (cosyntropin; Cortrosyn), 250 μg intravenously or intramuscularly.

Sample collection: Obtain samples for plasma cortisol at 0 and 30 minutes or at 0 and 60 minutes.

Possible side effects; contraindications: Rare allergic reactions have been reported.

Interpretation: A normal response is an increment in plasma cortisol of 7 μg/dL (0.19 μmol/L) and a peak level greater than 18 μg/dL (0.49 μmol/L).

Insulin Hypoglycemia Test

Method: Give nothing by mouth after midnight. Start an intravenous infusion with normal saline solution. Regular insulin is given intravenously in a dose sufficient to cause adequate hypoglycemia (blood glucose < 40 mg/dL). The dose is 0.1–0.15 unit/kg (healthy subjects); 0.2–0.3 unit/kg (obese subjects or those with Cushing's syndrome or acromegaly); 0.05 unit/kg (patients with suspected hypopituitarism).

Sample collection: Collect blood for glucose determinations every 15 minutes during the study. Samples of GH and cortisol are obtained at 0, 30, 45, 60, 75, and 90 minutes.

Possible side effects; contraindications: A physician must be in attendance. Symptomatic hypoglycemia (diaphoresis, headache, tachycardia, weakness) is necessary for adequate stimulation and occurs 20–35 minutes after insulin is administered in most patients. If severe central nervous system signs or symptoms occur, intravenous glucose (25–50 mL of 50% glucose) should be given immediately; otherwise, the test can be terminated with a meal or oral glucose. This test is contraindicated in the elderly or in patients with cardiovascular or cerebrovascular disease and seizure disorders.

Interpretation: Symptomatic hypoglycemia and a fall in blood glucose to less than 40 mg/dL (2.2 mmol/L) will increase GH to a maximal level greater than 10 ng/mL (454 pmol/L); some investigators regard an increment of 6 ng/mL (279 pmol/L) as normal. Plasma cortisol should increase to a peak level of at least 18 μg/dL (0.49 μmol/L).

Metyrapone Tests

Method:

Overnight test: Metyrapone is given orally between 11 and 12 PM with a snack to minimize gastrointestinal discomfort. The dose is 2 g for patients weighing less than 70 kg; 2.5 g for patients weighing 79–90 kg; and 3 g for patients weighing over 90 kg.

Three-day test: Twenty-four-hour urine collections are made for 3 consecutive days, and metyrapone, 750 mg, is given every 4 hours for 6 doses on the second day.

Sample Collection:

Overnight test: Blood for plasma 11-deoxycortisol and cortisol determinations is obtained at 8 AM the morning after metyrapone is given.

Three-day test: The 3 consecutive 24-hour urine samples are analyzed for 17-hydroxycorticosteroids and creatinine determinations.

Possible side effects; contraindications: Gastrointestinal upset may occur. Adrenal insufficiency may occur. Metyrapone should not be used in sick patients or those in whom primary adrenal insufficiency is suspected.

Interpretation:

Overnight test: Serum 11-deoxycortisol should increase to greater than 7 μg/dL (0.19 μmol/L). Cortisol should be less than 10 μg/dL (0.28 μmol/L) in order to ensure adequate inhibition of 11β-hydroxylation.

Three-day test: Urine 17-hydroxycorticosteroids should double on day 2 or 3.

Levodopa Test

Method: The patient should be fasting and at bed rest after midnight. Levodopa, 500 mg, is given by mouth.

Sample collection: Blood samples for plasma GH determinations are obtained at 0, 30, and 60 minutes.

Possible side effects; contraindications: Nausea and vomiting may occur 45–60 minutes after levodopa is given. This test is safer than the insulin hypoglycemia test in older patients.

Interpretation: A normal response is a maximal level of GH greater than 6 ng/mL (279 pmol/L); however, the peak response is usually more than 20 ng/mL (930 pmol/L).

Arginine Infusion Test

Method: The patient should be fasting after midnight. Give arginine hydrochloride, 0.5 g/kg intravenously, up to a maximum of 30 g over 30 minutes. Pretreatment with estrogen in postmenopausal women and in men can also be done.

Sample collection: Blood for plasma GH determinations is collected at 0, 30, 60, 90, and 120 minutes. Arginine infusion also stimulates insulin and glucagon.

Possible side effects; contraindications: Nausea and vomiting may occur. This test is contraindicated in patients with severe liver disease, renal disease, or acidosis.

Interpretation: The response is greater in women than in men. The lower limit of normal for the peak GH response is 6 ng/mL (279 pmol/L) in non-estrogen-treated patients and 10 ng/mL (465 pmol/L) in estrogen-treated patients and premenopausal women.

Glucose-Growth Hormone Suppression Test

Method: The patient should be fasting after midnight. Give glucose, 75–100 g orally.

Sample collection: GH and glucose should be determined at 0, 30, and 60 minutes after glucose administration.

Possible side effects; contraindications: Patients may complain of nausea after the large glucose load.

Interpretation: GH levels are suppressed to less than 5 ng/mL (232 pmol/L) in healthy subjects. Failure of adequate suppression or a paradoxical rise may be seen in acromegaly, starvation, protein-calorie malnutrition, and anorexia nervosa.

TRH Test

Method: Fasting is not required, but since nausea may occur, it is preferred. Give protirelin, 500 μg intravenously over 15–30 seconds. The patient should be kept supine, since slight hypertension or hypotension may occur. Protirelin (Thypinone, Relefact TRH) is supplied in vials of 500 μg, although 400 μg will evoke normal responses.

Sample collection: Blood for determination of plasma TSH, PRL, or GH (in the case of suspected acromegaly) is obtained at 0, 30, and 60 minutes; a 90-minute sample for TSH may be necessary in cases of suspected tertiary hypothyroidism. An abbreviated test utilizes samples taken at 0 and 30 minutes only.

Possible side effects; contraindications: No serious complications have been reported. Most patients complain of a sensation of urinary urgency and a metallic taste in the mouth; other symptoms include flushing, palpitations, and nausea. These symptoms occur within 1–2 minutes of the injection and last 5 minutes at most.

Interpretation: Normal TSH and PRL responses to TRH are outlined in Table 6–5. GH should not increase in healthy subjects.

GnRH Test

Method: The patient should be at rest but need not be fasting. Give GnRH (gonadorelin), 100 μg intravenously, over 15 seconds.

Sample collection: Blood samples for LH and FSH determinations are taken at 0, 30, and 60 minutes. Since the FSH response is somewhat delayed, a 90-minute specimen may be necessary.

Possible side effects; contraindications: Side effects are rare, and no contraindications have been found.

Interpretation: This response is dependent on sex and time of the menstrual cycle. Table 6–4 illustrates the mean maximal change in LH and FSH after GnRH administration. An increase of LH of 10–20 mIU/mL (10–20 IU/L) is considered to be normal; FSH usually responds more slowly and less markedly. FSH may not increase even in healthy subjects.

Clomiphene Test

Method: Clomiphene is administered orally. For women, give 100 mg daily for 5 days (being on day 5 of the cycle if the patient is menstruating); for men, give 100 mg daily for 7–10 days.

Sample collection: Blood for LH and FSH determinations is drawn before and after clomiphene is given.

Possible side effects; contraindications: This drug may, of course, stimulate ovulation, and women should be advised accordingly.

Interpretation: In women, LH and FSH levels peak on the fifth day to a level above the normal range. After the fifth day, LH and FSH levels decline. In men, LH should double after 1 week; FSH will also increase, but to a lesser extent. (See Table 6–4 for normal values.)

CRH Test

Method: CRH (1μg/kg) is given intravenously as a bolus injection.

Sample collection: Blood samples for ACTH and cortisol are taken at 0, 15, 30, and 60 minutes.

Possible side effects; contraindications: Flushing often occurs. Transient tachycardia and hypotension have also been reported.

Interpretation: The ACTH response is dependent on the assay utilized and occurs 15 minutes after CRH is administered. The peak cortisol response occurs at 30–60 minutes and is usually greater than 10 μg/dL (0.28 μmol/L).

GRH Test

Method: GRH (1 μg/kg) is given intravenously as a bolus injection.

Sample collection: Blood samples for GH are drawn at 0, 30, and 60 minutes.

Possible side effects; contraindications: Mild flushing and a metallic taste or smell occur in a few patients.

Interpretation: The range of normal responses is wide. Most patients have a peak GH response of greater than 10 ng/mL (465 pmol/L) at 30–60 minutes.

NEURORADIOLOGIC EVALUATION OF THE SELLA TURCICA

Intrasellar or parasellar disease is usually suspected on clinical grounds. Thus, symptoms of pituitary hormone excess or deficiency, headache, or visual disturbance may lead the clinician to consider a hypothalamic-pituitary disorder. Although accurate neuroradiologic assessment of the sella turcica is essential in confirming the existence and defining the extent of hypothalamic-pituitary lesions, the diagnosis of such lesions should be primarily endocrinologic and based on a thorough clinical and biochemical evaluation of pituitary function. This is because variability of sellar anatomy in the normal population may lead to false-positive interpretations. Furthermore, patients with pituitary microadenomas may have normal neuroradiologic studies. Roentgenographic studies of the sella must be interpreted in light of the fact that 10–20% of the general population harbor nonfunctional and asymptomatic pituitary microadenomas.

This section describes current neuroradiologic procedures; however, the development of magnetic resonance imaging (MRI) and high-resolution computed tomography with thin-slice (1.5-mm collimation) techniques have superseded other neuroradiologic tests in evaluation of the sella turcica.

Plain Films of the Sella Turcica

A. Radiologic Anatomy: The initial and most important radiographic examination of the sella is simply a coned-down lateral projection accompanied by a Caldwell frontal projection. These views provide the clinician with an impression of the size and shape of the sella. The tuberculum sellae, the anterior clinoid processes, the sphenoid sinus, the floor of the dorsum sellae, and the posterior clinoid processes can be easily identified (Fig 6–10). Although most neuroradiologists and endocrinologists rely on their overall impression of the sella, specific measurements can be made, and normal criteria have been established. The anteroposterior diameter (maximum distance from anterior concavity of the sella to the anterior rim of the dorsum) varies from 5 to 16 mm, with an average of 10 mm; the depth, measured as the greatest distance from the floor to a perpendicular line drawn between

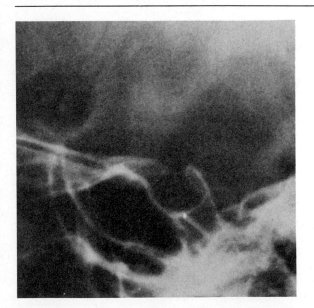
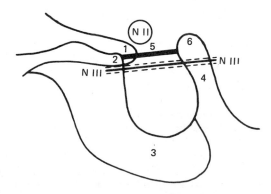

Figure 6–10. *Left:* Lateral radiograph of the normal sella turcica. (Reproduced, with permission, from Martin JB, Reichlin S, Brown GM: *Clinical Neuroendocrinology.* Davis, 1977.) *Right:* Diagram of the radiologic landmarks and relationships of the sella turcica and pituitary: (1) anterior clinoid process; (2) tuberculum sellae; (3) sphenoid sinus; (4) dorsum sellae; (5) diaphragma sellae; (6) posterior clinoid process; N II, optic chiasm; N III, oculomotor nerve lying lateral to the sella turcica. (Reproduced, with permission, from Bloch HJ, Joplin GF: Some aspects of the radiological anatomy of the pituitary gland and its relationship to surrounding structures. *Br J Radiol* 1959;**32**:527.)

the tuberculum sellae and the top of the dorsum sellae, has an upper limit of normal of 13 mm; the width (determined from the frontal projection) is normally 10–15 mm.

The volume of the sella can be calculated using the DiChiro formula (anteroposterior diameter $\times$ depth $\times$ width $\div$ 2). The mean volume of the normal sella is 600 mm^3; a volume that exceeds 1100 mm^3 is considered abnormal.

B. Variability of Sellar Shape: The normal sella may be oval, round, or flat. Pituitary tumors may produce focal erosion and distortion of the sella without increasing its volume; however, because of the variety of shapes seen in patients without clinical pituitary disease, such focal changes must be interpreted cautiously. Pituitary adenomas, which are predominantly lateral, may cause depression and expansion of only one side of the sellar floor, leading to a "double floor" appearance of the sella turcica on lateral projection.

C. Calcification: Calcification may also occur in the parasellar region. In older persons, the internal carotid artery may calcify, causing an arch of calcification in the center of the sella. Bridging calcification between the anterior and posterior clinoids occasionally occurs as a normal variant. Tumors such as craniopharyngiomas (70%) and parasellar meningiomas (30%) may calcify. In addition, pituitary adenomas that have undergone hemorrhagic necrosis may calcify, resulting in a "pituitary stone."

D. Tumors: Small pituitary tumors (microadenomas) do not increase the volume of the sella, and the size of the sella does not always correlate well with the pituitary size (eg, empty sella). Consequently, normal plain x-rays of the sella do not, by any means, prove or exclude a pituitary disorder. Nonetheless, the finding of an enlarged sella turcica on plain x-rays is a strong indication for further clinical investigation. The differential diagnosis of an enlarged sella turcica is discussed below.

High-Resolution Computed Tomography (Thin-Slice Technique)

The availability of high-resolution computed tomography with a thin-slice technique (1.5-mm collimation) using intravenous contrast media has altered the approach to intrasellar and parasellar disease. Invasive procedures such as arteriography or pneumoencephalography now have few, if any, applications in the diagnosis of pituitary disease. CT scanning permits precise visualization of the pituitary gland itself and can define small hypothalamic and pituitary lesions. In addition, nonosseous structures such as the pituitary stalk can be identified on CT scans reformatted in coronal and sagittal images (Fig 6–11).

A. Microadenomas: The superior margin of the normal pituitary gland is flat or concave, and the height of the gland ranges from 3 to 8 mm. The pituitary gland may occasionally be 10–12 mm in height in healthy menstruating young women. The presence of a convex superior margin with increased height of the gland is one of 2 major criteria used to diagnose pituitary microadenomas. The second finding is a focal alteration in the enhancement of the gland with intravenous contrast. Most pituitary adenomas appear as "low-density" areas when compared with the surrounding normal pituitary tissue; less commonly, they are contrast-enhancing.

B. Other Uses and Cautions: High-resolution CT scanning is also a valuable tool in the diagnosis of empty sella syndrome, determination of extrasellar extension of pituitary adenomas, and diagnosis of hypothalamic tumors and other parasellar lesions.

High-resolution CT scans must be interpreted with caution, since nonhomogeneous enhancement of the gland is demonstrated in almost 20% of patients who have had incidental high-resolution scans but no clinical pituitary disease. These abnormalities may, of course, represent the clinically insignificant pituitary abnormalities present in 15–20% of the general population, and they may also be due to small intrapituitary cysts, which usually occur in the pars intermedia. Artifacts within the sella turcica associated with the bones of the skull base may also result in misinterpretation of CT scans. Finally, the authors have seen many patients with pituitary microadenomas who have had normal high-resolution CT scans. Therefore, despite increased accuracy of neuroradiologic diagnosis, the presence or absence of a small pituitary tumor and the decision concerning its treatment must be based on the entire clinical picture.

Magnetic Resonance Imaging (MRI)

Magnetic resonance imaging will supersede the CT scan for diagnosis of hypothalamic-pituitary lesions, since it better defines the suprasellar cistern, cavernous sinuses, pituitary stalk, and optic chiasm. Imaging is performed in sagittal and coronal planes at 1.5–2 mm intervals. With this technique, lesions as small as 3–5 mm can be accurately visualized; with larger tumors, lateral or suprasellar extension can be easily documented. In addition, distortion of the optic nerves, optic chiasm, and pituitary stalk can be defined well. The use of the heavy-metal contrast agent gadolinium allows even more precise differentiation of the adenoma from normal anterior pituitary tissue and other adjacent structures.

NEURO-OPHTHALMOLOGIC EVALUATION

Although most patients with pituitary adenomas currently present with endocrine abnormalities, visual disturbances are a common feature of large pituitary tumors with suprasellar extension because of the close proximity of the pituitary to the optic chiasm, optic

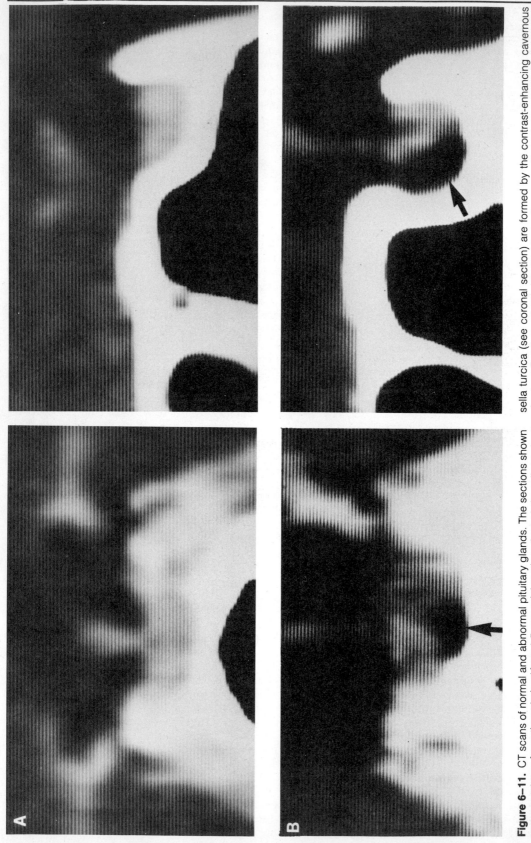

Figure 6–11. CT scans of normal and abnormal pituitary glands. The sections shown are computer re-formations derived from 1.5-mm axial sections through the sella turcica. Coronal re-formations are shown on the left and sagittal ones on the right. *A:* Normal pituitary gland. The upper border is flat; the pituitary stalk (seen on the coronal section) is midline; and the gland is relatively homogeneous in density. The lateral margins of the sella turcica (see coronal section) are formed by the contrast-enhancing cavernous sinuses. *B:* In a patient with Cushing's disease, a 3- to 4-mm pituitary adenoma is visualized as a low-density lesion in the anterior inferior portion of the anterior lobe (arrows).

nerves, and optic tracts. Thus, the evaluation of any patient with a known pituitary tumor or an enlarged sella should include careful visual examination. Serial visual field testing is also a valuable method of following the clinical progression of a pituitary lesion.

Visual Field Examination

Visual field examination can be performed at the bedside by confrontation or in the neuro-ophthalmology laboratory with more precise equipment such as the Goldmann or Tubinger perimeter. The use of finger movements is not an adequate method for bedside evaluation. The employment of a small (2- to 3-mm diameter) object—preferably red—affords a more sensitive index of loss of vision. Visual field testing with the Goldmann perimeter may identify a compressive lesion earlier than confrontation. In chiasmal lesions, the most common among pituitary tumors, a central field (within 30 degrees of fixation) may be affected earlier than peripheral fields.

Lateral Tumor Extension

In addition to causing visual field defects, large pituitary lesions may occasionally extend laterally into the cavernous sinus, compromising the function of the third, fourth, or sixth cranial nerve, leading to diplopia.

PITUITARY & HYPOTHALAMIC DISORDERS

Hypothalamic-pituitary lesions present with a variety of manifestations, including pituitary hormone hypersecretion and hyposecretion, sellar enlargement, and visual loss. The approach to evaluation should be designed to ensure early diagnosis at a stage when the lesions are amenable to therapy. All patients with hypothalamic-pituitary lesions should undergo a complete endocrine evaluation.

Etiology & Early Manifestations

In adults, the commonest cause of hypothalamic-pituitary dysfunction is a pituitary adenoma, of which the great majority are hypersecreting. Thus, the earliest symptoms of such tumors are due to endocrinologic abnormalities, and these precede sellar enlargement and local manifestations such as headache and visual loss, which are late manifestations seen only in patients with larger tumors or suprasellar extension.

In children, pituitary adenomas are uncommon; the most frequent structural lesions causing hypothalamic-pituitary dysfunction are craniopharyngiomas and other hypothalamic tumors. These also usually manifest as endocrine disturbances (low GH levels, delayed puberty, diabetes insipidus) prior to the development of headache, visual loss, or other central nervous system symptoms.

Common & Later Manifestations

A. Pituitary Hypersecretion: PRL is the hormone most commonly secreted in excess amounts by pituitary adenomas, and it is usually elevated in patients with hypothalamic disorders as well. Thus, PRL measurement is essential in evaluating patients with suspected pituitary disorders, and it should be obtained in patients presenting with galactorrhea, gonadal dysfunction, secondary gonadotropin deficiency, or enlargement of the sella turcica. Hypersecretion of GH or ACTH leads to the more characteristic syndromes of acromegaly and Cushing's disease (see below).

B. Pituitary Insufficiency: Although panhypopituitarism is a classic manifestation of pituitary adenomas, it is present in less than 20% of patients in current large series because of earlier diagnosis of these lesions.

At present, the earliest clinical manifestation of a pituitary adenoma in adults is hypogonadism secondary to elevated levels of PRL, GH, or ACTH and cortisol rather than to destruction of anterior pituitary tissue. Thus, patients with hypogonadism should first be screened with FSH/LH measurements to exclude primary gonadal failure (elevated FSH/LH) and those with hypogonadotropic hypogonadism should have serum PRL levels measured and be examined for clinical evidence of GH or ACTH and cortisol excess.

In children, short stature is the most frequent clinical presentation of hypothalamic-pituitary dysfunction; in these patients, GH deficiency should be considered.

TSH or ACTH deficiency is relatively unusual in current series of patients and usually indicates panhypopituitarism. Thus, in patients with hypothyroidism or hypoadrenalism, primary disorders of the thyroid or adrenal are excluded by the absence of elevated TSH or ACTH levels, and the patient should then undergo a complete assessment of pituitary function and neuroradiologic studies, since panhypopituitarism and large pituitary tumors are common in this setting. PRL measurement is again essential, since prolactinomas are the most frequent abnormalities in adults.

C. Enlarged Sella Turcica: Patients may present with enlargement of the sella turcica, which may be noted on radiographs performed for head trauma or on sinus series. These patients usually have either a pituitary adenoma or empty sella syndrome. Evaluation should include clinical assessment of pituitary dysfunction and measurements of PRL and thyroid and adrenal function. If pituitary function is normal, empty sella syndrome is likely; the diagnosis can be confirmed by MRI or CT scanning. Patients with clinical or laboratory evidence of pituitary dysfunction usually have a pituitary adenoma.

D. Visual Field Defects: Patients presenting with unexplained visual field defects or visual loss should be considered to have a pituitary or hypothalamic disorder until proved otherwise. The initial step in evaluation should be by MRI or CT scanning, which will reveal the tumor if one is present. These patients should also have PRL measurements and be assessed for anterior pituitary insufficiency, which is especially common with large pituitary adenomas.

E. Diabetes Insipidus: Diabetes insipidus is a common manifestation of hypothalamic lesions but is rare in primary pituitary lesions. The diagnosis is established as described in Chapter 9. In addition, all patients should undergo radiologic evaluation and assessment of anterior pituitary function.

EMPTY SELLA SYNDROME

Etiology & Incidence

The empty sella syndrome occurs when the subarachnoid space extends into the sella turcica, partially filling it with cerebrospinal fluid. This process causes remodeling and enlargement of the sella turcica and flattening of the pituitary gland. An empty sella may occur as a primary event resulting from congenital incompetence of the diaphragma sellae (Fig 6–12) or as a secondary phenomenon after radiation therapy, surgery, or pituitary infarction.

Primary empty sella syndrome is common, with an incidence in autopsy series ranging from 5 to 23%. It is the most frequent cause of enlarged sella turcica. An empty sella is also commonly seen after pituitary surgery or radiation therapy and may also occur following postpartum pituitary infarction (Sheehan's syndrome). In addition, pituitary tumors may undergo subclinical hemorrhagic infarction and cause contraction of the overlying suprasellar cistern downward into the sella. This phenomenon has been described in both PRL-secreting and GH-secreting pituitary adenomas. Therefore, the presence of an empty sella does not exclude the possibility of a coexisting pituitary tumor.

Pathogenesis

The pathogenesis of primary empty sella syndrome is uncertain. It has been postulated that increased cerebrospinal fluid pressure leads to herniation of arachnoid through the diaphragma sellae. A mesenchymal defect may be present in some patients, resulting in hypoplasia of the sellar diaphragm. A kindred has been described in which both primary empty sella syndrome and Rieger's anomaly of the anterior chamber of the eye (a developmental abnormality of mesenchymal origin involving the iris) occurred in an autosomal dominant fashion.

Clinical Findings

A. Symptoms and Signs: Most patients are middle-aged obese women. Many have systemic hypertension; benign intracranial hypertension may also occur. Although 48% of patients complain of headache, this feature may have only initiated the evaluation (ie, skull x-rays), and its relationship with the empty sella is probably coincidental. Serious clinical manifestations are uncommon. Spontaneous cerebrospinal fluid rhinorrhea has been reported, and visual field impairment may rarely occur.

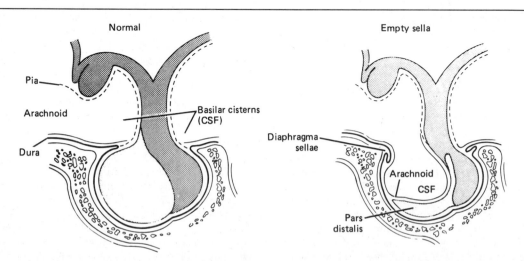

Figure 6–12. Representation of the normal relationship of the meninges to the pituitary gland (*left*) and the findings in the empty sella (*right*) as the arachnoid membrane herniates through the incompetent diaphragma sellae. (Reproduced, with permission, from Jordan RM, Kendall JW, Kerber CW: The primary empty sella syndrome: Analysis of the clinical characteristics, radiographic features, pituitary function, and cerebrospinal fluid adenohypophysial hormone concentrations. *Am J Med* 1977;**62**:569.)

B. Laboratory Findings: Tests of anterior pituitary function are almost always normal. This observation correlates well with histologic immunocytochemical studies of the pituitary gland in patients with the syndrome. Such studies have demonstrated that the remodeled pituitary gland contains adequate amounts of all 6 adenohypophyseal hormones. TSH, GH, and gonadotropin secretory reserves have rarely been reported to be impaired; however, pituitary hypofunction in such cases may result from subclinical pituitary ischemic damage followed by contraction of glandular tissue and a secondary empty sella.

Endocrine function studies should be performed to exclude pituitary hormone insufficiency or a hypersecretory pituitary adenoma.

Diagnosis

The diagnosis of primary empty sella syndrome can be confirmed by radiographic studies. Plain x-rays often show a symmetrically enlarged sella, but all degrees of sellar deformity have been seen. The plain x-ray cannot distinguish an empty sella from a pituitary adenoma. MRI or CT scanning provides a noninvasive means of establishing the presence of cerebrospinal fluid in the sellar contents.

HYPOTHALAMIC DYSFUNCTION

Hypothalamic tumors are the most common cause of hypothalamic dysfunction. Craniopharyngioma is the most common tumor in children, adolescents, and young adults. In older adults, primary central nervous system tumors and those arising from hypothalamic (epidermoid and dermoid tumors) and pineal structures (pinealomas) are more common. Other causes of hypothalamic-pituitary dysfunction are discussed below in the section on hypopituitarism.

Clinical Findings

A. Craniopharyngioma: The initial symptoms of craniopharyngioma in children and adolescents are predominantly endocrinologic; however, these manifestations are frequently unrecognized, and at diagnosis over 80% of patients have hypothalamic-pituitary endocrine deficiencies. These endocrine abnormalities may precede presenting symptoms by months or years; GH deficiency is most common, with about 50% of patients having growth retardation and approximately 70% decreased GH responses to stimulation at diagnosis. Gonadotropin deficiency leading to absent or arrested puberty is usual in older children and adolescents of pubertal age; TSH and ACTH deficiency is less common, and diabetes insipidus is present in about 15%.

Symptoms leading to the diagnosis are, unfortunately, frequently neurologic and due to the mass effect of the expanding tumor. Symptoms of increased intra-

cranial pressure such as headache and vomiting are present in about 42%; decreased visual acuity or visual field defects are the presenting symptoms in another 35%. Plain films of the skull reveal intrasellar or suprasellar calcification in 75% of these children. MRI or CT scans confirm the tumor in virtually all patients; in 95%, the tumor is suprasellar.

In adults, craniopharyngiomas have similar presentations; ie, the diagnosis is usually reached as a result of investigation of symptoms of increased intracranial pressure, headache, or visual loss. However, endocrine manifestations—especially hypogonadism, diabetes insipidus, or other deficiencies of anterior pituitary hormones—usually precede these late manifestations. Intrasellar or suprasellar calcification is less common in adults (for unknown reasons), but scans again readily demonstrate the tumors, which in adults are almost always both intrasellar and suprasellar.

B. Other Tumors: Other hypothalamic or pineal tumors and primary central nervous system tumors involving the hypothalamus have variable presentations in both children and adults. Thus, presentation is with headache, visual loss, symptoms of increased intracranial pressure, growth failure, various degrees of hypopituitarism, or diabetes insipidus. Endocrine deficiencies usually precede neurologic manifestations. Hypothalamic tumors in childhood may present with precocious puberty.

C. Other Manifestations of Hypothalamic Dysfunction: Lesions in the hypothalamus can cause many other abnormalities, including disorders of consciousness, behavior, thirst, appetite, and temperature regulation. These abnormalities are usually accompanied by symptoms of hypopituitarism and diabetes insipidus.

Somnolence can occur with hypothalamic lesions, as can a variety of changes in emotional behavior. Decreased or absent thirst may occur and predispose these patients to dehydration. When diminished thirst accompanies diabetes insipidus, fluid balance is difficult to control. Hypothalamic dysfunction may also cause increased thirst, leading to polydipsia and polyuria that may mimic diabetes insipidus. Obesity is common in patients with hypothalamic tumors because of hyperphagia, decreased satiety, and decreased activity. Anorexia and weight loss are unusual manifestations of these tumors.

Temperature regulation can also be disordered in these patients. Sustained or, less commonly, paroxysmal hyperthermia can occur following acute injury due to trauma, hemorrhage, or craniotomy. This problem usually lasts less than 2 weeks. Poikilothermia, the inability to adjust to changes in ambient temperature, can occur in patients with bilateral hypothalamic lesions. These patients most frequently exhibit hypothermia but can also develop hyperthermia during hot weather. A few patients manifest sustained hypothermia due to anterior hypothalamic lesions.

Diagnosis

Patients with suspected or proved hypothalamic tumors should have MRI or CT scans to determine the extent and nature of the tumor. Complete assessment of anterior pituitary function is necessary in these patients, since deficiencies are present in the great majority (see section on hypopituitarism below) and the evaluation will establish the requirements for replacement therapy. PRL levels should also be determined, since most hypothalamic lesions cause hyperprolactinemia either by hypothalamic injury or by damage to the pituitary stalk.

Treatment

Treatment depends upon the type of tumor. Since complete resection of craniopharyngioma is usually not feasible, this tumor is best managed by limited neurosurgical removal of accessible tumor and decompression of cysts, followed by conventional radiotherapy. Patients treated by this method have a recurrence rate of approximately 20%; when surgery alone is used, the recurrence rate approximates 80%.

Other hypothalamic tumors are also usually not surgically resectable. Therapy is usually primarily surgical to obtain a histologic diagnosis followed by conventional radiotherapy.

HYPOPITUITARISM

Hypopituitarism is usually a subtle clinical event with diverse causes. It is manifested by diminished or absent secretion of one or more pituitary hormones. The development of signs and symptoms is often slow and insidious, depending on the rate of onset and the magnitude of hypothalamic-pituitary damage—factors that are influenced by the underlying pathogenesis. Hypopituitarism is either a primary event caused by destruction of the anterior pituitary gland or a secondary phenomenon resulting from deficiency of hypothalamic stimulatory (or inhibitory) factors normally acting on the pituitary. Although provocative endocrine testing is essential in evaluating anterior pituitary gland function, it is not always possible (even with the use of hypothalamic releasing hormones) to distinguish between a pituitary and a hypothalamic lesion. Treatment and prognosis depend on the extent of hypofunction, the underlying cause, and the location of the lesion in the hypothalamic-pituitary axis.

Etiology

The etiologic considerations in hypopituitarism are diverse. As shown below and in Table 6–6, a helpful mnemonic device is the phrase "nine I's": Invasive, Infarction, Infiltrative, Injury, Immunologic, Iatrogenic, Infectious, Idiopathic, and Isolated. Most of these lesions may cause pituitary or hypothalamic failure (or both). Although it is not always possible to do so, establishing the precise cause of hypopitui-

Table 6–6. Hypopituitarism: Etiologic considerations. (The "nine I's.")

Invasive
 Large pituitary tumors
 Craniopharyngioma
 Metastatic tumors
 Primary central nervous system tumors (meningioma, chordoma, optic glioma; epidermoid, dermoid, pineal tumors)
 Carotid aneurysm
 Basal encephalocele
Infarction
 Postpartum necrosis (Sheehan's syndrome)
 Pituitary apoplexy
Infiltrative
 Sarcoidosis
 Hemochromatosis
 Histiocytosis X (Hand-Schüller-Christian disease, eosinophilic granuloma, Letterer-Siwe disease)
Injury
 Head trauma
 Child abuse
Immunologic
 Lymphocytic hypothysitis
Iatrogenic
 Surgery
 Radiation therapy
Infectious
 Mycoses, tuberculosis, syphilis
Idiopathic
 Familial
Isolated
 GH (dwarfism, emotional deprivation)
 LH, FSH (Kallmann's syndrome, weight loss, overtrained athletes, sickle cell anemia)
 TSH (chronic renal failure, pseudohypoparathyroidism)
 ACTH-LPH (lymphocytic hypophysitis, familial)
 PRL (pseudohypoparathyroidism)

tarism is helpful in determining treatment and prognosis.

A. Invasive: Space-occupying lesions cause hypopituitarism by destroying the pituitary gland or hypothalamic nuclei or by disrupting the hypothalamic-hypophyseal portal venous system. Large pituitary adenomas cause hypopituitarism by these mechanisms; however, small pituitary tumors—microadenomas (< 10 mm in diameter)—characteristically seen in the hypersecretory states (excess PRL, GH, ACTH) do not directly cause pituitary insufficiency. Thus, pituitary function may improve after the removal of large pituitary adenomas. Craniopharyngioma, the most common tumor of the hypothalamic-pituitary region in children, may impair pituitary function by its compressive effects. Primary central nervous system tumors, including meningioma, chordoma, optic glioma, epidermoid tumors, and dermoid tumors, may decrease hypothalamic-pituitary secretion by their mass effects. Metastatic lesions to this area are common (especially breast carcinoma) but rarely result in clinically obvious hypopituitarism. Anatomic malformations such as basal encephalocele and parasellar aneurysms cause hypothalamic-pituitary dysfunction and may enlarge the sella turcica and mimic pituitary tumors.

B. Infarction: Ischemic damage to the pituitary has long been recognized as a cause of hypopituitarism. In 1914, Simmonds reported pituitary necrosis in a woman with severe puerperal sepsis, and in 1937 Sheehan published his classic description of its occurrence following postpartum hemorrhage and vascular collapse. The mechanism for the ischemia in such cases is not certain. Hypotension along with vasospasm of the hypophyseal arteries is currently believed to compromise arterial perfusion of the anterior pituitary. During pregnancy, the pituitary gland may be more sensitive to hypoxemia because of its increased metabolic needs or more susceptible to vasoconstrictive influences because of the hyperestrogenic state. Some degree of hypopituitarism has been reported in 32% of women with severe postpartum hemorrhage. Other investigators have noted that the hypopituitarism does not always correlate with the degree of hemorrhage but that there is good correlation between the pituitary lesion and severe disturbances of the clotting mechanism (as in patients with placenta previa). Ischemic pituitary necrosis has also been reported to occur with greater frequency in patients with diabetes mellitus.

The extent of pituitary damage determines the rapidity of onset as well as the magnitude of pituitary hypofunction. The gland has a great secretory reserve, and more than 75% must be destroyed before clinical manifestations are evident. The initial clinical feature in postpartum necrosis may be failure to lactate after parturition; failure to resume normal menstrual periods is another clue to the diagnosis. However, the clinical features of hypopituitarism are often subtle, and years may pass before pituitary insufficiency is recognized following an ischemic insult.

Spontaneous hemorrhagic infarction of a pituitary tumor (pituitary apoplexy) frequently results in partial or total pituitary insufficiency. Pituitary apoplexy is often a fulminant clinical syndrome manifested by severe headache, visual impairment, ophthalmoplegias, meningismus, and an altered level of consciousness. Pituitary apoplexy is usually associated with a pituitary tumor; it may also be related to diabetes mellitus, radiotherapy, or open heart surgery. Acute pituitary failure with hypotension may result, and rapid mental deterioration, coma, and death may ensue. Emergency treatment with corticosteroids (see Chapter 12) and transsphenoidal decompression of the intrasellar contents may be lifesaving and may prevent permanent visual loss. Most patients who have survived pituitary apoplexy have developed multiple adenohypophyseal deficits, but infarction of the tumor in some patients may cure the hypersecretory pituitary adenoma and its accompanying endocrinopathy. Pituitary infarction may also be a subclinical event (silent pituitary apoplexy), resulting in improvement of pituitary hormone hypersecretion without impairing the secretion of other anterior pituitary hormones.

C. Infiltrative: Hypopituitarism may be the initial clinical manifestation of infiltrative disease processes such as sarcoidosis, hemochromatosis, and histiocytosis X.

1. Sarcoidosis—The most common intracranial sites of involvement of sarcoidosis are the hypothalamus and pituitary gland. At one time, the most common endocrine abnormality in patients with sarcoidosis was thought to be diabetes insipidus; however, many of these patients actually have centrally mediated disordered control of thirst that results in polydipsia and polyuria, which in some cases explains the abnormal water metabolism. Deficiencies of multiple anterior pituitary hormones have been well documented in sarcoidosis and are usually secondary to hypothalamic insufficiency. Granulomatous involvement of the hypothalamic-pituitary unit is occasionally extensive, resulting in visual impairment, and therefore may simulate the clinical presentation of a pituitary tumor.

2. Hemochromatosis—Hypopituitarism, particularly hypogonadotropic hypogonadism, is a prominent manifestation of iron storage disease—either idiopathic hemochromatosis or transfusional iron overload. Hypogonadism occurs in most such cases and is often the initial clinical feature of iron excess; complete iron studies should be obtained in any male patient presenting with unexplained hypogonadotropic hypogonadism. If the diagnosis is established early, hypogonadism in hemochromatosis may be reversible with iron depletion. Pituitary deficiencies of TSH, GH, and ACTH have also been documented but usually occur later in the course of the disease. The high incidence of hypothalamic-pituitary dysfunction in hemochromatosis requires careful documentation and serial evaluation, so that treatment (such as with corticosteroids) during periods of stress can be employed when indicated. Iron chelation therapy does not reverse pan hypopituitarism in hemochromatosis.

3. Histiocytosis X—Histiocytosis X, the infiltration of multiple organs by well-differentiated histiocytes, is often heralded by the onset of diabetes insipidus and anterior pituitary hormone deficiencies. The disorders in this category include Hand-Schüller-Christian disease, Letterer-Siwe disease, and eosinophilic granuloma of bone (eosinophilic infiltration predominates). Most histologic and biochemical studies have indicated that this infiltrative process involves chiefly the hypothalamus, and hypopituitarism occurs only as a result of hypothalamic damage.

D. Injury: Severe head trauma is an often-overlooked cause of anterior pituitary insufficiency even though diabetes insipidus is a well-described complication of closed head injury in children and adults. Posttraumatic anterior hypopituitarism may be due to injury to the anterior pituitary, the pituitary stalk, or the hypothalamus. Pituitary insufficiency with growth retardation has been described in battered children who suffer closed head trauma with subdural hematoma. Since the onset of posttraumatic hypopituitarism may be insidious, patients with serious head injuries, regardless of cause, require long-term observation for signs of impaired pituitary function.

E. Immunologic: Lymphocytic hypophysitis resulting in anterior hypopituitarism is a distinct entity, occurring in women usually during pregnancy or in the postpartum period. It may present as a mass lesion of the sella turcica with visual field disturbances simulating pituitary adenoma. An autoimmune process with extensive infiltration of the gland by lymphocytes and plasma cells destroys the anterior pituitary cells. These morphologic features are similar to those of other autoimmune endocrinopathies, eg, thyroiditis, adrenalitis, oophoritis, and orchitis. About 50% of patients with lymphocytic hypophysitis have other endocrine autoimmune disease, and circulating pituitary autoantibodies have been found in several cases. It is presently uncertain how this disorder should be diagnosed and treated. It must be considered in the differential diagnosis of women with pituitary gland enlargement and hypopituitarism during pregnancy or the postpartum period.

Lymphocytic hypophysitis may result in isolated hormone deficiencies (especially ACTH or prolactin). Consequently, women with this type of hypopituitarism may continue to menstruate while suffering from secondary hypothyroidism or hypoadrenalism.

F. Iatrogenic: Both surgical and radiation therapy to the pituitary gland may compromise its function. The anterior pituitary is quite resilient during transsphenoidal microsurgery, and despite extensive manipulation during the search for microadenomas, anterior pituitary function is usually preserved. The actual incidence of hypopituitarism following radiation therapy is unclear. The dose of conventional radiation therapy presently employed to treat pituitary tumors is 4500–5000 rads—considerably less than the 8000–10,000 rads required to ablate normal pituitary tissue. Nonetheless, follow-up studies of patients receiving radiation treatment for tumors disclose a high incidence of hypothalamic and pituitary insufficiency. Hypopituitarism in such patients is frequently accompanied by modest hyperprolactinemia (PRL 30–100 ng/mL [1363–4545 pmol/L]). Heavy particle (proton beam) irradiation for pituitary tumors results in a 20–50% incidence of hypopituitarism. In addition to radiotherapy directed at the pituitary or hypothalamus, irradiation of tumors of the head and neck (nasopharyngeal cancer, brain tumors) and prophylactic cranial irradiation in leukemia may also cause hypopituitarism. The clinical onset of pituitary failure in such patients is usually insidious and results from both pituitary and hypothalamic injury.

G. Infectious: Although many infectious diseases, including tuberculosis, syphilis, and mycotic infections, have been implicated as causative agents in pituitary hypofunction, anti-infective drugs have now made them rare causes of hypopituitarism. Tuberculous hypophysitis is usually accompanied by optic atrophy.

H. Idiopathic: In some patients with hypopituitarism, no underlying cause is found. These may be isolated (see below) or multiple deficiencies. Familial forms of hypopituitarism characterized by a small, normal, or enlarged sella turcica have been described. Both autosomal recessive and X-linked recessive inheritance patterns have been reported. The pathogenesis of these familial disorders is uncertain.

I. Isolated: Isolated (monotropic) deficiencies of the anterior pituitary hormones have been described.

1. GH deficiency–In children, congenital monotropic GH deficiency may be sporadic or familial and must be considered in the differential diagnosis of short stature. These children, who may experience fasting hypoglycemia, have a gradual deceleration in growth velocity after 6–12 months of age. Diagnosis must be based on failure of GH responsiveness to provocative stimuli and the demonstration of normal responsiveness of other anterior pituitary hormones. Monotropic GH deficiency and growth retardation have also been observed in children suffering severe emotional deprivation. This disorder is reversed by placing the child in a supportive psychosocial milieu. A more detailed description of GH deficiency and growth failure is provided in Chapter 8.

2. ACTH deficiency–Monotropic ACTH deficiency is rare and is manifested by the signs and symptoms of adrenocortical insufficiency. Lipotropin (LPH) deficiency has also been noted in such patients. The defect in these patients may be due to primary failure of the corticotrophs to release ACTH and its related peptide hormones or may be secondary to impaired secretion of CRH by the hypothalamus. Isolated GH deficiency, which may be a familiar disorder, can be diagnosed prenatally by estriol measurements. Most acquired cases of monotropic ACTH deficiency are due to lymphocytic hypophysitis.

3. Gonadotropin deficiency–Isolated deficiency of gonadotropins is not uncommon. Kallman's syndrome, an X-linked dominant disorder with incomplete penetrance, is characterized by an isolated defect in GnRH secretion associated with maldevelopment of the olfactory center with hyposmia or anosmia. Sporadic cases occur, and other neurologic defects such as color blindness and nerve deafness have been seen. Since anterior pituitary function is otherwise intact, young men with isolated hypogonadotropic hypogonadism develop a eunuchoid appearance; this is because lack of testosterone results in excessive growth of the limbs owing to failure of epiphyseal closure. In women, a state of hypogonadotropic hypogonadism manifested by oligomenorrhea or amenorrhea often accompanies weight loss, emotional or physical stress, and athletic training. Anorexia nervosa and marked obesity both result in hypothalamic dysfunction and impaired gonadotropin secretion. Hypothalamic hypogonadism has also been observed in overtrained male athletes. Sickle cell anemia also causes hypogonadotropic hypogonadism due to hypothalamic dysfunction and results in delayed puberty. Clomiphene treatment has been effective in such cases. Isolated gonadotropin deficiency may also be seen in the polyglandular autoimmune syndrome; this deficiency is related to selective pituitary gonadotrope failure from autoimmune hypophysitis. Other chronic illnesses, eg, poorly controlled diabetes and malnutrition, may result in gonadotropin deficiency. Isolated deficiencies of both LH and FSH without an obvious cause such as those described have been reported but are rare.

4. TSH deficiency–Monotropic TSH deficiency is rare and is caused by a reduction in hypothalamic TRH secretion (tertiary hypothyroidism). Some patients with chronic renal failure appear to have impaired TSH secretion.

5. Prolactin deficiency–PRL deficiency almost always indicates severe intrinsic pituitary damage, and panhypopituitarism is usually present. Deficiencies of TSH and PRL have been noted in patients with pseudohypoparathyroidism. Isolated PRL deficiency has been reported after lymphocytic hypophysitis.

Clinical Findings

The onset of pituitary insufficiency is usually gradual, and clinical features are related to the lack of individual pituitary hormones and their specific target gland secretion. The classic course of progressive hypopituitarism is an initial loss of gonadotropins followed by deficiencies of TSH, then ACTH, and finally PRL. Impairment of GH secretion is actually the most common abnormality in hypopituitarism, but this is, of course, clinically occult in adult patients.

A. Symptoms: Hypogonadism, manifested by amenorrhea in women and decreased libido or impotence in men, may antedate the clinical appearance of a hypothalamic-pituitary lesion.

Hypothyroidism caused by TSH deficiency generally stimulates the clinical changes observed in primary thyroid failure; however, it is usually less severe, and goiter is absent. Cold intolerance, dry skin, mental dullness, bradycardia, constipation, hoarseness, and anemia have all been observed; gross myxedematous changes are uncommon.

The lack of ACTH causes adrenocortical insufficiency, and its clinical features resemble those of primary adrenal failure. Weakness, nausea, vomiting, anorexia, fever, and postural hypotension may occur, although cardiovascular collapse as seen in Addison's disease is uncommon, since the renin-angiotensin system is usually intact. Again, these symptoms are less severe in secondary adrenal insufficiency and, because of their gradual onset, may go undetected for prolonged periods, becoming manifest only during periods of stress. Hypoglycemia aggravated by GH deficiency may occur with fasting and has been the initial presenting feature of some patients with isolated ACTH deficiency. Patients with type I (insulin-dependent) diabetes who develop hypopituitarism often have

a reduction in their insulin requirements. In contrast to the hyperpigmentation that occurs during states of ACTH excess (Addison's disease, Nelson's syndrome), depigmentation and diminished tanning have been described as a result of ACTH insufficiency. In addition, lack of ACTH-stimulated adrenal androgen secretion will cause a decrease in body hair if gonadotropin deficiency is also present.

The only symptom of PRL deficiency is failure of postpartum lactation.

B. Signs: Abnormal findings on physical examination may be subtle and require careful observation. Patients with hypopituitarism are not cachectic. A photograph of a cachectic patient with "Simmonds' syndrome" that appeared in some older textbooks of endocrinology caused confusion. That particular patient probably suffered from anorexia nervosa and was found to have a normal pituitary gland at postmortem examination.

Patients with pituitary failure are usually slightly overweight. The skin is fine, pale, and smooth, with fine wrinkling of the face. Body and pubic hair may be deficient or absent, and atrophy of the genitalia may occur. Postural hypotension, bradycardia, decreased muscle strength, and delayed deep tendon reflexes occur in more severe cases. Neuro-ophthalmologic abnormalities depend on the presence of a large intrasellar or parasellar lesion.

C. Laboratory Findings: These may include anemia (related to thyroid and androgen deficiency), hypoglycemia, hyponatremia (related to hypothyroidism and inappropriate water retention, not sodium loss), and low-voltage bradycardia on ECG. Hyperkalemia, which is common in primary adrenal failure, is not present.

Diagnosis

The diagnosis of anterior pituitary insufficiency must be established with provocative endocrine testing. However, these procedures should be preceded by a thorough clinical history and physical examination. For example, the presence of a normal menstrual cycle in a euthyroid woman is strong evidence against pituitary dysfunction, and further studies in such cases are usually not warranted. A diagnostic strategy for the evaluation of hypopituitarism is presented in Fig 6–13.

A. Assessment of Target Gland Function: If endocrine hypofunction is suspected, pituitary hormone deficiencies must be distinguished from primary failure of the thyroid, adrenals, or gonads. Basal determinations of each anterior pituitary hormone are useful only if compared to target gland secretion. Baseline laboratory studies should include thyroid function tests (T_4RIA, RT_3U, FT_4I) and determination of serum testosterone levels. Testosterone is a sensitive indicator of hypopituitarism in women as well as in men. In women, a substantial decrease in testosterone is commonly observed in pituitary failure related to hypofunction of

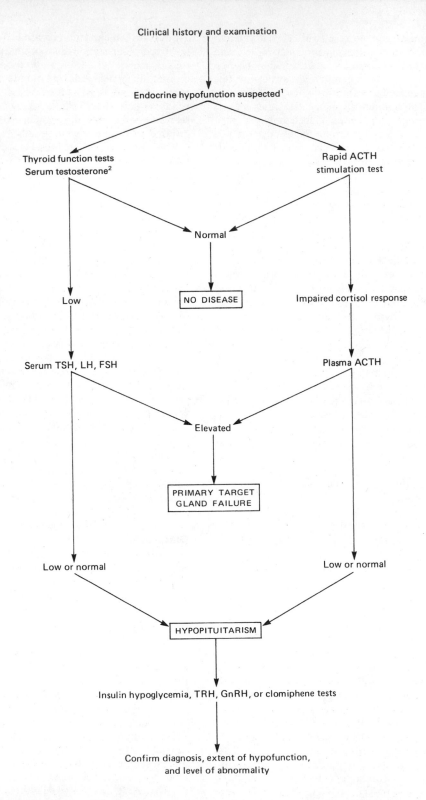

¹Evaluate GH in children (see text).
²Measure prolactin if hypogonadism suspected.

Figure 6–13. Diagnostic evaluation of hypothalamic-pituitary-target gland hypofunction.

the 2 endocrine glands responsible for its production—the ovary and the adrenal. Adrenocortical reserve should initially be evaluated by a rapid ACTH stimulation test.

B. Evaluation of Prolactin: Since hyperprolactinemia (discussed later), regardless of its cause, leads to gonadal dysfunction, serum PRL should be measured early in the evaluation of hypogonadism.

C. Differentiation of Primary and Secondary Hypofunction: Subnormal thyroid function as shown by appropriate tests, a low serum testosterone level, or an impaired cortisol response to the rapid ACTH stimulation test requires measurement of basal levels of specific pituitary hormones. In primary target gland hypofunction (such as polyglandular failure syndrome), TSH, LH, FSH, or ACTH will be elevated. Low or normal values for these pituitary hormones suggest hypothalamic-pituitary dysfunction.

D. Stimulation Tests: Provocative endocrine testing should then be employed to confirm the diagnosis; to assess the extent of hypofunction; and, when possible, to determine whether the abnormality is at the level of the hypothalamus or pituitary. Evaluation of the secretory reserve of the pituitary hormones has been discussed earlier. For convenience, a triple stimulation test combining simultaneous insulin hypoglycemia, TRH, and GnRH can be utilized to test the secretory capacity of all 6 major anterior pituitary hormones. Some investigators have also successfully infused CRH, GRH, TRH, and GnRH simultaneously as a means of assessing complete adenohypophyseal function.

Treatment

Appropriate therapy for hypopituitarism must include consideration of individual hormonal deficiencies as well as the extent of the deficiencies. Except in the case of GH, replacement therapy is provided by use of synthetic target gland hormones.

A. ACTH: Treatment of secondary adrenal insufficiency, like that of primary adrenal failure, must include glucocorticoid support (see Chapter 12). Hydrocortisone (20–30 mg/d), cortisone acetate (25–35 mg/d), prednisone (5–7.5 mg/d) orally in 2 or 3 divided doses provides adequate glucocorticoid replacement for most patients. The minimum effective dosage should be given in order to avoid iatrogenic hypercortisolism. Increased dosage is required during periods of stress such as illness, surgery, or trauma. Patients with only partial ACTH deficiency may need steroid treatment only during stress. A 2- or 3-fold increase in steroid dosage during the stressful situation should be recommended, followed by gradual tapering as the stress resolves. Unlike primary adrenal insufficiency, ACTH deficiency does not usually require mineralocorticoid therapy. Patients with adrenal insufficiency should wear medical alert bracelets so they may receive prompt treatment in case of emergency.

B. TSH: The decision to treat patients with second-

ary hypothyroidism must be based on clinical grounds and the circulating concentration of serum thyroxine (see Chapter 10). Since some patients with hypothyrotropic hypothyroidism have a normal TSH response to TRH, basal TSH levels and the TRH test should not be used as guidelines for thyroid replacement. The treatment of secondary and tertiary hypothyroidism is identical to that for primary thyroid failure. Levothyroxine sodium, 0.1–0.15 mg/d orally, is usually adequate. Response to therapy is monitored clinically and with measurement of serum thyroxine.

Caution must be urged in initiating thyroxine treatment in a patient with suspected hypoadrenalism. Since thyroid hormone replacement in patients with hypopituitarism may aggravate even partial adrenal insufficiency, the adrenal disorder should be treated first, followed by the judicious use of thyroxine.

C. Gonadotropins: The object of treatment of secondary hypogonadism is to replace sex steroids and restore gametogenesis (see Chapters 16 and 17).

1. Estrogens and progesterone—In women, estrogen replacement is essential. Adequate estrogen treatment will maintain secondary sex characteristics (eg, vulvar and vaginal lubrication), prevent osteoporosis, and abolish vasomotor symptoms, with an improvement in sense of well-being. Many estrogen preparations are available, but the optimal replacement dosage is unknown; the smallest dose that achieves the desired clinical effects should be used, eg, ethinyl estradiol, 0.02–0.05 mg orally daily; conjugated estrogens, 0.3–1.25 mg orally daily; or transdermal estradiol, 0.05–0.1 mg daily. Since long-term therapy with estrogen compounds increases the risk of endometrial carcinoma, estrogens should be withheld during the last 5–7 days of each month, and a progestin compound (eg, medroxyprogesterone, 10 mg orally) should be given during days 15–25 of the cycle to induce withdrawal bleeding and prevent endometrial hyperplasia.

2. Ovulation induction—Ovulation can often be restored in women with hypothalamic-pituitary dysfunction (see Chapter 17). In patients with gonadal failure of hypothalamic origin, clomiphene citrate causes a surge of gonadotropin secretion resulting in ovulation. Multiple births are a risk with this form of treatment. Combined treatment with FSH (human menopausal gonadotropins; menotropins; Pergonal) and LH (chorionic gonadotropin) can be utilized to provoke ovulation in women with intrinsic pituitary failure. This form of therapy is expensive, and multiple births are a risk. Pulsatile subcutaneous injections of GnRH with an infusion pump can also be used to induce ovulation and fertility in women with hypothalamic dysfunction.

3. Androgens in women—Because of a deficiency of adrenal androgens, some women with hypopituitarism have diminished libido despite adequate estrogen therapy. Small doses of long-acting androgens (testosterone enanthate, 25–50 mg intramuscularly every 4–8 weeks) may be helpful in restoring sexual activity without causing hirsutism.

4. Androgens in men–In men, testosterone replacement is essential to restore libido and potency, provide adequate beard growth and muscle strength, prevent osteopenia, and improve the sense of well-being. Adequate treatment consists of a long-acting intramuscular preparation such as testosterone enanthate. Three dosage schedules have proved efficacy: 300 mg every 3 weeks, 200 mg every 2 weeks, or 100 mg every week. Side effects, including aggressive sexual behavior, acne, gynecomastia, and fluid retention, are unusual and can be managed by lowering the dosage. Therapy should be withheld in adolescents as long as possible in order to prevent premature epiphyseal closure and ensure maximum linear growth. Replacement therapy with oral androgenic preparations should be avoided, since inadequate absorption results in poor androgenization, and serious side effects such as peliosis hepatis (blood-filled cysts within the hepatic parenchyma) may occur. Transdermal testosterone therapy has also been shown to be an effective and acceptable means of administering androgens. Preparations that use this new route of administration may be available soon.

5. Spermatogenesis–Spermatogenesis can be achieved in some patients with the combined use of chorionic gonadotropin and menotropins. If pituitary insufficiency is of recent onset, therapy with chorionic gonadotropin alone may restore both fertility and adequate gonadal steroid production. Pulsatile GnRH infusion pumps have also been used to restore fertility in male patients with secondary hypogonadism.

D. Growth Hormone: (See Chapter 8.) The recognition of Creutzfeldt-Jakob disease, a transmissible subacute degeneration of the central nervous system, in young patients who had received growth hormone derived from human pituitary glands has resulted in a discontinuation of such therapy. Fortunately, production of human growth hormone (hGH) has been accomplished by recombinant DNA technology so that the hormone is available for use in children with hypopituitarism. The identification of a subgroup of children with normal variant short stature (normal GH secretory capacity) who benefit from long-term administration of hGH may broaden the therapeutic horizons of biologically engineered growth hormone.

PITUITARY ADENOMAS

Advances in endocrinologic and neuroradiologic research in recent years have allowed earlier recognition and more successful therapy of pituitary adenomas. Prolactinomas are the most common type, accounting for about 60% of primary pituitary tumors; GH hypersecretion occurs in approximately 20% and ACTH excess in 10%. Hypersecretion of TSH, the gonadotropins, or alpha subunits is unusual. Nonfunctional tumors currently represent only 10% of all pituitary adenomas, and some of these may in fact be alpha subunit–secreting adenomas.

Early clinical recognition of the endocrine effects of excessive pituitary secretion, especially the observation that PRL excess causes secondary hypogonadism, has led to early diagnosis of pituitary tumors before the appearance of late manifestations such as sellar enlargement, panhypopituitarism, and suprasellar extension with visual impairment.

Pituitary **microadenomas** are defined as intrasellar adenomas less than 1 cm in diameter that present with manifestations of hormonal excess without sellar enlargement or extrasellar extension. Panhypopituitarism is rare, and such tumors are very successfully treated.

Pituitary **macroadenomas** are those larger than 1 cm in diameter and cause generalized sellar enlargement. Tumors 1–2 cm in diameter confined to the sella turcica can usually be successfully treated; however, larger tumors—and especially those with suprasellar, sphenoid sinus, or lateral extensions—are much more difficult to manage. Panhypopituitarism and visual loss increase in frequency with tumor size and suprasellar extension.

Treatment

Pituitary adenomas are treated with surgery, irradiation, or drugs to suppress hypersecretion by the adenoma or its growth. All patients with pituitary tumors should undergo endocrinologic evaluations before a method of treatment is decided upon. Details are outlined in subsequent sections.

The aims of therapy are to correct hypersecretion of anterior pituitary hormones, to preserve normal pituitary tissue secreting other anterior pituitary hormones, and to remove or suppress the adenoma itself. These objectives are currently achievable in most patients with pituitary microadenomas; however, in the case of larger tumors, multiple therapies are frequently required and may be less successful.

A. Surgical: Pituitary surgery is the initial therapy of choice at many centers, and the transsphenoidal microsurgical approach to the sella turcica is the procedure of choice; transfrontal craniotomy is required only in the occasional patient with massive suprasellar extension of the adenoma. In the transsphenoidal procedure, the surgeon approaches the pituitary from the nasal cavity through the sphenoid sinus, removes the anterior-inferior sellar floor, and incises the dura. The adenoma is selectively removed; normal pituitary tissue is identified and preserved. Success rates approach 90% in patients with microadenomas. Major complications, including postoperative hemorrhage, cerebrospinal fluid leak, meningitis, and visual impairment, occur in less than 5% and are most frequent in patients with large or massive tumors. Transient diabetes insipidus lasting a few days to 1–2 weeks occurs in approximately 15%; permanent diabetes insipidus is rare. A transient form of the syndrome of inappropriate secretion of vasopressin (antidiuretic hormone) (SIADH) with symptomatic hyponatremia occurs in 10% of patients within 5–10 days of transsphenoidal pituitary microsurgery. Surgical hypopituitarism is rare in patients with microadenomas but approaches 5–10% in patients with larger tumors. The perioperative management of such patients should include glucocorticoid administration in stress doses (see Chapter 12) and postoperative assessment of daily weight, fluid balance, and electrolyte status. Mild diabetes insipidus is managed by giving fluids orally; in more severe cases—urine output greater than 5–6 L/24 h—vasopressin therapy in the form of subcutaneous Pitressin (aqueous vasopressin) or intranasal DDAVP should be administered (see Chapter 9). SIADH is managed by fluid restriction.

B. Radiologic: Pituitary irradiation is usually reserved for patients with larger tumors who have had incomplete resection of large pituitary adenomas.

1. X-ray irradiation–Conventional irradiation using high energy sources, in total doses of 4000–5000 rads given in daily doses of 180–200 rads, is most commonly employed. The response to radiation therapy is slow, and 5–10 years may be required to achieve the full effect (see section on acromegaly). Treatment is ultimately successful in about 80% of acromegalics but only 15% of patients with Cushing's disease. The response rate in prolactinomas is not precisely known, but tumor progression is prevented in most patients. Morbidity during radiotherapy is minimal, though some patients experience malaise and nausea, and serous otitis media may occur. Rare late complications include damage to the optic nerves and chiasm, seizures, and radionecrosis of brain tissue. Hypopituitarism is common, and the incidence increases with time following radiotherapy—about 40–50% at 5–10 years.

2. Heavy particle irradiation–Heavy particle irradiation using alpha particles or protons is also used. Advantages of this technique are the ability to focus the radiation beam precisely; the smaller port allows larger doses (8000–12,000 rads) to be delivered to the sellar area and limits the radiation exposure of surrounding structures. Disadvantages are the limited availability, and the smaller radiation field precludes use of this technique in patients with tumors over 1.5 cm in diameter and in those with extrasellar extension. Responses to therapy are more rapid than with conventional irradiation and occur within 2 years in most patients. Successful responses are obtained in about 80% of patients with acromegaly or Cushing's disease. Experience with prolactinomas is limited. Neurologic damage and visual impairment are rare complications of heavy particle irradiation, but hypopituitarism occurs in 40–50% and will almost certainly increase with further follow-up.

C. Medical: Medical management of pituitary adenomas has become feasible with the availability of bromocriptine, a dopamine agonist. This drug is most successful in the treatment of hyperprolactinemia and is also useful in some patients with acromegaly or Cushing's disease. Octreotide acetate, a new somatostatin analogue, is being evaluated in the therapy of acromegaly and TSH-secreting adenomas. Specifics of the use of these and other medications are discussed below.

Posttreatment Follow-Up

Patients undergoing transsphenoidal microsurgery should be reevaluated 4–6 weeks postoperatively to document that complete removal of the adenoma and correction of endocrine hypersecretion have been achieved. Prolactinomas are assessed by basal PRL measurements, GH-secreting tumors by glucose suppression testing, and ACTH-secreting adenomas by measurement of urine free cortisol and the response to low-dose dexamethasone suppression (see below). Other anterior pituitary hormones—TSH, ACTH, and LH/FSH—should also be assessed as described above in the section on endocrine evaluation. In patients with successful responses, yearly evaluation should be done to watch for late recurrence; late hypopituitarism does not occur after microsurgery. MRI or CT scanning is not necessary in patients with normal postoperative pituitary function but should be utilized in patients with persisting or recurrent disease.

Follow-up of patients treated by pituitary irradiation is also essential, since the response to therapy may be delayed and the incidence of hypopituitarism increases with time. Yearly endocrinologic assessment of both the hypersecreted hormone and the other pituitary hormones is recommended.

1. PROLACTINOMAS

The clinical application of prolactin (PRL) assays has greatly expanded our understanding of pituitary disorders. Although the **galactorrhea-amenorrhea syndromes** were previously described, PRL measurement has greatly facilitated their early recognition and is a useful index of response to therapy.

PRL hypersecretion is the most common endocrine abnormality due to hypothalamic-pituitary disorders, and PRL is the hormone most commonly secreted in excess by pituitary adenomas. In addition, most chromophobe adenomas, which were previously classified as "nonfunctional" on the basis of routine histologic studies, have now been shown to be PRL-secreting adenomas.

The understanding that PRL hypersecretion causes not only galactorrhea but also gonadal dysfunction and the use of PRL measurements in screening such patients have permitted recognition of these PRL-secreting tumors before the development of sellar enlargement, hypopituitarism, or visual impairment.

Thus, plasma PRL should be measured in patients

Table 6–7. Indications for prolactin measurement.

Galactorrhea
Enlarged sella turcica
Suspected pituitary tumor
Hypogonadotropic hypogonadism
   Unexplained amenorrhea
   Unexplained male hypogonadism or infertility

with galactorrhea, suspected hypothalamic-pituitary dysfunction, or sellar enlargement and in those with unexplained gonadal dysfunction, including amenorrhea, infertility, decreased lidido, or impotence (Table 6–7).

Pathology

PRL-secreting pituitary adenomas arise most commonly from the lateral wings of the anterior pituitary, but with progression they fill the sella turcica and compress the normal anterior and posterior lobes. Tumor size varies greatly from microadenomas to large invasive tumors with extrasellar extension. Most patients have microadenomas, ie, tumors less than 1 cm in diameter at diagnosis. Prolactinomas frequently undergo spontaneous partial necrosis, and thus a partially empty sella turcica accompanies the pituitary adenoma in 30–40% of patients.

Prolactinomas usually appear chromophobic on routine histologic study, reflecting the inadequacy of the techniques used. The cells are small and uniform, with round or oval nuclei and scanty cytoplasm, and secretory granules are usually not visible with routine stains. The stroma contains a diffuse capillary network.

Electron microscopic examination shows that prolactinoma cells characteristically contain secretory granules that usually range from 100 to 500 nm and are spherical. Larger granules (400–500 nm), which are irregular or crescent-shaped, are less commonly seen. The cells show evidence of secretory activity, with a large Golgi area, nucleolar enlargement, and a prominent endoplasmic reticulum. Immunocytochemical studies of these tumors have confirmed that the secretory granules indeed contain PRL.

Clinical Findings

The clinical manifestations of PRL excess are the same regardless of the cause (see below). The classic features are galactorrhea and amenorrhea in women and galactorrhea and decreased libido or impotence in men. Although the sex distribution of prolactinomas is approximately equal, microadenomas are much more common in females, presumably because of earlier recognition of the endocrine consequences of PRL excess.

A. Galactorrhea: Galactorrhea occurs in less than half of patients with prolactinomas and is less common in men than in women. It is usually not spontaneous, or may be present only transiently or inter-

mittently; careful breast examination is required in most patients to demonstrate galactorrhea. The absence of galactorrhea despite markedly elevated PRL levels is probably due to concomitant deficiency of the gonadal hormones required to initiate lactation (see Chapter 20).

B. Gonadal Dysfunction:

1. In Women: Amenorrhea, oligomenorrhea with anovulation, or infertility is present in approximately 90% of women with prolactinomas. These menstrual disorders usually present concurrently with galactorrhea if it is present but may either precede or follow it. The amenorrhea is usually secondary and may follow pregnancy or oral contraceptive use. Primary amenorrhea occurs in the minority of patients who have onset of hyperprolactinemia during adolescence. The necessity of measuring PRL in patients with unexplained primary or secondary amenorrhea is emphasized by several studies showing that hyperprolactinemia occurs in as many as 20% of patients with neither galactorrhea nor other manifestations of pituitary dysfunction. A number of these patients have been shown to have prolactinomas.

Gonadal dysfunction in these women is due to interference with the hypothalamic-pituitary-gonadal axis by the hyperprolactinemia and except in patients with large or invasive adenomas is not due to destruction of the gonadotropin-secreting cells. This has been documented by the return of menstrual function following reduction of PRL levels to normal by drug treatment or surgical removal of the tumor. Although basal gonadotropin levels are frequently within the normal range despite reduction of sex steroid levels in hyperprolactinemic patients, PRL inhibits both the normal pulsatile secretion of LH and FSH and the midcycle LH surge, resulting in anovulation. The positive feedback effect of estrogen on gonadotropin secretion is also inhibited; in fact, patients with hyperprolactinemia are usually estrogen-deficient. PRL may also exert an effect directly on the ovary, although evidence suggests that its major influence is on the hypothalamic-pituitary axis by some mechanism not yet identified.

Estrogen deficiency in women with prolactinomas may be accompanied by decreased vaginal lubrication, other symptoms of estrogen deficiency, and osteopenia as assessed by bone densitometry. Other symptoms may include weight gain, fluid retention, and irritability. Hirsutism may also occur, accompanied by elevated plasma levels of dehydroepiandrosterone (DHEA) sulfate. Patients with hyperprolactinemia may also suffer from anxiety and depression. Treatment with bromocriptine has been shown to improve psychologic distress in such patients.

2. In Men: In men, PRL excess may also occasionally cause galactorrhea; however, the usual manifestations are those of hypogonadism. The initial symptom is decreased libido, which may be dismissed by both the patient and physician as due to psychosocial factors; thus, the recognition of prolactinomas in men is frequently delayed, and marked hyperprolactinemia (PRL > 200 ng/mL [9090 pmol/L]) and sellar enlargement are usual. Unfortunately, prolactinomas in men are often not diagnosed until late manifestations such as headache, visual impairment, or hypopituitarism appear; virtually all such patients have a history of sexual or gonadal dysfunction. Serum testosterone levels are low, and in the presence of normal or subnormal gonadotropin levels, PRL excess should be suspected as well as other causes of hypothalamic-pituitary-gonadal dysfunction (see section on hypopituitarism). Impotence also occurs in hyperprolactinemic males, and its cause is unclear, since testosterone replacement may not reverse it, if hyperprolactinemia is not corrected. Male infertility accompanied by reduction in sperm count is a less common initial complaint.

C. Tumor Progression: In general, the growth of prolactinomas is slow, and the natural history of microadenomas has not been well defined.

Differential Diagnosis

The many conditions associated with hyperprolactinemia are listed in Table 6–3. Pregnancy, hypothalamic-pituitary disorders, hypothyroidism, and drug ingestion are the most common causes. Careful history and examination are essential in all cases in order to determine the origin of PRL excess.

Hypothalamic lesions frequently cause PRL hypersecretion by decreasing the secretion of factors that tonically inhibit PRL release (eg, dopamine); the lesions are usually accompanied by panhypopituitarism. Similarly, traumatic or surgical section of the pituitary stalk leads to hyperprolactinemia and hypopituitarism. The cause and clinical features of hypothalamic lesions are discussed in previous sections.

Pregnancy leads to a physiologic increase in PRL secretion; the levels increase as pregnancy continues and may reach 200 ng/mL (9090 pmol/L) during the third trimester. Following delivery, basal PRL levels gradually fall to normal over several weeks but increase in response to breast feeding. Hyperprolactinemia persisting for 6–12 months or longer following delivery is an indication for evaluation for prolactinoma. PRL levels are also high in normal neonates.

Several systemic disorders lead to hyperprolactinemia. Primary hypothyroidism is a common cause, and measurement of thyroid function, including TSH, should be part of the evaluation. Primary hypothyroidism may even result in significant pituitary gland enlargement and so may be mistaken for a PRL-secreting pituitary tumor. The PRL response to TRH is usually exaggerated in these patients. PRL may also be increased in liver disease, particularly in patients with severe cirrhosis, and in patients with chronic renal failure.

PRL excess and galactorrhea may also be caused by breast disease, nipple stimulation, disease or injury to the chest wall, and spinal cord lesions. These disorders increase PRL secretion by stimulation of afferent neural pathways.

The most common cause of hyperprolactinemia is drug ingestion, and a careful history of drug intake must be obtained. Elevated PRL levels, galactorrhea, and amenorrhea may occur following estrogen therapy or oral contraceptive use, but their persistence should suggest prolactinoma. Many other drugs also cause increased PRL secretion and elevated plasma levels (Table 6–3). PRL levels are usually less than 100 ng/mL (4545 pmol/L), and the evaluation of these patients is primarily by discontinuance of the drug or medication and reevaluation after several weeks. In patients in whom drug withdrawal is not feasible, neuroradiologic studies, if normal, will usually exclude prolactinoma.

Diagnosis

A. General Evaluation: The evaluation of patients with galactorrhea or unexplained gonadal dysfunction with normal or low plasma gonadotropin levels should first include a history regarding menstrual status, pregnancy, fertility, sexual function, and symptoms of hypothyroidism or hypopituitarism. Current or previous use of medication, drugs, or estrogen therapy should be documented. Basal PRL levels, gonadotropins, thyroid function tests, and TSH levels should be established, as well as serum testosterone in men. Liver and kidney function should be assessed. A pregnancy test should be performed in women with recent onset of amenorrhea or galactorrhea.

Patients with galactorrhea but normal menses usually do not have hyperprolactinemia or prolactinomas. If the PRL level is normal, they may be reassured and followed with sequential PRL measurements. Those with elevated levels require further evaluation as described below.

B. Specific Diagnosis: When other causes of hyperprolactinemia have been excluded, the most likely cause of persisting hyperprolactinemia is prolactinoma, especially if there is associated hypogonadism. Currently available suppression and stimulation tests do not clearly distinguish PRL-secreting tumors from other causes of hyperprolactinemia. Therefore, the diagnosis must be established primarily by the assessment of basal PRL levels and neuroradiologic studies of the pituitary and sella turcica. In our experience, both hyperprolactinemia and a radiologic abnormality are required to establish the diagnosis of prolactinoma with certainty. Patients with large tumors and marked hyperprolactinemia usually present little difficulty. With very rare exceptions, basal PRL levels greater than 200 ng/mL (9090 pmol/L) are virtually diagnostic of prolactinoma. In addition, since there is a general correlation between the PRL elevation and the size of the pituitary adenoma, these patients usually have sellar enlargement and obvious macroadenomas. Similarly, if the basal PRL level is between 100 and

200 ng/mL (4545 and 9090 pmol/L), the cause is usually prolactinoma. These patients may have either micro- or macroadenomas; however, with basal levels of PRL greater than 100 ng/mL (4545 pmol/L), the PRL-secreting tumor is usually radiologically evident, and again the diagnosis is generally straightforward. Patients with mild to moderate hyperprolactinemia (20–100 ng/mL [909–4545 pmol/L]) present the greatest difficulty in diagnosis, since both PRL-secreting microadenomas and the many other conditions causing hyperprolactinemia (Table 6–3) cause PRL hypersecretion of this degree. In such patients, MRI or CT scanning should be performed and will frequently demonstrate a definite pituitary microadenoma, thus establishing the diagnosis. Scans showing only minor or equivocal abnormalities should be interpreted with caution, because of the high incidence of false-positive scans in the normal population (see neuroradiologic evaluation, above). Since the diagnosis cannot be either established or excluded in patients with normal or equivocal neuroradiologic studies, they require further evaluation or serial assessment (see below).

Treatment

Satisfactory control of PRL hypersecretion, cessation of galactorrhea, and return of normal gonadal function can be achieved in most patients with PRL-secreting microadenomas, although the choice of primary therapy (surgical or medical) remains controversial. In patients with hyperprolactinemia, ovulation should not be induced without careful assessment of pituitary anatomy and sella turcica size, since pregnancy may cause further expansion of these tumors as discussed below. All patients with PRL-secreting macroadenomas should be treated, because of the risks of further tumor expansion, hypopituitarism, and visual impairment. Patients with larger prolactinomas—over 2 cm in diameter, or basal PRL levels over 200 ng/mL (9090 pmol/L)—may require combined therapy with surgery, radiation, and bromocriptine or long-term suppression with bromocriptine alone.

Treatment for all patients with microadenomas is also recommended to prevent early osteoporosis secondary to persisting hypogonadism and to restore fertility. In addition, surgical or medical therapy is more successful in these patients than in those with larger tumors.

Patients with persisting hyperprolactinemia and hypogonadism and normal neuroradiologic studies—ie, those in whom prolactinoma cannot be definitely established—may be managed by observation if hypogonadism is of short duration. However, in patients whose hypogonadism has persisted for more than 1–2 years, bromocriptine should be used to suppress PRL secretion and restore normal gonadal function. In women with suspected or proved prolactinomas, replacement estrogen therapy is contraindicated because of the risk of tumor growth.

A. Surgical:

1. Transsphenoidal microsurgery–This is the surgical procedure of choice in patients with prolactinomas and is the preferred initial method of therapy in some institutions.

a. Microadenomas–In patients with microadenomas, success, as measured by restitution of normal PRL levels, normal menses, and cessation of galactorrhea, is achieved in 85–90% of cases. Success is most likely in patients with basal PRL levels under 200 ng/mL (9090 pmol/L) and a duration of amenorrhea of less than 5 years. In these patients, the incidence of surgical complications is less than 5%, and hypopituitarism is a rare complication. Thus, in this group of patients with PRL-secreting microadenomas, PRL hypersecretion can be corrected, gonadal function restored, and secretion of TSH and ACTH preserved. Recurrence rates vary considerably in reported series. In our experience, approximately 75% of patients have had long-term remissions, and 25% have had recurrences 5–10 years following surgery.

b. Macroadenomas–Transsphenoidal microsurgery is considerably less successful in restoring normal PRL secretion in patients with macroadenomas; many clinicians would treat these patients with bromocriptine alone. The surgical outcome is directly related to tumor size and the basal PRL level. Thus, in patients with tumors 1–2 cm in diameter without extrasellar extension and with basal PRL levels under 200 ng/mL (9090 pmol/L), transsphenoidal surgery is successful in about 80% of cases. In patients with higher basal PRL levels and larger tumors, the success rate—defined as complete tumor resection and restoration of normal basal PRL secretion—is about 25–50%. Although surgical results are relatively poor in this latter group of patients, surgery is recommended at many centers as the primary therapy in order to decompress vital structures such as the optic chiasm and to reduce tumor bulk and PRL hypersecretion. Additional therapy with bromocriptine or radiotherapy is required in the subsequent management of these patients (see below).

2. Transfrontal craniotomy–This procedure should be used only in patients with major suprasellar extension of tumor not accessible via the transsphenoidal route in whom decompression of vital structures is required. It must be followed by bromocriptine or radiation therapy, since residual tumor is virtually always present.

B. Radiologic: Conventional radiation therapy is reserved for patients with PRL-secreting macroadenomas who have persisting hyperprolactinemia following surgical treatment. In this group of patients, radiotherapy with 4000–5000 rads prevents further tumor expansion, though PRL levels usually do not fall into the normal range. Impairment of anterior pituitary function occurs in approximately 30–50% of patients. Conventional radiation therapy has not been used as initial treatment for patients with microadenomas, since experience is limited and the radiation-induced damage to gonadotropin-secreting cells may further impair fertility.

Experience with heavy particle irradiation in prolactinomas is limited.

C. Medical:

1. Bromocriptine–Bromocriptine (Parlodel; 2-bromo-α-ergocryptine mesylate) is a potent dopamine agonist that has been used extensively in the treatment of hyperprolactinemia. Bromocriptine stimulates dopamine receptors and has effects at both the hypothalamic and pituitary levels. It is effective therapy for a PRL-secreting pituitary adenoma and directly inhibits PRL secretion by the tumor. The dosage is 2.5–10 mg/d orally in divided doses. Side effects consisting of dizziness, postural hypotension, nausea, and occasionally vomiting are common at onset of therapy but usually resolve with continuation of the medication. They can usually be avoided by starting with a low dose and gradually increasing the dose over days to weeks until the PRL level is suppressed to the normal range. An example would be to give 1.25 mg at bedtime for 2 or 3 days and then increase to 2.5 mg; if tolerated, an additional 2.5 mg can be added in the morning. PRL levels should then be assessed. If they remain elevated, the dosage is gradually increased to a total of 7.5–10 mg/d. With these dosages, hyperprolactinemia is controlled in most patients; further increases in dosage are usually not warranted and are usually accompanied by increased side effects. Most patients tolerate doses of 2.5–10 mg without difficulty; however, in a minority, persisting postural hypotension and gastrointestinal side effects necessitate discontinuance of therapy.

a. Microadenomas–In patients with microadenomas, bromocriptine successfully reduces PRL levels to normal in over 90% of cases. In addition, correction of hyperprolactinemia allows recovery of normal gonadal function; ovulation and fertility are restored, so that mechanical contraception should be advised if pregnancy is not desired. Bromocriptine induces ovulation in most female patients who wish to become pregnant. In these patients with microadenomas, the risk of major expansion of adenoma during the pregnancy appears to be less than 5%; however, both the patient and the physician must be aware of this potential complication. Current data do not indicate an increased risk of multiple pregnancy, abortion, or fetal malformations in pregnancies induced by bromocriptine; however, the patient should be instructed to discontinue bromocriptine at the first missed menstrual period and obtain a pregnancy test.

At present, there is no evidence that bromocriptine causes permanent resolution of PRL-secreting microadenomas, and virtually all patients have resumption of hyperprolactinemia following discontinuation of therapy even when it has been continued for several years. Although no late toxicity has yet been reported other than the side effects noted above, questions about possible long-term risk and the indicated duration of therapy in such patients with microadenomas are currently unanswered.

b. Macroadenomas–Bromocriptine is effective in controlling hyperprolactinemia in patients with PRL-secreting macroadenomas even when basal PRL levels are markedly elevated. Bromocriptine may be used either as initial therapy or to control residual hyperprolactinemia in patients unsuccessfully treated with surgery or radiotherapy. Bromocriptine should not be used to induce ovulation and pregnancy in women with untreated macroadenomas, since the risk of tumor expansion and visual deficits in the later part of pregnancy is approximately 15–25%. These patients should be treated with surgery or radiotherapy prior to induction of ovulation with bromocriptine or by gonadotropin therapy.

Bromocriptine not only reduces PRL secretion in patients with macroadenomas but also reduces tumor size in about 70–80% of patients. Reduction of tumor size with bromocriptine may occur within days to weeks following institution of therapy. The drug has been used to restore vision in patients with major suprasellar extension and chiasmal compression. Tumor reduction in response to bromocriptine is sustained only as long as the medication is continued, and reexpansion of the tumor and recurrence of hyperprolactinemia may occur rapidly following discontinuation of therapy. The question of duration of therapy in patients with macroadenomas remains unanswered.

2. Pergolide–Pergolide mesylate is a long-acting ergot derivative with dopaminergic properties that has been shown to reduce hypersecretion and shrink most PRL-secreting macroadenomas. This new drug remains investigational. It is more potent than bromocriptine, requiring doses of 25–300 μg/d to treat hyperprolactinemia. The side effects of pergolide are similar to those of bromocriptine.

Management of Prolactinomas

The treatment of prolactinomas is controversial and depends on the wishes of the patient, the patient's plans for pregnancy and tolerance of medical therapy, and the availability of a skilled neurosurgeon.

A. Microadenomas: All patients should be treated to prevent tumor progression and osteopenia due to prolonged hypogonadism. Medical therapy with bromocriptine effectively restores normal gonadal function and fertility, and pregnancy carries only a small risk of tumor expansion. The major disadvantage of this treatment is the need for chronic therapy. In contrast, transsphenoidal adenectomy, either initially or after a trial of bromocriptine therapy, carries little risk when performed by an experienced neurosurgeon and offers a high probability of long-term remission.

B. Macroadenomas: Primary surgical therapy in

these patients frequently does not result in long-term remission, so medical therapy is being used more often, particularly when the patient's prolactin levels are greater than 200 ng/mL (9090 pmol/L) and the tumor is larger than 2 cm. Although transsphenoidal microsurgery will rapidly decrease tumor size and decompress the pituitary stalk, the optic chiasm, and the cavernous sinuses, both the tumor and the hyperprolactinemia will usually persist. Thus, these patients will require additional therapy with radiation or bromocriptine. Although tumor growth and prolactin secretion can be controlled by medical therapy, therapeutic failure can result from drug intolerance or poor compliance. Thus, all patients with prolactinomas should be followed up carefully.

2. ACROMEGALY & GIGANTISM

GH-secreting pituitary adenomas are second in frequency to prolactinomas and cause the classic clinical syndromes of acromegaly and gigantism.

The characteristic clinical manifestations are the consequence of chronic GH hypersecretion, which in turn leads to excessive generation of the somatomedins, the mediators of most of the effects of GH (see Chapter 7). Although overgrowth of bone is the classic feature, GH excess causes a generalized systemic disorder with deleterious effects on many systems and an increased mortality rate, though deaths are rarely due to the space-occupying or destructive effects of pituitary adenoma per se.

Acromegaly and gigantism are virtually always secondary to pituitary adenoma. Ectopic GRH secretion has been identified as another cause of GH hypersecretion and acromegaly in a few patients with carcinoid or islet cell tumors. Reports of intrapituitary GRH-secreting gangliocytomas in direct contiguity with GH-secreting somatotroph adenomas and a report of a GRH-secreting hypothalamic hamartoma in a patient with acromegaly provide a link between ectopic and eutopic GRH production. Ectopic secretion of GH per se is very rare.

In adults, GH excess leads to acromegaly, the syndrome characterized by local overgrowth of bone, particularly of the skull and mandible. Linear growth does not occur, because of prior fusion of the epiphyses of long bones. In childhood and adolescence, the onset of chronic GH excess leads to gigantism. Many of these patients have associated hypogonadism, which further delays epiphyseal closure, and the combination of somatomedin excess and hypogonadism leads to a striking acceleration of linear growth. In addition, most patients with gigantism also have features of acromegaly if GH hypersecretion persists through adolescence and into adulthood.

Pathology

Pituitary adenomas causing acromegaly are usually over 1 cm in diameter when the diagnosis is estab-

lished. These tumors arise from the lateral wings of the anterior pituitary; less than 20% are diagnosed as microadenomas.

GH-secreting adenomas are of 2 histologic types: densely and sparsely granulated. However, there appears to be no difference in the degree of GH secretion or clinical manifestations in these patients. About 15% of GH-secreting tumors also contain lactotrophs, and these tumors thus hypersecrete both GH and PRL.

Densely granulated adenomas are acidophilic by light microscopy using routine stains and are usually strongly positive when stained for GH by immunocytochemical techniques. Electron microscopy demonstrates that the cells are similar to normal somatotrophs; ie, they are spherical or oval, with uniform features, round or oval centrally located nuclei, and abundant cytoplasm. The numerous spherical GH-containing granules are electron-dense, ranging in size from 300 to 600 nm, with the majority measuring 350–450 nm.

The sparsely granulated adenomas are chromophobic by light microscopy, a feature that merely reflects the paucity of stainable secretory granules; they are indistinguishable from other chromophobe adenomas except by the demonstration of GH within them by immunocytochemistry. By electron microscopy, the cells do not resemble normal somatotrophs but have variable shape and size; pleomorphic, frequently crescent-shaped nuclei; and globular fibrous bodies within the cytoplasm. The secretory granules measure 100–250 nm, and fewer are present than in normal somatotrophs or densely granulated adenomas.

Etiology & Pathogenesis

Excessive pituitary GH secretion may be secondary to abnormal hypothalamic function, but current evidence suggest that it is a primary pituitary disorder in most cases. Pituitary adenomas are present in virtually all patients and are usually greater than 1 cm in diameter; hyperplasia alone is rare, and nonadenomatous anterior pituitary tissue does not exhibit somatotroph hyperplasia when examined histologically. In addition, there is a return of normal GH levels and dynamic control of GH secretion following selective removal of the pituitary adenoma.

Indirect evidence that acromegaly may be a hypothalamic disorder consisting of either increased release of GRH or decreased secretion of somatostatin is based largely on the findings of abnormal GH dynamics in these patients.

Pathophysiology

In acromegaly, GH secretion is increased and its dynamic control is abnormal. Secretion remains episodic; however, the number, duration, and amplitude of secretory episodes are increased, and they occur randomly throughout the 24-hour period. The characteristic nocturnal surge is absent, and there are abnormal responses to suppression and stimulation. Thus, glucose suppressibility is lost (see diagnosis, below), and GH stimulation by hypoglycemia is usually absent. TRH and GnRH may cause GH release, whereas these substances do not normally stimulate GH secretion. Dopamine and dopamine agonists such as bromocriptine and apomorphine, which normally stimulate GH secretion, paradoxically cause GH suppression in about 70–80% of patients with acromegaly.

Most of the deleterious effects of chronic GH hypersection are caused by its stimulation of excessive amounts of the somatomedins (see Chapter 7), and plasma levels of these compounds are increased in acromegaly. The growth-promoting effects of the somatomedins (DNA, RNA, and protein synthesis) lead to the characteristic proliferation of bone, cartilage, and soft tissues and increase in size of other organs to produce the classic clinical manifestations of acromegaly. The insulin resistance and carbohydrate intolerance seen in acromegaly appear to be direct effects of GH and not due to somatomedin excess.

Clinical Findings

The sex incidence of acromegaly is approximately equal; the mean age at diagnosis is approximately 40 years; and the duration of symptoms is usually 5–10 years before the diagnosis is established.

Acromegaly is a chronic disabling and disfiguring disorder with increased late morbidity and mortality if untreated. Although spontaneous remissions have been described, the course is slowly progressive in the great majority of cases—patients once thought to be "burned out" can almost invariably be shown to have continuing clinical manifestations and GH hypersecretion.

A. Symptoms and Signs: Early manifestations (Table 6–8) include soft tissue proliferation, with enlargement of the hands and feet and coarsening of the facial features. This is usually accompanied by increased sweating, oiliness of the skin, fatigue, and weight gain.

At diagnosis, virtually all patients have classic manifestations; acral and soft tissue changes are always resent. Bone and cartilage changes affect chiefly the face and skull (Fig 6–14). These changes include thickening of the calvarium; increased size of the frontal sinuses, which leads to prominence of the supraorbital ridges; enlargement of the nose; and downward and forward growth of the mandible, which leads to prognathism and widely spaced teeth. Soft tissue growth also contributes to the facial appearance, with coarsening of the features and facial and infraorbital puffiness. The hands and feet are predominantly affected by soft tissue growth; they are large, thickened, and bulky, with blunt, spadelike fingers (Fig 6–15) and toes. A bulky, sweaty handshake frequently suggests the diagnosis, and there are increases in ring, glove, and shoe sizes. There is generalized thickening of the skin, with increased oiliness and sweating. Acne, sebaceous cysts, and fibromata mollusca (skin

Table 6–8. Clinical manifestations of acromegaly in 100 patients.[1]

Manifestations of GH excess	
Acral enlargement	100[2]
Soft tissue overgrowth	100
Hyperhidrosis	88
Lethargy or fatigue	87
Weight gain	73
Paresthesias	70
Joint pain	69
Photophobia	46
Papillomas	45
Hypertrichosis	33
Goiter	32
Acanthosis nigricans	29
Hypertension	24
Cardiomegaly	16
Renal calculi	11
Disturbance of other endocrine functions	
Hyperinsulinemia	70
Glucose intolerance	50
Irregular or absent menses	60
Decreased libido or impotence	46
Hypothyroidism	13
Galactorrhea	13
Gynecomastia	8
Hypoadrenalism	4
Local manifestations	
Enlarged sella	90
Headache	65
Visual deficit	20

[1]Adapted from Tyrrell JB, Wilson CB: Pituitary syndromes. In: *Surgical Endocrinology: Clinical Syndromes.* Friesen SR (editor). Lippincott, 1978.
[2]Percentage of patients in whom these features were present.

tags and papillomas) are common, as is acanthosis nigricans of the axillae and neck and hypertrichosis in women.

These bony and soft tissue changes are accompanied by systemic manifestations, which include hyperhidrosis, heat intolerance, lethargy, fatigue, and increased sleep requirement. Moderate weight gain usually occurs. Paresthesias, usually due to carpal tunnel compression, occur in 70%; sensorimotor neuropathies occur uncommonly. Bone and cartilage overgrowth leads to arthralgias and in long-standing cases to degenerative arthritis of the spine, hips, and knees. Photophobia of unknown cause occurs in about half of cases and is most troublesome in bright sunlight and during night driving.

GH excess leads to generalized visceromegaly, clinically evident as thyromegaly and enlargement of the salivary glands. Enlargement of other organs is usually not clinically detectable.

Hypertension of unknown cause occurs in about 25% of patients and cardiomegaly in about 15%. Cardiac enlargement may be secondary to hypertension, atherosclerotic disease, or, rarely, to "acromegalic cardiomyopathy." Renal calculi occur in 11% secondary to the hypercalciuria induced by GH excess.

Other endocrine and metabolic abnormalities are common and may be due either to GH excess or to mechanical effects of the pituitary adenoma. Glucose

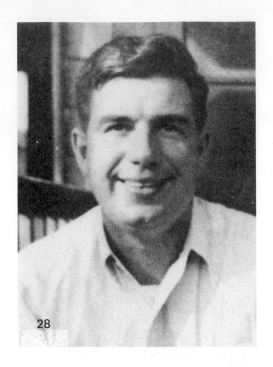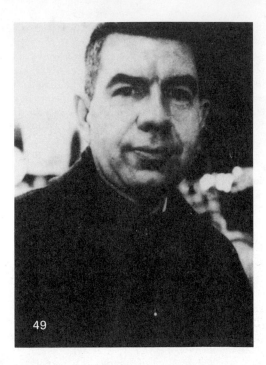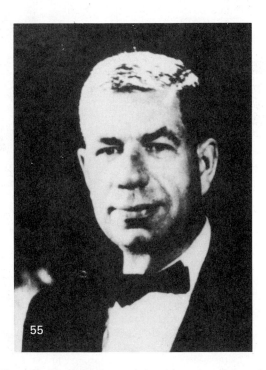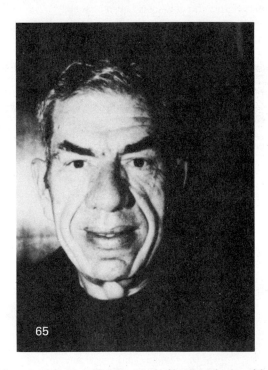

Figure 6–14. Serial photographs of an acromegalic patient at the ages indicated. Note the gradual increase in size of the nose, lips, and skin folds. (Reproduced, with permission, from Reichlin SR: Acromegaly. *Med Grand Rounds* 1982;1:9.)

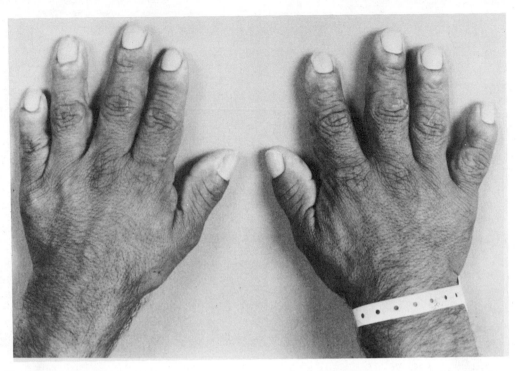

Figure 6–15. Markedly increased soft tissue bulk and blunt fingers in a middle-aged man with acromegaly.

intolerance and hyperinsulinism occur in 50% and 70%, respectively, owing to GH-induced insulin resistance. Overt clinical diabetes occurs in a minority, and diabetic ketoacidosis is rare. Hypogonadism occurs in 60% of female and 46% of male patients and is of multifactorial origin; tumor growth and compression may impair pituitary gonadotropin secretion, and associated hyperprolactinemia (see below) or the PRL-like effect of excessive GH secretion may impair gonadotropin and gonadal function. In men, low total plasma testosterone levels may be due to GH suppression of sex hormone–binding globulin (SHBG) levels; in these cases, plasma free testosterone levels may be normal, with normal gonadal function. With earlier diagnosis, hypothyroidism and hypoadrenalism due to destruction of the normal anterior pituitary are unusual and are present in only 13% and 4% of patients, respectively. Galactorrhea occurs in about 15% and is usually caused by hyperprolactinemia from a pituitary adenoma with a mixed cell population of somatotrophs and lactotrophs. Gynecomastia of unknown cause occurs in about 10% of men. Although acromegaly may be a component of multiple endocrine neoplasia (MEN) type I syndrome, it is distinctly unusual, and concomitant parathyroid hyperfunction or pancreatic islet cell tumors are rare.

When GH hypersecretion is present for many years, late complications occur, including progressive cosmetic deformity and disabling degenerative arthritis (which frequently requires operative treatment). In addition, the mortality rate is increased; after age 45, the death rate in acromegaly from cardiovascular and cerebrovascular atherosclerosis and respiratory diseases is twice that of the healthy population. Death rates are highest in patients with hypertension or clinical diabetes mellitus.

Manifestations of the pituitary adenoma are also common in acromegaly; eg, 65% of patients have headache. Although visual impairment was usually present in older series, it now occurs in only 15–20%, since most patients are now diagnosed because of the manifestations of GH excess.

B. Laboratory Findings: Postprandial plasma glucose may be elevated, and serum insulin is increased in 70%. Elevated serum phosphorus (due to increased renal tubular resorption of phosphate) and hypercalciuria appear to be due to direct effects of GH or somatomedins.

C. X-Ray Findings: Plain films (Fig 6–16) show sellar enlargement in 90% of cases. Thickening of the calvarium, enlargement of the frontal and maxillary sinuses, and enlargement of the jaw can also be seen. Radiographs of the hand show increased soft tissue bulk, "arrowhead" tufting of the distal phalanges, increased width of intra-articular cartilages, and cystic changes of the carpal bones. Radiographs of the feet show similar changes, and there is increased thickness of the heel pad (normal, < 22 mm).

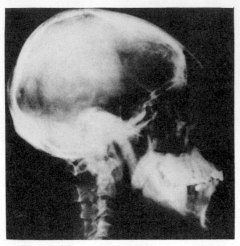
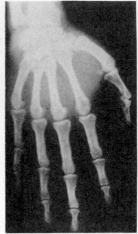
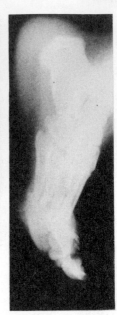

Figure 6–16. Radiologic signs in acromegaly: *Left:* Skull with enlarged sella turcica and frontal sinuses, thickening of the calvarium, and enlargement of the mandible. *Center:* Hand with enlarged sesamoid bone and increased soft tissue shadows. *Right:* Thickened heel pad. (Reproduced, with permission, from Levin SR: Manifestations and treatment of acromegaly. *Calif Med* [March] 1972;116:57.)

Diagnosis

Acromegaly is usually clinically obvious and can be readily confirmed by assessment of GH secretion; basal fasting GH levels (normal, 1–5 ng/mL [46.5–232 pmol/L]) are greater than 10 ng/mL in over 90% of patients and range from 5 ng/mL (232 pmol/L) to over 500 ng/mL (23,255 pmol/L), with a mean of approximately 50 ng/mL (2325 pmol/L). However, single measurements are not entirely reliable, because GH secretion is episodic in acromegaly and because other conditions may increase GH secretion (see below).

A. Glucose Suppression: Suppression with oral glucose is the simplest and most specific dynamic test for acromegaly. In healthy subjects, oral administration of 100 g of glucose causes a reduction of the GH level to less than 5 ng/mL (232 pmol/L) at 60 minutes. In acromegaly, GH levels may decrease, increase, or show no change; however, they do not decrease to less than 5 ng/mL (232 pmol/L), and this lack of response establishes the diagnosis.

B. Other Tests: Additional procedures that help establish or confirm the diagnosis are (1) GH stimulation with TRH; (2) the absence of a nocturnal GH surge; and (3) the paradoxic suppression of GH by levodopa, dopamine, bromocriptine, or apomorphine. These procedures are usually unnecessary except in patients with mild acromegaly who may have normal or only mildly elevated GH levels and equivocal responses to glucose suppression.

C. Somatomedin Measurement: Measurement of somatomedin-C (see Chapter 7) is a useful means of establishing a diagnosis of GH hypersecretion, although at present many methods lack specificity and measurements may not be clinically available. Somatomedin levels are elevated in virtually all patients with acromegaly (normal ranges vary widely in different laboratories). Although they confirm the diagnosis, a clear-cut advantage over GH suppression with glucose has yet to be established. Further experience may elucidate the role of somatomedin measurements; however, direct measurement of GH secretion, the product of the pituitary adenoma, will continue to be necessary in diagnosis and follow-up.

D. Tumor Localization: Radiographic localization of the pituitary adenoma causing acromegaly is usually straightforward (see Neuroradiologic Evaluation, above). In virtually all patients, tumor location and size can be shown by MRI or CT scanning; 90% have tumors over 1 cm in diameter that are readily visualized. In the rare patient with normal neuroradiologic studies, an extrapituitary ectopic source of GH or GRH should be considered. If the scans suggest diffuse pituitary enlargement or hyperplasia, ectopic GRH should also be suspected.

Differential Diagnosis

A. Other Causes of GH Hypersecretion: The presence of clinical features of GH excess, elevated GH secretion, and abnormal GH dynamics, together with the demonstration of a pituitary tumor by neuroradiologic studies, is diagnostic of acromegaly. However, other conditions associated with GH hypersecretion must be considered in the differential diagnosis: anxiety, exercise, acute illness, chronic renal failure, cirrhosis, starvation, protein-calorie malnutrition, anorexia nervosa, and type I (insulin-dependent) diabetes mellitus. Estrogen therapy may increase GH responsiveness to various stimuli. These conditions may be associated with abnormal GH suppressibility by glucose and by abnormal GH responsiveness to TRH; however, patients with these conditions do not have clinical manifestations of GH excess and are thus readily differentiated from patients with acromegaly.

B. Ectopic GH or GRH Secretion: There is a rare group of patients who have acromegaly due to ectopic secretion of GH or GRH and in whom clinical manifestations of acromegaly may be typical. This may occur in lung carcinoma, carcinoid tumors, and pancreatic islet cell tumors. These syndromes should be suspected in patients with a known extrapituitary tumor who have GH excess or in those with clinical and biochemical features of acromegaly who have radiologic procedures that show normal pituitary glands or that suggest diffuse pituitary enlargement or hyperplasia.

Treatment

All patients with acromegaly should undergo therapy to halt progression of the disorder and to prevent late complications. The objectives of therapy are removal or destruction of the pituitary tumor, reversal of GH hypersecretion, and maintenance of normal anterior and posterior pituitary function. These objectives are currently attainable in most patients, especially those with smaller tumors and only moderate GH hypersecretion. In patients with large tumors who have marked GH hypersecretion, several therapies are usually required to achieve normal GH secretion.

Various criteria exist for what constitutes an adequate response to therapy. Most authors agree that basal GH values under 5 ng/mL (232 pmol/L) indicate the return of normal GH secretion. The utility of somatomedin-C measurements is currently being evaluated, and preliminary results show that appropriate therapy lowers these values to normal.

The choice of initial therapy is between transsphenoidal microsurgery, radiotherapy, and medical management. Microsurgery is preferred because of its high success rate, rapid reduction of GH levels, the low incidence of postoperative hypopituitarism, and the low surgical morbidity rate. Conventional radiotherapy (x-ray radiation) is also successful, although a much longer period is required to reduce GH levels to normal, and heavy particle irradiation has limited availability. Medical management with bromocriptine has the disadvantage of requiring chronic therapy to suppress GH secretion, and it is generally used in patients who have not responded to surgery or irradia-

tion. Octreotide acetate, a long-acting somatostatin analogue, is currently being evaluated in the treatment of acromegaly.

A. Surgical: Transsphenoidal selective adenoma removal is the procedure of choice; craniotomy is necessary in the few patients in whom major suprasellar extension precludes the transsphenoidal approach. Successful reduction of GH levels is achieved in approximately 80% of patients. In those with small or moderate-sized tumors (< 2 cm), success is achieved in over 90%, whereas in those with larger tumors and basal GH levels greater than 50 ng/mL (2325 pmol/L)—and particularly in those with major extrasellar extension of the adenoma—successful responses occur in only 60–70%. Recurrence rates in those with a successful initial response are low (about 5% of patients at our institution). Surgical complications (discussed above) occur in less than 10%.

B. Radiologic: Conventional supervoltage irradiation in doses of 4500–5000 rads is successful in 60–80% of patients, although GH levels may not return to normal until several years after therapy. Thus, in one recent series, GH levels were under 10 ng/mL (465 pmol/L) in only 38% of patients at 2 years posttreatment; however, at 5 and 10 years, 73% and 81% had achieved such levels. The incidence of hypopituitarism is appreciable, and in this series hypothyroidism occurred in 19%, hypoadrenalism in 38%, and hypogonadism in approximately 50–60% of patients as a consequence of radiotherapy. Because of the prolonged delay in achieving reduction in GH levels, conventional radiotherapy is generally reserved for patients with persisting GH secretion following pituitary microsurgery.

Heavy particle irradiation is more rapidly effective than conventional irradiation, but because of the limitations of the field size, it can be used only in patients with smaller tumors and those in whom no extrasellar extension is present. About 80% of patients have GH levels under 10 ng/mL (465 pmol/L) at 5 years after irradiation, with most patients having a satisfactory response at 2 years. The incidence of hypopituitarism has been variously reported, but it appears to occur in approximately 40% of patients.

Therapy of acromegaly by radioactive implants within the sella turcica is limited to a few centers. Successful responses are achieved in about 70%; however, there is a significant incidence of hypopituitarism, cerebrospinal fluid rhinorrhea, and meningitis due to local radionecrosis. Because of these complications, the procedure has not gained wide acceptance.

C. Medical: Bromocriptine, a long-acting dopamine agonist, reduces GH levels in 60–80% of patients; however, only a few patients attain levels of 10 ng/mL (465 pmol/L) or less. In addition, although reduction in tumor size occurs in some patients, this therapy is suppressive only, and GH hypersecretion rapidly recurs upon discontinuation of the drug. For these reasons, bromocriptine is generally used in acromegalics in whom adequate reduction of GH levels has not been achieved with surgery or irradiation.

Octreotide acetate, a long-acting analogue of somatostatin, has been effective in the management of acromegaly. It reduces levels of growth hormone and somatomedin-C to normal in the majority of patients treated, and in some it has even caused tumor shrinkage. Effective doses appear to be in the range of 100–500 μg given by subcutaneous injection 3 times daily. The need for subcutaneous injection is a disadvantage, since chronic therapy is required. The long-term effects of this therapy are not yet known.

Response to Treatment

In patients with successful reduction in GH hypersecretion, there is cessation of bone overgrowth. In addition, these patients experience considerable clinical improvement, including reduction in soft tissue bulk of the extremities, decreased facial puffiness, increased energy, and cessation of hyperhidrosis, heat intolerance, and oily skin. Headache, carpal tunnel syndrome, arthralgias, and photophobia are also reversible with successful therapy. Glucose intolerance and hyperinsulinemia as well as hypercalciuria are also reversed in most cases.

In patients in whom operation is successful, reversal of clinical features is more rapid; decreased sweating and the onset of soft tissue regression may occur within a few days after surgery. The response to radiation therapy is much slower and occurs gradually over months to years.

Posttreatment Follow-Up

Patients undergoing surgery should be seen 4–6 weeks after the operation for assessment of GH secretion and pituitary function. Those with persisting GH hypersecretion should receive further therapy with radiation or bromocriptine. Patients with postoperative GH levels under 10 ng/mL (465 pmol/L) should have follow-up GH determinations at 6-month intervals for 2 years and yearly thereafter. Late hypopituitarism after surgery alone does not occur.

Patients treated with radiotherapy either primarily or following unsuccessful surgery should have biannual assessment of GH secretion and annual assessment of anterior pituitary function, since the incidence of late hypopituitarism is appreciable and increases with time following irradiation.

3. ACTH-SECRETING PITUITARY ADENOMAS: CUSHING'S DISEASE

In 1932, Harvey Cushing documented the presence of small basophilic pituitary adenomas in 6 to 8 patients with clinical features of adrenocortical hyperfunction. Years later, ACTH hypersecretion was identified from such tumors and found to be the cause of bilateral adrenal hyperplasia. Pituitary ACTH hypersecretion (Cushing's disease) is now recognized as the most common cause of spontaneous hypercortisolism (Cushing's syndrome) and must be distinguished from the other forms of adrenocorticosteroid excess—ectopic ACTH syndrome and adrenal tumors (see Chapter 12).

Pathology

ACTH-secreting pituitary tumors exist in virtually all patients with Cushing's disease. These tumors are usually benign microadenomas under 10 mm in diameter; 50% are 5 mm or less in diameter, and microadenomas as small as 1 mm have been described. These tumors in Cushing's disease are either basophilic or chromophobe adenomas and may be found anywhere within the anterior pituitary. Rarely, ACTH-secreting tumors are large, with invasive tendencies, and malignant tumors have occasionally been reported.

Histologically, the tumors are composed of compact sheets of uniform, well-granulated cells (granule size, 200–700 nm by electron microscopy) with a sinusoidal arrangement and a high content of ACTH and its related peptides (β-LPH, β-endorphin). A zone of perinuclear hyalinization (Crooke's changes) is frequently observed as a result of exposure of the corticotroph cells to prolonged hypercortisolism. A specific ultrastructural finding in these adenomas is the deposition of bundles of perinuclear microfilaments that encircle the nucleus; these are the ultrastructural equivalent of Crooke's hyaline changes seen on light microscopy. In contrast to the adenomas cells, ACTH content in the portion of the anterior pituitary not involved with the tumor is decreased.

Diffuse hyperplasia of anterior pituitary corticotrophs or adenomatous hyperplasia, presumed to result from hypersecretion of corticotropin-releasing hormone (CRH), occurs rarely.

The adrenal glands in Cushing's disease are enlarged, weighing 12–24 g (normal, 8–10 g). Microscopic examination shows a thickened cortex due to hyperplasia of both the zona reticularis and zona fasciculata; the zona glomerulosa is normal. In some cases, ACTH-secreting pituitary adenomas cause bilateral nodular hyperplasia; the adrenals show diffuse bilateral cortical hyperplasia and the presence of one or more nodules that vary from microscopic to several centimeters in diameter, with multiple small nodules being the most common. Occasionally, only a solitary nodule is observed on radiographic studies, and this entity may be confused with an autonomously functioning adrenal tumor (see Chapter 12).

Pathogenesis

The weight of current evidence is that Cushing's disease is a primary pituitary disorder and that hypothalamic abnormalities are secondary to hypercortisolism. Nonetheless, many authorities still believe that this disorder is the result of a primary central nervous system abnormality with excessive stimulation of anterior pituitary corticotrophs by CRH and secondary adenoma formation.

The endocrine abnormalities in Cushing's disease are as follows: (1) hypersecretion of ACTH, with bilateral adrenocortical hyperplasia and hypercortisolism; (2) absent circadian periodicity of ACTH and cortisol secretion; (3) absent responsiveness of ACTH and cortisol to stress (hypoglycemia or surgery); (4) abnormal negative feedback of ACTH secretion by glucocorticoids; and (5) subnormal responsiveness of GH, TSH, and gonadotropins to stimulation.

A primary central nervous system defect could explain these observed abnormalities in Cushing's disease as well as the occasional finding that certain pharmacologic agents such as cyproheptadine and bromocriptine inhibit ACTH release in a few patients with Cushing's disease.

However, evidence that Cushing's disease is a primary pituitary disorder is based on the high frequency of pituitary adenomas, the response to their removal, and the interpretation of hypothalamic abnormalities as being secondary to hypercortisolism. These findings suggest that ACTH hypersecretion arises from a spontaneously developing pituitary adenoma and that the resulting hypercortisolism suppresses the normal hypothalamic-pituitary axis and CRH release and thereby abolishes the hypothalamic regulation of circadian variability and stress responsiveness. There is in vitro evidence that the negative feedback effects of glucocorticoids are exerted directly on the pituitary tumor and that other pharmacologic agents such as vasopressin, cyproheptadine, and bromocriptine directly inhibit the ACTH-secreting adenoma. In addition, the abnormalities of GH, TSH, and gonadotropin secretion are also observed in exogenous Cushing's syndrome and are due to the hypercortisolism per se and not to a primary hypothalamic disorder.

Analysis of the response to therapy by pituitary microsurgery sheds some light on the pathogenesis of Cushing's disease. Selective removal of pituitary microadenomas by transsphenoidal microsurgery corrects ACTH hypersecretion and hypercortisolism in most patients. This suggests that the adenoma—not corticotroph hyperplasia—is responsible for the ACTH excess. Postoperatively, these patients experience transient ACTH deficiency with secondary hypoadrenalism. ACTH response to CRH is blunted immediately after complete removal of these tumors. The secretion of the other anterior pituitary hormones is not only preserved but enhanced once the microadenoma is removed. These findings, which suggest that the normal hypothalamic-pituitary axis is suppressed by the hypercortisolism, are supported by the in vitro demonstration of markedly decreased ACTH content in nonadenomatous pituitary tissue removed from patients with active Cushing's disease. After selective removal of the pituitary adenoma, the following return to normal: the circadian rhythmicity of

ACTH and cortisol, the responsiveness of the hypothalamic-pituitary axis to hypoglycemic stress, and the dexamethasone suppressibility of cortisol secretion. Thus, in these patients, there is no evidence for a persisting hypothalamic abnormality.

Clinical Findings

Cushing's disease presents with the signs and symptoms of hypercortisolism and adrenal androgen excess (see Chapter 12). The onset of these features is usually insidious, developing over months or years. Obesity (with predominantly central fat distribution), hypertension, glucose intolerance, and gonadal dysfunction (amenorrhea or impotence) are common features. Other common manifestations include moon facies, plethora, osteopenia, proximal muscle weakness, easy bruisability, psychologic disturbances, violaceous striae, hirsutism, acne, poor wound healing, and superficial fungal infections. Unlike patients with the classic form of ectopic ACTH syndrome, patients with Cushing's disease rarely have hypokalemia, weight loss, anemia, or hyperpigmentation. Virilization, observed occasionally in patients with adrenal carcinoma, is unusual in Cushing's disease. Clinical symptoms related to the ACTH-secreting primary tumor itself, such as headache or visual impairment, are rare because of early diagnosis and the small size of these adenomas.

The usual age range is 20–40 years, but Cushing's disease has been reported in infants and patients over 70. There is a female:male ratio of approximately 8:1. In contrast, the ectopic ACTH syndrome occurs more commonly in men (male:female ratio of 3:1).

Diagnosis

The initial step in the diagnosis of an ACTH-secreting pituitary adenoma is the documentation of endogenous hypercortisolism, which is confirmed by the presence of abnormal cortisol suppressibility to low-dose dexamethasone as well as an increased basal urine free cortisol or cortisol secretory rate. A more complete discussion of the diagnosis and differential diagnosis of Cushing's syndrome is presented in Chapter 12. The discussion here emphasizes the diagnosis of ACTH-secreting pituitary tumors.

The differentiation of an ACTH-secreting pituitary tumor from other causes of hypercortisolism must be based on biochemical studies, of which the measurement of basal plasma ACTH levels and the response to high-dose dexamethasone suppression testing are the most reliable.

A. ACTH Levels: Patients with Cushing's disease have normal or modestly elevated ACTH levels ranging from 40 to 200 pg/mL (8.8–44 pmol/L) (normal, 20–100 pg/mL [4.4–22.2 pmol/L]). Low levels (< 20 pg/mL [4.4 pmol/L]) are indicative of an autonomously secreting adrenal tumor, and levels greater than 200 pg/mL (44 pmol/L) suggest an ectopic ACTH-secreting neoplasm. Unfortunately, plasma

ACTH levels do not adequately differentiate pituitary from ectopic sources of ACTH hypersecretion. Thus, 30–40% of patients with the ectopic ACTH syndrome have ACTH levels (100–200 pg/mL [22.2–44 pmol/L]) that are in the range seen in Cushing's disease, and some patients actually have "normal" measurements (see Chapter 12).

B. Dexamethasone Suppression Tests: Although all patients with Cushing's syndrome have disordered regulation of glucocorticoid feedback at the hypothalamic-pituitary level (eg, failure of suppression with low-dose dexamethasone), some negative glucocorticoid feedback effect is maintained by ACTH-secreting pituitary tumors. Thus, administration of high-dose dexamethasone will suppress plasma or urine corticosteroids. The standard 2-day suppression test of Liddle requires administration of 2 mg of dexamethasone every 6 hours for 2 days. In patients with Cushing's disease, urine 17-hydroxycorticosteroids should fall to less than 50% of basal levels on the second day of dexamethasone therapy; failure of suppression indicates either an ectopic ACTH-secreting tumor or an adrenal neoplasm.

The rapid overnight high-dose dexamethasone test (see Chapter 12) is a reliable and simpler means of distinguishing ACTH-secreting pituitary tumors from other forms of endogenous hypercortisolism: The administration of 8 mg of dexamethasone at 11 PM will suppress plasma cortisol to less than 50% of baseline in Cushing's disease; failure of plasma cortisol to be suppressed indicates either ectopic ACTH syndrome or an adrenal tumor.

Caution must be urged in interpreting the results of these high-dose dexamethasone suppression tests, since they are not entirely specific. About 20–30% of patients with proved ACTH-secreting tumors fail to suppress basal urine steroids to less than 50% with the standard 2-day test, and some patients with ectopic ACTH syndrome (bronchial carcinoid; thymomas) do suppress with high-dose dexamethasone (see Chapter 12).

C. CRH Testing: CRH stimulation testing has recently been employed as a means of differentiating pituitary from ectopic causes of Cushing's syndrome. In patients with Cushing's disease, the administration of CRH causes a further increase in ACTH and cortisol levels. In contrast, patients with ectopic ACTH syndrome usually have no ACTH or cortisol responses to CRH. However, several exceptions to these typical responses have been observed.

D. Radiologic Procedures: Neuroradiologic techniques are not particularly useful in the localization of ACTH-secreting pituitary adenomas. Since these tumors average only 5 mm in diameter and exceed 1 cm in diameter in only 10% of cases, findings on plain films of the sella turcica are almost always normal.

High-resolution CT or MRI scanning of the sella turcica localizes pituitary adenomas in less than 50% of cases of ACTH-secreting pituitary adenomas. Both false-positive and false-negative findings occur—emphasizing again the importance of using clinical and biochemical techniques to establish the diagnosis of an ACTH-secreting microadenoma.

Roentgenographic studies of the adrenal glands in Cushing's disease must be interpreted with caution. CT scanning may demonstrate normal, enlarged, or asymmetric adrenal glands; and nodular adrenal hyperplasia secondary to an ACTH-secreting pituitary tumor may appear as a solitary adrenal mass and mimic an adrenal neoplasm. Radioactive iodocholesterol scanning of the adrenals is helpful in such cases, since it can usually differentiate between bilateral adrenocortical hyperfunction and a single adrenal tumor.

E. Petrosal Sinus ACTH Sampling: The studies that are employed for the differential diagnosis of ACTH-dependent Cushing's syndrome frequently cannot distinguish pituitary from ectopic ACTH hypersecretion, especially when the neoplasm is small or occult. Therefore, bilateral simultaneous petrosal sinus ACTH sampling with CRH stimulation of ACTH release is now the procedure of choice for patients with occult lesions. This study must be performed by a radiologist skilled in catheterization techniques. Petrosal sinus ACTH sampling may also lateralize the side of the lesion, thus assisting the surgeon in localizing the tumor.

Problems in Diagnosis

Patients with ectopic ACTH syndrome may be clinically indistinguishable from those with Cushing's disease, and the tumor in each may be radiologically occult. With the advent of specific therapy directed at pituitary microadenomas, establishing the presence or absence of a pituitary source of ACTH hypersecretion is essential. As noted above, selective venous ACTH sampling from the inferior petrosal sinus (pituitary venous effluent) is a useful aid in differential diagnosis.

Problems in diagnosis may also result from intermittent Cushing's disease. In this unusual form of the disorder, ACTH-cortisol hypersecretion fluctuates with periods of normal secretion, during which laboratory studies will be misleading. Proper biochemical confirmation may require repeated studies in these patients.

Treatment

The increasing clinical recognition of ACTH-secreting pituitary microadenomas and the clarification of their role in the pathogenesis of Cushing's disease have led to advances in treatment of this disorder. Sophisticated microsurgical techniques now permit removal of pituitary tumors by a transsphenoidal approach. A variety of other therapies—operative, radiologic, pharmacologic—are discussed below.

A. Surgical: Selective transsphenoidal resection of ACTH-secreting pituitary adenomas is the initial treatment of choice. Independent series from several centers have confirmed the efficacy of this procedure as well as its low morbidity rate and low incidence of surgical complications. The indication for this procedure is a secure biochemical diagnosis, as discussed earlier. Neuroradiologic procedures are employed preoperatively, but findings may be normal because of the small size of these tumors. In these patients, petrosal sinus ACTH sampling for ACTH should be performed before surgery, as noted above.

At operation, meticulous exploration of the intrasellar contents by an experienced neurosurgeon is required. The tumor, which is often found within the anterior lobe tissue, is selectively removed, and normal gland is left intact. If the tumor is too small to locate at surgery, total hypophysectomy may be performed in adult patients who are past the age of reproduction and whose biochemical diagnosis has been confirmed with selective venous ACTH sampling.

In about 85% of patients with microadenomas, selective microsurgery is successful in correcting hypercortisolism. Surgical damage to anterior pituitary function is rare, but most patients develop transient secondary adrenocortical insufficiency requiring postoperative glucocorticoid support until the hypothalamic-pituitary-adrenal axis recovers, usually in 6–18 months. Total hypophysectomy is necessary to correct hypercortisolism in another 10% of patients. In the remaining 5% of patients with microadenomas, selective tumor removal is unsuccessful. By contrast, transsphenoidal surgery is successful in only 25% of the 10–15% of patients with Cushing's disease with pituitary macroadenomas or in those with extrasellar extension of tumor.

Transient diabetes insipidus occurs in about 20% of patients, but other surgical complications (eg, hemorrhage, cerebrospinal fluid rhinorrhea, infection, visual impairment, permanent diabetes insipidus) are rare. Hypopituitarism occurs only in patients who undergo total hypophysectomy.

Before the introduction of pituitary microsurgery, bilateral total adrenalectomy was the preferred treatment of Cushing's disease and may still be employed in patients in whom other therapies are unsuccessful. Total adrenalectomy usually corrects hypercortisolism but produces permanent hypoadrenalism, requiring lifelong glucocorticoid and mineralocorticoid therapy. Morbidity is high and relates to poor wound healing, postoperative infection, pancreatic injury, and thromboembolic phenomena. In addition, the ACTH-secreting pituitary adenoma persists and may progress, causing hyperpigmentation and invasive complications (Nelson's syndrome; see below). Persistent hypercortisolism may occasionally follow total adrenalectomy as ACTH hypersection stimulates adrenal remnants or congenital rests. Attempts to transplant adrenal tissue

to a readily accessible location, such as the forearm, have been successful in only a few cases and may require several years before the transplant functions satisfactorily; recurrent hyperfunction may result.

B. Radiologic: In Cushing's disease, conventional irradiation in doses of 4500–5000 rads leads to biochemical and clinical improvement in only 15–25% of adults—although it can lead to improvement in as many as 80% of children. Adjunctive antiadrenal drug therapy has been used with some success, but the ultimate response to radiation therapy is often unsatisfactory, and prolonged drug therapy is required. Because of these low response rates, we do not recommend conventional irradiation as initial therapy.

Heavy particle irradiation, also used as initial therapy in patients with no extrasellar tumor extension, is currently available at only one center in the USA. Alpha particle irradiation is effective in controlling hypercortisolism in 80% of patients, with an incidence of hypopituitarism of approximately one-third. Proton beam therapy is effective in 65% of patients, with a similar incidence of hypopituitarism. Neurologic complications of both forms of therapy include visual loss and oculomotor paralysis. With both of these techniques, there is a lag period of 6–12 months or longer before cortisol secretion returns to normal.

Implantation of radioactive seeds (gold and yttrium) within the sella turcica has also been used in Cushing's disease. Such techniques have achieved a remission rate of 65%, with an additional 16% improved; however, the frequency of operative complications is high, and panhypopituitarism is common.

C. Medical: Drugs that inhibit adrenal cortisol secretion are useful in Cushing's disease, often as adjunctive therapy (see Chapter 12).

Ketoconazole, an imidazole derivative used as a broad-spectrum antimycotic agent, has been found to strongly inhibit adrenal steroid biosynthesis. It inhibits cytochrome P-450 enzymes, blocking the 14-demethylation of lanosterol to cholesterol, as well as inhibiting the cholesterol side chain cleavage and the 11-hydroxylase enzymes. In daily doses of 600–1200 mg, ketoconazole has been effective in the management of Cushing's syndrome. It is also less expensive than other antiadrenal medications. Hepatotoxicity is common, however, but may be transient.

Metyrapone, an 11β-hydroxylase inhibitor, and **aminoglutethimide,** which inhibits conversion of cholesterol to pregnenolone, have both been utilized to reduce cortisol hypersecretion. These drugs are expensive; their use is accompanied by increased ACTH levels that may overcome the enzyme inhibition; and both agents cause gastrointestinal side effects that may limit their effectiveness. More effective control of hypercortisolism with fewer side effects is obtained by combined use of these agents. Adequate data are not available on the long-term use of these drugs as the sole treatment of Cushing's disease. Thus, ketoconazole, metyrapone, and aminoglutethimide ordinarily are used while awaiting a response to therapy or in the preparation of patients for surgery.

The adrenolytic drug **mitotane** (Lysodren; *o,p'*-DDD) results in adrenal atrophy predominantly of the zonae fasciculata and reticularis. Remission of hypercortisolism is achieved in approximately 80% of patients with Cushing's disease, but most relapse after therapy is discontinued. Mitotane therapy is limited by the delayed response, which may take weeks or months, and by the frequent side effects, including sever nausea, vomiting, diarrhea, somnolence, and skin rash.

Pharmacologic inhibition of ACTH secretion in Cushing's disease has also been attempted. **Cyproheptadine,** a drug with antiserotonin, antihistamine, and anticholinergic effects, has had the widest use. Although a few well-documented cases of clinical and biochemical remission of Cushing's disease have been reported with its use, cyproheptadine causes unpleasant side effects (sedation, increase appetite, and weight gain) and is usually ineffective in treating ACTH-secreting pituitary adenomas. **Bromocriptine,** a dopamine agonist, has been reported to be effective in rare cases and should probably be reserved for those few patients who have hyperprolactinemia associated with Cushing's disease.

4. ACTH-SECRETING PITUITARY TUMORS FOLLOWING ADRENALECTOMY FOR CUSHING'S DISEASE: NELSON'S SYNDROME

The clinical appearance of an ACTH-secreting pituitary adenoma following bilateral adrenalectomy in patients with Cushing's disease was initially described by Nelson et al in 1958.

Pathogenesis
Based on current evidence, it now seems likely that Nelson's syndrome represents the clinical progression of a preexisting adenoma after the restraint of hypercortisolism on ACTH secretion and tumor growth is removed. That ACTH secretion in Cushing's disease is restrained by the circulating cortisol levels is demonstrated by its stimulation with metyrapone. Furthermore, the tumors in Nelson's syndrome are dexamethasone-suppressible, although larger doses may be required than with untreated Cushing's disease. Thus, following adrenalectomy, the suppressive effect of cortisol is no longer present, ACTH secretion increases, and the adenoma may progress.

Incidence
The incidence of Nelson's syndrome ranges from 10 to 78%, depending on what criteria are used for diagnosis (see Chapter 12). Pituitary irradiation before or after adrenalectomy does not prevent the development

of this syndrome. Approximately 30% of patients adrenalectomized for Cushing's disease develop classic Nelson's syndrome with progressive hyperpigmentation and an obvious ACTH-secreting tumor; another 50% develop evidence of a microadenoma without marked progression; and about 20% never develop a progressive tumor. The reasons for these differences in clinical behavior are uncertain, and they cannot be predicted prior to adrenal surgery. Continued examination, including plasma ACTH levels, visual fields, and sellar radiology, is required following bilateral adrenalectomy in patients with Cushing's disease.

Clinical Findings
The pituitary tumors in patients with classic Nelson's syndrome are among the most aggressive and rapidly growing of all pituitary tumors. These patients present with hyperpigmentation and with manifestations of an expanding intrasellar mass lesion. Visual field defects, headache, cavernous sinus invasion with extraocular muscle palsies, and even malignant changes with local or distant metastases may occur. Pituitary apoplexy may also complicate the course of these tumors.

Diagnosis
Plasma ACTH levels are markedly elevated, usually over 1000 pg/mL (222 pmol/L) and often as high as 10,000 pg/mL (2220 pmol/L). The sella turcica is enlarged on routine radiographs; CT or MRI scanning defines the extent of the tumor.

Treatment
Pituitary surgery, either by the transsphenoidal approach or by transfrontal craniotomy, is the initial mode of treatment. Complete resection is usually not possible, because of the large size of these tumors. Conventional radiotherapy alone is satisfactory in a minority of patients but is often employed postoperatively in patients with extrasellar extension.

5. THYROTROPIN-SECRETING PITUITARY ADENOMAS

Thyrotropin-secreting pituitary adenomas have been the subject of isolated case reports. Clinically, these rare tumors are usually manifested by hyperthyroidism with goiter in the presence of elevated TSH. Patients with TSH-secreting tumors are often resistant to routine ablative thyroid therapy, requiring large, often multiple doses of ^{131}I and several operations for control of thyrotoxicosis. Histologically, the tumors are chromophobe adenomas. They are often very large and cause visual impairment, which alerts the physician to a pituitary abnormality. Although a patient has been described whose massive TSH-secreting adenoma invaded the orbit, causing unilateral exophthalmos, most patients with these tumors do not have extrathyroidal systemic manifestations of Graves' disease (ophthalmopathy, dermopathy). Pituitary TSH hypersecretion in the absence of a demonstrable pituitary tumor has also been reported to cause hyperthyroidism in a few patients.

TSH dynamics are variable; TRH (protirelin) administration rarely stimulates TSH secretion from these tumors, nor do levodopa and bromocriptine suppress TSH as they do the TSH hypersecretion of primary hypothyroidism. The diagnosis is based on findings of hyperthyroidism with elevated TSH and neuroradiologic studies consistent with pituitary tumor. Differential diagnosis includes those equally rare patients with primary hypothyroidism (thyroid failure) who develop major hyperplasia of pituitary thyrotrophs with sellar enlargement and occasional suprasellar extension.

Treatment should be directed initially at the adenoma, with surgery or radiation therapy. If TSH hypersecretion persists, ablative treatment of the thyroid with either ^{131}I or surgery is necessary to achieve clinical remission of the thyrotoxic state.

Octreotide acetate, a long-acting somatostatin analogue, has been effective in decreasing TSH secretion from these tumors when given subcutaneously in doses similar to those used for the treatment of acromegaly (see above). Shrinkage of the tumor has also been observed. However, as mentioned previously, the long-term effects of this therapy are not yet known.

6. GONADOTROPIN-SECRETING PITUITARY ADENOMAS

Gonadotropin-secreting pituitary adenomas have been well documented in only a few patients. All reported cases have occurred in men; the majority hypersecreted only FSH, but tumors secreting both LH and FSH and a tumor secreting only LH have been described. Enlargement of the sella turcica has been noted in several patients with long-standing primary hypogonadism (eg, Klinefelter's syndrome). In most of these cases, a pituitary tumor was not proved histologically, and such sellar abnormalities probably reflect reactive pituitary enlargement and gonadotropin cell hyperplasia secondary to primary gonadal failure.

Gonadotropin-secreting pituitary adenomas are usually large chromophobe adenomas presenting with visual impairment and are often considered to be functionless before LH and FSH measurements are obtained. Testosterone levels may be low or elevated; in either case, the patients are frequently impotent or infertile. FSH and LH secretory dynamics are abnormal. GnRH may or may not stimulate gonadotropin release from these tumors, and testosterone administration results in subnormal or absent suppression. In addition, LH and FSH secretion in patients is often provoked by TRH, unlike the lack of stimulation observed in healthy individuals. The alpha subunit of the glycoprotein hormones is also secreted in excess from these tumors.

Therapy for gonadotropin-secreting adenomas has been directed at surgical removal. Because of their large size, adequate control of LH/FSH hypersecretion has not been achieved.

7. ALPHA SUBUNIT-SECRETING PITUITARY ADENOMAS

Excessive quantities of the alpha subunit of the glycoprotein pituitary hormones have been observed in association with the hypersecretion of many anterior pituitary hormones (TSH, GH, PRL, LH, FSH). Recently, however, pure alpha subunit hypersecretion has been identified in 2 male patients with large invasive chromophobe adenomas and partial panhypopituitarism. Isolated alpha subunit–secreting tumors may become increasingly recognized, and the determination of the alpha subunit may be a useful marker in patients with presumed "nonfunctioning" pituitary adenomas.

8. NONFUNCTIONAL PITUITARY ADENOMAS

Until recently, "nonfunctional" chromophobe adenomas represented approximately 80% of all primary pituitary tumors; however, with clinical application of radioimmunoassay of anterior pituitary hormones, these tumors currently account for only about 10% of all pituitary adenomas. Thus, the great majority of these chromophobe adenomas have now been documented to be PRL-secreting; a smaller number secrete TSH or the gonadotropins. The incidence of alpha subunit hypersecretion is currently under investigation, and it is likely that the increasing applications of such assays will further decrease the percentage of pituitary adenomas which are truly "nonsecreting."

Nonfunctional tumors are usually large when the diagnosis is established; headache and visual field defects are the usual presenting symptoms. However, endocrine manifestations are usually present for months to years before the diagnosis is made, with gonadotropin deficiency being the most common initial symptom. Hypothyroidism and hypoadrenalism are also common, but the symptoms are subtle and may be missed.

Evaluation should include CT or MRI scans and visual field testing; endocrine studies should include assessment of pituitary hormones and end-organ function to determine whether the adenoma is hypersecreting or whether hormonal replacement is needed.

Since these tumors are generally large, both surgery and radiation therapy are usually required to prevent tumor progression or recurrence. In the absence of an endocrine index of tumor hypersecretion such as PRL excess, serial scans at yearly intervals are required to assess the response to therapy and to detect possible recurrence.

REFERENCES

General

Besser GM (editor): The hypothalamus and pituitary. *Clin Endocrinol Metab* 1977;**6.** [Entire issue.]

Daughaday WH: The anterior pituitary. Chap 18, pp 568–613, in: *Williams Textbook of Endocrinology,* 7th ed. Wilson J, Foster DW (editors). Saunders, 1985.

Frohman LA: Diseases of the anterior pituitary. Chap 8, pp 247–337, in: *Endocrinology and Metabolism,* 2nd ed. Felig P et al (editors). McGraw-Hill, 1987.

Imura H (editor): *The Pituitary Gland.* Raven Press, 1985.

Martin JB, Reichlin S: *Clinical Neuroendocrinology,* 2nd ed. Davis, 1987.

ACTH: Cushing's Syndrome

Aron DC et al: Cushing's syndrome: Problems in diagnosis. *Medicine* 1981;**60:**25.

Aron DC et al: Cushing's syndrome: Problems in management. *Endocr Rev* 1982;**3:**229.

Aron DC, Findling JW, Tyrrell JB: Cushing's disease. *Endocrinol Metab Clin North Am* 1987;**16:**705.

Carey RM et al: Ectopic secretion of corticotropin-releasing factor as a cause of Cushing's syndrome: A clinical, morphologic, and biochemical study. *N Engl J Med* 1984;**311:**13.

Chrousos GP et al: Clinical applications of corticotropin-releasing factor. *Ann Intern Med* 1985;**102:**344.

Crapo L: Cushing's syndrome: A review of diagnostic tests. *Metabolism* 1979;**28:**955.

Cunningham SK et al: Normal cortisol response to corticotropin in patients with secondary adrenal failure. *Arch Intern Med* 1983;**143:**2276.

Findling JW, Aron DC, Tyrrell JB: Cushing's disease. In: *The Pituitary.* Imura H (editor). Raven Press, 1985.

Gold EM: The Cushing's syndromes: Changing views of diagnosis and treatment. *Ann Intern Med* 1979;**90:**829.

Krieger DT: *Cushing's Syndrome.* Springer-Verlag, 1982.

Landolt AM et al: Corticotrophin-releasing factor-test used with bilateral, simultaneous inferior petrosal sinus blood-sampling for the diagnosis of pituitary-dependent Cushing's disease. *Clin Endocrinol* 1986;**25:**687.

Lindholm J, Kehlet H: Reevaluation of the clinical value of the 30 min ACTH test in assessing the hypothalamic-pituitary-adrenocortical function. *Clin Endocrinol* 1987;**26:**53.

Mampalam TJ, Tyrrell JB, Wilson CB: Transsphenoidal microsurgery for Cushing's disease: A report of 216 cases. *Ann Intern Med* 1988;**109:**487.

Nelson DH, Meakin JW, Thorn GW: ACTH-producing pituitary tumors following adrenalectomy for Cushing's syndrome. *Ann Intern Med* 1960;**52:**560.

Orth DN et al: Effects of synthetic ovine corticotropin-releasing factor: Dose response of plasma adrenocorticotropin and cortisol. *J Clin Invest* 1983;**71:**587.

Pont A et al: Ketoconazole blocks adrenal steroid synthesis. *Ann Intern Med* 1982;**97:**370.

Streeten DH et al: Normal and abnormal function of the hypothalamic-pituitary-adrenocorticol system in man. *Endocr Rev* 1984;**5:**371.

Taylor AL, Fishman LM: Corticotropin-releasing hormone. *N Engl J Med* 1988;**319:**213.

Tyrrell JB et al: Cushing's disease: Selective transsphenoidal resection of pituitary microadenomas. *N Engl J Med* 1978;**298:**753.

Urbanic RC, George JM: Cushing's disease: Eighteen years' experience. *Medicine* 1981;**60:**14.

Vale W et al: Characterization of a 41-residue ovine hypothalamic peptide that stimulates secretion of corticotropin and β-endorphin. *Science* 1981;**213:**1394.

GH: Acromegaly

Alford FP, Baker HWG, Burger HG: The secretion rate of human growth hormone. 1. Daily secretion rates: Effects of posture and sleep. *J Clin Endocrinol Metab* 1973;**37:**515.

Barkan AL et al: Acromegaly due to ectopic growth hormone (GH)-releasing hormone (GHRH) production: Dynamic studies of GH and ectopic GHRH secretion. *J Clin Endocrinol Metab* 1986;**63:**1057.

Barnard LB et al: Treatment of resistant acromegaly with a long-acting somatostatin analogue (SMS 201-995). *Ann Intern Med* 1986;**105:**856.

Brown P et al: Potential epidemic of Creutzfeldt-Jakob disease from human growth hormone therapy. *N Engl J Med* 1985;**313:**728.

Clemmons DR et al: Evaluation of acromegaly by radioimmunoassay of somatomedin-C. *N Engl J Med* 1979;**301:**1138.

Frohman LA, Jansson JO: Growth hormone-releasing hormone. *Endocr Rev* 1986;**7:**223.

Hanew K et al: The spectrum of pituitary growth hormone responses to pharmacological stimuli in acromegaly. *J Clin Endocrinol Metab* 1980;**51:**292.

Lamberts SW: The role of somatostatin in the regulation of anterior pituitary hormone secretion and the use of its analogues in the treatment of human pituitary tumors. *Endocr Rev* 1989;**9:**417.

Melmed S et al: Pathophysiology of acromegaly. *Endocr Rev* 1983;**4:**271.

Melmed S et al: Pituitary tumors secreting growth hormone and prolactin. *Ann Intern Med* 1986;**105:**238.

Mims RB, Behune JE: Acromegaly with normal fasting growth hormone concentrations but abnormal growth hormone regulation. *Ann Intern Med* 1974;**81:**781.

Ross DA, Wilson CB: Results of transsphenoidal microsurgery for growth hormone-secreting pituitary adenoma in a series of 214 patients. *J Neurosurg* 1988;**68:**854.

Sano T et al: Growth hormone-releasing hormone-producing tumors: Clinical, biochemical, and morphological manifestations. *Endocr Rev* 1988;**9:**357.

Serri O et al: Acromegaly: Biochemical assessment of cure after long-term follow-up of transsphenoidal selective adenomectomy. *J Clin Endocrinol Metab* 1985;**61:**1185.

PRL: Prolactinoma

Carter JN et al: Prolactin-secreting tumors and hypogonadism in 22 men. *N Engl J Med* 1978;**299:**847.

Franz AG: Prolactin. *N. Engl J Med* 1978;**298:**201.

Greenspan SL et al: Osteoporosis in men with hyperprolactinemic hypogonadism. *Ann Intern Med* 1986;**104:**777.

Johnston DG et al: Hyperprolactinemia: Long-term effects of bromocriptine. *Am J Med* 1983;**75:**868.

Keye WR Jr et al: Amenorrhea, hyperprolactinemia, and pituitary enlargement secondary to primary hypothyroidism: Successful treatment with thyroid replacement. *Obstet Gynecol* 1976;**48:**697.

Keye WR Jr et al: Prolactin-secreting pituitary adenomas. 3. Frequency and diagnosis in amenorrhea-galactorrhea. *JAMA* 1980;**244:**1329.

Kirby RW, Kotchen TA, Rees ED: Hyperprolactinemia: A review of recent clinical advances. *Arch Intern Med* 1979;**139:**1415.

Kleinberg DL, Noel GL, Franz AG: Galactorrhea: A study of 235 cases, including 48 with pituitary tumors. *N Engl J Med* 1977;**296:**589.

Kleinberg DL et al: Pergolide for the treatment of pituitary tumors secreting prolactin or growth hormone. *N Engl J Med* 1983;**309:**704.

Klibanski A et al: Decreased bone density in hyperprolactinemic women. *N Engl J Med* 1980;**303:**1511.

Mehta AE, Reyes FI, Faiman C: Primary radiotherapy of prolactinomas: Eight- to 15-year follow-up. *Am J Med* 1987;**83:**49.

Molitch M: Hyperprolactinemia. *Med Grand Rounds* 1982;**1:**307.

Molitch ME: Pregnancy and the hyperprolactinemic woman. *N Engl J Med* 1985;**312:**1364.

Randall RV et al: Transsphenoidal microsurgical treatment of prolactin-producing pituitary adenomas: Results in 100 patients. *Mayo Clin Proc* 1983;**58:**108.

Serri O et al: Recurrence of hyperprolactinemia after selective transsphenoidal adenomectomy in women with prolactinoma. *N Engl J Med* 1983;**309:**280.

Spark RF et al: Bromocriptine reduces pituitary tumor size and hypersecretion. *JAMA* 1982;**247:**311.

Tolis G: Prolactin: Physiology and pathology. *Hosp Pract* (Feb) 1980;**15:**85.

Gonadotropins (LH/FSH)

Abraham GE et al: Simultaneous radioimmunoassay of plasma FSH, LH, progesterone, 17-hydroxyprogesterone, and estradiol-17β during the menstrual cycle. *J Clin Endocrinol Metab* 1972;**34:**312.

Beling CG et al: LH and FSH responses in normal males and females. Page 328 in: *The LH-Releasing Hormone*. Beling CG, Wentz AC (editors). Masson, 1980.

Hurley DM et al: Induction of ovulation and fertility in amenorrheic women by pulsatile low-dose gonadotropin-releasing hormone. *N Engl J Med* 1984;**310:**1069.

Jaffe RB, Monroe SE: Hormone interaction and regulation during the menstrual cycle. Chap 8, pp 219–247, in: *Frontiers in Neuroendocrinology*. Martin L, Ganong WF (editors). Raven Press, 1980.

McCann SM: Luteinizing hormone-releasing hormone. *N Engl J Med* 1977;**296:**797.

Ojeda SR et al. Recent advances in the endocrinology of puberty. *Endocr Rev* 1980;**1:**228.

Snyder PJ: Gonadotroph cell adenomas of the pituitary. *Endocr Rev* 1985;**6:**552.

TSH

Comi RJ et al: Response of thyrotropin-secreting pituitary adenomas to a long-acting somatostatin analogue. *N Engl J Med* 1987;**317:**12.

Jackson IMD: Thyrotropin-releasing hormone. *N Engl J Med* 1982;**306:**145.

Larsen PR: Thyroid-pituitary interaction: Feedback regulation of thyrotropin secretion by thyroid hormones. *N Engl J Med* 1982;**306:**23.

Segerson TP et al: Thyroid hormone regulates TRH biosynthesis in the paraventricular nucleus of the rat hypothalamus. *Science* 1987;**238:**78.

Snyder PJ, Utiger RD: Inhibition of thyrotropin response to thyrotropin-releasing hormone by small quantities of thyroid hormones. *J Clin Invest* 1972;**51:**2077.

Vagenakis AG et al: Recovery of pituitary thyrotropic function after withdrawal of prolonged thyroid-suppression therapy. *N Engl J Med* 1975;**293:**681.

Weintraub BD (moderator): Inappropriate secretion of thyroid-stimulating hormone. *Ann Intern Med* 1981;**95:**339.

Pituitary Function Testing & Neuroradiology

Abboud CF: Laboratory diagnosis of hypopituitarism. *Mayo Clin Proc* 1986;**61:**35.

Burrow GN et al: Microadenomas of the pituitary and abnormal sellar tomograms in an unselected autopsy series. *N Engl J Med* 1981;**304:**156.

Carroll BJ: Hypothalamic-pituitary function in depressive illness: Insensitivity to hypoglycaemia. *Br Med J* 1969;**3:**27.

Chambers EF et al: Regions of low density in the contrast-enhanced pituitary gland: Normal and pathologic processes. *Radiology* 1982;**144:**109.

Cohen KL: Metabolic, endocrine, and drug-induced interference with pituitary function tests: A review. *Metabolism* 1977;**26:**1165.

Feldman HA, Singer I: Endocrinology and metabolism in uremia and dialysis: A clinical review. *Medicine* 1974;**54:**345.

Glass AR et al: Endocrine function in human obesity. *Metabolism* 1981;**30:**89.

Gwinup G, Johnson B: Clinical testing of the hypothalamic-pituitary-adrenocortical system in states of hypo- and hypercortisolism. *Metabolism* 1975;**24:**777.

Kucharczyk W et al: Pituitary adenomas: High resolution MR imaging at 1.5 T. *Radiology* 1986;**161:**761.

Lufkin EG et al: Combined testing of anterior pituitary gland with insulin, thyrotropin-releasing hormone, and luteinizing hormone–releasing hormone. *Am J Med* 1983;**75:**471.

Mortimer CH et al: Luteinizing hormone and follicle stimulating hormone–releasing hormone test in patients with hypothalamic-pituitary-gonadal dysfunction. *Br Med J* 1973;**4:**73.

Sheldon WR Jr et al: Rapid sequential intravenous administration of four hypothalamic releasing hormones as a combined anterior pituitary function test in normal subjects. *J Clin Endocrinol Metab* 1985;**60:**623.

Snyder PJ et al: Diagnostic value of thyrotrophin-releasing hormone in pituitary and hypothalamic diseases: Assessment of thyrotrophin and prolactin secretion in 100 patients. *Ann Intern Med* 1974;**81:**751.

Valenta LJ et al: Diagnosis of pituitary tumors by hormone

assays and computerized tomography. *Am J Med* 1982;**172**:861.

Pituitary Adenomas

Branch CL, Laws ER Jr: Metastatic tumors of the sella turcica masquerading as primary pituitary tumors. *J Clin Endocrinol Metab* 1987;**65**:469.

Cook DM: Pituitary tumors: Current concepts of diagnosis and therapy. *West J Med* 1980;**133**:189.

Cusick JF, Hagen TC, Findling JW: Inappropriate secretion of antidiuretic hormone after transsphenoidal surgery for pituitary tumors. *N Engl J Med* 1984;**311**:36.

Lawrence JH et al: Treatment of pituitary tumors with heavy particles. Pages 253–262 in: *Diagnosis and Treatment of Pituitary Tumors*. Kohler PO, Ross GT (editors). Excerpta Medica, 1973.

Molitch ME (editor): Pituitary tumors: Diagnosis and management. *Endocrinol Metab Clin North Am* 1987;**16**:475.

Ridgway EC et al: Pure alpha-secreting pituitary adenomas. *N Engl J Med* 1981;**304**:1254.

Zervas NT, Martin JB: Management of hormone-secreting pituitary adenomas. *N Engl J Med* 1980;**302**:210.

Empty Sella Syndrome

Bergeron C, Kovacs K, Biilbao JM: Primary empty sella: A histologic and immunocytologic study. *Arch Intern Med* 1979;**139**:248.

Fleckman AM et al: Empty sella of normal size in Sheehan's syndrome. *Am J Med* 1983;**175**:585.

Jordan RM, Kendall JW, Kerber CW: The primary empty sella syndrome: Analysis of the clinical characteristics, radiographic features, pituitary function and cerebrospinal fluid adenohypophysial hormone concentrations. *Am J Med* 1977;**62**:569.

Hypopituitarism

Asa SL et al: Lymphocytic hypophysitis of pregnancy resulting in hypopituitarism: A distinct clinicopathologic entity. *Ann Intern Med* 1981;**95**:166.

Braunstein GD, Kohler PO: Pituitary function in Hand-Schuller-Christian disease: Evidence for deficient growth-hormone release in patients with short stature. *N Engl J Med* 1972;**1286**:1225.

Edwards DM, Clark JD: Posttraumatic hypopituitarism: Six cases and a review of the literature. *Medicine* 1986;**65**:281.

Males JL, Townsend JL, Schneider RA: Hypogonadotropic hypogonadism with anosmia—Kallmann's syndrome: A disorder of olfactory and hypothalamic function. *Arch Intern Med* 1973;**131**:501.

Purnell DC, Randall RV, Rynearson EH: Postpartum pituitary insufficiency (Sheehan's syndrome): Review of 18 cases. *Mayo Clin Proc* 1964;**139**:321.

Samaan NA et al: Hypopituitarism after external irradiation: Evidence of both hypothalamic and pituitary origin. *Ann Intern Med* 1975;**83**:771.

Schafer AL et al: Clinical consequences of acquired transfusional iron overload in adults. *N Engl J Med* 1981;**304**:319.

Schwabe AD (moderator): Anorexia nervosa. *Ann Intern Med* 1981;**94**:371.

Snyder PJ et al: Hypopituitarism following radiation therapy of pituitary adenomas. *Am J Med* 1986;**81**:457.

Stuart CA, Neelon FA, Lebovitz HE: Hypothalamic insufficiency: The cause of hypopituitarism in sarcoidosis. *Ann Intern Med* 1978;**88**:589.

Thomsett MJ et al: Endocrine and neurologic outcome in childhood craniopharyngioma: Review of effect of treatment in 42 patients. *J Pediatr* 1980;**97**:728.

Veldhuis JD, Hammond, JM: Endocrine function after spontaneous infarction of the human pituitary: Report, review, and reappraisal. *Endocr Rev* 1980;**1**:100.

Somatomedins

7

E. Martin Spencer, MD, PhD

Somatomedins are a family of structurally related polypeptide cellular growth factors that mediate the growth-promoting action of growth hormone (GH). As a group, somatomedins share the following common properties: GH is the primary regulator of their plasma level; all have insulinlike activity; they are mitogenic for chondrocytes, osteoblasts, and a variety of cells derived from extraskeletal tissues; and they are transported in plasma bound to one or more large carrier proteins.

History

Our present understanding of somatomedins results from a convergence of knowledge from 3 different areas of research: (1) the mediators of the growth-promoting actions of GH, (2) the nature of the nonsuppressible insulinlike activity in serum, and (3) the identity of serum factors that stimulate cellular multiplication in vitro. Eventually it became apparent that each area concerned a different property of somatomedins.

Salmon and Daughaday (1957) found that while GH in vivo stimulated the incorporation of sulfate into cartilage cells, it was inactive in vitro. They presented evidence for an active factor in serum under the control of GH that stimulated in vitro sulfate incorporation into cartilage and called this mediator of GH action "sulfation factor." Clinical studies verified that the serum level of "sulfation factor" was elevated in GH excess and that the low level in GH deficiency rose to normal with GH treatment. Further research demonstrated that "sulfation factor" also stimulated the synthesis of DNA, RNA, protein, and hydroxyproline in chondrocytes; promoted the multiplication of cultured cells in serum-free media; and had insulinlike activity in all tissues. In recognition of these properties, the limiting term "sulfation factor" was replaced in 1972 by the name somatomedin to reflect what was thought to be its primary function, the mediation of the growth-promoting effect of GH. Later, human serum was found to contain at least 2 somatomedins, based on their isoionic points: A (neutral) and C (basic).

While the mediator of GH action was being studied, Froesch et al (1963) were investigating the nature of the insulinlike activity in serum detected by bioassay

Acronyms Used in This Chapter	
BP-1	Somatomedin-binding protein 1
BP-3	Somatomedin-binding protein 3
BRL-MSA	Multiplication-stimulating activity from cultured buffalo rat liver cell media
cAMP	Cyclic adenosine monophosphate
cGMP	Cyclic guanosine monophosphate
GH	Growth hormone (somatotropin)
GRH	Growth hormone-releasing hormone
hPI	Human proinsulin
hPL	Human placental lactogen
hPM	Human placental membrane
IGF-I	Human insulinlike growth factor I (SM-C)
IGF-II	Human insulinlike growth factor II
mRNA	Messenger ribonucleic acid
MSA	Multiplication-stimulating activity
NSILA	Nonsuppressible insulinlike activity
NSILA-p	Nonsuppressible insulinlike activity precipitated by acid-ethanol
NSILA-s	Nonsuppressible insulinlike activity soluble in acid-ethanol
PDGF	Platelet-derived growth factor
PRL	Prolactin
SM-A	Neutral human somatomedin (primarily IGF-II)
SM-C	Basic human somatomedin (IGF-I)
TRH	Thyrotropin-releasing hormone
TSH	Thyroid-stimulating hormone (thyrotropin)

but not radioimmunoassay. The addition of excess insulin antibodies to serum revealed that about 90% of the total biologic insulinlike activity was unaffected. This activity was called nonsuppressible insulinlike activity (NSILA) and was found to consist of acid-ethanol soluble (NSILA-s) and precipitable (NSILA-p) fractions. NSILA-s was later found to possess the same properties as somatomedins. Two polypeptides were purified from human serum and sequenced. They were renamed insulinlike growth factors I and II (IGF-I and IGF-II). The former is identical with SM-C, and data now indicate that IGF-II is the major component and deaminated IGF-I the minor component of SM-A. (See Chemistry, below.)

Simultaneously with the research on somatomedins

and NSILA, Pierson and Temin (1972) were studying the factor in serum that was responsible for the multiplication of cells in tissue cultures. The activity present in calf serum that stimulated the multiplication of chicken embryo fibroblasts was called multiplication-stimulating activity (MSA). Another MSA was found to be produced by continuous cultures of buffalo rat liver cells and named BRL-MSA. (This name is often shortened to the general term MSA, but the most appropriate name, based on structural homology, is now rat IGF-II. [See Chemistry, below.]) MSA from both sources has activity typical of somatomedins and is included in this family of polypeptides.

For simplicity, this chapter will employ the general term somatomedin or somatomedins to refer to what are common properties of all the peptides in the group: SM-A, SM-C, IGF-I, IGF-II, and BRL-MSA. The general term somatomedin will also be used in describing experiments conducted with preparations containing unknown proportions of more than one somatomedin, making it impossible to assign that effect to a unique somatomedin. When information is available, the name of the specific somatomedin will be used. The acidic glial cell growth factor previously referred to as SM-B is not one of the somatomedins.

Measurement of Somatomedins

Somatomedin levels can be measured by bioassays, competitive binding assays, and radioimmunoassays (Table 7–1). The most frequently used bioassay procedure measures the incorporation of labeled sulfate into the glycosaminoglycans of cartilage. The classic method uses hypophysectomized rat costal cartilage, but cartilage from different species or the incorporation of ^{3}H-thymidine into cartilage can be used. Somatomedins can also be bioassayed by their insulinlike activity in the rat epididymal fat pad. The disadvantages of bioassays lie in their laboriousness, imprecision, and lack of specificity. They do not discriminate among the different somatomedins, and inhibitors and other hormones may influence results. Bioassays that reflect the mitogenic activity of somatomedins for cultured cells, such as chicken embryo fibroblasts and GH_3 pituitary cells, considerably improve the precision and are less time-consuming.

The popularity of competitive binding assays over bioassays stems from their substantially decreased variability, increased ease of operation, and lack of influence by inhibitors. The most widely used competitive binding assays employ either human placental membrane (hPM) fractions or the plasma carrier protein of somatomedins as receptors. These assays, like the bioassay, measure all somatomedins. However, because individual somatomedins cross-react to different degrees, an accurate total somatomedin content cannot be determined. Exceptions appear to be the rat placental and hepatic membrane-binding assays, which for practical purposes appear to measure IGF-II.

Radioimmunoassays have been developed for

Table 7–1. Tests for somatomedins.

	Measures	Specific for
Bioassays		
Hypophysecto-mized rat costal cartilage[1]	$^{35}SO_4$ uptake	All somatomedins
Embryonic chick pelvic cartilage	$^{35}SO_4$ uptake or ^{3}H-thymidine uptake	All somatomedins
Rat epidymal fat pad[1]	^{14}C incorporation from ^{14}C-glucose (insulinlike activity)	All somatomedins
GH_3 cells	Cell multiplication	All somatomedins
Chicken embryonic fibroblasts[1]	^{3}H-thymidine uptake or cell multiplication	All somatomedins
Competitive binding assays		
Human placental membrane[1]	Displacement of ^{125}I-labeled somatomedins	All somatomedins
Plasma carrier protein	Displacement of ^{125}I-labeled somatomedins	All somatomedins
Rat placental membrane	Displacement of ^{125}I-IGF-II	?IGF-II
Radioimmunoassays		
SM-C[1] (IGF-I)	Displacement of ^{125}I-SM-C/GF-I	SM-C (IGF-I)
IGF-II (SM-A)	Displacement of ^{125}I-IGF-II	IGF-II
BRL-MSA	Displacement of ^{125}I-BRL-MSA	BRL-mSA (rat IGF-II)

[1]Most commonly used.

SM-C (IGF-I), human IGF-II, and rat IGF-II (BRL-MSA). However, some problems still remain with their specificity and interpretation. A small amount of cross-reactivity usually occurs between the somatomedins. For example, Hall has reported an SM-A radioimmunoassay that has SM-C specificity. It is 10 times more sensitive to SM-C than to SM-A and exhibits the typical age dependency of SM-C rather than that of IGF-II. This effect is due to the use of the desamido form of SM-C, which like SM-A has a neutral isoionic point, for immunization and preparation of antisera.

The carrier protein complicates the measurement of the level of somatomedins in serum by hindering the access of bound somatomedin to the somatomedin receptor or antibody used in the assay and by competing for the labeled somatomedin. A probable exception to this is the rat cartilage sulfate uptake bioassay. In earlier work, laboratories measured plasma or serum directly; now most investigators remove the carrier protein prior to assay either by gel filtration or Sephadex chromatography in acid media or by acid-ethanol extraction. Some radioimmunoassays are still performed under nonequilibrium assay conditions (delayed addition of the labeled antigen) or use samples that have first been acidified and then lyophilized or incubated to eliminate the effect of the serum-binding protein. Radioimmunoassays that do not remove the carrier protein can still give qualitatively valid levels if a high-affinity antibody is used. Free somatomedin cannot yet be measured.

The results of assays for somatomedins are usually expressed as ng/mL of pure standard, or relative to a pool of normal sera arbitrarily assigned a value of 1 unit/mL. Normal values are established by each laboratory. The normal laboratory values for adults range from 0.5 to 1.6 units/mL in the hPM-radioreceptor assay and from 0.4 to 2 units/mL for the SM-C radioimmunoassay using purified radiolabeled SM-C as a tracer. Prepubertal children have lower values, while adolescents have higher values (see below). One unit of SM-C has been reported to average 200–250 ng by radioimmunoassay, and IGF-II has been found to be considerably higher—approximately 550 ng—by radioimmunoassay. However, the specific activity of the pure somatomedins was not tested in many previously used assay systems.

Chemistry

Two human somatomedins, IGF-I and IGF-II, have been sequenced, and both are structurally homologous with proinsulin. This undoubtedly explains the prominent insulinlike activity of somatomedins as well as the weak cellular proliferative action of insulin. This homology is also present at the genetic level, suggesting that the somatomedin and insulin genes evolved by duplication of and divergence from a common primitive gene, possibly the growth factor gene.

Like proinsulin, IGF-I and IGF-II are single polypeptide chains, cross-linked by 3 disulfide bonds. Fig 7–1 compares the sequence of the 3 peptides aligned for maximum homology with the common residues outlined. IGF-I and IGF-II consist of 70 and 67 residues, respectively, and have 62% homology. Twenty-six residues are identical between IGF-I and proinsulin and 25 between IGF-II and proinsulin. The 3 disulfide bonds occupy the same position in all 3 peptides. The IGFs have domains that correspond to the A and B "chain" regions and the C-peptide segment of proinsulin (Fig 7–1). The C-peptide regions of IGF-I and IGF-II are 12 and 8 residues, respectively, and have no sequence homology to the 35-residue C segment of proinsulin. The IGFs have an additional region, called the "D region," composed of a carboxy-terminal extension that is not found in proinsulin. This extension consists of 8 residues in IGF-I and 6 residues in IGF-II.

A theoretical model of the tertiary structure of IGF-I, constructed on the basis of its sequence homology with proinsulin, gave a 3-dimensional structure of IGF-I that corresponded closely to that for proinsulin and accommodated the shorter C-peptide region (Fig 7–2). By comparing the model for IGF-I to that for insulin, many of their similarities and differences could be explained. IGF-I cross-reacts with insulin receptors because the area concerned with binding insulin to the insulin receptor appears to have been conserved during evolution. The nonreactivity of insulin antibodies with IGF-I can be explained by the C-peptide region and carboxy-terminal extension of IGF blocking one antigenic region that is exposed in insulin and by significant amino acid substitutions at the second antigenic region.

Spencer, Ross, and Smith (1981) established that SM-C and IGF-I were identical. They also found that the major component in the SM-A (neutral) peak on isoelectric focusing was IGF-II, and a modified form of SM-C was a minor component (see below). Two minor uncharacterized peaks with somatomedinlike activity have been found in isoelectric focusing—one with an isoelectric point (pI) of 5.2 and the other with a pI of 9.5.

Two rat IGF-II (BRL-MSA) peptides with molecular weights of 8700 and 7500 have been purified from conditioned media of BRL cells. The sequence of the latter shows 93% homology with human IGF-II, with only 5 different residues. Three of these residues are in the C-peptide region and one is immediately adjacent to it. Immunologic evidence indicates that considerable amounts of IGF-II are present in fetal and neonatal rats. After the neonatal period, however, SM-C is essentially the only somatomedin present in rats. Rat SM-C differs from the human peptide by 3 residues.

Genetics

An analysis of the human genome indicates that the 2 somatomedin genes are single-copy genes. The sequence of one corresponds to SM-C/IGF-I and the other to IGF-II. The SM-C-like material contaminating the SM-A peak on isoelectric focusing is a desamido modification of SM-C. The other peaks at pI 9.5 and 5.2 may be modified forms—proforms, splicing variants, or genetic variants. A second rat IGF-II has been predicted from cDNA sequencing. This differs from the other rat IGF-II by one residue and from human IGF-II by only 4 residues. Bovine IGF-II is identical to human IGF-II. The SM-C/IGF-I gene has been localized to the long arm of chromosome 12 and the IGF-II gene to the short arm of Chromosome 11, adjacent to the insulin gene. Oncogenes have been identified in the proximity of both somatomedin genes.

The liver has the highest amount of somatomedin mRNA; the kidneys, heart, and brain also have high levels. However, most—if not all—cells have low levels of somatomedin mRNA: 3–6 copies per cell. These low levels may be used for normal "housekeeping" functions such as facilitating replication and differentiated functions.

Although the somatomedin genes are single-copy genes, multiple species of mRNA can be identified in tissues expressing these genes. The size of these mRNAs ranges from approximately 1–8 kb. The mechanisms involved in generating these transcripts

Region

B

	B10	B20	B30
hPI	Phe Val Asn Gln His Leu Cys Gly Ser His Leu Val Glu Ala Leu Tyr Leu Val Cys Gly Glu Arg Gly Phe Phe Tyr Thr Pro Lys Thr
IGF-I	Gly Pro Glu Thr Leu Cys Gly Ala Glu Leu Val Asp Ala Leu Gln Phe Val Cys Gly Asp Arg Gly Phe Tyr Phe Asn Lys Pro Thr
IGF-II	Ala Tyr Arg Pro Ser Glu Thr Leu Cys Gly Gly Glu Leu Val Asp Thr Leu Gln Phe Val Cys Gly Asp Arg Gly Phe Tyr Phe Ser Arg Pro Ala

C

hPI	Arg Arg Glu Ala Glu Asp Leu Gln Val Gly Gln Val Glu Leu Gly Gly Gly Pro Gly Ala Gly Ser Leu Gln Pro Leu Ala Leu Glu Gly Ser Leu Gln Lys Arg
IGF-I	Gly Tyr Gly Ser Ser Arg Arg Ala Pro Gln Thr
IGF-II	Ser Arg Val Ser Arg Arg Ser Arg

A

	A10	A20
hPI	Gly Ile Val Glu Gln Cys Cys Thr Ser Ile Cys Ser Leu Tyr Gln Leu Glu Asn Tyr Cys Asn
IGF-I	Gly Ile Val Asp Glu Cys Cys Phe Arg Ser Cys Asp Leu Arg Arg Leu Glu Met Tyr Cys Ala
IGF-II	Gly Ile Val Glu Glu Cys Cys Phe Arg Ser Cys Asp Leu Ala Leu Leu Glu Thr Tyr Cys Ala

D

hPI	
IGF-I	Pro Leu Lys Pro Ala Lys Ser Ala
IGF-II	Thr ----- Pro Ala Lys Ser Glu

Figure 7–1. Alignment of the amino acid sequences of insulinlike growth factors I and II (IGF-I and IGF-II) and human proinsulin (hPI). Symbols above hPI refer to the chain and residue number of insulin. The regions of the insulinlike molecules are listed in the column at right. A and B refer to the regions of hPI that give the classic A and B chains of insulin. C is the connecting peptide region, and D represents a C-terminal extension only in IGFs.

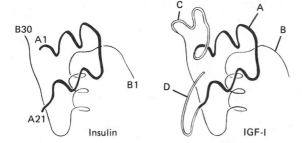

Figure 7–2. Three-dimensional representation of the structure of IGF-I based on model building and patterned after the known tertiary structure of insulin. *A, B, C,* and *D* represent different regions of the IGF-I molecule. Note the similarity of the *A* and *B* regions and the differences in the *C* and *D* areas in comparison with the insulin molecule. (Reproduced, with permission, from Blundell TL et al: Insulin-like growth factor: A model for tertiary structure accounting for immunoreactivity and receptor binding. *Proc Natl Acad Sci USA* 1978;75:180.)

include the use of alternative promoter, polyadenylation, and splicing sites. Differential expression of these mRNAs has been identified, but the significance of this is still unclear.

Physiology

A. Sites of Synthesis: All vertebrate species tested have somatomedin activity in serum. Contrary to the case with GH, they show very little species specificity when tested in cartilage, protein-binding, or receptor assays.

The liver is a site for production of SM-C, as shown by perfusion and cell culture studies with GH. IGF-II synthesis has been demonstrated in fetal rat livers. The somatomedins are the only hormones known to be produced by the liver. After synthesis, SM-C is not stored but is released into the plasma, which is the best source for its isolation. Many tissues can synthesize somatomedins, including fibroblasts, myoblasts, chondrocytes, osteoblasts, bone, brain, gastrointestinal epithelium, kidney, etc. Local production of somatomedins may be very important physiologically in that they may act in an autocrine or paracrine fashion, in contrast to circulating somatomedins, which act in an endocrine fashion. Several types of malignant and fetal cells have been found to express somatomedin mRNA and release somatomedins. Thus, somatomedins may play a role in malignancy and in fetal organogenesis.

The somatomedins are transported in plasma bound to high-molecular-weight carrier proteins that are also synthesized in the liver and tissues. The serum level of the carrier protein is also GH-dependent and tightly coupled with the level of somatomedins, for little unsaturated carrier protein or free somatomedin is present in serum. (See Somatomedin-Binding Proteins, below.)

B. Regulation of Synthesis: The major regulator of the SM-C (IGF-I) level in serum after birth is growth hormone (GH) while IGF-II is only weakly GH-dependent. GH administration to healthy subjects causes a rise in the serum SM-C value after 4–6 hours. SM-C exerts a negative feedback on GH release by stimulating hypothalamic somatostatin release and by a direct effect on the pituitary that blocks the action of growth hormone-releasing hormone (GRH).

Several other hormones affect the somatomedin level but not to the extent of GH (Table 7–2). The effects of most of these hormones on individual somatomedins is unknown, because in many cases assays measuring total somatomedins were used. Insulin stimulates somatomedin production based on hepatic perfusion studies, but both low and high somatomedin serum levels have been reported in diabetes mellitus. The small increase in somatomedin release by hypophysectomized rat livers perfused with insulin could have resulted just from improved metabolism, because nutritional factors, especially dietary protein, are major regulators of the serum somatomedin level. Human placental lactogen (hPL) has a moderate and thyroxine a weak stimulatory effect on somatomedin levels. The effects of estrogens are not completely understood. Estrogen administration in large doses to acromegalic subjects decreases the serum somatomedin activity by bioassay and by SM-C radioimmunoassay; this could result from decreased somatomedin synthesis, increased carrier protein synthesis (since this was not removed prior to assay), or increased catabolism.

Table 7–2. Effects of hormones on plasma somatomedin levels in humans.

Hormone	Effects and Remarks
GH	The most important regulator; stimulates SM-C levels more than those of IGF-II.
hPL	May stimulate somatomedin levels in the fetus.
Thyroxine	Causes weak increase in somatomedin levels.
Insulin	Stimulates SM-C levels.
PRL	Very weak stimulator. Maintains normal SM-C levels in hyperprolactinemic children with impaired GH responses.
Adrenal corticosteroids	Result depends on the method. Increases somatomedin levels by SM-C radioimmunoassay and hPM receptor assay, produces no effect on them by competitive protein-binding assay, and decreases them by some bioassays.
Testosterone	Does not appear to affect somatomedin levels.
Estrogen	Pharmacologic doses decrease SM-C levels and have an uncertain effect on IGF-II. Physiologic doses may increase somatomedin levels.
Progesterone	Increases SM-C levels.

However, physiologic levels of estrogen have been reported to stimulate or inhibit plasma SM-C levels. Adrenal corticosteroids increase the serum concentration of somatomedins when measured by hPM-radioreceptor assay and radioimmunoassay for SM-C. However, no effect has been noted by binding protein assay, and decreased levels are observed with some bioassays. In humans, an elevated prolactin (PRL) level has no effect on the serum somatomedin level measured by hPM-radioreceptor assay or SM-C radioimmunoassay. However, normal SM-C values have been reported in patients with hyperprolactinemia and GH deficiency due to large pituitary tumors; thus, high levels of PRL may exert a weak effect on SM-C in GH deficiency. In rodents, the action of PRL is confusing. Its administration to hypophysectomized rats has been reported both to have no effect and to elevate the serum somatomedin levels, unattended by growth. In contrast, PRL given to GH-deficient Snell dwarf mice stimulated both bioassayable somatomedin levels and growth. Rat liver perfusion studies have shown that PRL did not affect somatomedin synthesis when hypophysectomized animals were used, possibly because of the absence of PRL receptors. Curiously, when normal rat livers were used, PRL stimulated somatomedin activity at 11 AM but not at 3 PM.

C. Inhibitors: Inhibitors of the biologic action of somatomedins may have a major counterregulatory role, perhaps shunting nutrients from growth to more important functions during critical times. Inhibitors occur in both pathologic and normal states; at least one of these inhibitors is produced in the liver. Inhibitors of sulfate uptake have been found in diabetic or hypophysectomized rats and in malnourished humans. Normal rat serum contains a factor that inhibits somatomedin-stimulated thymidine but not sulfate incorporation into cartilage. Partial characterization has indicated that it has the properties of a pentose and nucleic acid. In addition, there appears to be a steroid and a peptide inhibitor. The peptide inhibitor may be a somatomedin-binding protein, but the mechanism of action of the other inhibitors is unknown.

D. Somatomedin-Binding Proteins: Two specific binding proteins regulate the biologic activity of somatomedins. Although no standard nomenclature exists, we refer to them as binding protein 1 (BP-1) and binding protein 3 (BP-3). Human BP-1 is a glycosylated, approximately 140 kd GH-dependent binding protein. Binding to BP-3 inactivates somatomedins, prolongs their half-life, and prevents the level of somatomedins from fluctuating as does the level of GH. BP-3 probably regulates the level of free, biologically active somatomedins, estimated to be about 1%, as well as transporting them. (Whether the transport is to or from tissues is unknown.) Recently an ELISA and an RIA have been developed to measure BP-3. The somatomedin BP-3 complex dissociates at pHs lower than 3.0, releasing active somatomedin, an acid-labile unit of 90 kd BP-3 complex, and an acid-stable binding unit of 50 kd (S50). Only S50 has been isolated; its sequence has been partially determined by Spencer et al. (With special procedures, smaller N-terminal binding fragments can be generated, eg, S15, S26.) Partially pure S50, which probably does not circulate, has been shown to maintain the properties of BP-3 —on binding, it reversibly inhibits the biologic activity of and prolongs the half-life of somatomedins.

Human BP-1 is also known as placental protein 12 and amniotic fluid-binding protein. It differs from BP-3 in molecular weight (28 kd), glycosylation, inverse GH dependency, immunologic reactivity, degree of unsaturation, binding constants, and relative affinity for SM-C and IGF-II. Its plasma level rises dramatically during the early morning hours, whereas the level of BP-3 does not fluctuate diurnally. The most striking difference between the 2 BPs is that BP-1 has been reported to associate with the cell membrane and stimulate the mitogenic effect of SM-C on fibroblasts and smooth muscle cells. (However, inhibitory effects have been reported in other cell systems.) Therefore, both BPs may be able to independently modulate somatomedin activity. Studies on wound healing indicate that BPs may be important in regulating the biologic activity of somatomedins. The binding protein may also have undiscovered functions, such as enzymatic activity analogous to that of the peptidases associated with nerve growth factor and epidermal growth factor.

All cells that synthesize somatomedins also synthesize a binding protein, except for one line of cultured hepatocytes that synthesizes only the binding protein. Genetic evidence indicates that the proteins and somatomedins originate from separate genes. However, BP-1 and BP-3 exhibit significant homology at their immunoreactive N-terminal ends. How the syntheses of somatomedin and BP-3 are coordinated so tightly is unknown.

E. Catabolism: Intravenously administered labeled somatomedin localizes primarily in the kidney. The proximal tubule has enzymes that degrade somatomedins, and insulin competes for this pathway. However, nephrectomy does not significantly alter the half-life of somatomedin, whereas it does alter that of insulin. Somatomedins can be recovered from urine. Hepatic metabolism does not seem to be an important mechanism for degradation of somatomedin.

Biologic Effects on Tissues

A. Metabolic Effects: In adipose tissue, somatomedins have the same metabolic actions as insulin but are one-sixteenth as potent. All somatomedins stimulate glucose transport, oxidation to CO_2, and incorporation into lipid. Somatomedins inhibit lipolysis and epinephrine-stimulated adenylate cyclase activity. In some tissues, basal adenylate cyclase activity is inhibited. The insulinlike actions of somatomedins are initiated by binding to the insulin receptor, not to the specific somatomedin receptor present on adipocytes.

In the rat diaphragm, somatomedins are equipotent with insulin. Both have an immediate stimulatory effect on the transport of amino acids and sugars. This effect does not require protein synthesis and is unaffected by phosphodiesterase inhibitors; it thus appears to operate via a mechanism different from that used by GH. However, both somatomedins and GH may be physiologically important for protein synthesis in muscle. In the perfused heart, somatomedin stimulates glucose uptake and lactic acid production.

Somatomedins stimulate chondrocyte DNA, RNA, protein, collagen, and proteoglycan synthesis. In fetal calvarial bone cells, somatomedins stimulate the synthesis of DNA, collagen, collagenase nondigestible protein, and glycogen.

B. Mitogenic Effects: Somatomedins are the major stimulators of animal growth. They act primarily on the skeletal tissues but also stimulate a wide variety of extraskeletal tissues to grow and differentiate. In addition, many fetal tissues (gut, brain, lung, heart, kidney) produce somatomedins and may autostimulate their growth or that of neighboring cells (autocrine and paracrine actions). The corollary is that the somatomedins can stimulate a wide variety of cultured cells to proliferate in serum-free media. The list includes several types of fibroblasts, myoblasts, smooth muscle cells, GH_3 pituitary cells, chondrocytes, testicular cells, vascular endothelium, osteoblasts, and thyroid cells. Although somatomedins have no direct effect on lymphocytes in serum-free media, they can potentiate concanavalin A-induced DNA synthesis, completely replacing the serum requirement for optimal mitogenic activity for mouse spleen lymphocytes and partially replacing that for human peripheral lymphocytes. Because somatomedin-deficient species do not have an immunologic defect, the measurable somatomedin in GH deficiency is presumably enough to maintain immunologic competence or cells involved in the immune response (eg, macrophages) transiently express a somatomedin gene. The immunologic defect previously reported in GH-deficient Snell mice was due to malnutrition and disappears with special attention to animal care.

C. Differentiated Functions in Organs: Evidence from several areas indicates that the somatomedins play a much larger biologic role than just growth promotion in tissues. The almost ubiquitous presence of cellular somatomedin mRNA and plasma membrane receptors is further evidence for this role. The most promising areas for investigation include the role of somatomedins in steroid and thyroid hormone synthesis and action. In addition to the gonads and the thyroid gland, other organs are also affected by somatomedins, as discussed in the following sections.

1. Vitamin D and Bones—SM-C mediates GH's stimulatory action on both the production of $1,25(OH)_2D$ from 25-OHD by renal 25-OHD 1α-hydroxylase and on renal phosphate reabsorption. In addition, the occurrence of a low plasma phosphorus level, which is a potent stimulator of the renal 1α-hydroxylase, requires SM-C. These interrelations between $1,25(OH)_2D$ and phosphorus indicate the important role of SM-C in bone formation.

2. Gonads—SM-C increases estrogen synthesis by synergizing with FSH to stimulate follicular aromatase activity. SM-C also strongly stimulates progesterone synthesis by acting on the P-450 side-chain cleavage enzyme. There is also evidence of local testicular and ovarian synthesis of SM-C, suggesting an autocrine or paracrine role for SM-C.

3. Adrenal and Thyroid Glands—SM-C potentiates the effect of ACTH on adrenal steroid synthesis and synergizes with TSH in stimulating the proliferation of thyroid follicular cells.

4. Wound Healing and Skin—SM-C probably plays a major role in wound healing, although this has not been conclusively established. Platelet alpha granules release SM-C into wounds at the earliest stage of healing. Actuated macrophages express somatomedin mRNA. During later stages of healing, SM-C levels in wound fluid approach those of plasma. This wound SM-C appears to be much more biologically active than comparable serum levels, probably because of a weaker association with binding proteins. Fibroblasts produce at least part of the wound SM-C during this phase of repair; the SM-C gene is expressed in actively proliferating fibroblasts.

SM-C acts as an autocrine stimulator of both fibroblast proliferation and collagen synthesis. When healing is completed, the SM-C gene is turned off by an unknown regulating factor. Platelet-derived growth factor (PDGF) might act as a regulating factor early in the healing process. GH is not essential to this process, because healing progresses normally in GH deficiency. The importance of anoxia and elevated wound lactate levels in healing is presently unclear.

Biologic Effects in Organisms

A. Growth Promotion: The Snell mouse, which is genetically deficient in GH, PRL, and TSH, was first used to demonstrate the growth-promoting properties of partially purified somatomedins. Administering pure somatomedins (SM-C and IGF-II) to hypophysectomized mice confirmed these results by stimulating demonstrable growth. Large amounts must be administered continuously because of the short half-life of somatomedins when given without BP-A. However, exogenously administered somatomedins cannot completely replace the effect of GH. GH and somatomedin effects differ consistently in growth stimulation and organ weights. Local production of somatomedins may be more efficient, or binding proteins may be necessary for targeting. Another possibility is that GH may be required to stimulate cellular differentiation.

B. Metabolic Effects: Somatomedins have been

shown to induce hypoglycemia in humans, pigs, and rats. On a molar basis, SM-C is about one-sixteenth as potent as insulin in producing hypoglycemia. In adrenalectomized rats, somatomedins produce even more prolonged hypoglycemia than does insulin and, in addition, lowers free fatty acids. Administration of somatomedins to normal rats stimulates the incorporation of ^{14}C-glucose into adipose tissue and diaphragm. Insulin does not further increase ^{14}C-glucose incorporation when maximally stimulated by somatomedins, so both somatomedin and insulin act on the same transport site. Somatomedins have also been shown to stimulate amino acid transport and incorporation into protein, and sulfate incorporation into cartilage and bone.

Mechanisms of Action

A. Receptors: Somatomedins, like other polypeptide hormones, bind to receptors on the cell surface, thereby triggering a programmed series of intracellular events. These events can be either immediate (transport), intermediate, or delayed. Specific somatomedin receptors have been found on chondrocytes, myoblasts, fibroblasts, osteoblasts, adipocytes, hPMs, lymphocytes, human lymphoblastic cells, and many other cell types. Two types of receptors, type 1 and type 2, have been identified by cross-linking ^{125}I-SM with cellular membranes and by cDNA sequencing. The same cell may contain both classes of receptors as well as insulin receptors. The type 1 somatomedin receptor is structurally homologous with the insulin receptor. Its molecular weight is more than 400 kd; it consists of 2 alpha-beta subunits of 210 kd connected by disulfide bonds. The affinities of IGF-II and insulin for this receptor are 10% and 1% of SM-C, respectively. The type 1 receptor is a protein kinase that autophosphorylates tyrosine residues and other intracellular proteins. The type 2 receptor is structurally different. It has a molecular weight of 220 kd and no subunits. It does not bind insulin and binds SM-C minimally if at all. The type 2 receptor is the same as the mannose-6-phosphate receptor, which appears to transport or target lysosomal enzymes. Currently, no evidence exists that the type 2 receptor mediates any IGF-II actions after birth. A recent theory suggests that the growth-promoting effects of somatomedins and insulin are generally mediated by the somatomedin receptors and the metabolic effects by the insulin receptor, but exceptions to this rule do exist.

B. Intracellular Mediators: The intracellular mediators of somatomedin actions have not been identified. Intracellular calcium may be involved, because calcium can stimulate the uptake of sulfate into cartilage and other growth factors are known to increase intracellular calcium. Protein phosphorylation could play a part, because the type 1 somatomedin receptor is a protein kinase. The role of cyclic nucleotides is controversial. Initial evidence suggested that somatome-

dins could lower cAMP levels by inhibiting adenylate cyclase. Subsequent studies questioned this mechanism because the response of basal and stimulated adenylate cyclase to somatomedins varied in different target tissues. Recent investigations have shown that somatomedins may in fact elevate intracellular cyclic nucleotide levels. cAMP-dependent or cAMP-independent protein kinases do not seem to be affected by somatomedins. Efforts to tie somatomedin actions to cGMP levels have not given convincing results. Since the actions of somatomedins can be immediate, intermediate, or delayed, a single mechanism may not explain all of them.

C. Intracellular Binding Sites: Intracellular binding sites for somatomedins have been found in hepatic membrane fractions and theoretically could be involved in somatomedin action. These binding sites are distributed differently from those for insulin. Because the liver is not a primary target organ for somatomedins, the function of intracellular membranous binding sites probably should be established in proliferating or differentiated cells sensitive to somatomedins. Intracellular incorporation of somatomedins may down-regulate somatomedin receptors or degrade somatomedins. Intracellular binding sites could even be recently synthesized receptors or binding proteins in transport.

Soluble somatomedin receptors have been identified in the cytosol of the liver, kidney, and placenta. The hepatic soluble receptors may have been shed after synthesis. Renal cytosol receptors appear to be involved in the catabolism of somatomedins, and those in the placenta may play a role in regulating fetal growth.

D. Factors Regulating the Cell Cycle: Somatomedins have been shown to be one of 2 types of factors controlling the growth of BALB/c3T3 and some other cells. The first type is a competence factor that prepares resting cells for DNA synthesis by stimulating their passage into the G_1 phase. However, cells will not exit from the G_1 phase and begin to synthesize DNA unless the second factor, called a progression factor, is present along with epidermal growth factor. Competence factors are platelet-derived growth factor and fibroblast growth factor, and the major progression factors are somatomedins. Recent evidence shows that platelet-derived growth factor up-regulates somatomedin cellular receptors during the cell cycle. This could explain the role of the competence factor.

E. Somatomedins and Growth Hormone as Dual Regulators of Cell Growth: Green, Morikawa, and Nixon (1985) have proposed a dual role for the growth-promoting action of GH. GH can act both directly, by stimulating differentiation of precursor cells; and indirectly, by stimulating somatomedin synthesis, which causes proliferation of the differentiated cells. Thus, both GH and somatomedins should be able to stimulate growth of certain tissues. This theory agrees with the findings of other investigators who have reported that direct epiphyseal injections of GH stimulate growth.

Clinical Considerations

A. Somatomedins and Fetal Growth: GH appears to have little or no role in regulating fetal growth, because GH-deficient and anencephalic children have normal birth weights. Nevertheless, somatomedins are easily measured in fetal sera before the 20th week of gestation. Somatomedin concentrations in human cord blood have generally correlated well with birth size. Fetal somatomedin levels may be regulated by placental lactogen or progesterone. However, local tissue synthesis is probably the most important determinant of fetal somatomedin levels. The GH-dependent 140,000-MW binding protein appears only after 32 weeks of gestation.

The relative proportion of IGF-II and SM-C in fetal life varies with the species studied, but the lack of GH dependency suggests that IGF-II may be the fetal somatomedin. This is supported by data showing that fetal rat sera have immunoreactive IGF-II levels 20–100 times higher than those in maternal rat sera and elevated IGF-II values by the rat placental membrane assay. This is consistent with the weak GH dependency of IGF-II. Further evidence that IGF-II is the fetal somatomedin is the preponderance of type 2 receptors in several fetal tissues and the development of high concentrations of these receptors late in gestation.

During the first part of pregnancy, the SM-C level in maternal serum (as measured by radioimmunoassay) may fall slightly, but in the last half of pregnancy it rises steadily to almost twice the normal value. At parturition, the increase correlates with the duration of gestation and with maternal levels of placental lactogen. IGF-II levels also rise during the last half of pregnancy. The stimulus for the maternal increase in SM-C and IGF-II levels is not GH, for both were observed to increase in a pregnant GH-deficient patient. In both this patient and in healthy patients, SM-C and IGF-II levels fall abruptly after delivery.

B. Normal Plasma Somatomedin Levels Throughout Life: In humans, the plasma level of SM-C is lowest at birth and rises progressively throughout childhood. The increase in somatomedin levels correlates with age and occasionally height but not with weight or growth velocity. The low level of SM-C at the time of the greatest growth rate may be partly explained by the increased sensitivity of young skeletal tissue to SM-C.

IGF-II levels are low for the first year of life and then abruptly rise to the adult level. In rats, the IGF-II level falls after birth and reaches adult values by day 25. At about this time the SM-C level begins to rise progressively.

Girls have been reported to have higher values of SM-C by radioimmunoassay than boys of the same age, and the pubertal spurt of SM-C in girls precedes that in boys by 1–2 years. After puberty, the plasma SM-C level falls to normal adult values, which are reportedly higher in women than in men. At menopause, the SM-C level declines in women over several years by an average of 30%. This level also declines in men—but approximately 20 years later, SM-C sensitivity to GH remains.

CONDITIONS ASSOCIATED WITH SHORT STATURE

GROWTH HORMONE DEFICIENCY

The clinical features and treatment of GH deficiency are described in Chapter 8. Growth hormone deficiency results in dwarfism. However, the birth weight of GH-deficient children is in the normal range; only later is their condition clinically manifested.

Affected children have low serum somatomedin levels by bioassay, competitive binding assay, and SM-C and IGF-II radioimmunoassays, but these tests must be interpreted by comparison with sera from healthy children of the same age because of the age dependence of somatomedin concentrations (Table 7–3). The SM-C radioimmunoassay is the best diagnostic measurement, followed by competitive binding assays. Bioassays are less specific. A low value of somatomedins by these assays is consistent with but not diagnostic of GH deficiency. In the absence of other conditions that

Table 7–3. Clinical indications for somatomedin determinations.

Condition	Usefulness of Somatomedin Levels
Acromegaly	To establish diagnosis (especially valuable when GH values are in the normal range) and to evaluate therapy.
Excessively tall stature	To differentiate gigantism due to GH excess from cerebral gigantism and normally tall stature.
GH deficiency	Strongly suggests diagnosis in a child with growth failure and no other cause for subnormal somatomedin.
Laron dwarfism	Elevated GH and low somatomedin levels, unresponsive to GH, required to establish the diagnosis.[1]
Biologically inactive GH	Low somatomedin levels, responsive to exogenous GH stimulation, required to make this diagnosis.[1]
Dwarfism due to resistance to somatomedins	Elevated somatomedin levels in the presence of normal GH values required to make the diagnosis.[1]

[1] After other causes of growth failure have been eliminated.

can also cause low values, eg, malnutrition, marasmus, chronic liver disease, hypothyroidism, and Laron type dwarfism, further studies are indicated. In an otherwise healthy child, low somatomedin values (especially by SM-C radioimmunoassay), with low or undetectable GH unresponsive to stimulation, is diagnostic of GH deficiency.

GH administration to hypopituitary subjects causes a detectable elevation of somatomedin levels as soon as 6 hours afterward; peak values are reached between 12 and 24 hours. Daily administration results in a progressive increase in somatomedin levels that reach a plateau after 4 days. Using sera freed of binding protein, the same result is obtained measuring somatomedin by either hPM-radioreceptor assay or SM-C radioimmunoassay. Although GH therapy almost always causes an elevation in somatomedin levels that may be dose-dependent, the somatomedin response to GH does not correlate with the resultant growth velocity. An occasional child will respond clinically to GH therapy but will not have a rise in SM-C or total somatomedin levels either acutely or after long-term therapy. In these children, GH also fails to induce the 140,000-MW binding protein. Because most of the somatomedin in serum is actually stored in association with this protein, synthesis and utilization of somatomedin could be normal in these children. Metabolic production rates of somatomedin would determine if this is the case.

LARON TYPE DWARFISM

Laron type dwarfism is a familial form of short stature phenotypically resembling GH deficiency. Somatomedin levels are low, but characteristically the immunoreactive GH level is elevated or occasionally normal. The endogenous GH of Laron dwarfs has normal immunoassay and receptor-binding activity. Exogenous GH fails to stimulate not only somatomedin generation but also the other metabolic actions of GH, such as lipolysis. In vitro, GH also fails to stimulate erythroid colony formation in bone marrow cultures of Laron dwarfs. Therefore, Laron dwarfs are considered to have defective GH receptors. Somatomedin therapy may be the only way to restore growth in these children if it can be demonstrated that somatomedins can mediate all the essential actions of GH.

BIOLOGICALLY INACTIVE GROWTH HORMONE SYNDROME

Eight children have been reported with this form of growth retardation. The physical appearance of 2 subjects has been described, and one had the typical features of pituitary dwarfism. Fasting serum GH concentrations and GH responses to provocative stimulation were usually increased. Although the endogenous GH appeared to be normal in several radioimmunoassays, radioreceptor activity was significantly decreased. In all cases, serum somatomedin levels were subnormal. Exogenous GH stimulated free fatty acid release, somatomedin levels, and growth. This evidence led to the conclusion that endogenous GH was abnormal in this syndrome. The consensus is that biologically inactive GH is a rare condition in spite of one report to the contrary. In this report, 38% of children with unexplained extreme growth failures, negative physical examinations, and normal GH levels (normal variant short stature) were found to have subnormal SM-C levels. Exogenous GH administration increased the SM-C level and stimulated growth. The major problem with the study was that the baseline growth of these children prior to therapy was much less than that found in children with GH deficiency; other factors were probably involved in causing their short stature.

CONGENITAL RESISTANCE TO SOMATOMEDINS

Two cases of growth retardation due to congenital resistance to somatomedins have been described. In one case, although the child had a normal serum GH level and response to provocative stimuli, the serum somatomedin level was strikingly elevated by bioassay, hPM-radioreceptor assay, and SM-C radioimmunoassay. Exogenous GH had no effect on the somatomedin level and growth. The patient's serum somatomedin was active in the bioassay and radioreceptor assay, so it appears that the patient's cells were not able to respond to somatomedin because of a receptor or postreceptor defect.

CHRONIC RENAL DISEASE

Children with chronic renal disease are severely growth-retarded, usually below the third percentile. The mechanism that causes short stature in such cases has not been established. GH and insulin levels are elevated. The somatomedin level measured by bioassay is low, and the SM-C level measured by radioimmunoassay is in the low normal range. However, somatomedin values determined by the hPM-radioreceptor assay are elevated into the acromegalic range. The cause of the elevation of somatomedin measured by radioreceptor assay is unknown. The low levels of SM-C by radioimmunoassay suggest that the hPM-radioreceptor assay is detecting another somatomedin, possibly IGF-II. This is substantiated by measurements with the rat placental membrane radioreceptor assay. Although the elevation of somatomedin levels is inversely related to the glomerular filtration rate, it probably does not reflect decreased catabolism, for this should not selectively affect one somatomedin.

Another explanation could be the presence of an interfering factor such as a binding protein; however, various extraction procedures applied to uremic sera have failed to alter the result. If an elevated somatomedin level exists in chronic renal disease, it is unassociated with growth stimulation or metabolic effects. This could be due to a circulating inhibitor or to down-regulation of the somatomedin receptor analogous to that of the insulin receptor in chronic renal insufficiency. Successful renal transplantation results in a decrease of the radioreceptor-active somatomedin level to normal. However, growth is still impaired, possibly owing to the required chronic glucocorticoid administration.

THALASSEMIA MAJOR

Growth retardation is frequently encountered in children with β-thalassemia, but plasma GH values and responses are normal. Bioassayable somatomedin levels are reportedly in the range of GH deficiency, and therapy for iron overload with deferoxamine was without effect. In contrast, we have found normal levels of somatomedin by hPM-radioreceptor assay and SM-C radioimmunoassay in a group with β-thalassemia. However, all our patients had normal stature. This may have been due to the therapy administered; hypertransfusion maintained hemoglobin levels higher than 11 g/dL, and deferoxamine therapy was begun early.

MISCELLANEOUS CONDITIONS

Low serum somatomedin concentrations have been found in the presence of elevated GH levels in **anorexia nervosa, marasmus,** and **malnutrition**. With successful therapy, the somatomedin level is normalized and growth returns in children. There is evidence for a plasma inhibitor in malnutrition.

Hyperadrenocorticism in children usually results in short stature. Somatomedin levels are low by most bioassays, and the success of alternate-day steroid therapy in minimizing growth failure has been correlated with an improved bioassayable serum somatomedin level. Elevated levels of somatomedin have been found in hyperadrenocorticism by the hPM-radioreceptor assay and the SM-C radioimmunoassay. This suggests that short stature in this condition may be due to a direct steroid effect on cartilage or to an inhibitor of the biologic activity of somatomedin. However, the binding proteins had not been removed from these samples. Competitive protein-binding assays on extracted samples revealed normal values.

Serum somatomedin values in **hypothyroidism** are lower than normal, and a comparison of pretreatment values with those measured after thyroid replacement therapy shows a significant difference. **Pygmies** are short because of an isolated defect in SM-C generation

that develops at puberty. GH and IGF-II levels are normal. GH administration fails to correct the SM-C levels and stimulate growth.

CONDITIONS ASSOCIATED WITH EXCESSIVE GROWTH

ACROMEGALY

The clinical features of acromegaly are discussed in Chapter 6. Somatomedin values are particularly valuable in the diagnosis and evaluation of therapy for acromegaly. Virtually all patients with acromegaly have elevated values by SM-C radioimmunoassay and competitive binding assays, whereas bioassay measurements frequently may be within the normal range. The reason for this discrepancy is not known. Somatomedin levels have the additional advantage of being relatively constant throughout the day, in contrast to the wide fluctuations in the level of GH. Thus, one or 2 somatomedin measurements in an appropriate clinical setting may substitute for several baseline GH determinations plus provocative and suppression tests.

Rarely, patients with clinical acromegaly have radioimmunoassayable GH levels in the normal range, a finding that may delay therapy. Although paradoxic responses to glucose suppression and TRH stimulation can usually be elicited, these are not diagnostic. However, in the cases the author has studied, all have had elevated somatomedin values by hPM-radioreceptor assay. SM-C radioimmunoassay should be just as effective.

The measurement of SM-C levels may be most useful in evaluating the efficacy of therapy for acromegaly. The successful removal of a GH-producing tumor results in a fall in the serum SM-C level within 4 days. Persistent elevation of the SM-C level is consistent with clinical findings of continued activity and indicates that additional therapy should be directed toward normalizing the serum SM-C level. When the serum SM-C value is used as a criterion for successful therapy, a basal GH level of persistently less than 2 ng/mL appears to be required before it can be reasonably concluded that all tumor has been removed or destroyed. Increased morbidity and mortality rates from pulmonary, cardiac, and other diseases in treated acromegalics are probably related to the failure of adequate therapy; previous goals were only to reduce the GH levels to less than 5 or 10 ng/mL.

EXCESSIVELY TALL STATURE

GH-producing tumors in childhood, when the epiphyses are actively proliferating, lead to exaggerated linear growth and gigantism. The typical features of acromegaly may not be obvious, but SM-C levels are elevated. The elevated SM-C levels of gigantism should not be confused with the normal pubertal increase in these values. Patients with cerebral gigantism have normal SM-C levels.

BECKWITH-WIEDEMANN SYNDROME

Beckwith-Wiedemann syndrome consists of visceromegaly, macroglossia, omphalocele, hyperinsulinism, and hypoglycemia. An increase in the bioassayable serum somatomedin level has been reported in a child born with this syndrome. The stimulus for the increased somatomedin level may be hyperinsulinism, because the plasma GH level is normal. The only treatment is to supply adequate calories to prevent hypoglycemia. In the reported case, with time, the hyperinsulinism, hypoglycemia, elevated somatomedin level, and abnormal growth returned to normal (see Chapter 8).

EXCESSIVE GROWTH IN POSTOPERATIVE PATIENTS WITH CRANIOPHARYNGIOMA

An occasional craniopharyngioma patient exhibits normal or even excessive postoperative growth despite GH levels undetectable by radioimmunoassay. In these cases, the somatomedin levels have been normal rather than low, and somatomedins may be responsible for the continued growth. The stimulus for the normal somatomedin level has never been satisfactorily explained. Prolactin (PRL) was initially suggested, but subsequent studies disproved this. Insulin is a more likely candidate, because these patients generally have hyperphagia and hyperinsulinism.

CONDITIONS RELATED TO THE METABOLIC ACTION OF SOMATOMEDINS

TUMOR HYPOGLYCEMIA

Hypoglycemia may occasionally be associated with non-insulin-producing tumors of the liver, the adrenal cortex, and the retroperitoneum. The pathophysiology of the hypoglycemia is not understood. Insulinlike activity has been isolated from the extracts of 2 tumors, and approximately half of patients have elevated serum somatomedin levels measured either by a rat liver membrane receptor assay or a rat placental membrane receptor assay, which has been reported to be specific for IGF-II. However, the radioimmunoassay for IGF-II, the hPM-radioreceptor assay, and the bioassay for insulinlike activity give normal values, while the radioimmunoassay for SM-C gives a low value. The cause of the spurious radioreceptor assay values is unknown, but increased IGF-II mRNA has recently been reported in some of these tumors.

DIABETES MELLITUS

Low serum values of bioassayable somatomedin were initially reported in untreated juvenile diabetics and a series of long-term untreated and treated diabetics of presumably mixed origin. Chemically induced diabetes in rats also produces a low serum somatomedin level. Decreased serum somatomedin levels or a somatomedin inhibitor could explain the poor growth of juvenile diabetics in spite of their hyperresponsiveness to GH. The author has observed that a group of lean, insulin-dependent, well-controlled diabetic patients had normal somatomedin levels by hPM radioreceptor assay. However, modestly elevated bioassayable somatomedin concentrations have been found in long-standing insulin-dependent diabetic patients. Others have noted in juvenile diabetic patients normal radioimmunoassayable SM-C levels that increased after improved control by continuous insulin infusion. Chronic exposure to excess GH stimulation may have elevated the plasma SM-C level and contributed to some of the vascular complications of diabetes. Elevated somatomedin levels have been noted in patients with diabetic retinopathy, and the author has observed a dramatic exacerbation of retinopathy associated with an increased plasma SM-C level. This effect is consistent with the ability of SM-C to stimulate proliferation of endothelial and mesangeal cells and fibroplasia.

RELATIONSHIP BETWEEN SOMATOMEDINS & CANCER

Human chondrosarcomas and fibrosarcomas were discovered to produce a factor with IGF-II-like binding activity and, by indirect evidence, to have receptors that bound IGF-II. Thus, these tumors may stimulate their own growth by the production of an autocrine hormone and thereby escape some of the body's growth-retarding mechanisms. Human breast cancers in continuous culture have been found to express SM-C mRNA, to release a peptide with SM-C-like radioimmunoreactivity, and to respond to exogenous SM-C with an increase in growth. This mechanism is probably operating in human breast cancers in vivo, because immunohistochemical data also indicate that human breast carcinomas produce SM-C, and hybridization studies indicate SM-C gene expression. Wilms' tumors, renal carcinomas, colon carcinomas, buffalo rat liver tumor cells, and other cancers have now been reported to express somatomedin genes. Chromosome studies have demonstrated the proximity of *ras* oncogenes to the somatomedin genes, a juxtaposition that may be important in carcinogenesis.

REFERENCES

Adams SO et al: Developmental patterns of insulin-like growth factor-I and -II synthesis and regulation in rat fibroblasts. *Nature* 1983;**302**:150.

Ashton IK, Matheson JA: Change in response with age of human articular cartilage to plasma somatomedin activity. *Calcif Tissue Int* 1979;**29**:89.

Atkison PR et al: Release of somatomedin-like activity by cultured WI-38 human fibroblasts. *Endocrinology* 1980;**106**:2006.

Blundell TL et al: Insulin-like growth factor: A model for tertiary structure accounting for immunoreactivity and receptor binding. *Proc Natl Acad Sci USA* 1978;**75**:180.

Clemmons DR, Underwood LE, Van Wyk JJ: Hormonal control of immunoreactive somatomedin production by cultured human fibroblasts. *J Clin Invest* 1981;**67**:10.

Daughaday WH, Mariz IK, Blethen SL: Inhibition of access of bound somatomedin to membrane receptor and immunobinding sites: A comparison of radioreceptor and radioimmunoassay of somatomedin in native and acid-ethanol–extracted serum. *J Clin Endocrinol Metab* 1980;**51**:781.

De Larco JE, Todaro GJ: A human fibrosarcoma cell line producing multiplication stimulating activity (MSA)-related peptides. *Nature* 1978;**272**:356.

D'Ercole AJ, Willson DF, Underwood LE: Changes in the circulating form of serum somatomedin-C during fetal life. *J Clin Endocrinol Metab* 1980;**51**:674.

Dull, TJ et al: Insulin-like growth factor II precursor gene organization in relation to insulin gene family. *Nature* 1984;**310**:777.

Froesch ER et al: Antibody-suppressible and non-suppressible insulin-like activities in serum and their physiologic significance. *J Clin Invest* 1963;**42**:1816.

Furlanetto RW: Nongrowth hormone dependent hormonal regulation of plasma somatomedin levels. Page 197 in: *Insulin-Like Growth Factors/Somatomedins: Basic Chemistry, Biology and Clinical Importance.* Spencer EM (editor). Walter de Gruyter, 1981.

Green H, Morikawa M, Nixon T: A dual effector theory of growth hormone action. *Differentiation* 1985;**29**:195.

Hintz RL, Liu F: Demonstration of specific plasma protein binding sites for somatomedin. *J Clin Endocrinol Metab* 1977;**45**:988.

Hintz RL, Liu F: A radioimmunoassay for insulin-like growth factor-II specific for the C-peptide region. *J Clin Endocrinol Metab* 1982;**54**:442.

Holder AT, Spencer EM, Preece MA: Effect of bovine growth hormone and a partially pure preparation of somatomedin on various growth parameters in hypopituitary dwarf mice. *J Clin Invest* 1981;**89**:275.

Howard GA, Spencer EM: Somatomedins A and C directly stimulate bone cell proliferation in vitro. In: *Endocrine Control of Bone and Calcium Metabolism.* Cohn DV et al (editors). Elsevier, 1984.

Jansen M et al: Sequence of cDNA encoding human insulin-like growth factor I. *Nature* 1983;**306**:609.

Kasuga M et al: Demonstration of two subtypes of insulin-like growth factor receptors by affinity cross-linking. *J Biol Chem* 1981;**256**:5305.

Knauer DJ, Smith GL: Inhibition of biological activity of multiplication-stimulating activity by binding to its carrier protein. *Proc Natl Acad Sci USA* 1980;**77**:7252.

Lanes R et al: Dwarfism associated with normal serum growth hormone and increased bioassayable, receptorassayable and immunoassayable somatomedin. *J Clin Endocrinol Metab* 1980;**50**:485.

Laron Z et al: Administration of growth hormone to patients with familial dwarfism with high plasma immunoreactive growth hormone: Measurement of sulfation factor, metabolic and linear growth responses. *J Clin Endocrinol Metab* 1971;**33**:332.

Moses AC et al: Increased levels of multiplication-stimulating activity, an insulin-like growth factor, in fetal rat serum. *Proc Natl Acad Sci USA* 1980;**77**:3649.

Pierson RW, Temin HM: The partial purification from calf serum of a fraction with multiplication-stimulating activity for chicken fibroblasts in cell culture and with nonsuppressible insulin-like activity. *J Cell Physiol* 1972;**79**:319.

Rudman D et al: Children with normal-variant short stature: Treatment with human growth hormone for six months. (2 parts.) *N Engl J Med* 1981;**305**:3, 123.

Salmon WD Jr, Daughaday WH: A hormonally controlled serum factor which stimulates sulfate incorporation by cartilage in vitro. *J Lab Clin Med* 1957;**49**:825.

Schlecter NL et al: Evidence suggesting that the direct growth-promoting effect of growth hormone on cartilage in vivo is mediated by local production of somatomedin. *Proc Natl Acad Sci USA* 1986;**83**:7932.

Schoenle E et al: Insulin-like growth factor I stimulates growth in hypophysectomized rats. *Nature* 1982;**206**:252.

Spencer EM: Lack of response of serum somatomedin to hyperprolactinemia in humans. *J Clin Endocrinol Metab* 1980;**50**:182.

Spencer EM, Mims R, Uthne KO: Somatomedin levels in patients with pituitary microadenomas. In: *Pituitary Microadenomas.* Faglia G, Giovanelli MA, McLeod RM (editors). Academic Press, 1980.

Spencer EM, Ross M, Smith B: The identity of human insulin-like growth factors I and II: Somatomedins C and A and homology with rat IGF I and II. Page 81 in: *Insulin-Like Growth Factors/Somatomedins: Basic Chemistry, Biology and Clinical Importance.* Spencer EM (editor). Walter de Gruyter, 1981.

Spencer EM, Uthne KO: The effect of somatomedin on adenylyl cyclase and guanylyl cyclase activity in various tissues. Page 37 in: *Somatomedins and Growth.* Giordano

G, Van Wyk JJ, Minuto F (editors). Academic Press, 1979.

Spencer EM, Uthne K, Arnold W: Growth impairment with elevated somatomedin levels in children with chronic renal insufficiency. *Acta Endocrinol* 1979;**91**:36.

Stiles CD et al: Dual control of cell growth by somatomedins and platelet derived growth factor. *Proc Natl Acad Sci USA* 1979;**76**:1279.

Tricoli JV et al: Location of insulin-like growth factor genes to human chromosomes 11 and 12. *Nature* 1984;**310**:784.

Growth

8

Dennis M. Styne, MD

Assessment of growth in stature is an essential part of the pediatric examination. Growth is an important index of physical and mental health and of the quality of the child's psychosocial environment; chronic problems in any of these areas may be reflected in a decreased growth rate. In this discussion, we will consider influences on normal growth, the normal growth pattern, the measurement of growth, and conditions that lead to disorders of growth.

NORMAL GROWTH

INTRAUTERINE GROWTH

The great changes that take place in the human fetus during intrauterine growth have been summarized by Pierson and Deschamps: From conception to delivery, fetal mass increases 44×10^7 times, compared to a 20-fold increase from birth to adulthood; length increases 3850 times to term, compared to a 3- to 4-fold increase from birth to adulthood. The determinants of normal prenatal growth are poorly understood, though many factors that lead to abnormal prenatal growth have been identified.

Endocrine Factors

Much research remains to be done before the endocrine factors influencing fetal growth will be completely elucidated.

A. Growth Hormone: Although fetal plasma values of growth hormone (GH) are higher than levels reported in most adult acromegalics, GH appears to have little influence on length at birth; infants with GH deficiency have normal birth lengths, and even those with anencephaly (who therefore lack hypothalamic releasing factors) have normal body lengths. Remarkably, when GH concentrations are high at birth, IGF-I concentrations are exceedingly low; a lack of growth hormone receptors before delivery may explain this paradox. Human chorionic

Acronyms Used in This Chapter	
ACTH	Adrenocorticotropic hormone
cAMP	Cyclic adenosine monophosphate
DNA	Deoxyribonucleic acid
GH	Growth hormone
GnRH	Gonadotropin-releasing hormone
GRH	Growth hormone-releasing hormone
hCG	Human chorionic gonadotropin
hCS	Human chorionic somatomammotropin
hGH	Human growth hormone
IGF	Human insulinlike growth factor (somatomedin)
IGF-I	Human insulinlike growth factor I
IGF-II	Human insulinlike growth factor II
IUGR	Intrauterine growth retardation
LH	Luteinizing hormone
LS	Lower segment
MSA	Multiplication-stimulating activity
NCHS	National Center for Health Statistics
PTH	Parathyroid hormone
RTA	Renal tubular acidosis
RWT	Roche, Warner, and Theisen method of height prediction
SS	Somatostatin
TBG	Thyroid hormone-binding globulin
TRH	Thyrotropin-releasing hormone
TSH	Thyroid-stimulating hormone (thyrotropin)
US	Upper segment

somatomammotropin (hCS), a placental hormone similar in structure to GH and prolactin, may not be essential to fetal growth, since mothers lacking the hCS gene have given birth to children with normal birth lengths.

B. Thyroid Hormone: The absence of thyroid hormone may have devastating effects on the mental development of a neonate, but hypothyroid newborns are of normal length. In fact, perhaps because of the longer duration of pregnancy in hypothyroid fetuses, the hypothyroid newborn may be longer than average.

C. Insulin: Excessive serum insulin concentrations may be associated with increased length in infants of diabetic mothers and in Beckwith-Wiedemann syndrome, characterized by neonatal hypoglycemia, neonatal gigantism, omphalocele, macroglossia, and hepatomegaly. Inadequate insulin production, found in transient neonatal diabetes mellitus, or insulin resistance, found in the leprechaun syndrome (Donohue syndrome), is associated with short newborn length.

D. Somatomedins (IGF-I and IGF-II): The role of somatomedins in prenatal growth in unclear. IGF-I is made in the placenta but appears to be quickly cleared from the plasma. IGF-II may play an important role, as suggested by the observation that serum MSA (multiplication-stimulating activity) and IGF-II levels are higher than IGF-I levels in fetal rats and fetal sheep, respectively. (MSA is chemically similar to IGF-II; see Chapter 7.) After birth, IGF-II values decrease and IGF-I values increase. The actual cellular effects of these factors may be unrelated to their serum levels, so the relationship of serum levels to clinical conditions must be inferred. Serum IGF-I values do correlate with newborn weight in normal infants. Laron's dwarfism, characterized by an inability to generate IGF-I, is associated with short birth length.

Maternal & Uterine Factors

Maternal factors, often expressed through the uterine environment, exert more influence on birth size than paternal factors. The height of the mother correlates better with fetal size than the height of the father. Worldwide, poor maternal nutrition is the most important condition leading to low birth weight and length; it also predisposes the infant to other serious health hazards after birth. Chronic maternal disease and eclampsia can also lead to poor fetal growth. Maternal alcohol ingestion has been shown to have severe adverse effects on fetal length and mental development and to predispose to other physical abnormalities such as microcephaly, mental retardation, midfacial hypoplasia, short palpebral fissures, wide-bridged nose, long philtrum, and narrow vermilion border of the lip. Abuse of other substances and chronic use of some medications (eg, phenytoin) can cause intrauterine growth retardation. Cigarette smoking causes not only retarded intrauterine growth but also decreased postnatal growth for as long as 5 years after parturition. Maternal infection—most commonly rubella, toxoplasmosis, and cytomegalovirus—leads to many developmental abnormalities as well as short birth length. Recently, congenital AIDS was noted to cause intrauterine growth retardation. In multiple births, the weight of each fetus is usually less than that of the average singleton. Uterine tumors or malformations may decrease fetal growth.

Because infants who are small for gestational age usually do not grow well after birth, any of the factors that cause low birth weight may ultimately have a deleterious effect on postnatal growth and final stature in adulthood. This is in contrast to infants with normal weight for gestational age. Premature infants usually recover to the range of normal height and weight for age by age 2 years. To do this, they must have growth rates that are higher than the average. Thus, a key point in assessing the patient with short stature is determining gestational age at birth and relating it to birth weight and length.

Chromosomal Abnormalities & Malformation Syndromes

Many chromosomal abnormalities that lead to malformation syndromes also cause poor fetal growth. Other malformation syndromes associated with a normal karyotype are characterized by intrauterine growth retardation, but in most cases endocrine abnormalities have not been noted. For further discussion, the reader is referred to other sources listed in the references at the end of this chapter.

POSTNATAL GROWTH

Although we have limited knowledge of the factors affecting prenatal growth, more is known about postnatal growth. Assessment of growth is, of course, easier after birth, and the effects of environmental manipulation and replacement of deficient hormones are easier to document in the child than in the fetus.

Postnatal growth in stature and weight follows a definite pattern in normal children (Figs 8–1 and 8–2). The highest overall growth rate is in the fetus; the highest postnatal growth rate occurs just after birth, followed by a slower growth rate in mid childhood (Figs 8–3 and 8–4). The striking increase in stature known as the pubertal growth spurt then follows, leading to a second peak of growth velocity. The final decrease follows, until the epiphyses fuse and growth ceases.

Endocrine Factors

A. Growth Hormone and Somatomedins: As discussed in Chapter 6, somatotropin, or growth hormone (GH), is regulated by hypothalamic somatostatin and growth hormone–releasing hormone (GRH). GH then stimulates somatomedin production, which has a direct influence on the growth of cartilage. In general, serum IGF-I varies with states of GH secretion—decreased in GH deficiency and elevated in acromegaly—but nutrition, chronologic age, and other genetic and metabolic factors can alter this relationship. The replacement of GH in hypopituitary dwarfism leads to striking improvement in growth and elevation of serum IGF-I and has clearly demonstrated the importance of the GH-somatomedin axis in postnatal growth. Plasma somatomedin values are age-dependent. Values are lowest in the neonate, and levels in children are lower than those in adults. Acromegalic levels are reached during puberty, although peak somatomedin values do not closely correlate chronologically with peak height velocity.

B. Thyroid Hormone: Although hypothyroid newborns are not short, they manifest exceedingly poor

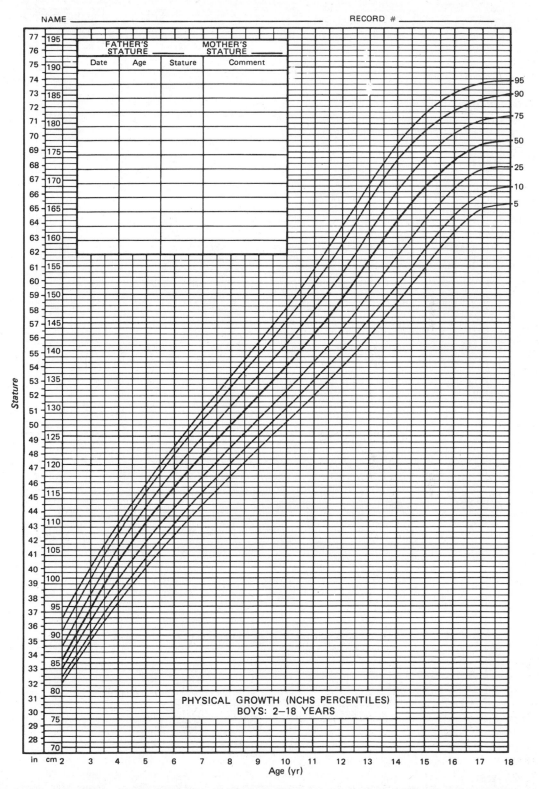

Figure 8–1. Growth chart for boys in the USA. (Redrawn and reprinted with permission of Ross Laboratories, Columbus, OH 43216. © 1980 Ross Laboratories. Sources of data: 1976 study of the National Center for Health Statistics [NCHS; Hyattsville, MD]; Hamill PVV et al: Physical growth: National Center for Health Statistics percentiles. *Am J Clin Nutr* 1979;**32:**607.)

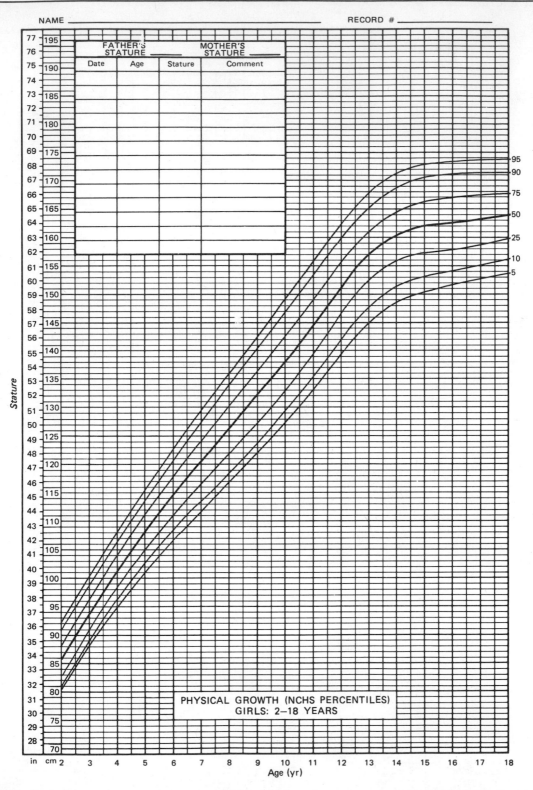

Figure 8–2. Growth chart for girls in the USA. (Redrawn and reprinted with permission of Ross Laboratories, Columbus, OH 43216. © 1980 Ross Laboratories. Sources of data: 1976 study of the National Center for Health Statistics [NCHS; Hyattsville, MD]; Hamill PVV et al: Physical growth: National Center for Health Statistics percentiles. *Am J Clin Nutr* 1979;**32**:607.)

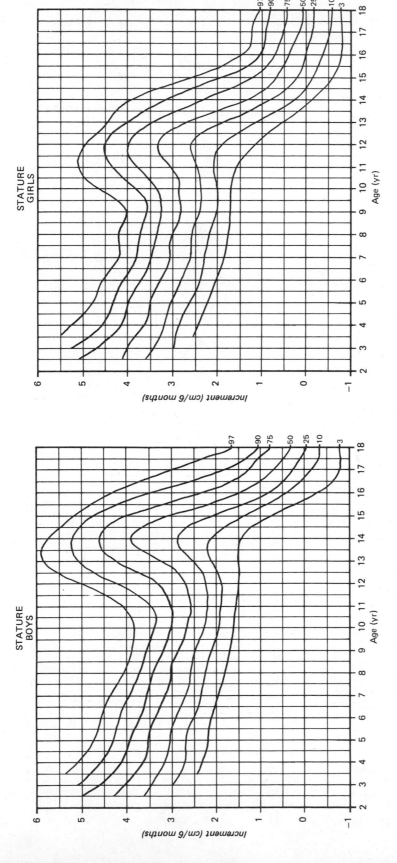

Figures 8–3 and 8–4. Incremental growth charts for boys (Fig 8–3) and girls (Fig 8–4). Height velocity measured over a period of at least 6 months can be compared with the percentiles on the right axis of the charts. (Redrawn and reprinted with permission of Ross Laboratories, Columbus, OH 43216. © 1981 Ross Laboratories. Sources of data: Longitudinal studies of the Fels Research Laboratories [Yellow Springs, OH]; Roche AF, Himes JH: Incremental growth charts. *Am J Clin Nutr* 1980;**33**:2041.)

growth soon after birth if untreated. Acquired hypothyroidism can also lead to a markedly decreased growth rate. Bone age advancement is severely delayed, usually more so than in GH deficiency. The upper to lower segment ratio (Fig 8–7) is also elevated and therefore delayed, owing to poorer limb growth than trunk growth.

C. Sex Steroids: Gonadal steroids exert an important influence on the pubertal growth spurt, while absence of these factors is not important in prepubertal growth. Gonadal and adrenal sex steroids in excess can cause a sharp increase in growth rate as well as the premature appearance and progression of secondary sexual features. If unabated, increased sex steroids will cause advancement of skeletal age, premature epiphyseal fusion, and short adult stature.

D. Glucocorticoids: Cortisone or its analogues in excess can stop growth. The absence of glucocorticoids has little effect on growth if the individual is clinically well in other respects.

Other Factors

A. Genetic Factors: Genetic factors can influence final height. Good correlation is found between mid

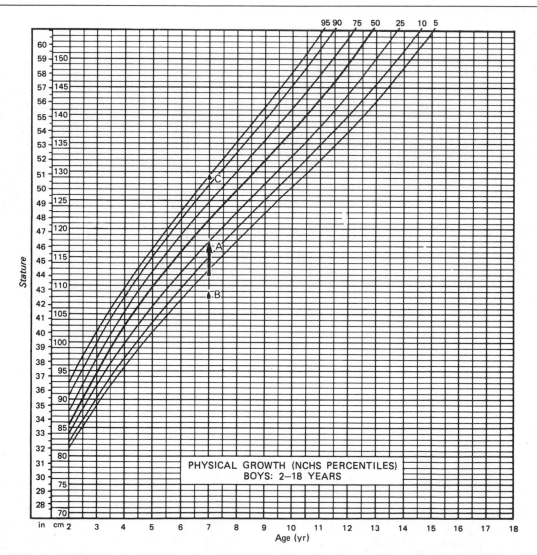

Figure 8–5. Adjustment of height based on mid parental stature (Table 8–1). Charts of 3 boys, each 7 years of age. *A* is below the 5th percentile, with a height of 112 cm; taking his mid parental stature of 158 cm into consideration, his adjusted height of 118 cm (arrow) is at the 25th percentile, suggesting that he is short because of familial tendency. *B* is far below the 5th percentile, with a height of 108 cm; his mid parental height of 166 cm causes his adjusted height to rise only 1 cm, suggesting that familial factors may not be the cause of his short stature. The converse is shown by *C*, whose height is 129 cm (95th percentile); mid parental height is 172 cm and adjusted height is equal to measured height, suggesting that the cause of his tall stature is probably not familial.

parental height and the child's height between 3 and 18 years of age; appropriate charts and tables have been developed to display this (Figs 8–5 and 8–6; Tables 8–1 and 8–2).

B. Socioeconomic Factors: Worldwide, the most common cause of short stature is poverty and its effects. Thus, poor nutrition, poor hygiene, and poor health have effects on growth both before and after birth. In people of the same ethnic group and in the same geographic location, variations in stature are often attributable to these factors. For example, studies have shown that Japanese born and reared in North America were taller than Japanese-born immigrants to North America. Conversely, when socioeconomic factors are equal, the differences in average height between various ethnic groups are probably genetic.

C. Nutritional Factors: The influence of malnutrition accounts for much of the socioeconomic discrepancy in height noted above, but malnutrition may occur in the midst of plenty and must always be suspected in disorders of growth. Other factors may be blamed for poor growth when nutritional deficiencies are actually responsible. For example, Sherpas were previously thought to have short stature owing to the fact that they live on the slopes of Mouth Everest, but nutritional supplementation was recently demonstrated to

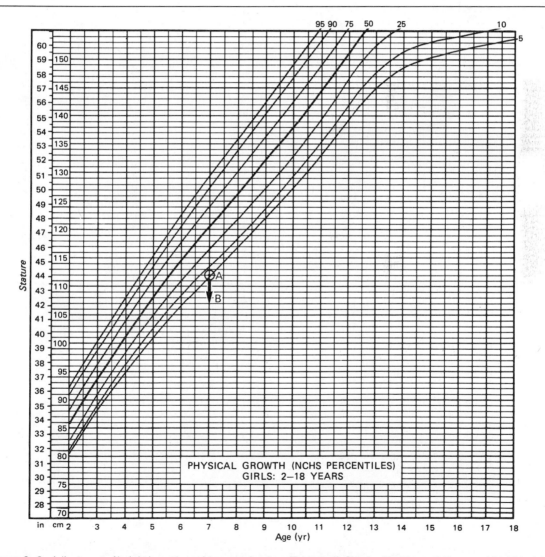

Figure 8–6. Adjustment of height based on mid parental stature (Table 8–2). Charts of 2 girls, each 7 years old, with height of 112 cm (5th percentile). *A* has a mid parental stature of 168 cm, and her adjusted height is unchanged, suggesting that genetic influences do not explain her short stature. *B* has a mid parental stature of 178 cm, causing her adjusted height (arrow) to fall 5 cm, suggesting that her short stature is more severe than suspected from the original growth chart and that genetic influences are certainly not the cause.

Table 8–1. Parent-specific adjustments (cm) for stature of boys from 3 to 18 years of age.[1]

Age (yr)	Stature (cm)	Mid Parental Stature (cm)																	
		150	152	154	156	158	160	162	164	166	168	170	172	174	176	178	180	182	184
3	86.0– 87.9	7	6	5	5	4	3	2	1	1	0	−1	−2	−3	−3	−4	−5	−6	−7
	88.0– 97.9	8	7	6	5	4	4	3	2	1	0	−1	−1	−2	−3	−4	−5	−5	−6
	98.0–106.9	8	8	7	6	5	4	4	3	2	1	0	0	−1	−2	−3	−4	−4	−5
4	90.0– 93.9	7	6	5	4	4	3	2	1	0	−1	−1	−2	−3	−4	−5	−5	−6	−7
	94.0–103.9	8	7	6	5	4	3	3	2	1	0	−1	−1	−2	−3	−4	−5	−6	−6
	104.0–112.9	8	8	7	6	5	4	3	3	2	1	0	−1	−1	−2	−3	−4	−5	−6
5	96.0–103.9	8	7	6	5	4	3	2	1	0	0	−1	−2	−3	−4	−5	−6	−7	−8
	104.0–113.9	9	8	7	6	5	4	3	2	1	0	0	−1	−2	−3	−4	−5	−6	−7
	114.0–122.9	9	9	8	7	6	5	4	3	2	1	0	0	−1	−2	−3	−4	−5	−6
6	102.0–111.9	8	7	7	6	5	4	3	2	1	0	−1	−2	−3	−4	−5	−6	−7	−8
	112.0–121.9	9	8	7	7	6	5	4	3	2	1	0	−1	−2	−3	−4	−5	−6	−7
	122.0–130.9	10	9	8	7	6	6	5	4	3	2	1	0	−1	−2	−3	−4	−5	−6
7	108.0–117.9	9	8	7	6	5	4	3	2	1	0	−1	−2	−4	−5	−6	−7	−8	−9
	118.0–127.9	10	9	8	7	6	5	4	3	2	1	0	−1	−2	−4	−5	−6	−7	−8
	128.0–136.9	12	10	9	8	7	6	5	4	3	2	1	0	−1	−2	−4	−5	−6	−7
8	114.0–115.9	10	9	8	6	5	4	3	2	1	−1	−2	−3	−4	−5	−6	−8	−9	−10
	116.0–125.9	11	9	8	7	6	5	4	2	1	0	−1	−2	−3	−5	−6	−7	−8	−9
	126.0–135.9	12	10	9	8	7	6	5	3	2	1	0	−1	−2	−4	−5	−6	−7	−8
	136.0–144.9	13	12	10	9	8	7	6	5	3	2	1	0	−1	−2	−4	−5	−6	−7
9	120.0–121.9	11	9	8	7	6	4	3	2	1	0	−2	−3	−4	−5	−7	−8	−9	−10
	122.0–131.9	11	10	9	8	6	5	4	3	1	0	−1	−2	−3	−5	−6	−7	−8	−10
	132.0–141.9	12	11	10	9	7	6	5	4	2	1	0	−1	−2	−4	−5	−6	−7	−9
	142.0–150.9	13	12	11	10	8	7	6	5	4	2	1	0	−1	−3	−4	−5	−6	−7
10	124.0–127.9	11	10	9	7	6	5	3	2	1	−1	−2	−3	−5	−6	−7	−9	−10	−11
	128.0–137.9	12	11	10	8	7	6	4	3	2	0	−1	−2	−4	−5	−6	−8	−9	−10
	138.0–147.9	13	12	11	9	8	7	5	4	3	1	0	−1	−3	−4	−5	−7	−8	−9
	148.0–158.9	14	13	12	11	9	8	7	5	4	3	1	0	−1	−3	−4	−5	−7	−8
11	128.0–133.9	12	10	9	8	6	5	4	2	1	0	−2	−3	−5	−6	−7	−9	−10	−11
	134.0–143.9	12	11	10	8	7	6	4	3	2	0	−1	−2	−4	−5	−6	−8	−9	−10
	144.0–153.9	14	12	11	10	8	7	5	4	3	1	0	−1	−3	−4	−5	−7	−8	−9
	154.0–162.9	15	13	12	11	9	8	7	5	4	3	1	0	−2	−3	−4	−6	−7	−8
12	132.0–141.9	12	10	9	8	6	5	4	2	1	0	−2	−3	−4	−6	−7	−8	−10	−11
	142.0–151.9	13	11	10	9	7	6	5	3	2	1	−1	−2	−3	−5	−6	−7	−9	−10
	152.0–161.9	13	12	11	9	8	7	5	4	3	1	0	−1	−2	−4	−5	−6	−8	−9
	162.0–170.9	14	13	12	10	9	8	6	5	4	2	1	0	−2	−3	−4	−6	−7	−8
13	136.0–139.9	12	10	9	8	6	5	4	2	1	−1	−2	−3	−5	−6	−7	−9	−10	−12
	140.0–149.9	12	11	10	8	7	6	4	3	1	0	−1	−3	−4	−6	−7	−8	−10	−11
	150.0–159.9	13	12	10	9	8	6	5	4	2	1	−1	−2	−3	−5	−6	−7	−9	−10
	160.0–169.9	14	13	11	10	8	7	6	4	3	2	0	−1	−3	−4	−5	−7	−8	−9
	170.0–178.9	15	13	12	11	9	8	6	5	4	2	1	0	−2	−3	−5	−6	−7	−9
14	142.0–145.9	13	11	10	8	7	5	4	2	1	−1	−2	−4	−5	−7	−8	−10	−11	−13
	146.0–155.9	14	12	11	9	8	6	5	3	1	0	−2	−3	−5	−6	−8	−9	−11	−12
	156.0–165.9	15	13	11	10	8	7	5	4	2	1	−1	−2	−4	−5	−7	−8	−10	−11
	166.0–175.9	15	14	12	11	9	8	6	5	3	2	0	−1	−3	−4	−6	−7	−9	−11
	176.0–184.9	16	15	13	12	10	9	7	6	4	3	1	−1	−2	−4	−5	−7	−8	−10
15	148.0–151.9	14	13	11	9	7	6	4	2	0	−1	−3	−5	−7	−8	−10	−12	−14	−15
	152.0–161.9	15	14	12	10	8	7	5	3	1	0	−2	−4	−6	−7	−9	−11	−13	−14
	162.0–171.9	17	15	13	11	10	8	6	4	3	1	−1	−3	−4	−6	−8	−10	−11	−13
	172.0–181.9	18	16	14	13	11	9	7	6	4	2	0	−1	−3	−5	−7	−8	−10	−12
	182.0–190.9	19	17	16	14	12	10	9	7	5	3	2	0	−2	−4	−5	−7	−9	−11
16	156.0–163.9	17	15	13	11	9	7	5	3	1	−1	−3	−5	−7	−9	−11	−13	−16	−18
	164.0–173.9	19	17	15	13	10	8	6	4	2	0	−2	−4	−6	−8	−10	−12	−14	−16
	174.0–183.9	21	19	17	15	12	10	8	6	4	2	0	−2	−4	−6	−8	−10	−12	−14
	184.0–192.9	23	21	19	17	14	12	10	8	6	4	2	0	−2	−4	−6	−8	−10	−12
17	162.0–165.9	17	15	13	11	9	7	4	2	0	−2	−4	−7	−9	−11	−13	−15	−17	−20
	166.0–175.9	20	17	15	13	11	9	6	4	2	0	−2	−4	−7	−9	−11	−13	−15	−18
	176.0–185.9	22	20	18	16	13	11	9	7	5	3	0	−2	−4	−6	−8	−11	−13	−15
	186.0–194.9	25	23	20	18	16	14	12	9	7	5	3	1	−1	−4	−6	−8	−10	−12
18	160.0–165.9	18	16	13	11	9	6	4	2	0	−3	−5	−7	−10	−12	−14	−17	−19	−21
	166.0–175.9	20	18	16	13	11	9	7	4	2	0	−3	−5	−7	−10	−12	−14	−17	−19
	176.0–185.9	23	21	19	16	14	12	9	7	5	3	0	−2	−4	−7	−9	−11	−14	−16
	186.0–194.9	26	24	22	19	17	15	12	10	8	6	3	1	−1	−4	−6	−8	−11	−13

[1]See footnote for Table 8–2.

Table 8–2. Parent-specific adjustments (cm) for stature of girls from 3 to 18 years of age.[1]

Age (yr)	Stature (cm)	Mid Parental Stature (cm)																	
		150	152	154	156	158	160	162	164	166	168	170	172	174	176	178	180	182	184
3	82.0– 83.9	6	5	4	4	3	2	1	1	0	−1	−1	−2	−3	−3	−4	−5	−6	−6
	84.0– 93.9	6	6	5	4	3	3	2	1	1	0	−1	−1	−2	−3	−4	−4	−5	−6
	94.0–102.9	7	7	6	5	4	4	3	2	2	1	0	−1	−1	−2	−3	−3	−4	−5
4	92.0– 93.9	6	6	5	4	3	3	2	1	0	0	−1	−2	−3	−3	−4	−5	−6	−7
	94.0–103.9	7	6	6	5	4	3	2	2	1	0	−1	−1	−2	−3	−4	−4	−5	−6
	104.0–112.9	8	7	7	6	5	4	3	3	2	1	0	0	−1	−2	−3	−3	−4	−5
5	100.0–101.9	8	7	6	5	4	3	2	1	1	0	−1	−2	−3	−4	−5	−5	−6	−7
	102.0–111.9	8	7	6	6	5	4	3	2	1	0	−1	−1	−2	−3	−4	−5	−6	−7
	112.0–120.9	9	8	7	7	6	5	4	3	2	1	1	0	−1	−2	−3	−4	−5	−6
6	106.0–109.9	9	8	7	6	5	4	3	2	1	0	−1	−2	−3	−4	−5	−6	−7	−8
	110.0–119.9	9	9	8	7	6	5	4	3	2	1	0	−1	−2	−3	−4	−5	−6	−7
	120.0–128.9	11	10	9	8	7	6	5	4	3	2	1	0	−1	−2	−3	−4	−5	−6
7	112.0–117.9	9	8	7	6	5	4	3	2	1	0	−1	−2	−3	−4	−5	−6	−7	−8
	118.0–127.9	10	9	8	7	6	5	4	3	2	1	0	−1	−2	−3	−4	−5	−6	−7
	128.0–136.9	11	10	9	8	7	6	5	4	3	2	1	0	−1	−2	−3	−4	−5	−6
8	116.0–123.9	9	8	7	6	5	4	3	2	1	0	−1	−2	−3	−4	−5	−6	−8	−9
	124.0–133.9	10	9	8	7	6	5	4	3	2	1	0	−1	−2	−3	−4	−5	−7	−8
	134.0–142.9	11	10	9	8	7	6	5	4	3	2	1	0	−1	−2	−3	−4	−6	−7
9	122.0–131.9	10	9	8	7	6	5	3	2	1	0	−1	−2	−3	−4	−5	−6	−7	−9
	132.0–141.9	11	10	9	8	7	6	4	3	2	1	0	−1	−2	−3	−4	−5	−7	−8
	142.0–150.9	12	11	10	9	8	6	5	4	3	2	1	0	−1	−2	−3	−5	−6	−7
10	126.0–127.9	10	9	7	6	5	4	3	2	1	0	−1	−2	−3	−5	−6	−7	−8	−9
	128.0–137.9	10	9	8	7	6	5	4	2	1	0	−1	−2	−3	−4	−5	−6	−7	−8
	138.0–147.9	11	10	9	8	6	5	4	3	2	1	0	−1	−2	−3	−4	−5	−7	−8
	148.0–158.9	12	10	9	8	7	6	5	4	3	2	1	0	−1	−3	−4	−5	−6	−7
11	130.0–133.9	10	9	8	6	5	4	3	2	1	0	−1	−2	−3	−4	−6	−7	−8	−9
	134.0–143.9	10	9	8	7	6	5	4	3	1	0	−1	−2	−3	−4	−5	−6	−7	−8
	144.0–153.9	11	10	9	7	6	6	4	3	2	1	0	−1	−2	−3	−5	−6	−7	−8
	154.0–162.9	11	10	9	8	7	6	5	4	3	1	0	−1	−2	−3	−4	−5	−6	−7
12	134.0–139.9	10	9	8	7	6	5	3	2	1	0	−1	−3	−4	−5	−6	−7	−8	−10
	140.0–149.9	11	10	9	7	6	5	4	3	2	0	−1	−2	−3	−4	−6	−7	−8	−9
	150.0–159.9	12	10	9	8	7	6	5	3	2	1	0	−1	−3	−4	−5	−6	−7	−8
	160.0–168.9	12	11	10	9	8	6	5	4	3	2	0	−1	−2	−3	−4	−5	−7	−8
13	140.0–145.9	10	9	8	7	6	4	3	2	1	0	−1	−3	−4	−5	−6	−7	−8	−10
	146.0–155.9	11	10	9	7	6	5	4	3	2	0	−1	−2	−3	−4	−6	−7	−8	−9
	156.0–165.9	12	10	9	8	7	6	5	3	2	1	0	−1	−3	−4	−5	−6	−7	−8
	166.0–174.9	12	11	10	9	8	6	5	4	3	2	1	−1	−2	−3	−4	−5	−7	−8
14	146.0–149.9	10	9	8	6	5	4	3	2	1	0	−1	−3	−4	−5	−6	−7	−8	−9
	150.0–159.9	11	9	8	7	6	5	4	3	1	0	−1	−2	−3	−4	−5	−7	−8	−9
	160.0–169.9	11	10	9	8	7	6	5	3	2	1	0	−1	−2	−3	−5	−6	−7	−8
	170.0–178.9	12	11	10	9	8	6	5	4	3	2	1	0	−2	−3	−4	−5	−6	−7
15	146.0–151.9	10	9	8	7	5	4	3	2	1	−1	−2	−3	−4	−5	−6	−8	−9	−10
	152.0–161.9	11	10	9	7	6	5	4	3	1	0	−1	−2	−3	−4	−6	−7	−8	−9
	162.0–171.9	12	11	10	8	7	6	5	4	2	1	0	−1	−2	−4	−5	−6	−7	−8
	172.0–180.9	13	12	11	9	8	7	6	5	3	2	1	0	−1	−3	−4	−5	−6	−7
16	146.0–151.9	11	10	8	7	6	5	3	2	1	−1	−2	−3	−4	−6	−7	−8	−10	−11
	152.0–161.9	12	10	9	8	7	5	4	3	2	0	−1	−2	−4	−5	−6	−7	−9	−10
	162.0–171.9	13	12	10	9	8	6	5	4	3	1	0	−1	−3	−4	−5	−6	−8	−9
	172.0–180.9	14	13	11	10	9	7	6	5	4	2	1	0	−2	−3	−4	−5	−7	−8
17	148.0–153.9	11	10	9	7	6	5	3	2	1	0	−2	−3	−4	−6	−7	−8	−10	−11
	154.0–163.9	12	11	10	8	7	6	4	3	2	0	−1	−2	−4	−5	−6	−8	−9	−10
	164.0–173.9	13	12	11	9	8	7	5	4	3	1	0	−1	−3	−4	−5	−6	−8	−9
	174.0–182.9	14	13	12	10	9	8	6	5	4	2	1	0	−1	−3	−4	−5	−7	−8
18	148.0–149.9	10	9	8	7	5	4	3	2	1	−1	−2	−3	−4	−6	−7	−8	−9	−10
	150.0–159.9	11	10	8	7	6	5	4	2	1	0	−1	−3	−4	−5	−6	−7	−9	−10
	160.0–169.9	12	11	9	8	7	6	4	3	2	1	0	−2	−3	−4	−5	−6	−8	−9
	170.0–178.9	13	11	10	9	8	7	5	4	3	2	1	−1	−2	−3	−4	−5	−7	−8

[1]These figures can be used to adjust measured stature to account for parental heights. The average of the mother's and father's heights (mid parental stature) is calculated, and the column closest to the figure is selected. The intersection of a row containing the child's age and height range with the column showing the mid parental height is noted, and the adjustment figure is read from the chart. If the figure has no sign, it is added to the child's height (cm). If there is a negative sign, the number is subtracted from the measured height (cm). The adjusted height is read from the chart in Fig 8–1 (boys) or Fig 8–2 (girls) to determine in what percentile the adjusted height falls. If the child is short but the height percentile adjusted for mid parental height is closer to the 50th percentile, the child probably has inherited a familial tendency toward short stature. If the adjusted height percentile remains low, the child's height is probably inappropriate for the genetic potential of the family, and diagnostic studies may be indicated for an organic cause of short stature. (Reprinted with permission of Ross Laboratories, Columbus, OH 43216 © 1983 Ross Laboratories. Source of data: Himes JH, Roche AF, Thissen D: *Parent-Specific Adjustments for Assessment of Recumbent Length and Stature.* Vol 13 of: *Monographs in Paediatrics.* Karger, 1981.)

increase stature in this group. The developed world places a premium on appearance, so significant numbers of children, primarily teenagers, voluntarily decrease their caloric intake even if they are not obese; this factor may account for numerous cases of poor growth. Chronic disease, which hampers adequate nutrition, often leads to short stature. For example, bronchopulmonary dysplasia decreases growth to some degree because it increases metabolic demands; improved nutrition will increase growth in these patients. In infants, feeding problems resulting from inexperience of parents may account for poor growth. Deliberate starvation of children by parents is an extreme form of child abuse that may be first discovered because of poor growth.

D. Psychologic Factors: Aberrant intrafamilial dynamics, psychologic stress, or psychiatric disease can inhibit growth either by altering endocrine function or by secondary effects on nutrition. The terms psychosocial dwarfism and maternal deprivation denote conditions due to these factors.

E. Chronic Disease: Even apart from the effects of poor nutrition, various chronic systemic diseases can interfere with growth. For example, congestive heart failure and asthma, if uncontrolled, are associated with decreased stature; in some cases, final height is in the normal range because growth continues over a longer period of time. Abnormalities of any organ system can decrease growth rate.

Catch-Up Growth

Correction of growth-retarding disorders may be temporarily followed by an abnormally high growth rate as the child approaches normal height for age. This catch-up growth will occur after initiation of therapy for hypothyroidism and GH deficiency, after correction of glucocorticoid excess, and after appropriate treatment of many chronic diseases. Catch-up growth is usually short-lived and is followed by a more average growth rate.

MEASUREMENT OF GROWTH

Accurate measurement of height is an extremely important aspect of the physical examination of children and adolescents. The onset of a chronic disease may often be determined by an inflection point in the growth chart. In other cases, a detailed growth chart will indicate a normal constant growth rate in a child observed to be short for age. If careful growth records are kept, a diagnosis of constitutional delay in growth and adolescence may be made in such a patient; without previous measurements, the child might be subjected to unnecessary diagnostic testing.

Height

The growth charts in most common use indicate the 5th and 95th percentiles as the outer limits of normal.

This still leaves 10 out of 100 healthy children outside of these boundaries, and it is both unnecessary and impractical to evaluate 10% of the population. Instead, the examining physician should accurately determine which short children warrant further evaluation and which ones (and their parents) require only reassurance that the child is healthy. Figs 8–1 and 8–2 furnish data necessary to evaluate height of children at various ages.

Pathologic short stature is usually far below the 5th percentile, but a diagnosis of pathologic short stature should not be based on a single measurement. Serial measurements are required because they allow determination of **growth velocity,** which is a more sensitive index of the growth process than a single determination. A very tall child who develops a postnatal growth problem will not fall below the 5th percentile in height for some time but will fall below the mean in growth velocity soon after the onset of the disorder. As Figs 8–3 and 8–4 indicate, growth velocity varies at different ages, but as a rough guide, a growth rate of less than 4.5 cm per year between age 4 years and the onset of puberty is abnormal. In children under 4 years of age, variations in growth velocity are more difficult to interpret. Healthy newborns tend to be clustered in length measurements (partially owing to difficulties in obtaining accurate measurements). In the ensuing months and years, the child's height will enter the channel on the growth chart in which it will continue throughout childhood. Thus, a child whose height is at the mean at birth and falls to the 10th percentile at 1 year of age and to the 5th percentile by 2 years of age may in fact be healthy in spite of crossing standard deviation lines in the journey to a growth channel at the 5th percentile. Although the growth rate may decrease during these years, it should not be less than the 3rd percentile. A steeper decrease in growth rate may be a sign of disease. When a question of abnormal growth arises, previous measurements are always helpful; every physician treating children should record length or height as well as weight at every office visit. Height and growth velocity should be determined in relation to the standards for the child's age on a graph chart.

Relation to Mid Parental Height

There is a positive correlation between mid parental height (the average of the heights of both parents) and the stature of a child. This may be taken into account with special charts (Tables 8–1 and 8–2), which indicate the number of centimeters to add or subtract from a child's height to adjust for parental heights when interpreting height for age. An abnormal height is below the 5th percentile for chronologic age when corrected for mid parental height by this chart.

Technique of Measurement

Length and height must be measured accurately. Hasty measurements derived from marks made at an infant's foot and head while the infant is squirming on the examining table are useless. Infants must be measured on a firm horizontal surface with a permanently attached rule, a stationary plate perpendicular to the rule for the head, and a movable perpendicular plate for the feet. One person should hold the head stable while another makes sure the knees are straight and the feet firm against the movable plate. Children over age 2 are measured standing up but cannot be accurately measured on the measuring rod that projects above the common weight scale; the rod is too flexible, and the scale footplate will in fact drop lower when the patient stands on it. Instead, height should be measured with the child standing with heels at the wall, ankles together, and knees and spine straight against a vertical metal rule permanently attached to an upright board or wall. Height is measured at the top of the head by a sliding perpendicular plate (or square wooden block). A Harpenden stadiometer is a mechanical measuring device capable of accurate measurement. Standing height is less than supine length, and it is essential to record the position of measurement each time; shifting from supine height at 2 years to standing height at 2½ years can falsely suggest an inadequate growth rate over that 6-month period. Standing height is an average of 1.25 cm less than supine height. Using the available sitting height standards can provide an alternative to determining the upper to lower segment ratio; sitting height reflects truncal growth without influence from the extremities. A new technique called knemometry can be used to determine the growth of a lower extremity over a period of a few weeks, thereby allowing the evaluation of several short courses of therapy expected to influence growth over a relatively short period. This technique is presently used for research, however, and is not widely available.

In addition to height or length, other significant measurements include (1) the frontal occipital head circumference; (2) horizontal arm span (between the outspread middle fingertips with the patient standing against a flat backboard); and (3) the upper segment (US) to lower segment (LS) ratio. For the latter, the LS is measured from the top of the symphysis pubis vertically to the floor with the patient standing straight, and the US is determined by subtracting the LS from the height measurement using the techniques noted above. (Normal standard US:LS ratios are shown in Fig 8–7.) It is preferable to measure in the metric system, since the smaller gradations make measurements more accurate by eliminating the tendency to round off numbers.

Height & Growth Rate Summary

In summary, we may consider 3 criteria for pathologically short stature: (1) height well below the 5th percentile for chronologic age; (2) growth rate below the 3rd percentile for chronologic age; and (3) height below the 5th percentile for chronologic age when corrected for mid parental height.

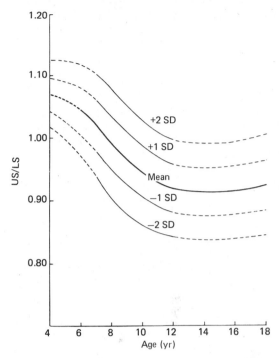

Figure 8–7. Normal upper to lower segment (US/LS) ratios, based on findings in 1015 white children. Values are slightly lower for black children. (Reproduced, with permission, from McKusick V: *Hereditable Disorders of Connective Tissue,* 4th ed. Mosby, 1972.)

Weight

The assessment of weight is similar to that of height, except that weight is more difficult to mismeasure than stature. The measured weight should be plotted for age on standard graphs developed by the National Center for Health Statistics (NCHS), which are available from baby food companies. The variation in the weights of children in the USA makes it difficult to compare percentiles of height with percentiles of weight. Weight-for-height charts from the NCHS (often included on the charts that show height and weight) are a better way to determine whether the patient's weight is appropriate.

SKELETAL (BONE) AGE

Skeletal development is a reflection of physiologic maturation. For example, menarche is better correlated with a skeletal age of 13 years than with a given chronologic age. Skeletal age also affords an indication of remaining growth available to a child and can be used to predict height in adulthood. However, skeletal age is not a definitive diagnostic factor in any disease; it can assist in diagnosis only when considered along with other aspects.

Table 8-3. The RWT method for predicting adult stature.[1]

Tables of Multipliers for Boys

Age Yrs	Mos	Recumbent length	Weight	Midparental stature	Skeletal age	Adjustment factor
1	0	0.966	0.199	0.606	-0.673	1.632
1	3	1.032	0.086	0.580	-0.417	-1.841
1	6	1.086	-0.016	0.559	-0.205	-4.892
1	9	1.130	-0.106	0.540	-0.033	-7.528
2	0	1.163	-0.186	0.523	0.104	-9.764
2	3	1.189	-0.256	0.509	0.211	-11.618
2	6	1.207	-0.316	0.496	0.291	-13.114
2	9	1.219	-0.369	0.485	0.349	-14.278
3	0	1.227	-0.413	0.475	0.388	-15.139
3	3	1.230	-0.450	0.466	0.410	-15.729
3	6	1.229	-0.481	0.458	0.419	-16.081
3	9	1.226	-0.505	0.451	0.417	-16.228
4	0	1.221	-0.523	0.444	0.405	-16.201
4	3	1.214	-0.537	0.437	0.387	-16.034
4	6	1.206	-0.546	0.431	0.363	-15.758
4	9	1.197	-0.550	0.424	0.335	-15.400
5	0	1.188	-0.551	0.418	0.303	-14.990
5	3	1.179	-0.548	0.412	0.269	-14.551
5	6	1.169	-0.543	0.406	0.234	-14.106
5	9	1.160	-0.535	0.400	0.198	-13.672
6	0	1.152	-0.524	0.394	0.161	-13.267
6	3	1.143	-0.512	0.389	0.123	-12.901
6	6	1.135	-0.499	0.383	0.085	-12.583
6	9	1.127	-0.484	0.378	0.046	-12.318
7	0	1.120	-0.468	0.373	0.006	-12.107
7	3	1.113	-0.451	0.369	-0.034	-11.948
7	6	1.106	-0.434	0.365	-0.077	-11.834
7	9	1.100	-0.417	0.361	-0.121	-11.756
8	0	1.093	-0.400	0.358	-0.167	-11.701
8	3	1.086	-0.382	0.356	-0.217	-11.652
8	6	1.079	-0.365	0.354	-0.270	-11.592
8	9	1.071	-0.349	0.353	-0.327	-11.498
9	0	1.063	-0.333	0.353	-0.389	-11.349
9	3	1.054	-0.317	0.353	-0.455	-11.118
9	6	1.044	-0.303	0.355	-0.527	-10.779
9	9	1.033	-0.289	0.357	-0.605	-10.306
10	0	1.021	-0.276	0.360	-0.690	-9.671
10	3	1.008	-0.263	0.363	-0.781	-8.848
10	6	0.993	-0.252	0.368	-0.878	-7.812
10	9	0.977	-0.241	0.373	-0.983	-6.540

Tables of Multipliers for Girls

Age Yrs	Mos	Recumbent length	Weight	Midparental stature	Skeletal age	Adjustment factor
1	0	1.087	-0.271	0.386	0.434	21.729
1	3	1.112	-0.369	0.367	0.094	20.684
1	6	1.134	-0.455	0.349	-0.172	19.957
1	9	1.153	-0.530	0.332	-0.374	19.463
2	0	1.170	-0.594	0.316	-0.523	19.131
2	3	1.183	-0.648	0.301	-0.625	18.905
2	6	1.195	-0.693	0.287	-0.690	18.740
2	9	1.204	-0.729	0.274	-0.725	18.604
3	0	1.210	-0.757	0.262	-0.736	18.474
3	3	1.215	-0.777	0.251	-0.729	18.337
3	6	1.217	-0.791	0.241	-0.711	18.187
3	9	1.217	-0.798	0.232	-0.684	18.024
4	0	1.215	-0.800	0.224	-0.655	17.855
4	3	1.212	-0.797	0.217	-0.626	17.691
4	6	1.206	-0.789	0.210	-0.600	17.548
4	9	1.199	-0.777	0.205	-0.582	17.444
5	0	1.190	-0.761	0.200	-0.571	17.398
5	3	1.180	-0.742	0.197	-0.572	17.431
5	6	1.168	-0.721	0.193	-0.584	17.567
5	9	1.155	-0.697	0.191	-0.609	17.826
6	0	1.140	-0.671	0.190	-0.647	18.229
6	3	1.124	-0.644	0.189	-0.700	18.796
6	6	1.107	-0.616	0.188	-0.766	19.544
6	9	1.089	-0.587	0.189	-0.845	20.489
7	0	1.069	-0.557	0.189	-0.938	21.642
7	3	1.049	-0.527	0.191	-1.043	23.011
7	6	1.028	-0.498	0.192	-1.158	24.602
7	9	1.006	-0.468	0.194	-1.284	26.416
8	0	0.938	-0.439	0.196	-1.418	28.448
8	3	0.960	-0.411	0.199	-1.558	30.690
8	6	0.937	-0.384	0.202	-1.704	33.129
8	9	0.914	-0.359	0.204	-1.853	35.747
9	0	0.891	-0.334	0.207	-2.003	38.520
9	3	0.868	-0.311	0.210	-2.154	41.421
9	6	0.845	-0.289	0.212	-2.301	44.415
9	9	0.824	-0.269	0.214	-2.444	47.464
10	0	0.803	-0.250	0.216	-2.581	50.525
10	3	0.783	-0.233	0.217	-2.710	53.548
10	6	0.766	-0.217	0.217	-2.829	56.481
10	9	0.749	-0.203	0.217	-2.936	59.267

Years	Months	Recumbent length	Weight	Midparental stature	Skeletal age	Adjustment factor
11	0	0.960	−0.231	0.378	−1.094	−5.010
11	3	0.942	−0.222	0.384	−1.211	−3.206
11	6	0.923	−0.213	0.390	−1.335	−1.113
11	9	0.902	−0.206	0.397	−1.464	1.273
12	0	0.881	−0.198	0.403	−1.597	3.958
12	3	0.859	−0.191	0.409	−1.735	6.931
12	6	0.837	−0.184	0.414	−1.875	10.181
12	9	0.815	−0.177	0.418	−2.015	13.684
13	0	0.794	−0.170	0.421	−2.156	17.405
13	3	0.773	−0.163	0.422	−2.294	21.297
13	6	0.755	−0.155	0.422	−2.427	25.304
13	9	0.738	−0.146	0.418	−2.553	29.349
14	0	0.724	−0.136	0.412	−2.668	33.345
14	3	0.714	−0.125	0.401	−2.771	37.183
14	6	0.709	−0.112	0.387	−2.856	40.738
14	9	0.709	−0.098	0.367	−2.922	43.869
15	0	0.717	−0.081	0.342	−2.962	46.403
15	3	0.732	−0.062	0.310	−2.973	48.154
15	6	0.756	−0.040	0.271	−2.949	48.898
15	9	0.792	−0.015	0.223	−2.885	48.402
16	0	0.839	−0.014	0.167	−2.776	46.391

Years	Months	Recumbent length	Weight	Midparental stature	Skeletal age	Adjustment factor
11	0	0.736	−0.190	0.216	−3.029	61.841
11	3	0.724	−0.179	0.214	−3.108	64.123
11	6	0.716	−0.169	0.211	−3.171	66.093
11	9	0.711	−0.159	0.206	−3.217	67.627
12	0	0.710	−0.151	0.201	−3.245	68.670
12	3	0.713	−0.143	0.193	−3.254	69.140
12	6	0.720	−0.136	0.184	−3.244	68.966
12	9	0.733	−0.129	0.173	−3.214	68.061
13	0	0.752	−0.121	0.160	−3.166	66.339
13	3	0.777	−0.113	0.144	−3.100	63.728
13	6	0.810	−0.105	0.127	−3.015	60.150
13	9	0.850	−0.085	0.106	−2.915	55.522
14	0	0.898	−0.083	0.083	−2.800	49.781

The RWT method predicts the height of an individual at 18 years of age; after this age the average total increase in stature is 0.6 cm for girls and 0.8 cm for boys.

The RWT method predicts the height of an individual at 18 years of age; after this age the average total increase in stature is 0.6 cm for girls and 0.8 cm for boys.

Recumbent length is measured in cm (add 1.25 cm to the standing height, without shoes, if that is available). Weight is measured in kg. The *midparental height* is calculated by adding the standing height of each parent in cm (without shoes) and dividing by two; if the parents' heights are unknown, in the USA a height of 174.5 cm can be substituted for the father's height or 162 cm for the mother's height. The skeletal age is determined from an x-ray of the left wrist and hand comparing it to the Greulich and Pyle atlas.

A prediction is made by:

1. Recording the child's data as noted below.
2. Finding the multipliers from the charts on these pages, making sure the positive and negative signs are retained for the calculations.
3. Multiplying the data by the multipliers, taking note of the positive or negative sign.
4. Adding the products to the adjustment factor, taking note of the sign of the factor: the result is a prediction of the height at 18 years of age.

DATA		MULTIPLIERS		PRODUCTS
Recumbent length (cm)	×	_____	=	_____
Weight (kg)	×	_____	=	_____
Midparental stature (cm)	×	_____	=	_____
Skeletal age (years)	×	_____	=	_____
Adjustment factor for age		_____	= +/−	_____
Predicted height at age 18 years (cm)			=	_____

[1]Modified and reproduced, with permission, from Roche AF, Wainer H, Thissen D: The RWT method for the prediction of adult stature. *Pediatrics* 1975;**56**:1026, as modified in Styne DM: Growth Disorders. Page 99 in: *Handbook of Clinical Endocrinology.* Fitzgerald PA (editor). Jones Medical Publications, 1986.

Bone age is determined by comparing the appearance of epiphyses or shapes of bones on a radiograph to an atlas demonstrating normal skeletal maturation for various ages. The Greulich and Pyle atlas of radiographs of the left hand and wrist is most commonly used for comparison with patients' radiographs. The development of various bones, the time of appearance of epiphyses, and the stage of fusion of epiphyses are evaluated to determine the degree of skeletal maturation. Any skeletal age more than 2 SD above or below the mean for chronologic age is out of the normal range. Other methods of skeletal age determination such as Tanner and Whitehouse maturity scoring are less widely used in the USA.

For newborn infants, knee and foot radiographs are compared to an appropriate skeletal age atlas; for late pubertal children, just before epiphyseal fusion, the knee atlas will reveal whether any growth remains or whether the epiphyses are fused.

Height may be predicted by determining skeletal age and height at the time the radiograph was taken and consulting the Bayley-Pinneau tables in the Greulich and Pyle skeletal atlas of the hand. The Roche, Warner, and Theisen (RWT) method of height prediction uses patient weight and mid parental height, in addition to the variables noted above, to calculate predicted height (Table 8–3). Height prediction by any method becomes more accurate as the child approaches the time of epiphyseal fusion.

DISORDERS OF GROWTH
(Table 8–4)

SHORT STATURE DUE TO NONENDOCRINE CAUSES

There are many causes of poor childhood growth and short adult height. The following discussion covers only the more common conditions, emphasizing those that might be included in an endocrinologic differential diagnosis.

1. CONSTITUTIONAL SHORT STATURE

Constitutional short stature is not a disease but rather a variation from normal for the population. It has been considered a disorder of the pace of development. It is characterized by moderate short stature (usually not far below the 5th percentile), thin habitus, and retardation of skeletal age. The family history often includes similarly affected members and delayed puberty.

All other causes of decreased growth must be ruled out. The patient may be considered physiologically (but not mentally) delayed in development. Characteristic growth patterns include normal birth length and height, with a gradual decrease in percentiles of height for age by 2 years. Onset of puberty is usually delayed for chronologic age but normal for skeletal age. Adult height is in the normal or low normal range. Sometimes the final height is less than the predicted height because growth is less than expected during puberty (see Fig 18–8).

2. GENETIC SHORT STATURE

Short stature may also occur in a familial pattern without retarded bone age or delay in puberty; this is considered "genetic" short stature. Affected children are closer to the mean after correction for mid parental height on the normal population growth charts (Fig 8–5 and 8–6). Adult height depends on the mother's and father's heights. Patients with the combination of constitutional short stature and genetic short stature are quite noticeably short due to both factors and are the patients most likely to seek evaluation.

3. INTRAUTERINE GROWTH RETARDATION

The small-for-gestational-age infant will often follow a lifelong pattern of short stature; in comparison, appropriate-for-gestational-age premature infants will usually catch up to the normal range of height and weight by 1–2 years of age. Intrauterine growth–retarded infants have fewer cells at birth than do appropriate-for-gestational-age infants; this disparity continues throughout childhood. Bone age, age at onset of puberty, and yearly growth rate are normal, and the patients are characteristically thin. Within this grouping are many distinctive genetic or sporadically occurring syndromes. The most common example is Russell-Silver dwarfism, characterized by small size at birth, triangular facies, a variable degree of asymmetry of extremities, and clinodactyly of the fifth finger.

Intrauterine infections with CMV, rubella, toxoplasmosis, and, now, HIV are noted to cause IUGR. Furthermore, maternal drug usage, either illicit, eg, cocaine, or legally prescribed, eg, phenytoin, may cause IUGR. Reports of other syndromes in small-for-gestational-age infants can be found in sources listed in the bibliography.

4. SYNDROMES OF SHORT STATURE

Many syndromes have short stature as one of their characteristic features. Some include intrauterine growth retardation and some do not. Common ones are described briefly below.

Laurence-Moon-Biedl syndrome, Prader-Willi syn-

Table 8–4. Causes of abnormalities of growth.

Short Stature	**Short Stature (cont'd)**
I. Nonendocrine causes:	**II. Endocrine disorders:**
A. Constitutional short stature.	A. GH deficiency and its variants–
B. Genetic short stature.	1. Congenital GH deficiency–
C. Intrauterine growth retardation.	a. With midline defects.
D. Syndromes of short stature–	b. With other pituitary hormone deficiencies.
1. Turner's syndrome and its variants.	c. Isolated GH deficiency.
2. Noonan's syndrome (pseudo-Turner's syndrome).	d. Pituitary agenesis.
3. Prader-Willi syndrome.	2. Acquired GH deficiency–
4. Laurence-Moon-Biedl syndrome.	a. Hypothalamic-pituitary tumors.
5. Other autosomal abnormalities and dysmorphic syndromes.	b. Histocytosis X.
E. Chronic disease–	c. Central nervous system infections.
1. Cardiac disorders–	d. Head injuries.
a. Left-to-right shunt.	e. GH deficiency following cranial irradiation.
b. Congestive heart failure.	f. Central nervous system vascular accidents.
2. Pulmonary disorders–	g. Hydrocephalus.
a. Cystic fibrosis.	h. Empty sella syndrome.
b. Asthma.	3. Variants of GH deficiency–
3. Gastrointestinal disorders–	a. Laron's dwarfism–syndrome of increased GH and decreased IGF-I.
a. Malabsorption (eg, celiac disease).	b. Biologically inactive GH.
b. Disorders of swallowing.	c. Pygmies.
4. Hepatic disorders.	d. Neurosecretary dysfunction.
5. Hematologic disorders–	B. Psychosocial dwarfism.
a. Sickle cell anemia.	C. Hypothyroidism.
b. Thalassemia.	D. Glucocorticoid excess (Cushing's syndrome)–
6. Renal disorders–	1. Endogenous.
a. Renal tubular acidosis.	2. Exogenous.
b. Chronic uremia.	E. Pseudohypoparathyroidism.
7. Immunologic disorders–	F. Disorders of vitamin D metabolism.
a. Connective tissue disease.	G. Diabetes mellitus.
b. Juvenile rheumatoid arthritis.	H. Diabetes insipidus, untreated.
c. Chronic infection.	**Tall Stature**
8. Central nervous system disorders.	**I. Nonendocrine causes:**
9. Malnutrition–	A. Constitutional tall stature.
a. Decreased availability.	B. Genetic tall stature.
b. Fad diets.	C. Syndromes of tall stature–
c. Voluntary dieting.	1. Cerebral gigantism.
d. Anorexia nervosa.	2. Marfan's syndrome.
e. Anorexia of cancer or chemotherapy.	3. Homocystinuria.
10. Skeletal dysplasias.	4. Beckwith-Wiedemann syndrome.
11. Juvenile rheumatoid arthritis.	5. XYY syndrome.
	6. Klinefelter's syndrome.
	II. Endocrine disorders:
	A. Pituitary gigantism.
	B. Sexual precocity.
	C. Thyrotoxicosis.
	D. Infants of diabetic mothers.

drome, hypothyroidism, glucocorticoid excess, pseudohypoparathyroidism, and GH deficiency combine obesity with short stature. Moderately obese but otherwise normal children without these conditions tend to have slightly advanced bone age and physiologic maturation with increased stature during childhood and early onset of puberty. Thus, short stature in a chubby child must be considered to have an organic cause until proved otherwise.

Turner's Syndrome & Its Variants

While classic Turner's syndrome of 45,XO gonadal dysgenesis (see Chapter 18) is often correctly diagnosed, it is not always appreciated that any phenotypic female with short stature may have a variant of Turner's syndrome. Thus, a karyotype determination should be done for every short girl if no other cause for short stature is found (see Chapters 17, 18, and 19).

Noonan's Syndrome (Pseudo-Turner's Syndrome)

This syndrome shares several phenotypic characteristics of Turner's syndrome, but the karyotype is 46,XX in the female or 46,XY in the male, and other features clearly differentiate it from Turner's syndrome; pseudo-Turner's syndrome is an autosomal dominant disorder (see Chapters 16 and 19).

Prader-Willi Syndrome

This condition is characterized by infantile hypotonia, acromicria (small hands and feet), mental retardation, almond-shaped eyes, and extreme obesity.

Glucose intolerance and delayed puberty are characteristic. This syndrome is associated with abnormalities of chromosome 15 in approximately 50% of affected cases (see Chapter 19).

Laurence-Moon-Biedl Syndrome

This syndrome of retinitis pigmentosa, polydactyly, and obesity is also associated with poor growth and delayed puberty. It is inherited as an autosomal recessive disorder (see Chapter 19).

Autosomal Karyotypic Disorders & Syndromes

Numerous autosomal karyotypic disorders and syndromes of dysmorphic children with or without mental retardation are characterized by short stature. Often the key to diagnosis is the presence of several major or minor physical abnormalities that indicate the need for karyotype determination. Other abnormalities may include unusual body proportions, such as short extremities, leading to aberrant upper to lower segment ratios, and arm spans quite discrepant from stature. Some conditions, such as trisomy 21 (Down's syndrome), are quite common, while others are rare. Details of these syndromes can be found in references listed at the end of the chapter.

Skeletal Dysplasias

There are more than 100 known types of genetic skeletal dysplasias (osteochondrodysplasias). Often they are noted at birth because of short limbs or trunk, but some are only diagnosed after a period of growth. The most common condition is autosomal dominant achondroplasia. This condition is characterized by short extremities, a large head with a prominent forehead and a depressed nasal bridge, and lumbar lordosis in later life. Adult height is quite short, with a mean of 132 cm for males and 123 cm for females. No therapy is known; growth hormone treatment has not been used for the skeletal dysplasias because it may exacerbate some of the abnormalities of bone development.

5. CHRONIC DISEASE

Severe chronic disease of any organ system can cause poor growth in childhood and adolescence. In many cases, there will be adequate physical findings by the time of consultation to permit diagnosis; in some cases, however—most notably celiac disease and regional enteritis—short stature and decreased growth may precede obvious signs of malnutrition or gastrointestinal disease. Patients with chronic disease are usually thin, and poor nutrition may be part of the cause of short stature. In some cases, growth is only delayed; eg, in asthma, children develop slowly but ultimately reach their predicted heights. In others, growth can be increased by improved nutrition; patients with gastrointestinal disease, kidney disease, or

cancer may benefit from nocturnal parenteral nutritional infusions. Cystic fibrosis combines several causes of growth failure: lung disease impairs oxygenation and predisposes to chronic infections, gastrointestinal disease decreases nutrient availability, and late-developing abnormalities of the endocrine pancreas cause symptoms of diabetes mellitus. Children with congestive heart failure due to either a variety of congenital heart diseases or acquired myocarditis grow poorly unless successfully treated with medications or surgery; however, patients with cyanotic heart disease experience little or no deficit in growth. Patients with chronic hematologic diseases, such as sickle cell anemia or thalassemia, often have poor growth, delayed puberty, and short adult stature. Juvenile rheumatoid arthritis may compromise growth either before or after therapy.

The 2 forms of renal tubular acidosis (RTA), proximal and distal, may both cause short stature. Proximal RTA causes bicarbonate wasting at normal or low plasma bicarbonate concentrations; patients have hypokalemia, alkaline urine pH, severe bicarbonaturia, and later acidemia. The condition may be inherited or sporadic or secondary to many metabolic or medication-induced disorders. Distal RTA is caused by the inability to acidify the urine; it may occur in sporadic or familial patterns or be acquired as a result of metabolic disorders or medication therapy. Distal RTA is characterized by hypokalemia, hypercalciuria, and occasional hypocalcemia. The administration of bicarbonate is the primary therapy for either RTA, and correct treatment can substantially improve growth rate.

Hemoglobin, white blood cell count, erythrocyte sedimentation rate, serum carotene and folate levels, plasma bicarbonate levels, and liver and kidney function should be assessed in short but otherwise apparently healthy children before endocrine screening tests are done. Urinalysis should be performed, with attention to specific gravity (to rule out diabetes insipidus) and ability to acidify urine (to evaluate possible renal tubular acidosis). A list of some chronic diseases causing short stature is presented in Table 8–4.

6. MALNUTRITION (OTHER THAN CHRONIC DISEASE)

Malnutrition not due to chronic disease is the most common worldwide cause of short stature. This diagnosis is based on historical and physical findings, particularly the dietary history. Food faddism and anorexia nervosa, as well as voluntary dieting due to "fear of obesity," can cause poor growth. Infection with parasites, such as *Ascaris lumbricoides* or *Giardia,* can decrease growth. Specific nutritional deficiencies can have particular effects upon growth. For example, severe iron deficiency can cause a thin habitus as well as growth retardation. Zinc deficiency (although probably overinvoked as a cause of growth retardation) can cause anorexia, decreased growth, and delayed puberty, usually in the presence of chronic systemic disease or infection. There are no simple laboratory tests for diagnosis of malnutrition, although somatomedin levels are low in malnutrition as well as in GH deficiency.

7. DRUGS

Children with hyperactivity (or those incorrectly diagnosed as such) are frequently treated with dextroamphetamine or methylphenidate. These agents can decrease weight gain, possibly because of decreased appetite and growth rate. Discontinuing therapy temporarily, usually during vacations from school, allows some catch-up growth in weight and height but will not necessarily repair the deficit completely. These drugs must be used in moderation and only in children who definitely need them.

Exogenous glucocorticoids are a common cause of poor growth. They are discussed below.

SHORT STATURE DUE TO ENDOCRINE DISORDERS

1. GROWTH HORMONE DEFICIENCY & ITS VARIANTS (Table 8–5)

Current concepts of endocrine regulation of growth propose that GH stimulates growth through intermediary substances, the **somatomedins** (see above and Chapter 7).

Chromosome 17 contains a cluster of 5 genes of the growth hormone gene family. The GH-N gene codes for the 22K growth hormone molecule that is most plentiful; GH-V codes for a product that is normally untranslated. hCS-A and hCS-B code for the hCS molecule and are expressed at various times during gesta-

Table 8–5. Postulated disorders of hGH release and action.

Site of Defect	Clinical Condition
Hypothalamus	Idiopathic GH deficiency due to decreased GRH secretion; hypothalamic tumors.
Pituitary gland	Dysplasia, trauma, surgery, or tumor of the pituitary gland. Production of an abnormal GH molecule in "biologically inactive GH syndrome." Absence of the gene for GH production (type IA GH defiency).
Sites of somatomedin production	Laron's dwarfism with high GH and low somatomedin concentrations (GH receptor defect). Pygmies with normal GH, low IGF-I, and normal IGF-II concentrations.
Cartilage	Glucocorticoid-induced growth failure. Resistance to IGF-I.

tion, while the hCS-L gene appears to be an unexpressed pseudogene.

Earlier theories suggested the liver as the major source of plasma somatomedin that affects cartilage, but recent studies show that many organs produce somatomedin. In fact, somatomedin may be an autocrine or paracrine factor that influences its own cell of origin or neighboring cells. Recombinant DNA technology has increased the supply of these growth factors, and they are being used to determine the direct effects of somatomedins.

The incidence of GH deficiency is estimated to approach 1:4000 in European populations, so the disorder should not be considered rare. Most patients with idiopathic GH deficiency apparently lack GRH, and some have been shown to have adequate pituitary somatotropes; thus, long-term treatment of these patients with GRH can improve growth. Patients with pituitary tumors or those rare patients with congenital absence of the pituitary gland lack somatotrophs. Several kindreds have been described that lack the 7.6 kB region of the GH-N gene responsible for producing the secretory product.

Before 1986, the only clinical method of treatment for GH deficiency was replacement with human GH (hGH) from cadaver donors. In early 1985, three cases of neurologic disease were diagnosed in patients who had received natural hGH 10–15 years before. At least 2 of the 3 cases were diagnosed as having Creutzfeldt-Jakob disease, and the possibility arose that prions contaminating a donor's pituitary gland were transmitted to the GH-deficient patients and caused their death. While no proof of such transmission is available at this writing and despite the fact that newer methods of purifying hGH instituted in 1977 probably would remove such agents, natural growth hormone from all sources has been removed from distribution until the issue can be resolved. Recombinant DNA technology has been applied to the production of GH from *Escherichia coli* or mammalian cell culture, and such methods account for the world's current supply of growth hormone. Although other forms are under study, commercial growth hormone is currently available in the 191-amino-acid natural-sequence form (somatropin) and the 192-amino-acid methionyl form (somatrem). Thus, GH is now available in virtually unlimited amounts, allowing innovative treatment regimens not previously possible owing to scarce supplies; however, this also produces the potential for abuse of GH in athletes or even in children of normal size whose parents wish them to be taller than average.

GRH has been isolated from pancreatic GH-releasing tumor, sequenced, and synthesized. Hypothalamic GRH has the same structure as GRH from the pancreatic tumors. GRH has potential in the diagnosis of GH deficiency; in experimental studies, GH-deficient patients have demonstrated lower or absent GH secretion after administration of GRH. In numerous studies, episodic doses of GRH have restored GH secretion, somatomedin production, and growth in children with idiopathic GH deficiency. Continuous infusion of GRH has also increased endogenous GH secretion, and intranasal insufflation of GRH is currently being studied. These studies using GRH further demonstrate that GH deficiency is primarily a disease of the hypothalamus, not of the pituitary gland.

Insulinlike growth factor I (somatomedin C) is now produced by recombinant DNA technology and has been shown to increase the growth of rodents. Although no long-term human treatment program has yet been reported, IGF-I may be another useful treatment for short stature, particularly in Laron dwarfism (and possibly pygmies) where no other treatment is possible. Growth disturbances due to disorders of GH release or action are shown in Table 8–5.

Congenital Growth Hormone Deficiency

Congenital GH deficiency is associated with normal birth length but a decrease in growth rate soon after birth. The disorder can be identified by careful measurement in the first year and becomes more obvious by 1–2 years of age. Patients with classic GH deficiency will have short stature, obesity with immature facial appearance, immature high-pitched voice, and some delay in skeletal maturation. Males with GH deficiency may have microphallus, especially if the condition is accompanied by gonadotropin-releasing hormone (GnRH) deficiency (Fig 8–8). GH deficiency in the neonate or child can also lead to symptomatic hypoglycemia and seizures; if ACTH deficiency is also present, the hypoglycemia is usually more severe. The differential diagnosis of neonatal hypoglycemia in a full-term infant who has not sustained birth trauma must include neonatal hypopituitarism. If microphallus (in a male subject) or optic hypoplasia is noted, the diagnosis of congenital GH deficiency is likely. Congenital GH deficiency is also statistically correlated with breech delivery; whether the abnormal presentation causes hypothalamic damage at birth or whether the hypopituitarism contributes to the abnormal fetal position is not clear. Intelligence is normal in GH deficiency unless repeated or severe hypoglycemia has compromised brain development. When thyrotropin-releasing hormone (TRH) deficiency is also present, there may be additional signs of hypothyroidism. Secondary or tertiary hypothyroidism is not generally associated with mental retardation, but a few cases of isolated TRH deficiency and severe mental retardation have been reported. Less severe forms of partial GH deficiency have also been described.

Congenital GH deficiency may occur along with midline anatomic defects. Optic hypoplasia with visual defects ranging from nystagmus to blindness has been described in association with variable hypothalamic deficiency, including diabetes insipidus; absence of the septum pellucidum may also be found on CT or MRI scan in about half of patients with this condition.

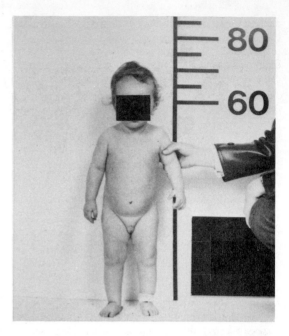

Figure 8–8. A 12-month-old boy with congenital hypopituitarism. He had hypoglycemic seizures at 12 hours of age. At 1 year, he had another hypoglycemic seizure (plasma glucose, 25 mg/dL) associated with an episode of otitis media, and it was noted that his penis was quite small. He was referred for evaluation because of these findings. At 12 months, length was 66.5 cm (−2 SD) and weight was 8.5 kg (−3 SD). The penis was less than 1.5 cm long, and both testes were descended (each 1 cm in diameter). Plasma GH did not rise above 1 ng/mL after arginine and levodopa testing. (No insulin was given because of the history of hypoglycemia.) LH rose only from 8.6 to 11.7 mIU/mL* after administration of GnRH, 100 μg. Serum thyroxine was low (T$_4$, 6.6 μg/dL; T$_4$ index, 1.5), and after administration of 200 μg of protirelin (TRH), serum TSH rose with a delayed peak characteristic of tertiary hypothyroidism. Plasma ACTH rose only to 53 pg/mL after metyrapone. Thus, he had GH, ACTH, GnRH, and TRH deficiency. He was given 6 doses of 2000 units of chorionic gonadotropin (hCG) intramuscularly over 2 weeks, and plasma testosterone rose to 62 ng/dL. He was then treated with 25 mg of testosterone enanthate every month for 3 months, and his phallus enlarged to 3.5 × 1.2 cm without significant advancement of bone age. With hGH therapy (0.1 unit/kg intramuscularly every other day), he grew at a greater than normal rate for 12 months (catch-up growth), and growth then continued at a normal rate.

*1 ng of LH (preparation LER 960) = 7.8 mIU.

Cleft palate or other forms of oral dysraphism may be associated with GH deficiency; thus, such children may need more than nutritional support to improve their growth. Children with a single maxillary incisor and GH deficiency have been described. Congenital absence of the pituitary, often found in an autosomal recessive pattern, leads to severe hypopituitarism, including hypoglycemia and hypopituitarism; affected patients have shallow development or absence of the sella turcica.

Hereditary GH deficiency has been described in several kindreds. Recent biochemical techniques have defined the defect in some families. Type IA GH deficiency is inherited in an autosomal recessive pattern; unlike those with classic sporadic GH deficiency, some of these children have been described with somewhat short birth lengths. While they do initially respond to exogenous hGH administration, they soon develop high antibody titers that stop the effect of the therapy; however, one reported kindred continued to grow and did not develop blocking antibodies. DNA analysis proved that these patients lack the gene for hGH production. Type IB patients have autosomal recessive GH deficiency but no such gene depletion; type II patients have autosomal dominant GH deficiency; and type III patients have X-linked GH deficiency.

Acquired Growth Hormone Deficiency

Onset of GH deficiency in late childhood or adolescence, particularly if accompanied by other pituitary hormone deficiencies, may be due to a hypothalamic-pituitary tumor. The presence of posterior pituitary deficiency in addition to anterior pituitary deficiency makes this even more likely. Conditions that may cause acquired GH deficiency—craniopharyngiomas, germinomas, gliomas, etc—are described in Chapters 6 and 19. Histiocytosis X was previously considered a common cause of GH deficiency, but recent evidence suggests that this combination occurs rarely.

The empty sella syndrome is more frequently associated with hypothalamic-pituitary abnormalities in childhood than in adulthood; thus, GH deficiency may be found in affected patients. Some patients, predominantly boys, with constitutional delay in growth and adolescence may have transient GH deficiency before the actual onset of puberty; when testosterone concentrations begin to increase in these patients, GH secretion and growth rate also increase.

Cranial irradiation of the hypothalamic-pituitary region to treat head tumors or acute lymphoblastic leukemia may result in GH deficiency 6–24 months later, owing to radiation-induced hypothalamic (or possibly pituitary) damage. Such patients must be carefully observed for growth failure after irradiation. Some of these patients receive spinal irradiation, which may impair upper body growth and cause a higher upper to lower segment ratio, and others may receive gonadal irradiation (or chemotherapy), which impairs gonadal function and leads to the absence of onset or progression of puberty and of the pubertal growth spurt.

Variants of Growth Hormone Deficiency

Other disorders of GH production or action have been reported that are not manifested in the classic manner of GH deficiency.

Laron's dwarfism is characterized by high plasma GH and low plasma somatomedin concentrations. Growth rate does not increase and somatomedin values do not rise when exogenous hGH is administered. The defect is due to inability to produce somatomedin in response to growth hormone because of impaired GH receptors. It is inherited as an autosomal recessive disorder.

Patients have been reported with radioimmunoassayable but **biologically inactive GH** and low somatomedin values. Treatment with exogenous hGH improves their growth rate and causes a rise in somatomedin levels. The defect may be due to production of an abnormal GH molecule that reacts in radioimmunoassay studies but exerts no biologic activity in the patient. The incidence of this disorder is not known, but it is probably rare. Some patients with this diagnosis may have neurosecretory dysfunction, as noted below.

Several very short, poorly growing children with delayed skeletal maturation, normal GH and somatomedin values, and no signs of organic disease have responded to GH therapy with increased growth rates equal to those of patients with bona fide GH deficiency. These patients may have a variation of constitutional delay in growth or genetic short stature, but a subtle abnormality of GH secretion is possible.

Pygmies have normal plasma GH, low IGF-I, and normal IGF-II concentrations. They do not respond to exogenous GH with improved growth rate or a rise in IGF-I. They have a congenital inability to produce IGF-I, which is of greater importance in stimulating growth than is IGF-II. Pygmy children have appropriate prepubertal growth but lack a pubertal growth spurt, suggesting that IGF-I is essential to attain a normal peak growth velocity.

Diagnosis of Growth Hormone Deficiency

Because basal values of GH are low in both normal children and GH-deficient patients, the diagnosis of GH deficiency rests upon demonstration of an inadequate rise of serum GH after provocative stimuli. The various radioimmunoassay systems complicate this by varying widely in their measurements of the same blood sample; a sample may repeatedly measure 15 ng/mL in one assay but only 6 ng/mL in another. The lack of a national standard for GH radioimmunoassays has forced each laboratory to carefully establish normal responses for GH secretion, and the physician must be aware of the standards of the laboratory being used.

The very concept of growth hormone testing provides a further complication. While a patient who does not secrete GH in response to standard challenges is generally considered to be GH deficient, a normal GH response to these tests may not rule out GH deficiency. Except for sleep studies, testing should occur after an overnight fast; carbohydrate ingestion will suppress GH response, as will the presence of obesity. Because

10% or more of healthy children will not have an adequate rise in GH with one test of GH reserve, several methods of assessing GH reserve are necessary. Serum GH values should rise during stage III–IV sleep (usually 90 minutes after onset of sleep) or after 10 minutes of vigorous exercise. After an overnight fast, GH levels should also rise in response to arginine infusion (0.5 g/kg body weight [up to 20 g] over 30 minutes), oral levodopa (125 mg for up to 15 kg body weight, 250 mg for up to 35 kg, or 500 mg for over 35 kg), or clonidine (0.15 mg/m² orally). Side effects of levodopa include several hours of nausea; those of clonidine include some drop in blood pressure and drowsiness. Regular procedure used to include the administration of propranolol before the test to attempt to increase the GH response to secretagogues; this procedure is less utilized now because of difficulties in test interpretation.

GH levels also rise after acute hypoglycemia due to insulin administration; this test carries a risk of seizure if the blood glucose level drops excessively. An insulin tolerance test may be performed if dextrose infusion is available for emergency use, if the patient can be continuously observed by a physician, and if the patient has no history of previous hypoglycemic seizures. The patient must have a normal glucose concentration at the beginning of the test. Regular insulin, 0.075–0.1 unit/kg in saline, may be given as a bolus. In 20–40 minutes, a 50% drop in blood glucose will occur and a rise in serum GH and cortisol should follow. Glucose should be monitored, and an intravenous line must be maintained for emergency dextrose infusion in case the patient becomes unconscious or has a hypoglycemic seizure. If dextrose infusion is necessary, it is imperative that blood glucose not be raised above the normal range, since hyperosmolarity has been reported from overzealous glucose replacement. (See Chapter 6.) New techniques are available for the measurement of urinary GH and IGF-I concentrations; such tests may aid in the diagnosis of growth disorders.

Patients with **GH neurosecretory dysfunction** have been described who respond to pharmacologic stimuli (levodopa, clonidine, and insulin) but not to physiologic stimuli such as exercise or sleep; these patients may have decreased 24-hour secretion of hGH (or integrated concentrations of hGH) compared to healthy subjects, similar to GH-deficient patients. The true status of such patients and the role of 24-hour GH monitoring are still controversial; secretagogue testing remains the standard for the diagnosis of GH deficiency, but even pharmacologic testing cannot always determine which patients truly need GH therapy.

Somatomedin values will be low in most GH-deficient subjects, but, as noted above, short patients with normal somatomedin concentrations have been reported who require GH treatment for improvement of growth rate. In addition, starvation will lower somatomedin values in healthy children and incorrectly suggest GH deficiency. Children with psychosocial dwarfism, who need family therapy or foster home placement rather than GH therapy, have low GH and IGF-I concentrations and appear to have growth hormone deficiency. Likewise, patients with constitutional delay in adolescence will have low IGF-I values for chronologic age but normal values for skeletal age. The determination of both IGF-II and IGF-I levels may improve the reliability of somatomedin results in predicting GH deficiency. Also, formic acid extraction of serum on a sephadex column yields IGF-I concentrations that are more closely related to growth rate and stature than are IGF-I determinations done by direct radioimmunoassay. Thus, somatomedin determinations are not infallible in the diagnosis of GH deficiency. They must be interpreted with regard to nutrition and psychosocial status and skeletal ages.

The above discussion indicates that although pharmacologic tests of GH secretion and plasma somatomedin values will usually indicate who has true GH deficiency, the diagnosis will remain in doubt in some cases. This should not lead to the conclusion that all short children should receive GH therapy. Only very short children (height well below the 5th percentile) who grow very slowly (growth velocity below the 3rd percentile for age) with delayed bone ages meticulously studied in research protocols have been shown to benefit from hGH therapy in the absence of proved GH deficiency. Children meeting less stringent criteria have also been treated with GH, producing some increase in growth rate, but it is not yet clear whether this increases adult height. Furthermore, in the absence of classic GH deficiency, no clearly recognized measurement can predict which short child is likely to respond to GH therapy before it is instituted.

Treatment of Growth Hormone Deficiency

A. Hormonal Replacement: GH-deficient children require biosynthetic somatropin (natural-sequence GH) at a dose of 0.1 mg/kg body weight, or somatrem (methionyl GH) at a dose of 0.05–0.1 mg/kg body weight 3 times per week during the period of active growth. Various administration schedules are under study, and the daily administration of GH in amounts equal to the total weekly dose received under the 3-times-per-week schedule also appears to increase growth. The increase in growth rate (Figs 8–9, 8–10, and 8–11) is most marked during the first year of therapy. Older children with bone ages over 10 years do not respond as well and may require larger doses. One study showed that cyproheptadine can increase the rate of growth produced by GH treatment by improving the patient's nutritional status.

Antibodies to GH are present in measurable quantities in the serum of children receiving GH. While antibodies are more frequent in those treated with somatrem than somatropin, a high titer of blocking

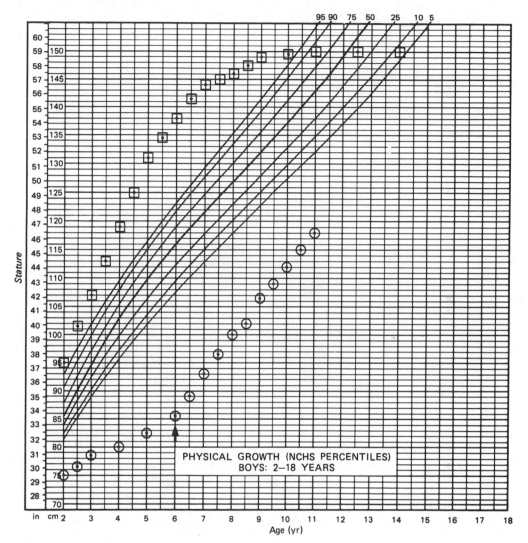

Figure 8–9. Examples of abnormal growth charts. Squares (□) represent the growth pattern of a child (such as patient A in Fig 8–11) with precocious sexual development and early excessive growth leading to premature closure of the epiphyses and cessation of growth. Circles (○) represent growth of a boy (such as patient B in Fig 8–11) with GH deficiency who showed progressively poorer growth until 6 years of age, when he was treated with hGH (***arrow***), after which catch-up growth occurred.

antibodies with significant binding capacity is rare and only a few patients are reported to have temporarily ceased growing on methionyl GH therapy.

GH exerts anti-insulin effects. Although clinical diabetes is not a reported result of GH therapy, the long-term effects of a small rise in glucose in an otherwise healthy child are unknown. Another potential risk is the tendency to slipped capital femoral epiphyses, although it is not clear that this occurs more frequently in treated than untreated patients. The occurrence of 5 cases of leukemia in young adults previously treated with growth hormone in Japan has led to epidemiologic studies, but because this phenomenon has not

been reported in other countries, it may be a random cluster event. GH does not increase the recurrence rate of tumors existing before therapy; thus, patients with craniopharyngiomas, for example, may receive GH if indicated after the disease is clinically stable. Usually clinicians wait 1 year after tumor therapy before starting tumor patients on GH therapy. Organomegaly and skeletal changes like those found in acromegaly are potential side effects of excessive GH therapy.

B. Psychologic Management and Outcome: Research into the psychologic outcome of patients with short stature has been criticized for variable investigation methods and lack of controlled studies.

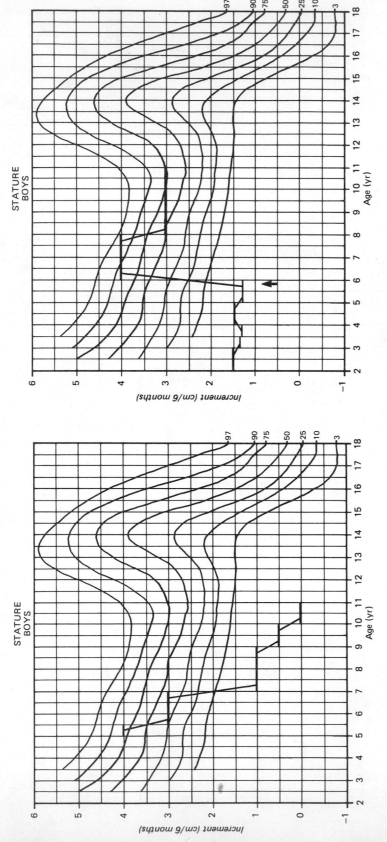

Figure 8–10. Two examples of abnormal growth plotted on a height velocity chart. **A:** The plot is taken from the data recorded as squares in Fig 8–9, describing a patient with precocious puberty, premature epiphyseal closure, and cessation of growth. **B:** The plot is taken from the data recorded as circles in Fig 8–9, describing a patient with GH deficiency who was treated with hGH (arrow) at age 6. Initial catch-up growth is noted for 2 years, with a lower (but normal) velocity of growth following.

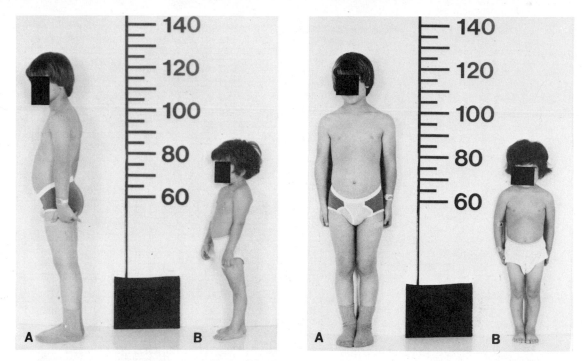

Figure 8–11. Two boys demonstrating extremes of growth. The boy at left in each photograph (**A**) has precocious puberty due to a central nervous system lesion. At 4 4/12 years, he was 125.1 cm tall, which is 5 SD above the mean. (A normal 4-year-old is 101.5 cm tall.) His testes measured 2 × 3.5 cm each, his penis 9.8 × 2.8 cm. He was muscular and had acne and a deep voice. His bone age was 10 years, testosterone 480 ng/dL, and the rise of LH after 100 μg of GnRH was 23.4 mIU/mL, which is pubertal. His brain CT scan revealed a hamartoma of the tuber cinereum. The boy at right (**B**) at 4 2/12 years was 85 cm tall, which is 4.5 SD below the mean. He had the classic physical and historical characteristics of idiopathic GH deficiency, including early growth failure and a cherubic appearance. His plasma GH values did not rise after provocative testing.

Children with growth hormone deficiency have been the most studied; they are reported to have more passive personality traits than do healthy children. Such patients have delayed emotional maturity and suffer from infantilization from parents, teachers, and peers. Their academic achievement is generally substandard even if their intelligence is normal; this has been attributed to the delayed emotional maturity or poor body image, both situations fostered by short stature. However, many of these children have been held back in school because of their size without regard to their academic abilities. Some patients retain a body image of short stature even after normal height has been achieved with treatment. Depression and suicidal behavior can occur in affected adolescents because of short stature and delayed development. Thus, the way that GH-deficient individuals are perceived by their world appears to be of primary importance in their psychologic outcome; our "heightist" society values physical stature and equates it with the potential for success, a belief that is not lost on the patients. A supportive environment in which they are not allowed to act younger than their age or to occupy a "special place" in the family is recommended. Psychologic help is indicated in severe cases of maladjustment.

2. PSYCHOSOCIAL DWARFISM (Fig 8–12)

Children with psychosocial dwarfism present with poor growth, potbelly, immature appearance, and bizarre eating and drinking habits. Parents may report that the affected child begs for food from neighbors, forages in garbage cans, and drinks from toilet bowls. As a rule this tragic condition occurs in only one of several children in a family. Careful questioning reveals a disordered family situation in which the child is ignored or severely disciplined. Caloric deprivation or physical battering may or may not be a feature of the history.

These children have functional hypopituitarism. Testing will often reveal GH deficiency at first, but after the child is removed from the home, GH function quickly returns to normal. Diagnosis rests upon improvement in behavior or catch-up growth in the hospital or in a foster home. Separation from the family is therapeutic, but the prognosis is guarded. Family psychotherapy may be beneficial.

Growth disorder due to abnormal parent-child interaction in a younger infant is called maternal deprivation. Caloric deprivation due to parental neglect

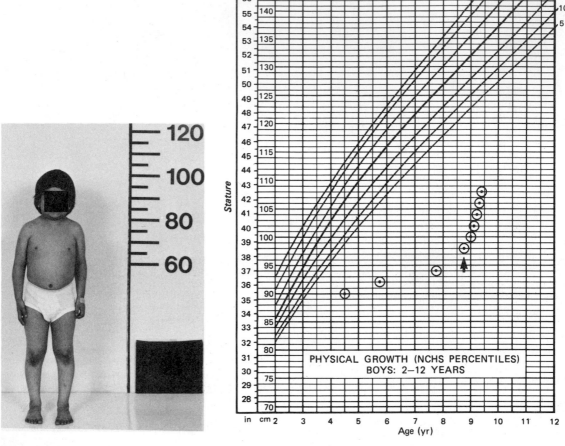

Figure 8–12. Photograph and growth chart of a 9 1/12-year-old boy with psychosocial dwarfism. He had a long history of poor growth (<3 cm/yr). The social history revealed that he was given less attention and punished more frequently than his 7 sibs. He ate from garbage cans and begged for food, although he was not completely deprived of food at home. When the photograph was taken (at 9 1/12 years), he was 99 cm tall (−7 SD) and weighed 14.7 kg (−3 SD). His bone age was 5 years, with growth arrest lines visible. Serum thyroxine was 7.8 μg/dL. Peak serum GH varied from nondetectable to 8 ng/mL on different provocative tests between age 6 years and 8 7/12 years. He was placed in a hospital chronic care facility (**arrow**) for a 6-month period and grew 9 cm, which projects to a yearly growth velocity of 18 cm. On repeat testing, the peak serum GH was 28 ng/mL.

may be of greater significance in this younger age group. Even in the absence of nutritional restriction or full-blown psychosocial dwarfism, constant negative interactions within a family may inhibit the growth of a child.

3. HYPOTHYROIDISM

Thyroid hormone deficiency decreases growth rate and skeletal development and, if onset is at or before birth, leads to mental retardation. Screening programs for the diagnosis of congenital hypothyroidism have been instituted all over the world, and early treatment following diagnosis in the neonatal period will mark-edly reduce growth failure and mental retardation caused by severe primary hypothyroidism. The more subtle forms of congenital or acquired hypothyroidism in older children (eg, lymphocytic thyroiditis) may lead to growth failure in later life. Characteristics of hypothyroidism are a decreased growth rate and short stature, retarded bone age, and an increased upper to lower segment ratio for chronologic age.

Hypothyroidism cannot be diagnosed solely on the basis of a low plasma total T_4 value; an indication of a low free T_4 value or low free T_4 index is necessary to rule out the relatively frequent cases (one in 10,000) of thyroid hormone–binding globulin (TBG) deficiency, which will artifactually lower total T_4 values into the hypothyroid range. If a test of TBG levels (such as a resin T_3 uptake or plasma TBG concentration) is obtained along with the total T_4, this diagnostic trap can be avoided. Since the majority of cases of hypothyroidism are primary, elevated TSH levels will confirm the diagnosis of bona fide hypothyroidism.

4. CUSHING'S SYNDROME

Excess glucocorticoids (either exogenous or endogenous) will often lead to decreased growth rate before obesity and other signs of Cushing's syndrome develop. The underlying disease may be bilateral adrenal hyperplasia due to abnormal ACTH-cortisol regulation in Cushing's disease, adrenal adenomas, or adrenal carcinoma. The appropriate diagnosis may be missed if urinary cortisol and 17-hydroxycorticosteroid determinations are not interpreted on the basis of the child's body size or if inappropriate doses of dexamethasone are used for testing (appropriate doses are 20 μg/kg/d for the low-dose and 80 μg/kg/d for the high-dose suppression test). Furthermore, daily variations in cortisol production necessitate several urinary or plasma cortisol determinations before Cushing's disease can be appropriately diagnosed or ruled out. Exogenous sources of glucocorticoids that cause poor growth may be oral corticosteroids used to treat asthma or even overzealous use of topical corticosteroid ointments or creams. These iatrogenic cases of Cushing's syndrome, if resolved early, may allow catch-up growth and so may not affect final height. Thus, an accurate history of prior medications is important in diagnosis. Growth failure in Cushing's syndrome may be due to decreased peripheral effect of somatomedin on growing cartilage or decreased GH secretion due to hypothalamic-pituitary effects of elevated glucocorticoid concentrations. Treatment of the underlying disorder (eg, transsphenoidal microadenectomy for Cushing's disease) will restore growth rate to normal (catch-up growth may occur initially) if epiphyseal fusion has not occurred.

5. PSEUDOHYPOPARATHYROIDISM

Pseudohypoparathyroidism is a rare disorder consisting of a characteristic phenotype and chemical signs of hypoparathyroidism, with elevated circulating PTH levels and failure of target tissues to respond to PTH. Children with pseudohypoparathyroidism are short and chubby, with characteristic round faces, short fourth and fifth metacarpal bones, and mental retardation. Serum calcium is low and serum phosphorus is high (as in hypoparathyroidism), but plasma PTH is high. The defect is in the guanyl nucleotide-sensitive regulatory protein that couples PTH-occupied receptors to adenylate cyclase. Thus, administration of PTH fails to induce a rise in nephrogenous cAMP or an increase in urinary phosphorus. A rare variant of this disorder (pseudohypoparathyroidism type II) occurs in which administration of PTH produces a rise in nephrogenous cAMP but fails to induce an increase in phosphorus excretion, suggesting a defect distal to the receptor–adenylate cyclase complex. Treatment with high-dose vitamin D or physiologic replacement with 1,25 OH vitamin D and calcium, as well as phosphate-binding agents, will correct the biochemical defects and control hypocalcemic seizures, but it will not improve stature or mentation.

Children with the pseudohypoparathyroid phenotype but with normal circulating levels of calcium, phosphate, and PTH have pseudopseudohypoparathyroidism. They require no calcium or vitamin D therapy. (See Chapter 11.)

6. DISORDERS OF VITAMIN D METABOLISM

Short stature and poor growth are features of rickets in its obvious and more subtle forms. The disease may be vitamin D deficiency due to inadequate oral intake, fat malabsorption, inadequate sunlight exposure, anticonvulsant therapy, or renal or hepatic disease. Classic findings include bowing of the legs, chest deformities (rachitic rosary), and characteristic radiographic findings associated with decreased serum calcium and phosphate levels and elevated serum alkaline phosphatase levels. Vitamin D dependency may be diagnosed when vitamin D is required in doses far higher than necessary to resolve vitamin D deficiency. Short stature may be associated with rickets in renal disorders with hypophosphatemia due to a defect in renal reabsorption of phosphate; examples are Fanconi's syndrome (including cystinosis and other inborn errors of metabolism) and renal tubular acidosis.

When treatment is effective in these disorders (eg, vitamin D for vitamin D deficiency or alkali therapy for appropriate types of renal tubular acidosis), growth rate will improve. In the Williams syndrome of infantile hypercalcemia, elfin facies, supravalvular aortic stenosis, and mental retardation, patients have IUGR and severely reduced childhood and adult height. (See Chapter 11.)

7. DIABETES MELLITUS

Remarkably, early studies of children with insulin-dependent diabetes mellitus demonstrated a taller than average height at the time of diagnosis. Once the disorder is treated, growth depends a great deal on the efficacy of the therapy. Well-controlled diabetes mellitus is compatible with normal growth; poorly controlled diabetes often causes slow growth. However, even with good control, there is evidence that a child with diabetes mellitus will reach an adult height lower than predicted. With the relatively recent advent of home blood glucose monitoring, the present generation of well-treated children with diabetes may fare better, but such data are not yet available. Another factor that may decrease growth rate in children with diabetes mellitus is the increased incidence of Hashimoto's thyroiditis; yearly thyroid function screening is advisable as the peripubertal period approaches. Liver and spleen enlargement in a poorly controlled short diabetic child is indicative of Mauriac's syndrome, which is rarely seen now owing to improved diabetic care. The cause of this syndrome may be poor nutritional status. Growth hormone concentrations are higher in children with diabetes, and this factor may play a role in complications of diabetes mellitus. IGF-I concentrations tend to be normal or low, depending upon glucose control, but judging from the elevated GH, the stimulation of IGF-I by GH may be blocked in these children. (See Chapter 22.)

8. DIABETES INSIPIDUS

Polyuria and polydipsia due to inadequate vasopressin (neurogenic diabetes insipidus) or inability of the kidney to respond to vasopressin (nephrogenic diabetes insipidus) will lead to poor caloric intake and decreased growth. With appropriate treatment (see Chapter 9), the growth rate should return to normal. Acquired neurogenic diabetes insipidus may herald a hypothalamic-pituitary tumor, and growth failure may be due to associated GH deficiency.

THE DIAGNOSIS OF SHORT STATURE

As previously stated, an initial decision must be made about whether a child is pathologically short or simply distressed because his or her height is not as close to the 50th percentile as desired by the patient or the parents. Performing unnecessary tests is expensive and may be a source of long-term concern to the parents—a concern that could have been avoided by appropriate reassurance. Alternatively, missing a diagnosis of pathologic poor growth may cause the patient to lose inches of final height.

If a patient's stature, growth rate, or height adjusted for mid parental height is sufficiently decreased to warrant evaluation, an orderly approach to diagnosis will eliminate unnecessary laboratory testing. The medical history will provide invaluable information regarding intrauterine course and toxin exposure, birth size and the possibility of birth trauma, mental and physical development, symptoms of systemic diseases (Table 8–4), abnormal diet, and family heights and ages at which pubertal maturation occurred. Evaluation of psychosocial factors affecting the family and the relationship of parents and child can be carried out during the history-taking encounter. Often the diagnosis can be made at this point.

On physical examination, present height—measured without shoes on an accurate measuring device—and weight should be plotted and compared with any previous data available. If no past heights are available, a history of changes in clothing and shoe sizes or a need to lengthen skirts or pants may reflect prior growth. Questions about how the child's stature compares with that of his or her peers and whether the child's height has always been in the same relationship to that of classmates are useful. One of the most important features of the evaluation process is to determine height velocity and compare the child's growth rate with the normal growth rate for age. Adjustment for mid parental height is calculated and nutritional status determined. Arm span, head circumference, and upper to lower segment ratio are measured. Physical stigmas of syndromes or systemic diseases are evaluated. Neurologic examination is essential.

If no specific diagnosis emerges from the physical examination, a set of laboratory evaluations may prove useful. Complete blood count, urinalysis, and serum electrolyte measurements may reveal anemia, abnormalities of hepatic or renal disease (including concentration defects), glucose intolerance, acidosis, calcium disorder, or other electrolyte disturbances. Age-adjusted values must be used, since the normal ranges of serum alkaline phosphatase and phosphorus values is higher in children than in adults. A sedimentation rate, serum carotene, or antigliadin or antireticulin antibody determination may indicate connective tissue disease, Crohn's disease, or malabsorption. Determination of total T_4, TSH, and resin T_3 uptake or free T_4 is appropriate. Skeletal age evaluation will not make a diagnosis; however, if the study shows delayed bone age, the possibility of constitutional delay in growth, hypothyroidism, or GH deficiency must be considered. A somatomedin level, if normal for age, would speak against classic GH deficiency or malnutrition; if low, it must be considered in relation to skeletal age, nutritional status, and general health status. Elevated 24-hour urinary 17-hydroxycorticosteroids (normal, < 4.5 mg/m^2 [12.4 μm/m^2]) and free cortisol (normal, < 60 μg/m^2 [0.166 μm/m^2]) signify Cushing's syndrome. If a hypothalamic pituitary disorder is suspected, a skull x-ray or CT or MRI scan is indicated. Serum prolactin may be elevated in cases of hypothalamic disorder.

If no diagnosis is apparent after all of the above have been considered and evaluated, more detailed procedures, such as provocative testing for GH deficiency, are indicated. It must be emphasized that a long and expensive evaluation is not indicated until it is likely that psychologic or nutritional factors are not at fault. Likewise, if a healthy-appearing child presents with borderline short stature, normal growth rate, and short familial stature, a period of observation may be more appropriate than laboratory tests.

TALL STATURE DUE TO NONENDOCRINE CAUSES

1. CONSTITUTIONAL TALL STATURE

A person who has been taller than his or her peers and is growing at a velocity within the normal range for bone age, has a moderately advanced bone age, and has no signs of the disorders listed below may be considered to be constitutionally advanced. Predicted final height will usually be in the normal adult range. There may be a history of a close relative who was taller than his or her peers during childhood but who eventually reached normal adult height.

Exogenous obesity in an otherwise healthy child will usually lead to moderate advancement of bone age, slightly increased growth rate, and tall stature in childhood. Puberty will be in the early range of normal, and adult stature will be normal according to genetic influence. As a rule, obesity and short stature should be considered an indication of a potential organic disorder or syndrome.

2. GENETIC TALL STATURE

Children with exceptionally tall parents have a tendency to reach a height above the normal range. The child will be tall for his or her age, will grow at a high normal rate, and the bone age will be close to chronologic age, leading to a tall height prediction. Children with tall stature have been noted to have growth hormone secretory patterns somewhat reminiscent of acromegaly; eg, GH levels have increased after TRH administration.

Occasionally, children will be concerned about being too tall as adults. These worries are more common in girls and will sometimes be of greater concern to the parents than to the patient. Final height can be limited by promoting early epiphyseal closure with estrogen in girls or testosterone in boys. Such therapy should not be undertaken without careful consideration of the risks involved, especially those of high-dose estrogen therapy. Testosterone therapy has been associated with decreasing HDL cholesterol levels as well as causing the onset and progression of acne fulminans, even after therapy has been withdrawn. Estrogen carries the theoretic risk of causing thrombosis, ovarian cysts, and galactorrhea, but few complications have been reported. High-dose estrogen therapy may decrease final height by as much as 4.5–7 cm, although this is only an estimated decrease based upon the predicted final height. Such therapy will be less effective if not started 3–4 years before epiphyseal fusion. Some studies suggest that bromocriptine will decrease growth rate in children with tall stature, but other studies have not confirmed this.

3. SYNDROMES OF TALL STATURE

Cerebral Gigantism

The syndrome of rapid growth in infancy, prominent forehead, high-arched palate, sharp chin, and hypertelorism (Sotos' syndrome) is not associated with GH excess. Mentation is usually impaired. The growth rate decreases to normal in later childhood, but stature remains tall.

Marfan's Syndrome

Arachnodactyly (Marfan's syndrome) is an autosomal dominant abnormality of connective tissue exhibiting variable penetrance. This condition may be diagnosed by characteristic physical manifestations of tall stature, long thin fingers, hyperextension of joints, and superior lens subluxation. Pectus excavatum and scoliosis may be noted. Furthermore, aortic or mitral regurgitation or aortic root dilation may be present and aortic dissection or rupture may ultimately occur. In patients with this syndrome, arm span exceeds height, and the upper to lower segment ratio is quite low owing to long legs.

Homocystinuria

Patients with homocystinuria have an autosomal recessive deficiency of cystathionine beta-synthetase and phenotypes similar to those of patients with Marfan's syndrome. Additional features of homocystinuria include mental retardation, increased incidence of seizures, osteoporosis, inferior lens dislocation, and increased urinary excretion of homocystine with increased plasma homocystine and methionine but low plasma cystine. Thromboembolic phenomenona may precipitate a fatal complication. This disease is treated by restricting dietary methionine and, in responsive patients, administering pyridoxine.

Beckwith-Wiedemann Syndrome

This syndrome of the large newborn with omphalocele, macroglossia, hypoglycemia with hyperinsulinism due to pancreatic hyperplasia, fetal adrenocortical cytomegaly, and large kidneys with medullary dysplasia is also associated with increased growth in childhood.

XYY Syndrome

Patients with one (47,XYY) or more (48,XYYY) extra Y chromosomes achieve greater than average adult heights. They have normal birth lengths but higher than normal growth rates. Excess GH secretion has not been documented.

Klinefelter's Syndrome

Patients with Klinefelter's syndrome (see Chapter 16) tend toward tall stature, but this is not a constant feature.

TALL STATURE DUE TO ENDOCRINE DISORDERS

1. PITUITARY GIGANTISM

If a GH-secreting pituitary adenoma occurs before epiphyseal fusion, the result will be excessive linear growth rather than just the acral overgrowth characteristic of acromegaly. Height velocity will be abnormally rapid, and other somatic signs that occur in acromegaly may be found in addition to increased stature (see Chapter 6). Elevated fasting GH and somatomedin concentrations are diagnostic.

2. SEXUAL PRECOCITY

Early onset of secretion of estrogens or androgens will lead to abnormally increased height velocity. Because bone age is advanced, there will be the paradox of the tall child who, because of early epiphyseal closure, is short as an adult. The conditions include complete and incomplete sexual precocity (including virilizing congenital adrenal hyperplasia) (Figs 8–9, 8–10, and 8–11).

3. THYROTOXICOSIS

Excessive thyroid hormone due to overproduction or overtreatment with thyroxine will lead to increased growth, advanced bone age, and, if occurring in early life, craniosynostosis. If the condition remains untreated, final height will be reduced.

4. INFANTS OF DIABETIC MOTHERS

Glucose intolerance of pregnancy (gestational diabetes) or diabetes mellitus causes large birth size and neonatal hypoglycemia due to pancreatic hyperplasia. With adequate support, postnatal growth and glucose metabolism become normal a few weeks after birth.

REFERENCES

Normal Growth

Elwood PC et al: Growth of children from 0–5 years: With special reference to mothers' smoking in pregnancy. *Ann Hum Biol* 1987;**14:**543.

Hamill PVV et al: Physical growth: National Center for Health Statistics percentiles. *Am J Clin Nutr* 1979;**32:**607.

Himes JH, Roche AF, Thissen D: *Parent-Specific Adjustments for Assessment of Recumbent Length and Stature.* Vol 13 of: *Monographs in Paediatrics.* Karger, 1981.

Kaplan SL: Normal and abnormal growth. Pages 83–104 in: *Pediatrics,* 17th ed. Rudolph A, Hoffman JIE (editors). Appleton-Century-Crofts, 1982.

Pierson M, Deschamps J-P: Growth. In: *Pediatric Endocrinology.* Job J-C, Pierson M (editors). Wiley, 1981.

Preece, MA: The insulinlike growth factors. In: *Current Concepts in Pediatric Endocrinology.* Styne DM, Brook GG (editors). Elsevier, 1987.

Roche AF, Himes JH: Incremental growth charts. *Am J Clin Nutr* 1980;**33:**2041.

Roche AF, Wainer H, Thissen D: The RWT method for the prediction of adult stature. *Pediatrics* 1975;**56:**1027.

Smith DW: Growth and its disorders. Vol 15 of: *Major Problems in Clinical Pediatrics.* Schaffer AJ, Markowitz M (editors). Saunders, 1977.

Smith DW et al: Shifting linear growth during infancy: Illustration of genetic factors in growth from fetal life through infancy. *J Pediatr* 1976;**89:**225.

Styne DM: Growth. In: *Pediatric Endocrinology for the House Officer.* Styne DM (editor). Williams & Wilkins, 1988.

Tanner JM, Whitehouse RH: Clinical longitudinal standards for height, weight, height velocity, weight velocity, and stages of puberty. *Arch Dis Child* 1976;**51:**170.

US Department of Health, Education, and Welfare, Public Health Service: *NCHS Growth Curves for Children: Birth–18 Years, United States.* Publication No. (PHS) 78-1650. Series 11, No. 165, 1977.

Wales JK, Milner RD: Knemometry in assessment of linear growth. *Arch Dis Child* 1987;**62:**166.

Short Stature

Ad Hoc Committee on Growth Hormone Usage, The Lawson Wilkins Pediatric Endocrine Society, and Committee on Drugs: Growth hormone in the treatment of children with short stature. *Pediatrics* 1983;**72:**891.

Albertsson-Wikland K: The effect of human growth hormone injection frequency on linear growth rate. *Acta Paediatr Scand [Suppl]* 1987;**337:**110.

Albini CH et al: Quantitation of urinary growth hormone in children with normal and abnormal growth. *Pediatr Res* 1988;**23:**89.

Aynsley-Green A, Zachmann M, Prader A: Interrelation of the therapeutic effects of growth hormone and testosterone on growth in hypopituitarism. *J Pediatr* 1976;**89:**992.

Bierich JR: Treatment by hGH of constitutional delay of growth and adolescence. *Acta Paediatr Scand [Suppl]* 1986;**325:**71.

Borges JLC et al: Stimulation of growth hormone and somatomedin-C in idiopathic GH-deficient subjects by intermittent, pulsatile administration of synthetic human pancreatic tumor growth hormone–releasing factor–40. *J Clin Endocrinol Metab* 1984;**59:**1.

Braga S et al: Familial growth hormone deficiency resulting from a 7.6 kb deletion within the growth hormone gene cluster. *Am J Med Genet* 1986;**25**:443.

Brown P: Human growth hormone therapy and Creutzfeldt-Jakob disease: A drama in three acts. *Pediatrics* 1988;**81**:85.

Clarren, SK, Smith DW: The fetal alcohol syndrome. *N Engl J Med* 1978;**298**:1063.

Clayton PE, Price DA, Shalet SM: Growth hormone state after completion of treatment with growth hormone. *Arch Dis Child* 1987;**62**:222.

Clayton PE et al: Does growth hormone cause relapse of brain tumours? *Lancet* 1987;**1**:711.

Dean HJ, Bishop A, Winter JS: Growth hormone deficiency in patients with histiocytosis X. *J Pediatr* 1986;**109**:615.

Friesen HG: Raben Lecture 1980: A tale of stature. *Endocrine Rev* 1980;**1**:309.

Furlanetto RW, Underwood LE, Van Wyk JJ: Estimation of somatomedin-C levels in normals and patients with pituitary disease by radioimmunoassay. *J Clin Invest* 1977;**60**:648.

Groll A et al: Short stature as the primary manifestation of coeliac disease. *Lancet* 1980;**2**:1097.

Harris DA et al: Somatomedin-C in normal puberty and in true precocious puberty before and after treatment with a potent luteinizing hormone–releasing hormone agonist. *J Clin Endocrinol Metab* 1985;**61**:152.

Harrison HE, Harrison HC: *Disorders of Calcium and Phosphate Metabolism in Childhood and Adolescence.* Vol 19 of: *Major Problems in Clinical Pediatrics.* Schaffer AJ, Markowitz M (editors). Saunders, 1979.

Hintz RL et al: Plasma somatomedin and growth hormone values in children with protein-calorie malnutrition. *J Pediatr* 1978;**92**:153.

Horner JM, Thorsson AV, Hintz RL: Growth deceleration patterns in children with constitutional short stature: An aid to diagnosis. *Pediatrics* 1978;**62**:529.

Johnson JD et al: Hypoplasia of the anterior pituitary and neonatal hypoglycemia. *J Pediatr* 1973;**82**:634.

Jones KL: *Smith's Recognizable Patterns of Human Malformation.* Saunders, 1988.

Kaplan SL, Grumbach MM: Pathophysiology of GH deficiency and other disorders of GH metabolism. Pages 45–55 in: *Problems in Pediatric Endocrinology.* La Cauza C, Root AW (editors). Academic Press, 1980.

Kaplan SL et al: Clinical studies with recombinant-DNA-derived methionyl human growth hormone in growth hormone deficient children. *Lancet* 1986;**1**:697.

Kaplowitz PB, Jennings S: Enhancement of linear growth and weight gain by cyproheptadine in children with hypopituitarism receiving growth hormone therapy. *J Pediatr* 1987;**110**:140.

Kowarski AJ et al: Growth failure with normal serum RIA-GH and low somatomedin activity: Somatomedin restoration and growth acceleration after exogenous GH. *J Clin Endocrinol Metab* 1978;**47**:461.

Kurzner SI et al: Growth failure in bronchopulmonary dysplasia: Elevated metabolic rates and pulmonary mechanics. *J Pediatr* 1988;**112**:73.

Laron Z: Syndrome of familial dwarfism and high plasma immunoreactive growth hormone. *Isr J Med Sci* 1974;**10**:1247.

Levitsky LL: Growth and pubertal pattern in insulin-dependent diabetes mellitus. *Semin Adolesc Med* 1987;**3**:233.

Lippe B: Turner syndrome: A recognizable cause of adolescent short stature. *Semin Adolesc Med* 1987;**3**:365.

Lovinger RD, Kaplan SL, Grumbach MM: Congenital hypopituitarism associated with neonatal hypoglycemia and microphallus: Four cases secondary to hypothalamic hormone deficiencies. *J Pediatr* 1975;**87(Part 2)**:1171.

Miller WL, Kaplan SL, Grumbach MM: Child abuse as a cause of post-traumatic hypopituitarism. *N Engl J Med* 1980;**302**:724.

Norman C: Virus scare halts hormone research. *Science* 1985;**228**:1176.

Phillips JA III: Genetic diagnosis: Differentiating growth disorders. *Hosp Pract* (April) 1985;**20**:85.

Powell GF, Brasel JA, Blizzard RM: Emotional deprivation and growth retardation simulating idiopathic hypopituitarism. *N Engl J Med* 1967;**276**:1271.

Powell GF et al: Emotional deprivation and growth retardation simulating idiopathic hypopituitarism. 2. Endocrinologic evaluation of the syndrome. *N Engl J Med* 1967;**276**:1279.

Prader A, Tanner JM, von Harnack GA: Catch-up growth following illness or starvation. *J Pediatr* 1963;**62**:646.

Pugliese MI et al: Fear of obesity: A cause of short stature and delayed puberty. *N Engl J Med* 1983;**309**:513.

Quattrin T et al: Quantitation of urinary somatomedin-C in children with normal and abnormal growth. *J Clin Endocrinol Metab* 1987;**65**:1168.

Richards GE et al: Delayed onset of hypopituitarism: Sequelae of therapeutic irradiation of central nervous system, eye, and middle ear tumors. *J Pediatr* 1976;**89**:553.

Rickard KA et al: The value of nutrition support in children with cancer. *Cancer* 1987;**58(Suppl 8)**:1904.

Reiter EO et al: Variable estimates of serum growth hormone concentrations by different radioassay systems. *J Clin Endocrinol Metab* 1988;**66**:68.

Rivarola MA et al: Phenotypic heterogeneity in familial isolated growth hormone deficiency type I-A. *J Clin Endocrinol Metab* 1984;**59**:34.

Roche AF: Growth assessment in abnormal children. *Kidney Int* 1978;**14**:369.

Rogol AD et al: Growth hormone release in response to human pancreatic tumor growth hormone–releasing hormone–40 in children with short stature. *J Clin Endocrinol Metab* 1984;**59**:580.

Rosenfeld RG, Northcraft GB, Hintz RL: A prospective, randomized study of testosterone treatment of constitutional delay of growth and development in male adolescents. *Pediatrics* 1982;**69**:681.

Safer DJ, Allen RP, Barr E: Growth rebound after termination of stimulant drugs. *J Pediatr* 1975;**86**:113.

Sanders JE et al: Growth and development following marrow transplantation for leukemia. *Blood* 1986;**68**:1129.

Schechter J, Kovacs K, Rimoin D: Isolated growth hormone deficiency: Immunocytochemistry. *J Clin Endocrinol Metab* 1984;**59**:798.

Shohat M et al: Childhood asthma and growth outcome. *Arch Dis Child* 1987;**62**:63.

Silver HK, Finkelstein M: Deprivation dwarfism. *J Pediatr* 1967;**7**:317.

Sipponen P et al: Familial syndrome with panhypopituitarism, hypoplasia of the hypophysis, and poorly developed sella turcica. *Arch Dis Childhood* 1978;**53**:664.

Sklar CA et al: Hormonal and metabolic abnormalities associated with central nervous system germinoma in children and adolescents and the effect of therapy: Report of 10 patients. *J Clin Endocrinol Metab* 1981;**52**:9.

Smith PJ et al: Nocturnal pulsatile growth hormone-releasing hormone treatment in growth hormone deficiency. *Clin Endocrinol* 1986;**25**:35.

Spiliotis BE et al: Growth hormone neurosecretory dysfunction. *JAMA* 1984;**251**:2223.

Styne DM, Grumbach MM: Puberty in the male and female: Its physiology and disorders. Pages 313–384 in: *Reproductive Endocrinology,* 2nd ed. Yen SSC, Jaffe RB (editors). Saunders, 1986.

Styne DM et al: Treatment of Cushing's disease in childhood and adolescence by transsphenoidal microadenomectomy. *N Engl J Med* 1984;**310**:889.

Takano K et al: Plasma growth hormone (GH) response to GH-releasing factor in normal children with short stature and patients with pituitary dwarfism. *J Clin Endocrinol Metab* 1984;**58**:236.

Tanner JM, Lejarraga H, Cameron N: The natural history of the Silver-Russell syndrome: A longitudinal study of thirty-nine cases. *Pediatr Res* 1975;**9**:611.

Tanner JM et al: The effect of human growth hormone treatment for 1 to 7 years on the growth of 100 children with growth hormone deficiency, low birth weight, inherited smallness, Turner's syndrome and other complaints. *Arch Dis Child* 1971;**46**:745.

Tanner JM et al: Relative importance of growth hormone and sex steroids for the growth at puberty of trunk length, limb length, and muscle width in growth hormone–deficient children. *J Pediatr* 1976;**89**:1000.

Thomsett MJ et al: Endocrine and neurologic outcome in childhood craniopharyngioma: Review of effect of treatment in 42 patients. *J Pediatr* 1980;**97**:728.

Thorner MO et al: Acceleration of growth in two children treated with human growth hormone–releasing factor. *N Engl J Med* 1985;**312**:2.

Underwood LE, D'Ercole AJ, Van Wyk JJ: Somatomedin-C and the assessment of growth. *Pediatr Clin North Am* 1980;**27**:771.

Van Vliet G et al: Growth hormone can increase growth rate in short normal children: Evaluation of the somatomedin-C generation test in the assessment of children with short stature. *N Engl J Med* 1983;**309**:1016.

Zapf J, Walter H, Froesch ER: Radioimmunological determination of insulin-like growth factors I and II in normal subjects and in patients with growth disorders and extrapancreatic tumor hypoglycemia. *J Clin Invest* 1981;**68**:1321.

Tall Stature

Conte FA, Grumbach MM: Epidemiological aspects of estrogen use: Estrogen use in children and adolescents: A survey. *Pediatrics* 1978;**62(Suppl)**:1091.

Costin G, Fefferman RA, Kogut MD: Hypothalamic gigantism. *J Pediatr* 1973;**83**:419.

Schwarz HP, Joss EE, Zuppinger KA: Bromocriptine treatment in adolescent boys with familial tall stature: A pair-matched controlled study. *J Clin Endocrinol Metab* 1987;**65**:136.

Wettenhall HNB, Cahill C, Roche AF: Tall girls: A survey of 15 years of management and treatment. *J Pediatr* 1975;**86**:602.

Posterior Pituitary Gland

9

David J. Ramsay, DM, DPhil

The posterior pituitary gland secretes 2 potent nonapeptides: vasopressin and oxytocin. **Vasopressin** (antidiuretic hormone [ADH]) has important effects on urine flow and thus on water balance. In the presence of vasopressin, the average adult human can produce a urine concentrated to 1200 mosm/kg of water at a flow of approximately 0.5 mL/min. In the absence of vasopressin, as in diabetes insipidus, urine flow may be as high as 15–20 mL/min at a concentration of 30 mosm/kg of water. Vasopressin is also a potent vasoconstrictor agent, and the implications of this action for control of circulation are just beginning to be appreciated.

Oxytocin has important contractile effects on smooth muscle. In particular, it causes contraction of the myoepithelial cells that line the ducts of the mammary gland, thus causing milk ejection, and initiates contractions of the appropriately primed uterus.

ANATOMY

The posterior pituitary gland, or neurohypophysis, develops as a downgrowth from the hypothalamus (Fig 9–1). It consists of fibers and endings of the hypothalamoneurohypophyseal nerve tract and contains many blood vessels, including capillary sinusoids. Humans have approximately 100,000 such nerve fibers in the tracts. The nerve terminals are characterized by a series of repeated swellings along the nerve fiber varying from 1 to 50 μm in thickness.

PHYSIOLOGY

The 2 peptides secreted by the posterior pituitary gland into the bloodstream, arginine vasopressin and oxytocin, each contain 9 amino acids. They are characterized by a ring structure with a disulfide (S–S) linkage (Fig 9–2). In humans, as in most mammals, arginine vasopressin is the peptide associated with urinary concentration. Lysine vasopressin is the form of the peptide in the pig and is much less active in humans, though it has been used therapeutically. Ar-

---

Acronyms Used in This Chapter

ACTH	Adrenocorticotropic hormone
ADH	Antidiuretic hormone (vasopressin)
CRH	Corticotropin-releasing hormone
DDAVP	Desmopressin acetate; 1-desamino-8-D-arginine vasopressin
SIADH	Syndrome of inappropriate secretion of vasopressin (antidiuretic hormone)

---

ginine vasopressin has a molecular weight of 1084 and is basic, with an isoelectric point of 10.9.

Oxytocin is a less basic peptide with a molecular weight of 1007. In vertebrates, there is a whole family of similar peptides with various amino acid configurations that exert effects on water metabolism and blood pressure. Vasotocin, which is a combination of the structures of vasopressin and oxytocin, has various species-specific effects including water absorption in the kidney and constriction of smooth muscle in the female reproductive tract.

Synthesis

Vasopressin and oxytocin to be secreted into the circulation are manufactured in large cell bodies situated mainly in the supraoptic and paraventricular nuclei. The synthesis of the 2 peptides is associated with synthesis of 2 specific binding proteins called **neurophysins.** One molecule of neurophysin I binds one molecule of oxytocin, and one molecule of neurophysin II binds one molecule of vasopressin. Common genetic mechanisms are involved in the synthesis of the peptide and of the neurophysin. For example, the Brattleboro rat, a strain deficient in vasopressin, does not make neurophysin II, although normal quantities of neurophysin I are present. The nucleotide sequences of bovine arginine vasopressin–neurophysin II and oxytocin–neurophysin I precursors have been determined from cloned cDNA, proving the common precursor hypothesis. The precursors have been termed propressophysin and prooxyphysin.

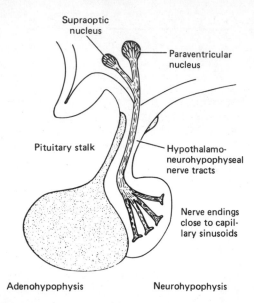

Figure 9–1. The hypothalamoneurohypophyseal system.

Secretion & Transport

Neurophysin-peptide combination, often referred to as neurosecretory material, is transported along the axons of the hypothalamoneurohypophyseal nerve tract at a rate of 2–3 mm/h. Complexes are then stored in the nerve terminals in granules. The peptide is released into the bloodstream following electrical activation of the cell bodies of the nerve tract. For example, intracellular recording techniques have shown groups of neurons that respond to stimuli such as hyperosmolality and certain baroreceptor reflexes. At the nerve terminal, the process of secretion appears to involve the influx of calcium across the membrane. Secretion then proceeds by a process of exocytosis, with release of peptide and associated neurophysin into the bloodstream. The granule membrane is reclaimed by the cell following coating and microvesicle formation.

Extension of Magnocellular System

Oxytocin- and vasopressin-containing neurons project to regions other than the neurohypophysis. The supraoptic nucleus is fairly homogeneous and consists

Cys — Tyr — Ile — Gln — Asn — Cys — Pro — Leu — Gly — NH₂

Oxytocin

Cys — Tyr — Phe — Gln — Asn — Cys — Pro — Arg — Gly — NH₂

Arginine vasopressin

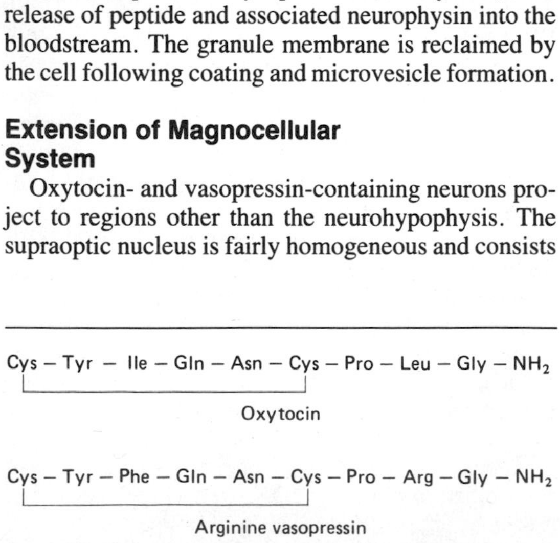

Figure 9–2. Structures of oxytocin and vasopressin.

of cell bodies of magnocellular neurons that contain oxytocin or vasopressin and project mainly to the neurohypophysis. This magnocellular projection, which is called the **hypothalamoneurohypophyseal system,** subserves the neuroendocrine function and accounts for the oxytocin and vasopressin in peripheral blood. In addition to containing some magnocellular neurons, the paraventricular nucleus contains many smaller (parvocellular) cell bodies. Parvocellular cell bodies are also found in the bed nucleus of the stria terminalis, the suprachiasmatic nucleus, and other sites. Parvocellular neurons are widely distributed and appear to be involved in integration of central autonomic functions. There are groups of cells that contain oxytocin and vasopressin in other parts of the hypothalamus. Other peptides such as corticotropin-releasing hormone (CRH) and somatostatin have also been localized in parvocellular neurons.

Vasopressin-containing fibers in the paraventricular nucleus project into the zona externa of the median eminence. The release of vasopressin from these terminals allows entry of the peptides into the hypophyseal–portal vascular system and may be connected with the ability of vasopressin to stimulate ACTH secretion. There are caudal projections from parvocellular neurons of vasopressin and oxytoxin fibers to the brain stem, the nucleus of the solitary tract, the dorsal motor nucleus of the vagus, and throughout the substantia gelatinosa and intermediolateral gray matter of the spinal cord. Projections of vasopressin-containing and neurophysin II–containing neurons have been identified in the choroid plexus of lateral ventricles. The oxytocin and vasopressin present in cerebrospinal fluid may originate from nerve endings that do not project to the neurohypophysis (see Chapter 5).

VASOPRESSIN

Vasopressin has many actions, as shown in Table 9–1. Vasopressin acts through 2 major types of receptors, termed V_1 and V_2, that have different ligand specificities and cellular mechanisms of action. The V_1 receptors mediate vascular smooth muscle contraction and stimulate prostaglandin synthesis and liver glyconeogenolysis. Activation of these receptors increases phosphatidylinositol breakdown, thus causing cellular calcium mobilization. The V_2 receptors, which produce the renal actions of vasopressin, activate guanyl nucleotide regulatory proteins (G proteins) and stimulate the generation of cAMP (see Chapter 1).

Renal Actions

The most important actions of vasopressin are those on the kidney. The major action of vasopressin is to

Table 9–1. Actions of vasopressin.

Target Organ	Type of Receptor	Action
Kidney glomerulus:	V_1	Mesangial cell contraction and ↓ glomerular capillary ultrafiltration coefficient.
Vasa recta	V_1	↓ Medullary blood flow.
Cortical and outer medullary collecting tubules	V_2	↑ Water permeability and NaCl reabsorption.
Inner medullary (papillary) collecting tubules	V_2	↑ Water and urea permeability.
Thick ascending limb of loop of Henle	V_2	↑ Na^{2+}, Cl^-, K^+ reabsorption.
Juxtaglomerular cells	V_1	Suppression of renin release.
Cardiovascular system:		
Arterioles	V_1	Constriction.
Blood vessel baroreceptors	V_2 ?	Sensitization of baroreflex via area postrema.
	V_1 ?	Desensitization of baroreflex via vasopressin released in brain.
Liver	V_1	↑ Glyconeogenolysis.
Adenohypophysis	V_1	↑ ACTH release.
Brain	?	Enhanes passive avoidance behavior.

increase the water permeability of the collecting duct epithelium. The luminal membrane of the collecting duct epithelial cell governs the permeability of that epithelium to water. In the absence of vasopressin, permeability of the epithelium to water is very low; and, although the presence of vasopressin markedly increases permeability, vasopressin must first attach to receptors on the peritubular side of the cell to exert this action. Vasopressin-sensitive adenylate cyclase is then stimulated, resulting in the generation of cyclic nucleotides within the cell. The sequence of intermediate events is not so clear, but it probably involves activation of the protein kinase system. These intracellular events lead to an increase in the water permeability of the luminal membrane by increasing the number of narrow aqueous channels with radii of about 0.2 nm. Diffusion of water through the membrane is enhanced, and thus the transcellular flow of water is also enhanced. Such changes may involve considerable reorganization of membrane structure—perhaps even microtubule and microfilament formation.

The collecting ducts convey urine from the distal tubule and connecting tubule to the renal pelvis. As the collecting ducts traverse the medulla, the urine passes regions of ever-increasing osmolality up to a maximum in the healthy human of 1200 mosm/kg of water at the tip of the papilla. In the presence of vasopressin, collecting duct fluid equilibrates with this hyperosmotic environment, and urine osmolality approaches that of medullary interstitial fluid. Vas-

opressin also increases the permeability of the papillary collecting duct epithelium to urea. Thus, in the presence of vasopressin, urine flow is low and urine osmolality is approximately 1200 mosm/kg; in its absence, urine flow is high (15–20 mL/min) and urine osmolality approaches 30 mosm/kg.

Cardiovascular Actions

The direct action of vasopressin on V_1 receptors in peripheral arterioles tends to increase blood pressure. However, vasopressin buffers its own hypertensive action by increasing the sensitivity of baroreceptor reflexes. This buffering, which requires an intact area postrema, is accomplished with efferent mechanisms such as bradycardia and inhibition of sympathetic nerve activity. These actions of vasopressin may be important during hypovolemia when plasma vasopressin levels are very high and maintaining tissue perfusion is critical.

Other Actions

The physiologic significance of the other actions of vasopressin listed in Table 9–1 is less clear. The actions of vasopressin released in the brain on cardiovascular function and on behavior particularly require elucidation.

CONTROL OF WATER BALANCE

Water Requirements

Water balance is controlled by an integrated system that involves precise regulation of water intake via thirst mechanisms and control of water output via vasopressin secretion. Table 9–2 lists the major sources of fluid losses from the human body in temperate environments. Thus, the average individual loses 2.5–3 L of water per day and must take in that amount in order to maintain balance. Given free access to water, total human body water rarely varies by more than 1–2%. Approximately 1.2 L of the water necessary to maintain balance is taken in food or is provided by oxidative metabolism. The remainder is ingested as water or other fluid beverages.

Concentration of Urine

The capacity of the kidney to produce a concentrated urine plays an important part in maintenance of water balance. Animals eat a diet that produces os-

Table 9–2. Routes of loss of water in an average adult human.

	mL/24 h
Urine	1500
Skin	600
Lungs	400
Feces	100
	2600

motically active material which is excreted in urine and thus requires water in which to be excreted. The more concentrated the urine the kidney can produce, the less water is required in order to excrete those solutes. It is not surprising, therefore, that the evolutionary appearance of peptides that can affect water transport coincided with the development of amphibians.

The importance of urinary concentration is demonstrated in Table 9–2. The average human receiving a normal diet excretes 1.5 L of urine per day at an osmolality of approximately 600 mosm/kg of water, ie, twice the concentration of plasma. Without the capacity to concentrate urine, 3 L of water at a concentration of 300 mosm/kg would have to be excreted, and extra amounts of water would have to be provided in the diet. During negative water balance, the urine volume may be reduced to 600 mL/d at a maximum urinary concentration of 1200 mosm/kg. This capacity to concentrate the urine 4 times more than plasma is of extreme importance, since otherwise it would be necessary to provide very large quantities of water in the diet. Animals in arid environments may concentrate urine up to 5 times more than humans and without that capacity would be unable to survive.

Urinary concentration mechanisms can reduce but not completely prevent loss of water in the urine. Even if an individual is maximally concentrating urine, obligatory fluid loss is still considerable. This situation is exacerbated in a warm environment, where many liters of fluid may be lost to maintain a constant temperature via sweating. The only way to bring body fluid back to normal is by increasing water intake. It is not surprising that many similarities exist between mechanisms involved in the control of thirst and vasopressin secretion.

Control of Thirst & Vasopressin Secretion

Two major mechanisms are involved in the control of thirst and vasopressin secretion: cellular dehydration and extracellular dehydration.

A. Cellular Dehydration: Cellular dehydration occurs when extracellular fluid osmolality is increased by a solute that cannot penetrate cell membranes. As the osmolality in intracellular and extracellular fluids is equalized by the passage of water across cell membranes, any increase in extracellular fluid osmolality will cause water to be withdrawn from cells. Verney, in a classic 1947 paper, proposed that osmoreceptor cells were present in the anterior hypothalamus and that when extracellular fluid osmolality increased, all cells—including these hypothesized hypothalamic osmoreceptors—became dehydrated, thus providing the signal for secretion of vasopressin. This theory has now received substantial experimental support. The effect of increasing plasma osmolality in conscious dogs prepared with exteriorized carotid loops on drinking is shown in Fig 9–3. Increasing the osmolality by approximately 10 mosm/kg with a solution of hyper-

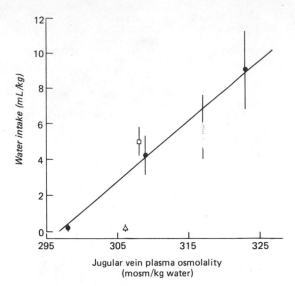

Figure 9–3. Relationship between water intake and jugular vein plasma osmolality. Central osmolality was increased selectively by infusing hypertonic sodium chloride into carotid loops in trained conscious dogs (●). Infusion of hypertonic sucrose was equally effective (□), whereas hypertonic urea (△) did not stimulate drinking. (Data from Wood RJ, Rolls BJ, Ramsay DJ: *Am J Physiol* 1977;**323**:88.)

tonic sodium chloride or hypertonic sucrose stimulates drinking, whereas solutions of urea and glucose—solutes that penetrate cell membranes and therefore will not cause osmotic withdrawal of water from cells—have no effect on drinking. Fig 9–4 shows the relationship between plasma vasopressin concentration and osmolality in human subjects during dehydration. Increases of only 1% in plasma osmolality cause stimulation of water intake and vasopressin secretion.

Experiments on conscious goats have suggested that the central osmoreceptors are sensitive to sodium concentration rather than to osmolality. Furthermore, the receptors are reportedly situated in a periventricular site and thus are sensitive to the composition of the cerebrospinal fluid rather than that of the plasma. Although there is some evidence for this hypothesis in ruminants, experiments in rats and dogs have failed to provide evidence for the existence of specific sodium receptors in these species. Moreover, it appears that the osmoreceptors must be situated in an area of the brain where the blood-brain barrier is deficient and thus is influenced by the composition of plasma rather than that of the cerebrospinal fluid. In fact, lesions of the organum vasculosum of the lamina terminalis, one of the circumventricular organs, prevent drinking and vasopressin secretion in response to increased plasma osmolality in the normal physiologic range, although responses to hypovolemia are normal. Although electrical activity of magnocellular neurons in the supraoptic nucleus is sensitive to changes in osmolality, the

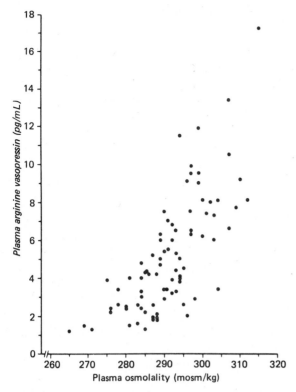

Figure 9–4. Relationship between plasma vasopressin concentration and plasma osmolality in humans during dehydration. (Reproduced, with permission, from Hammer M, Ladefoged J, Olgaard K: *Am J Physiol* 1980;**238**:313.)

effects on vasopressin secretion, but reductions larger than 10% cause a marked stimulation of vasopressin secretion. Indeed, values over 100 pg/mL are not uncommon. These high plasma circulating levels of vasopressin do not appear to significantly affect water conservation, since maximum urinary concentration is reached at much lower plasma levels of vasopressin. However, the high levels of vasopressin secretion following depletion may be important in maintaining blood pressure, acting via the vasoconstrictor function of vasopressin.

C. Interaction of Osmolality and Volume: The pathways involved in hypovolemic stimulation of thirst and vasopressin secretion are still not clear. Two major mechanisms have been proposed, and there is evidence that both are involved. Reductions in blood volume may be sensed by low-pressure receptors in the left and right atria and in the pulmonary circulation. More severe hypovolemia resulting in reduction in blood pressure may be sensed by the arterial baroreceptors. Electrophysiologic evidence shows that information from both low- and high-pressure baroreceptor areas in the circulation is transmitted to magnocellular cells in the hypothalamus (see Fig 5–4). In addition to this direct reflex pathway, the renin-angiotensin system may be involved. In all animal species that have been studied, including humans, angiotensin II is an effective dipsogen. In addition, particularly in the presence of a raised plasma osmolality, angiotensin may stimulate vasopressin secretion. Hypovolemia stimulates renin secretion and angiotensin formation reflexly. The relative roles of the

organum vasculosum of the lamina terminalis is essential for normal osmotic release of vasopressin and stimulation of thirst.

The relationship between plasma vasopressin concentration and plasma osmolality in humans is presented in Fig 9–4. Although controversy exists about some points at the lower end of the relationship and about whether the relationship is best represented in a linear or a logarithmic form, the exquisite sensitivity of vasopressin release to changing plasma osmolality is obvious. With plasma vasopressin concentrations of 5–6 pg/mL, the urine is maximally concentrated. Thus, in terms of water conservation, Fig 9–4 represents the physiologic range of variations in plasma vasopressin in humans.

B. Extracellular Fluid Dehydration: Both drinking and vasopressin secretion may be stimulated by contraction of the extracellular fluid volume without a change in osmolality, This is referred to as extracellular fluid dehydration. Phenomena such as hemorrhage that reduce extracellular fluid volume result in both drinking and vasopressin secretion. Fig 9–5 demonstrates the relationship between reduction in blood volume and plasma concentrations of vasopressin. Small decreases in volume have minimal

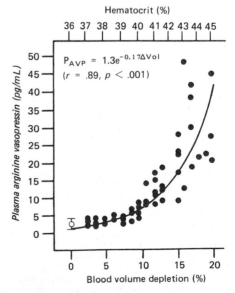

Figure 9–5. Relationship of plasma vasopressin to isosmotic reductions in blood volume in rats. (Reproduced, with permission, from Dunn FL et al: *J Clin Invest* 1973;**52**:3212.)

direct baroreceptor input and angiotensin mechanisms in the responses to extracellular dehydration have yet to be determined.

The normal day-to-day regulation of water balance therefore involves interaction between osmotic and volume stimuli. In the case of vasopressin secretion, the fall in extracellular fluid volume sensitizes the release of vasopressin to a given osmotic stimulus. Thus, for a given increase in plasma osmolality, the increase in plasma vasopressin concentration will be greater in hypovolemic than in normovolemic states.

In dehydration, an increase in plasma osmolality results in withdrawal of fluid from cells. Thus, the reduction in total body water is shared equally between intracellular and extracellular fluid compartments. The increase in plasma osmolality and the reduction of extracellular fluid volume act synergistically to stimulate vasopressin release. In salt depletion, however, plasma vasopressin concentrations remain constant or even slightly elevated in spite of a fall in plasma osmolality. Hypovolemia in this situation, as a result of osmotic movements of water from the extracellular into the intracellular fluid space, appears to provide the sensitizing influence.

Thirst mechanisms also involve interactions between extracellular fluid volume and osmolality. During periods of dehydration, increased plasma osmolality provides approximately 70% of the increased thirst drive, and the remaining 30% is due to hypovolemia. In salt depletion, the situation is less clear, but the normal or increased drinking that has been observed in experimental animals has been attributed to the associated hypovolemia.

Satiety

Dehydrated animals have a remarkable capacity to take in the appropriate volume of water to repair the deficit. It has been demonstrated that dogs deprived of water for various periods of time drink just the volume of water needed to repair the deficit within 5 minutes. All animals have this capacity, though some species usually take longer to ingest the required amount of fluid. If drinking ceases before the ingested fluid has been completely absorbed by the intestine, mechanisms other than restoration of volume and composition of extracellular fluid to normal must be involved. These include oropharyngeal and gastric distention factors and perhaps the participation of receptors in the liver. Similar inhibitory influences affect vasopressin secretion. Following voluntary rehydration in dehydrated animals (including humans), plasma vasopressin secretion returns to normal before redilution of the body fluids has been completed.

DIABETES INSIPIDUS

Diabetes insipidus is characterized by the passage of copious amounts of very dilute urine. The disease is due either to failure of the neurohypophysis to secrete adequate quantities of vasopressin (neurogenic diabetes insipidus; also called pituitary, central, or vasopressin-sensitive diabetes insipidus) or failure of the kidney to respond to circulating vasopressin (nephrogenic diabetes insipidus). The loss of large volumes of dilute urine leads to both cellular and extracellular dehydration. Therefore, the disease is associated with polydipsia.

Classification

A. Neurogenic Diabetes Insipidus: The major causes of neurogenic diabetes insipidus are shown in Table 9–3. Operations in the region of the hypothalamus and pituitary gland—eg, removal of chromophobe adenoma—form an important group. Temporary impairment of posterior pituitary function is generally associated with pituitary surgery. Any damage to the hypothalamoneurohypophyseal nerve tracts will result in retrograde degeneration of the fiber tracts that have been interrupted. However, permanent diabetes insipidus will not develop unless over 80% of the pathways have been destroyed.

Idiopathic diabetes insipidus may occur at any age after infancy and may affect both sexes. In this condition, the number of vasopressin-containing fibers in the nuclei, nerve tracts, and posterior pituitary is reduced. Familial diabetes insipidus, which appears in infancy, is a much more rare disorder. It is also associated with sparsity of vasopressin-containing fibers. The other causes of diabetes insipidus involve mechanical disturbances to the pituitary or hypothalamus. Supra- or intrasellar tumors may be primary or secondary. A variety of infiltrative, vascular, autoimmune, and infectious causes complete this group. In partial neurogenic diabetes, vasopressin secretion is not completely absent, but plasma arginine vasopressin concentrations are inappropriately low for the plasma osmolality.

B. Nephrogenic Diabetes Insipidus: In this group of diseases (Table 9–4), circulating levels of vasopressin are normal or elevated, but the renal response is suppressed. These can result from a variety of forms of chronic renal disease, particularly those preferentially affecting the medulla and collecting duct system. Thus, if medullary disease (eg, from pyelonephritis) prevents formation of a medullary concentra-

Table 9–3. Causes of neurogenic diabetes insipidus.

Hypophysectomy, complete or partial.
Surgery to remove suprasellar tumors.
Idiopathic.
Familial.
Tumors and cysts (intra- and suprasellar).
Histiocytosis.
Granulomas.
Infections.
Interruption of blood supply.
Autoimmune.

Table 9–4. Causes of nephrogenic diabetes insipidus.

Chronic renal disease: Any renal disease that interferes with collecting duct or medullary function, eg, chronic pyelonephritis.
Hypokalemia.
Protein starvation.
Hypercalcemia.
Sickle cell anemia.
Sjögren's syndrome.
Drugs, eg, lithium, fluoride, methoxyflurane anesthesia, demeclocycline (Declomycin), colchicine.
Congenital defect.
Familial.

tion gradient, urine passing through the collecting duct system cannot become concentrated.

Chronic potassium deficiency leading to hypokalemia is associated with reduction in urinary concentrating capacity. This is partly due to lack of medullary hypertonicity and may be exacerbated by increased medullary production of prostaglandins, thus inhibiting vasopressin action. The neuropathy associated with hypercalcemia generally affects the medullary portions of the kidney first, and this leads to lack of urinary concentration. Drugs such as lithium carbonate and demeclocycline greatly reduce the sensitivity of the renal tubule to vasopressin by their inhibitory effect on vasopressin-sensitive renal medullary adenylate cyclase. Congenital nephrogenic diabetes insipidus is a rare condition caused by a defect in the response of the renal tubule to vasopressin; it is often associated with insensitivity of medullary adenylate cyclase to vasopressin. It is most common in males with a family history of transmission through apparently healthy females, though cases have recently been reported in females.

Psychogenic Polydipsia

Psychogenic polydipsia, or **potomania,** involves greatly increased drinking, usually in excess of 5 L of water per day, leading to dilution of the extracellular fluid, inhibition of vasopressin secretion, and water diuresis. This type of compulsive water drinking may be associated with a number of psychologic disturbances, so it must be carefully distinguished from polydipsia due to tumors and other diseases affecting the hypothalamus and interfering with normal drinking pathways.

Differential Diagnosis

It is important to distinguish both types of diabetes insipidus and psychogenic polydipsia from other common causes of polyuria. In general, other forms of polyuria involve osmotic or solute diuresis. For example, in diabetes mellitus, increased excretion of glucose and other solutes requires excretion of increased volumes of water. In osmotic diuresis, the osmolality of the urine tends toward that of plasma. In sharp contrast, the osmolality of the urine in diabetes insipidus and psychogenic polydipsia is very low when compared with that of plasma. Thus, a urine specific gravity less than 1.005 (osmolality < 200 mosm/kg of water) will generally rule out polyuria due to osmotic diuresis. After a careful history has been taken, focusing on patterns of drinking and urination behavior and the family history, a series of investigations should be instituted to distinguish between the 2 types of diabetes insipidus and psychogenic polydipsia. The physiologic principles are set forth in Table 9–5, and the actual procedures are summarized in Table 9–6.

A. Plasma and Urine Osmolality: The first test is to take plasma and urine samples simultaneously for estimation of osmolality. Since in both forms of diabetes insipidus the primary problem is inappropriate water diuresis, the urine will be less concentrated than plasma, whereas the plasma osmolality will be higher than normal. In psychogenic polydipsia, dilute plasma will be associated with the production of dilute urine.

B. Water Deprivation: The next step is to examine the effect of water deprivation on urine osmolality under supervision. Supervision is necessary both because the patient with psychogenic polydipsia will go to great lengths to obtain water and because the patient with complete diabetes insipidus may become dangerously dehydrated very rapidly. The patient should be weighed and denied access to water and each voided urine sample measured for specific gravity or osmolality (or both). Whereas the healthy individual will soon reduce urine flow to 0.5 mL/min at a concentra-

Table 9–5. Results of diagnostic studies in various types of polyuria.

	Neurogenic Diabetes Insipidus	Nephrogenic Diabetes Insipidus	Psychogenic Polydipsia
Random plasma osmolality	↑	↑	↓
Random urine osmolality	↓	↓	↓
Urine osmolality during mild water deprivation	No change	No change	↑
Urine osmolality during nicotine or hypertonic saline	No change	No change	↑
Urine osmolality following vasopressin intravenously	↑	No change	↑
Plasma vasopressin	Low	Normal or high	Low

Table 9–6. Differential diagnosis of diabetes insipidus.

Procedure	Interpretation
Measure plasma and urine osmolality.	A urine osmolality less than that of plasma is consistent with neurogenic or nephrogenic diabetes insipidus; if both urine and plasma are dilute, that is consistent with psychogenic polydipsia.
Dehydration test: If serum osmolality is less than 295 mosm/kg, allow no fluids for 12–18 hours. Measure body weight, urine flow, urine specific gravity, urine and plasma osmolality every 2 hours. Terminate study if body weight falls more than 3%.	A rise in urine osmolality above that of plasma osmolality indicates psychogenic polydipsia. Urine specific gravity less than 1.005 (or 200 mosm/L) indicates either neurogenic or nephrogenic diabetes insipidus.
Measure serum vasopressin at conclusion of dehydration test.	Normal or high vasopressin level usually indicates nephrogenic diabetes insipidus.
Inject 5 units of aqueous vasopressin or 1 μg DDAVP subcutaneously. Measure urine flow and urine and plasma osmolality	Rise in urine osmolality above that of plasma osmolality indicates neurogenic diabetes insipidus; failure of urine osmolality to rise indicates nephrogenic diabetes insipidus.

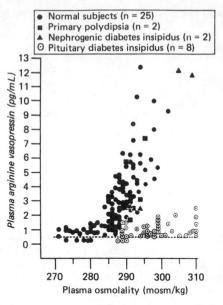

Figure 9–6. Effect of dehydration on plasma vasopressin concentration in normal subjects and patients with polyuria. Note that patients with neurogenic (pituitary) diabetes insipidus cannot increase plasma vasopressin concentration with dehydration, in contrast to patients with psychogenic polydipsia and nephrogenic diabetes insipidus. (Reproduced, with permission, from Robertson GL et al: *J Clin Invest* 1973;**52**:2346.)

tion greater than that of plasma, the patient with diabetes insipidus will maintain a high urine flow at a specific gravity less than 1.005 (200 mosm/kg of water). A period of 18 hours is usually ample to confirm the diagnosis. The test should be terminated if the body weight falls by more than 3%, since serious consequences of dehydration may ensue. Patients with psychogenic polydipsia will always increase urine osmolality to values greater than those of plasma.

C. Vasopressin Test: Once the diagnosis of diabetes insipidus is established, the vasopressin-insensitive (nephrogenic) disease must be distinguished from the vasopressin-sensitive (neurogenic) form. This is done by injection of aqueous vasopressin (Pitressin) or desmopressin acetate (DDAVP). Give 5 units Pitressin subcutaneously or 1 μg DDAVP intravenously, intramuscularly, or subcutaneously, and measure urine osmolality after 1 hour; patients with neurogenic diabetes insipidus will show an increase in urine osmolality to values above that of plasma. Such patients will not show a completely normal response to vasopressin following a single injection. To increase the sensitivity of this test, some clinicians prefer to inject vasopressin following the period of mild water deprivation. Under these circumstances, the patient with neurogenic diabetes insipidus will always show urinary concentration.

D. Vasopressin Radioimmunoassays: Sensitive radioimmunoassays for vasopressin are available that allow plasma vasopressin to be measured either from random plasma samples, with infusions of hyperosmotic saline, or during the water deprivation test. Patients with nephrogenic diabetes insipidus secrete normal quantities of vasopressin following water deprivation, allowing a clear distinction to be made from neurogenic forms of diabetes insipidus (Fig 9–6). Patients with partial neurogenic diabetes insipidus show a smaller than normal increase in plasma vasopressin concentration following dehydration or infusion of hypertonic saline.

E. Influence of Endocrine Disease: The diagnosis of neurogenic diabetes insipidus is sometimes difficult to make in the presence of anterior pituitary disease. Low or absent levels of glucocorticoids or thyroid hormone reduce the solute load to the kidney and thus reduce urine flow. Patients with normal plasma levels of vasopressin but hyposecretion of adrenal glucocorticoids will retain a water load. Thus, even if diabetes insipidus is present, coincident thyroid or adrenal insufficiency may mask the polyuria. A history of a prior endocrine disorder should instigate appropriate diagnostic investigation.

Treatment

A. Neurogenic Diabetes Insipidus:

1. Treatment of Choice—At present, the drug of choice is DDAVP, a synthetic analogue of vasopressin prepared in aqueous solution containing 0.1 mg/mL. It is administered intranasally via a calibrated plastic catheter in doses of 5–20 μg (0.05–0.2 mL) every 12 hours. This agent provides excellent control of polyuria and polydipsia in patients with pituitary diabetes insipidus. Serum osmolality must be monitored at regular intervals (initially every 1–2 weeks, later every 3 months) to be certain that the dose is appropriate. For patients who cannot tolerate intranasal therapy, DDAVP can be given subcutaneously in a single dose of 1–2 μg/d. Alternatively, some patients can be treated with a number of oral agents, including chlorpropamide (Diabinese), clofibrate (Atromid-S), and carbamazepine (Tegretol). Thiazide diuretics may also be used as a supplement. These oral regimens are useful in some patients with either severe or partial neurogenic diabetes insipidus. However, these drugs may have undesirable side effects such as hypoglycemia, myalgia, or serious hematologic toxicity. Thus, DDAVP is clearly the treatment of choice for neurogenic diabetes insipidus.

2. Older Methods–Older methods of treatment include the following:

Vasopressin in oil (Pitressin Tannate in oil), 5 units intramuscularly, is given every 2–3 days. This material is difficult to suspend, irregularly absorbed, and produces "peaks" and "valleys" in its effect.

Lypressin (Diapid) is a pure synthetic vasopressin administered by intranasal spray. It is effective for only a few hours, so that it must be administered at least every 4–6 hours.

B. Nephrogenic Diabetes Insipidus: The underlying disorder should be treated if possible. It is important to recognize familial disease early, since infants are particularly susceptible to brain damage due to dehydration. Diuretics are helpful, along with dietary salt restriction if necessary. Prostaglandin synthesis inhibitors may also be useful. The objective is to maintain the patient in a state of mild sodium depletion and reduce the solute load on the kidney, thus enhancing proximal tubular reabsorption. Reduction in distal tubular flow allows some sodium concentration to take place and minimizes loss of water. Patients with partial sensitivity to vasopressin may be treated with large doses of desmopressin acetate (up to 40 μg/4 h intranasally).

SYNDROME OF INAPPROPRIATE VASOPRESSIN SECRETION (SIADH)

A number of diseases are associated with a plasma vasopressin concentration that is inappropriately high for that plasma osmolality. Thus, water retention accompanies normal water intake, leading to hyponatremia and hypo-osmolality. The urine is usually more concentrated than plasma. Sodium balance is essentially normal. It is important to rule out renal and endocrine disorders and drug effects that diminish the kidney's capacity to dilute the urine. The syndrome is termed **syndrome of inappropriate secretion of vasopressin (antidiuretic hormone),** or **SIADH.** The clinical picture can be produced experimentally by giving high doses of vasopressin to a healthy subject receiving normal to high fluid intake. Water restriction in patients suspected of having SIADH will result in plasma osmolality and sodium concentration returning to normal.

Causes of SIADH

The causes of SIADH are outlined in Table 9–7. A number of malignant neoplasms are associated with ectopic production of vasopressin, leading to high plasma vasopressin levels. Bronchogenic carcinomas are particularly apt to be associated with SIADH. Tumors at other sites such as the pancreas and duodenum have also been shown to produce vasopressin. A number of nonmalignant pulmonary diseases such as tuberculosis are associated with high plasma vasopressin concentrations. Tuberculous lung tissue has been shown to contain assayable levels of vasopressin. However, it is not known whether all types of lung disease causing SIADH do so by producing ectopic vasopressin or by stimulation of pituitary vasopressin.

Many different types of central nervous system disorders are associated with increased vasopressin secretion, leading to the clinical picture of SIADH. Temporary causes of SIADH include surgical trauma, anesthesia, pain, and anxiety. A number of drugs implicated in vasopressin release are discussed in the section on diabetes insipidus. Endocrine disorders such as adrenal insufficiency, myxedema, and anterior pituitary insufficiency may be associated with SIADH secondary to hypovolemia and impaired renal excretion of free water. All of these factors—particularly with fluid loading—can lead to hyponatremia and hypo-osmolality.

Types of Osmoregulatory Defects

Serial measurements of serum arginine vasopressin in patients with SIADH were used by Robertson et al to describe 4 patterns of osmoregulatory defects in this syndrome. Type A, found in 20% of patients, is characterized by large irregular changes in plasma arginine vasopressin completely unrelated to serum osmolality.

Table 9–7. Conditions associated with SIADH.

Malignant lung disease, particularly bronchogenic carcinoma.
Nonmalignant lung disease, eg, tuberculosis.
Tumors at other sites (especially lymphoma, sarcoma), eg, duodenum, pancreas, brain, prostate, thymus.
Central nervous system trauma and infections.
Drugs that stimulate vasopressin release, eg, clofibrate, chlorpropamide, and other drugs such as thiazides, carbamazepine, phenothiazines, vincristine, cyclophosphamide.
Endocrine diseases: adrenal insufficiency, myxedema, anterior pituitary insufficiency.

This erratic and irregular secretion of arginine vasopressin can be associated with both malignant and nonmalignant disease. Type B is found in about 35% of patients and is associated with secretion of arginine vasopressin that is excessive but proportionate to osmolality. In these patients, the osmotic control of arginine vasopressin secretion appears to be either set at a low level or abnormally sensitive to changes in serum osmolality. Type C, found in 35% of patients, is characterized by a high basal level of arginine vasopressin that rises even higher with a rise in serum osmolality. Type D, found in only 10% of patients, represents a different type of problem. Arginine vasopressin is normally suppressed in hypovolemic states and rises normally with increase in osmolality. Thus, SIADH in these patients may be associated with a change in renal sensitivity to serum arginine vasopressin. Thus far, the pattern of arginine vasopressin abnormality cannot be correlated with the pathology of the syndrome.

Treatment

The treatment of SIADH depends upon the underlying cause. A patient with drug-induced SIADH is treated by withholding the drug. The treatment of SIADH in a patient with bronchogenic carcinoma is more complicated, however, and the prognosis is poor. Treatment aims to return plasma osmolality to normal without causing further expansion of the extracellular fluid compartment, as would occur following infusion of hyperosmotic solutions.

A. Fluid Restriction: The simplest form of treatment is fluid restriction, although in the long term the excessive thirst associated with this treatment may be difficult to manage.

B. Diuretics: If plasma osmolality is low and rapid correction is required, diuretics such as furosemide or ethacrynic acid can be employed. These agents prevent the concentration gradient in the medulla from building up and thus decrease the effectiveness of vasopressin. Because diuresis is accompanied by significant urinary losses of potassium, calcium, and magnesium, these electrolytes should be replaced by intravenous infusion.

C. Other Methods: In an emergency situation with severe hyponatremia, hypertonic saline, ie, 3% saline, administered intravenously at a rate of 0.1 mL/kg/min, will increase plasma sodium and osmolarity. However, this must be done with great caution, since fluid overload may precipitate heart failure, central pontine myelinolysis, or circulatory collapse. Drugs (mentioned earlier in this chapter) that reduce the effect of vasopressin on the kidney may be useful. Demeclocycline (Declomycin), 1–2 g/d orally, causes a reversible form of diabetes insipidus, countering the effect of SIADH. However, it is nephrotoxic, and renal function (blood urea nitrogen and creatinine) must be monitored carefully. Lithium carbonate has a similar effect, but therapeutic doses are so close to the toxic dose that this drug is rarely useful.

VASOPRESSIN ANTAGONISTS

Improved understanding of structure-activity relationships has made it possible to synthesize agonists and antagonists of neurohypophyseal peptides. Two groups of peptides have been synthesized that antagonize the V_1 and V_2 receptors. Further refinement of specific antagonists for specific receptors should lead to the development of powerful therapeutic tools.

OXYTOCIN

Oxytocin has a profound effect on uterine smooth muscle. It increases both the frequency and the duration of action potentials during each burst of firing. Thus, administration of oxytocin may initiate contractions in a quiescent uterus or increase the strength and frequency of muscle contractions in an active uterus. The presence of estrogen enhances the action of oxytocin on uterine smooth muscle. Estrogen acts by reducing the membrane potential of smooth muscle cells, thus lowering the threshold of excitation. Toward the end of pregnancy, as estrogen levels become higher, the membrane potential of uterine smooth muscle cells thus becomes less negative, rendering the uterus at full term more sensitive to oxytocin. The number of oxytocin receptors in the uterus also increases at this time. Activation of oxytocin receptors causes cellular calcium to be mobilized through polyphosphatidylinositol hydrolysis.

Female Reproductive System Actions

A. Parturition: Oxytocin is involved in the process of parturition. As the fetus enters the birth canal, the lower segment of the uterus, the cervix, and then the vagina are dilated. Dilatation of these regions causes reflex release of oxytocin into the bloodstream. Strong uterine contractions are initiated, causing further descent of the fetus, further distention, and further release of oxytocin. However, the precise role of oxytocin in the initiation of labor in humans is still not clear. Patients with diabetes insipidus caused by hypothalamic tumors—and thus a presumed absence of oxytocin secretion—may have normal deliveries, or there may be an increased incidence of forceps deliveries and cesarean sections. The complex neuroendocrine relationships involved in parturition are not yet fully understood.

B. Lactation: Oxytocin is also involved in lactation. Stimulation of the nipple area produces a neurohumoral reflex involving the secretion of oxytocin. Oxytocin causes contraction of the myoepithelial cells lining the mammary ducts and the ejection of milk contained within them. The milk ejection reflex is essential if the infant is to obtain adequate quantities of milk. The milk ejection reflex may also be conditioned by events related to the infant, such as crying or arrival of the scheduled feeding time. Stress has a potent inhibitory influence on the milk ejection reflex, an event that depends upon central inhibition of oxytocin release in the hypothalamus.

Other Actions

A number of stimuli that also release vasopressin—such as increased plasma osmolality and hypovolemia—cause oxytocin secretion. Since oxytocin is an effective natriuretic agent, particularly at low rates of urine flow, it may be involved in the regulation of sodium balance. This proposed role for oxytocin remains to be elucidated.

REFERENCES

Bartter FC, Schwartz WB: The syndrome of inappropriate secretion of antidiuretic hormone. *Am J Med* 1967;**42:**790.

Bie P: Osmoreceptors, vasopressin, and control of renal water excretion. *Physiol Rev* 1980;**60:**961.

Cross BA, Leng G (editors): The neurohypophysis: Structure, function and control. *Prog Brain Res* 1983;**60:**1. [Entire issue.]

Cowley AW, Liard JF, Ausiello DA: *Vasopressin.* Raven Press, 1988.

Land H et al: Deduced amino-acid sequence from the bovine oxytocin–neurophysin I precursor cDNA. *Nature* 1983;**302:**342.

Land H et al: Nucleotide sequence of cloned cDNA encoding bovine arginine vasopressin–neurophysin II precursor. *Nature* 1982;**295:**299.

Lauson HD: Metabolism of the neurohypophysial hormones. Section 7 in: *Handbook of Physiology.* Vol 4. American Physiological Society, 1974.

Miller M et al: Recognition of partial defects in antidiuretic hormone secretion. *Ann Intern Med* 1970;**73:**721.

Moses AM, Scheinman SJ, Oppenheim A: Marked hypotonic polyuria resulting from nephrogenic diabetes insipidus with partial sensitivity to vasopressin. *J Clin Endocrinol Metab* 1984;**59:**1044.

Robertson GL, Athar S, Shelton RL: Osmotic control of vasopressin function. In: *Disturbances in Body Fluid Osmolality.* Andreoli TE, Grantham JJ, Rector FC Jr (editors). American Physiological Society, 1977.

Robertson GL, Berl T: Pathophysiology of water metabolism. In: *The Kidney.* Brenner BM, Rector FC Jr (editors). Saunders, 1986.

Robinson AG: DDAVP in the treatment of central diabetes insipidus. *N Engl J Med* 1976;**294:**507.

Russell JT, Brownstein MJ, Gainer H: Biosynthesis of vasopressin, oxytocin, and neurophysins: Isolation and characterization of two common precursors (propressophysin and prooxyphysin). *Endocrinology* 1980;**107:**1880.

Schrier RW (editor): *Vasopressin.* Raven Press, 1985.

Schrier RW, Berl T, Anderson RJ: Osmotic and non-osmotic control of vasopressin release. *Am J Physiol* 1979;**236:**321.

Swanson LW, Sawchenko PE: Hypothalamic integration: Organization of the paraventricular and supraoptic nuclei. *Annu Rev Neurosci* 1983;**6:**269.

Thrasher TN, Keil LC, Ramsay DJ: Lesions of the organum vasculosum of the lamina terminalis (OVLT) attenuate osmotically-induced drinking and vasopressin secretion in the dog. *Endocrinology* 1982;**110:**1837.

Thrasher TN et al: Satiety and inhibition of vasopressin secretion in dehydrated dogs. *Am J Physiol* 1981;**240:**394.

Thrasher TN et al: Thirst and vasopressin release in the dog: An osmoreceptor or sodium receptor mechanism? *Am J Physiol* 1980;**238:**333.

Verney EB: The antidiuretic hormone and the factors which determine its release. *Proc R Soc Lond* 1947;**135:**25.

Vokes TJ, Robertson GL: Disorders of antidiuretic hormone. *Endocrinol Metab Clin North Am* 1988;**17:**28.

Zerbe RL, Robertson GL: A comparison of plasma vasopressin measurements with a standard indirect test in the differential diagnosis of polyuria. *N Engl J Med* 1981;**305:**1539.

10

Thyroid Gland

Francis S. Greenspan, MD, & Basil Rapoport, MB, ChB

Thyroid hormones (thyroxine, T_4; triiodothyronine, T_3) (Fig 10–1) play a vital role in fetal development, and throughout life they influence metabolic processes in almost all tissues. The thyroid gland is the only significant source of T_4. While the gland does produce some T_3, which is biologically more active than T_4, most T_3 in humans is produced extrathyroidally from T_4.

The thyroid gland is unique among the endocrine organs in 2 important ways: (1) It maintains a large store of hormone, and (2) it requires iodide for hormone synthesis.

ANATOMY OF THE THYROID

Gross Anatomy

The thyroid consists of a left and right lobe connected (in humans) by an isthmus at the approximate level of the cricoid cartilage (Fig 10–2). The adult thyroid weighs 15–20 g, and assessment of its size is important in clinical evaluation of thyroid function. The thyroid is derived from the embryonic thyroglossal duct, which is a midline invagination at the junction of the anterior two-thirds and posterior one-third of the tongue. A remnant of the thyroglossal duct may be observed as a pyramidal thyroid lobe, inserting into the isthmus or into the medial aspect of one of the lobes.

In palpating the thyroid gland, it is important to note the following: (1) The thyroid lobes are largely covered by the sternohyoid and sternothyroid muscles. Enlargement of the thyroid is limited superiorly by the sternothyroid attachment to the thyroid cartilage, but the thyroid gland, when enlarged, can extend superolaterally beneath the sternocleidomastoid. (2) The thyroid moves upward with the larynx on swallowing. (3) The cricoid cartilage is a landmark for the isthmus. (4) Pyramidal lobe enlargement is a good indication of diffuse rather than local abnormality of the thyroid.

Histology

The basic functional unit of the thyroid is the follicle, a hollow sphere of cells, 15–500 μm in diameter,

Acronyms Used in This Chapter

ATP	Adenosine triphosphate
BMR	Basal metabolic rate
cAMP	Cyclic adenosine monophosphate
cDNA	Complementary deoxyribonucleic acid
CPK	Creatine phosphokinase
DIHPPA	Diiodohydroxyphenylpyruvic acid
DIT	Diiodotyrosine
FSH	Follicle-stimulating hormone
hCG	Human chorionic gonadotropin
HLA	Human leukocyte antigen
LATS	Long-acting thyroid stimulator
LDH	Lactate dehydrogenase
LH	Luteinizing hormone
MIT	Monoiodotyrosine
MRI	Magnetic resonance imaging
mRNA	Messenger ribonucleic acid
PBI	Protein-bound iodine
PTH	Parathyroid hormone
RAIU	Radioactive iodine uptake
RIA	Radioimmunoassay
TBG	Thyroid hormone–binding globulin
TBI	TSH binding inhibition
TBPA	Thyroxine-binding prealbumin
TDA	TSH displacement assay
TETRAC	Tetraiodothyroacetic acid
TRH	Thyrotropin-releasing hormone
TRIAC	Triiodothyroacetic acid
TSH	Thyroid-stimulating hormone (thyrotropin)
TSI	Thyroid-stimulating immunoglobulin

surrounded by a basement membrane. The wall of the follicle is a single layer of thyroid cells. A few adjacent parafollicular cells (C cells) are larger, clearer on staining, and secrete calcitonin (Fig 10–3A). The follicular cells are cuboidal when quiescent and columnar when active (Figs 10–3B and 10–3C). The follicular lumen contains colloid, a viscous gel that is primarily a store of thyroglobulin secreted by the thyroid cells. This store is sufficient for about 100 days of normal thyroid hormone secretion. The follicles are surrounded by a rich capillary network. Blood flow through the thyroid is very high (about 5 mL/g/min) and may be audible with a stethoscope (bruit) when the thyroid is overactive and flow is increased. Networks of sympathetic and parasympathetic nerves also surround the follicles. Their significance is unclear, however, and they do not appear to play a major role in the regulation of thyroid hormone synthesis and secretion.

PHYSIOLOGY OF THE THYROID

IODIDE METABOLISM

Adequate ingestion of iodide is a prerequisite for the normal synthesis of thyroid hormones by the thyroid. While the dietary intake of iodide may vary widely, thyroidal secretion of iodine in the form of thyroid hormones is relatively stable. The homeostatic mechanisms at play will be discussed below. The major sources of dietary iodide are water, iodated bread, iodinated salt, and, increasingly, medications, disinfectants, and x-ray contrast material. In addition, kelp, available in health food stores, is being ingested with increasing frequency in the USA.

A typical daily dietary intake of iodide in the USA is now about 500 μg. Iodide is almost completely absorbed in the gastrointestinal tract, where it enters the inorganic iodide pool in the extracellular fluid (Fig 10–4). In the presence of normal renal function, inorganic iodide in the extracellular fluid is rapidly cleared, with

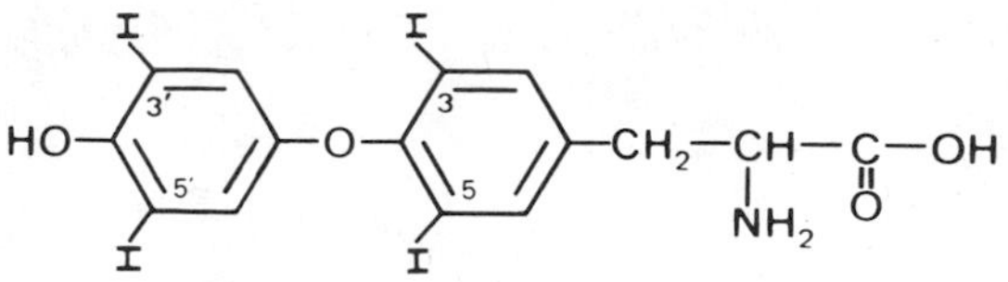

$3,5,3',5'$-Tetraiodothyronine
(thyroxine, T_4)

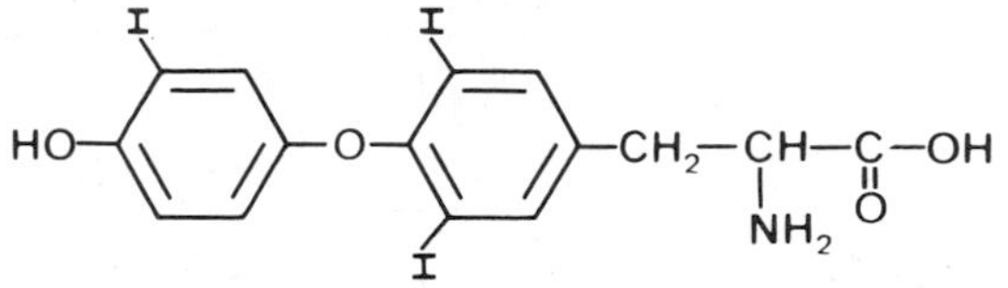

$3,5,3'$-Triiodothyronine (T_3)

Figure 10–1. Chemical structures of thyroxine (T_4) and triiodothyronine (T_3).

a half-life of about 2 hours. Besides dietary iodide, there are 2 other smaller sources contributing to the extracellular fluid iodide pool: (1) iodide released by the deiodination of thyroid hormones in the peripheral tissues (about 60 μg/d) and (2) the release ("leak") of inorganic iodide by the thyroid (about 10–50 μg/d).

The only 2 significant pathways of iodide clearance from the extracellular fluid are the kidneys and the thyroid. Since the thyroid is able to regulate the net amount of iodide it clears from the extracellular fluid (see below), taking up only as much as is needed

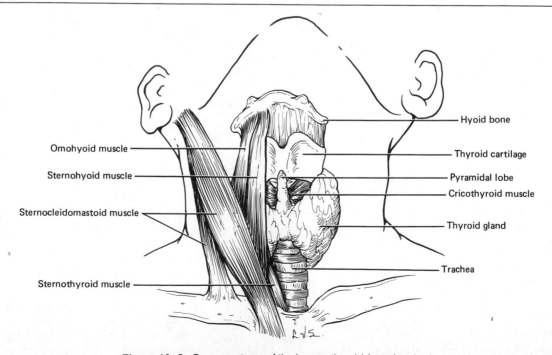

Figure 10–2. Gross anatomy of the human thyroid (anterior view).

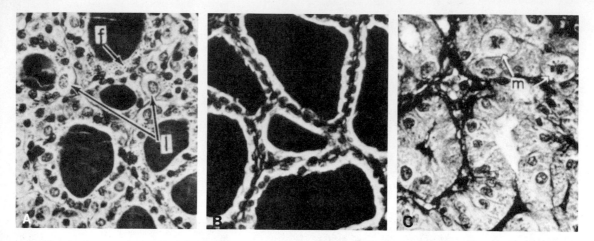

Figure 10–3. *A:* Normal rat thyroid. A single layer of cuboidal epithelial cells surrounds PAS-positive material in the follicular space (colloid). The larger, lighter-staining cells indicated by the arrows (l) are C cells that produce calcitonin. F = follicular cells. *B:* Inactive rat thyroid several weeks after hypophysectomy. The follicular lumens are larger and the follicular cells flatter. *C:* Rat thyroid under intensive TSH stimulation. The animal was fed an iodine-deficient diet and injected with propylthiouracil for several weeks. Little colloid is visible. The follicular cells are tall and columnar. Several mitoses (m) are visible. (Reproduced, with permission, from Halmi NS in: *Histology.* Greep RO, Weiss L [editors]. McGraw-Hill, 1973.)

(about 75 μg/d) for thyroid hormone synthesis, it follows that when the dietary intake of iodide increases, the fractional uptake of extracellular fluid iodide by the thyroid decreases and the proportionate urinary excretion of iodide increases. Conversely, when iodide intake is reduced, the proportionate uptake of extracellular fluid iodide by the thyroid is increased. This is clinically important, because the percentage uptake of radioactive iodide by the thyroid is a useful index of thyroid function (Fig 10–5). In the USA, particularly since the iodation of bread, the radioactive iodide uptake (RAIU) by the thyroid gland in normal subjects has decreased from about 20–50% of the ingested dose at 24 hours to about 5–25%. RAIU is generally higher

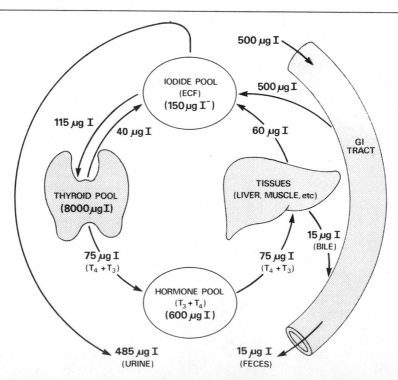

Figure 10–4. Iodine metabolism. The values indicated are representative of those that might be found in a healthy subject ingesting 500 μg of iodine a day. The actual iodine intake varies considerably among different individuals.

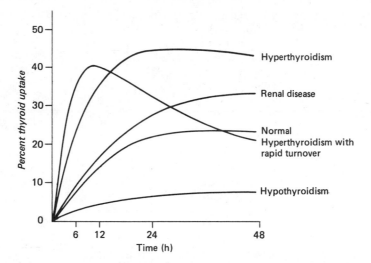

Figure 10–5. Typical radioactive iodine uptake (RAIU) curves over 48 hours in patients with normal and abnormal thyroid function. (Reproduced, with permission, from DeGroot LJ, Stanbury JB: *The Thyroid and Its Diseases.* Wiley, 1975.)

in hyperthyroidism and lower in hypothyroidism, although there are exceptions. Measurement of urinary iodide excretion may be useful clinically if it is suspected that the patient has ingested excess iodide.

The largest iodine pool in the body is the slowly turning over thyroid pool (approximately 1% per day; faster in hyperthyroidism). This pool is almost entirely organic iodine in the form of iodinated thyroglobulin stored as colloid within the thyroid follicular lumen.

The thyroid secretes about 75 μg of organic iodine per day in the form of thyroid hormones (chiefly T_4, with a small amount of T_3). Secreted thyroid hormones enter a pool of thyroid hormones, mainly intravascular, bound to thyroid hormone–binding proteins. The iodine content of this hormonal pool is about 600μg. Cellular uptake of thyroid hormones from this pool is approximately 75 μg of iodine per day in the euthyroid individual. Of this 75 μg of thyroid hormone iodine, about 60 μg reenters the extracellular fluid iodide pool following intracellular enzymatic deiodination of the thyroid hormones. The remainder (15 μg) is conjugated in the liver to the glucuronide and sulfate forms and excreted in the bile and subsequently in the stool. In humans, there is very little enterohepatic recirculation of thyroid hormone.

THYROID HORMONE SYNTHESIS

Thyroglobulin

Thyroglobulin, the precursor of all thyroid hormones, is a very large glycoprotein molecule that is the major protein in the follicular luminal colloid. About 75% of the weight of the entire thyroid gland consists of this protein, though the proportion varies widely depending on the physiologic demands on the gland (Figs 10–3B and 10–3C).

Thyroglobulin is a heterogeneous substance that ex-

ists in multiple forms. The most prevalent form and the major precursor for thyroid hormones is a 19S molecule with a molecular weight of 660,000. Ultracentrifugation of thyroglobulin also reveals a small fraction with a sedimentation coefficient of 27S, believed to be a dimer of 19S thyroglobulin. The 19S molecule can in turn dissociate into two 12S components, particularly when the thyroglobulin is poorly iodinated. Studies of the translation of thyroglobulin messenger RNA (mRNA) and the sequencing of this mRNA from a complementary DNA (cDNA) library show that thyroglobulin is synthesized as the 12S subunit.

Human thyroglobulin contains approximately 110 tyrosine residues. These residues are iodinated and ultimately form the thyroid hormones. The relative number of tyrosines in thyroglobulin is not higher than in many other proteins. The propensity of thyroglobulin for iodination is determined instead by its proximity to a very efficient iodination mechanism in the thyroid cell as well as by its tertiary structure, which facilitates iodination. Only a small proportion of the tyrosine residues in thyroglobulin—those that are closest to the surface of the globular molecule—are available for iodination. In geographic areas of iodine sufficiency, a thyroglobulin molecule will contain an average of about 7 molecules of monoiodotyrosine (MIT) and 5 of diiodotyrosine (DIT). In addition, an average of 2 molecules of T_4 will be present, each representing the coupling of 2 molecules of DIT. On average, every third molecule of thyroglobulin will contain one molecule of T_3, formed by the coupling of one DIT with one MIT.

The degree of thyroglobulin iodination varies depending upon the availability of iodide and the efficiency of the iodinating mechanism (see below). Poorly iodinated thyroglobulin contains a relatively high MIT/DIT ratio, which in turn favors increased T_3

synthesis relative to T_4. This is presumably of adaptive significance in that during periods of iodide insufficiency, available iodide is utilized more efficiently by synthesizing a more active hormone. In addition, there is evidence that decreased thyroglobulin iodine content produces a more loosely folded molecule that is more susceptible to proteolysis within the thyroid and will therefore also lead to greater efficiency in the generation of biologically active thyroid hormones.

The mechanism of synthesis of thyroglobulin (Fig 10–6) is the same as that of other glycoproteins (see Chapter 1, Fig 1–4). After transcription and processing of thyroglobulin mRNA has taken place, the mRNA is translated by ribosomes in the rough endoplasmic reticulum. The thyroglobulin polypeptide chain is extruded into the lumen of the endoplasmic reticulum. During transport to the Golgi apparatus, thyroglobulin is progressively glycosylated. The molecules are packaged into exocytotic vesicles in the Golgi apparatus. These vesicles fuse with the plasma membrane at the apical border of the follicular cell and release their contents into the follicular lumen. The membrane incorporated into the plasma membrane by this process is believed to recycle by the formation of endocytotic vesicles during the process of hormone secretion (see below).

The exact site of thyroglobulin iodination is not established with certainty, but evidence suggests that iodination occurs at the apical (follicular) surface of the thyroid cell. This is based on (1) the autoradiographic localization of radioiodinated thy-

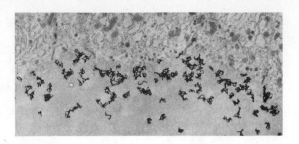

Figure 10–7. Evidence that iodination of thyroglobulin occurs at or near the apical (follicular) border of the thyroid cell. The figure depicts electron-microscopic autoradiography of part of a rat thyroid cell 30–40 seconds after the administration of sodium ^{125}I to the animal in vivo. The radioactive iodine is represented on a photographic emulsion layer by the silver grains. Few radioactive iodine molecules are localized over the thyroid cell itself, but there are many at the junction of the thyroid cell and the follicular colloid. (× 7000.) (Reproduced, with permission, from Ekholm R: *Endocrinology*. DeGroot LJ et al [editors]. Grune & Stratton, 1979.)

roglobulin a few seconds after exposure of the thyroid to radioactive iodine (Fig 10–7), (2) the demonstration of the enzyme necessary for thyroglobulin iodination at the site by histochemical means, and (3) the indication by molecular cloning of thyroid peroxidase that the protein has a transmembrane domain consistent with its being a cell surface enzyme.

The process of thyroglobulin biosynthesis and exocytosis into the follicular lumen is believed to be under the dominant control of TSH. TSH stimulates both the transcriptional and translational processes, resulting in increased thyroglobulin and thyroid peroxidase synthesis. TSH also rapidly stimulates the exocytosis (extrusion into the follicular lumen) of preformed thyroglobulin.

Thyroglobulin is not the only protein that may be iodinated within the thyroid gland, and other proteins such as albumin may occasionally be iodinated. This, however, occurs to a significant degree only in the abnormal thyroid gland. Because other molecules lack the unique tertiary structure of thyroglobulin necessary for the efficient coupling of iodotyrosines, their iodination does not lead to adequate biologically active thyroid hormone synthesis. Excess iodoalbumin production may be detected by a disproportionately high organic iodine concentration in serum relative to the amount of thyroid hormone present.

Iodide Transport

Iodide is actively transported ("trapped") from the extracellular fluid into the thyroid follicular cell (Fig 10–8). Once within the cell, inorganic iodide may either be incorporated into protein ("organified") or diffuse back into the extracellular fluid. At equilibrium, the inorganic iodide concentration ratio between the thyroid cell and the serum (T:S iodide gradient) repre-

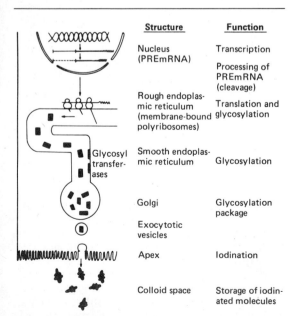

Structure	Function
Nucleus (PREmRNA)	Transcription
	Processing of PREmRNA (cleavage)
Rough endoplasmic reticulum (membrane-bound polyribosomes)	Translation and glycosylation
Smooth endoplasmic reticulum	Glycosylation
Golgi	Glycosylation package
Exocytotic vesicles	
Apex	Iodination
Colloid space	Storage of iodinated molecules

Glycosyl transferases

Figure 10–6. Synthesis of thyroglobulin. See text for details. (Reproduced, with permission, from Dumont J, Vassart G: *Endocrinology*. DeGroot LJ et al [editors]. Grune & Stratton, 1979.)

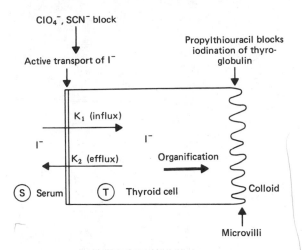

Figure 10–8. The iodide transport mechanism in the thyroid cell. K_1 is the rate constant for iodide being transported from the serum into the thyroid cell and K_2 the diffusion of inorganic iodide from the thyroid cell back into the serum. The iodide transport mechanism involves only inorganic iodide (I^-). $SCN^- $ = thiocyanate; ClO_4^- = perchlorate.

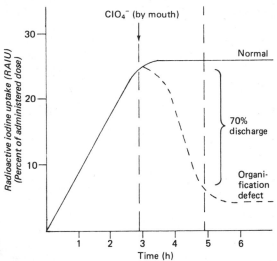

Figure 10–9. Perchlorate discharge of thyroidal inorganic iodine. Two to 3 hours after administration of a tracer dose of radioactive iodide, perchlorate is administered orally, blocking further active transport of iodide into the thyroid cell. In the normal subject (solid line), no significant decrease in radioactivity is detectable over the thyroid gland. In the representative example shown by the dashed line, there is a significant discharge of thyroidal iodide, indicating that iodide organification has been incomplete. ClO_4^- = perchlorate.

sents the balance between iodide influx and efflux. It is important to realize that organic iodine, such as iodinated thyroglobulin, does not contribute to this iodide gradient. In the normal thyroid gland, inorganic iodide is organified almost immediately upon entering the cell, so that a high T:S inorganic iodide gradient is not detectable. However, if iodide organification is blocked (see below), a T:S iodide ratio as high as 500:1 has been observed in the mouse thyroid in vitro.

Other structurally related anions such as SCN^-, BF_4^-, NO_3^-, and ClO_4^- competitively inhibit iodide transport. The latter (perchlorate) is used clinically on occasion to evaluate the iodide organification mechanism (Fig 10–9). If the thyroidal iodide organification mechanism is inefficient, inorganic iodide transported into the cell will accumulate. Perchlorate given a few hours after administration of a tracer amount of radioiodide blocks further iodide influx, but passive diffusion of inorganic iodide from the cell back into the extracellular fluid continues. Patients with faulty organification mechanisms have an abnormal "discharge" of radioactivity from the thyroid as it is released back into the extracellular fluid. This is detected by a decrease in radioactivity in the neck. The normal thyroid discharges little of the administered radioiodide with ClO_4^-, because it is readily organified and no longer able to leak out into the serum.

Tissues other than the thyroid also have an active transport mechanism for iodide. These include gastric mucosa, salivary glands, and the choroid plexus. However, unlike the thyroid, these tissues have a minimal capacity for iodide organification and storage of organic iodine. The active process of I^- concentration against an electrochemical gradient is energy-dependent, requiring oxidative metabolism. Because cardiac glycosides inhibit thyroidal I^- transport, there is much interest in the possible role of Na^+-K^+ ATPase activity in the iodide transport mechanism. Sodium increases I^- influx and inhibits I^- efflux. However, the exact relationship between this enzyme, sodium transport, and the iodide transport mechanism is presently unclear.

Iodide Organification
(Fig 10–10)

Once within the thyroid cell, inorganic iodide is rapidly oxidized by thyroid peroxidase in the presence of H_2O_2 into a reactive intermediate that is then incorporated into the tyrosine residues of acceptor proteins, mainly thyroglobulin. Thyroid peroxidase is a membrane-bound hemoprotein that is relatively unstable and difficult to purify. Molecular cloning studies indicate that human thyroid peroxidase contains 933 amino acids. In its glycosylated form, its molecular weight is 107,000. Concurrent molecular cloning of the thyroid microsomal antigen (see below) indicates that this antigen is, at least in part, thyroid peroxidase. The exact nature of the reactive oxidized iodide intermediate that binds to acceptor proteins is unknown. Although I_2 (iodine) has been considered,

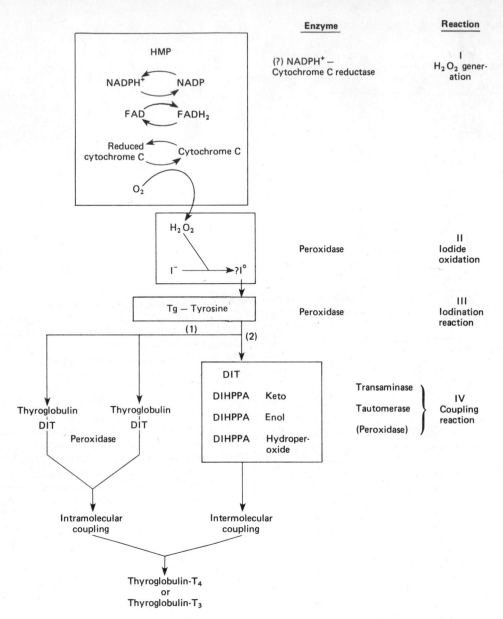

	Enzyme	Reaction
	(?) NADPH$^+$ – Cytochrome C reductase	I H$_2$O$_2$ generation
	Peroxidase	II Iodide oxidation
	Peroxidase	III Iodination reaction
	Transaminase Tautomerase (Peroxidase)	IV Coupling reaction

Figure 10–10. Present concepts of thyroglobulin iodination. See text for details. HMP = hexose monophosphate pathway; NADP = nicotinamide adenine dinucleotide phosphate; NADPH$^+$ = reduced form of NADP; FAD = flavin adenine dinucleotide; FADH$_2$ = reduced form of FAD; I$^-$ = iodide; I° = iodine free radical; Tg = thyroglobulin; DIT = diiodotyrosine; DIHPPA = diiodohydroxyphenylpyruvic acid. (Slightly modified and reproduced, with permission, from Rapoport B, DeGroot LJ: *Semin Nucl Med* 1971;1:265.)

more acceptable alternatives include a sulfenyl iodide or possibly the I° free radical.

The exact mechanism of thyroid H$_2$O$_2$ generation is also unknown, but it is probably dependent on reduced pyridine nucleotide oxidation. NADPH–cytochrome C reductase is believed to be involved in thyroidal H$_2$O$_2$ production in that a specific antibody against this enzyme is able to inhibit thyroglobulin iodination in

vitro by a thyroid particulate (microsomal) preparation.

As mentioned previously, the site of thyroglobulin iodination is most likely to be apical plasma membrane. Still being investigated, however, are the role of the thyroid peroxidase–like material that is demonstrable histochemically within the interior of the thyroid cell (such as in the Golgi apparatus) and the possible role in iodide organification of multiple pools of intracellular iodide differing in their rates of turnover.

Iodotyrosine Coupling

Iodinated tyrosine residues in thyroglobulin combine to form iodothyronines. Thus, DIT couples with DIT to form thyroxine and MIT with DIT to form triiodothyronine. The exact mechanism by which this coupling reaction occurs is unknown. Two theories currently exist (Fig 10–10): intramolecular coupling and intermolecular coupling. In the former, 2 peptide-linked DIT molecules couple while still part of the thyroglobulin polypeptide chain—a process that may involve generation of free radicals of DIT. In intermolecular coupling, there is evidence that DIT is liberated from thyroglobulin and in turn converted into its pyruvic acid analogue diiodohydroxyphenylpyruvic acid (DIHPPA) by tyrosine transaminase. After conversion to its enol form and subsequent oxidation by H_2O_2 and thyroid peroxidase to the DIHPPA hydroperoxide, this intermediate then couples with DIT present within the thyroglobulin molecule to form thyroxine. While this issue remains unsettled, it is clear that thyroid peroxidase plays an important role in the coupling process as well as in initial iodotyrosine formation. Thyroid peroxidase therefore catalyzes all steps in the synthesis of iodothyronines. DIT may itself have a stimulatory effect on iodotyrosine coupling, but the mechanism by which this occurs is poorly understood.

A defect in the coupling mechanism results in diminished T_4 and T_3 formation from DIT and MIT. This may be related to inadequate concentrations of precursor iodotyrosines or to a defect in the enzymes responsible for coupling. As an example of the first possibility, in iodine deficiency, poorly iodinated thyroglobulin contains fewer iodotyrosine molecules overall and more MIT relative to DIT. There may therefore be insufficient DIT residues to permit adequate T_4 formation. As a corollary, there is a proportionate increase in T_3 production relative to T_4. This may represent an adaptive mechanism to environmental iodine deficiency in that T_3 is biologically more potent than T_4. While thyroid peroxidase is important in the coupling mechanism, it is not clearly established whether a deficiency in this enzyme or some abnormality in its action is responsible for the apparent cou-

pling defect very rarely observed in the human thyroid. The difficulty in determining this is that decreased thyroid peroxidase activity also leads to decreased thyroglobulin iodination, with less MIT and DIT available for coupling.

A number of related drugs are used clinically to treat hyperthyroidism by decreasing thyroid hormone synthesis (Fig 10–11). The thionamide drugs, including methimazole and propylthiouracil, inhibit thyroid peroxidase-catalyzed iodination of thyroglobulin. These drugs may also specifically inhibit the iodotyrosine coupling reaction independently of inhibition of iodotyrosine generation. Propylthiouracil, unlike methimazole, inhibits iodotyrosine coupling in vitro.

THYROID HORMONE SECRETION

Thyroglobulin is stored extracellularly in the follicular lumen. Therefore, as a prerequisite for thyroid hormone secretion into the blood, thyroglobulin must first reenter the thyroid cell and undergo proteolysis. A small quantity of intact thyroglobulin enters the circulation, some by way of the lymphatics. This leakage can be increased when the thyroid cells are damaged, such as occurs in thyroiditis, hyperthyroidism, or papillary or follicular thyroid carcinoma.

Autoradiographic studies show that newly iodinated thyroglobulin is stored adjacent to the epithelial border. Continuing synthesis may produce concentric lamellae of colloid with older thyroglobulin in the center. It follows, therefore, that the most recently iodinated thyroglobulin may be the first to be secreted. This has been called the "last come, first served" principle. Not all follicles in the thyroid are of the same size, and their thyroglobulin turnover rates vary considerably. The smaller follicles turn over their contents at a faster rate. Processing of thyroglobulin by the thyroid cell and secretion of the thyroid hormones into the circulation occur in the following sequence (Fig 10–12): (1) Pseudopods from the apical cell surface extend into the colloid in the follicular lumen, and large colloid droplets enter the cytoplasm by endocytosis. Each colloid droplet is enclosed in membrane derived from the apical cell border. Endocytosis of the colloid is dependent on the addition of membrane to

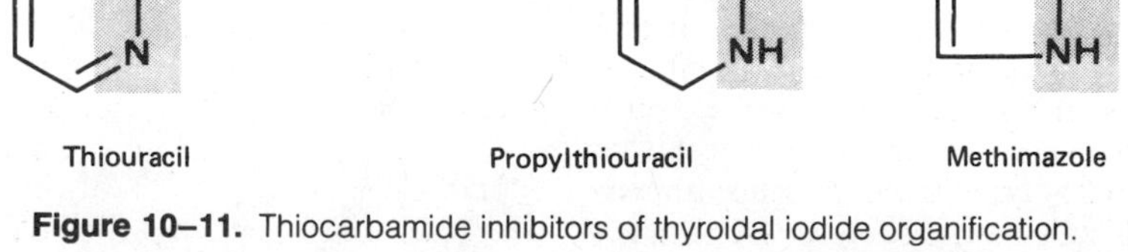

Thiouracil   Propylthiouracil   Methimazole

Figure 10–11. Thiocarbamide inhibitors of thyroidal iodide organification.

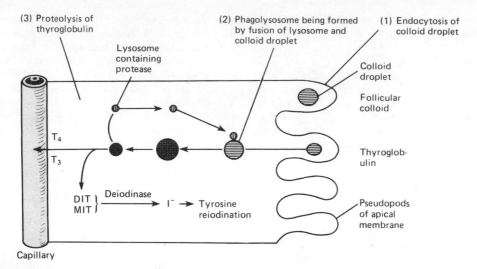

Figure 10–12. Schematic representation of thyroid hormone secretion. See text for details. (Slightly modified and reproduced, with permission, from Rapoport B, DeGroot LJ: *Semin Nucl Med* 1971;**1**:265.)

the apical surface of the cell that occurs during exocytosis of thyroglobulin—ie, there is membrane recycling. (2) Electron-dense lysosomes migrate apically, meet the incoming colloid droplets, and fuse with them to produce phagolysosomes. The phagolysosomes continue their migration toward the basal aspect of the cell, during which time they become smaller and more dense as the lysosomal proteases hydrolyze the thyroglobulin. (3) T_4 and, to a much lesser degree, T_3, liberated from thyroglobulin by the proteolytic process, pass from the phagolysosome into the blood by a mechanism that is presently unknown, possibly diffusion. Most of the liberated iodotyrosines (MIT and DIT) are deiodinated by iodotyrosine deiodinase, releasing free iodide. This iodide is partly reutilized for thyroglobulin iodination, but some diffuses out into the circulation (iodide leak).

Microtubules and microfilaments may play an important role in these steps, presumably by regulating organelle movement. Thus, colchicine and cytochalasin B, which disrupt microtubular and microfilament function, respectively, inhibit thyroid hormone secretion.

Pharmacologic doses of iodide acutely reduce thyroid hormone secretion by an unknown mechanism, possibly by inhibiting thyroid cAMP generation. This slight effect on hormone secretion is clinically insignificant in the normal thyroid. In the hyperfunctioning thyroid, however, iodide has a marked inhibitory effect on hormone secretion that is clinically useful. Continued iodide administration usually inhibits thyroid hormone secretion for only a few weeks. The reason for the escape from this inhibitory effect is not known (and must not be confused with escape from the Wolff-Chaikoff block, discussed below). Lithium acts in a manner similar to iodide; this may explain the adverse effects of lithium on the thyroid (hypothyroidism and goiter) when it is used as a psychotherapeutic drug.

In addition to the iodotyrosines, which are rapidly deiodinated by NADPH-dependent flavoprotein deiodinase within the thyroid, some T_4 released from thyroglobulin may also undergo intrathyroidal monodeiodination to T_3. The quantitative significance of this source of T_3 is uncertain. In the normally functioning thyroid gland, however, the secretion of T_3 (whether synthesized de novo or derived from T_4) is relatively small (see below). The deiodination of iodotyrosines and the reutilization of this iodide are very important in the efficient utilization of iodide by the thyroid. This is because perhaps 80% of the iodide in thyroglobulin is in the form of iodotyrosines, which, once secreted into the blood, are rapidly lost in the urine. There is evidence that intrathyroidal iodide released from iodotyrosines exists in a pool separate from iodide entering the thyroid cell directly from the extracellular fluid.

REGULATION OF THYROID FUNCTION

Thyroid hormone synthesis and secretion are regulated by extrathyroidal (thyrotropin) and intrathyroidal (autoregulatory) mechanisms. Although thyrotropin (TSH) is the major modulator of thyroid activity, the importance of autoregulation is receiving increasing recognition.

TSH

TSH is a glycoprotein (MW 28,000; 15% carbohydrate) secreted by specialized cells (thyrotrophs) in the

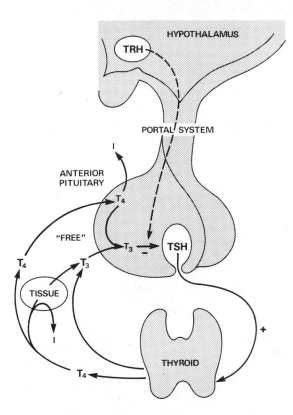

Figure 10–13. The hypothalamic-hypophyseal-thyroid axis. TRH produced in the hypothalamus reaches the thyrotrophs in the anterior pituitary by the hypothalamic-hypophyseal portal system and enhances secretion of TSH by altering the set point of T_3 inhibition of TSH secretion. In the pituitary, it is primarily T_3 that inhibits TSH secretion. T_4 undergoes monodeiodination to T_3 both in the peripheral tissues and in the pituitary itself.

anterior pituitary. TSH consists of 2 polypeptide chains. The alpha chain is nearly identical to the alpha chains of LH, FSH, and chorionic gonadotropin (hCG). TSH specificity is determined by the uniquely different beta chain, which is critical for recognition of the TSH receptor. TSH biologic activity is present only when the 2 chains are combined. The half-life of TSH in plasma is very short (about an hour).

TSH secretion by the pituitary is modulated by thyroid hormone in a negative feedback regulatory mechanism (Fig 10–13). At the pituitary, it is primarily T_3, produced locally by the monodeiodination of T_4, that inhibits TSH secretion. T_3 also inhibits the transcriptional activity of the TSH subunit genes. The pituitary is therefore the only site where monodeiodination of T_4 to T_3 is a prerequisite for the expression of T_4 metabolic activity. Thyroid hormones reduce TRH mRNA levels in the hypothalamus, suggesting that T_3 acts both on the pituitary and the hypothalamus. In hypothyroidism, there is decreased suppression of TSH secretion, and serum TSH levels are higher than normal.

The measurement by radioimmunoassay of high TSH levels in serum is very important clinically in the diagnosis of primary thyroid failure.

The "thermostat" setting of the thyroid hormone–TSH feedback loop is modulated by a tripeptide, TSH-releasing hormone (TRH) (Fig 10–14). This factor is present throughout the brain and indeed in other organs, but it is present at highest concentration in the hypothalamus. Hypothalamic production and release of TRH are controlled by poorly understood neural pathways from higher brain centers (see Chapter 5). TRH reaches the anterior pituitary from the hypothalamus via the hypothalamic-hypophyseal portal system. After binding to specific receptors on the thyrotroph, TRH increases TSH synthesis and secretion.

Current evidence suggests that TRH stimulates TSH release via the phosphatidylinositol pathway by stimulating the release of intracellular calcium and so a burst of TSH. TSH is secreted in pulses with an amplitude of about 0.6 μU/mL and a frequency of about 6 per 24 hours. In addition, TSH secretion is affected by circadian rhythm; it peaks at 1–2 μU/mL between 10 PM and 2 AM. This cyclic secretion is related to neither the cyclic secretion of ACTH nor sleep. The hypothalamus probably controls both the cyclic and pulsatile secretion of TSH. T_3, T_4, dexamethasone, dopamine, and its agonist bromocriptine all inhibit both the cyclic and pulsatile secretion of TSH. As noted above, T_3 inhibits transcription of TRH mRNA; the mechanism of inhibition by dopamine or dexamethasone is still uncertain. Since TRH is widely distributed throughout the nervous system, and since some studies have shown an association between TRH administration and mood elevation, this tripeptide may act as a neurotransmitter in addition to regulating TSH secretion.

The acute injection of a bolus of synthetic TRH (200–500 μg) rapidly increases TSH secretion (Fig 10–15). This response is of clinical value, particularly in the diagnosis of thyrotoxicosis. In this situation, despite TRH stimulation, TSH secretion remains suppressed by the high (even minimally elevated) thyroid hormone levels (Fig 10–15). However, other influences such as glucocorticoids and starvation may also reduce the TSH response to TRH stimulation. TRH

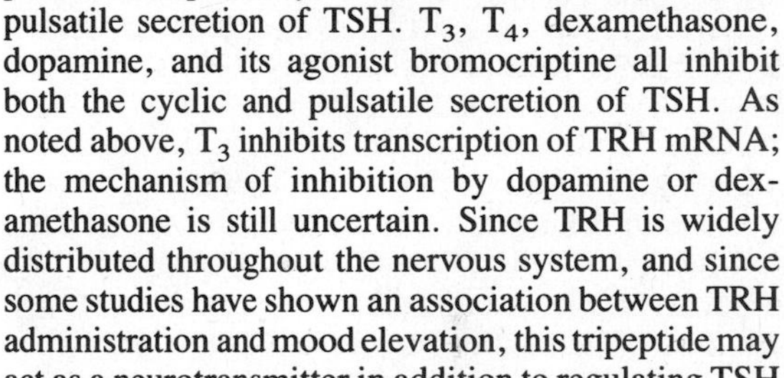

(pyro)Glu-His-Pro-(NH$_2$)

Figure 10–14. Chemical structure of thyrotropin-releasing hormone (TRH).

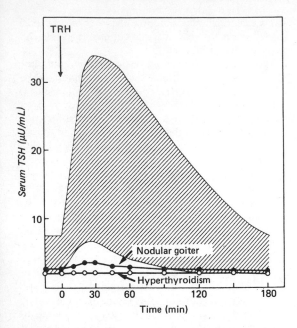

Figure 10–15. Typical serum TSH responses to TRH in patients with hyperthyroidism or toxic nodular goiter. The hatched area indicates normal range. (Reproduced, with permission, from Utiger RD: *The Thyroid,* 4th ed. Werner SC, Ingbar SH [editors]. Harper & Row, 1978.)

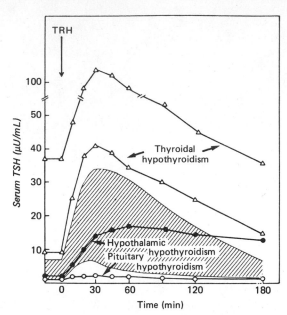

Figure 10–16. Typical serum TSH responses to TRH in patients with thyroid (primary), pituitary (secondary), and hypothalamic (tertiary) hypothyroidism. The hatched area indicates the normal range. (Reproduced, with permission, from Utiger RD: *The Thyroid,* 4th ed. Werner SC, Ingbar SH [editors]. Harper & Row, 1978.)

stimulation is also valuable in the diagnosis of the very rare condition known as tertiary (hypothalamic) hypothyroidism, which is distinguished from secondary (pituitary) hypothyroidism by the presence of a TSH response to TRH in the former but not in the latter (Fig 10–16). The TRH test is of little clinical value in primary (thyroidal) hypothyroidism, where the high serum TSH level even before TRH injection is diagnostic and the exaggerated TSH response provides little additional information (Fig 10–16).

Acute injection of TRH also stimulates prolactin release by the pituitary, but it is not clear whether this is physiologically important. In some patients with hypothyroidism, however, serum prolactin levels may be elevated. Dopaminergic stimuli such as levodopa reduce both the prolactin and TSH response to TRH stimulation. In addition, levodopa acutely depresses the elevated TSH levels in primary hypothyroidism. It is unlikely, however, that TRH is the sole releasing factor for both TSH and prolactin, because their secretion may be dissociated under certain circumstances. For example, the nocturnal elevation in prolactin and the acute prolactin response to suckling are not associated with changes in TSH secretion.

Actions of TSH on the Thyroid

TSH has many effects on the thyroid, the net result of which is increased thyroid hormone secretion.

(1) Most TSH actions are produced by binding to specific thyroid plasma membrane receptors with the subsequent stimulation of adenylate cyclase activity and cAMP generation.

(2) TSH affects the iodide transport mechanism in a biphasic manner. There is an initial acute (4-hour) decrease in the iodide thyroid:serum (T:S) ratio. This effect is also produced in vitro by cAMP and reflects an increased rate of I^- efflux. After 4 hours of continued TSH stimulation, the iodide T:S ratio increases as the iodide transport mechanism is enhanced in a process dependent on new protein synthesis.

(3) TSH (and cAMP) stimulate iodide organification (incorporation of iodide into thyroglobulin) primarily by increasing H_2O_2 generation. Exocytosis of thyroglobulin into the follicular lumen is also increased.

(4) Acute TSH stimulation (1–2 minutes) increases pseudopod formation at the apical cell border, followed by endocytosis of colloid, phagolysosome formation, and the subsequent secretion of thyroid hormones (Fig 10–12). As mentioned above, these effects are blocked by colchicine and cytochalasin, which disrupt the cytoskeletal system.

(5) Chronic TSH stimulation increases thyroid transcriptional and translational activity and ultimately produces hyperplasia and goiter.

(6) Many other effects of TSH on thyroid intermediary metabolism have been described, including increased glucose oxidation (primarily via the pentose phosphate pathway), phospholipid turnover, and in-

creased precursor uptake into thyroid cells. Not all of these effects are produced by cAMP, and some may involve activation of the phosphatidylinositol pathway and subsequently protein kinase C.

Other Thyroid Stimulators

Other stimulators of cAMP generation, particularly epinephrine and prostaglandins, can increase thyroid hormone secretion under experimental conditions. These agents mimic many (not all) of the effects of TSH. In the case of catecholamines, autonomic nerve endings have been demonstrated adjacent to the thyroid follicular cells, and they may play a role in the regulation of thyroid function. However, their role is most likely a minor one.

Thyroid Autoregulation

The thyroid is able to regulate its uptake of iodide and thyroid hormone synthesis by intrathyroidal mechanisms independent of TSH—ie, these regulatory mechanisms occur even in hypophysectomized animals.

A. Wolff-Chaikoff Block: When increasing amounts of I^- are given to experimental animals, inhibition of iodide organification occurs at a critical level of intrathyroidal inorganic I^- (Fig 10–17). Thy-

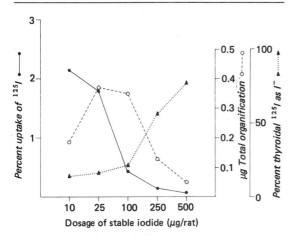

Figure 10–17. The Wolff-Chaikoff block. As increasing doses of iodide are administered to rats, there is an initial increase in iodide organification. At a critical concentration, however, higher doses of iodide given to the animals block iodide organification. The effect of increasing doses of iodide on thyroid hormone synthesis is therefore biphasic. Concomitantly with the increase in the organification block, the intracellular inorganic iodide concentration rises. As the amount of stable iodide injected is increased, there is a decrease in thyroidal uptake of radioactive iodide. (Reproduced, with permission, from DeGroot LJ, Stanbury JB: *The Thyroid and Its Diseases*, 4th ed. Wiley, 1975.)

roglobulin iodination and thyroid hormone synthesis subsequently decrease. This is known as the Wolff-Chaikoff block.

The normal thyroid gland escapes from the Wolff-Chaikoff block—and hypothyroidism does not ensue—because of intrathyroidal feedback inhibition of the iodide transport mechanism by an as yet unidentified organic iodine intermediate; ie, the ability of the thyroid to trap iodide and to maintain a high T:S ratio is reduced. Because of diminished active iodide transport, the intrathyroidal inorganic I^- concentration then declines and the "brakes" come off the organification block. A new equilibrium now exists in which thyroid hormone is synthesized at the same rate as before the excess iodide load. The fractional thyroid uptake of iodide from the extracellular fluid is, however, reduced. Conversely, in iodide insufficiency, the iodide transport mechanism becomes more active (independent of TSH) and there is a greater fractional uptake of iodide from the plasma perfusing the thyroid gland. This is reflected in an increased radioactive iodine uptake. In some thyroid diseases (eg, Hashimoto's thyroiditis), escape from the Wolff-Chaikoff block does not occur, and hypothyroidism (iodide myxedema) ensues.

B. Sensitivity to TSH: The thyroid is able to "sense" its organic iodide content and alter its sensitivity to TSH stimulation. For example, when animals receiving a high-iodide diet are injected with TSH, they develop less of a goiter than do iodide-deficient animals injected with the same amount of TSH. An important set point for this, as well as for the iodide transport mechanism, may be at the level of adenylate cyclase. Thus, an organic iodide intermediate also inhibits the cAMP response to TSH stimulation. Autoregulation by organic iodine of thyroid cellular amino acid and glucose transport has also been recognized. Whether these inhibitors are all the same remains to be determined.

C. Thyroid Hormone Secretion: The Wolff-Chaikoff block must be distinguished from the rapid and transient decrease in thyroid hormone secretion induced by iodide, especially in hyperthyroidism. This involves inhibition of lysosomal activity and thyroglobulin endocytosis by iodide, resulting in decreased T_3 and T_4 release. Although the iodide organification block occurs rapidly, its clinical effects are more delayed because follicular thyroid hormone stores must first be depleted before thyroid hormone secretion declines. On the other hand, in susceptible individuals, a block in hormone secretion can lower serum hormone levels even with full follicular stores of thyroid hormone.

D. Other Examples of Autoregulation: During periods of iodide insufficiency, the ratio of T_3 to T_4 secreted by the thyroid is increased. Since T_3 is more potent than T_4, the thyroid is therefore able to utilize available iodide more efficiently when the supply is limited. Poorly iodinated thyroglobulin is also more susceptible to proteolysis into thyroid hormones than is heavily iodinated thyroglobulin.

THYROID HORMONES IN PLASMA

Plasma Binding Proteins

Thyroid hormones (T_4 and T_3) in plasma are largely bound to protein. Only about 0.04% of the T_4 and 0.4% of the T_3 circulate "free" in the unbound state. The present concept is that only the free hormones enter cells, produce their biologic effects, and are in turn metabolized. Only the free hormone regulates the pituitary feedback mechanism (Fig 10–13). A dynamic equilibrium exists between the plasma and intracellular free hormone pools. Protein-bound thyroid hormones are therefore a very large reservoir that is slowly drawn upon as the free hormone dissociates from the binding proteins and enters the cells (Fig 10–18). Thyroid secretion is precisely regulated to replenish the metabolized thyroid hormones. This maintains a constant level of free hormone. Very little thyroid hormone is lost in the urine, because protein binding minimizes glomerular filtration. Metabolites of T_4 and T_3, however, are very poorly bound to plasma proteins and are therefore rapidly excreted in the urine.

There are 3 major thyroid hormone–binding proteins in plasma. The hormone-carrying capacity of these proteins can be determined by adding radioactive hormone to serum and subjecting it to electrophoresis (Fig 10–19).

A. Thyroid Hormone–Binding Globulin (TBG): TBG is a monomeric glycoprotein. It is the thyroid hormone–binding protein at lowest concentration in plasma (1–2 mg/dL). Each molecule has a single binding site for T_4 or T_3. Despite its very low concentration, it is the protein with the highest affinity for thy-

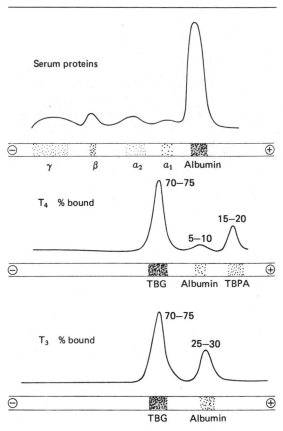

Figure 10–19. Diagrammatic representation of the distribution of radioactive T_4 and T_3 among serum thyroid hormone–binding proteins. *Top:* Paper electrophoretic pattern of serum proteins. *Middle:* Radioactive T_4 was added to serum and was then subjected to paper electrophoresis. The peaks represent the mobility of radioactive T_4 bound to different serum proteins. TBG, thyroid hormone–binding globulin; TBPA, thyroxine–binding prealbumin. *Bottom:* Radioactive T_3 was added to serum and subjected to paper electrophoresis. The peaks indicate the relative distribution of protein-bound radioactive T_3. The figures above each peak indicate the relative hormone distribution among the binding proteins in a normal adult. (Reproduced, with permission, from Rosenfield RL et al: *Pediatric Nuclear Medicine.* James AE Jr, Wagner HN Jr, Cooke RE [editors]. Saunders, 1974.)

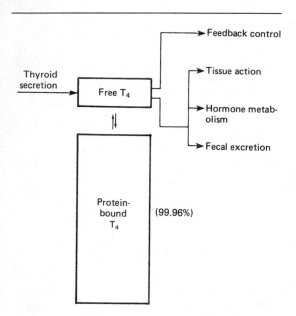

Figure 10–18. Representation of free T_4 (and free T_3) as the biologically active hormone at the level of the pituitary and the peripheral tissues. Most of the thyroid hormones circulating in plasma are protein-bound and have no biologic activity. This pool of bound hormone is in equilibrium with the free hormone pool. (Reproduced, with permission, from DeGroot LJ, Stanbury JB: *The Thyroid and Its Diseases,* 4th ed. Wiley, 1975.)

roid hormones ($T_4 > T_3$) and therefore carries most (70%) of the bound thyroid hormones. When fully saturated, it can carry about 20 μg of T_4 per deciliter.

B. Thyroxine-Binding Prealbumin (TBPA): TBPA is present at intermediate concentration in plasma (25 mg/dL). TBPA binds essentially no T_3. Even though its concentration in plasma is 20 times that of TBG, TBPA binds much less T_4 than TBG, because it has a much lower affinity for T_4. Thus, about 20% of T_4 plasma is bound to TBPA—in contrast to approximately 70% of T_4 bound to TBG.

C. Albumin: Albumin has the lowest affinity for T_4 and T_3. However, it binds significant amounts of thyroid hormone (approximately 10% of T_4 and 30% of T_3), because it is present in plasma at very high concentration (about 3500 mg/dL).

D. Kinetics of Thyroid Hormone Interaction With Plasma Binding Proteins: T_4 and T_3 bind reversibly with each binding protein according to the **law of mass action.** For example, in the case of T_4,

$$(T_4) + (TBG) \rightleftharpoons (TBG\text{-}T_4) \qquad \dots (1)$$

where (T_4) represents free (unbound) T_4, (TBG) is TBG not containing T_4, and (TBG-T_4) is T_4 bound to TBG (all in molar concentrations). At equilibrium, the rate of association of T_4 and TBG to form TBG-T_4 is the same as the dissociation of TBG-T_4 into its individual components. Thus,

$$kT_4 = \frac{(TBG\text{-}T_4)}{(T_4)\,(TBG)} \qquad \dots (2)$$

where kT_4 is the association constant for the interaction of T_4 with TBG.

From equation (2),

$$(T_4) = \frac{(TBG\text{-}T_4)}{kT_4\,(TBG)} \qquad \dots (3)$$

A similar relationship exists for each of the 3 major binding proteins, with their different affinities for T_4 (or T_3), as well as their different absolute concentrations. The free T_4 concentration in serum containing all of these binding proteins is the sum of the values in the numerator (equation 3) for each protein divided by the sum of the respective denominators.

It can therefore be seen from equation (3) that an increase in the concentration of a particular binding protein will initially result in a decrease in the free T_4 concentration (Fig 10–20). In the presence of a normal hypothalamic-pituitary-thyroid axis, there will be a compensatory increase in thyroid hormone secretion until the serum free T_4 level returns to normal. Under these conditions, the normal free T_4 concentration is now associated with an increase in the total (protein-bound) T_4. Daily free T_4 production and clearance rates are the same in both the "initial" and "new"

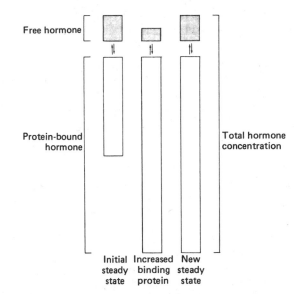

Figure 10–20. The effect of an increase in thyroid hormone–binding protein concentration on the free and protein-bound hormone concentrations. The initial increase in binding protein concentration (as may occur with estrogen administration) increases the amount of bound hormone and transiently decreases the free hormone concentration. There follows a transient increase in thyroid hormone secretion under the stimulus of TSH to replenish the free hormone pool. Another contributing factor is a transient decrease in the metabolic clearance rate of thyroid hormone. A new steady state is attained in which the free hormone secretion, metabolism, and plasma concentration are the same as initially except that the free hormone is now in equilibrium with a larger pool of bound hormone. In subjects receiving thyroid hormone medication, the same daily dose of thyroid hormone is necessary to maintain euthyroidism irrespective of the size of the bound hormone pool.

conditions despite the fact that total plasma T_4 concentrations are different.

Because of the high affinity of the binding proteins for thyroid hormones, the concentrations of free T_4 and T_3 in plasma are negligible compared to the concentrations of protein-bound hormones. The former values can therefore be ignored in expressing the total thyroid hormone concentration in plasma. If the thyroid hormone concentration increases to the point of saturation for TBG (approximately 20 μg T_4 per deciliter), as may occur in hyperthyroidism, any further increase in total serum T_4 concentration is accompanied by a much larger increase in free T_4.

In the converse situation, if the concentration of thyroid hormone–binding protein in plasma is decreased, or if hormonal binding to the proteins is inhibited by, for example, a pharmacologic agent (see below), there is an initial transient increase in the serum free T_4 concentration. This suppresses TSH secretion, and thyroid hormone secretion is consequently reduced. With continued utilization of thyroid hormone by the tissues, the free thyroid hormone level decreases to the normal "euthyroid" level. At equilibrium, the normal free hormone level is now associated with a decreased total (protein-bound) hormone concentration.

The binding of thyroid hormones to plasma binding proteins may vary considerably. Low or high TBG levels are uncommon genetic traits that can produce abnormal levels in total hormone concentrations, with the free (metabolically active) hormone levels remaining normal. In addition, a variety of diseases and pharmacologic agents can either decrease the amount of binding protein present in plasma or influence the binding of thyroid hormones to a normal concentration of binding proteins (Table 10–1). Because of the high affinity of TBG for T_4 and T_3, alterations in its concentration have a much greater effect on serum total hormone concentrations than do alterations in TBPA or albumin concentrations.

THYROID HORMONE METABOLISM

T_4 is the major secretory product of the normal thyroid. The major pathway of T_4 metabolism is via the progressive deiodination of the molecule. As shown in Fig 10–21, the initial deiodination of T_4 may occur in

Table 10–1. Factors influencing the concentration of protein-bound thyroid hormones in serum.

A. Increased TBG Concentration:
   1. Congenital.
   2. Hyperestrogenic states (pregnancy, estrogen treatment).
   3. Diseases (acute infectious hepatitis, hypothyroidism).
B. Decreased TBG Concentration:
   1. Congenital.
   2. Drugs (androgenic steroids, glucocorticoids).
   3. Major systemic illness (protein malnutrition, nephrotic syndrome, cirrhosis, hyperthyroidism).
C. Drugs Affecting Thyroid Hormone Binding to Normal Concentrations of Binding Protein:
   1. Phenytoin (Dilantin).
   2. Salicylates.
   3. Phenylbutazone.
   4. Mitotane (Lysodren, o,p'-DDD).
   5. Heparin.

the outer ring, producing T_3 ($3,3',5$-T_3); or in the inner ring, producing reverse T_3 (rT_3; $3,3',5'$-T_3). Less than 20% of total T_3 is produced in the thyroid (Fig 10–22). The remaining 80–90% is derived from outer (phenolic) ring monodeiodination of T_4 in the peripheral tissues. T_4 and T_3 in the plasma are metabolized by the peripheral tissues and subsequently excreted. Although the catabolic products of T_4 are generally less biologically active than the parent compound, some metabolites do have biologic activity and, as in the

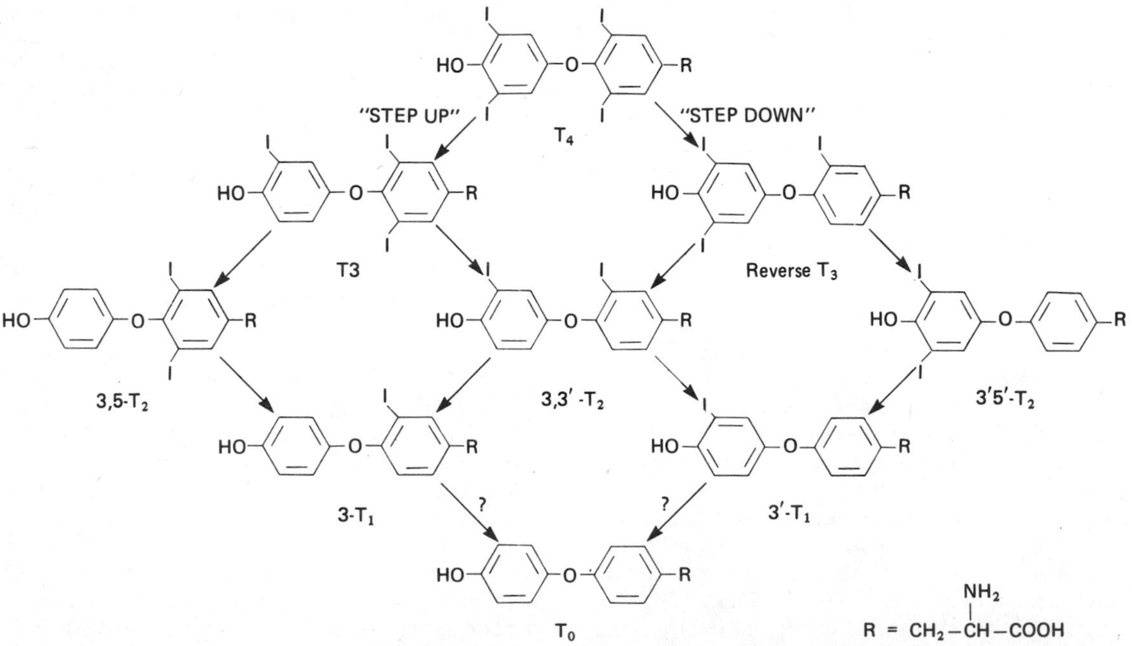

Figure 10–21. The deiodinative pathway of thyroxine metabolism. The monodeiodination of T_4 to T_3 represents a "step up" in biologic potency, whereas the monodeiodination of T_4 to reverse T_3 has the opposite effect. Further deiodination of T_3 essentially abolishes hormonal activity.

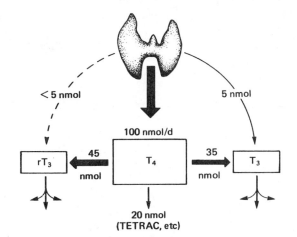

100 nmol/d

Figure 10–22. Major pathways of thyroxine metabolism in normal adult humans. Rates are expressed in nmol/24 h and are approximations based upon available data. 100 nmol of T_4 is equivalent to approximately 75 μg. rT_3, reverse T_3; TETRAC, tetraiodothyroacetic acid. (Reproduced, with permission, from Cavalieri RR, Rapoport B: Impaired peripheral conversion of thyroxine to triiodothyronine. *Ann Rev Med* 1977;**28**:5765.)

case of T_3, even exceed the biologic potency of T_4 (Table 10–2). It should be noted that data on the bioactivity of compounds other than T_4 and T_3 are based on difficult and inaccurate assays and should be regarded merely as approximations. Almost all (95%) of the reverse T_3 (rT_3) in the plasma is derived from the inner ring monodeiodination of T_4 in the peripheral tissues. Both T_3 and rT_3 are then deiodinated further to the diiodothyronines (T_2) and then to monoiodothyronines. Reverse T_3 and the 3 different T_2 metabolites are essentially biologically inactive and are cleared rapidly from the plasma.

There are 2 separate outer ring deiodinases that convert T_4 to T_3 (and rT_3 to 3,3'-T_2). The major differences between these 2 enzymes (iodothyronine 5'-deiodinase type I and type II) are outlined in Table 10–3.

Because conversion of T_4 to T_3 represents a "step up" in biologic activity whereas conversion of T_4 to rT_3 has the opposite effect (Fig 10–21), the conversion of T_4 to T_3 or rT_3 by inner or outer ring iodothyronine deiodinase is a pivotal regulatory step in determining thyroid hormone biologic activity. It has been proposed that T_4 is a biologically inactive prohormone and that its apparent biologic activity is dependent upon intracellular conversion to T_3. However, other than in the pituitary, all evidence indicates that T_4 itself has intrinsic biologic activity.

The kinetics of T_4, T_3, and rT_3 production, distribution, and clearance are shown in Table 10–4, which indicates typical values that may be seen in a euthyroid human. Because of its greater binding affinity to plas-

ma proteins, chiefly TBG, the distribution of T_4 is largely restricted to the intravascular volume; ie, T_4 has the smallest distribution volume and the largest pool size. Because of the large plasma pool of T_4 relative to its rate of utilization, the plasma T_4 reservoir turns over relatively slowly. T_3 and, to a greater degree, rT_3 are more loosely bound to plasma proteins and are therefore distributed in a larger volume and cleared more rapidly.

The tissues that concentrate the most thyroid hormone are liver, kidney, and muscle. Brain, spleen, and gonads take up little thyroid hormone. This variation in uptake by different tissues parallels the metabolic effects of T_4 on oxygen consumption in vitro.

How thyroid hormones enter peripheral tissue cells is uncertain. It was believed to be a passive diffusion process, but the possibility that there may be specific thyroid hormone receptors on the cell surface and active transport of thyroid hormone into cells is under active investigation. Once within the cell, thyroid hormones either remain free in the cytoplasm or are associated with low-affinity cytosol receptors or high-affinity nuclear and mitochondrial receptors.

In addition to the deiodinative pathways of T_4 metabolism, minor metabolic pathways of uncertain importance include the following:

(1) Oxidative deamination of the iodothyronines into their acetic acid derivatives, eg, tetraiodothyroacetic acid (TETRAC) and triiodothyroacetic acid (TRIAC) (Table 10–2). These compounds retain some biologic activity, but their relative physiologic importance is uncertain.

(2) Phenolic conjugation into glucuronide or sulfate derivatives. The former occurs mainly in the liver and the latter mainly in the kidney. Glucuronide conjugates of T_4 are excreted into the bile and thence in feces. In humans, there is little enterohepatic circulation of thyroid hormone conjugates.

(3) Decarboxylation of thyroxine to thyroxamine.

(4) Cleavage of the ether link between the 2 phenol rings of the iodothyronines.

As mentioned above, 80–90% of T_3 production is from the monodeiodination of T_4 to T_3 (Fig 10–22). This conversion of T_4 to T_3 utilizes approximately 30–40% of the secreted T_4. Virtually all rT_3 (95%) is produced by the monodeiodination of T_4, and this represents another 40% of the T_4 secreted by the thyroid. The remaining 20% of secreted T_4 is excreted in the feces or urine, either in the free form or as conjugates.

A variety of conditions and pharmacologic agents reduce the rate of T_4 monodeiodination to T_3 (Table 10–5). This may lead to decreased serum T_3 concentrations. The clinical status of a patient is therefore very important in interpreting the significance of a low serum T_3 level. In acute illness or starvation, the low serum T_3 value is usually associated with an elevated serum rT_3 concentration. This reflects primarily decreased rT_3 clearance rather than increased rT_3 production. While rT_3 clearly has little or no agonist ac-

Table 10–2. Chemical structures and biologic activity of thyroid hormones.

	Hormone	Common Name	Biologic Activity
	L-3,5,3′,5′-Tetraiodothyronine	L-Thyroxine; T_4	100
	L-3,5,3′-Triiodothyronine	T_3	300–800
	L-3,3′,5′-Triiodothyronine	Reverse T_3; rT_3	< 1
	DL-3,3′-Diiodothyronine	$3,3'$-T_2	< 1–3
	DL-3,5-Diiodothyronine	$3,5$-T_2	7–11
	DL-3′,5′-Diiodothyronine	$3'5'$-T_2	0
	L-3,5,3′,5′-Tetraiodothyroacetic acid	Tetrac	? 10–50
	L-3,5,3′-Triiodothyroacetic acid	Triac	? 25–35

Table 10-3. Differences between iodothyronine 5'-deiodinase type I and type II.

	Type I	Type II
Tissue (primary localization)	Liver, kidney, muscle	Brain, pituitary, brown adipose tissue, and skin
Inhibition by propylthiouracil	Yes	No
Substrate affinity	$rT_3 > T_4$	$T_4 = rT_3$
Enzyme kinetics	Ping-pong	Sequential
Influence of hypothyroidism	Decreased	Increased

Table 10-5. Conditions or factors associated with decreased conversion of T_4 to T_3.

1. Fetal life.
2. Caloric restriction.
3. Hepatic disease.
4. Major systemic illness.
5. Drugs:
   Propylthiouracil.
   Glucocorticoids.
   Propranolol (mild effect).
   Iodinated x-ray contrast agents (iopanoic acid, ipodate sodium).

tivity, it may act as a counterhormone to reduce the metabolic activity of more active thyroid hormones.

THYROID HORMONE ACTIONS

Administration of T_4 or T_3—or the pathologic or iatrogenic absence of these hormones—produces general effects on intermediary metabolism and has particular effects on specific organ systems.

Effects on Fetal Development

Thyroid hormones are critically important in fetal development, particularly of the neural and skeletal systems. Thus, intrauterine hypothyroidism leads to cretinism (mental retardation and dwarfism). Maternal thyroid hormones do not cross the placenta in sufficient quantity to maintain fetal euthyroidism, and the fetus is therefore dependent upon hormones synthesized by its own thyroid gland from about 11 weeks' gestation (see below).

Effects on Oxygen Consumption & Heat Production

The basal metabolic rate (O_2 consumption, at rest, by the whole animal) increases in hyperthyroidism and decreases in hypothyroidism. Severe hyperthyroidism is occasionally associated with fever and severe hypothyroidism with hypothermia. Postnatally, thyroid hormones increase O_2 consumption in all tissues except the brain, spleen, and testis. Compared to the effects of TSH on thyroid hormone secretion, most thyroid hormone actions on peripheral tissues are induced relatively slowly over a period of hours or days. For example, T_4 administration to hypothyroid patients does not increase oxygen consumption until 24–48 hours after administration. T_3 acts more rapidly than T_4 but still over a period of hours (Fig 10–23).

Cardiovascular Effects

Thyroid hormones have marked chronotropic and inotropic effects on the heart. Low cardiac output with bradycardia and slow myocardial contraction and relaxation are characteristic of hypothyroidism. The reverse occurs in hyperthyroidism. The force of contraction in hypothyroidism is normal.

Sympathetic Effects

Many thyroid hormone effects, particularly on the cardiovascular system, are similar to those induced by catecholamines. Hyperthyroid patients are more sen-

Table 10-4. Representative iodothyronine kinetic values in a euthyroid human.

	T_4	T_3	rT_3
Serum levels			
Total, μg/dL (nmol/L)	8 (103)	0.12 (1.84)	0.04 (0.51)
Free, ng/dL (pmol/L)	2.1 (27)	0.28 (4.3)	0.24 (3.69)
Body pool, μg (nmol)	800 (1023)	46 (70.7)	40 (61.5)
Distribution volume (L)	10	38	98
Metabolic clearance rate (MCR) (L/d)	1	22	90
Production (disposal) rate. MCRX serum concentration, μg/d (nmol/d)	80 (103)	26 (34)	36 (46)
Half-life in plasma ($t_{1/2}$) (days)	7	1	0.2

(**Note**: T_4 μg/dL × 12.87 = nmol/L; T_3 μg/dL × 15.38 = nmol/L)

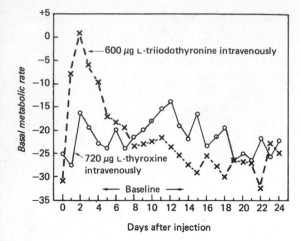

Figure 10–23. Basal metabolic rates after injection of equimolar amounts of T_3 and T_4 in a hypothyroid individual. (Reproduced, with permission, from Blackburn C et al: Calorigenic effects of single intravenous doses of L-triiodothyronine and L-thyroxine in myxedematous persons. *J Clin Invest* 1954;33:819.)

sitive to catecholamines. Thyroid hormones increase the number of catecholamine receptors in heart muscle cells. Hepatocyte receptors are unaffected. Thyroid hormones may also amplify catecholamine action at a postreceptor site. Beta-adrenergic inhibition reverses some features of clinical hyperthyroidism, such as eyelid retraction and tachycardia. However, other thyroid hormone actions—eg, effect on O_2 consumption—are not prevented by beta-adrenergic blockade. Thyroid hormone action is clearly distinct from catecholamine action, but their exact interrelationship remains to be elucidated.

Pulmonary Effects

Thyroid hormones are necessary for normal hypoxic and hypercapnic drive to the respiratory centers. Hypoventilation with hypoxia and hypercapnia is a consequence of severe hypothyroidism and may require artificial ventilation.

Hematopoietic Effects

Thyroid hormones increase erythropoiesis, possibly because of increased O_2 utilization by tissues leading to increased erythropoietin production. Thyroid hormones also increase 2,3-diphosphoglycerate concentrations in erythrocytes, allowing increased O_2 dissociation from hemoglobin and thereby increasing O_2 availability to the tissues. In hypothyroidism, the reverse occurs, and decreased tissue O_2 consumption leads to decreased erythropoietin production and an "adaptive" anemia.

Endocrine Effects

Thyroid hormones generally increase the metabolism and clearance of various hormones and phar-

macologic agents. For example, steroid hormone clearances are increased, leading to compensatory increases in production rates. Thus, administration of thyroid hormones will increase cortisol production and clearance, but the plasma cortisol concentration remains unchanged. Serum prolactin levels are increased in about 40% of patients with primary hypothyroidism. When present, this abnormality is corrected by treatment with thyroid hormone. Insulin requirements in diabetics are frequently increased in hyperthyroidism. The growth hormone response to stimuli such as hypoglycemia is reduced in primary hypothyroidism. Thyroid hormones are necessary for normal LH and FSH secretion. In hypothyroidism, anovulation and menstrual disturbances—particularly menorrhagia—may occur. Decreased renal free water clearance in hypothyroidism may be secondary to enhanced vasopressin activity but is more apt to be related to altered intrarenal hemodynamics. Finally, PTH action may be diminished in hypothyroidism.

Musculoskeletal Effects

Thyroid hormones have a potent stimulatory effect on bone turnover, increasing both bone formation and resorption. This is associated with increased urinary hydroxyproline excretion. Hypercalcemia is occasionally observed in severe hyperthyroidism. Thyroid hormones increase the rate of muscle relaxation as measured by elicitation of the deep tendon reflexes. This is of clinical value in diagnosing hypothyroidism.

THYROID HORMONE ACTION AT THE MOLECULAR LEVEL

Actions of thyroid hormones have been described at different intracellular sites. The relative importance of these sites is still controversial, however.

RNA Transcription

There is considerable evidence that free T_4 and T_3 enter tissue cells and bind to specific receptors in nuclear acidic proteins associated with chromatin. This is followed by increased RNA transcriptional activity. The physiologic importance of these nuclear binding sites is suggested by their high affinity constant, which is compatible with the prevailing plasma levels of free thyroid hormones. In addition, there is a good correlation between the binding of various analogues of thyroid hormones to nuclear receptors in liver and their metabolic potency. The thyroid hormone receptor, which was recently cloned, shows homology with the *erb*-A oncogene. The receptor belongs to a family of receptors that includes those for the steroid hormones and vitamins A and D. There appear to be at least 2 distinct thyroid hormone receptor genes that code for receptors that function differently in different tissues. The physiologic significance of these different receptor forms remains to be determined. The exact mechanism by which thyroid hormone binding to nuclear protein receptors leads to increased transcriptional activity is uncertain, but thyroid hormone bound to its receptor appears to interact with hormone regulatory elements in responsive genes.

Protein Translation

T_4 and T_3 increase detectable new protein synthesis in vitro within 5 hours. This effect presumably follows an increase in mRNA levels for some proteins, but may also occur by posttranscriptional mechanisms. For example, correlation of the induction by thyroid hormones of different enzymes such as mitochondrial malic enzyme and cytosolic α-glycerophosphate dehydrogenase with their respective mRNAs provides evidence for posttranscriptional effects of thyroid hormones.

Cell Membrane

Thyroid hormones markedly stimulate plasma membrane Na^+-K^+ ATPase activity, which is coupled to Na^+ and K^+ transport across the plasma membrane. This increases ATP utilization. Since a large portion of the O_2 consumption by the entire organism is for maintenance of this transport system, the stimulating effect of thyroid hormone on the basal metabolic rate may be related to this effect.

Thyroid hormones also have acute (within minutes) effects on the plasma membrane of cells such as lymphocytes in that they increase the intracellular transport of glucose and amino acids. The physiologic importance of this phenomenon has not been established.

Mitochondria

It now seems unlikely that thyroid hormones increase oxygen consumption by uncoupling mitochondrial oxidative phosphorylation, leading to inefficient energy utilization. ATP synthesis may be increased as a secondary phenomenon—eg, in response to increased ATP utilization in association with increased Na^+ and K^+ transport activity. Nevertheless, mitochondrial receptors of high affinity for thyroid hormones have been described, and their importance in mitochondrial function is being investigated.

Effects on Intermediary Metabolism

Thyroid hormones alter the metabolism of carbohydrates, fats, and proteins. However, these effects are probably secondary to the mechanisms described above. Cholesterol synthesis and degradation are both increased by thyroid hormones. Since the latter effect predominates, the serum cholesterol level declines in thyroid overactivity and vice versa. Thyroid hormone–induced effects on cholesterol metabolism may be secondary to increased beta-lipoprotein degradation. This may also account for the alteration in serum carotene that parallels the alteration in serum cholesterol. Lipolysis is also increased by thyroid hormones, possibly by enhancing the response to catecholamine stimulation. Glycogenolysis and gluconeogenesis are increased by thyroid hormones, presumably in relation to regeneration of ATP consumed—eg, by increased Na^+-K^+ ATPase activity. Thyroid hormones increase insulin requirements in diabetics. This may be related to increased insulin degradation or clearance rather than to alterations in carbohydrate metabolism.

PHYSIOLOGIC CHANGES IN THYROID FUNCTION

Thyroid Function in the Fetus

Thyroglobulin synthesis begins during the fifth week of intrauterine life, and the iodide transport mechanism becomes active at approximately 12 weeks. During pregnancy, the fetal thyroid is under the control of the fetal hypothalamus and pituitary. Maternal thyroid hormones in their active form can cross the placenta only to a slight extent. A contributing factor to this phenomenon may be that 5′ deiodinase is very active in placental tissue. Thus, athyreotic fetuses have detectable but low (hypothyroid) thyroid hormone concentrations.

At maturity, the human fetus has a slightly increased serum TSH and free thyroxine concentration. However, the serum T_3 level is very low—in the range noted in adults during starvation and acute illness. Similarly, the rT_3 concentration is elevated. Immediately after birth, there is a transient increase in TSH secretion, and serum T_3, T_4, and rT_3 levels revert to nearly normal within the first few days and approach normal adult levels during the first year of life.

Thyroid Function in Pregnancy

Serum TBG levels increase approximately 2-fold during pregnancy. A new equilibrium is reached in which the total thyroid hormone concentrations are twice normal but free hormone levels remain normal (see Fig 20–1). Radioactive iodine uptake increases during pregnancy, and the thyroid may increase slightly in size, because of increased renal clearance of iodide and perhaps because of increased iodide utilization by the fetus. The placenta produces a glycoprotein hormone with very weak thyrotropic activity. It is unclear whether this is human chorionic gonadotropin (hCG) itself or another closely related compound that is extracted from the placenta together with hCG. Recent evidence suggests the latter. In normal pregnancy, this substance has little or no effect on thyroid function.

Changes In Thyroid Function With Aging

Although serum T_3 levels are reported to decrease slightly with aging, this observation has been questioned, because elderly persons are more susceptible to a variety of illnesses that may reduce serum T_3 production from T_4 and therefore reduce the average T_3 level in the group. Whether an age-related decrease in T_3 occurs or not, thyroid function in old people appears to be normal as shown by the TSH response to TRH stimulation (see Chapter 29).

TESTS OF THYROID FUNCTION

Thyroid function tests may be classified as those that (1) measure concentrations of hormones or biologically inactive products secreted by the thyroid gland; (2) directly examine the function of the thyroid gland; (3) test the effects of thyroid hormones on peripheral tissues; (4) evaluate the hypothalamic-pituitary-thyroid axis; and (5) identify and measure pathologic substances in blood not usually present in healthy subjects.

MEASUREMENT IN BLOOD OF PRODUCTS SECRETED BY THE THYROID

Measurement of T_4

Older methods for the estimation of serum content of T_4 involved measurement of the iodine content of serum protein (protein bound iodine, or PBI), or the iodine content of a butanol extract of serum protein (butanol extractable iodine, or BEI). These nonspecific tests were replaced by a competitive binding assay that used the displacement of T_4 from TBG. All of these tests have now been replaced by immunoassay using highly specific T_4 antibodies. T_4 in serum is chemically dissociated from endogenous TBG and measured by displacement from the antibody with labeled T_4; the T_4 label may be isotopic (^{125}I), fluorescent, or detected by enzymatic assay. The results are quantified by comparing them with known T_4 standards. This method can be automated, allowing a large number of assays to be done with minimum technician time. The normal range for T_4 in adults is 5–12 µg/dL (64–154 nmol/L).

The total T_4 concentration in serum does not always reflect the metabolic status. As described previously (Table 10–1), thyroid hormone-binding protein concentrations may be altered in a variety of conditions. This alters total T_4 levels but does not alter the metabolically important free T_4 concentrations. Certain drugs—commonly phenytoin and salicylates—interfere with the binding of T_4 to serum proteins. For this reason, combining the estimated total serum T_4 with an indirect measurement of the free T_4 concentration is clinically useful (see below).

Measurement of Free T_4 Index & Free T_4

Direct measurement of serum free T_4 by dialysis is difficult because of its very low concentration. One method is to add radiolabeled T_4 to serum in a dialysis bag, measure the percent of radioactivity dialyzed, and multiply this by the previously determined total T_4 to obtain the free T_4 level (Fig 10–24). Although new, ingenious assays for the measurement of free T_4 in serum have been developed, many clinicians still depend on assays that provide an approximation of the absolute free T_4 concentration expressed as free T_4 index (FT$_4$I). Radiolabeled T_3 or T_4 is first added to the serum to be tested and allowed to equilibrate with unlabeled endogenous hormone. An aliquot is then added to either a resin or Sephadex—substances that bind free thyroid hormone with high affinity and therefore compete with serum binding proteins for the free hormone. The resin is then rinsed and counted for radioactivity to determine what percentage of the total radioactivity has been adsorbed. The percentage uptake of radioactive T_3 by the resin will be greater when there is less binding of the radioactive T_3 to serum binding proteins. Conversely, if serum binding proteins are increased, as in pregnancy, the percentage uptake of radioactive T_3 by the resin will decrease. More T_3 than T_4 binds to resin because T_3 binds with lower affinity to endogenous binding proteins. The assay using radiolabeled T_3 is therefore more practical than the one using T_4 (Fig 10–24).

Multiplication of the resin or Sephadex uptake value by the previously determined total T_4 concentration provides an index of the effective free T_4 concentration independent of changes in hormone binding capacity in serum. However, this is not a true free T_4 measurement but merely an index of this measurement. Direct measurement of free T_4 levels by dialysis has demonstrated a reasonable proportionality between the true free T_4 level and the free T_4 index, thereby establishing the clinical usefulness of the latter. It may seem confusing that the free T_4 index (FT$_4$I) can be measured with radioactive T_3 ("resin T_3 uptake test," or RT$_3$U). However, the test assesses the capacity for serum proteins to bind thyroid hormones and either T_3 or T_4 may be used. Currently, T_4 is used more commonly, and protein binding is determined with fluorescein- or enzyme-labeled T_4; in this procedure the activity of the label changes when the T_4 is bound to protein so that protein binding may be determined directly without using resin to separate "free" from "bound" hormone. The protein binding uptake is called the T_4 uptake (T_4U) and is expressed in "uptake units" with one as the normal midpoint. The FT$_4$I is obtained by dividing the total T_4 by the T_4U. The FT$_4$I can be expressed in either arbitrary units that vary with the laboratory or as an "adjusted T_4"; the T_4 level is adjusted upward if protein binding is low (eg, as in renal disease) or downward if protein binding is ele-

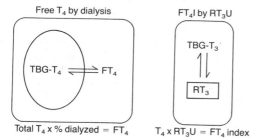

Figure 10–24. Comparison of free T_4 by dialysis and free T_4 index. *Left:* The left panel illustrates one method of determining free T_4, which is to calculate the product of the percent of dialyzed isotopically labeled T_4 and the total T_4. *Right:* The right panel illustrates the use of the resin T_3 uptake method to determine the free T_4 index by calculating the product of the percent of isotopically labeled T_3 adsorbed by the resin and the total T_4. See text for details. TBG T_4 = T_4 bound to TBG; FT_4 = Free T_4; RT_3U = Resin T_3 uptake; FT_4 index = Free thyroxine index.

vated (eg, as in pregnancy). In the euthyroid individual, if the FT_4I is expressed as an "adjusted T_4," the numerical range for the T_4 and the FT_4I will be the same.

In most instances, the FT_4I will establish the thyroid metabolic status of the patient. However, the FT_4I will be inappropriately low in patients on replacement therapy with triiodothyronine (T_3, Cytomel) or in patients with toxic nodules or early Graves' disease where hyperthyroidism is associated with relative overproduction of T_3 but not T_4 (T_3 thyrotoxicosis). Phenytoin is unique because it may lower the FT_4I as well as the total T_4 even though patients remain clinically euthyroid by all other available criteria. This may be partly due to increased hepatic metabolism of T_4, which causes about a 20% drop in total and free T_4. T_3 and TSH levels remain normal. The FT_4I may be inappropriately low in acute or chronic illness. This may be due to a circulating inhibitor of T_4-TBG binding or to a change in the TBG molecule itself. In these very sick patients, a direct measure of free T_4 will be normal or high and serum TSH will usually be normal, enabling the clinician to rule out hypothyroidism.

Occasionally, the FT_4I will be inappropriately high. An example of this is the rare condition of peripheral resistance to thyroid hormones. In addition, during acute illness, euthyroid patients may rarely present with an elevated FT_4I; however, the total T_3 is subnormal and TSH is normal, ruling out hyperthyroidism (see below).

A clinical method for the direct measurement of FT_4 would be very useful. However, many of the commercially available FT_4 methods are susceptible to the same problems (eg, artifacts present in systemic illness) that influence the interpretation of the FT_4I.

Measurement of T_3 & Free T_3 Index

The T_3 concentration in serum in generally measured by radioimmunoassay using highly specific T_3 antisera. The direct measurement of T_3 should not be confused with the resin T_3 uptake test, which does not measure the serum T_3 level (see above). T_3 measurement is more useful for diagnosing hyperthyroidism than hypothyroidism, because in hyperthyroidism the increase in T_3 secretion is proportionately greater than the increase in T_4 secretion. The normal ratio of T_3 in ng/dL to T_4 in μg/dL is usually less than 20 (eg, T_3 120 ng/dL; T_4 8 μg/dL, T_3/T_4 ratio = 15). In hyperthyroidism, this ratio is usually over 20, and in T_3 thyrotoxicosis, the ratio will be very high. In mild hypothyroidism, however, the serum T_3 level does not fall to the same degree as does the T_4, because TSH stimulation increases the relative secretion of T_3. Thus, many patients with hypothyroidism will have normal serum T_3 levels but markedly depressed serum T_4. Occasionally, when a very ill patient has a slightly elevated free T_4 index, measurement of the total T_3 is of great value in excluding hyperthyroidism. In a wide variety of acute and chronic illnesses, the serum total T_3 level is suppressed because of decreased conversion of T_4 to T_3 (Table 10–5, and see above).

Like the total T_4 level, the total T_3 concentration is influenced by changes in the concentration of serum binding proteins. Thus, just as the high total T_4 in a pregnant patient is difficult to interpret without determining the free T_4 index, so must a high total T_3 level in this situation be interpreted with caution. A free T_3 index can be calculated as the product of the RT_3U and the total T_3, thus correcting for the concentration of binding protein.

Reverse T_3 (rT_3) can be measured in serum by radioimmunoassay. The normal range in adults is approximately 25–75 ng/dL (0.39–1.15 nmol/L). This is approximately one-third of the total T_3 concentration. Reverse T_3 can be used to differentiate hypothyroidism from chronic illness because rT_3 levels are reduced in hypothyroidism and elevated in chronic illness. However, this differential diagnosis can be made by TSH determination (see below) so rT_3 is rarely measured.

Measurement of Thyroglobulin

Thyroglobulin is measured in serum by radioimmunoassay. The presence of endogenous thyroglobulin autoantibodies can interfere with the test and so, if present, they should be separated from the serum before testing. The concentration of thyroglobulin in normal serum is 10–40 ng/mL (10–40 μg/L). It is elevated in conditions of thyroid overactivity, such as hyperthyroidism, which increase its secretion as well as that of thyroid hormones. Elevated thyroglobulin levels are found in patients with large multinodular goiters, in proportion to the volume of thyroid tissue, or with thyroiditis, either acute or chronic, when it is released due to tissue damage. Determination of serum thyroglobulin has been most useful clinically in the follow-up of patients with papillary or follicular thyroid carcinome after total thyroidectomy. Following total thyroidectomy, the level of serum thyroglobulin should be low, usually below 10 ng/dL (10 μg/L). A rise in serum thyroglobulin indicates the presence of metastatic thyroid carcinoma. In patients with existing metastases, an increase in the concentration of serum thyroglobulin usually indicates progression of the disease, and vice versa.

EVALUATION OF THYROID GLAND SIZE AND IODINE METABOLISM

Radioactive Iodine Uptake (RAIU)

The rationale for this test was described in the section on iodide metabolism. Sodium ^{123}I is administered orally, and a gamma scintillation counter is used to measure radioactivity over the area of the thyroid after 24 hours. This interval is chosen because the tracer uptake is near maximum at 24 hours. An earlier measurement at 4 or 6 hours is usually taken as well, because in situations of high iodine turnover, the uptake at 6 hours may be higher than at 24 hours. Such situations include severe thyrotoxicosis and early primary thyroid failure (such as Hashimoto's thyroiditis), where a small remnant of functional thyroid under TSH stimulation is releasing newly synthesized hormone very rapidly without a long period of storage.

Occasionally, thyrotoxicosis may be associated with a very low or absent RAIU, an important diagnostic indicator. Examples of low RAIU thyrotoxicosis include (1) subacute thyroiditis, (2) "spontaneously resolving hyperthyroidism" as a phase of Hashimoto's thyroiditis, (3) thyrotoxicosis factitia, (4) struma ovarii, (5) excessive iodide intake (jodbasedow effect), and (6) ectopic functional thyroid metastasis after total thyroidectomy.

Perchlorate Discharge

The efficiency of the thyroid organification mechanism may be tested by giving $KClO_4$, 0.5 gm in solution orally, 2–3 hours after oral administration of radioiodide, and observing its effect on the RAIU (Fig 10–9). In subjects with a normal organification mechanism, ClO_4^- blocks further uptake of radioiodide by the thyroid but does not discharge more than 5% of the accumulated iodide in the next hour. Conversely, if iodide organification is incomplete, ClO_4^- blocks further I^- transport, but diffusion of I^- out of the cell continues. This is seen as discharge of radioactivity from the gland. A positive test may be observed in (1) congenital iodide organification defects, (2) some cases of Hashimoto's thyroiditis, (3) Graves' disease

previously treated with ^{131}I, and (4) patients being treated with inhibitors of iodide organification such as methimazole or propylthiouracil. Although this test is rarely used clinically, it can be very helpful in understanding the pathophysiology of the above illnesses.

Thyroid Imaging

The size and shape and some features of the internal structure of the thyroid may be assessed by a wide variety of thyroid imaging techniques. Their clinical application will be discussed in greater detail in subsequent sections of this chapter. However, they may be summarized as follows:

A. Radionuclide Scanning: After the administration of radioactive iodide—eg, sodium ^{123}I—an image of the thyroid may be obtained using an appropriate scanning apparatus. With the rectilinear scanner, the scanner moves in a matrix over the patient's neck, and the radioactivity at each point is recorded as a dot on paper or x-ray film (Fig 10–25). The advantage of this scan is that it accurately represents the size of the thyroid and accurately localizes palpable thyroid abnormalities. On the other hand, its resolution is relatively poor, and it takes considerable time for the scan to be completed.

Over recent years, the pinhole collimated gamma camera (scintillation camera) has moved to the fore. The field of the gamma camera is relatively large and encompasses the entire thyroid. This allows the thyroid to be rapidly scanned without moving the camera. The data are usually recorded on Polaroid film (Fig 10–26). Besides speed, the major advantage of this method is increased resolution.

^{99m}Tc pertechnetate is also concentrated by the thyroid and can be used for imaging with high resolution. Unlike radioactive iodine, this isotope is not organi-

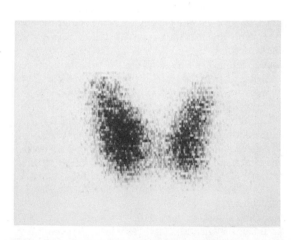

Figure 10–25. Rectilinear thyroid sodium ^{123}I scan performed 6 hours after the ingestion of 100 μCi of sodium ^{123}I. (Courtesy of RR Cavalieri.)

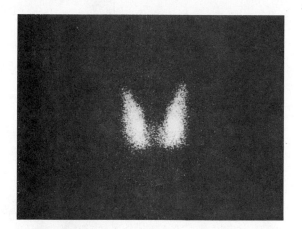

Figure 10–26. Scintiphoto (pinhole collimator) thyroid scan performed 6 hours after the ingestion of 100 μCi of sodium ^{123}I. (Courtesy of RR Cavalieri.)

fied and stored, and the scan is therefore performed very shortly (eg, 20 minutes) after isotope administration. Advantages of this scan in addition to its speed include the fact that it is not interfered with by drugs that block iodide organification. Occasionally, however, thyroid nodules that are "cold" with sodium ^{123}I are not identified with ^{99m}Tc pertechnetate.

B. Fluorescent Scanning: The fluorescent scan provides an image of the distribution of nonradioactive, stable iodine within the thyroid. An approximate quantitation can also be made of the thyroidal iodine store. No radioisotope is administered. An external source of ^{241}Am is directed at the thyroid, resulting in the emission of x-rays by thyroid molecules. By selectively recording emitted 28.5 keV x-rays specific for iodine, an image of the intrathyroidal iodine distribution can be formed. The scan is similar in appearance to the rectilinear radioactive iodine scan (Fig 10–25). The advantage of the fluorescent scan is that it does not require radioactive iodine administration, and the thyroid may be imaged even if the RAIU is zero, such as when the patient is taking exogenous thyroid hormones. Thus, it can be used to determine whether thyroid tissue is absent or when it is present but not trapping radioiodine.

C. Ultrasonography: The application of this technique is similar to that for other organs. Its major use is to differentiate between cystic and solid thyroid lesions that may both appear to be "cold" on radionuclide scanning.

D. Magnetic Resonance Imaging (MRI): The thyroid gland is clearly visualized by MRI scan. The MRI scan has been extremely useful for evaluating the extent of both posterior and substernal thyroid enlargement. It has also been useful for checking patients with thyroid carcinomas for metastatic involvement deep in the neck or the mediastinum.

TESTS OF THE EFFECTS OF THYROID HORMONES ON PERIPHERAL TISSUES

The ultimate test of whether a patient is experiencing the effects of too much or too little thyroid hormone is not a measurement of hormone concentration in the blood or of the size and functional activity of the thyroid but of the effect of thyroid hormones on the peripheral tissues. Unfortunately, no simple, reproducible, and specific tests are available to do this.

Many years ago thyroid hormones were discovered to increase heat production and oxygen consumption, and so measurement of basal oxygen consumption to calculate basal heat production, or **basal metabolic rate (BMR),** was one of the first methods used to evaluate thyroid status. However, the test is insensitive and nonspecific and is rarely used today.

The speed of muscle contraction and relaxation is also related to thyroid status—muscle reflexes are brisk in hyperthyroidism and slowed in hypothyroidism. The speed of relaxation of the Achilles tendon reflex can be measured by a simple apparatus called the **photomotogram.** The half-relaxation time in the healthy individual is 230–350 ms. However, the normal and hyperthyroid or hypothyroid states overlap considerably, so that the test is of limited diagnostic value. The **Q–Kd Interval** measures the interval between the initiation of the QRS complex on the ECG and the arrival of the pulse wave in the brachial artery as measured by the Korotkoff sound. Although the rate of myocardial contraction is increased in hyperthyroidism and decreased in hypothyroidism, these ranges overlap considerably with the normal range, which limits the clinical usefulness of this test. Thyroid hormones influence the concentration of numerous tissue and blood compounds as well as the activity of many different enzymes. For example, serum cholesterol is usually elevated in hypothyroidism and decreased in hyperthyroidism, and serum creatine phosphokinase (CPK) and lactic dehydrogenase (LDH) may also be increased in hypothyroidism. However, none of these biochemical changes are sufficiently specific or sensitive for clinical diagnostic use.

EVALUATION OF THE HYPOTHALAMIC-PITUITARY-THYROID AXIS

Measurement of Serum TSH

The effects of T_3 and T_4 on pituitary TSH secretion have been described above. The early radioimmunoassays of TSH were able to detect the elevated levels in hypothyroidism, but were not sensitive enough to detect the suppressed levels in hyperthyroidism. The production of monoclonal antibodies to human TSH allowed the development of immunoassays for TSH that are sensitive enough to both accurately measure nor-

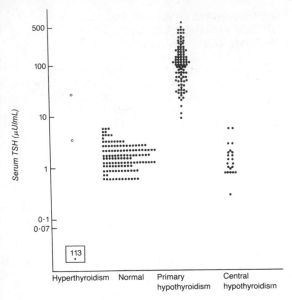

Figure 10–27. Serum TSH concentrations in normal (133) subjects, untreated overt hyperthyroidism (115), primary (96) and central (22) hypothyroidism. Undetectable values were observed in all hyperthyroid subjects excluding two patients (open circle) with hyperthyroidism due to TSH-secreting pituitary tumor. Note logarithmic scale for TSH. (Reproduced, with permission, from Martino E, et al, *Clin Endocrinol* 1986;**24**:141.)

mal circulating TSH levels and detect suppressed levels (Fig 10–27). The normal range for serum TSH is 0.5–5 μU/mL (0.5–5 mU/L). In hyperthyroidism due to Graves' disease, toxic nodular goiter, or high-dose thyroxine therapy, TSH levels are usually suppressed or undetectable, except in the rare situation of hyperthyroidism due to a TSH-secreting pituitary tumor. Serum TSH is also low in patients with pituitary insufficiency. In primary hypothyroidism, TSH levels are markedly elevated. In hypothyroidism due to hypothalamic disease, TSH levels may be in the normal range, but after injection of TRH response is blunted and delayed (Fig 10–16). Note that corticosteroids and dopamine inhibit TSH secretion, which will modify the interpretation of serum TSH levels in patients taking these drugs.

The ultrasensitive technique for measuring serum TSH levels has become the most sensitive, convenient, and specific test for the diagnosis of both hypothyroidism and hyperthyroidism. Indeed, a suppressed TSH level correlates very well with an impaired pituitary response to TRH, and simple measurement of serum TSH has replaced the TRH test in the diagnosis of hyperthyroidism.

Thyrotropin-Releasing Hormone (TRH) Test

The TRH test may be regarded as a test of the metabolic effects of the thyroid hormones on peripheral tissues, in this case, the thyrotrophs. In hyperthyroidism, the TSH response to TRH is dampened or abolished, and in primary hypothyroidism the maximum response is enhanced (Figs 10–15 and 10–16). The TRH response is slightly greater in females than in males. A normal response is a 2- to 5-fold increase over basal serum TSH 15–30 minutes after intravenous injection of 500 μg of TRH. With the ultrasensitive TSH method, in euthyroid individuals, TSH should increase more than 6 μU/mL (6 mU/L) at 30–45 minutes. (see Table 6–5).

The TRH test is the only test available to distinguish between secondary (pituitary) and tertiary (hypothalamic) hypothyroidism (Fig 10–16). In the former, TSH response to TRH is decreased or absent. In the latter, despite low serum TSH levels in association with low serum T_4 and T_3 levels, TSH response to injected TRH is adequate but sometimes delayed.

TSH Stimulation and Suppression Tests

The TSH stimulation test involved intramuscular administration of bovine TSH followed by determination of RAIU. Originally devised to determine the degree of thyroid reserve in hypothyroidism, this test has been superseded by direct measurement of the endogenous TSH level in serum. The TSH suppression test involves suppression of endogenous TSH by oral administration of T_3 followed by measurement of RAIU. This was originally used to detect autonomous thyroid function, as in Graves' disease or in autonomously functioning thyroid nodules. However, autonomous thyroid function can easily be diagnosed by the demonstration of thyroid RAIU in the presence of a suppressed serum TSH, so that the suppression test is rarely indicated.

MEASUREMENT OF PATHOLOGIC THYROID AUTOANTIBODIES

Thyroglobulin Autoantibodies and Thyroid Microsomal (Thyroid Peroxidase) Autoantibodies

Many of these antibodies are present in the serum of patients with autoimmune thyroid disease, while some are present in other thyroid conditions. The clinical value of their measurement will be discussed in subsequent sections of this chapter. These antibodies were originally assayed by a hemagglutination technique, but now they are usually measured by immunoradiometric assay. The lower limit of detectability varies with the method and the laboratory.

Thyroid-Stimulating Immunoglobulins (TSI)

Thyroid-stimulating immunoglobulin (TSI) is an autoantibody against the TSH receptor on the surface of the thyroid cell. It may mediate the thyrotoxicosis of Graves' disease (see below). It was discovered when serum from patients with Graves' disease was injected into animals pretreated with radioiodine, and radioiodine was discharged from the gland. It acted like TSH but had a long duration of action, so that it was initially called **long-acting thyroid stimulator (LATS).** The assay in mice was laborious and insensitive. It has been replaced by the **thyroid cAMP assay.** Serum—or IgG—from a patient with Graves' disease is tested for its ability to stimulate cAMP generation in human thyroid tissue—either slices or thyroid cells cultured in monolayers. The disadvantage of the slice assay is the need for fresh human thyroid tissue. Cultured thyroid cells provide a continuous source of material and have allowed the development of a sensitive, specific, and readily available test for TSI. It is positive in about 90% of patients with Graves' disease and undetectable in healthy subjects or patients with Hashimoto's thyroiditis (without concurrent Graves' ophthalmopathy), nontoxic goiter, and toxic nodular goiter. Thus, it can be of great value in the diagnosis of autoimmune Graves' disease in euthyroid patients with ophthalmopathy, and it may be useful to predict neonatal Graves' disease in the newborn of a mother with active or past Graves' disease.

A **TSH binding inhibition (TBI)** assay has been developed to simplify the above bioassay. This assay involves the binding of radiolabeled bovine or human TSH to human thyroid plasma membranes. This binding is inhibited to varying degrees by sera or IgG from patients with active Graves' disease. It is not a measure of TSI, since it does not measure biologic activity. While this assay is convenient and has a low false-negative rate, it is plagued by false-positive results. Thus, a wide variety of nonspecific interfering substances, such as thyroglobulin, inhibit TSH binding. In addition, results of the TSI and the TBI assay using the same test sera correlate poorly.

DISORDERS OF THE THYROID

Patients with thyroid disease will usually complain of (1) thyroid enlargement, or goiter; (2) symptoms of thyroid deficiency, or hypothyroidism; (3) symptoms of thyroid hormone excess, or hyperthyroidism; or (4) complications of a specific form of hyperthyroidism, Graves' disease, which may present with striking prominence of the eyes (exophthalmos) or, rarely, thickening of the skin over the lower legs (thyroid dermopathy).

The **history** should include evaluation of symptoms related to the above complaints, discussed in more detail below. Exposure to ionizing radiation in child-

hood has been associated with an increased incidence of thyroid disease, including cancer. Iodide ingestion in the form of kelp or iodide-containing cough preparations may induce goiter, hypothyroidism, or hyperthyroidism. Lithium carbonate, used in the treatment of manic-depressive psychiatric disorder, can also induce hypothyroidism and goiter. Residence in an area of low dietary iodide is associated with iodine-deficiency goiter, or "endemic goiter." Although dietary iodide is generally adequate in developed countries, there are still areas low in natural iodine (ie, developing countries in Africa, Asia, South America, and inland mountainous areas). Finally, the family history should be explored with particular reference to goiter, hyperthyroidism, or hypothyroidism, as well as immunologic disorders such as diabetes, rheumatoid disease, pernicious anemia, or myasthenia gravis, which may be associated with an increased incidence of thyroid disease. Multiple endocrine neoplasia type IIa (Sipple's syndrome) with medullary carcinoma of the thyroid gland is an autosomal dominant condition.

Physical examination of the thyroid gland is illustrated in Fig 10–28. The thyroid is firmly attached to the anterior trachea midway between the sternal notch and the thyroid cartilage; it is often easy to see and to palpate. The patient should have a glass of water for comfortable swallowing. There are 3 maneuvers: (1) With a good light coming from behind the examiner, have the patient swallow a sip of water. Observe the gland as it moves up and down. Enlargement and nodularity can often be noted. (2) Palpate the gland anteriorly. Gently press down with one thumb on one side of the gland to rotate the other lobe forward, and palpate as the patient swallows. (3) Palpate the gland from behind the patient with the middle 3 fingers on each lobe while the patient swallows. An outline of the gland can be traced on the skin of the neck and measured (Fig 10–28D). Nodules can be measured in a similar way. Thus, changes in the size of the gland or in nodules can be followed.

Each lobe of the normal thyroid gland measures about 2 cm in vertical dimension and about 1 cm in horizontal dimension above the isthmus. An enlarged thyroid gland has been called **goiter** (derived from French; ultimately from Latin *guttur* "throat"). Generalized enlargement is termed **diffuse goiter;** irregular or lumpy enlargement is called **nodular goiter.**

HYPOTHYROIDISM

Hypothyroidism is a clinical syndrome resulting from a deficiency of thyroid hormones, which in turn results in a generalized slowing down of metabolic processes. Hypothyroidism in infants and children results in marked slowing of growth and development, with serious permanent consequences including mental retardation. Hypothyroidism with onset in adulthood causes a generalized slowing down of the orga-

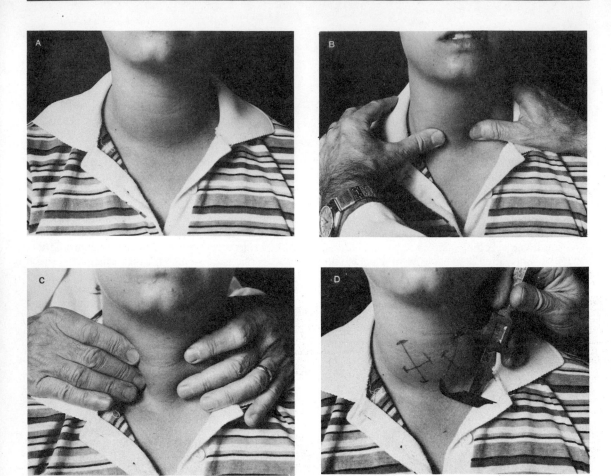

Figure 10–28. Examination of the thyroid gland. *A:* Observe the neck, especially as the patient swallows. *B:* Examine from the front, rotating the gland slightly with one thumb while palpating the other lobe with the other thumb. *C:* Examine from behind, using 3 fingers and the same technique. *D:* The size of each lobe or of thyroid nodules can be measured by first drawing an outline on the skin.

nism, with the deposition of glycosaminoglycans in intracellular spaces, particularly in skin and muscle, producing the clinical picture of **myxedema.** The symptoms of hypothyroidism in adults are largely reversible with therapy.

Etiology
(Table 10–6)

Hypothyroidism may be classified in a number of ways. It may be primary (thyroid failure), secondary (to pituitary TSH deficit), or tertiary (due to hypothalamic deficiency of TRH); or there may be an abnormality of the thyroxine (T_4) receptor in the cell, inducing peripheral resistance to the action of thyroid hormones. Hypothyroidism can also be classified as goitrous or nongoitrous, but this is probably unsatisfactory since Hashimoto's thyroiditis may produce hypothyroidism with or without goiter. The incidence of various causes of hypothyroidism will vary depending on geographic and environmental factors

Table 10–6. Etiology of hypothyroidism.

Primary:
1. Hashimoto's thyroiditis:
   a. With goiter.
   b. "Idiopathic" thyroid atrophy, presumably end-stage autoimmune thyroid disease, following either Hashimoto's thyroiditis or Graves' disease.
2. Radioactive iodine therapy for Graves' disease.
3. Subtotal thyroidectomy for Graves' disease or nodular goiter.
4. Excessive iodide intake (kelp, radiocontrast dyes).
5. Subacute thyroiditis.
6. Rare causes in the USA:
   a. Iodide deficiency.
   b. Other goitrogens such as lithium; antithyroid drug therapy.
   c. Inborn errors of thyroid hormone synthesis.

Secondary: Hypopituitarism due to pituitary adenoma, pituitary ablative therapy, or pituitary destruction.
Tertiary: Hypothalamic dysfunction (rare).
Peripheral resistance to the action of thyroid hormone.

such as dietary iodide and goitrogen intake, the genetic characteristics of the population, and the age distribution of the population (pediatric or adult). The causes of hypothyroidism, listed in the approximate order of their frequency in an adult population in the USA, are presented in Table 10–6.

Hashimoto's thyroiditis is probably the most common cause of hypothyroidism. In younger patients, it is more likely to be associated with goiter; in older patients, the gland may be totally destroyed by the immunologic process, and the only trace of the disease will be a persistently positive test for thyroid microsomal autoantibodies. Similarly, the end stage of Graves' disease may be hypothyroidism. This is accelerated by destructive therapy such as administration of radioactive iodine or subtotal thyroidectomy. Thyroid glands involved in autoimmune disease are particularly susceptible to excessive iodide intake (eg, ingestion of kelp tablets, iodide-containing cough preparations, or the antiarrhythmic drug amiodarone) or administration of iodide-containing radiographic contrast media. The large amounts of iodide block thyroid hormone synthesis, producing hypothyroidism with goiter in the patient with an abnormal thyroid gland; the normal gland usually "escapes" from the iodide block (see above). Although the process may be temporarily reversed by withdrawal of iodide, the underlying disease will often progress, and permanent hypothyroidism will usually supervene. Hypothyroidism may occur during the late phase of subacute thyroiditis; this is usually transient, but it is permanent in about 10% of patients. Iodide deficiency is rarely a cause of hypothyroidism in the USA but may be more common in developing countries. Certain drugs can block hormone synthesis and produce hypothyroidism with goiter; at present, the most common pharmacologic cause of hypothyroidism (other than iodide) is lithium carbonate, used for the treatment of manic-depressive states. The antithyroid drugs propylthiouracil and methimazole in continuous dosage will do the same. Inborn errors of thyroid hormone synthesis will result in severe hypothyroidism if the block in hormone synthesis is complete or will result in mild hypothyroidism if the block is partial.

Pituitary and hypothalamic deficiencies as causes for hypothyroidism are quite rare and are usually associated with other symptoms and signs. Peripheral resistance to thyroid hormones is extremely rare, occurs in families, and is characterized by high serum concentrations of T_4 and T_3, goiter, and features of hypothyroidism rather than hyperthyroidism.

Pathogenesis

Thyroid hormone deficiency affects every tissue in the body, so that the symptoms are multiple. Pathologically, the most characteristic finding is the accumulation of glycosaminoglycans—mostly hyaluronic acid—in interstitial tissues. Accumulation of this hydrophilic substance accounts for the interstitial edema that is particularly evident in the skin, heart muscle, and striated muscle. The accumulation is due not to excessive synthesis but to decreased destruction of glycosaminoglycans.

Clinical Presentations & Findings

A. Newborn Infants (Cretinism): The term cretinism was originally applied in endemic goiter areas to infants with mental retardation, short stature, a characteristic puffy appearance of the face and hands, and (frequently) deaf mutism and pyramidal tract signs (Fig 10–29). In the USA, neonatal screening programs have revealed that approximately one out of 4000 neonates will have a low T_4 and elevated TSH, indicative of primary neonatal hypothyroidism. This may be due to failure of the thyroid to descend during embryonic development from its origin at the base of the tongue to its usual site in the lower anterior neck, which results in an "ectopic thyroid" gland that functions poorly. Another cause of neonatal hypothyroidism is placental transfer of thyroid antibodies in a mother with Hashimoto's thyroiditis, which results in blocking of TSH action or antibody-related immune destruction of the fetal thyroid. Rare causes of neonatal hypothyroid-

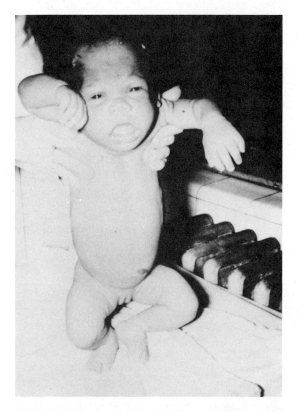

Figure 10–29. A 9-month-old infant with hypothyroidism (cretinism). Note the puffy face, protuberant abdomen, umbilical hernia, and muscle weakness (infant cannot sit up unassisted).

ism include administration during pregnancy of iodides, antithyroid drugs, or radioactive iodine for thyrotoxicosis.

The symptoms of hypothyroidism in newborns include respiratory difficulty, cyanosis, jaundice, poor feeding, hoarse cry, umbilical hernia, and marked retardation of bone maturation. The proximal tibial epiphysis and distal femoral epiphysis are present in almost all full-term infants with a body weight of over 2500 g. Absence of these epiphyses strongly suggests hypothyroidism. Because early treatment is essential to prevent permanent mental retardation, neonatal screening programs have been introduced to measure serum T_4 or TSH: A serum T_4 under 6 μg/dL or a serum TSH over 30 μU/mL is indicative of neonatal hypothyroidism. The diagnosis can then be confirmed by radiologic evidence of retarded bone age.

B. Children: Hypothyroidism in children is characterized by retarded growth and evidence of mental retardation. In the adolescent, precocious puberty may occur, and there may be enlargement of the sella turcica in addition to short stature. This is not due to pituitary tumor but probably to pituitary hypertrophy associated with excessive TSH production.

C. Adults: In adults, the common features of hypothyroidism include easy fatigability, coldness, weight gain, constipation, menstrual irregularities, and muscle cramps. Physical findings include a cool, dry skin, puffy face and hands, hoarse, husky voice, and slow reflexes (Fig 10–30). Reduced conversion of carotene

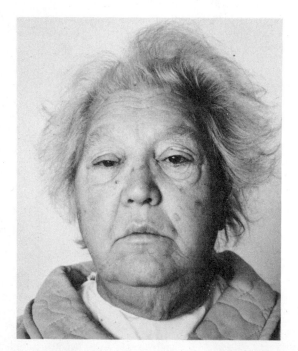

Figure 10–30. Hypothyroidism in adult (myxedema). Note puffy face, puffy eyes, frowsy hair, and dull and apathetic appearance.

to vitamin A and increased blood levels of carotene may give the skin a yellowish color.

Cardiovascular signs include bradycardia and cardiac enlargement; the enlargement may be due in part to interstitial edema and left ventricular dilatation but is often due to pericardial effusion (Fig 10–31). The ECG reveals low voltage of QRS complexes and P and T waves, with improvement on therapy. The degree of pericardial effusion can easily be determined by echocardiography. Cardiac output is reduced, although congestive heart failure and pulmonary edema are rarely noted. Although there is controversy about whether myxedema induces coronary artery disease, there is evidence that coronary artery disease is more common in patients with hypothyroidism, particularly in older patients. For this reason, it is important to start levothyroxine replacement therapy in myxedematous patients over age 50 with very small doses, increasing the dose slowly over a period of several months.

Pulmonary function in adult hypothyroidism is characterized by shallow, slow respirations and impaired ventilatory responses to hypercapnia or hypoxia. This feature is important in the development of myxedema coma.

Intestinal peristalsis is markedly slowed, resulting in chronic constipation and occasionally severe fecal impaction.

Renal function is impaired, with decreased glomerular filtration rate and impaired ability to excrete a water load. This predisposes the myxedematous patient to water intoxication if excessive free water is administered.

There are at least 4 mechanisms that may contribute to **anemia** in patients with hypothyroidism: (1) impaired hemoglobin synthesis as a result of thyroxine deficiency; (2) iron deficiency from increased iron loss with menorrhagia, as well as impaired intestinal absorption of iron; (3) foliate deficiency from impaired intestinal absorption of folic acid; and (4) pernicious anemia, with vitamin B_{12}-deficient megaloblastic anemia. The pernicious anemia is often part of a spectrum of autoimmune diseases: myxedema due to chronic thyroiditis, with thyroid autoantibodies present; pernicious anemia with parietal cell autoantibodies present; diabetes mellitus with islet cell autoantibodies present; adrenal insufficiency with adrenal autoantibodies present; etc (see Chapter 28).

Many patients complain of symptoms referable to the **neuromuscular system,** eg, severe muscle cramps, paresthesias, and muscle weakness.

Central nervous system symptoms may include chronic fatigue, lethargy, and inability to concentrate.

Hypothyroidism impairs peripheral metabolism of estrogens, with altered FSH and LH secretion, resulting in anovulatory cycles and infertility. This may also be associated with severe menorrhagia.

Patients with myxedema are usually quite placid but can be severely depressed or even extremely agitated ("myxedema madness").

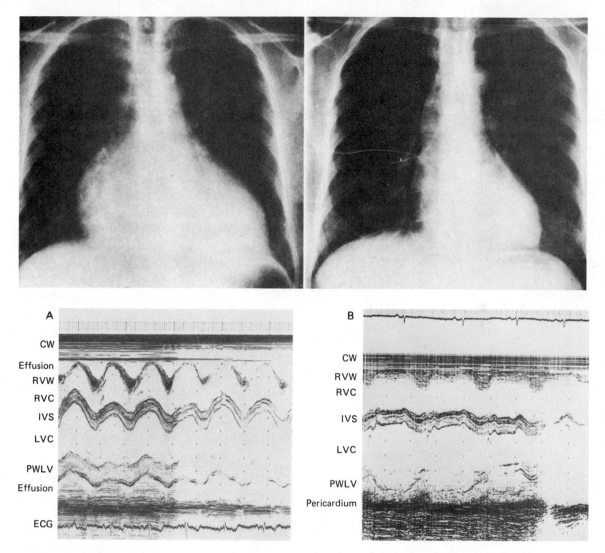

Figure 10–31. *Top:* Chest x-ray studies of patient with hypothyroid cardiomyopathy. *Left:* Before therapy, showing pronounced cardiomegaly. *Right:* Six months after institution of thyroxine therapy, the heart size has returned to normal. (Reproduced, with permission, from Reza MJ, Abbasi AS: Congestive cardiomyopathy in hypothyroidism. *West J Med* 1975;**123**:228.) *Bottom:* Echocardiogram of a 29-year-old woman with hypothyroidism *(A)* before and *(B)* after 2 months of therapy with levothyroxine sodium (Synthroid). CW = chest wall; RVW = right ventricular wall; RVC = right ventricular cavity; IVS = interventricular septum; LVC = left ventricular cavity; PWLV = posterior wall left ventricle. Note disappearance of pericardial effusion following levothyroxine therapy. (Reproduced, with permission, from Sokolow M, McIlroy MB: *Clinical Cardiology,* 4th ed. Lange, 1986.)

Diagnosis

The laboratory diagnosis of hypothyroidism is not difficult (Fig 10–32). A low serum T_4, low free thyroxine index, low free thyroxine, and elevated serum TSH are characteristic of primary hypothyroidism. Serum T_3 levels are variable and may be within the normal range. A positive test for thyroid autoantibodies suggests underlying Hashimoto's thyroiditis. In patients with pituitary myxedema, the FT_4I or FT_4 will be low but serum TSH will not be elevated. To differentiate pituitary from hypothalamic disease, the TRH test is most helpful (Fig 10–16). An elevated basal TSH level with excessive response indicates primary hypothyroidism. Absence of TSH response to TRH indicates pituitary deficiency. A partial or "normal" response indicates that pituitary function is intact but that a defect exists in hypothalamic secretion of TRH. Since pituitary or hypothalamic hypothyroidism is rare, TRH tests are usually unnecessary in the diagnosis of hypothyroidism.

The patient may be taking thyroid medication (levothyroxine or desiccated thyroid tablets) when first

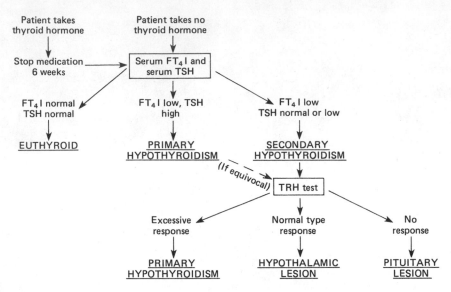

Figure 10–32. Diagnosis of hypothyroidism. Either free thyroxine (FT_4) or free thyroxine index (FT_4I) may be used with TSH for evaluation.

seen. A palpable thyroid gland and a positive test for thyroid autoantibodies would suggest underlying Hashimoto's thyroiditis, in which case the medication should be continued. If antibodies are absent, the medication should be withdrawn for 6 weeks and determinations made for FT_4I or FT_4 and for TSH. The 6-week period of withdrawal is necessary because of the long half-life of thyroxine (8 days) and to allow the pituitary gland to recover after a long period of suppression. The pattern of recovery of thyroid function after withdrawal of T_4 is noted in Fig 10–33. In hypothyroid individuals, TSH becomes markedly elevated at 5–6 weeks and T_4 remains subnormal, whereas both are normal after 6 weeks in euthyroid controls.

In patients with hypothyroidism, a delay in muscle contraction and relaxation is usually evident on physical examination, particularly in the biceps reflex. The speed of contraction and partial relaxation of the Achilles tendon reflex can be measured by the "photomotogram" (see above). Improvement in reflex contraction and relaxation time will coincide with the clinical response to appropriate therapy.

The clinical picture of fully developed myxedema is usually quite clear, but the symptoms and signs of mild hypothyroidism may be very subtle. Patients with hypothyroidism will at times present with unusual features—neurasthenia with symptoms of muscle cramps, paresthesias, and weakness; anemia; disturbances in reproductive function, including infertility, delayed puberty, or menorrhagia; idiopathic edema or pleuropericardial effusions; retarded growth; obstipation; chronic rhinitis or hoarseness due to edema of nasal mucosa on vocal cords; and severe depression progressing to emotional instability or even frank paranoid psychosis. In such cases, the diagnostic studies

outlined above will confirm or rule out hypothyroidism as a contributing factor.

Complications

A. Myxedema Coma: Myxedema coma is the end stage of untreated hypothyroidism. It is characterized by progressive weakness, stupor, hypothermia, hypoventilation, hypoglycemia, hyponatremia, water intoxication, shock, and death. Although rare now, in the future it may occur more frequently in association with the increasing use of radioiodine for the treatment of Graves' disease, with resulting permanent hypothyroidism. Since it occurs most frequently in older patients with underlying pulmonary and vascular disease, the mortality rate is extremely high.

The patient (or a family member if the patient is comatose) may recall previous thyroid disease, radioiodine therapy, or thyroidectomy. The medical history is of gradual onset of lethargy progressing to stupor or coma. Examination shows bradycardia and marked hypothermia, with body temperature as low as 24 °C (75 °F). The patient is usually an obese elderly woman with yellowish skin, a hoarse voice, a large tongue, thin hair, puffy eyes, ileus, and slow reflexes. There may be signs of other illnesses such as pneumonia, myocardial infarction, cerebral thrombosis, or gastrointestinal bleeding.

Laboratory clues to the diagnosis of myxedema coma include lactescent serum, high serum carotene, elevated serum cholesterol, and increased cerebrospinal fluid protein. Pleural, pericardial, or abdominal effusions with high protein content may be present. Serum tests will reveal a low T_4(RIA), low FT_4I, and usually a markedly elevated TSH. Thyroidal radioactive iodine uptake is low, and thyroid autoantibodies

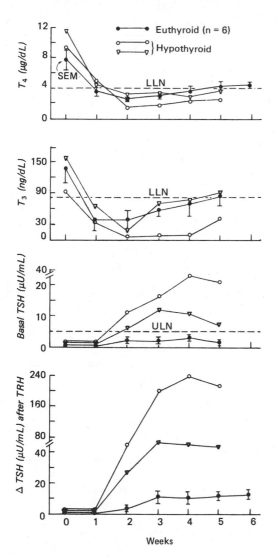

Figure 10–33. Changes in T_4, T_3, TSH, and TRH response following abrupt withdrawal of suppressive thyroxine therapy. Note that in euthyroid individuals the T_4 may not return to normal until 6 weeks after withdrawal of therapy and that serum TSH is never elevated. In hypothyroid patients, TSH may be elevated as early as 2 weeks after withdrawal of therapy, and TRH response is exaggerated. LLN = lower limit of normal; ULN = upper limit of normal. (Reproduced, with permission, from Wood LC: Controversial questions in thyroid disease. Workshop in the Thyroid, American Thyroid Association, Nov 1979, as adapted from Vagenakis AG et al: Recovery of pituitary thyrotropic function after withdrawal of prolonged thyroid suppression therapy. *N Engl J Med* 1975;**293**:681.)

are usually strongly positive, indicating underlying thyroiditis. The ECG shows sinus bradycardia and low voltage. If laboratory studies are not readily available, which is frequently the case, the diagnosis must be made clinically.

The pathophysiology of myxedema coma involves 3 major aspects: (1) CO_2 retention and hypoxia, (2) fluid and electrolyte imbalance, and (3) hypothermia. CO_2 retention has long been recognized as an integral part of myxedema coma and had been attributed to such factors as obesity, heart failure, ileus, immobilization, pneumonia, pleural or peritoneal effusions, central nervous system depression, and weak chest muscles. However, Zwillich et al have demonstrated that the ventilatory responses to hypoxia are markedly depressed in patients with myxedema, as are the ventilatory responses to hypercapnia. These authors suggest that the failure of the myxedema patient to respond to hypoxia or hypercapnia may be associated with hypothermia. Thyroid hormone therapy in patients with myxedema markedly improves the ventilatory response to hypoxia. Because of the impaired ventilatory drive, assisted respiration is almost always necessary in patients with myxedema coma. The major fluid and electrolyte disturbance is water intoxication due to the syndrome of inappropriate secretion of vasopressin (SIADH). This presents as hyponatremia and is managed by water restriction. Hypothermia is frequently not recognized, because the ordinary clinical thermometer only goes down to about 34 °C (94 °F); a laboratory type thermometer that registers a broader scale must be used to obtain accurate body temperature readings. Active rewarming of the body is contraindicated, because it may induce vasodilatation and vascular collapse. A rise in body temperature is a useful indication of therapeutic effectiveness of thyroxine.

Other disorders that may precipitate myxedema coma include heart failure, pulmonary edema, pleural or peritoneal effusions, ileus, and anemia. Adrenal insufficiency occurs occasionally in association with myxedema coma, but it is relatively rare and usually associated with either pituitary myxedema or concurrent autoimmune adrenal insufficiency (Schmidt's syndrome). Drug intoxication is quite common, and myxedema coma that develops in the hospital may be precipitated by administration of sedatives or narcotics. Seizures, bleeding episodes, hypocalcemia, or hypercalcemia may be present.

It is important to differentiate pituitary myxedema from primary myxedema. In pituitary myxedema, adrenal insufficiency may be present, and adrenal replacement is essential. Clinical clues to the presence of pituitary myxedema include a history of amenorrhea or impotence and physical evidence of scanty pubic or axillary hair. Laboratory findings will usually reveal normal serum cholesterol and normal or low pituitary TSH levels. On skull x-ray, the sella turcica may be enlarged. The treatment of myxedema coma is discussed below.

B. Myxedema With Heart Disease: Hypothyroidism has a direct effect upon the myocardium, causing interstitial edema, nonspecific myofibrillary swelling, and pericardial effusion, manifested by bradycardia and diminished cardiac output. These

Table 10–7. Equivalence and cost of preparations available for the treatment of hypothyroidism.

	Average Daily Adult Dose (mg/d)	Approximate Daily Cost[1]	Comment
Levothyroxine (T$_4$)	0.15	$0.14	Best preparation.
Liothyronine sodium (T$_3$)	0.05	0.16	Difficult to monitor. Multiple doses required.
Desiccated thyroid	90	0.07	Variable potency.
Thyroglobulin	90	0.06	Difficult to monitor.
Liotrix (T$_4$/T$_3$ mixture)	(a) T$_4$ 0.075, T$_3$ 0.019 (b) T$_4$ 0.09, T$_3$ 0.023	0.27	Two different formulas.

[1]Data from: *Redbook Update* (Dec) 1988;**7**.

complications are usually completely reversible with appropriate therapy.

C. Myxedema With Coronary Artery Disease: Since myxedema frequently occurs in older persons, it is often associated with underlying coronary artery disease. In this situation, the low levels of circulating thyroid hormone actually protect the heart against increased demands that would result in increasing angina pectoris or myocardial infarction. Correction of the myxedema must be done very cautiously in order not to provoke arrhythmia, angina, or acute myocardial infarction. In some patients, coronary bypass surgery to improve coronary circulation is needed before full replacement therapy can be instituted.

Treatment

Hypothyroidism is treated with levothyroxine, which is available in pure form and is stable and inexpensive (Table 10–7). Levothyroxine is converted in the body in part to T$_3$, so that both hormones become available even though only one is administered. Desiccated thyroid is unsatisfactory because of its variable hormone content, and triiodothyronine (as liothyronine) is unsatisfactory because of its rapid absorption, short half-life, and transient effects. The half-life of levothyroxine is about 8 days, so it need be given only once daily. Although only 60–80% of the preparation is absorbed, blood levels are easily monitored by following the free thyroxine index and serum TSH levels. Replacement doses of levothyroxine in adults range from 0.05 to 0.2 mg/d, with a mean of 0.125 mg/d. In infants under 1 year of age, the dose of levothyroxine is about 6 μg/kg/d; in older children (2–12 years), the dose is about 2–4 μg/kg/d; and in adults, the dose is about 1.7 μg/kg/d, or about 0.8 μg/lb/d. For TSH suppression, which is used to treat patients with nodular goiters or cancers of the thyroid gland, the average dose of levothyroxine is about 2.2 μg/kg/d (1 μg/lb/d).

Treatment of Complications

A. Myxedema Coma: Myxedema coma is an acute medical emergency and should be treated in the intensive care unit. Blood gases must be monitored regularly, and the patient usually requires intubation and me-

chanical ventilation. Associated illnesses such as infections must be sought and treated by appropriate therapy. Intravenous fluids should be administered with caution, and excessive free water intake must be avoided.

Because patients with myxedema coma absorb all drugs poorly, it is imperative to give levothyroxine intravenously. Holvey et al pointed out that these patients have marked depletion of serum thyroxine and a large number of empty binding sites on thyroxine-binding globulin and therefore should receive an initial loading dose of thyroxine intravenously, followed by a small daily intravenous dose. An initial dose of 300–400 μg of levothyroxine is administered intravenously, followed by 50 μg of levothyroxine intravenously daily. The clinical guides to improvement are a rise in body temperature and the return of normal cerebral and respiratory function. If the patient is known to have had normal adrenal function before the coma, adrenal support is probably not necessary. If, however, no data is available, the possibility of concomitant adrenal insufficiency (due to autoimmune adrenal disease or pituitary insufficiency) does exist, so full adrenal support should be administered, eg, hydrocortisone hemisuccinate 100 mg intravenously followed by 50 mg intravenously every 6 hours, tapering the dose over 7 days.

When giving levothyroxine intravenously in large doses, there is an inherent risk of precipitating angina, heart failure, or arrhythmias in older patients with underlying coronary artery disease. Thus, this type of therapy is not recommended for ambulatory patients with myxedema; it is better to start slowly and build up the dose as noted above.

B. Myxedema With Heart Disease: In longstanding hypothyroidism or in older patients, particularly those with cardiovascular disease, it is imperative to start treatment slowly. Levothyroxine is given in a dosage of 0.025 mg/d for 2 weeks, increasing by 0.025 mg every 2 weeks until a daily dose of 0.1 or 0.125 mg is reached. It usually takes about 2 months for a patient to come into equilibrium on full dosage. In these patients, the heart is very sensitive to the level of circulating thyroxine, and if angina pectoris or cardiac arrhythmia develops, it is essential to reduce the dose of thyroxine immediately. In younger patients, or patients with mild disease, full replacement may be started immediately.

Course & Prognosis

The course of untreated myxedema is one of slow deterioration leading eventually to myxedema coma and death. With appropriate treatment, however, the long-term prognosis is excellent. Because of the long half-life (7 days) of thyroxine, it takes time to establish equilibrium on a fixed dose. Therefore, it is important to monitor the free thyroxine index and TSH levels every 4–6 weeks until a normal balance is reached. Thereafter, the patient must be maintained on replacement therapy for life, with free thyroxine index and TSH monitoring about once a year.

The mortality rate of myxedema coma was about 80% at one time. The prognosis has been vastly improved by recognition of the importance of mechanically assisted respiration and the use of intravenous levothyroxine. At present, the outcome probably depends upon how well the underlying disease problems can be managed.

HYPERTHYROIDISM & THYROTOXICOSIS

Thyrotoxicosis is the clinical syndrome that results when tissues are exposed to high levels of circulating thyroid hormone. In most instances, thyrotoxicosis is due to hyperactivity of the thyroid gland, or hyperthyroidism. Occasionally, thyrotoxicosis may be due to other causes such as excessive ingestion of thyroid hormone or excessive secretion of thyroid hormone from ectopic sites. The various forms of thyrotoxicosis are listed in Table 10–8. These syndromes will be discussed individually below.

1. DIFFUSE TOXIC GOITER (Graves' Disease)

Graves' disease is the most common form of thyrotoxicosis and may occur at any age, more commonly in females than in males. The syndrome consists of one or more of the following features: (1) thyrotoxicosis, (2) goiter, (3) ophthalmopathy (exophthalmos), and (4) dermopathy (pretibial myxedema).

Table 10–8. Conditions associated with thyrotoxicosis.

1. Diffuse toxic goiter (Graves' disease).
2. Toxic adenoma (Plummer's disease).
3. Toxic multinodular goiter (Marine-Lenhart syndrome).
4. Subacute thyroiditis.
5. Hyperthyroid phase of Hashimoto's thyroiditis.
6. Thyrotoxicosis factitia.
7. Rare forms of thyrotoxicosis: ovarian struma, metastatic thyroid carcinoma (follicular), hydatidiform mole, TSH-secreting pituitary tumor.

Etiology

The cause of Graves' disease is not known. There is a strong familial predisposition in that about 15% of patients with Graves' disease have a close relative with the same disorder, and about 50% of relatives of patients with Graves' disease have circulating thyroid autoantibodies. Females are involved about 5 times more commonly than males. The disease may occur at any age, with a peak incidence in the 20- to 40-year age group. Human leukocyte antigen (HLA) typing has indicated an increased frequency of HLA-B8 and DR3 in Caucasian, HLA-Bw35 in Japanese, and HLA-Bw46/Bw40 in Chinese patients with Graves' disease and in their relatives, indicating a genetic factor in the pathogenesis of the disease.

Pathogenesis

Graves' disease is currently viewed as an autoimmune disease in which T lymphocytes become sensitized to antigens within the thyroid gland and stimu-

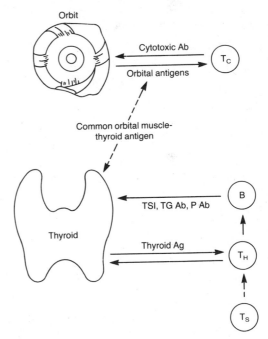

Figure 10–34. One theory of the pathogenesis of Graves' disease. There is a defect in suppressor T lymphocytes (T_S) that allows helper T lymphocytes (T_H) to stimulate B lymphocytes (B) to synthesize thyroid autoantibodies. The thyroid-stimulating immunoglobulin (TSI) is the driving force for thyrotoxicosis. The inflammatory process in the orbital muscles may be due to sensitization of cytotoxic T lymphocytes (T_C), or killer cells, to orbital antigens in association with cytotoxic antibodies. The thyroid and the eye may be linked by a common antigen in thyroid and orbital muscle. It is not yet clear what triggers this immunologic cascade. (Tg Ab = thyroglobulin antibody; P Ab = Peroxidase or microsomal antibody; Ag = Antigen; Ab = antibody)

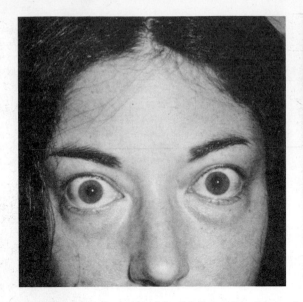 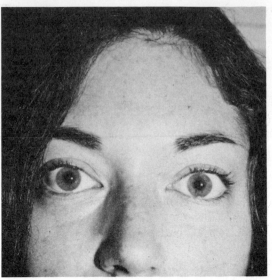

Figure 10–35. Patient with mild ophthalmopathy of Graves' disease. *Left:* Before radioactive iodine therapy. Note white sclera visible above and below the iris as well as mild periobital edema. *Classification* (see Table 10–9): class 1, mild; class 2, mild: class 3, mild. *Right:* After radioactive iodine therapy. Marked improvement is noted.

late B lymphocytes to synthesize antibodies to these antigens (Fig 10–34). One such antibody may be directed against the TSH receptor site in the thyroid cell membrane and has the capacity to stimulate the thyroid cell to increased growth and function. This antibody has been called thyroid-stimulating immunoglobulin (TSI). (Initially it was called long-acting thyroid stimulator; see LATS, above.) The presence of this circulating antibody is positively correlated with active disease and with relapse of the disease. It is not clear what "triggers" the acute episode. There may be a defect in immunoregulation that causes the failure of "suppressor" T lymphocyte function, allowing "helper" T lymphocytes to stimulate B lymphocytes to produce immunoglobulins directed against the thyroid gland, some of which would have the capacity to stimulate the thyroid gland as TSI. The pathogenesis of ophthalmopathy may involve cytotoxic lymphocytes (killer cells) and cytotoxic antibodies sensitized to an antigen in both orbital muscle and thyroid tissue. The inflammation of the muscle causes enlargement of the muscles, proptosis of the globes, and diplopia as well as redness, congestion, and conjunctival and periorbital edema. (Figs 10–35 and 10–36). The pathogenesis of thyroid dermopathy (pretibial myxedema) and the rare subperiosteal inflammation has not yet been clarified.

The symptoms of thyrotoxicosis that suggest a catecholamine-excess state include tachycardia, tremor, sweating, lid lag, and stare. Circulating levels of epinephrine are normal; thus, the body may be hyperreactive to catecholamines in this state. This reaction may be due in part to a thyroid hormone-mediated increase in cardiac catecholamine receptors.

Clinical Findings

A. Symptoms and Signs: In younger individuals, common manifestations include palpitations, nervousness, easy fatigability, hyperkinesia, diarrhea, excessive sweating, and preference for cold. There is often marked weight loss without loss of appetite. Thy-

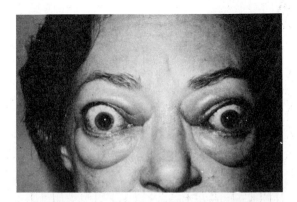

Figure 10–36. Severe ophthalmopathy of Graves' disease. Note marked periorbital edema, injection of corneal blood vessels, and proptosis. There was also striking limitation of upward and lateral eye movements and reduced visual acuity. *Classification* (see Table 10–9): class 1, severe; class 2, severe; class 3, severe; class 4, severe; class 5, none; class 6, mild.

roid enlargement, thyrotoxic eye signs (see below), and mild tachycardia commonly occur. In children, rapid growth with accelerated bone maturation often occurs. In older patients, cardiovascular and myopathic manifestations often predominate. Muscle weakness and loss of muscle mass may be so severe that the patient cannot rise from a chair without assistance. In patients over the age of 60, the most common presenting complaints are palpitation, dyspnea on exertion, tremor, nervousness, and weight loss.

The eye signs of Graves' disease have been classified by the American Thyroid Association as noted in Table 10–9. Note that this classification utilizes the mnemonic "NO SPECS." Class 1 involves spasm of the upper lids associated with active thyrotoxicosis and usually resolves spontaneously when the thyrotoxicosis is adequately controlled. Classes 2 through 6 represent true infiltrative disease involving orbital muscles and orbital tissues (Figs 10–35 and 10–36). Class 2 represents soft tissue involvement with periorbital edema, congestion or redness of the conjunctiva, and swelling of the conjunctiva (chemosis). Class 3 represents proptosis as measured by the Hertel exophthalmometer. This instrument is illustrated in Fig 10–37A. It consists of 2 prisms with a scale, mounted on a bar. The prisms are placed on the lateral orbital ridges, and the distance from the orbital ridge to the anterior cornea is measured on the scale (Fig 10–37B). The upper limits of normal according to race are listed in the footnote to Table 10–9. Class 4 represents muscle involvement. The muscle most commonly involved in the infiltrative process is the inferior rectus, with involvement impairing upward gaze. The muscle second most commonly involved is the medial rectus, with involvement impairing lateral gaze. Class 5 represents corneal involvement (keratitis), and class 6 repre-

Table 10–9. Classification of eye changes in Graves' disease.[1]

Class	Definition
0	No signs or symptoms.
1	Only signs, no symptoms. (Signs limited to upper lid retraction, stare, lid lag.)
2	Soft tissue involvement (symptoms and signs).
3	Proptosis (measured with Hertel exophthalmometer).[2]
4	Extraocular muscle involvement.
5	Corneal involvement.
6	Sight loss (optic nerve involvement).

[1]Reproduced, with permission, from Werner SC: Classification of the eye changes of Graves' disease. *J Clin Endocrinol Metab* 1969;**29**:782 and 1977;**44**:203.
[2]Upper limits of normal according to race: Oriental, 18mm; white, 20 mm; black, 22 mm. Increase in proptosis of 3–4 mm is mild involvement; 5–7 mm, moderate involvement; and over 8 mm, severe involvement. Other classes can be similarly graded as mild, moderate, or severe.

sents loss of vision from optic nerve involvement. Infiltrative ophthalmopathy is due to infiltration of the extraocular muscles with lymphocytes and edema fluid in an acute inflammatory reaction. This produces muscle enlargement with proptosis, periorbital edema, chemosis, and congestion of the conjunctiva (Fig 10–36). In addition, the impaired muscle movement results in diplopia. Ocular muscle enlargement has been demonstrated in orbital CT scans (Fig 10–38). When muscle swelling occurs posteriorly, toward the apex of the orbital cone, the optic nerve is compressed, which may cause loss of vision.

Thyroid dermopathy consists of thickening of the skin, particularly over the lower tibia, due to accumulation of glycosaminoglycans (Fig 10–39). It is relatively rare, occurring in about 2–3% of patients with Graves' disease. It is usually associated with ophthalmopathy. The skin is markedly thickened and

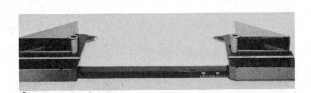
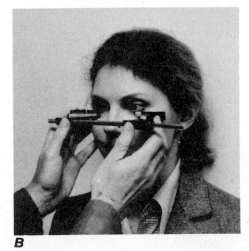

A   **B**

Figure 10–37. *A:* Hertel exophthalmometer. *B:* Proper use of the exophthalmometer. The edges of the instrument are placed on the lateral orbital ridges, and the distance from the orbital bone to the anterior cornea is read on the scale contained within the prisms.

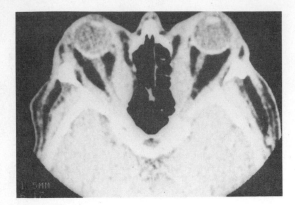

Figure 10–38. Orbital CT scan in a patient with severe ophthalmopathy and visual failure. Note the marked enlargement of extraocular muscles posteriorly, with compression of the optic nerve at the apex of the orbital cone.

cannot be picked up between the fingers. Sometimes dermopathy involves the entire lower leg and may extend onto the feet. Bony involvement (osteopathy), with subperiosteal bone formation and swelling, is particularly evident in the metacarpal bones (Fig 10–40).

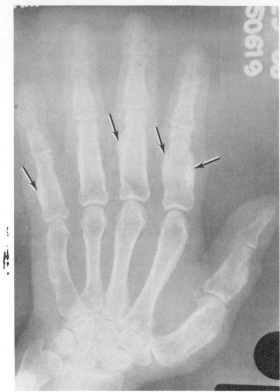

Figure 10–40. X-ray of hand of patient with thyroid osteopathy. Note marked periosteal thickening of the proximal phalanges.

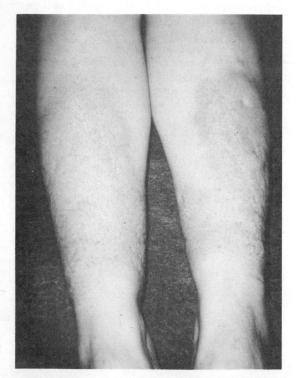

Figure 10–39. Dermopathy of Graves' disease. Marked thickening of the skin is noted, usually over the pretibial area. Thickening will occasionally extend downward over the ankle and the dorsal aspect of the foot but almost never above the knee.

This too is a relatively rare finding. A more common finding in Graves' disease is separation of the nail from its bed, or onycholysis (Fig 10–41).

B. Laboratory Findings: These have been reviewed in the Tests of Thyroid Function section above. Essentially, the combination of an elevated FT_4I and a suppressed TSH diagnoses hyperthyroidism. In early and recurrent Graves' disease, T_3 may be secreted in excess before T_4, so that the serum T_4 may be normal while the T_3 is elevated. Thus, if TSH is suppressed and FT_4I is not elevated, serum T_3 should be measured. Thyroid autoantibodies are usually present, particularly TSI. This may be a useful diagnostic test in the "apathetic" hyperthyroid patient, or in the patient who presents with unilateral exophthalmos without obvious signs of Graves' disease. Radioiodine uptake is helpful to rule out low uptake hyperthyroidism, which may occur as a phase of subacute or Hashimoto's thyroiditis; this type of hyperthyroidism frequently resolves spontaneously. The ^{123}I or technetium scan may be helpful to clarify the size of the gland and to detect the presence of "hot" or "cold" nodules. Since the ultrasensitive TSH test will detect TSH suppression, the TRH test and the TSH suppression test (see above) are rarely indicated. Echography,

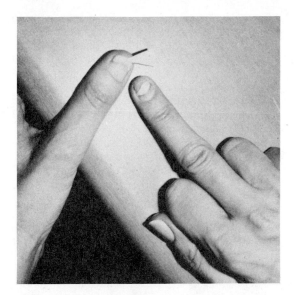

Figure 10–41. Onycholysis (separation of the nail from its bed) in Graves' disease usually resolves spontaneously as the patient improves.

CT, and MRI scans of the orbit have revealed muscle enlargement in most patients with Graves' disease even when there is no clinical evidence of ophthalmopathy. In patients with clinical evidence of ophthalmopathy, orbital muscle enlargement is frequently striking (Fig 10–38).

Differential Diagnosis

Graves' disease occasionally presents in an unusual or atypical fashion, in which case the diagnosis may not be obvious. Marked muscle atrophy may suggest severe myopathy that must be differentiated from primary neurologic disorder. Older patients with Graves' disease may present with symptoms of heart involvement, especially refractory atrial fibrillation or heart failure. This is characterized by high-output heart failure or chronic atrial fibrillation relatively insensitive to digoxin. Finally, patients with Graves' disease may present with infertility and amenorrhea as the primary symptoms. In all of these instances, the diagnosis of Graves' disease can usually be made with the above clinical and laboratory studies.

In the recently recognized syndrome called "familial dysalbuminemic hyperthyroxinemia," an abnormal albumin is present in serum that preferentially binds T_4 but not T_3. This results in elevation of serum T_4 and FT_4I, but free T_4, T_3, and TSH are normal. It is important to differentiate this euthyroid state from hyperthyroidism. In addition to the lack of clinical features of hyperthyroidism, a normal serum T_3 and TSH level and a normal TRH response will rule out Graves' disease or toxic nodular goiter.

Complications

Thyrotoxic crisis ("thyroid storm") is the acute exacerbation of all of the symptoms of thyrotoxicosis, often presenting as a syndrome that may be of life-threatening severity. Occasionally, thyroid storm may be mild and present simply as an unexplained febrile reaction after thyroid surgery in a patient who has been inadequately prepared. More commonly, it occurs in a more severe form, after surgery, radioactive iodine therapy, or parturition in a patient with inadequately controlled thyrotoxicosis, or during a severe, stressful illness or disorder such as uncontrolled diabetes, trauma, acute infection, severe drug reaction, or myocardial infarction. The clinical manifestations of thyroid storm are marked hypermetabolism and excessive adrenergic response. Fever ranges from 38 to 41 °C (from 100 to 106 °F) and is associated with flushing and sweating. There is marked tachycardia, often with atrial fibrillation and high pulse pressure and occasionally with heart failure. Central nervous system symptoms include marked agitation, restlessness, delirium, and coma. Gastrointestinal symptoms will include nausea, vomiting, diarrhea, and jaundice. A fatal outcome will be associated with heart failure and shock.

Originally, "dumping" of stored thyroxine and triiodothyronine was believed to be responsible for thyroid storm. Careful studies have revealed that the serum levels of T_4 and T_3 in patients with thyroid storm are not higher than in thyrotoxic patients without this condition. There is no evidence that thyroid storm is due to excessive production of triiodothyronine. There is evidence that in thyrotoxicosis the number of binding sites for catecholamines increases, so that heart and nervous tissues have increased sensitivity to circulating catecholamines. In addition, there is decreased binding to TBG, with elevation of free T_3 and T_4. The present theory is that in this setting, with increased binding sites available for catecholamines, an acute illness, infection, or surgical stress triggers an outpouring of catecholamines which, in association with high levels of free T_4 and T_3, precipitate the acute problem.

The most striking clinical diagnostic feature of thyrotoxic crisis is hyperpyrexia out of proportion to other findings. Laboratory findings include elevated serum T_4, FT_4I, and T_3 by radioimmunoassay, as well as a suppressed TSH.

Treatment

Although autoimmune mechanisms are responsible for the syndrome of Graves' disease, management has been largely directed toward controlling the hyperthyroidism. Three good methods are available: (1) antithyroid drug therapy, (2) surgery, and (3) radioactive iodine therapy.

A. Antithyroid Drug Therapy: In general, antithyroid drug therapy is most useful in young patients with small glands and mild disease. The drugs (propylthiouracil or methimazole) are given until the disease undergoes spontaneous remission. This occurs in 20–40% of patients treated for 6 months to 15 years. Although this is the only therapy that leaves an intact thyroid gland, it does require a long period of observation, and the incidence of relapse is high, perhaps 60–80% even in selected patients. Antithyroid drug therapy is generally started with large divided doses; when the patient becomes clinically euthyroid, maintenance therapy may be achieved with a lower single morning dose. A common regimen consists of giving propylthiouracil, 100–150 mg every 6 hours initially, and then in 4–8 weeks reducing the dose to 50–200 mg once or twice daily. Propylthiouracil has one advantage over methimazole in that it partially inhibits the conversion of T_4 to T_3, so that it is effective in bringing down the levels of activated thyroid hormone more quickly. However, methimazole has a longer duration of action and is more useful if a single daily dose is desirable. A typical program would start with a 40-mg dose of methimazole each morning for 1–2 months; this dose would then be reduced to 5–20 mg each morning for maintenance therapy. The laboratory tests of most value in monitoring the course of therapy are serum FT_4I and TSH.

1. Duration of Therapy–The duration of therapy with antithyroid drugs in Graves' disease is quite variable and can range from 6 months to 20 years or more. A sustained remission may be predicted in about 80% of treated patients in the following circumstances: (1) The thyroid gland returns to normal size. (2) The disease can be controlled on a relatively small dose of antithyroid drugs. (3) TSI is no longer detectable in the serum. (4) The thyroid gland becomes normally suppressible following the administration of liothyronine.

2. Reaction to Drugs–Reactions to antithyroid drugs most commonly involve either a rash (about 5% of patients) or agranulocytosis (about 0.5% of patients). The rash may frequently be managed by simple addition of antihistamines and is not necessarily an indication for discontinuing the medication unless it is severe and generalized. Agranulocytosis is an indication for immediate cessation of antithyroid drug therapy, institution of appropriate antibiotic therapy, and shifting to an alternative type of therapy. Agranulocytosis is usually heralded by sore throat and fever. Thus, all patients receiving antithyroid drugs are instructed that if sore throat or fever develops, they should immediately stop taking the drug and see a physician, who should obtain a white count and differential count. Cholestatic jaundice, hepatocellular toxicity, and acute arthralgia are rare side effects but require cessation of drug therapy when they do occur.

B. Surgical Treatment: Subtotal thyroidectomy is the treatment of choice for patients with very large glands or multinodular goiters.

The patient is prepared with antithyroid drugs until euthyroid (about 6 weeks). In addition, starting 2 weeks before the day of operation, the patient is given saturated solution of potassium iodide, 5 drops twice daily. This regimen has been shown empirically to diminish the vascularity of the gland and to simplify surgery.

There is disagreement about how much thyroid tissue should be removed. Total thyroidectomy is usually not necessary unless the patient has severe progressive ophthalmopathy (see below). However, if too much thyroid tissue is left behind, the disease will relapse. Most surgeons leave 2–3 g of thyroid tissue on either side of the neck. Many patients require thyroid supplementation following thyroidectomy for Graves' disease.

Hypoparathyroidism and recurrent laryngeal nerve injury occur as complications of surgery in about 1% of cases.

C. Radioactive Iodine Therapy: Therapy with sodium ^{131}I is the preferred treatment for most patients over age 21. In many patients without underlying heart disease, radioactive iodine may be given immediately in a dosage of 80–120 µCi/g of thyroid weight estimated on the basis of physical examination and sodium ^{123}I rectilinear scan. The dosage is corrected for iodine uptake according to the following formula:

$$80–120 \text{ µCi/g} \times \frac{\text{Estimated weight of gland in grams}}{} \times \frac{100}{\text{24-Hour radioactive iodine uptake (\%)}} = \text{Dose in µCi}$$

In patients with underlying heart disease, severe thyrotoxicosis, or large glands (> 100 g), it is desirable to achieve a euthyroid state before radioactive iodine is started. These patients are treated with antithyroid drugs (as above) until they are euthyroid; medication is then stopped for 5–7 days; radioactive iodine uptake is then determined and a scan is done; and a dose of 100–150 µCi/g of estimated thyroid weight is calculated on the basis of this uptake. A slightly larger dose is necessary in patients previously treated with antithyroid drugs. Following the administration of radioactive iodine, the gland will shrink and the patient will usually become euthyroid over a period of 6–12 weeks.

The major complication of radioactive therapy is hypothyroidism, which ultimately develops in 80% or more of patients who are adequately treated. However, this complication may indeed be the best assurance that the patient will not have a recurrence of hyperthyroidism. Serum free thyroxine index and TSH levels should be followed, and if they show the development of hypothyroidism, prompt replacement therapy with levothyroxine, 0.05–0.2 mg daily, is instituted.

Hypothyroidism may occur after any type of therapy for Graves' disease and may occasionally be the outcome of "burned-out" Graves' disease. Accordingly, all patients with Graves' disease require lifetime follow-up to be certain that they remain euthyroid.

D. Other Medical Measures: During the acute phase of thyrotoxicosis, beta-adrenergic blocking agents are extremely helpful. Propranolol, 10–40 mg every 6 hours, will control tachycardia, hypertension, and atrial fibrillation. This drug is gradually withdrawn as serum thyroxine levels return to normal. Adequate nutrition, including multivitamin supplements, is essential. Barbiturates accelerate T_4 metabolism, and phenobarbital may be helpful both for its sedative effect and to lower T_4 levels. Sodium ipodate or iopanoic acid (Oragrafin or Telepaque) has been shown to inhibit both thyroid hormone synthesis and release as well as peripheral conversion of T_4 to T_3. Thus, in a dosage of 1 g daily, this drug may help to rapidly restoring the euthyroid state. It leaves the gland saturated with iodide, so it should not be used before ^{131}I therapy or antithyroid drug therapy with propylthiouracil or methamizole.

Treatment of Complications

A. Thyrotoxic Crisis: Thyrotoxic crisis (thyroid storm) requires vigorous management. Propranolol, 1–2 mg slowly intravenously or 40–80 mg every 6 hours orally, is extremely helpful in controlling the severe cardiovascular symptoms. In the presence of severe heart failure or asthma, one can use reserpine, 1 mg intramuscularly every 6 hours, or guanethidine, 1–2 mg/kg in divided doses orally daily. Hormone release is retarded by the administration of sodium iodide, 1 g intravenously over a 24-hour period, or saturated solution of potassium iodide, 10 drops twice daily. Sodium ipodate, 1 g daily given intravenously or orally, may be used instead of sodium iodide. Hormone synthesis is blocked by the administration of propylthiouracil, 250 mg every 6 hours. The conversion of T_4 to T_3 is partially blocked by the combination of propranolol and propylthiouracil and the administration of hydrocortisone hemisuccinate, 50 mg intravenously every 6 hours. Supportive therapy includes a cooling blanket and acetaminophen to help control fever. Aspirin is probably contraindicated, because of its tendency to bind to TBG and displace thyroxine, rendering more thyroxine available in the free state. Fluids, electrolytes, and nutrition are important. For sedation, phenobarbital is probably best because it accelerates the peripheral metabolism and inactivation of thyroxine and triiodothyronine, ultimately bringing these levels down. Oxygen, diuretics, and digitalis are indicated for heart failure. Finally, it is essential to treat the underlying disease process that may have precipitated the acute exacerbation. Thus, antibiotics, anti-allergy drugs, and postoperative care are indicated for management of these problems. As an extreme measure (rarely needed) to control thyrotoxic crisis, plasmapheresis or peritoneal dialysis may be used to remove high levels of circulating thyronines.

B. Ophthalmopathy: Management of ophthalmopathy due to Graves' disease involves treatment of thyroid disease. In the opinion of one of the authors (FSG), total surgical excision of the thyroid gland or total ablation of the thyroid gland with radioactive iodine is indicated. Although there is controversy over the need for total ablation, removal or destruction of the thyroid gland certainly prevents exacerbations and relapses that may worsen residual ophthalmopathy. Keeping the patient's head elevated will diminish periorbital edema. For the severe acute inflammatory reaction, a short course of corticosteroid therapy is frequently effective, eg, prednisone, 100 mg daily orally in divided doses for 7–14 days, then every other day for 6–12 weeks. If corticosteroid therapy is not effective, external x-ray therapy to the retro-orbital area may be helpful. The dose is usually 2000 rads in 10 fractions given over a period of 2 weeks. The lens and anterior chamber structures must be shielded.

In very severe cases with threat to vision, orbital decompression can be used. One type of orbital decompression involves the transantral approach through the maxillary sinus, removing the floor and the lateral walls of the orbit. In the alternative anterior approach, the orbit is entered under the globe and portions of the floor and the walls of the orbit are removed. Both approaches have been extremely effective, and exophthalmos can be reduced by 5–7 mm in each eye by these techniques. After the acute process has subsided, the patient is frequently left with double vision or lid abnormalities due to muscle fibrosis and contracture. These can be corrected by cosmetic lid surgery or eye muscle surgery.

Thyrotoxicosis & Pregnancy

Thyrotoxicosis during pregnancy presents a special problem. Radioactive iodine is contraindicated, because it crosses the placenta freely and may injure the fetal thyroid. Two good alternatives are available. If the disease is detected during the first trimester, the patient can be prepared with propylthiouracil, and subtotal thyroidectomy can be performed safely during the mid trimester. It is essential to provide thyroid supplementation during the balance of the pregnancy. Alternatively, the patient can be treated with antithyroid drugs throughout the pregnancy, postponing the decision regarding long-term management until after delivery. The dosage of antithyroid drugs must be kept to the minimum necessary to control symptoms, because these drugs cross the placenta and may affect the function of the fetal thyroid gland. If the disease can be controlled by initial doses of propylthiouracil of 300 mg or less and maintenance doses of 50–150 mg/d, the likelihood of fetal hypothyroidism is extremely small. The free thyroxine index should be maintained in the upper range of normal by appropriately reducing the propylthiouracil dosage. Supplemental thyroxine is not necessary. Breast feeding is not contraindicated, because propylthiouracil is not concentrated in the milk.

Graves' disease may occur in the newborn infant. There seem to be 2 neonatal forms of the disease. In both types, the mother has a current or recent history of Graves' disease. In the first type, the child is born small, with weak muscles, tachycardia, fever, and frequently respiratory distress or neonatal jaundice. Examination reveals an enlarged thyroid gland and occasionally prominent, puffy eyes. The heart rate is rapid, temperature is elevated, and heart failure may ensue. Laboratory studies reveal an elevated FT_4I, a markedly elevated T_3, and usually a low TSH—in contrast to normal infants who have elevated TSH at birth. Bone age may be accelerated. TSI is often found in the serum of both the infant and the mother. The pathogenesis of this syndrome is thought to involve transplacental transfer of TSI from mother to fetus, with subsequent development of thyrotoxicosis. The disease is self-limited and subsides over a period of 4–12 weeks, coinciding with the fall in the child's TSI. Therapy includes propylthiouracil in a dose of 5–10 mg/kg/d (in divided doses at 8-hour intervals); strong iodine (Lugol's) solution, 1 drop (8 mg potassium iodide) every 8 hours; and propranolol, 2 mg/kg/d in divided doses. In addition, adequate nutrition, antibiotics for infection if present, sedatives if necessary, and supportive therapy are indicated. If the child is very toxic, corticosteroid therapy (prednisone, 2 mg/kg/d) will partially block conversion of T_4 to T_3 and may be helpful in the acute phase. The above medications are gradually reduced as the child improves and can usually be discontinued by 6–12 weeks.

A second form of neonatal Graves' disease occurs in children from families with a high incidence of Graves' disease. Symptoms develop more slowly and may not be noted until the child is 3–6 months old. This syndrome is thought to be a true genetic inheritance of defective lymphocyte immunoregulation. It is much more severe, with a 20% mortality rate and evidence of persistent brain dysfunction even after successful treatment. The hyperthyroidism may persist for months or years and requires prolonged therapy.

Maternal sera may contain TSH-blocking antibodies that can cross the placenta and produce transient hypothyroidism in the infant. This condition may need to be treated with T_4 supplementation for a short time.

Course & Prognosis

In general, the course of Graves' disease is one of remissions and exacerbations over a protracted period of time unless the gland is destroyed by surgery or radioactive iodine. Although some patients may remain euthyroid for long periods after treatment, many eventually develop hypothyroidism. Lifetime follow-up is therefore indicated for all patients with Graves' disease.

2. OTHER FORMS OF THYROTOXICOSIS

Toxic Adenoma
(Plummer's Disease)

Thyrotoxicosis may develop because of a single adenoma, usually a follicular adenoma, hypersecreting

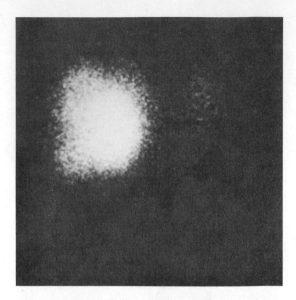

Figure 10–42. Toxic nodule of the right lobe of the thyroid gland as it appears on 99mTc pertechnetate scan. Note that the left lobe of the gland has been almost completely suppressed. (Courtesy of JM Lowenstein.)

T_3 and T_4. These lesions start out as a "hot nodule" on the thyroid scan, slowly increase in size, and gradually suppress the other lobe of the thyroid gland (Fig 10–42).

The typical patient is an older individual (usually over 40) who has noted recent growth of a longstanding thyroid nodule. Symptoms of weight loss, weakness, shortness of breath, palpitation, tachycardia, and heat intolerance are noted. Eye signs are almost never present. Physical examination reveals a definite nodule on one side, with very little thyroid tissue on the other side. Laboratory studies usually reveal suppressed TSH and marked elevation in serum T_3 levels, with only borderline elevation of thyroxine levels. The scan reveals that the nodule is "hot." Toxic adenomas are almost always follicular adenomas and almost never malignant. They are easily managed by administration of antithyroid drugs such as propylthiouracil, 100 mg every 6 hours, or methimazole, 10 mg every 6 hours, followed by unilateral lobectomy; or with radioactive iodine. Sodium 131I in doses of 20–30 mCi is usually required to destroy the benign neoplasm. Radioactive iodine is preferable for smaller toxic nodules, but larger ones are best managed by operation.

Toxic Multinodular Goiter
(Marine-Lenhart Syndrome)

This disorder occurs in older patients with long-standing multinodular goiter. Ophthalmopathy is extremely rare. Clinically, the patient presents with tachycardia, heart failure, or arrhythmia and sometimes weight loss, nervousness, tremors, and sweating. Laboratory studies reveal suppressed TSH and a striking elevation in serum T_3 levels, with less striking elevation in serum T_4 levels. Radioiodine scan reveals multiple functioning nodules in the gland or occasionally an irregular, patchy distribution of radioactive iodine (Fig 10–43).

Hyperthyroidism in patients with multinodular goiters can often be precipitated by the administration of iodides (jodbasedow effect, or iodide-induced hyperthyroidism). It was at first thought that jodbasedow effect occurred only in iodine-deficient geographic areas and that administration of iodides supplied the "building blocks" for hypersecretion of T_4 and T_3. However, Vagenakis et al have reported that 4 out of 8 patients with nontoxic goiters who lived in a high-iodine area (Boston) and who received 5 drops of saturated solution of potassium iodide daily developed hyperthyroidism. Thus, large doses of iodide can induce hyperthyroidism in any patient with a nontoxic goiter regardless of the geographic locality.

The antiarrhythmic drug amiodarone has caused hypothyroidism or hyperthyroidism to develop in certain patients. Hyperthyroidism in very sick cardiac patients can be difficult to manage, because the iodide-loaded gland cannot be treated with ^{131}I and these patients are poor operative risks. Antithyroid drugs are effective but take a long time to deplete the gland of stored hormone. If possible, administration of the drug should be stopped and the patient treated with antithyroid drugs and other antiarrhythmics until radioiodine can be used.

The management of the toxic nodular goiter is also difficult. Ideally, subtotal thyroidectomy would be the treatment of choice, but these patients are often poor operative risks. Alternatively, fairly large doses of radioactive iodine can be given, but the multinodular goiter will not be destroyed, and repeated doses of radioactive iodine may be necessary. Antithyroid drugs are effective only to induce a temporary euthyroid state. They should be used prior to surgery or radioactive iodine therapy to diminish the stress of these procedures. Propranolol may be helpful to control the cardiac problems.

Subacute Thyroiditis

This entity will be discussed in a separate section, but it should be mentioned here that thyroiditis may present with an acute release of T_4 and T_3 with symptoms of thyrotoxicosis. The typical patient is a young person with a history of malaise and complaints of neck pain, tachycardia, weight loss, and sweating. The thyroid gland is large and slightly tender. Laboratory findings reveal suppressed TSH, elevated free thyroxine index and serum T_3 but a very low radioactive iodine uptake, often less than 1%. The erythrocyte sedimentation rate is usually markedly elevated. This disease will usually subside spontaneously, although the patient may require propranolol to control cardiovascular symptoms and aspirin for local pain and discomfort.

Hashimoto's Thyroiditis

Hashimoto's thyroiditis can also go through an acute phase with increased T_3 and T_4 release, producing transient hyperthyroidism. This too is associated with suppressed TSH, high T_3 and T_4 levels, and very low radioactive iodine uptake. It is important to differentiate Hashimoto's thyroiditis from true Graves' disease, since the former will resolve spontaneously and does not require surgery, antithyroid drug therapy, or radioactive iodine. In most cases, propranolol is the only therapy required.

Thyrotoxicosis Factitia

This is a psychoneurotic disturbance in which excessive amounts of thyroxine or thyroid hormone are ingested, usually for purposes of weight control. The individual is often someone connected with medicine to whom thyroid medication is easily available. Features of thyrotoxicosis, including weight loss, nervousness, palpitation, tachycardia, and tremor, may be present, but no goiter or eye signs. Characteristically, TSH is suppressed, the serum T_4 and T_3 levels are elevated, and radioactive iodine uptake is nil. Management requires careful discussion of the hazards of long-term thyroxine therapy, particularly cardiovascular damage and muscle wasting. Formal psychotherapy may be necessary.

Rare Forms of Thyrotoxicosis

A. Struma Ovarii: In this syndrome, teratoma of the ovary contains thyroid tissue, and the thyroid tissue becomes hyperactive. Mild features of thyrotoxicosis

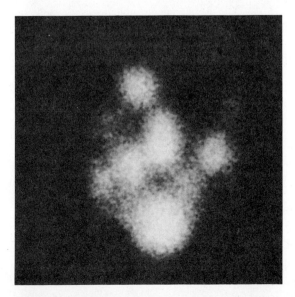

Figure 10–43. Toxic multinodular goiter as it appears on 99mTc pertechnetate scan. Note multiple functioning thyroid nodules. (Courtesy of JM Lowenstein.)

result, such as weight loss and tachycardia, but there is no evidence of goiter or eye signs. Free thyroxine index and serum T_3 are usually mildly elevated, serum TSH is suppressed, and the radioiodine uptake in the neck will be nil. Body scan reveals uptake of radioiodine in the pelvis. The disease is curable with removal of the teratoma.

B. Thyroid Carcinoma: Carcinoma of the thyroid, particularly follicular carcinoma, may concentrate radioactive iodine, but only rarely does it retain the ability to convert this iodide into active hormone. Only a few cases of metastatic thyroid cancer have presented with hyperthyroidism. The clinical picture consists of weakness, weight loss, and palpitation, without goiter or ophthalmopathy. Body scan reveals areas of uptake usually distant from the thyroid, eg, bone or lung. Treatment with large doses of radioactive iodine may destroy the metastatic deposits.

C. Hydatidiform Mole: Hydatidiform mole produces chorionic gonadotropin, which has intrinsic TSH-like activity. This may induce thyroid hyperplasia, increased iodine turnover, suppressed TSH, and mild elevation of serum T_4 and T_3 levels. It is rarely associated with overt thyrotoxicosis and is totally curable by removal of the mole.

D. Syndrome of Inappropriate TSH Secretion: A group of patients have recently been reported with elevated serum immunoreactive TSH in association with elevated serum free thyroxine values. This has been called the "syndrome of inappropriate TSH secretion." Two types of problems are found: (1) TSH-secreting pituitary adenoma and (2) nonneoplastic pituitary hypersecretion of TSH.

Patients with TSH-secreting pituitary adenomas usually present with mild thyrotoxicosis and goiter, usually with amenorrhea. There are no eye signs of Graves' disease. Study reveals elevated total and free serum T_4 and T_3. Serum TSH, usually undetectable in Graves' disease, is elevated. There is no response to TRH, and the increased radioactive iodine uptake is not suppressible with exogenous thyroid hormone. Visual field examination may reveal temporal defects, and CT or MRI scan of the sella reveals a pituitary tumor. Management usually involves control of the thyrotoxicosis with antithyroid drugs and removal of the pituitary tumor via transsphenoidal hypophysectomy. If the tumor cannot be completely removed, it may be necessary to treat residual tumor with radiation therapy and to control thyrotoxicosis with radioactive iodine.

Nonneoplastic pituitary hypersecretion of TSH is essentially a form of pituitary (and occasionally peripheral) resistance to T_3 and T_4. Thus, increasing levels of T_3 and T_4 fail to suppress pituitary TSH secretion, and TSH pours out. Patients with only pituitary resistance to T_3 and T_4 present with goiter and hyperthyroidism, elevated free T_4, elevated TSH, normal response to TRH, and a normal response to T_3 suppression. These patients act as if the pituitary set point for

T_3 suppression is higher than normal. Patients with both pituitary and peripheral resistance to thyroid hormones will present with goiter, elevated T_3 and T_4, and elevated TSH, but they are euthyroid or mildly hypothyroid. This syndrome is familial and has been called **Refetoff's syndrome.** A defect in the β thyroid hormone receptor gene has been found in some of these patients.

Management of these syndromes is difficult. If the patient is hypothyroid or euthyroid, T_3 therapy may maintain a euthyroid state and reduce TSH. In the hyperthyroid patient, bromocriptine may lower TSH and control thyrotoxic symptoms. Long-acting somatostatin analogues have effectively controlled the disease in some patients.

NONTOXIC GOITER

Etiology

Nontoxic goiter usually represents enlargement of the thyroid gland from TSH stimulation, which in turn results from inadequate thyroid hormone synthesis. Table 10–10 lists some of the causes of nontoxic goiter.

Iodine deficiency was the most common cause of nontoxic goiter or "endemic goiter"; with the widespread use of iodized salt and the introduction of iodides into fertilizers, animal feeds, and food preservatives, iodide deficiency in developed countries is relatively rare. The only remaining areas of endemic goiter are in inland, undeveloped regions such as the Himalayas, the Andes, Central Africa, and New Guinea. It does not exist in the USA. Estimated optimal iodine requirements for adults are in the range of 150–300 μg/d. In endemic goiter areas, the daily urinary excretion of iodine falls below 50 μg/d; in areas where iodine is extremely scarce, excretion falls below 20 μg/d. The mechanism for goiter formation is thought to be low iodine intake, impaired hormone formation, increased TSH secretion, and hyperplasia of thyroid cells.

Dietary goitrogens are a rare cause of goiter, and of these the most common is iodide itself. Large doses of iodides used (for example) in the treatment of chronic pulmonary disease may in susceptible individuals produce goiter and hypothyroidism. Withdrawal of iodide reverses the process. Other goitrogens include lithium carbonate, used for the treatment of manic-depressive

Table 10–10. Etiology of nontoxic goiter.

1. Iodine deficiency.
2. Goitrogen in the diet.
3. Hashimoto's thyroiditis.
4. Subacute thyroiditis.
5. Inadequate hormone synthesis due to inherited defect in thyroidal enzymes necessary for T_4 and T_3 biosynthesis.
6. Inherited deficiency in T_4 receptor in cell membrane (rare).
7. Neoplasm, benign or malignant.

psychosis, and some vegetable foodstuffs such as thio-glucosides, found in cabbage, and goitrin, found in certain roots and seeds. Cyanogenic glycosides found in cassava can release thiocyanates that may cause goiter, particularly in the presence of iodide deficiency. The role of these vegetable goitrogens in the production of goiter is not clearly established.

Thyroid enlargement may occur in adolescents, particularly at the time of menarche, or as a result of pregnancy or ingestion of oral contraceptive drugs. Many of these patients have underlying chronic lymphocytic thyroiditis (Hashimoto's thyroiditis), which is the real cause of the goiter. Hashimoto's thyroiditis is a common illness, particularly in women. Hormone synthesis is impaired, and thyroid enlargement develops. In subacute thyroiditis, thyroid enlargement occurs in association with acute inflammatory changes, presumably due to viral infection (see below).

Nontoxic goiter may be due to impaired hormone synthesis resulting from genetic deficiencies in enzymes necessary for hormone biosynthesis (thyroid dyshormonogenesis). These effects may be complete, resulting in a syndrome of cretinism with goiter; or partial, resulting in nontoxic goiter with mild hypothyroidism. At least 5 separate biosynthetic abnormalities have been reported: (1) impaired transport of iodine; (2) deficient peroxidase with impaired oxidation of iodide to iodine and failure to incorporate iodine into thyroglobulin; (3) impaired coupling of iodinated tyrosines to triiodothyronine or tetraiodothyronine; (4) absence or deficiency of iodotyrosine deiodinase, so that iodine is not conserved within the gland; and (5) excessive production of metabolically inactive iodoprotein by the thyroid gland. This may involve impaired or abnormal thyroglobulin synthesis. In all of these syndromes, impaired production of th̶ mones presumably results in TS̶ formation.

Finally, thyroid enlargement lesion, such as adenoma, or to a carcinoma.

Pathogenesis

The pathogenetic mechanism of to dyshormonogenesis involves fi plasia, followed by focal hyperplasia hemorrhage, and finally the developm of focal hyperplasia. Studer has show perplasia usually involves a clone of c may not be able to pick up iodine or s roglobulin. Thus, the nodules will var̶ nodules that can concentrate iodine to "c that cannot, and from colloid nodules that size thyroglobulin to microfollicular nodul not. Initially the hyperplasia is TSH depe later the nodules become TSH independent, mous. Thus, a diffuse nontoxic TSH-depend progresses over a period of time to a multinod̶ toxic TSH-independent goiter.

Clinical Findings

A. Symptoms and Signs: Patients with nontoxic goiter usually present with thyroid enlargement, which may be diffuse or multinodular. The gland may be relatively firm but is often extremely soft. Over a period of time, the gland becomes progressively larger, so that in long-standing multinodular goiter, huge goiters may develop and extend inferiorly to present as substernal goiter. The patient may complain of pressure symptoms in the neck, particularly on moving the head upward or downward, and of difficulty in swallowing. Vocal cord paresis is rare. There may be symptoms of mild hypothyroidism, but most of these patients are euthyroid. Thyroid enlargement represents compensated hypothyroidism.

B. Laboratory Findings: Laboratory studies will reveal a low or normal free thyroxine index and, usually, normal levels of TSH. At the time the studies are made, the patient should be in equilibrium or balance, so that TSH levels are not elevated. In patients with dyshormonogenesis due to abnormal iodoprotein synthesis, PBI may be elevated out of proportion to serum T_4, because of secretion of nonhormonal organic iodide compounds.

C. Scan Studies: Isotope scanning usually reveals a patchy uptake, frequently with focal areas of increased uptake corresponding to "hot" nodules. Radioactive iodine uptake may be suppressible on administration of thyroid hormones such as liothyronine. Echography may reveal cystic changes in one or of the nodules, representing previous h necrosis.

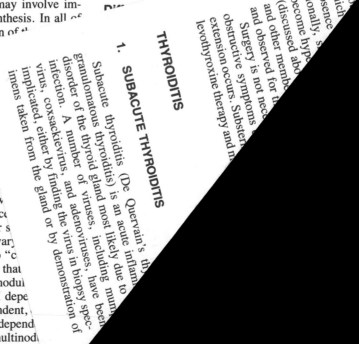

levo which absence sionally, s become hype (discussed ab and other memb and observed for t

Surgery is not nece obstructive symptoms extension occurs. Subster levothyroxine therapy and n

THYROIDITIS

1. SUBACUTE THYROIDITIS

Subacute thyroiditis (De Quervain's th̶ granulomatous thyroiditis) is an acute inflam̶ disorder of the thyroid gland most likely due to infection. A number of viruses, including mum virus, coxsackievirus, and adenoviruses, have been implicated, either by finding the virus in biopsy specimens taken from the gland or by demonstration of

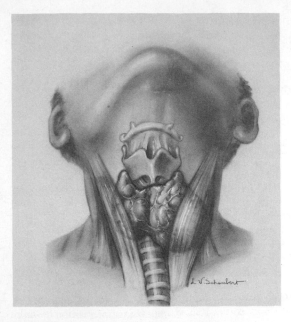

Figure 10–44. Multinodular goiter at the time of surgery. The asymmetric enlargement and the nodularity are apparent, as is the rightward deviation of the trachea resulting from marked enlargement of the lobe.

size of the mass with resulting pressure symptoms may require subtotal thyroidectomy.

Course & Prognosis

Patients with nontoxic goiter must usually take thyroxine for life. They should avoid iodides, may induce either hyperthyroidism or, in the of thyroxine therapy, hypothyroidism. Occa-ingle adenomas or several adenomas will rplastic and produce toxic nodular goiter ve). Nontoxic goiter is often familial, rs of the family should be examined e possible development of goiter. ssary for nontoxic goiter unless evelop or marked substernal al goiter does not respond to ust be removed surgically.

roiditis, matory viral ps

rising titers of viral antibodies in the blood during the course of the infection. Pathologic examination reveals moderate thyroid enlargement and a mild inflammatory reaction involving the capsule. Histologic features include destruction of thyroid parenchyma and the presence of many large phagocytic cells, including giant cells.

Clinical Findings

A. Symptoms and Signs: Subacute thyroiditis usually presents with fever, malaise, and soreness in the neck, which may extend up to the angle of the jaw or toward the ear lobes on one or both sides of the neck. Initially, the patient may have symptoms of hyperthyroidism with palpitations, agitation, and sweats. There is no ophthalmopathy. On physical examination, the gland is exquisitely tender, so that the patient will object to pressure upon it. There are no signs of local redness or heat suggestive of abscess formation. Clinical signs of toxicity, including tachycardia, tremor, and hyperreflexia, may be present.

B. Laboratory Findings: Laboratory studies will vary with the course of the disease. Initially, FT_4I and T_3 are elevated, whereas serum TSH and thyroid radioactive iodine uptake are extremely low. The erythrocyte sedimentation rate is markedly elevated, sometimes as high as 100 mm/h by the Westergren scale. Thyroid autoantibodies are usually not detectable in serum. As the disease progresses, T_4 and T_3 will drop, TSH will rise, and symptoms of hypothyroidism are noted. Later, radioactive iodine uptake will rise, re-

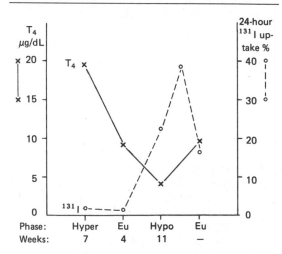

Figure 10–45. Changes in serum T_4 and radioactive iodine uptake in patients with subacute thyroiditis. In the initial phase, serum T_4 is elevated and the patient may have symptoms of thyrotoxicosis, but radioactive iodine uptake is markedly suppressed. The illness may pass through phases of euthyroidism and hypothyroidism before remission. (Data adapted, with permission, from Woolf PD, Daly R: Thyrotoxicosis with painless thyroiditis. *Am J Med* 1976;**60**:73.)

flecting recovery of the gland from the acute insult (Fig 10–45).

Differential Diagnosis

Subacute thyroiditis can be differentiated from other viral illnesses by the involvement of the thyroid gland. It is differentiated from Graves' disease by the presence of low thyroid radioiodine uptake when T_3 and T_4 levels are elevated.

Treatment

In most cases, only symptomatic treatment is necessary, eg, aspirin, 0.6 g 4 times daily. If pain, fever, and malaise are disabling, a short course of corticosterioids such as prednisone, 20 mg 3 times daily for 7–10 days, may be necessary to reduce the inflammation. Therapy with thyroid hormones, either levothyronine, 25 μg 3 times daily, or levothyroxine, 0.2 mg once daily, may be necessary during the hypothyroid phase of the illness in order to prevent reexacerbation of the disease induced by the rising TSH levels. In most patients, complete recovery occurs, but in about 10% of cases permanent hypothyroidism ensues and long-term thyroxine therapy is necessary.

Course & Prognosis

Subacute thyroiditis usually resolves spontaneously over weeks or months. Occasionally, the disease may begin to resolve and then suddenly get worse, sometimes involving first one lobe of the thyroid gland and then the other. Exacerbations occur when the T_4 levels have fallen, TSH has risen, and the gland is starting to recover function. Rarely, the course may extend over several years, with repeated bouts of inflammatory disease.

2. CHRONIC (HASHIMOTO'S) THYROIDITIS

Chronic thyroiditis (Hashimoto's thyroiditis, lymphocytic thyroiditis) is probably the most common cause of hypothyroidism and goiter in the USA. It is certainly the major cause of goiter in children and in young adults and is probably the major cause of "idiopathic myxedema," which represents an end stage of Hashimoto's thyroiditis with total atrophy of the gland. **Riedel's struma** is probably a variant of Hashimoto's thyroiditis with extensive fibrosis extending outside the gland and involving overlying muscle and surrounding tissues. Riedel's struma presents as a stony hard mass that must be differentiated from thyroid cancer.

Etiology & Pathogenesis

Hashimoto's thyroiditis is thought to be an autoimmune disease that involves a defect in "suppressor" T cells. In this disease, "helper" T cells stimulate B lymphocytes to produce autoantibodies to thyroidal antigens, including microsomal and thyroglobulin autoantibodies. During the early phases of Hashimoto's thyroiditis, thyroglobulin autoantibodies are markedly elevated, and microsomal autoantibodies are not so high. Later, thyroglobulin autoantibodies may disappear, but the microsomal autoantibodies will be present for many years. Pathologically, huge numbers of lymphocytes infiltrate the thyroid gland, totally destroying normal thyroidal architecture. Lymphoid follicles and germinal centers may actually be formed. The follicular epithelial cells are frequently enlarged and contain a basophilic cytoplasm (Hurthle cells). Destruction of the gland results in a fall in serum T_3 and T_4 levels and a rise in TSH. Initially, TSH may maintain adequate hormonal synthesis by the development of thyroid enlargement or goiter, but in many cases the gland fails, and hypothyroidism with or without goiter ensues.

Hashimoto's thyroiditis is part of a spectrum of thyroid diseases that includes Graves' disease at one end and idiopathic myxedema at the other (Fig 10–46). It is familial and may be associated with other autoimmune diseases such as pernicious anemia, adrenocortical insufficiency, idiopathic hypoparathyroidism, myasthenia gravis, and vitiligo. **Schmidt's syndrome** consists of Hashimoto's thyroiditis, idiopathic adrenal insufficiency, hypoparathyroidism, diabetes mellitus, ovarian insufficiency (rarely), and candidal infections. Schmidt's syndrome represents destruction of multiple endocrine glands on an autoimmune basis (see Chapter 28).

Clinical Findings

A. Symptoms and Signs: Hashimoto's thyroiditis usually presents with goiter in a patient who is euthyroid or has mild hypothyroidism. The sex distribu-

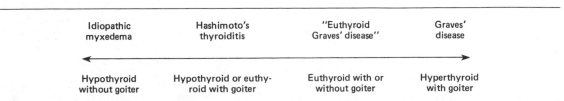

Idiopathic myxedema	Hashimoto's thyroiditis	"Euthyroid Graves' disease"	Graves' disease
Hypothyroid without goiter	Hypothyroid or euthyroid with goiter	Euthyroid with or without goiter	Hyperthyroid with goiter

Figure 10–46. Spectrum of autoimmune disease of the thyroid gland. The clinical manifestations of autoimmune disease of the thyroid gland range from idiopathic myxedema, through nontoxic goiter, to diffuse toxic goiter, or Graves' disease. At times one can see progression of autoimmune disease from one form to another in the same patient.

tion is about 4 females to one male. The process is painless, and the patient may be unaware of the goiter unless it becomes very large.

B. Laboratory Findings: There are multiple defects in iodine metabolism. Peroxidase activity is decreased, so that organification of iodine is impaired. This can be demonstrated by a positive perchlorate discharge test. In addition, iodination of metabolically inactive protein material occurs, so that there will be a disproportionately high serum PBI compared to serum T_4. Radioiodine uptake may be high, normal, or low. Circulating thyroid hormone levels are usually normal or low, and if low, TSH will be elevated.

The most striking laboratory finding is the high titer of autoantibodies to thyroidal antigens in the serum. Thyroglobulin and microsomal autoantibody tests are strongly positive in most patients with Hashimoto's thyroiditis.

An additional diagnostic test that may be helpful is the fine needle aspiration biopsy. With this technique, biopsy samples will reveal a heavy infiltration of lymphocytes as well as the presence of Hurthle cells on the smear.

Differential Diagnosis

Hashimoto's thyroiditis must be differentiated from other causes of nontoxic goiter. This is best done by antibody studies and if necessary by fine needle aspiration biopsy.

Complications & Sequelae

The major complication of Hashimoto's thyroiditis is progressive hypothyroidism. Although only 10–15% of young patients presenting with goiter and hypothyroidism seem to progress to permanent hypothyroidism, the high incidence of permanent hypothyroidism in older patients with positive antibody tests and elevated TSH levels suggests that long-term treatment is desirable. Rarely, a patient with Hashimoto's thyroiditis may develop lymphoma of the thyroid gland, but whether the 2 conditions are causally related is not clear. Thyroid lymphoma is characterized by rapid growth of the gland despite continued thyroid hormone therapy; the diagnosis of lymphoma must be made by surgical biopsy.

There is no evidence that adenocarcinoma of the thyroid gland occurs more frequently in patients with Hashimoto's thyroiditis, but the 2 diseases—chronic thyroiditis and carcinoma—can coexist in the same gland. Cancer must be suspected when a solitary nodule or thyroid mass grows or fails to regress while the patient is receiving maximal tolerated doses of thyroxine. Fine needle aspiration biopsy may be helpful in differential diagnosis.

Treatment

Treatment consists of giving levothyroxine, 0.1–0.25 mg daily. These doses are slightly higher than physiologic replacement in an effort to suppress TSH and allow regression of the goiter. Surgery is rarely indicated.

Course & Prognosis

Without treatment, Hashimoto's thyroiditis may progress from goiter and hypothyroidism to myxedema. The myxedema is totally corrected by adequate thyroxine therapy. Because Hashimoto's thyroiditis may be a part of a syndrome of multiple autoimmune diseases, the patient should be followed for other illnesses such as pernicious anemia, adrenal insufficiency, hypothyroidism, or diabetes mellitus.

Hashimoto's thyroiditis may go through periods of activity when large amounts of T_4 and T_3 are released or "dumped," resulting in symptoms of thyrotoxicosis. This syndrome, which has been called **spontaneously resolving hyperthyroidism,** is characterized by low radioiodine uptake. However, it can be differentiated from subacute thyroiditis in that the gland is not tender, the erythrocyte sedimentation rate is not elevated, autoantibodies to thyroidal antigens are strongly positive, and fine needle aspiration biopsy reveals lymphocytes and Hurthle cells. Therapy is symptomatic, usually requiring only propranolol, until symptoms subside; T_4 supplementation may then be necessary.

Since Hashimoto's thyroiditis is part of a spectrum of autoimmune thyroid disease that includes Graves' disease, patients with Hashimoto's thyroiditis may develop true Graves' disease, occasionally with severe ophthalmopathy or dermopathy. The chronic thyroiditis may blunt the severity of the thyrotoxicosis, so that the patient may present with eye or skin complications of Graves' disease without marked thyrotoxicosis, a syndrome often called euthyroid Graves' disease. The thyroid gland will invariably be nonsuppressible, and this, plus the presence of thyroid autoantibodies, will help to make the diagnosis. The ophthalmopathy and dermopathy are treated as if thyrotoxic Graves' disease were present.

3. OTHER FORMS OF THYROIDITIS

The thyroid gland may be subject to acute abscess formation in patients with septicemia or acute bacterial endocarditis. Abscesses cause symptoms of pyogenic infection, with local pain and tenderness, swelling, and warmth and redness of the overlying skin. Needle aspiration may be helpful to confirm the diagnosis and identify the organism. Treatment includes antibiotic therapy and occasionally incision and drainage. A thyroglossal duct cyst may become infected and present as acute suppurative thyroiditis. This too will respond to antibiotic therapy and occasionally incision and drainage.

Ionizing radiation can induce both acute and chronic thyroiditis. Thyroiditis may occur acutely in patients treated with large doses of radioiodine and may be associated with release of thyroid hormones and an acute thyrotoxic crisis. Such an occurrence is extremely rare, however; the authors have seen only 2 cases in several thousand patients treated for Graves' disease with radioactive iodine.

External radiation was used many years ago for the treatment of benign conditions such as severe acne and chronic tonsillitis or adenoiditis. This treatment was frequently associated with the development of focal thyroiditis and at times with hypothyroidism, nodular goiter, and thyroid cancer. If cancer can be ruled out by physical examination and other studies, patients with radiation-induced goiter or hypothyroidism should be treated with long-term thyroxine therapy as described above in the discussion of Hashimoto's thyroiditis (see below and Table 10–13).

EFFECTS OF ACUTE & CHRONIC ILLNESS ON THYROID FUNCTION

The effects of thyroid hormone are controlled by a number of factors, including the following: (1) T_3 and T_4 feedback on TSH secretion; (2) autoregulation of hormone synthesis, depending on iodide availability; (3) peripheral metabolism of T_4, with activation by conversion to T_3 or inactivation by conversion to rT_3; and (4) the binding equilibrium between serum thyroid-binding proteins and tissue receptors. Acute and chronic illnesses have striking effects on these systems, particularly the peripheral metabolism of T_4 to T_3.

The peripheral metabolism of T_4 is diagrammed in Fig 10–21. Activation of the inner ring deiodinase accelerates conversion of T_4 to rT_3 and conversion of T_3 to $3,3'-T_2$, markedly lowering the circulating level of T_3. This occurs physiologically in the fetus and pathologically in circumstances of carbohydrate re-

striction, as in malnutrition, starvation, anorexia nervosa, and diabetes mellitus (Table 10–5). Among the drugs that tend to lower the circulating levels of T_3, corticosteroids, amiodarone, and iodinated dyes are the most effective and propylthiouracil and propranolol are relatively weak. Finally, acute illness such as myocardial infarction, febrile illness, trauma, burns, and surgery, as well as chronic illness—especially chronic liver disease, chronic renal disease, and cancer in advanced stages—also inhibit conversion of T_4 to T_3. These conditions result in what has been called the low T_3 syndrome.

Low T_3 Syndromes

Low T_3 syndrome is characterized by normal or slightly elevated T_4, low T_3, increased rT_3, and a normal TSH. Typical findings are presented in Fig 10–47. Data from normal, "sick," and hypothyroid individuals are compared. The "sick" patients have relatively normal serum T_4, compared with true hypothyroid patients, who have a very low T_4. T_3 is low in both "sick" and hypothyroid patients, but rT_3 is elevated in the "sick" group in comparison with both the normal and the hypothyroid groups. TSH is markedly elevated in the hypothyroid patients and normal in the "sick" patients. Further evidence that the "sick" patients are not hypothyroid can be obtained by the TRH test, which is normal in "sick" patients and hyperresponsive in hypothyroid patients (Fig 10–16).

A group of patients have been reported with a **low T_3, low T_4 syndrome.** Generally, they are much sicker and are usually in the intensive care unit. Indeed, the presence of both low T_3 and low T_4 has been associated with high mortality rates and poor outcomes. This syndrome is characterized by low T_4, low T_3, high rT_3, normal TSH, and usually an impaired response to TRH. Typical findings are presented in Fig 10–48. Note that T_4 and T_3 are low, but reverse T_3 is markedly

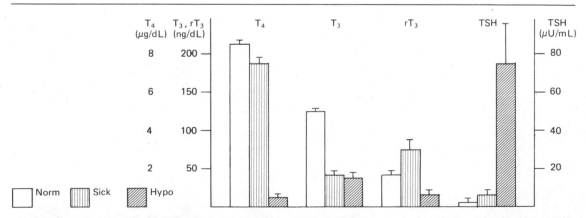

Figure 10–47. Low T_3 syndrome. Note that euthyroid sick patients have normal T_4, low T_3, elevated rT_3, and normal TSH, compared to normal and hypothyroid patients. (Reproduced, with permission, from Chopra IJ et al: Misleading low free thyroxine index and usefulness of reverse triiodothyronine measurements in nonthyroidal illness. *Ann Intern Med* 1979;**90**:905.)

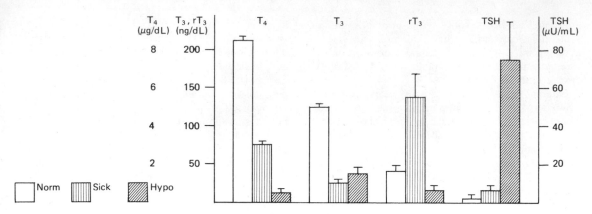

Figure 10–48. Low T_3, low T_4 syndrome. Note that very sick patients have low T_4, low T_3, elevated rT_3, and normal TSH, compared with normal and hypothyroid patients. (Reproduced, with permission, from Chopra IJ et al: Misleading low free thyroxine index and usefulness of reverse triiodothyronine measurements in nonthyroidal illness. *Ann Intern Med* 1979;**90**:905.)

elevated, and TSH is normal, in contrast to findings in hypothyroid patients. It is not clear why patients with this syndrome are not hypothyroid. However, a greater percentage of T_4 appears to be free in these patients, so that the actual level of free T_4 was increased. This was not detected by the free thyroxine index; it was only detected by dialysis measurements. To account for these findings, it has been postulated that an inhibitor of T_4-binding to thyroid-binding proteins is present in the serum of these patients.

The clinical implications of these observations are important. The presence of low T_3 in milder diseases and low T_4 and low T_3 in very severe diseases suggests that these findings are related to the severity of the disease process.

A. Differential Diagnosis: It is essential to rule out hyperthyroidism in low T_3 syndrome with elevated T_4 and to rule out hypothyroidism in both syndromes. Failure to treat hypothyroidism in the presence of other illness could be catastrophic. In low T_3 syndrome, the normal T_4, elevated rT_3, and normal TSH will rule out hypothyroidism. Occasionally, T_4 may be slightly elevated, perhaps to compensate for the low T_3. In this case, patients may be confused with hyperthyroid patients but can be differentiated by the low T_3 and normal TSH and TRH tests. The FT_4I may not adequately reflect the level of free T_4 in severely ill patients, and direct determination of free T_4 may be necessary to clarify the thyroid status.

B. Management: Patients with these syndromes should not be treated with thyroid hormones to restore normal blood levels, since there is no evidence that treatment with T_3 or T_4 will be helpful and there are many reasons why such treatment might be hazardous. It is thought that these aberrations of thyroid hormone metabolism are an adaptive mechanism that may in some way protect the organism from excessive metabolic activity in the presence of serious illness. Certainly, one should correct any caloric or carbohydrate

deprivation and treat the underlying illness, which will usually be accompanied by a return of thyroid hormone metabolism to normal.

THYROID NODULES & THYROID CANCER

In 95% of cases, thyroid cancer presents as a nodule or lump in the thyroid. In occasional instances, particularly in children, enlarged cervical lymph nodes will be the first sign of the disease, although on careful examination a small primary focus in the form of a thyroid nodule can usually be felt. Rarely, distant metastasis in lung or bone is the first sign of thyroid cancer.

Thyroid nodules are extremely common, particularly among women. The prevalence of thyroid nodules in the USA has been estimated to be about 4% of the adult population, with a female : male ratio of 4:1. In young children, the incidence is less than 1%; in persons aged 11–18 years, about 1.5%; and in persons over age 60, about 5%.

In contrast to thyroid nodules, thyroid cancer is a rare condition—0.004% per year according to the Third National Cancer Survey. Thus, most thyroid nodules are benign, and it is important to identify those that are likely to be malignant.

1. BENIGN THYROID NODULES

Etiology
Benign conditions that can produce nodularity in the thyroid gland are listed in Table 10–11. They include focal areas of chronic thyroiditis, a dominant portion of a multinodular goiter, or a cyst involving either thyroid tissue, parathyroid tissue, or thyroglossal duct remnants. Other benign conditions include agenesis of

Table 10–11. Etiology of benign thyroid nodules.

1. Focal thyroiditis.
2. Dominant portion of multinodular goiter.
3. Thyroid, parathyroid, or thyroglossal cysts.
4. Agenesis of a thyroid lobe.
5. Postsurgical remnant hyperplasia or scarring.
6. Postradioiodine remnant hyperplasia.
7. Benign adenomas:
    a. Follicular:
        Colloid or macrofollicular.
        Fetal.
        Embryonal.
        Hurthle cell.
    b. Rare: Teratoma, lipoma, hemangioma.

one lobe of the thyroid, with hypertrophy of the other lobe presenting as a mass in the neck. It is usually the left lobe of the thyroid that fails to develop, and the hypertrophy occurs in the right lobe. Scarring in the gland following surgery—or regrowth of the gland after surgery or radioiodine therapy—can present with nodularity. Finally, benign neoplasms in the thyroid include follicular adenomas such as colloid or macrofollicular adenomas, fetal adenomas, embryonal adenomas, and Hurthle cell or oxyphil adenomas. Rare types of benign lesions include teratomas, lipomas, and hemangiomas. Except for thyroid hyperplasia of the right lobe of the gland in the presence of agenesis of the left lobe—and some follicular adenomas—all of the above lesions present as "cold" nodules on isotope scanning.

Differentiation of Benign & Malignant Lesions

Risk factors that predispose to benign or malignant disease are set forth in Table 10–12 and discussed below.

A. History: A family history of goiter suggests benign disease, as does residence in an area of endemic goiter. However, a family history of medullary carcinoma or a history of recent thyroid growth, hoarseness, dysphagia, or obstruction strongly suggests cancer.

Probably the most important historical feature is exposure to ionizing radiation. The incidence of thyroid lesions after irradiation is summarized in Table 10–13. As little as 6.5 rads to the thyroid gland received during the radiation treatment of tinea capitis has been reported to cause cancer in 0.11% of exposed children; the incidence of thyroid cancer in sibling controls was 0.02%. Radiation therapy to the thymus was used many years ago for the treatment of respiratory problems or poor growth in infants. The thyroid received dosages of 100–400 rads, and the incidence of thyroid cancer attributed to this source ranged from 0.5 to 5%. X-ray therapy to the neck and chest given to children or adolescents for acne, tonsillitis, adenoiditis, otitis media, or skin lesions with thyroid doses ranging from 200 to 1500 rads produced nodular goiter with an incidence of around 27% and thyroid cancer with an incidence of 5–7%. These tumors developed 10–40 years after radiation was administered, with a peak incidence at 20–30 years. Radiation fallout with a thyroid dose of 700–1400 rads has produced nodular goiter in approximately 40% of patients exposed and thyroid cancer in about 6%. However, radioiodine therapy, which exposes the thyroid to a dosage of around 10,000 rads, was rarely associated with the development of thyroid cancer, presumably because the thyroid gland is largely destroyed by these doses of radioiodine so that—although the incidence of postradiation hypothyroidism is high—the incidence of thyroid cancer is extremely low.

Table 10–12. Risk factors useful in distinguishing benign from malignant thyroid lesions.

	More Likely Benign	More Likely Malignant
History	Family history of benign goiter. Residence in endemic goiter area.	Family history of medullary cancer of thyroid. Previous therapeutic irradiation of head or neck. Recent growth of nodule. Hoarseness, dysphagia, or obstruction.
Physical characteristics	Older woman. Soft nodule. Multinodular goiter.	Child, young adult, male. Solitary, firm nodule clearly different from rest of gland ("dominant nodule"). Vocal cord paralysis, firm lymph nodes, distant metastases.
Serum factors	High titer of thyroid autoantibodies.	Elevated serum calcitonin. Elevated serum thyroglobulin (?).
Scanning techniques ^{123}I or ^{99m} TcO$_4$	"Hot nodule."	"Cold nodule."
Echo scan	Cyst (pure).	Solid or semicystic.
Biopsy (needle)	Benign appearance on cytologic examination.	Malignant or suggestion of malignancy.
Levothyroxine therapy (0.2 mg/d or more for 3 months or longer)	Regression.	No regression.

Table 10–13. Thyroid lesions after irradiation.

| Areas Treated | Estimated Dose to Thyroid (rads) | Incidence (%) | | Source |
		Nodular Goiter	Cancer	
Scalp	6.5	. . .	0.11	Modan et al (1974)
Thymus Total group	119	1.8	0.8	Hemplemann et al (1975)
Subgroup	399	7.6	5.0	
Neck, chest	807	27.2	5.7	Favus et al (1975)
	180–1500	26.2	6.8	Refetoff et al (1975)
Radiation fallout	<50	. . .	0.4	Parker et al (1974)
	>50	. . .	6.7	Sampson et al (1969)
	175 (γ) and 700– 1400 (β)	39.6	5.7	Conrad et al (1970)
131I therapy	±10,000	0.17	0.08	Dobyns et al (1974)

Ninety percent of patients with radiation-induced thyroid cancer develop papillary carcinoma; the remainder develop follicular carcinoma. Medullary carcinoma and anaplastic carcinomas have been rare following radiation exposure. Data from several large series suggest that the incidence of cancer in a patient who presents with a solitary cold nodule of the thyroid gland and a history of therapeutic radiation of the head, neck, or chest is around 50%.

B. Physical Characteristics: Physical characteristics associated with a low risk for thyroid cancer include older age, female sex, soft thyroid nodules, and the presence of a multinodular goiter. Individuals at higher risk for thyroid cancer include children, young adults, and males. A solitary firm or dominant nodule that is clearly different from the rest of the gland increases the risk of malignancy. Vocal cord paralysis, enlarged lymph nodes, and suspected metastases are strongly suggestive of malignancy.

C. Serum Factors: A high titer of thyroid autoantibodies in serum is associated with a low risk of thyroid cancer and suggests chronic thyroiditis as the cause of thyroid enlargement. However, an elevated serum calcitonin, particularly in patients with a family history of medullary carcinoma, strongly suggests the presence of thyroid cancer. Elevated serum thyroglobulin titers may be associated with metastatic follicular or papillary thyroid carcinoma but are usually not helpful in determining the nature of the thyroid nodule.

D. Scanning Techniques: Scanning procedures can be used to identify "hot" or "cold" nodules, ie, those that take up more or less radioactive iodine than surrounding tissue. Hot nodules are almost never malignant, whereas cold ones may be. Scintillation camera photographs with ^{99m}Tc pertechnetate give the best resolution (Fig 10–49). Echo scans can distinguish cystic and solid lesions. A pure cyst is almost never malignant. Lesions that have internal echoes or are solid on echo scan may be benign or malignant. CT scanning or magnetic resonance imaging (MRI) may be helpful in defining substernal extension or deep thyroid nodules in the neck.

E. Needle Biopsy: The major advance in management of the thyroid nodule in recent years has been the fine needle aspiration biopsy. Large needle aspiration biopsies of the thyroid for diagnostic purposes were in use from about 1930, but Soderstrom in 1952 introduced the technique of fine needle aspiration biopsy. Since then, fine needle biopsy has been widely used. With this technique, a 23- or 25-bore needle is used, and the diagnosis relies on cytologic rather than histologic examination. It is nontraumatic, simple, easily repeated, and very acceptable to the patient.

Fine needle aspiration biopsy clearly separates thyroid nodules into 3 groups:

1. Malignant thyroid nodules–The technique is almost 100% diagnostic.

2. Follicular neoplasms–About 15% of these lesions are malignant, and about 85% are benign. Some follicular neoplasms may be hot; most of them are cold.

3. Benign thyroid nodules–The rate of false-negative results with fine needle aspiration biopsy is about 4%. Results are accurate in about 96% of cases, as demonstrated by subsequent surgery or long-term follow-up of patients with lesions originally reported to be benign.

F. Suppressive Therapy: Benign lesions may undergo spontaneous involution and regression, and some may be sufficiently TSH dependent to shrink on thyroxine therapy. One study found no significant difference in nodule size (confirmed by thyroid sonography) between thyroxine- and placebo-treated controls during a 6-month period. In both groups, about half of the benign nodules decreased in size. However, malignant lesions are unlikely to regress either spontaneously or on T_4 therapy.

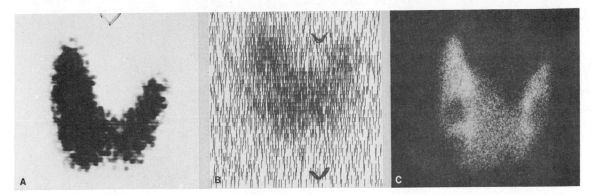

Figure 10–49. Demonstration of resolution obtained utilizing different scanning techniques: *A:* ¹²³I scintiscan with rectilinear scanner. *B:* Fluorescent scan with rectilinear scanner. *C:* ⁹⁹ᵐTc pertechnetate scan with the pinhole collimated gamma camera. Note the presence of 2 "cold" nodules, one in each lobe of the thyroid, easily detected in *C* but not clearly delineated in the other 2 scans. The lesion in the right lobe was palpable, about 1 cm in diameter, and was shown to be follicular carcinoma on needle biopsy. The lesion in the left lobe was either a metastatic tumor or a second primary follicular carcinoma. (Courtesy of MD Okerlund.)

Management of Thyroid Nodules

A decision matrix for the management of a thyroid nodule is outlined in Fig 10–50. A patient with a thyroid nodule should have a fine needle aspiration biopsy as the initial screening test for a thyroid mass. If the nodule is malignant, the patient is referred directly to the surgeon. If the cytologic report shows that the nodule is benign, the patient is given thyroxine, and if the lesion regresses, the patient is maintained on thyroxine indefinitely at a dose sufficient to suppress serum TSH. If there is no regression, the lesion is biopsied again, or if it grows or changes in consistency, it may be excised. In patients who are reported to have follicular neoplasms, scanning is employed. If the scan reveals the nodule to be hot, the patient is simply observed, at times with thyroxine therapy. If the lesion is cold and there is an increased chance of malignancy (large lesion over 2 cm in diameter, firm nodule, young patient), the patient might be referred directly to the surgeon. If the risk is low (small lesion 1 cm or less in diameter, soft nodule, older patient), the patient is given thyroxine. If thyroxine does not induce regression in the latter case, the lesion should probably be excised.

There are 2 groups that represent special problems: patients with thyroid cysts and patients who have received radiation therapy. Although thyroid cysts are almost always benign, occasionally cancer is found in the wall of the cyst. For this reason, recurrent cysts should be studied with ultrasonography, and if there is evidence of a septated lesion or growth in the wall of the lesion, the lesion should be surgically removed. In patients who have received radiation therapy, there may be multiple lesions, some benign and some malignant. Therefore, in the presence of a cold nodule in a patient who has had radiation exposure, surgery is recommended directly.

If this protocol is followed, there will be a marked reduction in surgery for benign thyroid nodules, and the incidence of malignancy at the time of surgery will be about 40%. The cost savings is enormous, since unnecessary surgery is eliminated and the cost of thyroid nodule "workup" is cut in half. In addition, there is no delay in making the diagnosis and referring the patient with thyroid cancer for appropriate therapy.

2. THYROID CANCER

Pathology

The types and approximate frequency of malignant thyroid tumors are listed in Table 10–14.

A. Papillary Carcinoma: Papillary carcinoma of the thyroid gland usually presents as a firm, solitary, "cold," "solid" nodule clearly different from the rest of the gland. In multinodular goiter, the cancer will be a "dominant nodule"—larger, firmer, and (again) clearly different from the rest of the gland. About 10% of papillary carcinomas, especially in children, present with enlarged cervical nodes, but careful examination will usually reveal a "cold" nodule in the thyroid. Rarely, there will be hemorrhage, necrosis, and cyst formation in the malignant nodule, but on echo scan clearly defined internal echoes will differentiate the semicystic malignant lesion from the nonmalignant "pure cyst." Finally, papillary carcinoma may be found incidentally as a microscopic focus of cancer in the middle of a gland removed for other reasons such as Graves' disease.

Microscopically, the tumor consists of single layers

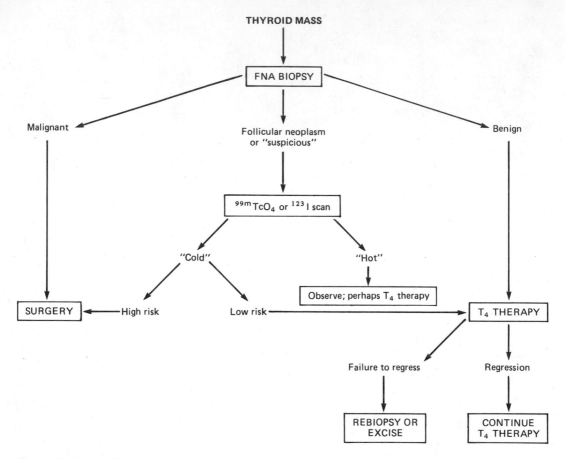

Figure 10–50. Decision matrix for workup of a thyroid nodule. See text for details. FNA = fine needle aspiration.

of thyroid cells arranged in vascular stalks, with papillary projections extending into microscopic cyst-like spaces. The nuclei of the cells are large and pale and frequently contain clear, glassy intranuclear inclusion bodies. About 40% of papillary carcinomas form laminated calcified spheres, often at the tip of a papillary projection, called "psammoma bodies." These are usually diagnostic of papillary carcinoma. These cancers usually extend by intraglandular metastasis and by local lymph node invasion. They grow very slowly and remain confined to the thyroid gland and local lymph nodes for many years. In older patients, they may become more aggressive and invade locally into muscles

Table 10–14. Approximate frequency of malignant thyroid tumors.

Papillary carcinoma (including mixed papillary and follicular)	75%
Follicular carcinoma	16%
Medullary carcinoma	5%
Undifferentiated carcinomas	3%
Miscellaneous (including lymphoma, fibrosarcoma, squamous cell carcinoma, malignant hemangioendothelioma, teratomas, and metastatic carcinomas)	1%

and trachea. In later stages, they can spread to the lung. Death is usually due to local disease, with invasion of deep sectors in the neck; less commonly, death may be due to extensive pulmonary metastases. In some older patients, a slowly growing papillary carcinoma will begin to grow rapidly and convert to undifferentiated or anaplastic carcinoma. This "late anaplastic shift" is another cause of death from papillary carcinoma. Many papillary carcinomas secrete thyroglobulin, which can be used as a marker for recurrence or metastasis of the cancer.

B. Follicular Carcinoma: Follicular carcinoma is characterized by the maintenance of small follicles, although colloid formation is poor. Indeed, follicular carcinoma may be indistinguishable from follicular adenoma except by capsular or vascular invasion. The tumor is slightly more aggressive than papillary carcinoma and can spread either by local invasion of lymph nodes or by blood vessel invasion with distant metastases to bone or lung. Microscopically, the cells are cuboidal, with large nuclei arranged around follicles that frequently contain colloid. These tumors often retain the ability to concentrate radioactive iodine, to form thyroglobulin, and, rarely, to synthesize T_3 and T_4. Thus, the rare "functioning thyroid cancer" is almost always a follicular carcinoma. This characteristic makes these tumors more likely to respond to radioactive iodine therapy. In untreated patients, death is due to local extension or to distant bloodstream metastasis with extensive involvement of bone, lungs, and viscera.

A variant of follicular carcinoma is the "Hurthle cell" carcinoma, characterized by large individual cells with pink-staining cytoplasm filled with mitochondria. They behave like follicular cancer except that they rarely take up radioiodine. Mixed papillary and follicular carcinomas behave more like papillary carcinoma. Most follicular carcinomas secrete thyroglobulin, and this feature can be used to follow the course of disease.

C. Medullary Carcinoma: Medullary cancer is a disease of the C cells (parafollicular cells) derived from the ultimobranchial body and capable of secreting calcitonin, histaminase, prostaglandins, serotonin, and other peptides. Microscopically, the tumor consists of sheets of cells separated by a pink-staining substance that has characteristics of amyloid. This material stains with Congo red. Amyloid consists of chains of calcitonin laid down in a fibrillary pattern—in contrast to other forms of amyloid, which may have immunoglobulin light chains or other proteins deposited in a fibrillary pattern.

Medullary carcinoma is somewhat more aggressive than papillary or follicular carcinoma but not as aggressive as undifferentiated thyroid cancer. It extends locally into lymph nodes and into surrounding muscle and trachea. It may invade lymphatics and blood vessels and metastasize to lungs and viscera. Calcitonin secreted by the tumor is a marker for medullary carcinoma and can be used both to discover the tumor and to follow its cure or recurrence. About two-thirds of medullary carcinomas are familial, and about one-third are isolated instances of the cancer. The familial tumors may be associated with multiple endocrine neoplasia type IIa (Sipple's syndrome), characterized by medullary carcinoma, pheochromocytomas, and parathyroid adenomas; or they may be associated with type IIb, characterized by medullary carcinoma, pheochromocytomas, and multiple neuromas of the tongue, lips, and bowel (see Chapter 28). At times, only the medullary carcinoma is familial, and no other endocrine glands are involved. If medullary carcinoma is diagnosed, it is important that all family members be screened for possible medullary carcinoma. The best screening test is measurement of serum calcitonin after pentagastrin and calcium stimulation (see Chapter 11).

D. Undifferentiated (Anaplastic) Carcinoma: Undifferentiated thyroid gland tumors include small cell, giant cell, and spindle cell carcinomas. They usually occur in older patients with a long history of goiter in whom the gland suddenly—over weeks or months—begins to enlarge and produce pressure symptoms, dysphagia, or vocal cord paralysis. Death from massive local extension usually occurs within 6–36 months. These tumors are very resistant to therapy.

E. Miscellaneous Types:

1. Lymphoma–The only type of rapidly growing thyroid cancer that is responsive to therapy is the lymphoma, which may develop as a part of a generalized lymphoma or may be primary in the thyroid gland. Thyroid lymphoma occasionally develops in a patient with long-standing Hashimoto's thyroiditis and may be difficult to distinguish from chronic thyroiditis. It is characterized by lymphocyte invasion of thyroid follicles and blood vessel walls, which helps to differentiate thyroid lymphoma from chronic thyroiditis. If there is no systemic involvement, the tumor may respond dramatically to radiation therapy.

2. Metastatic thyroid cancer–Many systemic cancers metastasize to the thyroid gland, including cancers of the breast and kidney, bronchogenic carcinoma, and malignant melanoma. The primary site of involvement is usually obvious. Occasionally, the diagnosis is made by needle biopsy or open biopsy of a rapidly enlarging cold thyroid nodule. The prognosis is that of the primary tumor.

Management of Thyroid Cancer (Fig 10–51)

A. Papillary and Follicular Carcinoma: Lobectomy is satisfactory for small (< 2 cm) papillary and follicular thyroid carcinomas, but near-total thyroidectomy is required for larger lesions or for cancers with evidence of extrathyroidal extension. Modified neck dissection is indicated if there is evidence of lymph node metastases. Prophylactic neck dissections are not recommended.

Radioidine scan and therapy are indicated for patients with large papillary or follicular carcinomas (> 2 cm) or with evidence of intra- or extrathyroidal extension. Postoperatively, the patient receives liothyronine (Cytomel), 75–100 μg daily in divided doses for about 3 months; the medication is then stopped for 2 weeks and the patient is placed on a low-iodine diet. The patient is scanned at 24 and 72 hours after a dose of 2–5 mCi of ^{131}I. Liothyronine is used for replacement therapy because it is cleared from the blood rapidly; after 2 weeks off therapy, TSH levels are sufficiently high to obtain good scanning studies. If there is evidence of residual radioactive iodine uptake in the neck or elsewhere, radioactive iodine (^{131}I) is effective treatment. The scan is repeated at intervals of 6–12 months until no further uptake is observed; the patient is then maintained on maximum replacement therapy with levothyroxine, 0.15–0.3 mg daily, to suppress serum TSH to undetectable levels.

Follow-up at intervals of 6–12 months should include careful examination of the neck for recurrent masses. If a lump is noted, needle biopsy examination is indicated to confirm or rule out cancer. Serum thyroglobulin will usually be undetectable after total thyroidectomy and levothyroxine therapy. A rise in serum

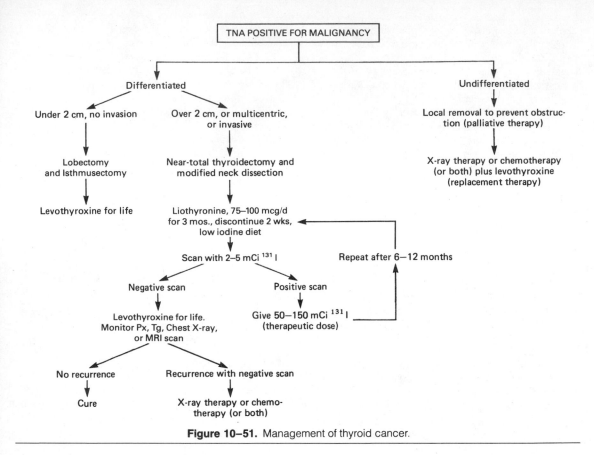

Figure 10–51. Management of thyroid cancer.

thyroglobulin suggests recurrence of thyroid cancer. Chest x-ray or MRI scan every 2–3 years may reveal local or pulmonary metastases, although a rising serum thyroglobulin concentration is a more sensitive indicator. If the patient does develop a mass in the neck, a rise in serum thyroglobulin, or a mass on chest x-ray or MRI scan, ^{131}I scan should be repeated following the technique outlined above. If the lesions concentrate ^{131}I, this may be useful in treatment; if they do not concentrate ^{131}I, local excision or local x-ray therapy may be useful. For recurrences that cannot be managed by these modalities, chemotherapy should be considered.

B. Medullary Carcinoma: Patients with medullary carcinoma should be followed in a similar way, except that the marker for recurrent medullary cancer is serum calcitonin. Carcinoembryonic antigen (CEA) is also a useful marker for medullary carcinoma. Histaminase and other peptides are also secreted by these tumors, but assays for these substances are not generally available. If a patient has a persistently elevated serum calcitonin concentration after total thyroidectomy and regional node dissection, MRI scan of the neck and chest or selective venous catheterization and sampling for serum calcitonin may reveal the location of the metastases. If this fails to localize the lesion (as is often the case), the patient must be followed until the

metastatic lesion shows itself as a palpable mass or a shadow on the chest x-ray or MRI scan. Metastatic medullary carcinoma cannot be treated with ^{131}I; therefore, initial thorough surgical excision and levothyroxine therapy are best. Chemotherapy for medullary carcinoma has not been effective.

C. Anaplastic Carcinoma: Anaplastic carcinoma of the thyroid has a very poor prognosis. Treatment consists of isthmusectomy (to confirm the diagnosis and to prevent tracheal compression) and palliative x-ray therapy. Thyroid lymphomas are quite responsive to x-ray therapy; giant cell, squamous cell, spindle cell, and anaplastic carcinomas are unresponsive. Chemotherapy is not very effective for anaplastic carcinomas. Doxorubicin (Adriamycin), 75 mg/m² as a single injection or divided into 3 consecutive daily injections repeated at 3-week intervals, has been useful in some patients with disseminated thyroid cancer unresponsive to surgery, TSH suppression, or radiation therapy. This drug is quite toxic; side effects include cardiotoxicity, myelosuppression, alopecia, and gastrointestinal symptoms.

D. X-Ray Therapy: Local x-ray therapy has been useful in the treatment of solitary metastatic lesions, particularly follicular or papillary tumors, that do not concentrate radioactive iodine. It is particularly effective in isolated nonfunctional bone metastases.

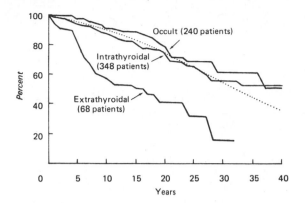

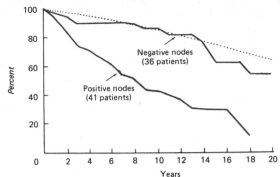

Figure 10–52. Papillary carcinoma. Survivorship curves for occult, intrathyroidal, and extrathyroidal lesions. Dotted line is curve for normal persons of comparable age and sex. (Reproduced, with permission, from Woolner LB et al: Long term survival rates. In: *Thyroid Cancer.* Vol 12. Hedinger CE [editor]. UICC Monograph Series. Springer-Verlag, 1969.)

Figure 10–54. Medullary carcinoma. Survivorship curves for patients with metastatic involvement of cervical lymph nodes at time of initial surgery and those without such involvement. Dotted line is curve for normal persons of comparable age and sex. (Reproduced, with permission, from Woolner LB et al: Long term survival rates. In: *Thyroid Cancer.* Vol 12. Hedinger CE [editor]. UICC Monograph Series. Springer-Verlag, 1969.)

Prognosis

Papillary carcinoma of the thyroid (the most common type) may exist as a microscopic focus in the gland. The incidence of microscopic foci of thyroid cancer at autopsy has varied from 4% in several series in the USA to as high as 25% in persons of Japanese descent living in the Hawaiian Islands. The lesion does not shorten life and is probably of no clinical significance. Woolner et al have shown that in patients with "occult" or microscopic papillary carcinoma—or small intrathyroidal papillary carcinoma—the sur-

vival rate is about the same as that of individuals without thyroid cancer. However, if there is evidence of extrathyroidal extension of the cancer, life expectancy is markedly affected (Fig 10–52). Similarly, in persons with small, noninvasive follicular carcinoma, the survival rate does not differ from that of control groups; whereas in the case of follicular carcinoma that has invaded blood vessels or in which there is evidence of extrathyroidal extension, survival is poor (Fig 10–53). Medullary carcinoma shows a similar pattern, with good survival for intrathyroidal small lesions and impaired survival for patients with extrathyroidal extension (Fig 10–54). Patients with anaplastic carcinomas have a very poor prognosis; almost all are dead within 3 years (Fig 10–55).

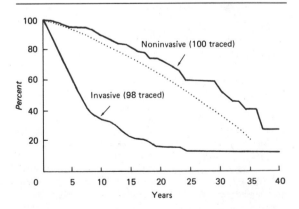

Figure 10–53. Follicular carcinoma. Survivorship curves (6 operative deaths excluded) for patients with slight or equivocal capsular invasion and those with moderate or marked invasion (including recurrent and inoperable tumors). Dotted line is curve for normal persons of comparable age and sex. (Reproduced, with permission, from Woolner LB et al: Long term survival rates. In: *Thyroid Cancer.* Vol 12. Hedinger CE [editor]. UICC Monograph Series. Springer-Verlag, 1969.)

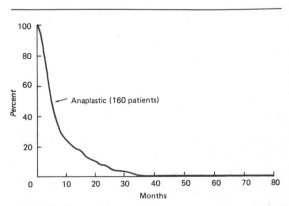

Figure 10–55. Anaplastic carcinoma. Survivorship curve, plotted in months. (Reproduced, with permission, from Woolner LB et al: Long term survival rates. In: *Thyroid Cancer.* Vol 12. Hedinger CE [editor]. UICC Monograph Series. Springer-Verlag, 1969.)

Other factors related to prognosis in patients with papillary or follicular carcinoma are:

1. Age at diagnosis: Patients over 40 generally have a worse prognosis than younger patients.

2. Sex: Males have a poorer survival rate than females.

3. Size of primary tumor: Over 4 cm has a worse prognosis.

4. Degree of differentiation of the primary tumor: The less well differentiated tumors produce a poor prognosis.

5. Extent of local spread at time of initial surgery:

Local invasion has a worse prognosis than nodal involvement.

6. Extent of initial surgery: Although young patients with small lesions of papillary carcinoma may do well after lobectomy, near-total thyroidectomy and modified neck dissection if nodes are positive yield the best survival rates.

7. Postoperative ^{131}I therapy for residual tumor: This greatly improves the prognosis.

8. Postoperative T_4 therapy with TSH suppression: This also improves the prognosis.

REFERENCES

Thyroid Physiology & Tests

Bilezikan JP, Loeb JN: The influence of hyperthyroidism and hypothyroidism on α- and β-adrenergic receptor systems and adrenergic responsiveness. *Endocr Rev* 1983;**4**:378.

DeGroot LJ, Niepomniszcze H: Biosynthesis of thyroid hormone: Basic and clinical aspects. *Metabolism* 1977;**26**:665.

Gershengorn MC: Mechanism of thyrotropin-releasing hormone stimulation of pituitary hormone secretion. *Annu Rev Physiol* 1986;**48**:515.

Greenspan SL et al: Pulsatile secretion of thyrotropin in man. *J Clin Endocrinol Metab* 1986;**63**:661.

Hay ID, Klee GG: Thyroid dysfunction in diagnostic evaluation of endocrine disorders. *Endocrinol Metab Clin North Am* 1988;**17**:473.

Ingbar SH: Autoregulation of the thyroid: Response to idoide excess and depletion. *Mayo Clin Proc* 1972;**47**:814.

Jackson IM: Thyrotropin-releasing hormone. *N Engl J Med* 1982;**306**:145.

Krenning EP et al: Strategy of thyroid-function testing: A comparative study using TT_4, FT_4I, various FT_4, and IRMA-TSH kits. *J Endocrinol Invest* 1986;**9(Suppl 4)**:95.

Magnusson RP et al: Molecular cloning of the complementary deoxribonucleic acid for human thyroid peroxidase. *Mol Endocrinol* 1987;**1**:856.

Martino E et al: Human serum thyrotrophin measurement by ultrasensitive immunoradiometric assay as a first-line test in the evaluation of thyroid function. *Clin Endocrinol* 1986;**24**:141.

Morley JE: Neuroendocrine control of thyrotropin secretion. *Endocr Rev* 1981;**2**:396.

Oppenheimer JH et al: Advances in our understanding of thyroid hormone action at the cellular level. *Endocr Rev* 1987;**8**:288.

Roti E et al: The placental transport, synthesis and metabolism of hormones and drugs which affect thyroid function. *Endocr Rev* 1983;**4**:131.

Samuels HH et al: Regulation of gene expression by thyroid hormone. *J Clin Invest* 1988;**81**:957.

Wall JR (editor): Autoimmune thyroid disease. *Endocrinol Meta Clin North Am* 1987;**16**:229.

Wolff J: Iodide goiter and the pharmacologic effects of excess idoide. *Am J Med* 1969;**47**:101.

Wolff J, Chaikoff IL: Plasma inorganic iodide as a homeostatic regulator of thyroid function. *J Biol Chem* 1948;**174**:555.

Hypothyroidism

Bastenie PA, Bonnyns M, Vanhaelst L: Natural history of primary myxedema. *Am J Med* 1985;**79**:91.

Becker C: Hypothyroidism and atherosclerotic heart disease: Pathogenesis, medical management, and the role of coronary artery bypass surgery. *Endocr Rev* 1985;**6**:432.

Fisher DA et al: Results of screening one million North American infants. *J Pediatr* 1979;**94**:700.

Hennessey JV et al: L-Thyroxine dosage: A reevaluation of therapy with contemporary preparations. *Ann Intern Med* 1986;**105**:11.

Holvey DN et al: Treatment of myxedema coma with intravenous thyroxine. *Arch Intern Med* 1964;**113**:89.

Lazarus JH, Hall R (editors): Hypothyroidism and goitre. *Bailliere Clin Endocrinol Metab* 1988;**2**:531. [Entire issue.]

Robuschi G et al: Hypothyroidism in the elderly. *Endocr Rev* 1987;**8**:142.

Santos AD et al: Echocardiographic characterization of the reversible cardiomyopathy of hypothyroidism. *Am J Med* 1980;**68**:675.

Symons RG, Murphy LJ: Acute changes in thyroid function tests following ingestion of thyroxine. *Clin Endocrinol* 1983;**19**:539.

van der Gaag RD, Drexhage HA, Dussault JH: Role of maternal immunoglobulins blocking TSH-induced thyroid growth in sporadic forms of congenital hypothyroidism. *Lancet* 1985;**1**:246.

Zwillich CW et al: Ventilatory control in myxedema and hypothyroidism. *N Engl J Med* 1975;**292**:662.

Hyperthyroidism

Bradley EL III, DiGirolamo M, Tarcan Y: Modified subtotal thyroidectomy in the management of Graves' disease. *Surgery* 1980;**87**:623.

Burrow GN: The management of thyrotoxicosis in pregnancy. *N Engl J Med* 1985;**313**:562.

Char DH: *Thyroid Eye Disease.* Williams & Wilkins, 1985.

Cooper DS: Which antithyroid drug? *Am J Med* 1986;**80**:1165.

Gorman CA, Robertson JS: Radiation dose in the selection of ^{131}I or surgical treatment for toxic thyroid adenoma. *Ann Intern Med* 1978;**89**:85.

Graham GD, Burman KD: Radioiodine treatment of Graves' disease: An assessment of its potential risks. *Ann Intern Med* 1986;**105**:900.

Ikram H: The nature and prognosis of thyrotoxic heart disease. *Q J Med* 1985;**54**:19.

Jacobson DH, Gorman CA: Diagnosis and management of endocrine ophthalmopathy. *Med Clin North Am* 1985;**69**:973.

Lamberg BA et al: Antithyroid treatment of maternal hyperthyroidism during lactation. *Clin Endocrinol* 1984;**21**:81.

Laurberg P et al: Goitre size and outcome of medical treatment of Graves' disease. *Acta Endocrinol* 1986;**111**:39.

Marcocci C et al: Orbital cobalt irradiation combined with retrobulbar or systemic corticosteroids for Graves' ophthalmopathy: A comparative study. *Clin Endocrinol* 1987;**27**:33.

Matsuura N et al: TSH-receptor antibodies in mothers with Graves' disease and outcome in their offspring. *Lancet* 1988;**1**:14.

Murakami M et al: Studies of thyroid function and immune parameters in patients with hyperthyroid Graves' disease in remission. *J Clin Endocrinol Metab* 1988;**66**:103.

Rapoport B et al: Clinical experience with a human thyroid cell bioassay for thyroid-stimulating immunoglobulin. *J Clin Endocrinol Metab* 1984;**58**:332.

Ruiz M et al: Familial dysalbuminemic hyperthyroxinemia, a syndrome that can be confused with thyrotoxicosis. *N Engl J Med* 1982;**306**:635.

Streeten DH et al: Prevalence, natural history, and surgical treatment of exophthalmos. *Clin Endocrinol* 1987;**27**:125.

Toft AD (editor): Hyperthyroidism. *Clin Endocrinol Metab* 1985;**14**:299 [Entire issue.]

Volpé R: Immunoregulation in autoimmune thyroid disease. (Editorial.) *N Engl J Med* 1987;**316**:44.

Wang YS et al: Long-term treatment of Graves' disease with iopanoic acid (Telepaque). *J Clin Endocrinol Metab* 1987;**65**:679.

Syndrome of Inappropriate TSH Secretion

Comi RJ et al: Response of thyrotropin-secreting pituitary adenomas to a long-acting somatostatin analogue. *N Engl J Med* 1987;**317**:12.

Gharib H et al: The spectrum of inappropriate pituitary thyrotropin secretion associated with hyperthyroidism. *Mayo Clin Proc* 1982;**57**:556.

Nontoxic Goiter

Greenspan FS: Medical treatment of nodular goiters. In: *Endocrine Surgery of the Thyroid and Parathyroid Glands.* Clark OH (editor). Mosby, 1985.

Stanbury JB, Metzel BS (editors): *Endemic Goiter and Endemic Cretinism.* Wiley, 1980.

Studer H, Ramelli F: Simple goiter and its variants: Euthyroid and hyperthyroid multinodular goiters. *Endocr Rev* 1982;**5**:40.

Thyroiditis

Hamburger JI: The various presentations of thyroiditis: Diagnostic considerations. *Ann Intern Med* 1986;**104**:219.

Hay ID: Thyroiditis: A clinical update. *Mayo Clin Proc* 1985;**60**:836.

Nikolai TF et al: Lymphocytic thyroiditis with spontaneously resolving hyperthyroidism (silent thyroiditis). *Arch Intern Med* 1980;**140**:478.

Tunbridge WM et al: The spectrum of thyroid disease in a community: The Whickham survey. *Clin Endocrinol* 1977;**7**:481.

Effects of Chronic Illness on Thyroid Function

Chopra IJ et al: Serum thyroid hormone-binding inhibitor in nonthyroidal illness. *Metabolism* 1986;**35**:152.

Chopra IJ et al: Thyroid function in nonthyroidal illness. *Ann Intern Med* 1983;**98**:946.

Engler D, Burger AG: The deiodination of the iodothyronines and of their derivatives in man. *Endocr Rev* 1984;**5**:151.

Faber J et al: Pituitary-thyroid axis in critical illness. *J Clin Endocrinol Metab* 1987;**65**:315.

Hamblin PS et al: Relationship between thyrotropin and thyroxine changes during recovery from severe hypothyroxinemia of critical illness. *J Clin Endocrinol Metab* 1986;**62**:717.

Wehmann RE et al: Suppression of thyrotropin in the low-thyroxine state of severe nonthyroidal illness. *N Engl J Med* 1985;**312**:546.

Thyroid Nodules & Thyroid Cancer

Gharib H et al: Suppressive therapy with levothyroxine for solitary thyroid nodules: A double-blind controlled clinical study. *N Engl J Med* 1987;**317**:70.

Goolden AW: The indications for ablating normal thyroid tissue with ^{131}I in differentiated thyroid cancer. *Clin Endocrinol* 1985;**23**:81.

Hamilton TE, van Belle G, LoGerfo JP: Thyroid neoplasia in Marshall Islanders exposed to nuclear fallout. *JAMA* 1987;**258**:629.

Lowhagen T et al: Aspiration Biopsy Cytology (ABC) in tumors of the thyroid gland suspected to be malignant. *Surg Clin North Am* 1979;**59**:3.

Mazzaferri EL: Papillary and follicular thyroid cancer: A selective approach to diagnosis and treatment. *Annu Rev Med* 1981;**32**:73.

Miller JM, Hamburger JI, Kim S: Diagnosis of thyroid nodules: Use of fine-needle aspiration and needle biopsy. *JAMA* 1979;**241**:481.

Pacini F et al: Diagnostic value of a single serum thyroglobulin determination on and off thyroid suppressive therapy in the follow-up of patients with differentiated thyroid cancer. *Clin Endocrinol* 1985;**23**:405.

Roher HD, Clark OH (editors): *Thyroid Tumors.* Vol 19 of: *Progress in Surgery.* Farthmann EH (editor). Karger, 1988.

Rojeski MT, Gharib H: Nodular thyroid disease: Evaluation and management. *N Engl J Med* 1985;**313**:428.

Samaan NA et al: Impact of therapy for differentiated carcinoma of the thyroid: An analysis of 706 cases. *J Clin Endocrinol Metab* 1983;**56**:1131.

Sampson RJ et al: Thyroid carcinoma in Hiroshima and

Nagasaki. I. Prevalence of thyroid carcinoma at autopsy. *JAMA* 1979;**209:**65.

Sarkar SK et al: Subsequent fertility and birth histories of children and adolescents treated with ^{131}I for thyroid cancer. *J Nucl Med* 1976;**17:**460.

Schlumberger M et al: Differentiated thyroid carcinoma in childhood: Long-term follow-up of 72 patients. *J Clin Endocrinol Metab* 1987;**65:**1088.

Schlumberger M et al: Long-term results of treatment of 283 patients with lung and bone metastases from differentiated thyroid carcinoma. *J Clin Endocrinol Metab* 1986;**63:**960.

Schneider AB et al: Radiation-induced thyroid carcinoma: Clinical course and results of therapy in 296 patients. *Ann Intern Med* 1986;**105:**405.

Simpson WJ et al: Papillary and follicular thyroid cancer: Prognostic factors in 1578 patients. *Am J Med* 1987;**83:**479.

Watson RG et al: Invasive Hürthle cell carcinoma of the thyroid: Natural history and management. *Mayo Clin Proc* 1984;**59:**851.

Wells SA Jr et al: Early diagnosis and treatment of medullary thyroid carcinoma. *Arch Intern Med* 1985;**145:**1248.

Werner B et al: Multimodal therapy in anaplastic giant cell thyroid carcinoma. *World J Surg* 1984;**8:**64.

The Calciotropic Hormones & Metabolic Bone Disease

11

Claude D Arnaud, MD, & Felix O Kolb, MD

EXTRACELLULAR & BONE MINERAL HOMEOSTASIS

A highly integrated and complex endocrine system maintains calcium, phosphate, and magnesium homeostasis in all vertebrates. It involves an interplay between the actions of 2 polypeptide hormones, parathyroid hormone (PTH) and calcitonin (CT), and a sterol hormone, 1,25-dihydroxycholecalciferol, or $1,25(OH)_2D_3$.* Biosynthesis and secretion of the polypeptide hormones are regulated by a negative feedback mechanism that involves the activity of ionic calcium in the extracellular fluid (Fig 11–1). The biosynthesis of $1,25(OH)_2D_3$ from the major circulating metabolite of vitamin D, 25-hydroxycholecalciferol ($25OHD_3$), takes place in the kidney and is regulated by PTH and CT, as well as by the extracellular fluid concentrations of calcium and phosphate. Other hormones, such as insulin, cortisol, growth hormone (GH), thyroxine, epinephrine, estrogen, testosterone, somatomedin, and inorganic phosphate, together with some compounds not yet identified and certain physical phenomena, undoubtedly have roles in modifying and regulating organ responses to PTH, CT, and $1,25(OH)_2D_3$.

PTH, CT, and $1,25(OH)_2D_3$ regulate the flow of minerals into and out of the extracellular fluid compartment through their actions on intestine, kidney, and bone (Table 11–1; Fig 11–2). The target cells of these organs function as a cellular barrier between the extracellular fluid compartment and the intestinal

---

*The nomenclature of the calciotropic hormones and vitamin D metabolites discussed in this chapter is generally in agreement with the recommendations of the Endocrine Society and conforms to the editorial practices of the *Journal of Clinical Endocrinology and Metabolism*. Note especially the following: vitamin D_3 = cholecalciferol; vitamin D_2 = ergocalciferol; 25-hydroxycholecalciferol = $25OHD_3$; 25-hydroxyergocalciferol = $25OHD_2$; 1,25-dihydroxycholecalciferol (often written $1\alpha,25$-dihydroxy . . . in other texts) = $1,25(OH)_2D_3;24,25$-dihydroxycholecalciferol = $24,25(OH)_2D_3$. A few others of lesser importance are mentioned briefly in the section entitled Vitamin D.

Acronyms Used in This Chapter

ACTH	Adrenocorticotropic hormone
ATP	Adenosine triphosphate
cAMP	Cyclic adenosine monophosphate
CGRP	Calcitonin gene-related peptide
CT	Calcitonin
DER (DEX)	Dual-energy radiography
DPA	Dual-photon absorptiometry
GFR	Glomerular filtration rate
GH	Growth hormone
Gpp (NH)p	5'-Guanyl-imidodiphosphate
HAM	Hypoparathyroidism–Addison's disease–mucocutaneous candidiasis (syndrome)
iCT	Immunoreactive calcitonin
iPTH	Immunoreactive parathyroid hormone
MEDAC	Multiple endocrine deficiency–autoimmune–candidiasis (syndrome)
MEN	Multiple endocrine neoplasia
MRI	Magnetic resonance imaging
OAF	Osteoclast-activating factor
PRL	Prolactin
PTH	Parathyroid hormone
QCT	Quantitative computer-assisted tomography
RNA	Ribonucleic acid

---

lumen, the renal tubular lumen, and the bone fluid compartment (adjacent to mobilizable bone mineral) (Fig 11–3). These target cells are highly specialized for solute transport against a concentration gradient and thus are often described as being polarized.

Role of Parathyroid Hormone
Target Tissues

Under normal circumstances, PTH prevents serum calcium from falling below physiologic concentrations by stimulating calcium movement from intestinal and renal tubular lumina and from the bone fluid compartment into the blood. Whereas its effects on bone and kidney are direct, PTH acts indirectly on the intestine, through the mediation of vitamin D. The hormone

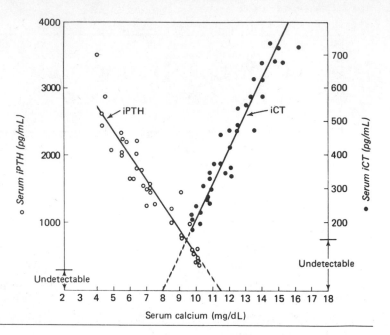

Figure 11–1. Plasma immunoreactive PTH (iPTH) and CT (iCT) as a function of plasma total calcium in pigs given EDTA to decrease plasma calcium or given calcium infusions to increase plasma calcium. Note that as serum calcium increases, serum iPTH falls and serum iCT rises; as serum calcium decreases, the reverse occurs. ($r = -0.942$ for iPTH and 0.964 for iCT; p for both is <.001.) (Reproduced, with permission, from Arnaud CD et al, in: *Calcitonin: Proceedings of the Second International Symposium.* Taylor S [editor]. Heinemann, 1969.)

stimulates (directly and through its hypophosphatemic effects) the conversion of $25OHD_3$ to $1,25(OH)_2D_3$ in the kidney via a $25OHD_3$ 1α-hydroxylase in the mitochondria of the renal tubule. The $1,25(OH)_2D_3$ thus formed stimulates intestinal calcium absorption. PTH also prevents serum phosphate levels from rising above normal physiologic concentrations by increasing renal tubular excretion of phosphate. This regulatory action is important because phosphate, like calcium, is also released into the blood by PTH-induced bone resorption. This function can be particularly appreciated in patients with end-stage renal failure associated with severe hyperparathyroidism. These patients develop hyperphosphatemia because large quantities of phosphate are released from bone, and the kidney can no longer excrete them.

Role of Calcitonin

Calcitonin prevents abnormal increases in both serum calcium and serum phosphate. It decreases the translocation of calcium from the renal tubule and bone fluid compartment into the blood and thus can be considered as a counterregulator of PTH. The effects of CT on vitamin D metabolism and on the intestinal absorption of calcium are uncertain.

Integrated Actions of PTH, CT, & $1,25(OH)_2D_3$

It is likely that PTH and CT regulate the entry of calcium into polarized cells of the surface membrane of bone and the renal tubular lumen. $1,25(OH)_2D_3$ acts primarily to maintain the cellular calcium transport system in the intestine, which causes the active

Table 11–1. Actions of major calcium-regulating hormones.

	Bone	Kidney	Intestine
Parathyroid hormone (PTH)	Increases resorption of calcium and phosphate.	Increases reabsorption of calcium; decreases reabsorption of phosphate; increases conversion of $25OHD_3$ to $1,25(OH)_2D_3$; decreases reabsorption of bicarbonate.	No direct effects.
Calcitonin (CT)	Decreases resorption of calcium and phosphate.	Decreases reabsorption of calcium and phosphate. Questionable effect on vitamin D metabolism.	No direct effects.
Vitamin D	Maintains Ca^{2+} transport system.	Decreases reabsorption of calcium.	Increases absorption of calcium and phosphate.

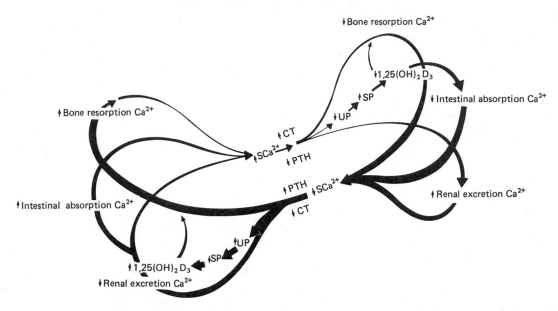

Figure 11–2. Regulation of calcium homeostasis. Three overlapping control loops interlock and relate to one another through the level of blood concentrations of ionic calcium, PTH, and CT. Each loop involves a calciotropic hormone target organ (bone, intestine, kidney). The limbs on the left depict physiologic events that increase the blood concentration of calcium (SCa²⁺), and the limbs on the right, events that decrease this concentration. UP = urine phosphorus, SP = serum phosphorus. See text for detailed descriptions. (Modified and reproduced, with permission, from Arnaud CD: *Fed Proc* 1978;**37**:2558.)

extrusion of calcium against a concentration gradient from the interior of the cell (ionized calcium concentration = 10^{-7} to 10^{-6} mol/L), across the antiluminal membrane, and into the extracellular fluid (ionized calcium concentration = 10^{-3} mol/L) (Fig 11–4). Thus, the calciotropic hormones, especially PTH and $1,25(OH)_2D_3$, are interdependent. The renal production of $1,25(OH)_2D_3$ depends upon the prevailing concentration of PTH in the blood, and the ability of PTH to increase plasma calcium depends upon a calcium transport system maintained by $1,25(OH)_2D_3$.

Interrelationship of Calcium & the Calciotropic Hormones

The relationships among the several components involved in maintaining mineral homeostasis are illustrated in Figure 11–2. Each of the 3 overlapping

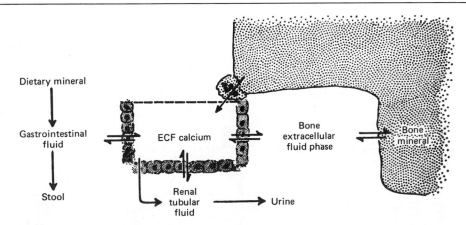

Figure 11–3. Cellular barrier separating the extracellular fluid compartment from the intestinal and renal tubular lumina and from the bone fluid compartment. PTH, CT, and $1,25(OH)_2D_3$ act on those cells (directly or indirectly) to regulate the flow of calcium into and out of the extracellular fluid (ECF) compartments. (See Fig 11–2.) (Reproduced, with permission, from Rasmussen H et al: *Fed Proc* 1979;**29**:1190.)

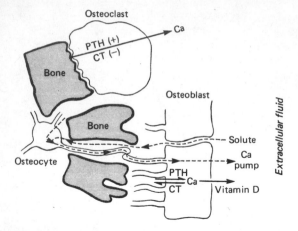

Figure 11–4. Relationships among calciotropic hormones, bone cells, and calcium transport. Bone crystal is represented by the shaded areas. The osteoclast, with an active "ruffled border," is shown resorbing bone—a process stimulated by PTH (+) and inhibited by CT (−). The "osteoblasts" (perhaps better called "surface osteocytes") are not forming bone but are actively extruding calcium from the bone fluid (between cells and crystals) under the influence of hormones. Processes connecting deep osteocytes are shown participating in transport of calcium (dotted arrows).

feedback loops involves one of the target organs of the calciotropic hormones and the 4 controlling elements, ie, plasma calcium, PTH, CT, and $1,25(OH)_2D_3$. The left limbs of the loops depict physiologic events that increase plasma calcium, and the right limbs, events that decrease plasma calcium. Under physiologic conditions, there are small fluctuations in plasma calcium. Decreases in plasma calcium increase PTH secretion and decrease CT secretion. These changes in hormone secretion lead to increased bone resorption, decreased renal excretion of calcium, and increased intestinal calcium absorption via PTH stimulation of $1,25(OH)_2D_3$ production (left side of Fig 11–2). As a consequence of these events, plasma calcium rises slightly above its physiologic concentrations, inhibiting PTH secretion and stimulating CT secretion. These changes in plasma hormone concentrations decrease bone resorption, increase renal excretion of calcium, and decrease intestinal absorption of calcium (right side of Fig 11–2), causing plasma calcium to fall below the physiologic level. This sequence of events probably occurs within milliseconds, so that plasma calcium is maintained at physiologic levels within minimal oscillation. The "butterfly" scheme in Figure 11–2 not only demonstrates the relationships among elements that control mineral homeostasis under physiologic conditions but also suggests how potential pathogenic mechanisms and adaptive responses elicited by disease or treatment would operate in this system.

Plasma Calcium & Phosphate

A. Calcium: The circulating forms of calcium and phosphorus and their normal ranges are shown in Fig 11–5. Calcium is distributed in 3 major fractions: ionized, protein-bound, and complexed. The ionized fraction (Ca^{2+}), which is the only biologically active form, constitutes 46–50% of the total calcium. The protein-bound fraction, roughly equivalent to the ionized fraction in amount, is biologically inert. However, the calcium bound to albumin (80%) and globulin (20%) is an important source of readily available Ca^{2+}; since the binding of calcium to these proteins obeys the mass-law equation, calcium can dissociate from its binding sites as a first line of defense against hypocalcemia. Moreover, hyperproteinemia (eg, hyperglobulinemia in myelomatosis) can increase, and hypoproteinemia (eg, hypoalbuminemia in cirrhosis of liver and nephrosis) can decrease total plasma calcium without changing the concentration of ionized calcium. Formulas such as the following have been developed to estimate the percentage of calcium bound to the plasma proteins based on the differential binding affinities of albumin and globulin:

$$\text{\% protein-bound } Ca^{2+} = 8 \times \text{albumin (g/dL)} + 2 \times \text{globulin (g/dL)} + 3$$

Such formulas permit the calculation of diffusible calcium (see below) by subtracting protein-bound from total calcium. Estimates of this type can be inadequate, however, especially in patients with low plasma protein concentrations. The only means of accurately determining the plasma concentration of ionized calcium in hypo- or hyperproteinemic states is to measure it

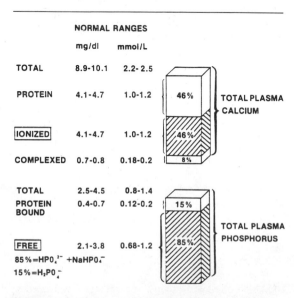

Figure 11–5. Distribution and normal ranges of calcium and phosphorus in the plasma.

directly using an ion-sensitive electrode procedure. The fraction of calcium that is complexed to organic (eg, citrate) and inorganic (eg, phosphate or sulfate) acids is small (approximately 8%) and, like the ionized fraction, it is ultrafiltrable (diffusible). Complexed calcium probably has little quantitative importance as a reservoir for ionized calcium, but excessive complexing of calcium with phosphate may contribute to the decrease in plasma ionized calcium observed in states of hyperphosphatemia such as may exist in chronic renal failure.

The normal distribution for the serum calcium (Fig 11–5) is small 1.2 mg/dL) compared to the total serum calcium (8.9–10.1 mg/dL), and the same is true for the ionized fraction. Assuming that plasma protein concentrations are normal, values for total calcium below 8.9 mg/dL reflect clinically significant hypocalcemia, and values above 10.1 mg/dL reflect hypercalcemia. In recent years, serum calcium has been measured with reasonable accuracy in most clinical laboratories. However, stored plasma samples may yield artifactual decreases in circulating calcium concentrations, and contaminated serum samples may yield artifactual increases. Thus, in order to obtain reliable measurements of calcium, it is important to use fresh serum and to eliminate sources of contamination (eg, chalk writing boards) from the laboratory.

The plasma calcium concentration varies little in spite of major changes in dietary calcium because of the adaptive alterations made by the endocrine system regulating this mineral (Fig 11–2). Minor diurnal changes (decreases in the afternoon) have been recorded. In addition, plasma calcium decreases with age in men but not in women, probably owing to a decrease in the serum albumin in men. Total (but not ionized) serum calcium also decreases in pregnancy; this change may be due to the decrease in the serum albumin concentration in this condition.

1. Hypocalcemia–Hypocalcemia produces a myriad of symptoms; severe hypocalcemia can result in tetany and, possibly, convulsions (see Hypoparathyroidism).

2. Hypercalcemia–Hypercalcemia can produce functional changes in most organ systems, and these changes may lead to a variety of symptoms and objective findings (see Hyperparathyroidism).

B. Phosphorus: Only 15% of the plasma phosphate is bound to proteins in the blood (Fig 11–5). The rest is ultrafiltrable and consists mainly of free HPO_4^{2-} and $NaHPO_4^-$ (85%), with free $H_2PO_4^-$ making up the remainder (15%). By convention, plasma phosphate is expressed in terms of the amount of elemental phosphorus measured.

Compared with calcium concentration, phosphorus concentration has a wider range of normal plasma values (2.5–4.5 mg/dL) (Fig 11–5). Moreover, increases or decreases in dietary phosphorus are promptly reflected in corresponding increases or decreases in

serum phosphorus and urinary phosphorus excretion. Marked diurnal variations in serum and urinary phosphorus excretion occur (both may as much as double in the afternoon and evening), even in fasting subjects. These variations are caused in part by diurnal changes in plasma cortisol. Serum phosphorus concentrations in young children are almost double those in adults, and in women they increase slightly with age. The reason for these differences in children and in aging women is poorly understood but may be associated with the increased bone turnover present in both of these groups.

Serum phosphorus can be measured accurately and precisely in most laboratories. However, artifactually high levels may be obtained if (1) serum extracts or dialysates are exposed to acid longer than is prescribed (resulting in the hydrolysis of organic compounds containing phosphorus), or (2) hemolyzed serum is used (red blood cells contain phosphorus).

1. Hypophosphatemia–Acute respiratory alkalosis, the administration of a large quantity of carbohydrate, and the administration of insulin all cause a rapid decrease in serum phosphorus. Severe hypophosphatemia (<1.5 mg/dL) may occur during the treatment of diabetic ketoacidosis or during forced nutrition of undernourished patients and can cause both skeletal myopathy and cardiomyopathy. Hypophosphatemia may lead to rhabdomyolysis, as evidenced by increases in serum creatine phosphokinase. The levels of 2,3-diphosphoglyceric acid and adenosine triphosphate (ATP) in erythrocytes may also decrease; the decrease in 2,3-diphosphoglyceric acid in turn may decrease oxygen delivery to tissues, and the decrease in ATP may cause hemolytic anemia. Chronic moderate hypophosphatemia frequently results in osteomalacia or rickets, as seen in X-linked hypophosphatemia, a genetic disorder (see Osteomalacia). Generally, restoration of serum phosphate concentrations to normal levels corrects the abnormal organ function caused by hypophosphatemic conditions, except in X-linked hypophosphatemic rickets, which requires individualized treatment regimens.

2. Hyperphosphatemia–Acute, severe hyperphosphatemia—as might be induced by intravenous phosphate infusion—can cause hypocalcemia severe enough to result in tetany and even death. The less severe hyperphosphatemia induced by phosphate ingestion rarely causes symptoms; however, if patients have associated disorders in which there is a tendency toward hypocalcemia (eg, mild hypoparathyroidism or chronic renal failure), frank hypocalcemia may be precipitated.

Interrelationship of Plasma Calcium & Phosphate

The physiologic importance of the relationship between the circulating concentrations of ionized calcium and diffusible (free) phosphate is poorly understood, especially with regard to the formation and dissolution of amorphous calcium phosphate [Ca$_3$(PO$_4$)$_2$] and hydroxyapatite [Ca$_{10}$(PO$_4$)$_6$(OH)$_2$] in bone. However, available evidence indicates that the ion product of normal plasma concentrations of calcium and phosphate (the calcium × phosphate product) is considerably higher than that necessary to form these 2 compounds. Thus, compared with bone, plasma is supersaturated with calcium and phosphate, and this can be considered an important driving force in bone mineralization. The positive effect of vitamin D on bone mineralization is probably indirect and resides in its ability to maintain the calcium × phosphate product in the normal range by increasing absorption of calcium and phosphate in the gut and resorption of calcium and phosphate from bone (Fig 11–2).

The biologic significance of the calcium × phosphate product has been questioned in recent years, but it is important to recognize that products below 20 mg/dL (0.7 mmol/L) usually reflect a mineralization defect in bone, and products above 70 mg/dL (2.2 mmol/L) reflect a propensity toward soft tissue calcification. There are exceptions to these numerical guidelines, but short of directly measuring changes in bone formation in bone biopsy specimens or changes in calcium content in soft tissues, determining the calcium × phosphate product may provide the best indirect indication of the presence of these pathologic changes.

Calcium & Phosphate Economy

The quantitative aspects of calcium and phosphorus metabolism under conditions of metabolic balance (dietary intake equal to urinary and fecal excretion) are illustrated in Figures 11–6 and 11–7, respectively. The amounts of dietary calcium and phosphate required to maintain metabolic balance vary with the physiologic need for these minerals, the ability of the intestine to absorb them, and the ability of the kidneys to conserve them.

Normally, young adults (ages 21–35 years) require a dietary intake of 12–15 mg/kg/d of calcium and 15–20 mg/kg/d of phosphorus. During periods of rapid skeletal growth (eg, in children or during the development of the fetal skeleton in pregnant women) these requirements may double or triple. In adults aged 50 years and older, calcium requirements tend to increase because the efficiency of intestinal calcium absorption declines. Postmenopausal women and most elderly men need to ingest approximately 50% more calcium than do young adults. Unfortunately, even this level of dietary calcium may not compensate for the inefficient

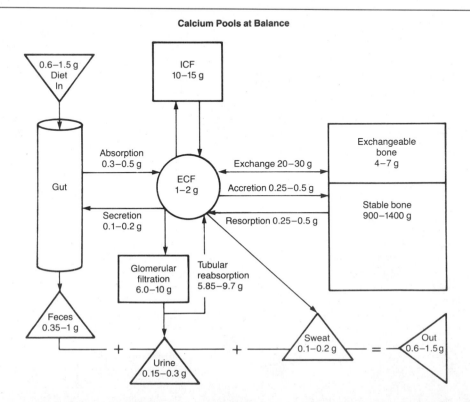

Figure 11–6. Normal distribution of calcium in the body. ICF = intracellular fluid, ECF = extracellular fluid.

Phosphorus Pools at Balance

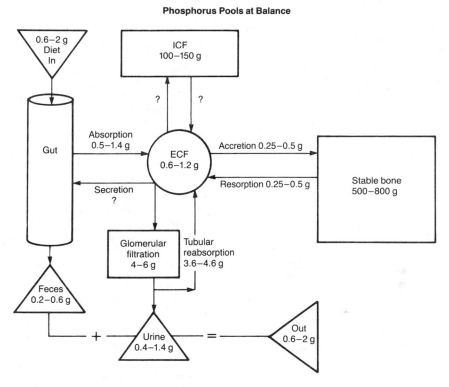

Figure 11–7. Normal distribution of phosphorus in the body. ICF = intracellular fluid, ECF = extracellular fluid.

intestinal absorption of calcium in many elderly persons.

Dietary deprivation of calcium or phosphorus induces adaptive changes in the production and secretion of the calciotropic hormones that minimize the development of negative metabolic balance of calcium and phosphate ions. Like most adaptive mechanisms in biology, these changes are beneficial when applied over a relatively short period of time but, when applied chronically, they can have destructive effects of considerable consequence. In the case of calcium, only 30–50% of ingested calcium is normally absorbed (Fig 11–6). With decreased intake, serum calcium decreases slightly, and the sequence of events depicted in the left limbs of the feedback loops in Figure 11–2 is activated. In severe, chronic dietary calcium deficiency in normal subjects, PTH stimulates an increase in plasma $1,25(OH)_2D_3$ levels, which can increase fractional intestinal calcium absorption up to 75%. It also reduces renal calcium excretion to low levels, but this response is quantitatively less important because of the relatively small percentage of filtered calcium excreted. Such changes reduce the overall consequences of this perturbation on overall body calcium economy. However, this adaptive response is offset by the development of chronic hyperparathyroidism, a condition that can induce progressive bone demineralization (see Primary Hyperparathyroidism).

Whereas the intestine plays the major role in the body's adaptation to a dietary deficiency of calcium, the kidney plays the major role in maintaining phosphate balance during dietary deficiency of phosphorus. This is because 70–80% of dietary phosphorus is normally absorbed and practically all (80% or more) of absorbed phosphorus is excreted by the kidney (Fig 11–7). Thus, any increase in intestinal absorption of phosphorus in response to dietary deficiency would have little influence in preventing a negative balance, but a decrease in renal excretion of phosphorus by only 50%, for example, would have an effect comparable to that of almost tripling dietary intake. Reductions of this magnitude and greater occur rapidly and are sustained for long periods in response to dietary deficiency of phosphorus. The mechanism (or mechanisms) involved in this response is not entirely understood. The hypophosphatemia that occurs in phosphate deficiency is associated with increased production of $1,25(HO)_2D_3$, increased intestinal absorption of calcium, mild hypercalcemia and a decrease in PTH secretion (Fig 11–2, left, middle limb), increased renal tubular reabsorption of phosphate, and hypophosphaturia. However, it is well established that efficient renal phosphate conservation in response to dietary phosphate deprivation occurs in parathyroidectomized animals; this finding casts doubt upon the hypothesis that the calciotropic hormone response to phosphorus deprivation alone is responsible for the observed hypophosphaturia in hypophosphatemia.

Magnesium Homeostasis

Magnesium is the major intracellular divalent cation. Its extracellular concentration is normally maintained within a reasonably narrow range (1.5–2.2 mg/dL), but, whereas diets low in calcium do not lead to appreciable hypocalcemia, dramatic decreases in serum magnesium can be observed in humans whose diets are deficient in magnesium for as little as one week. Thus, despite the presence of appreciable stores of magnesium in cells and bone, it is not readily available; serum concentrations of magnesium are greatly dependent upon adequate dietary supplies and normal intestinal absorption.

Increased renal conservation of magnesium is an almost immediate response to dietary deficiency of magnesium. This response is thought to be due to an effect of PTH on the renal tubule similar to that which PTH exerts on the renal tubular reabsorption of calcium. Like hypocalcemia, mild to moderate hypomagnesemia stimulates PTH secretion, albeit to a lesser extent, indicating the presence of at least the rudiments of a negative feedback system that can potentially maintain extracellular magnesium homeostasis. The feedback system is complicated, however, because severe hypomagnesemia (<1 mg/dL) inhibits both PTH secretion and action, causing hypocalcemia and hyperphosphatemia (see Hypoparathyroidism).

PARATHYROID HORMONE

Structure & Biosynthesis

PTH is an 84-amino-acid, linear polypeptide with a molecular weight of 9500. Its biosynthesis and intracellular processing are complex (Fig 11–8). The original gene product of the parathyroid cell is a 115-amino-acid precursor called preproparathyroid hormone (preproPTH). The hydrophobic 23-amino-acid "pre" sequence acts to bind the polyribosome-precursor complex to the endoplasmic reticulum, providing access to the cisternal space and, presumably, to the enzyme ("clipase") that removes the "pre" sequence, leaving the 90-amino-acid proPTH structure. The proPTH is converted to PTH in the Golgi apparatus by proteolytic removal ("tryptic clipase") of the remaining 6-amino-terminal amino acid sequence. Here, the 84-amino-acid polypeptide is readied for secretion either in a secretory granule or in its free form. There is no evidence that either of the PTH precursor molecules or the "pre" or "pro" peptide sequences normally find their way into the circulation. In contrast to the rapid regulation of PTH *secretion,* PTH *biosynthesis* is only slowly influenced by changes in concentration of extracellular ionic calcium.

Intracellular stores of PTH may be regulated by a degradative pathway that is stimulated by high and inhibited by low extracellular calcium. Not only may this degradative pathway provide an important mechanism for regulating PTH economy, but the fragments of the hormone produced during intracellular degradation and secreted from the cell may also provide a major source of the multiple immunoreactive forms of PTH known to circulate in the blood (see below).

The amino acid sequences of bovine, porcine, and human PTH have been determined (Fig 11–9). The differences among them prevent complete immunologic cross-reactivity. This probably accounts for the difficulties in developing radioimmunoassays for the measurement of human PTH using antisera directed against bovine or porcine peptides. All of the structural information required for full biologic activity of native 84-amino-acid PTH lies in the 34 amino acids at the amino terminus. The active fragments of the bovine and human hormones, multiple fragments of the mid and carboxyl regions of the bovine and human hormones, and recently the full sequence of human parathyroid hormone have been synthesized and are available for investigational use. Studies of the mid- and carboxy-region fragments have shown them to be biologically inert.

Control of Secretion

PTH is rapidly released from the parathyroid gland in response to decreases in the plasma ionic calcium. It acts on kidney and bone and indirectly on intestine to restore the concentration of this cation to just above the normal set point (Fig 11–1), which in turn inhibits secretion of the hormone. This negative feedback cycle is depicted in Figure 11–2. The concentration of extracellular ionic calcium is the major regulator of PTH secretion. Other factors influence secretion only indirectly through increasing or decreasing extracellular ionic calcium. The effects of extracellular magnesium concentrations on secretion are qualitatively similar to but physiologically less important than those induced by ionic calcium. Paradoxically, severe, prolonged hypomagnesemia markedly inhibits secretion of PTH and may be associated with hypocalcemia (see above). Known direct PTH secretagogues of questionable physiologic importance include beta-adrenergic agonists, prostaglandins, and histamine. These agents, as well as decreased ionic calcium, stimulate the production of cyclic 3′,5′-adenosine monophosphate (cAMP) in parathyroid cells in vitro. cAMP may be an important mediator of parathyroid cell secretagogues, but intracellular calcium itself and the phosphoinositol-diacyl-glycerol system play important roles in regulating PTH secretion.

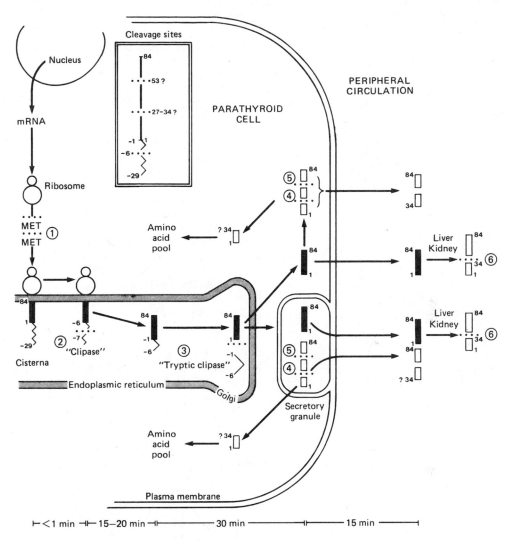

Figure 11–8. Proposed intracellular pathway of the biosynthesis of PTH. The initial product of synthesis on the ribosomes, preproPTH, is converted into proPTH by removal of ① the NH$_2$-terminal methionyl residues (methionyl aminopeptidase) and ② the NH$_2$-terminal sequence (−29 through −7) of 23 amino acids (by "clipase") during synthesis and within seconds afterward, respectively. The conversion of preproPTH to proPTH probably occurs during transport of the polypeptide into the cisterna of the rough endoplasmic reticulum. By 20 minutes after synthesis, proPTH reaches the Golgi region and is converted into PTH by ③ removal of the NH$_2$-terminal hexapeptide. PTH is either stored in secretory granules or released into the cell cytoplasm, where it remains until it is released into the circulation in response to a fall in the blood concentration of calcium. The intact PTH, PTH(1–84), undergoes at least 2 cleavages while in the secretory granule (and possibly in the cytoplasm) ④ and ⑤. These cleavages generate amino-, mid-, and carboxy-region fragments. The mid- and carboxy-region fragments are secreted into the circulation along with PTH(1–84), whereas the amino-region fragments are further degraded by the cell. The PTH(1–84) released into the circulation undergoes metabolic degradation in the liver and kidney ⑥, and this adds to the pool of circulating fragments. The time required for these events to occur is shown. (Modified and reproduced, with permission, from Habener JF et al: *Recent Prog Horm Res* 1977;**33**:287.)

Metabolism & Circulating Forms

Circulating PTH is heterogeneous, consisting of the intact 84-amino-acid polypeptide and multiple fragments of the hormone (Fig 11–10). These fragments are derived from the mid and carboxyl regions of the hormone molecule and thus are likely to be biologically inert. There is no convincing evidence that biologically active fragments are secreted by the parathyroid gland or that they are present in the circulation. The relative quantities of intact PTH and its fragments in serum are not known precisely at present, but there are more circulating fragments than intact hormone.

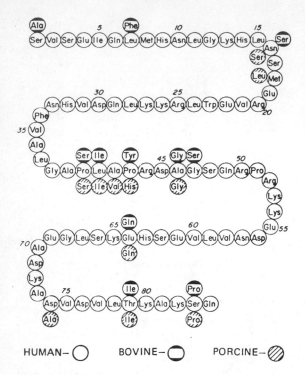

Figure 11–9. Parathyroid hormone. The figure shows the structure of human PTH and indicates at which positions the amino acid residues differ for bovine and porcine PTH. (From Keutmann HT et al: *Biochemistry* 1978;**17**:5723.)

This difference is due primarily to the longer survival time of the fragments in the circulation (see Fig 11–10 legend). The fragments are derived both by release from the parathyroid gland and from the degradative metabolism of intact 84-amino-acid PTH (liver and kidney); the quantitative importance of these sources is uncertain.

Biologically active PTH normally circulates in the blood at extremely low concentrations (<50 pg/mL). It is likely that there are individual, constitutionally dependent "set point" values for plasma ionic calcium above which glandular secretion rates are decreased and below which they are increased. However, the steady-state levels of PTH and the size of the glands are probably determined primarily by the degree to which the parathyroid glands must adapt to individual, chronic, environmentally induced changes in the plasma level of ionic calcium (eg, dietary calcium and phosphate). In normal humans (Fig 11–11), as in lower animals (Fig 11–1), there is an inverse relationship between the fasting levels of serum calcium and serum immunoreactive PTH.

Actions

The major function of PTH is to correct hypocalcemia. As Figure 11–2 shows, it performs this function by (1) conservation of calcium by the kidney, (2) release of calcium from bone, (3) enhanced absorption of calcium from the gut (indirectly via vitamin D), and (4) reduction in plasma phosphate.

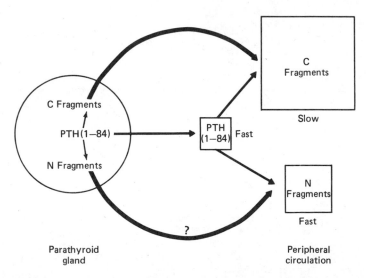

Figure 11–10. Metabolic alterations in PTH(1–84) that result in its immunoheterogeneity in gland extracts and biologic fluids. This scheme is based on study of abnormal parathyroid tissue and hyperparathyroid serum. Data on normal glands and serum are not available. An uncertain proportion of intraglandular PTH(1–84) is proteolytically cleaved into amino-region fragments (N fragments) and carboxy-region fragments (C fragments). All of these PTH molecular species are released into the circulation (approximately 80% PTH[1–84] and 20% fragments). Once in the circulation, PTH(1–84) undergoes proteolytic cleavage in liver and kidney, generating N and C fragments that are added to the circulating pool of hormone fragments. The rate of disappearance of C fragments from the circulation is slow ($t_{1/2}$ 20–40 minutes), whereas that of PTH(1–84) and of N fragments is fast ($t_{1/2}$ < 10 minutes). These differences in metabolic turnover probably account for the large pool of C fragments and small pools of PTH(1–84) and N fragments in the blood under steady-state conditions (see text). (Reproduced, with permission, from DiBella FP et al: Page 338 in: *Excerpta Medica Int Cong Ser* No 421, 1977.)

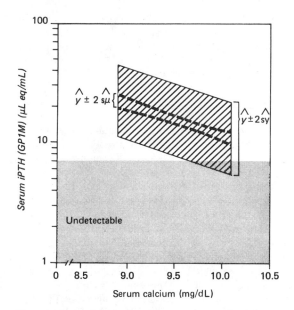

Figure 11–11. Serum immunoreactive PTH (iPTH) (log scale) as a function of total serum calcium in 150 normal human subjects ($r = -0.424$; $p < .001$). $y \pm 2\,s\mu$ = mean ± 2 SEM; $y \pm 2\,sy$ = mean ± 2 SD. GP1M is the antiserum (mid region) used in the radioimmunoassay. (Reproduced, with permission, from Purnell D et al: *Am J Med* 1974;**56**:801.)

A. Effects of PTH on Kidney: PTH acts on the kidney (1) to increase renal tubular reabsorption of calcium and magnesium and (2) to increase phosphate and bicarbonate excretion by inhibiting their proximal tubular resorption. These latter effects have several important indirect effects on the homeostasis of extracellular calcium. Hormone-induced bicarbonaturia tends to produce acidosis, which decreases the ability of circulating albumin to bind calcium, thus increasing ionic calcium by physicochemical means. Hormone-induced phosphaturia ensures that the increased release of phosphate from bone, which occurs obligately during hormone-induced calcium mobilization from bone, does not produce hyperphosphatemia. Increased serum phosphate would tend to complex calcium and thereby counteract the physiologic effect of PTH to increase plasma ionic calcium.

The most important indirect effect of the phosphaturic action of the hormone is illustrated in the intestinal feedback loop in Figure 11–2. PTH, either directly or indirectly by its hypophosphatemic action, stimulates renal tubular $25OHD_3$ 1α-hydroxylase to convert the major circulating metabolite of cholecalciferol, $25OHD_3$, to its major biologically active metabolite, $1,25(OH)_2D_3$. This latter compound acts directly on intestinal mucosal cells to increase calcium absorption and on bone to increase resorption.

In the process of stimulating adenylate cyclase in renal tubular cells (see below), PTH increases urinary

excretion of cAMP. Presumably, cAMP is released into the tubular fluid following its intracellular synthesis. Urinary cAMP is increased by administration of other hormones, including epinephrine and glucagon, but its renal production and excretion are almost entirely due to PTH. It can therefore be used as an indirect measure of PTH secretion or action, as noted below.

B. Effects of PTH on Bone: PTH increases the net release of calcium and phosphate from bone into extracellular fluid (Fig 11–4). This is a direct result of the hormone's effect on the differentiation or activities of bone cells (osteogenic precursors, osteoblasts, osteoclasts, and osteocytes). These events appear to depend upon a permissive effect of $1,25(OH)_2D_3$, but the precise cellular mechanism of this important hormonal relationship is poorly understood. The physiology and pathophysiology of mineral metabolism demonstrate a wide range of interactions between PTH (tropic) and vitamin D (permissive), and these interactions will be noted below in the sections on hypoparathyroidism, hyperparathyroidism, and metabolic bone disease.

Mechanisms of Action

PTH binds to specific plasma membrane receptors of target cells. These occupied receptors interact with a guanyl nucleotide-regulated membrane-bound protein that in turn activates membrane-bound adenylate cyclase to convert ATP to cAMP (Fig 11–12). cAMP, by virtue of its ability to initiate a cascade of enzyme-activated intracellular phosphorylations, is considered to be one of possibly several intracellular "second messengers" responsible for mediating the final expression of the action of the hormone. The details of these enzyme activations and the manner in which they relate to discrete effects of the hormone are unknown. Other potential second messengers of PTH (eg, calcium itself) that might act in concert with or modulate the actions of cAMP are currently being investigated.

Information concerning the structural requirements for the action of PTH at the site of its receptor is rapidly becoming available. The region of the molecule essential for receptor binding is the amino acid sequence 25–30, and for receptor activation, the 1–7 sequence. Recently, 2 analogues of bovine PTH that are truncated at the amino terminus have been developed. One of these is [8]Nle-[18]Nle-[34]Tyr-bPTH(3–34)amide, or bPTH(3–34)amide. This analogue has both agonist and antagonist properties in vitro. It binds to PTH receptors in the kidney to the same degree as bPTH(1–34) but is much less potent in converting the receptor to the high-affinity state necessary to activate adenylate cyclase (Fig 11–12). Although bPTH(3–34)amide acts as an antagonist in vitro, it fails to antagonize concomitantly administered PTH in vivo. The other analogue, [34]Tyr-bPTH(7–34)amide, has antagonist but no agonist properties in vitro. It antagonizes PTH in vivo, but

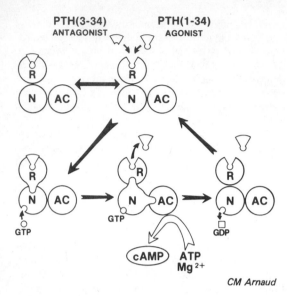

PTH(3-34) ANTAGONIST   **PTH(1-34)** AGONIST

CM Arnaud

Figure 11–12. Mechanism of PTH action on membrane-bound adenylate cyclase. PTH(1–34) is the biologically active PTH agonist 8Nle-18Nle-23Tyr-bPTH(1–34)amide, and PTH(3–34) is the biologically inactive PTH antagonist 8Nle-18Nle-34Tyr-bPTH(3–34)amide. Both of these are capable of binding to the PTH receptor (R). However, only PTH(1–34) is capable of converting the receptor to a high-affinity state, so that guanyl nucleotide regulatory protein (N) can be stimulated to bind guanosine triphosphate (GTP). The binding of GTP to N converts R to a low-affinity state, inducing dissociation of PTH(1–34) *and* the formation of an N-adenylate cyclase (AC) complex, leading to the activation of this enzyme and the increased production of intracellular cAMP. In contrast, the binding of PTH(3–34) to R does not change the affinity of R; consequently, R cannot interact with N or induce activation of adenylate cyclase.

large doses are required, possibly owing to the fact that its ability to bind to PTH receptors is weak. In spite of this, the development of this analog represents an important advance in the effort to design a PTH antagonist that can rapidly reverse hypercalcemia in patients with severe hyperparathyroidism.

Assay in Biologic Fluids

The major tool for measuring PTH in biologic fluids has been radioimmunoassay. Values for serum iPTH have varied from laboratory to laboratory because of the differences in the preparations used as standards and in the specificity of the antisera. Therefore, interpretation of serum iPTH values has required knowledge of the normal range for each assay system. Until recently, most radioimmunoassays of human PTH have used 125I-labeled bovine PTH as the radioligand and cross-reacting antisera directed against porcine or bovine PTH. The use of new preparations of synthetic human PTH or its fragments has helped to minimize

some of the inconsistencies. However, variations in the specificities of antisera used in different assays will continue to result in different iPTH values for the same serum sample. Such differences reflect true differences in the concentrations of the various forms of circulating PTH.

At present, all available antisera that have sufficiently high affinity for PTH to be useful in radioimmunoassays are multivalent and contain antibodies directed at multiple regions of the PTH molecule. Whereas antisera directed primarily against the mid or carboxyl region of the PTH molecule recognize both inactive mid- or carboxy-region fragments and intact biologically active PTH, antisera directed against the amino region recognize only amino-region fragments and intact PTH. Because the quantities of mid- and carboxy-region fragments in the circulation are greater than those of amino-region fragments or intact PTH, values for serum iPTH are higher in mid- and carboxy-region assays than in amino-region assays.

Mid- and carboxy-region assays have provided surprisingly good diagnostic tools in the evaluation of patients suspected of having parathyroid disease, even though the resulting values for serum iPTH primarily reflect circulating biologically inactive hormone (ie, mid- and carboxy-region fragments). This is fortunate because the concentration of intact PTH in the circulation are so low that, with rare exception, they are beyond the sensitivity limits of all the amino-region radioimmune assays.

Two-site immunoradiometric or chemiluminometric assays for circulating intact PTH have been reported as having a clinical diagnostic potential similar to that of mid- and carboxy-region assays except that, as expected, patients with chronic renal failure have relatively lower values compared to normal subjects than when mid- and carboxy-region assays are used. Because of the high sensitivity and ease with which such assays can be performed, it is likely that they will replace classic radioimmunoassay procedures.

Until recently, bioassays for PTH lacked sufficient sensitivity for the study of circulating PTH. This obstacle has now been overcome by 2 novel approaches. One is cytochemical bioassay that is based on the PTH-specific stimulation of glucose 6-phosphate dehydrogenase in guinea pig renal slices. This assay is extremely sensitive, measuring femtogram amounts of PTH. Its disadvantage is its technical complexity. The other assay, which is more convenient, uses a nonhydrolyzable analogue of guanosine triphosphate—ie, 5′-guanyl-imidodiphosphate, or Gpp(NH)p—to greatly augment the sensitivity of adenylate cyclase to PTH in canine kidneys in vitro. In the presence of Gpp(NH)p, as little as 10 pg/mL of intact PTH elicits significant stimulation. However, even with this sensitivity, the measurement of PTH in normal serum requires the immunoextraction of 3 mL of serum.

CALCITONIN

Structure & Biosynthesis

Calcitonin (CT), a 32-amino-acid polypeptide with a molecular weight of 3700 and a disulfide bridge between residues 1 and 7 (Fig 11–13), is biosynthesized and secreted by the ultimobranchial (parafollicular, "C") cells. Human CT is cleaved from a high-molecular-weight precursor that also contains 2 other peptides, katacalcin and calcitonin gene-related peptide (CGRP). These peptides circulate in normal subjects in roughly equimolar relationship to CT and, like CT, are secreted in excess in medullary carcinoma of the thyroid. The physiologic roles of these peptides are not known, but CGRP is a potent vasodilator.

The ultimobranchial cells develop from neural crest tissue during embryonic life. They form a discrete organ in submammalian vertebrates called the ultimobranchial gland. In the mammal, the anlage of the cells merges with the embryonic thyroid gland, ultimately becoming dispersed in the central region of each lobe (of the thyroid gland), adjacent to the follicular cells.

The amino acid sequences of CT from many species (porcine, bovine, human, rat, salmon, eel) have been determined (Fig 11–13). They are different enough so that immunologic cross-reactivity between them is in-

complete. In fact, radioimmunoassay of human CT was not possible until synthetic human CT became available so that specific antibodies directed against it could be used. The entire CT molecule is required for full biologic activity, as is the intact 1–7 disulfide bridge. Salmon CT has an amino acid sequence markedly different from those of mammalian CTs and is about 30 times more potent. Synthetic salmon and human CTs are commercially available and can be used for treatment of metabolic bone disease (see Osteoporosis and Paget's Disease, below).

Control of Secretion

CT is rapidly released by the "C" cells in response to small increases in plasma ionic calcium. It acts on kidney and bone to restore the level of this cation to just below a normal set point, which in turn inhibits secretion of the hormone (Fig 11–2). CT thus is a physiologic antagonist of PTH. The hormones act in concert to maintain the normal concentration of ionic calcium in extracellular fluid (Fig 11–2).

There is a positive correlation between plasma calcium and plasma immunoreactive CT (iCT) in normal subjects when plasma calcium is increased above the normal range (by oral calcium ingestion) (Fig 11–14). Induced hypercalcemia causes an increase in plasma iCT in about 40–60% of normal women and 70–80%

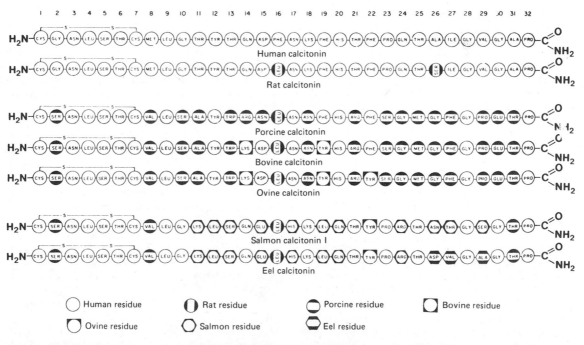

Figure 11–13. Amino acid sequence of CTs. Note the similarity between human and rat CT and the substantial differences in amino acid sequence from the porcine, bovine, and ovine CTs. Salmon and eel CTs are actually more similar to human CT than are hormones from ungulates. In the 7 amino acids in the N-terminal ring, the only substitution is serine for glycine. (Modified and reproduced, with permission, from Hirsch PF: *J Exp Zool* 1971;**178**:139.)

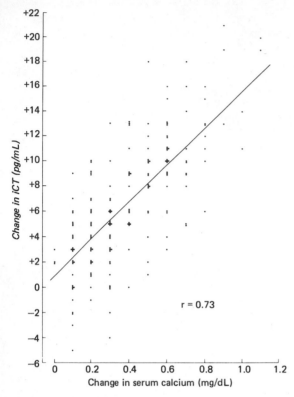

Figure 11–14. Changes in iCT plotted against corresponding changes in serum calcium after calcium ingestion. The data represent the responses of 10 subjects to each of 3 different oral calcium doses. (Reproduced, with permission, from Austin LA et al: *J Clin Invest* 1979;**64**:1721.)

of normal men. Although pentagastrin injection also increases plasma iCT, it is unlikely that gastrin is a physiologic CT secretagogue. Other CT secretagogues of unknown physiologic significance include glucagon, beta-adrenergic agonists, and alcohol.

Metabolism & Circulating Forms

CT exists in several molecular forms both in ultimobranchial tissue and in plasma. In contrast to PTH, however, the major circulating species are not hormone fragments but consist of as many as 4 or 5 immunoreactive forms with molecular weights larger than 32-amino-acid CT. It is likely that some of these forms are polymers of CT with interchain disulfide molecular linkages. The different antisera used in radioimmunoassays recognize these forms differently, and therefore the normal range for plasma CT must be established for each assay. The plasma concentrations of monomeric iCT are extremely low (<50 pg/mL).

Actions

The importance of CT in the calcium homeostasis of adult humans is not established. An excess or deficien-

cy of PTH or vitamin D produces dramatic clinical disorders. In contrast, an excess or deficiency of CT, as occurs in medullary thyroid carcinoma or postthyroidectomy, respectively, produces few discernible and no serious abnormalities of mineral metabolism. The basal plasma levels of CT and its responsiveness to induced hypercalcemia or pentagastrin injection are lower in women than in men. In adult humans, CT may function primarily to restrain the bone resorptive effects of PTH.

When bone turnover rates are high, CT administration rapidly produces hypocalcemia and hypophosphatemia. These effects are largely due to decreased bone resorption secondary to inhibition of activities of bone-resorbing cells (osteoclasts). CT also increases urinary calcium and phosphate, but its action on the kidney is transient and variable. Current evidence does not support a direct effect of CT on the intestinal absorption of calcium. However, several recent reports suggest that the hormone may have a negative influence on the renal production of $1,25(OH)_2D_3$. Such an effect would be consistent with the concept of CT as a physiologic antagonist of PTH.

Mechanisms of Action

CT receptors have been demonstrated in renal tubular cells and osteoclasts. The hormone stimulates adenylate cyclase in bone and kidney in some species (human and rat), but whether cAMP is a major intracellular mediator of CT action has not been established.

Assay in Biologic Fluids

The major tool for measuring CT in biologic fluids has been radioimmunoassay. Antibodies against human CT generally cross-react with rat CT, but antibodies against porcine or bovine CT cross-react poorly with human and rat CT. Although iCT in human plasma is heterogeneous, synthetic human CT is generally used as an assay standard. As with PTH, most antisera to human CT are multivalent, and assays using them measure the different circulating forms of CT differently. Thus, as noted above, the normal ranges for plasma iCT vary from laboratory to laboratory.

The single most important factor determining the clinical utility of a CT radioimmunoassay is its sensitivity. This is because many patients with CT-secreting medullary cancers of the thyroid gland have normal basal levels of plasma iCT and can be identified only with provocative tests (ie, calcium infusion, pentagastrin injection; see below). An assay that cannot measure basal levels of iCT cannot demonstrate an abnormal increase in plasma iCT.

Since the introduction of the original rat hypocalcemic assay for CT, there has been little progress in the development of convenient bioassays for this hormone. Although CT receptors have been demonstrated, radioreceptor assays are too insensitive for the measurement of CT in biologic fluids.

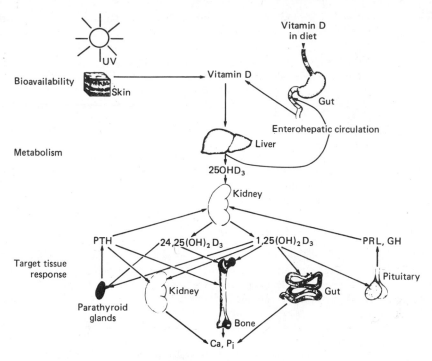

Figure 11–15. The vitamin D endocrine system. **Bioavailability:** Vitamin D is made available to the body by photogenesis in the skin and by absorption from the intestine. Part of the intestinal absorption involves endogenous vitamin D products secreted in bile (enterohepatic circulation). **Metabolism:** Vitamin D must be hydroxylated first in the liver to $25OHD_3$ and then in the kidney to $1,25(OH)_2D_3$ and $24,25(OH)_2D_3$. Other metabolites and other tissues capable of metabolizing the vitamin D metabolites are known. **Target tissue response:** The 3 principal target tissues are kidney, bone, and intestine, but the parathyroid glands and the anterior pituitary may also be target tissues. Their hormone products (PTH, PRL, and GH) help regulate vitamin D metabolism in the kidney, and PTH, at least, also has independent effects on the regulation of calcium and phosphate homeostasis in bone and kidney. (Reproduced, with permission, from Bikle DD: *Advances in Internal Medicine,* 1982. Year Book, 1982.)

VITAMIN D

Physiology, Metabolism, & Action

It is now firmly established that vitamin D and its metabolites are sterol hormones and that their metabolism and mechanism of action have much in common with those of the other steroid hormones (Fig 11–15). Vitamin D_3 (cholecalciferol) is primarily synthesized in the skin by ultraviolet irradiation of 7-dehydrocholesterol. Vitamin D_2 (ergocalciferol), which is used to fortify dairy products, is produced by ultraviolet irradiation of the plant sterol ergosterol.

A. Activation of Vitamin D: The parent compound, vitamin D, essentially lacks biologic activity and requires metabolic transformation to attain potency.

1. 25-Hydroxylation–The first step in this activation (Fig 11–15) involves 25-hydroxylation by microsomal enzymes—a process that occurs chiefly in the liver. This conversion does not appear to be tightly regulated, and the circulating concentration of 25-hydroxycholecalciferol ($25OHD_3$),* estimated to be

*See the footnote at the beginning of this chapter for a comment on the nomenclature of vitamin D metabolites.

about 30 ng/mL in normal individuals, is primarily a function of the bioavailability of vitamin D. Therefore, it is subject to both seasonal and regional variation, owing to differences in both diet and sunlight exposure. $25OHD_3$ is the most abundant circulating form of the hormone, and it is transported in serum bound to a specific globulin (vitamin D–binding protein), as are the other vitamin D metabolites.

2. 1α-Hydroxylation–The next step in the bioactivation of vitamin D, 1α-hydroxylation of $25OHD_3$, occurs in the mitochondria of the renal tubules. This hydroxylation is tightly regulated and constitutes the rate-limiting step in the production of the active metabolite, $1,25(OH)_2D_3$.* Production of $1,25(OH)_2D_3$ is controlled by a number of regulators in accordance with the body's mineral requirements. Hypophosphatemia and hypocalcemia appear to be the primary stimuli for activating renal 1α-hydroxylase. The stimulus created by low calcium levels is probably mediated by PTH, which stimulates 1α-hydroxylase activity either directly or by its hypophosphatemic effects (Figs 11–2 and 11–15). Evidence that CT inhibits the activity of 1α-hydroxylase is less strong. In addition, $1,25(OH)_2D_3$ may regulate its own synthesis directly or by suppressing the parathyroid glands, where receptors for this metabolite have been reported.

B. Concentrations of Vitamin D Metabolites: In normal individuals, $1,25(OH)_2D_3$ is estimated to circulate at concentrations as low as 30 pg/mL. This metabolite is more rapidly cleared from plasma than its more abundant precursor, $25OHD_3$, and is about 100 times more potent in stimulating intestinal calcium absorption. It is thus generally considered to be the major biologic effector of the vitamin D endocrine system. However, the fact that $25OHD_3$ circulates in concentrations 1000 times greater than $1,25(OH)_2D_3$ suggests that $25OHD_3$ may have intrinsic biologic importance as well.

C. Other Hydroxylation Pathways: Hydroxylation of $25OHD_3$ to $24,25(OH)_2D_3$ occurs mainly in the kidney and represents an alternative metabolic fate for $25OHD_3$. The regulation of this pathway generally appears to be reciprocal to that leading to $1,25(OH)_2D_3$: for example, PTH stimulates production of $1,25(OH)_2D_3$ but suppresses that of $24,25(OH)_2D_3$. At present, the physiologic importance of $24,25(OH)_2D_3$ is unclear. It may be involved in normal bone formation, but it is more likely that 24-hydroxylation represents the initial step in the metabolic elimination of $25OHD_3$. Additional vitamin D metabolites have been identified, including $25,26(OH)_2D_3$, $1,24,25(OH)_3D_3$, $1,25,26(OH)_3D_3$, and $25OH-26,23$-lactone. Excretion of vitamin D metabolites occurs primarily in the bile, and evidence has been presented for enterohepatic circulation of both $25OHD_3$ and $1,25(OH)_2D_3$.

Role of Vitamin D

It is generally accepted that the principal physiological role of vitamin D is to increase plasma levels of calcium and phosphate and thus maintain conditions favorable for bone mineralization. The most extensively studied physiologic action of $1,25(OH)_2D_3$, however, is its role in facilitating the absorption of calcium and phosphate by the intestine, and much of our knowledge concerning the molecular mechanism of action of vitamin D has been derived from studies of the intestinal cell. Intestinal cytosolic receptors for $1,25(OH)_2D_3$ have been demonstrated; they function to translocate the hormone into the cell nucleus, where the association of the hormone-receptor complex with chromatin influences transcription and promotes the production of at least one new protein, calcium-binding protein, which is presumed to facilitate transcellular calcium transport. According to this view, vitamin D acts as a classic steroid hormone; however it has also been suggested that the hormone may have cellular actions independent of de novo protein synthesis.

$1,25(OH)_2D_3$ receptors have also been demonstrated in bone, parathyroid glands, pancreas, pituitary, placenta, and other tissues. It is possible, therefore, that vitamin D acts directly on these tissues. Vitamin D may also have a role, as yet poorly defined, in muscle function. The recent identification of several additional target organs for $1,25(OH)_2D_3$, such as the hematolymphopoietic tissue, suggests a role far beyond its known importance in mineral metabolism. Some lymphomas and granulomatous disorders such as sarcoidosis may show ectopic production of $1,25(OH)_2D_3$ from its precursors, which may explain the hypercalcemia observed in these disorders. $1,25(OH)_2D_3$ may also have a regulatory role in connection with bone marrow stem cells and their progeny, including cells of T lymphocyte lineage.

Assay in Biologic Fluids

Two general approaches using radiolabeled vitamin D derivatives have been developed for measurement of the various vitamin D sterols in vitro: competitive protein-binding analysis and radioimmunoassay. The sensitive technique of competitive protein-binding analysis takes advantage of naturally occurring specific proteins that have high affinity for the vitamin D metabolites and are present either in serum (vitamin D-binding protein) or in intestinal target cells (vitamin D receptors). Both of these techniques involve competition in vitro between a radioligand and the vitamin D sterol of interest for available sites on the binding protein. Antisera for use in radioimmunoassays are developed against immunogenic derivatives of the vitamin D sterol molecule.

Existing competitive protein-binding assays and radioimmunoassays are not inherently specific for a single circulating vitamin D metabolite, because other closely related vitamin D metabolites compete to some extent for available binding sites on the binding protein or antibody. Furthermore, other components of blood, including plasma proteins and lipids, may cause nonspecific interference. To increase the specificity and sensitivity of the assays, it is necessary to first extract the vitamin D sterols from plasma using a suitable lipophilic solvent and then isolate the particular metabolite of interest chromatographically (using Sephadex LH-20 followed by high-pressure liquid chromatography). Simplified, rapid fractionation techniques that have been introduced recently should make the measurement of $25OHD_3$ and $1,25(OH)_2D_3$ more convenient.

A sensitive bioassay for $1,25(OH)_2D_3$ has been developed using the hormone's ability to mobilize calcium in embryonic bone organ cultures in vitro as an index of activity. This assay is comparable in sensitivity to competitive protein-binding assays and radioimmunoassays, but the procedure is tedious and requires experience to perform.

DISORDERS OF PARATHYROID FUNCTION

HYPOPARATHYROIDISM

Deficient secretion of PTH is characterized clinically by symptoms of neuromuscular hyperactivity and biochemically by hypocalcemia, hyperphosphatemia, and diminished to absent circulating iPTH.

Etiology

There are 3 major categories of PTH-deficient hypoparathyroidism: surgical, idiopathic, and functional.

Surgical hypoparathyroidism is the most common type. It may occur after any surgical procedure in which the anterior neck is explored, including thyroidectomy, removal of abnormal parathyroid glands, and excision of malignant neck lesions. Parathyroid glands need not actually be removed for hypoparathyroidism to ensue; in such cases, it is presumed that the blood supply to the parathyroid glands has been interrupted. Surgical hypoparathyroidism is relatively unusual (0.5–1%) when experienced surgeons perform neck explorations and when such procedures are quick and easy; however, the incidence increases alarmingly with surgical inexperience or with prolonged, extensive procedures requiring frequent blood vessel ligation.

Idiopathic hypoparathyroidism is a broad category of disorders undoubtedly with more than one cause. It can be divided into 2 subcategories depending on the age at onset: that occurring at an early age and that occurring late in life. Aside from congenital absence of the glands (as in DiGeorge's syndrome), the syndromes occurring at an early age are of genetic origin, usually with an autosomal recessive mode of transmission. This type of hypoparathyroidism is termed "multiple endocrine deficiency–autoimmune-candidiasis (MEDAC) syndrome" or "juvenile familial endocrinopathy" or "hypoparathyroidism–Addison's disease–mucocutaneous candidiasis (HAM) syndrome" (see Chapter 27). Circulating autoantibodies specific for parathyroid and adrenal tissue are frequently present but correlate poorly with clinical manifestations. Candidiasis is usually the first problem to appear (early childhood) and is resistant to both local antifungal measures and treatment of endocrine deficiencies. Hypoparathyroidism generally occurs about 4 years after the onset of candidiasis, at a mean age of 9 years, and Addison's disease about 5 years later, at a mean age of 14 years. Pernicious anemia (with autoantibodies to parietal cells and intrinsic factor), ovarian failure, and autoimmune thyroiditis with hypothyroidism and di-

abetes mellitus also occur in this category of patients. Sporadic cases of MEDAC syndrome have been reported; in most of these cases, patients are seen at a later age, and some have hypoparathyroidism only.

The late-onset form of idiopathic hypoparathyroidism occurs sporadically without circulating glandular autoantibodies. Except for rare instances of hemochromatotic and metastatic involvement, the cause of parathyroid gland destruction in these cases is unknown.

Functional hypoparathyroidism occurs in patients who have undergone long periods of hypomagnesemia. Such patients include those with selective defects in gastrointestinal magnesium absorption, generalized gastrointestinal malabsorption, or alcoholism. Since magnesium is required for PTH release from the glands, serum iPTH is characteristically low or undetectable. Hypocalcemia is also present. Treatment with magnesium salts is followed within minutes by an increase in serum iPTH and, ultimately, by restoration of eucalcemia. Magnesium is probably also required for the peripheral action of PTH, and hypocalcemia in patients with functional hypoparathyroidism may be partly due to failure of the hormone to act normally on its target tissues.

Less well understood is the neonatal hypoparathyroidism in infants of mothers with primary hyperparathyroidism. It is thought that in utero exposure to maternal hypercalcemia results in prolonged suppression of fetal parathyroid glands and failure of the parathyroid glands to respond to hypocalcemic stimuli after birth.

Pathology

Although it has not been documented, it is likely that small remnants of viable parathyroid tissue are present in many patients with surgical hypoparathyroidism. Patients with MEDAC syndrome may have lymphocytic infiltration and fibrosis of glands. In the few patients with late-onset idiopathic hypoparathyroidism who have been examined, fatty infiltration, fibrosis, and atrophy have been found.

Long-standing cases of hypoparathyroidism have characteristic soft tissue calcifications in the lens and basal ganglia of the brain. All types of bone cells are diminished, and both formation and resorption surfaces in bone are decreased.

Pathologic Physiology

The pathophysiologic and biochemical consequences of parathyroid gland removal can be appreciated by referring to the "butterfly" diagram (Fig 11–2). In this disease, the right limbs of the 3 feedback loops predominate, with (1) decreased bone resorption; (2) decreased renal phosphate excretion, increased serum phosphate, decreased $1,25(OH)_2D_3$, and decreased intestinal absorption of calcium; and (3) increased renal excretion of calcium for the prevailing serum concentration of calcium. There is hypocalcemia and usually hyperphosphatemia, if dietary phosphate intake has been normal. Urinary calcium is usually low unless eucalcemia has been restored with treatment. In the latter case, urinary calcium is generally higher than it was before the development of hypoparathyroidism, and it occasionally reaches hypercalciuric levels. Nephrogenous cAMP is decreased (Fig 11–22), but it increases promptly following administration of PTH.

Hypocalcemia and alkalosis (due to decreased bicarbonate excretion; see above), if sufficiently severe, cause increased neuromuscular excitability with consequent tetany and, rarely convulsions. Chronic hypocalcemia per se may also cause (1) basal ganglia calcification and occasional extrapyramidal neurologic syndromes; (2) papilledema and increased intracranial pressure; (3) psychiatric disorders; (4) skin, hair, and fingernail abnormalities; (5) candidal infections; (6) inhibition of normal dental development; (7) lenticular cataracts; (8) intestinal malabsorption; (9) prolongation of the QT and ST intervals of the ECG; (10) in rare cases, 2:1 heart block and, even more rarely, heart failure requiring digitalis and diuretics; and finally (11) increased serum concentrations of creatine phosphokinase and lactic dehydrogenase.

Classification

Parfitt has divided clinical hypoparathyroidism into 5 categories based primarily on the concentration of serum calcium. Grades 1 and 2 represent patients with no hypocalcemia and inconstant spontaneous hypocalcemia, respectively; grades 3, 4, and 5 represent patients whose serum calcium is below 8.5, 7.5, and 6.5 mg/dL, respectively. The clinical manifestations of hypoparathyroidism depend upon the severity and chronicity of the hypocalcemia.

Clinical Features

A. Neuromuscular Manifestations: In general, the rate of decrease in serum calcium appears to be the major determinant for development of neuromuscular complications (see below) of hypocalcemia. Thus, complications are most likely to occur within 1–2 days after parathyroidectomy, when serum calcium decreases acutely, and at serum calcium values that may be considerably higher (eg, 8 mg/dL) than might be found in patients who have had severe hypocalcemia (eg, 6 mg/dL) for long periods. Immediately after neck surgery in the region of the parathyroid glands, and for several days afterward, it is important to observe patients carefully for the development of the clinical signs (see below) heralding tetany rather than to rely on the absolute level of serum calcium.

Nerves exposed to low concentrations of calcium show decreased thresholds of excitation, repetitive responses to a single stimulus, reduced accommodation, and, in extreme cases, continuous activity. Such abnormal neural function occurs spontaneously in both sensory and motor fibers in hypocalcemic states and gives rise to neuromuscular manifestations.

1. Paresthesias–Numbness and tingling may occur around the mouth, in the tips of the fingers, and sometimes in the feet.

2. Tetany–An attack of tetany usually begins with prodromal paresthesias and is followed by spasms of the muscles of the extremities and face. The hands (Fig 11–16), forearms, and, less commonly, the feet become contorted in a characteristic way. First, the thumb is strongly adducted, followed by flexion of the metacarpophalangeal joints, extension of the interphalangeal joints (fingers together), and flexion of the wrist and elbow joints. This somewhat grotesque spastic condition, although quite painful when full-blown, is more alarming than dangerous.

3. Hyperventilation–Because of the alarm resulting from tetany, patients may hyperventilate and secrete increased amounts of epinephrine. Hyperventilation causes hypocapnia and alkalosis, which in turn worsen hypocalcemia by causing increased binding of ionic calcium to plasma proteins. Prolonged hyperventilation in normal subjects can lower serum ionic calcium and produce tetany, but great care should be exercised in attributing such findings to hyperventilation alone.

4. Adrenergic symptoms–Increased epinephrine secretion produces further anxiety, tachycardia, sweating, and peripheral and circumoral pallor.

5. Convulsions–Patients with hypoparathyroidism may have convulsions. Convulsions are much more common in young people with the disease and are of 2 types: one is a more generalized form of tetany followed by prolonged tonic spasms; the other is a typical epileptiform seizure (grand mal, jacksonian, focal, or petit mal). The latter type is associated with electroencephalographic findings typical of epilepsy. Because restoration of eucalcemia results in a decrease

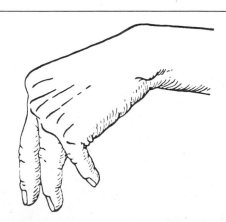

Figure 11–16. Position of hand in hypocalcemic tetany (Trousseau's sign). (Reproduced, with permission, from Ganong WF: *Review of Medical Physiology,* 12th ed. Lange, 1985.)

in the number of seizures without improvement in the electroencephalographic findings associated with seizures, it is thought that hypocalcemia lowers the excitation threshold of preexisting epilepsy. The characteristic electroencephalographic changes associated with hypocalcemia disappear after restoration of eucalcemia. Laryngeal spasm with obstruction may occur during tetany and may precipitate seizures because of hypoxia. The relatively unusual finding of papilledema and increased intracranial pressure resulting from hypocalcemia in association with convulsions mimics the clinical picture of brain tumor.

6. Signs of latent tetany—Latent tetany can be detected by several relatively specific physical signs. **Chvostek's sign** is elicited by tapping the facial nerve just anterior to the ear lobe, just below the zygomatic arch, or between the zygomatic arch and the corner of the mouth. The response ranges from twitching of the lip at the corner of the mouth to twitching of all of the facial muscles on the stimulated side. Simple twitching at the corner of the mouth occurs in 25% of normal subjects, but more extensive muscle contraction (ala nasi and orbital muscles) is a reliable sign of latent tetany.

Trousseau's sign (Fig 11–16) should be sought with a sphygmomanometer cuff. The cuff is inflated to above systolic blood pressure for at least 2 minutes while the hand is observed carefully. A positive response consists of the development of typical carpal spasm (Fig 11–16), with relaxation occurring 5–10 seconds after the cuff is deflated. An apparent spasm that disappears instantly may not be significant. Trousseau's sign is the most reliable sign of latent tetany, and serial tests for it should be performed and the results recorded in the immediate postoperative period after anterior neck surgery.

7. Extrapyramidal signs—Extrapyramidal neurologic syndromes, including classic parkinsonism, occur in patients with chronic hypoparathyroidism. Such manifestations are presumed to be related in some way to the calcification of the basal ganglia that is present in most patients. Many untreated patients without extrapyramidal syndromes are unduly sensitive to the dystonic side effects of phenothiazine drugs, suggesting that basal ganglion calcification may have more general pathologic importance than was once believed. Successful treatment of hypocalcemia may improve the neurologic disorder and is sometimes associated with decreases in basal ganglion calcification on x-ray.

B. Other Clinical Manifestations:

1. Posterior lenticular cataract—This is the most common sequela of hypoparathyroidism. Cataracts must be present and growing for 5–10 years before visual impairment occurs. Fully mature cataracts in hypoparathyroidism are confluent and produce total opacity of the lens. Such cataracts are different from senile cataracts, which are frequently confined to one segment of the lens. Successful treatment of hypo-

calcemia generally halts the progression of cataracts, and in rare cases the opacities may diminish in size.

2. Cardiac manifestations—Prolongation of the QT interval in the ECG (corrected for rate) is associated with hypocalcemia. Resistance to digitalis, hypotension, and refractory congestive heart failure with cardiomegaly may occur; these are reversed by normalization of the serum calcium.

3. Dental manifestations—Abnormalities in enamel formation, delayed or absent dental eruption, and defective dental root formation with short or blunted roots indicate that hypocalcemia was present during childhood.

4. Malabsorption syndrome—Intestinal malabsorption with steatorrhea is uncommon in hypoparathyroidism but may be present in patients with long-standing untreated disease. It is presumed to be due to decreased serum calcium because it is reversed by successful treatment of hypocalcemia but not by a gluten-free diet. Management is difficult because treatment of hypoparathyroidism largely depends on the ability to increase calcium transport across a normal gastrointestinal tract with drugs.

Diagnosis

A. Serum Calcium: Detection of hypoparathyroidism depends upon being alert to its possible presence in certain clinical situations. Accurate annual measurements of serum calcium are indicated (1) in patients who have had anterior neck surgery or (2) in those suspected of having MEDAC syndrome. Cutaneous candidiasis, cataracts, incidentally discovered calcifications of the basal ganglia, convulsions, numbness and tightening of the fingers, facial muscle spasm (spontaneous or self-induced), delayed dentition, and developmental retardation are all indications for prompt serum calcium measurement.

B. Serum Phosphorus: In the absence of renal failure, the diagnosis of hypoparathyroidism is virtually certain if hypocalcemia and hyperphosphatemia are found. Some patients, however, may be relatively phosphate-depleted because of dietary restriction, malabsorption, or the ingestion of aluminum hydroxide gels. In patients who have undergone parathyroidectomy for primary hyperparathyroidism, osseous avidity for minerals may be so great as to actually produce hypophosphatemia. In the first instance, the exclusion of nonparathyroid disorders as the cause of hypocalcemia becomes important. In the second, the question arises whether hypocalcemia is due to the hypoparathyroidism or to "bone hunger" alone.

C. Serum iPTH: In both circumstances, measurement of serum iPTH is crucial for the correct diagnosis. Increased values in a range appropriate to the degree of hypocalcemia would essentially exclude the presence of hypoparathyroidism and suggest end-organ resistance to PTH (pseudohypoparathyroidism, vitamin D deficiency, vitamin D dependency) or secondary hyperparathyroidism due to such disorders as dietary deficiency of calcium, intestinal malabsorption of calcium, or excessive intake of drugs containing absorbable phosphate (eg, neutral phosphate in the treatment of X-linked hypophosphatemic rickets).

An undetectable serum iPTH confirms the diagnosis of hypoparathyroidism if the assay technique used is sensitive enough to measure serum iPTH in the large majority of normal subjects. Serum iPTH may be detectable in some patients with hypoparathyroidism if the assay employed is very sensitive. Presumably, these patients have grade 1 parathyroid insufficiency. However, it is important to recognize that such low values may be due to nonspecific effects of serum per se in radioimmunoassays that do not adequately control for this factor.

Patients with functional hypoparathyroidism due to hypomagnesemia also have low to undetectable levels of serum iPTH. Identification of these individuals depends upon the measurement of serum magnesium and the demonstration that treatment with magnesium salts restores eucalcemia and increases serum iPTH.

Treatment

A. Therapeutic Difficulties: Theoretically, the most appropriate therapy for hypoparathyroidism would be physiologic replacement of PTH. There are practical limitations to this approach, including the need to administer the hormone parenterally and the current high cost of suitable commercial human PTH preparations. Such treatment might become feasible in the future for patients poorly controlled by conventional regimens.

Because of the absence of PTH and the consequent hyperphosphatemia, $25OHD_3$ 1α-hydroxylase, the renal enzyme that converts $25OHD_3$ to $1,25(OH)_2D_3$, is relatively inactive in patients with hypoparathyroidism. Thus, little if any circulating $25OHD_3$ is converted to $1,25(OH)_2D_3$, and there are low to undetectable serum levels of this metabolite. In fact, hypoparathyroid patients are for this reason resistant to pharmacologic doses of vitamin D.

Although lowering of serum phosphate levels with diets low in phosphate (ie, restricting dairy products and meat) and oral aluminum hydroxide gels (to bind intestinal phosphate) might be expected to increase the conversion of $25OHD_3$ to $1,25(OH)_2D_3$, such treatment has received little attention. Rather, treatment with pharmacologic doses of ergocalciferol or its more potent analog dihydrotachysterol, in combination with oral calcium, has been the mainstay of treatment. Severe hypercalcemia is often a complication of this treatment if serum calcium is not monitored frequently. Serum calcium should be measured weekly at the initiation of treatment with vitamin D, then monthly during dosage adjustment, and at least every 3 months during long-term follow-up. A single episode of vitamin D intoxication can irreversibly impair renal function. Furthermore, toxicity can persist for weeks to months because of the effective tissue storage of vitamin D and its circulating metabolite $25OHD_3$. Treatment of vitamin D intoxication is similar to that described for severe hypercalcemia (discussed below). Hydration is most important, and in some patients corticosteroids (60 mg prednisone or 300 mg cortisone daily in 4 divided doses), which appear to antagonize vitamin D action, are necessary.

B. Emergency Measures for Tetany: Tetany due to hypoparathyroidism requires emergency treatment with intravenous calcium. The aim is to prevent laryngeal stridor and convulsions. After a patent airway is assured, 10–20 mL of a 10% solution of calcium gluconate (90 mg elemental calcium per 10 mL) should be given slowly (not more than 10 mL/min) until symptoms are relieved or until serum calcium rises above 7 mg/dL. Hypercalcemia is to be avoided; maintaining calcium at levels between 7.5 and 9 mg/dL is adequate. Caution should be exercised in patients taking digitalis, because calcium potentiates the action of this drug on the heart; electrocardiographic monitoring is thus necessary during intravenous calcium therapy for these patients. Therapy with vitamin D should be initiated as soon as possible (see below). It may be necessary to maintain serum calcium at levels that prevent tetany for several days before vitamin D becomes effective. This is accomplished with the combined administration of oral and intermittent intravenous calcium. Oral calcium is begun as soon as possible, starting with 200 mg of elemental calcium (as calcium carbonate, 40% calcium) every 2 hours and gradually increasing to 500 mg every 2 hours if necessary. If serum calcium falls below 7.5 mg/dL after 6 hours of the combined regimen, a continuous calcium infusion should be started. Five hundred milliliters of 5% glucose and water containing 10 mL of 10% calcium gluconate is given over 6 hours initially, with the quantity of calcium increased in increments of 5 mL every 6 hours until satisfactory control is achieved. Anticonvulsive agents (phenytoin, phenobarbital, etc) may be helpful in management of patients with convulsions resistant to calcium therapy and should be given as soon as such resistance is suspected. Phenothiazine drugs should be avoided because they may induce severe dyskinesia.

C. Severe Hypocalcemia ("Hungry Bone" Syndrome): In patients with hyperparathyroidism and bone disease who have undergone successful excision of one or more hyperfunctioning parathyroid glands, hypocalcemia my be profound and resistant to treatment ("hungry bone" syndrome). As much as 10 g of elemental calcium administered intravenously by infusion over 24 hours may be required to increase serum calcium above 7.5 mg/dL. Such patients are notoriously resistant to vitamin D, but responses are regularly achieved with $1,25(OH)_2D_3$ (calcitriol [Rocaltrol]) in doses ranging from 0.5 to 2 μg daily or with parathyroid hormone (300–1000 units intramuscularly or intravenously). The manufacture of parathyroid extract has been discontinued, but synthetic human PTH(1–34) is now available.

D. Severe Hypoparathyroidism: Most patients with grades 4 and 5 hypoparathyroidism require some form of long-term vitamin D treatment (Table 11–2). Success is usually achieved with the regimen suggested by Parfitt: dihydrotachysterol (Hytakerol), 4 mg/d as a single dose for 2 days, then 2 mg/d for 2 days, then 1 mg/d, adjusting this dose as required by serum calcium measurements (1 mg is equivalent to about 120,000 USP units or 3 mg of vitamin D_2). Ideally, serum calcium should be maintained between 8.5 and 9 mg/dL. This leaves a margin for an increase in serum calcium to levels that are not dangerous. The major advantage of dihydrotachysterol is its relatively rapid onset of action and short half-life. With regard to the latter, hypercalcemia due to inadvertent overdoses of dihydrotachysterol is relieved within 1–3 weeks after the drug is discontinued, whereas toxicity from vitamin D_2 persists for 6–18 weeks. Dihydrotachysterol offers another advantage in that parathyroid function can be tested relatively soon after withdrawal of the drug. Hypocalcemia within 2 weeks of withdrawal strongly suggests the persistence of hypoparathyroidism. The disadvantage of dihydrotachysterol is that it is more expensive than ergocalciferol.

1. Ergocalciferol (vitamin D_2)–The most commonly available FDA-approved vitamin D preparation is ergocalciferol, or vitamin D_2 (Table 11–2). In initiating treatment with this drug, it is important to prevent hypercalcemia. This can be accomplished consistently by giving small doses in the beginning (0.6 mg/d, or 25,000 units/d) and increasing them gradually after steady-state levels of serum calcium are achieved at each dosage level. However, restoration of eucalcemia in this way sometimes requires an inordinately long time, and it is recommended that high doses (1.25–2.5 mg/d, or 50,000–100,000 units/d) be given early, tapering to 0.6–1.25 mg/d as serum calcium concentrations approach 9 mg/dL. Most patients can be managed successfully with 1.25–2.5 mg/d. The occasional patient who requires more than 3.75 mg/d (150,000 units/d) is a candidate for the shorter-acting analogs or metabolites of vitamin D.

More information is becoming available concerning the long-term management of hypoparathyroidism with the cholecalciferol metabolites calcifediol (Calderol) and calcitriol (Rocaltrol). Both appear to be effective and pharmacologically superior to ergocalciferol with respect to rapidity of onset and termination of action, but—except in patients who are particularly difficult to manage—neither seems to offer major advantages over dihydrotachysterol, and both are even more expensive than dihydrotachysterol. The initiation and termination of action appear to be faster for calcitriol than for dihydrotachysterol. Calcitriol has been approved by the FDA for the treatment of hypoparathyroidism.

2. Calcium–Since the major action of vitamin D preparations is to increase intestinal calcium absorption, dietary calcium must be adequate during treatment of hypoparathyroidism. This can be achieved with a total (dietary and supplemental) intake of 1 g or more daily in patients under age 40 and 2 g in patients over age 40. Supplements can be provided by administering calcium as the gluconate, lactate, chloride, or carbonate salt. There are disadvantages for each. Calcium gluconate and lactate tablets contain relatively small quantities of elemental calcium, so that large numbers of tablets must be given. Calcium chloride tablets contain large quantities of calcium but tend to produce gastric irritation. Calcium carbonate (eg, Tums, Oscal) is preferred for most patients. Calcium citrate has been recommended for patients with hypercalciuria, because urinary excretion of the citrate ion may be prophylactic against the development of renal lithiasis.

E. Moderate Hypoparathyroidism: Patients with grade 3 hypoparathyroidism may require only calcium supplementation (1–5 g daily) and moderate degrees of phosphate restriction (combined with aluminum hydroxide gels) to maintain serum calcium in the desired range of 8.5–9 mg/dL. This avoids the risk of vitamin D intoxication and should be tried in appropriate circumstances.

Complications

Aside from hypercalcemia, hypercalciuria may be a complication of successful treatment. Hypercalciuria

Table 11–2. Vitamin D preparations used in the treatment of hypoparathyroidism.

	Potency[1]	How Supplied	Daily Dose (Range)	Time Required for Toxic Effects to Subside
Ergocalciferol (ergosterol, vitamin D_2)	40,000 USP units/mg.	Capsules of 25,000 and 50,000 units; solution, 500,000 units/mL	25,000–200,000 units.	6–18 weeks.
Dihydrotachysterol (Hytakerol)	120,000 USP units/mg.	Tablets of 0.125, 0.2, and 0.4 mg.	0.2–1 mg.	1–3 weeks.
Calcifediol (Calderol)	. . .	Capsules of 20 and 50 μg.	20–200 μg.	3–6 weeks.
Calcitriol (Rocaltrol)	. . .	Capsules of 0.25 and 0.5 μg.	0.25–5 μg.	1/2–2 weeks.

[1]Number of units of vitamin D provided by 1 mg of the preparation.

develops because PTH is no longer maintaining normal renal tubular reabsorption of calcium (Fig 11–2). Accurate measurement of 24-hour urine calcium is therefore necessary to avert possible renal stone formation as serum calcium approaches normal levels during calcium and vitamin D treatment. Thiazide diuretics, which increase renal tubular reabsorption of calcium, may be useful in such cases and may have the added advantage of partially restoring eucalcemia. In fact, such treatment has been used successfully without vitamin D in the management of mild hypoparathyroidism.

Prognosis

Long-term restoration of serum calcium to normal or nearly normal ranges usually results in improvement in most manifestations of surgical and idiopathic hypoparathyroidism, including the ocular, neurologic, and dermatologic disorders and associated candidiasis. Unfortunately, the latter appears to persist in MEDAC syndrome, and resolution usually can be achieved only with iodoquinol or with systemic amphotericin B (alone or combined with transfer factor) therapy. Improved surgical techniques and the use of parathyroid autotransplantation in surgery for disorders requiring extensive removal of thyroid or parathyroid tissue may lower the incidence of permanent hypoparathyroidism. Early diagnosis of latent hypoparathyroidism with adequate long-term treatment will lead to a lower incidence of late complications.

PSEUDOHYPOPARATHYROIDISM & PSEUDOPSEUDOHYPO-PARATHYROIDISM

Pseudohypoparathyroidism is a rare familial disorder characterized by target tissue resistance to PTH, hypocalcemia, increased parathyroid gland function, and a variety of congenital defects in the growth and development of the skeleton, including short stature and short metacarpal and metatarsal bones. Patients with pseudopseudohypoparathyroidism have the developmental defects without the biochemical abnormalities of pseudohypoparathyroidism. There are also patients with pseudohypoparathyroidism who have target tissue resistance to the hormone but no developmental abnormalities, and others with developmental abnormalities who experience spontaneous cure of biochemical abnormalities. There are even patients who have developmental abnormalities and clinical hypoparathyroidism in the face of typical osteitis fibrosa cystica. This syndrome is known as pseudohypohyperparathyroidism.

Etiology

Clearly, the complex abnormalities mentioned in the foregoing paragraph cannot be ascribed to a single underlying biochemical defect. Although abnormal target tissue responses to PTH may be the basic disorder, it is likely that defects in any one of a number of limiting steps, from receptor binding of the hormone to final expression of the cellular actions of PTH, could be involved.

At present, the only proved biochemical defect of this type is one in which the guanyl nucleotide–sensitive regulatory protein that couples PTH-occupied receptors to adenylate cyclase is decreased by half in the red blood cells of some patients with pseudohypoparathyroidism (Fig 11–12). In such patients, this defect appears to produce resistance to several other hormones that apparently exert their actions by stimulating the production of increased cellular cAMP (vasopressin, glucagon). Other possible mechanisms, as yet largely untested, include secretion of a biologically inert form of PTH, circulating inhibitors of PTH action, an intrinsic abnormality of PTH receptors, autoantibodies to the PTH receptor, a defect in adenylate cyclase, a specific and defined disturbance in the process by which PTH alters the distribution of ions across membranes, and abnormalities of cellular protein kinases or other hormone-dependent enzymes.

Patients with pseudohypoparathyroidism generally fail to respond normally to the administration of large doses of PTH with an increase in urinary phosphate excretion and in nephrogenous cAMP (type I). A few patients have normal cAMP responses but diminished phosphate responses (type II), whereas others (rarely) may have the reverse. Studies describing these apparently paradoxic findings imply that cAMP may not be involved in all of the biologic actions of PTH. However, these results could also be explained in other ways, including (1) the possibility that urinary excretion of cAMP does not accurately reflect all of the cAMP-related cellular events critical to PTH action and (2) the likelihood that only small changes in intracellular cAMP are required for PTH action.

Serum levels of $1,25(OH)_2D_3$ have been reported to be low in pseudohypoparathyroidism, and defective conversion of $25OHD_3$ to $1,25(OH)_2D_3$ has therefore been suggested as the mechanism involved in abnormal mineral homeostasis in these patients. This argument is supported by reports of success in restoring serum calcium and urinary phosphate excretion to normal levels with administration of $1,25(OH)_2D_3$, but again, other explanations are probably more valid. There is evidence that generation of increased renal tubular cAMP is involved in stimulation of 1α-hydroxylation of $25OHD_3$. If such is the case, one could postulate that normal tissue responsiveness to PTH is necessary for production of $1,25(OH)_2D_3$, and its absence in pseudohypoparathyroidism would account for the low levels of serum $1,25(OH)_2D_3$ in this disease. Furthermore, administration of $1,25(OH)_2D_3$ might be expected to increase the responsiveness of bone to PTH in patients with deficient production of $1,25(OH)_2D_3$ simply because the hypercalcemic action of PTH depends on the presence of biologically active metabolites of vitamin D. Finally, the phosphaturia induced in pseudohypoparathyroidism by $1,25(OH)_2D_3$ administration could be due to the restoration of eucalcemia; it is well known that phosphaturia occurs when serum calcium is restored toward normal in patients with surgical hypoparathyroidism.

Genetic Basis of Pseudohypoparathyroidism

Although pseudohypoparathyroidism is inherited, its mode of transmission is unclear. The 2:1 female:male ratio of occurrence suggests an X-linked dominant mechanism; however, it is difficult to explain how the developmental defects of pseudohypoparathyroidism can be inherited in the absence of abnormalities in the adenylate cyclase system. Furthermore, 4 cases of male-to-male transmission of the developmental defects have been recorded.

Incidence

Pseudohypoparathyroidism and pseudopseudohypoparathyroidism are rare. Most cases are concentrated in a few centers in the USA.

Pathologic Physiology

Qualitatively, the biochemical findings in patients with pseudohypoparathyroidism are identical to those observed in patients with surgical or idiopathic hypoparathyroidism, except that in most patients serum

iPTH is increased appropriately for the degree of hypocalcemia. The pathophysiology of the disease is best understood by reference to Fig 11–2. PTH action is blocked in all 3 of the left limbs of the target tissue feedback loops. The results (in the right limbs) are (1) decreased bone resorption, caused by decreased bone cell responsiveness to PTH; (2) increased serum phosphate, caused by decreased renal tubular responsiveness to the phosphaturic effects of PTH and decreased production of $1,25(OH)_2D_3$ with decreased intestinal calcium absorption; and (3) increased renal excretion of calcium for the degree of hypocalcemia, which is caused again by decreased renal tubular responsiveness to the hypocalciuric effects of PTH. The consequent hypocalcemia stimulates PTH secretion. There is no good explanation for the hypocalcemia in patients with pseudohypohyperparathyroidism who (paradoxically) have osteitis fibrosa cystica and elevated levels of alkaline phosphatase (see below).

In patients with pseudohypoparathyroidism who are hypocalcemic, the parathyroid glands are hyperplastic.

Clinical Features

Most of the symptoms and signs of pseudohypoparathyroidism are the same as those of surgical hypoparathyroidism and idiopathic hypoparathyroidism and are due almost entirely to chronic hypocalcemia. However, there are certain unique developmental features. Many patients are mentally retarded, short and

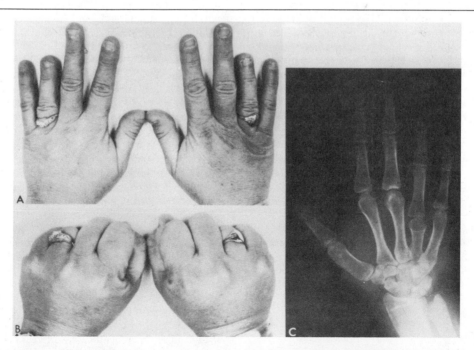

Figure 11–17. Hands of a patient with pseudohypoparathyroidism. **A:** Note the short fourth finger. **B:** Note the "absent" fourth knuckle. **C:** Film shows the short fourth metacarpal. (Reproduced, with permission, from Potts JT: Page 1359 in: *The Metabolic Basis of Inherited Disease,* 4th ed. Stanbury JB, Wyngaarden JB, Fredrickson DS [editors]. McGraw-Hill, 1978.)

stocky, and obese with rounded faces. Many have one or more short metacarpal or metatarsal bones, which is manifested by formation of a dimple over the head of the involved metacarpals on making a fist. The fingers (especially the fourth and fifth) may be short (Fig 11–17). The calvarium is thickened in one-third of patients, and there may be delayed dentition, defective enamel, and absence of teeth. There may also be exostoses, ectopic ossification, coxa vara or coxa valga, bowing of the radius, tibia, and fibula, and hypothyroidism.

Diagnosis

The diagnosis of pseudohypoparathyroidism is likely when the developmental abnormalities described above are present. When serum calcium and phosphorus are normal in such a patient, the diagnosis of pseudopseudohypoparathyroidism is almost certain, although some of the same abnormalities may be present (occasionally) in patients with Turner's, Gardner's, or basal cell nevus syndrome. If hypocalcemia and hyperphosphatemia are present, the diagnosis of pseudohypoparathyroidism is likely. Increased serum iPTH and markedly diminished phosphaturic and nephrogenous cAMP responses to PTH distinguish pseudohypoparathyroidism from surgical, idiopathic, or functional hypoparathyroidism in patients with equivocal signs or absence of developmental abnormalities. If the serum phosphorus is normal or low in a hypocalcemic patient, secondary hyperparathyroidism due to vitamin D or dietary calcium deficiency or to intestinal malabsorption of calcium must be excluded. Measurement of serum $25OHD_3$ should be helpful in the first instance, and dietary history or analysis in the second. The third (intestinal malabsorption) may present difficulties because hypocalcemia per se may produce malabsorption, and unless magnesium deficiency is present, patients with primary intestinal malabsorption usually have increased levels of serum iPTH. Therapeutic tests are needed in this situation. When successful treatment of malabsorption with a gluten-free diet restores eucalcemia, the diagnosis is probably gluten-sensitive enteropathy. If correction of hypocalcemia with a regimen used in the treatment of hypoparathyroidism cures the malabsorption syndrome, pseudohypoparathyroidism is a likely diagnosis.

Treatment

The treatment of pseudohypoparathyroidism is identical to that for hypoparathyroidism. No therapy is usually necessary for pseudopseudohypoparathyroidism.

PRIMARY HYPERPARATHYROIDISM

Primary hyperparathyroidism represents an overlapping group of syndromes that are caused by excessive, relatively uncontrolled secretion of PTH by one or more hyperfunctioning parathyroid glands. Hypercalcemia, the biochemical hallmark of the disorder, fails to inhibit gland activity in the normal manner. Most patients today are relatively asymptomatic and are detected by routine measurements of serum calcium. Symptoms, when present, can be remarkably varied and vague. The classic presentation of nephrolithiasis, osteitis fibrosa cystica, and soft tissue calcification is rare today.

Etiology

The cause of primary hyperparathyroidism is unknown. A genetic factor may be involved, since several families have been described in which the disease is inherited as an autosomal dominant trait. In this regard, a factor with parathyroid mitogenic activity has been reported in the plasma of patients with this genetic disease. Investigations of the incidence of thyroid carcinoma in patients who have had neck irradiation have shown a greater than expected number of cases of primary hyperparathyroidism, implicating this factor as one possible underlying cause. However, it is difficult to interpret such studies because there is little information about the general incidence and natural history of primary hyperparathyroidism.

Calcium infusions in hyperparathyroid patients with mild hypercalcemia incompletely suppress serum iPTH. This strongly suggests that increased hormone secretion in these patients is due, at least in part, to a set point error in the level of ionic calcium at which abnormal tissue is suppressed. This defect has been directly confirmed in vitro. Isolated parathyroid cells from hyperfunctioning glands require higher concentrations of calcium in the medium to decrease PTH secretion than do cells obtained from normal glands.

Incidence

Routine automated measurement of serum calcium has vastly increased detection of primary hyperparathyroidism. In one recent, well-controlled study, the annual rate of disease detection was 3.5 times greater after the introduction of routine screening of serum calcium than it was before. The incidence of primary hyperparathyroidism increases dramatically in both men and women after age 50; it is 2–4 times more common in women. In a careful epidemiologic study, the age-adjusted incidence was estimated to be 42 per 100,000. However, studies of selected patient populations (with most patients over 40 years of age) have revealed as many as 1/1000 to 1/200 patients with the disease.

Pathology

A. Parathyroid Glands: Histologically, abnormal parathyroid glands from patients with primary hyperparathyroidism have been characterized as being hyperplastic, adenomatous, or malignant. Unfortunately, controlled studies of histologic interpretations by pathologists have shown that it is difficult or impossible to distinguish between adenomas and hyperplasia. Furthermore, abnormal but nonmalignant parathyroid tissue may, in rare cases, have many of the histologic features of malignant tissue. Thus, to classify parathyroid lesions, it is generally necessary to rely on gross pathologic features observed during surgery. The surgeon determines the number, size, and gross appearance of abnormal glands present. The pathologist then determines whether biopsy specimens are parathyroid tissue. Single-gland involvement ("adenoma") occurs in about 80% of patients with hyperparathyroidism and multiple-gland involvement ("hyperplasia") in about 20%. The diagnosis of true carcinoma of the gland is based on a combination of gross appearance of the lesion, histologic features, and, ultimately, the biologic behavior of the abnormal tissue. Less than 2% of hyperfunctioning glands are malignant. Familial primary hyperparathyroidism and the hyperparathyroidism associated with multiple endocrine neoplasia almost always involve multiple glands. Abnormal parathyroid glands usually weigh 0.2–2 g (27–75 mg is normal) and have a characteristic yellow-red color and "bulging" appearance in situ. Occasionally, very large glands (> 10 g) are observed. The severity of the clinical manifestations—especially the degree of hypercalcemia—is generally proportionate to the quantity of hyperfunctioning tissue. The predominant cell type in most abnormal glands is the chief cell; it can be arrayed in sheets or cords or may appear in follicles. So-called water-clear cells and oxyphilic cells may be admixed, and in rare cases one of these may predominate. There is no question that the chief cell synthesizes and secretes PTH. The functions of the water-clear and oxyphilic cells are unknown.

B. Bone: In virtually all patients with primary hyperparathyroidism, histomorphometric analysis of bone biopsies of the iliac crest shows the effects of excess PTH on bone. These effects include increased bone resorption surfaces, increased numbers of osteoclasts, osteocytic osteolysis, and, in moderate to severe cases, marrow fibrosis. Only far-advanced disease is associated with classic bone cysts and fractures. These patients have a mineralization defect characterized by large quantities of unmineralized collagen and disorganized (woven rather than lamellar) bone.

C. Kidney: About 20–30% of patients have nephrolithiasis, which is frequently complicated by pyelonephritis. Gross nephrocalcinosis or calcification of the renal papillae is unusual, but microscopic examination of kidneys with special calcium stains has sometimes revealed peritubular and tubular calcifications at autopsy. The incidence of such soft tissue calcification in patients with mild to moderate disease is unknown. However, it may be relatively frequent, since chondrocalcinosis and calcific tendinitis can be demonstrated on x-rays in 7.5–18% of cases.

D. Other Organs: Calcification of other organs such as stomach, lung, and heart and blood vessels has been observed in patients with hyperparathyroid crisis (serum calcium > 15 mg/dL).

E. Muscle: Myopathy is relatively common in primary hyperparathyroidism, and muscle biopsy may show neuropathic atrophy of both type I and type II muscle fibers. These histologic changes parallel clinical, neurologic, and neuromuscular dysfunction.

Pathologic Physiology

As might be expected, the constant, incompletely controlled release of PTH from hyperfunctioning parathyroid tissue causes exaggerated physiologic responses in target organs.

A. Hypercalcemia: Because the excess PTH stimulates the transport of calcium into the blood from the intestinal and renal tubular lumina as well as from bone (Fig 11–2), the intestine and kidney are unable to correct the hypercalcemia. Thus, patients with primary hyperparathyroidism, in contrast to those with other (nonparathyroid) hypercalcemic diseases, lack the first lines of defense against hypercalcemia, increased renal and intestinal loss of calcium. Early in the course of the disease, when serum calcium values are less than 11.5 mg/dL (2.88 mmol/L) (normal range, 8.9–10.1 mg/dL [2.23–2.53 mmol/L]), urinary calcium can be relatively low for the degree of hypercalcemia. It is only when serum calcium values are greater than 12 mg/dL (3 mmol/L), when the renal tubular mechanism for resorbing calcium is overwhelmed, or when there is an unrelated decrease in the renal tubular capacity to resorb calcium, that the kidney's adaptive mechanism for correcting hypercalcemia becomes operative and hypercalciuria develops. Unfortunately, this chronic adaptation (hypercalciuria), along with other changes in urine composition that occur in primary hyperparathyroidism (eg, increased pH due to bicarbonaturia), contributes to the urolithiasis and urinary tract infections that are so common in these patients.

Many patients with primary hyperparathyroidism have decreased renal tubular reabsorption of phosphate, hyperphosphaturia, and hypophosphatemia. In normal people or in patients with a diminished capacity to convert $25OHD_3$ to $1,25(OH)_2D_3$, the renal tubular effects of PTH aid mineral homeostasis by stimulating $1,25(OH)_2D_3$ production and by clearing from the blood phosphate that was removed from bone during resorption of calcium. However, in patients with primary hyperparathyroidism, hypercalcemia is aggravated by the increased production of $1,25(OH)_2D_3$ and by a decrease in the amount of serum phosphate available to form complexes with serum ionic calcium.

B. Calcium in Soft Tissues: Other mechanisms for correcting hypercalcemia are required as the disease progresses. These generally result in a "trade-off" between a decrease in serum calcium and the development of organ disease. One such mechanism is the deposition of calcium in soft tissues that occurs because the normal solubility product of $Ca^{2+} \times$

$PO_4{}^{3-}$ in serum (approximately 40) is exceeded. This may cause joint pain due to calcific tendinitis and chondrocalcinosis, or it may compromise renal function (secondary to nephrocalcinosis).

C. Vitamin D Deficiency: Another adaptive mechanism is the development of vitamin D deficiency, which may render patients with even severe hyperparathyroidism eucalcemic or nearly so. In this instance, a patient with only marginal stores of vitamin D may develop vitamin D deficiency because of the long-term increase in the conversion of $25OHD_3$ to $1,25(OH)_2D_3$ that is caused by the increased circulating levels of PTH. Such patients may have severe osteomalacia.

D. Increased Degradation of PTH: A final adaptive mechanism may be a hypercalcemia-induced increase in the degradation of biologically active forms of PTH peripherally (eg, in the liver and possibly the kidney) and in parathyroid tissue itself. Evidence in support of such effects of ionic calcium is available in both animals and humans. Thus, it is possible that plasma calcium per se may not only regulate PTH secretion but may also be important in determining the relative quantities of biologically active PTH and inactive hormone fragments in the circulation. The one adaptive mechanism that might be expected to play an important role in correcting the hypercalcemia of primary hyperparathyroidism is increased secretion of CT. However evidence indicates that this does not occur in most patients; and in some patients (particularly women), CT reserve actually appears to be diminished.

E. Hyperchloremic Acidosis: Patients with primary hyperparathyroidism generally have mild to moderate hyperchloremic acidosis. This is due chiefly to excess PTH, which decreases the urinary concentration of hydrogen ion and increases urinary bicarbonate excretion. These effects also tend to aggravate existing hypercalcemia, first by impairing the ability of blood albumin to bind ionic calcium and secondly by increasing the dissolution of bone mineral.

F. Increased Urinary cAMP: Urinary cAMP is increased in as many as 80% of patients with primary hyperparathyroidism. This presumably reflects an increase in PTH-stimulated renal cell adenylate cyclase activity. Interestingly, some studies indicate that the phosphaturic and cAMP responses to exogenously administered PTH are blunted in patients with primary hyperparathyroidism, suggesting a state of refractoriness or "desensitization" of one or more of the cellular components responsible for these effects. This "desensitization" and the increase in urinary cAMP excretion have been used as diagnostic tests for the presence of hyperparathyroidism (see below).

G. Osteitis Fibrosa Cystica: Patients with radiologic evidence of osteitis fibrosa cystica frequently have increased serum concentrations of the bone isoenzyme of alkaline phosphatase. This bone enzyme is produced by osteoblasts and probably is one of several enzymes involved in osseous mineralization. These patients also excrete greater than normal quantities of hydroxyproline in their urine. This amino acid is unique to collagen, the major structural protein in bone. Such combined increases in serum alkaline phosphatase and urinary excretion of hydroxyproline have been interpreted as gross reflections of increased bone turnover in primary hyperparathyroidism.

Clinical Features

A. Symptoms: Patients with primary hyperparathyroidism are usually asymptomatic or have nonspecific symptoms such as weakness and easy fatigability. When symptoms do occur, they can generally be attributed to one of 2 causes: (1) hypercalcemia with associated hypercalciuria or (2) osteitis fibrosa cystica.

1. Hypercalcemia and associated hypercalciuria–The symptoms attributable to hypercalcemia involve a number of systems: (1) central nervous system: impaired mentation, loss of memory for recent events, emotional lability, depression, anosmia, somnolence, and even coma; (2) neuromuscular: weakness (especially of the proximal musculature); (3) rheumatologic: joint pain due to associated gout, intraarticular deposition of calcium pyrophosphate crystals (pseudogout), calcific tendinitis, and chondrocalcinosis; (4) dermatologic: pruritus, probably due to metastatic calcification in the skin; (5) gastrointestinal: anorexia, nausea, vomiting, dyspepsia, and constipation; and (6) renal: polyuria, nocturia, renal colic due to lithiasis, nephrocalcinosis that sometimes leads to renal failure, and associated symptoms of uremia. All of these abnormalities are related to the degree of elevation of ionic calcium in extracellular fluid, but the correlation is a crude one. One patient may be severely incapacitated at a level of serum calcium that produces only moderate symptoms in another.

Severe pancreatitis and intractable peptic ulcer have been observed in individual patients with primary hyperparathyroidism and are thought to be due to hypercalcemia. However, the evidence that these disorders occur with increased frequency in primary hyperparathyroidism is weak. Hypertension occurs with increased frequency, even in patients with mild hyperparathyroidism, but its cause is unknown.

2. Osteitis fibrosa cystica–Symptomatic bone disease (osteitis fibrosa cystica) is now unusual. Patients may complain of diffuse bone pain or, very rarely, may have a pathologic fracture through a bone cyst.

B. Signs: Most patients show no signs of the disorder. Such signs as are present are usually confined to the neuromuscular system or to organ systems in which soft tissue calcification is present. Neurologic abnormalities are nonspecific and include impaired mentation, mental depression, psychosis, hypoactive deep tendon reflexes, joint hyperextensibility, sensory loss for perception of pain and vibration, proximal muscle weakness (particularly the thighs), abnormal tongue movements (resembling fasciculations), lingual atrophy, ataxic gait, and abnormally strong (hard) fingernails.

1. Soft tissue calcification–Soft tissue calcification can result in arthritis (chondrocalcinosis or calcific tendinitis), conjunctivitis (conjunctival calcium phosphate crystals), and "band keratopathy," which is characterized by deposition in the cornea of opaque calcium phosphate in vertical lines parallel to and within the ocular limbus, usually laterally (3 o'clock and 9 o'clock). "Band keratopathy" can best be seen by slit lamp examination. It is rare in hyperparathyroidism unless serum phosphate is also elevated (eg, after the onset of renal failure).

2. Enlarged glands–It is seldom possible to palpate enlarged parathyroid glands. A nodule felt in the neck of a patient with primary hyperparathyroidism is much more likely to be in the thyroid than in the parathyroid gland.

3. Bone tenderness and deformities–Rarely, patients may exhibit bone tenderness on examination.

Bone deformities, fractures through an osteoclastic cyst, the presence of an epulis (brown tumor of the jaw), and "pseudoclubbing" due to collapsed terminal phalanges have been described even more rarely.

C. X-Ray Findings: The most specific and frequent radiographic sign of osteitis fibrosa cystica is subperiosteal bone resorption. This is best demonstrated in magnified fine-grain industrial x-rays of the fingers (especially the index finger). An example from a patient with severe primary hyperparathyroidism is shown in Figure 11–18A. Note the radial surface of the distal phalanx, where the cortex is almost completely resorbed, leaving only fine wisps of cortical bone. Other radiographic manifestations of the disease range from generalized osteopenia to bone cysts ("brown tumors") and erosion of distal phalangeal tufts or the distal ends of clavicles. Severe osteitis fibrosa cystica involving the skull is shown in Figure 11–18B.

Soft tissue calcifications (eg, calcific tendinitis, chondrocalcinosis, nephrocalcinosis, pulmonary calcifications) may be incidental findings on routine films. The latter 2 can be well demonstrated with scanning techniques using radioactively labeled diphosphonate compounds.

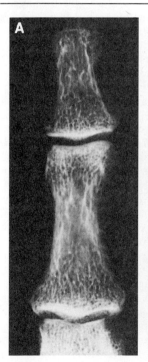
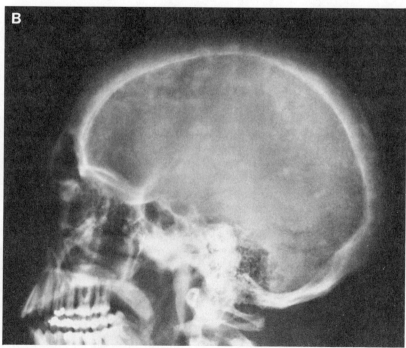

Figure 11–18. _A:_ Magnified x-ray of index finger on fine-grain industrial film showing classic subperiosteal resorption in a patient with severe primary hyperparathyroidism. Note the left (radial) surface of the distal phalanx, where the cortex is almost completely resorbed, leaving only fine wisps of cortical bone. **_B:_** Skull x-ray from a patient with severe secondary hyperparathyroidism due to prolonged end-stage renal disease. Extensive areas of demineralization alternate with areas of increased bone density, resulting in an exaggerated picture of the "salt and pepper" skull x-ray, which used to be a classic finding in primary hyperparathyroidism. This is rarely seen now and cannot be visualized easily in x-ray reproductions. Although it is difficult to appreciate at this magnification, the dental lamina dura is absent, another classic x-ray finding in severe hyperparathyroidism. (Both films courtesy of H Genant.)

Nephrocalcinosis is rarely seen on x-ray, but nephrolithiasis is common. The stones are usually radiopaque (ie, calcium oxalate and calcium phosphate stones) and can be seen on plain films. Renal sonograms or nephrotomograms are helpful in identifying, localizing, and measuring them. This latter procedure is important in determining the "activity" of the stone disease. An increase in stone diameter with time can be taken as evidence of "active" stone disease and is probably an indication for treatment of hyperparathyroidism. Primary hyperparathyroidism may also be associated, although less commonly, with uric acid stones (not radiopaque). Thus, renal sonography x-ray examination of the urinary tract with contrast material is also important.

Differential Diagnosis

In general, the major problem in the differential diagnosis of primary hyperparathyroidism is distinguishing it from other conditions associated with hypercalcemia (Table 11–3). Thiazide diuretic therapy and nonhematologic malignant diseases are the most common ones. Less common but equally important are (1) hematologic malignant diseases involving bone (myeloma, lymphoma, leukemia); (2) granulomatous diseases (sarcoidosis, tuberculosis, berylliosis); (3) endocrine disorders, including thyrotoxicosis and acute adrenal insufficiency; (4) familial hypocalciuric hypercalcemia (benign familial hypercalcemia); (5) intoxication with calcium, vitamin D, vitamin A, or lithium; (6) extensive skeletal immobilization (eg, in a spica body cast) in normal young people and prolonged bed rest in patients with osteolytic or metabolic bone disease; and (7) idiopathic hypercalcemia of infancy. More than one cause of hypercalcemia may coexist in the same patient (eg, hyperparathyroidism and sarcoidosis).

A. Pathogenesis of Hypercalcemia: Hypercalcemic disorders can be divided into those due to excess PTH and those due to other factors. Only primary hyperparathyroidism and a large subgroup of nonhematologic malignant diseases fall into the first category. The remainder fall into the second category and are characterized by suppression of PTH secretion.

B. Nonparathyroid Hypercalcemia: The underlying causes of hypercalcemia in the conditions in the second category are varied and, for the most part, uncertain. They will not be discussed here except to show how they can be excluded from the differential diagnosis of primary hyperparathyroidism. The most important ones are the hypercalcemia of cancer and familial hypocalciuric hypercalcemia.

1. Hypercalcemia of cancer–It is unlikely that a bony metastasis produces chronic hypercalcemia simply by physical displacement of bone. Rather, malignant tumors probably produce the same osteolytic humoral factors after metastasis to bone as they do before. These factors include PTH-like substances, prostaglandins, and osteoclast-activating factor (OAF). It is presumed that any one or a combination of these humors might be secreted systemically by parent tumors or released by bony metastases in sufficient quantities to stimulate local osteolysis and produce hypercalcemia. There is little question that OAF is involved in the production of hypercalcemia in patients with hematologic cancers, especially multiple myeloma. Until recently, it was thought that hypercalcemia in patients with nonhematologic cancers was, in large part, due to ectopic secretion of prostaglandins, but studies with inhibitors of prostaglandin synthesis have shown that plasma calcium rarely falls after their administration. This finding suggests that prostaglandins are relatively unimportant in the production of hypercalcemia in cancer.

Fuller Albright in 1941 postulated that PTH was responsible for solid-tumor hypercalcemia in some patients. In the absence of renal failure, many of these patients have the same degree of hypophosphatemia as patients with moderate to severe primary hyperparathyroidism. Normal (80%) to increased (20%) values for serum iPTH have been reported by some laboratories in as many as 70–80% of hypercalcemic patients with nonhematologic cancers. Serum values for iPTH in patients with primary hyperparathyroidism and equal degrees of hypercalcemia are much higher than in patients with the hypercalcemia of cancer. Yet, nephrogenous cAMP excretion in many patients with cancer-associated hypercalcemia is the same as or greater than that in patients with primary hyperparathyroidism. This paradox led to a search for compounds—in cancer tissue or released into the medium of cultured cancer cells—that bind to the PTH receptor and stimulate adenylate cyclase in PTH target tissues. This search was rewarded by the identification and chemical characterization of a bioactive peptide that resembles PTH in its N-terminal amino acid sequence but is totally dissimilar in its carboxyl sequence. For a complete discussion of the role this peptide may play in the humoral hypercalcemia of cancer, see Chapter 27.

Table 11–3. Differential diagnosis of hypercalcemia.

Due to increased serum PTH
Primary and "tertiary" hyperparathyroidism
Some nonhematologic malignant diseases
Not due to increased serum PTH
Drug-induced hypercalcemia (thiazides, furosemide, vitamin D, calcium, vitamin A, lithium)
Granulomatous diseases (sarcoidosis, tuberculosis, berylliosis)
Genetic diseases (familial hypocalciuric hypercalcemia)
Immobilization
"Idiopathic" hypercalcemia
Some nonhematologic malignant diseases
Malignant hematologic diseases
Nonparathyroid endocrine diseases (Addison's disease, hyper- and hypothyroidism)

2. Familial hypocalciuric hypercalcemia (familial benign hypercalcemia)—This syndrome is probably the second most important disorder in the differential diagnosis of primary hyperparathyroidism. It is inherited as an autosomal dominant trait and is characterized usually by asymptomatic or mild hypercalcemia, hypocalciuria, mild hypermagnesemia (variably present), and normal to low levels of serum iPTH. Parathyroid exploration in a number of patients has shown either normal parathyroid glands or equivocal "hyperplasia," and subtotal parathyroidectomy has consistently failed to restore eucalcemia. Recent studies have shown that the nephrogenous cAMP responses to exogenous and endogenous PTH are greater in patients with familial hypocalciuric hypercalcemia than in normal subjects or in patients with primary hyperparathyroidism. These observations suggest that the hypercalcemia in this familial syndrome may be partly due to renal hypersensitivity to the hypocalciuric effects of PTH. However, the persistence of increased renal tubular reabsorption of calcium after parathyroidectomy and the notable absence of the characteristic sequelae of primary hyperparathyroidism (eg, renal stones and osteitis fibrosa cystica) indicate that tissue hypersensitivity to PTH is probably not the sole cause of the disorder. It is likely that this disorder involves an abnormal parathyroid gland "set point" sensitivity to extracellular ionic calcium (as in lithium hypercalcemia).

Severe parathyroid hyperplasia may occur in infants born of parents with this syndrome. Thus, measurement of serum calcium is indicated in all such infants. Hypercalcemia associated with findings compatible with hyperparathyroidism (increased serum iPTH) should be treated promptly by subtotal parathyroidectomy.

Diagnosis

The presence of hypercalcemia is established when at least 3 measurements of total serum calcium are greater than normal. Venous blood should be drawn in the morning under fasting conditions with minimal venous stasis. The usual normal range for the total serum calcium is 8.9–10.1 mg/dL (2.23–2.53 mmol/L). Laboratories reporting a wider normal range (eg, 9–11 mg/dL [2.25–2.75 mmol/L]) may have based it on measurements of serum calcium in subjects not documented as normal or may have a significant problem with calcium contamination. The latter is frequently due to use of a conventional chalkboard (chalk contains calcium) in the laboratory or to use of contaminated test tubes when drawing blood. Such sources of error must be eliminated, since large numbers of patients with mild hypercalcemia (eg, 10.1–11 mg/dL [2.53–2.75 mmol/L]) will go undetected if the normal range for serum calcium is too wide. In the case of laboratory contamination, wide swings in serum calcium in individual subjects will be observed, leading to diagnostic confusion and to waste of patient and laboratory resources in the further investigation of artifactual hypercalcemia.

Freshly drawn blood specimens adjusted for pH must be used for measurements of serum ionic calcium. In practice, since most calcium is bound to serum albumin, a rough estimate of true calcium can be made by adding or subtracting 0.8 mg/dL (0.2 mmol/L) for each g/dL of albumin that is above or below normal. Special formulas and nomograms are also available. The QT interval in the ECG is shortened (adjusted for heart rate) when serum ionic calcium is significantly elevated.

A. Review of History of Present Illness: Hypercalcemia generally reflects serious underlying disease that may not have been suspected during the initial evaluation. Because of this, the patient with hypercalcemia should first have a repeat history and physical examination with specific objectives in mind. These include detailed evaluations of duration of illness, drug intake, the possible presence of non–mineral-related endocrine disease, a history of nephrolithiasis with documentation (old x-rays), symptoms of cancer, a family history of endocrine and mineral disorders, and the possible presence of palpable lymph nodes or masses, skin pigmentation or lesions (metastases), and thyromegaly, hepatomegaly, or splenomegaly.

1. Nephrolithiasis and body weight—Illness of long duration associated with nephrolithiasis and maintenance of normal weight favors a diagnosis of primary hyperparathyroidism; illness of short duration associated with weight loss without nephrolithiasis favors a nonparathyroid cause of hypercalcemia, particularly cancer.

2. Thiazide drugs—A history of thiazide intake might explain an increase in serum calcium to 11 mg/dL (2.75 mmol/L), but higher values usually indicate that this drug has merely increased the hypercalcemia of another condition (eg, mild primary hyperparathyroidism).

3. Lithium—Lithium carbonate, as administered for a bipolar affective disorder, can cause an increase in serum calcium to 11.5 mg/dL (2.88 mmol/L). The mechanism of this action is likely a drug-induced increase in the parathyroid gland "set point" for suppression by extracellular calcium.

4. Vitamin D intake—This may not have been elicited in the initial history. Vitamin D can cause severe hypercalcemia in adults when taken in doses exceeding 50,000 units/d. Furthermore, patients with any disorder that causes hypercalcemia may be abnormally sensitive to vitamin D. Thus, intake of less than 50,000 units/d may aggravate existing hypercalcemia in sarcoidosis and primary hyperparathyroidism; what may appear initially to be a severe form of the primary disorder may prove ultimately to be relatively mild when vitamin D intake is curtailed.

5. Calcium Intake—Excess calcium intake (< 5 g/d) in the form of calcium carbonate antacids can cause severe hypercalcemia in susceptible individuals, especially when coupled with additional intake of alkali (bicarbonate) ("milk alkali syndrome"). This condition is rare in its pure form. Most patients actually have underlying primary hyperparathyroidism and are taking calcium carbonate and alkali for associated gastric hyperacidity.

6. Family History–The family history may contain important clues to the correct diagnosis and treatment of a hypercalcemic patient. It is essential to inquire about the presence of hypercalcemia, nephrolithiasis, neck exploration, metabolic bone disease, intractable peptic ulcer disease, and endocrine tumors in family members, since primary hyperparathyroidism occurs as part of several familial multiple endocrine neoplasia (MEN) syndromes (see Chapter 28). There are few distinctive laboratory findings in the syndrome of familial hypocalciuric hypercalcemia, and a definitive diagnosis can be made only by documenting hypercalcemia in the patient's immediate relatives. A history of unsuccessful parathyroid surgery in more than one hypercalcemic relative is unfortunately characteristic of this condition. It is helpful if the surgeon is given information regarding possible multiple endocrine neoplasia or familial hyperparathyroidism before neck exploration is undertaken. Multiple parathyroid gland enlargement ("hyperplasia") is almost certain to be present in both of these conditions, and subtotal parathyroidectomy (removal of 3½ glands) rather than single-gland removal would be indicated. Finally, mothers of infants with severe neonatal tetany should be suspected of having primary hyperparathyroidism.

B. Radioimmunoassay of Parathyroid Hormone: There has been a revolutionary change in the laboratory investigation of hypercalcemia in recent years owing to the development of sensitive and specific radioimmunoassays for serum PTH. Whereas patients were once extensively evaluated for nonparathyroid disorders that could cause hypercalcemia, the trend now is to use serum iPTH and calcium measurements to assign patients either to a group likely to benefit from surgical resection of parathyroid lesions or to one that requires further diagnostic evaluation for the cause of hypercalcemia (Fig 11–19).

1. iPTH in primary hyperparathyroidism–The results of a study using sensitive radioimmunoassay technique for measuring serum PTH that is specific for the mid (43–68) region of the molecule in the diagnosis of primary hyperparathyroidism are illustrated in Figure 11–20. Ninety percent of patients with surgically proved disease had serum iPTH values that exceeded the upper limit of normal, and 10% had values that were in the upper range of normal but inappropriately high for the total calcium concentration in the same serum sample. Not shown are serum iPTH values in patients with nonparathyroid hypercalcemia (eg, sarcoidosis, vitamin D intoxication). These are low or undetectable except in ectopic hyperparathyroidism due to nonparathyroid cancer (see below) or in patients with coexisting primary hyperparathyroidism.

Thus, it is possible, by measuring calcium and iPTH in a single morning fasting serum sample, to correctly categorize 80–90% of hypercalcemic patients who may benefit from resection of hyperfunctioning parathyroid glands and a similar percentage of patients who have nonparathyroid hypercalcemia and require further study. The practical advantages of using serum iPTH as the principal laboratory probe to "triage" hypercalcemic patients are obvious. In most patients with primary hyperparathyroidism, a correct diagnosis can be made in an outpatient setting, eliminating the costs and inconveniences of hospitalization and the repeated indirect tests required to make a less definitive diagnosis by exclusion.

2. iPTH in hypercalcemia of cancer–Values of serum iPTH measured with a carboxy-region assay are much lower for a given serum calcium in hyperparathyroidism due to nonparathyroid cancer (ectopic) than in primary hyperparathyroidism (Fig 11–21). Values obtained using amino-terminal specific radioimmunoassays or the recently introduced immunoradiometric assays are even lower. Irrespective of the mechanisms involved, the relationships shown in Figure 11–21 help to indicate how a physician should manage hypercalcemic and hypophosphatemic patients suspected but not proved to have cancer (eg, those with weight loss, anemia, and high erythrocyte sedimentation rates). If serum calcium values are over 12.5 mg/dL (3.13 mmol/L) and serum iPTH is within the normal range or only slightly increased, more intensive efforts should be made to identify a neoplastic lesion and to follow the patient with medical treatment. If the situation is not clarified after 6–12 months, the patient should be reevaluated for the presence of primary hyperparathyroidism (Fig 11–19).

C. Serum and Urine Biochemistry: Several serum and urine measurements may be helpful in assigning hypercalcemic patients to parathyroid or nonparathyroid categories. Hyperphosphatemia in the absence of severe renal failure favors a nonparathyroid cause. Hypophosphatemia, when dietary phosphate is adequate and when oral phosphate-binding agents are not being ingested, favors primary hyperparathyroidism but is frequently present in ectopic hyperparathyroidism. Increased serum chloride favors primary hyperparathyroidism. Increased serum alkaline phosphatase is more common in patients with cancer than in those with primary hyperparathyroidism and, in the absence of radiographic evidence of osseous hyperparathyroidism, should suggest the possibility of ectopic hyperparathyroidism. Globulin abnormalities in serum protein electrophoresis point toward multiple myeloma or sarcoidosis, but increases in gamma globulin that disappear after parathyroidectomy have been observed in primary hyperparathyroidism. Although increases in the erythrocyte sedimentation rate and anemia have been recorded in primary hyperparathyroidism, these findings suggest a nonparathyroid cause of hypercalcemia, particularly cancer.

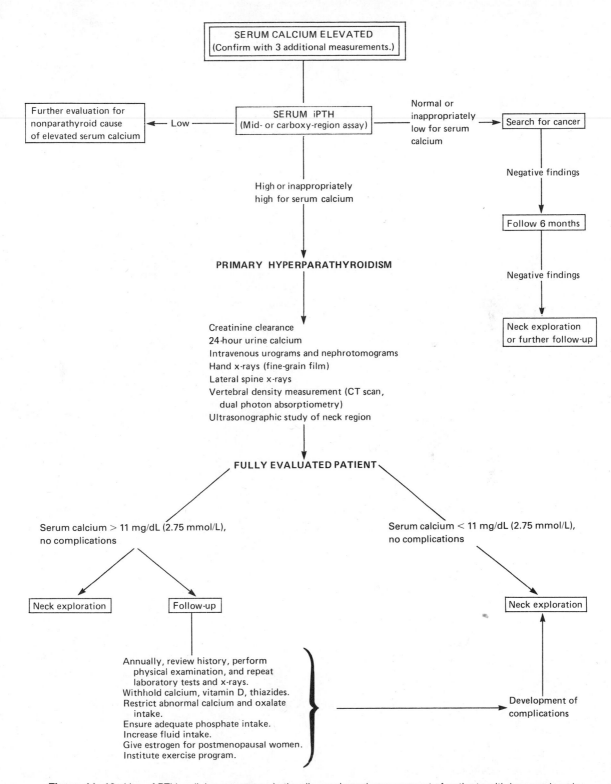

Figure 11–19. Use of PTH radioimmunoassay in the diagnosis and management of patients with hypercalcemia.

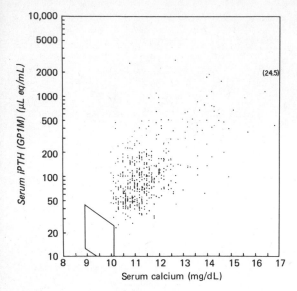

Figure 11–20. Serum iPTH values as a function of serum calcium concentration in 450 patients with surgically proved primary hyperparathyroidism. The area enclosed by the solid lines represents the normal range ±2 SD for serum iPTH and serum calcium. Note that there is a 10% overlap of serum iPTH with the normal range and that over 95% of normal sera and all hyperparathyroid sera have measurable iPTH. Formal discriminate analysis of serum iPTH and serum calcium distinguishes all hyperparathyroid patients from normal subjects. GP1M specifies the antiserum used in the assay. (Reproduced, with permission, from Arnaud CD et al: Page 19 in: *Excerpta Medica Int Cong Ser* No 346, 1975.)

Measurement of urine calcium in hypercalcemic patients is generally useful only when it is low. This finding may be the only clue to familial hypocalciuric hypercalcemia. Because of the therapeutic importance of making this diagnosis (ie, avoiding neck exploration), measurement of 24-hour urine calcium is recommended in the routine evaluation of any hypercalcemic patient before exploration is performed.

D. Nephrogenous cAMP: About 40–50% of the cAMP excreted in the urine is derived from renal tubular cells. Its production and cellular release into the urine are almost entirely under the control of PTH. This component of urinary cAMP can be accurately estimated and is termed nephrogenous cAMP. Since it is above normal in about 80% of patients with primary hyperparathyroidism (Fig 11–22) and in a large proportion of patients with ectopic hyperparathyroidism, it is not helpful in distinguishing between these 2 common disorders. However, because low levels of nephrogenous cAMP are present in patients who have nonparathyroid hypercalcemia but not cancer, the test may be useful in patients with equivocal increases in serum iPTH. In such patients, a low level of nephrogenous cAMP would suggest that the serum iPTH value was artifactual and would argue against primary hyperparathyroidism, whereas a normal or increased level would confirm the validity of the serum iPTH value and favor this condition.

E. Other Diagnostic Tests: The glucocorticoid suppression test may be used in unusual situations when the results of all of the tests discussed above are equivocal. It is based on the observation that the hypercalcemia of conditions such as vitamin D intoxication,

Figure 11–21. Relationship between serum iPTH (as measured by a mid-region assay) and serum calcium in patients with primary hyperparathyroidism (black dots) and hypercalcemic patients with cancer (open dots). Note that for a given serum calcium value, serum iPTH is lower in patients with cancer. In 5 of 105 patients with cancer, serum iPTH was undetectable (open triangles). Area enclosed with solid lines indicates normal range ±2 SD for serum iPTH and serum calcium. GP1M is the antiserum used in the assay. (Reproduced, with permission, from Benson RC Jr et al: *Am J Med* 1974; 56:823.)

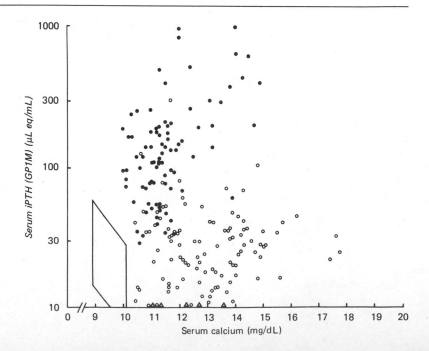

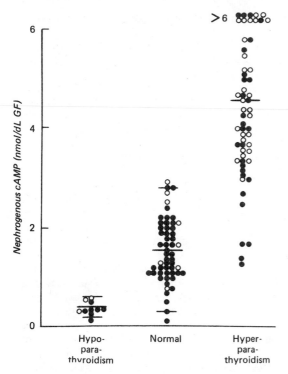

Figure 11–22. Nephrogenous cAMP, expressed as a function of glomerular filtration rate, in control subjects and patients with primary hyperparathyroidism. The open circles represent the subjects and patients with renal impairment (mean creatinine clearance < 80 mL/min). Closed circles represent subjects with normal renal function. The longer horizontal bars represent the mean values; shorter bars show ±2 SD. GF = glomerular filtrate. (Reproduced, with permission, from Broadus AE et al: *J Clin Invest* 1977;**60**:771.)

sarcoidosis, lymphoproliferative syndromes, and myeloma generally responds to the administration of 50–100 mg of cortisone or 40–60 mg of prednisone given daily in divided doses for 10 days, as shown by a decrease in serum calcium. This response is unusual in primary or ectopic hyperparathyroidism. However, results should be interpreted cautiously, since the mechanisms involved in steroid-induced suppression of hypercalcemia are poorly understood, and variables other than steroids (eg, hydration) may influence the level of serum calcium during the test. A positive test result (ie, a significant decrease in serum calcium) is a contraindication to neck exploration and signals the need for investigation for a nonparathyroid cause of hypercalcemia. A negative test result would be consistent with a diagnosis of primary or ectopic hyperparathyroidism.

Other diagnostic tests used rarely include measurements of phosphate clearance (increased in primary hyperparathyroidism) and of urinary cAMP after PTH administration (usually decreased in primary hyper-

parathyroidism, most likely because of a "desensitization" mechanism).

F. Radiographs: It is essential to obtain high-quality x-rays of the hands on fine-grain industrial film in all patients whose hypercalcemia is a diagnostic problem. Although the finding of definitive subperiosteal bone resorption is relatively unusual (occurring in about 8–10% of patients with primary hyperparathyroidism), it is diagnostic of hyperparathyroidism and probably represents the most reliable and readily available evidence that neck exploration is needed in patients with severe, life-threatening hypercalcemia.

G. Preoperative Localization of Abnormal Parathyroid Tissue: Abnormal parathyroid tissue that is causing primary hyperparathyroidism will be discovered and excised in over 90% of initial neck explorations performed by a competent parathyroid surgeon. Thus, there is no need for invasive procedures to localize glandular tissue prior to first surgery except under very unusual circumstances (see below).

With the exception of ultrasonography, localization procedures are generally reserved for patients whose first neck exploration was not successful or who suffer recurrent disease. These procedures can be divided into noninvasive and invasive. Noninvasive procedures include esophagography, ultrasonography, magnetic resonance imaging (MRI), computed tomography, and scanning with ^{201}Tl plus ^{99m}Tc. Invasive procedures include arteriography, differential venous catheterization with measurement of iPTH in the serum samples obtained, and needle aspiration of a mass localized by ultrasonography.

1. Esophagography–Esophagography may occasionally identify a relatively large parathyroid gland deep in the tracheoesophageal groove that was inadvertently missed on first exploration because of its aberrant shape. However, the procedure is usually unrewarding.

2. Ultrasonography, MRI, computed tomography, and scanning with ^{201}Tl plus ^{99m}Tc–Ultrasound technology has improved so rapidly that it is now possible to identify parathyroid lesions in the neck as small as 1 cm in diameter. Further technologic development in this area is expected, and routine ultrasound evaluation prior to initial neck exploration has become accepted practice. Because lesions can be identified in real time with this procedure, it has been possible to obtain needle aspiration biopsies of them. With use of routine and immunohistologic procedures and either immunoassays or bioassays of extracts of aspirated tissue, lesions located by ultrasonography can be identified as parathyroid in origin, thus giving the surgeon a histologic diagnosis preoperatively.

Whereas ultrasonography is generally not useful in identifying mediastinal lesions, MRI or computed tomography should be employed routinely with ultrasonography and esophagography in the patient harboring one or more missed or recurrent parathyroid lesions.

^{201}Tl is avidly concentrated by parathyroid tissue; when it is used in combination with ^{99m}Tc scans of the neck to identify thyroid tissue, parathyroid lesions can be effectively localized. However, the incidence of false-positive and false-negative results obtained with this procedure is a matter of concern. Both false-positive and false-negative results have also been obtained using ultrasonography, MRI, and computed tomography, and at their present stage of development, it is prudent to use more than one of these procedures in patients with recurrent hyperparathyroidism and in patients whose first neck explorations were unsuccessful.

These procedures may also help in the diagnosis of a severely hypercalcemic patient who has not undergone previous neck exploration. In such a case, identification of a mass lesion in a location consistent with normal or aberrant parathyroid tissue strongly suggests the presence of primary hyperparathyroidism and argues for early neck exploration, even before serum iPTH has been measured.

3. Thyroid arteriography–Of the invasive procedures, thyroid arteriography is most useful to the surgeon when a lesion is identified. However, as with the noninvasive procedures, the results are specific only in the sense that the location of an identified lesion is consistent with that of a normal or aberrant parathyroid gland. Neurologic complications such as transient occipital blindness and hemiplegia have been recorded; therefore, the procedure should be avoided in patients at risk for neurovascular disease. Use of small quantities of contrast medium by a radiologist with long experience in the technique minimizes the risk of complications.

4. Selective venous catheterization–Ideally, differential catheterization of the neck and mediastinal veins for the purpose of obtaining serum for iPTH analysis should be performed after veins have been identified by arteriography. The procedure is simple if a lesion has been identified by arteriography. If arteriography has not identified a lesion, all of the accessible small veins of the neck and mediastinum should be entered and sampled. It is often difficult to obtain blood from small veins because the lumina are obstructed by the catheter tip. The blood in the larger veins may be easier to aspirate, but the blood flow is so great that "step-up" increases in serum iPTH can be obliterated even if the catheter tip is near a small vein draining a parathyroid tumor. Venous catheterization studies must be interpreted with caution; because of the distortion in venous anatomy produced by individual variation, previous surgery, and venous anastomoses, the best result that can be obtained is usually lateralization of a parathyroid lesion. In general, less than a 2-fold "step-up" should be ignored unless all other values for iPTH are almost identical. It is important to recognize that significant increases in iPTH have been recorded in sera draining normal parathyroid glands. This finding argues against the use of differential venous sampling in the initial diagnosis of hyperparathyroidism.

Natural History of Hyperparathyroidism

The natural history of primary hyperparathyroidism is not well understood. This is because most patients in whom the diagnosis is made undergo neck exploration and removal of the abnormal glands and are cured.

A large proportion of patients have "biochemical" hyperparathyroidism—ie, only a slightly increased serum calcium (10.1–11 mg/dL [2.53–2.75 mmol/L]) and no clinical manifestations of the disease. A study of 150 such patients at the Mayo Clinic showed that a minority (10–30%) will develop a more severe form of the disease within 5 years, but no clinical or biochemical measurement was predictive of such progression.

It is presumed that patients with mild to moderately severe primary hyperparathyroidism started with the "biochemical" form of the disease. However, some of these patients attain a degree of disease stability; some have been observed for as long as 10–15 years without apparent progression. Except for a few who progress to severe disease, the remaining patients in this group probably have slow progression with gradual development of osteopenia and deterioration of renal function. Patients with severe primary hyperparathyroidism (serum calcium > 15 mg/dL [3.75 mmol/L]) will almost certainly die of the complications sooner or later unless the disease is diagnosed and appropriately treated.

Resection of benign parathyroid lesions is usually curative. Recurrences are rare in patients with single-gland disease but relatively common in multiple-gland disease. It is unclear whether successful surgical treatment restores impaired renal function. Stone formation generally ceases unless factors other than primary hyperparathyroidism are operative. There have been anecdotal reports of relief of severe psychiatric symptoms after removal of abnormal parathyroid glands. All but the more severe forms of osteitis fibrosa cystica improve within months and resolve completely within a year after parathyroidectomy. Recent studies suggest that surgical treatment of hyperparathyroidism in patients with postmenopausal or senile osteoporosis results in improvement of osteopenia. This is important because as many as 8–10% of patients with age-related osteopenia have increased circulating levels of iPTH and may suffer from some form of curable hyperparathyroidism.

Treatment of Hypercalcemia
A. Medical Treatment:
1. Chronic moderately severe hypercalcemia (serum calcium 12–15 mg/dL)–Medical management of diseases causing nonparathyroid hypercalcemia generally results in prompt resolution of this biochemical abnormality. Far-advanced malignant disorders (solid or hematologic tumors) are exceptions,

and long-term chronic treatment of cancer-related hypercalcemia in such cases is a therapeutic challenge. There is no satisfactory protocol for managing this problem, and it is a fertile area for pharmacologic research.

a. Glucocorticoids—Glucocorticoids have been the major resource for treatment of hypercalcemia associated with hematologic malignant neoplasms. They should be given in relatively high doses (eg, prednisone, 60–120 mg/d given orally in divided doses) and for relatively long periods (1 month) before the treatment is considered a failure. Bisphosphonate drugs are gradually replacing glucocorticoids in the treatment of this important complication of hematologic malignant neoplasms (see below).

b. Mithramycin—Mithramycin (Plicamycin), a toxic antibiotic that inhibits bone resorption, may be useful in the treatment of hypercalcemia due to both hematologic and solid malignant neoplasms. The usual dosage is 25 μg/kg by intravenous push. When hypercalcemia recurs, this same dose may be given again, provided platelet counts have not been dangerously suppressed and renal function has not become impaired. Lower doses (10–15 μg/kg) have been used successfully with fewer side effects. The lower dose is preferred if repeated doses are necessary.

c. Phosphate—Oral phosphate may be used as an antihypercalcemic agent in patients who have not been taking glucocorticoids. (The combination of oral phosphate and glucocorticoids occasionally induces nephrolithiasis, although the cause is unknown.) Either neutral phosphate or potassium phosphate may be given in doses as high as 2–4 g/d orally in divided doses. Initial doses should be relatively low (1–2 g of elemental phosphorus as phosphate per day orally in divided doses every 6 hours), because of gastrointestinal side effects; these disappear with time. Serum calcium, phosphate, and creatinine should be measured regularly to determine if phosphate treatment is effective and to detect the possible development of hyperphosphatemia or renal function impairment. Compliance can be assessed by measurement of 24-hour urine phosphorus. In general, decreases in serum calcium during phosphate therapy do not occur unless serum phosphate concentrations increase. Increases in serum phosphorus above 5 mg/dL should be avoided because of the danger of inducing extraskeletal calcifications. Phosphate therapy can be used as a temporary measure during diagnostic studies. Phosphate therapy may cause hypokalemia, requiring administration of potassium supplements.

d. Calcitonin—Although it would seem rational to use CT, normal doses (100 units/d) have been disappointing. However, good results have been obtained with high doses of CT (400–1000 units every 12 hours) or with CT plus glucocorticoids (CT, 100 units twice daily, and prednisone, 60 mg daily).

e. Estrogen—Because estrogens decrease bone resorption and serum calcium in postmenopausal osteoporosis, estrogens have been used successfully to lower serum calcium in primary hyperparathyroidism. In the absence of contraindications (eg, personal or family history of uterine or breast cancer), maintenance doses (eg, 0.625–1.25 mg conjugated estrogens [Premarin, etc]) should be given to all postmenopausal patients with primary hyperparathyroidism under medical management.

f. Intravenous disodium etidronate—This drug has been used successfully in the acute treatment of hypercalcemia. It is administered intravenously, in a dose of 7.5 mg/kg in 250 mL saline over 2 hours for 3 successive days.

g. Other agents—Based on the presence of both adrenergic and histamine receptors on parathyroid cells, alpha- and beta-adrenergic blockers and cimetidine have been tried in primary hyperparathyroidism, with generally negative results.

2. Acute severe hypercalcemia (serum calcium > 15 mg/dL)—The medical therapy of acute severe hypercalcemia is quite different from that of chronic moderate hypercalcemia. Treatment should be started as soon as severe hypercalcemia has been detected, because the condition is life-threatening.

a. Hospitalization—If possible, the patient should remain ambulatory, since immobilization may increase serum calcium in some patients. Serum calcium, magnesium, sodium, and potassium must be monitored every 2–4 hours. In patients with heart disease who are in danger of developing heart failure from volume overload, central venous pressure should be monitored so that appropriate measures can be taken if the pressure increases.

b. Calcium restriction—Dietary calcium should be restricted immediately, and all drugs that might cause hypercalcemia (thiazides, vitamin D, etc) should be discontinued.

c. Reduction of digitalis—If the patient is taking digitalis, it may be wise to reduce the dose because the hypercalcemic patient may be more sensitive to the toxic effects of this drug. Ideally, the patient should be admitted to an intensive care unit for electrocardiographic monitoring while antihypercalcemic measures are being instituted. Beta-adrenergic blocking agents are useful in protecting the heart against the adverse effects of severe hypercalcemia, especially serious arrhythmias.

d. Hydration and diuretics—The mainstay of therapy is a regimen of hydration with saline solutions plus diuresis with furosemide or ethacrynic acid. The objective is to increase the urinary excretion of calcium rapidly, thus decreasing the exchangeable calcium pool and the serum calcium concentration. Saline is given to increase sodium excretion, since sodium clearance and calcium clearance parallel one another during water or osmotic diuresis. Furosemide inhibits the tubular reabsorption of calcium and aids in maintaining diuresis. Approximately 4–6 L of isotonic saline should be given intravenously daily, along with

20–100 mg of furosemide intravenously every 1–2 hours or 10–40 mg of ethacrynic acid intravenously every 1–2 hours. Such a regimen should increase urinary calcium to 500–1000 mg/d and lower serum calcium by 2–6 mg/dL after 24 hours.

e. Potassium and magnesium depletion and dehydration–These complications of therapy must be anticipated and appropriate replacement therapy instituted early.

f. Maintenance regimen–After serum calcium has decreased to a reasonably safe level (< 13 mg/dL), a chronic regimen may be instituted. This should consist of furosemide (40–160 mg/d orally) or ethacrynic acid (50–200 mg/d orally), sodium chloride tablets (400–600 meq/d orally), and at least 3 L of fluid per day. Serum calcium, magnesium, and potassium should be monitored daily at first and then weekly when serum calcium has stabilized. Magnesium and potassium should be replaced as necessary.

g. Other drugs–Two other drugs are used in patients with severe hypercalcemia.

(1) Mithramycin–Mithramycin is given in 2–4 doses of 10–15 μg/kg intravenously on alternate days early in the course of treatment of acute hypercalcemia. It is probably unwise to give mithramycin if primary hyperparathyroidism is suspected, because the patient is likely to require surgery and mithramycin can cause marked thrombocytopenia. Patients receiving mithramycin should be followed carefully with platelet counts, serum creatinine, and liver function tests because of its possible toxicity to the liver, kidney, and marrow.

(2) Intravenous disodium etidronate–This drug is effective in many patients and is safer than mithramycin (Plicamycin). It is given in 2–4 doses of 10–15 μg/kg intravenously on alternate days. Several other bisphosphonates exist that are as effective as etidronate, but they are not yet available in the USA.

B. Surgery for Removal of Abnormal Parathyroid Tissue: Surgical treatment should be considered in all patients with an established diagnosis of primary hyperparathyroidism. It is not clear that the biochemical form of the disease necessarily progresses to the stage at which clinically significant sequelae develop. However, most of these patients have histologic evidence of hyperparathyroidism on bone biopsy. Age is not a contraindication to neck exploration. Indeed, it is better to perform elective parathyroidectomy and manage hypercalcemia in that way than to deal with it later as a complication of another serious illness (eg, myocardial infarction).

1. Indications for surgery–In the long-term follow-up of biochemical hyperparathyroidism commented upon earlier, a group of arbitrary criteria were developed as indications for neck exploration (Table 11–4): (1) serum calcium higher than 11 mg/d; (2) radiographic evidence of metabolic bone disease; (3) active nephrolithiasis; (4) demonstration of decreased

Table 11–4. Categories of treatment for patients with primary hyperparathyroidism.

Criteria	Preferred Treatment

1. One or more of the following:
  Serum calcium > 11 mg/dL.
  Osteitis fibrosa cystica.
  Progressive osteopenia.
  Metabolically active nephro-
    lithiasis.
  Decreased renal function.
  Intractable peptic ulcer.
  Pancreatitis.
  Serious psychiatric disease.
  Severe hypertension.
	Surgical removal of parathyroid lesion.

2. Unsuccessful surgery, or recurrence with manifestations noted in category 1.	Surgical removal of parathyroid lesion; preoperative localization may be indicated.
3. Serum calcium <11 mg/dL. Abnormal serum iPTH. Absence of manifestations noted in category 1.	Surgical removal of parathyroid lesion or medical management (see text).
4. Surgery contraindicated.	Medical management for hypercalcemia and prevention of nephrolithiasis (see text).

renal function; and (5) development of one or more "complications" of hyperparathyroidism such as serious psychiatric disease, peptic ulcer that is resistant to treatment, pancreatitis, and severe hypertension. In any patient in whom long-term medical management of the disease is planned, certain studies should be obtained routinely (Fig 11–19). *At a minimum,* these should include a yearly history and physical examination, serum calcium, creatinine clearance, and bone mineral content of the spine and radius; x-rays of the hand on fine-grain industrial film to detect subperiosteal bone resorption; and a plain film of the abdomen to detect renal calcifications. If inactive nephrolithiasis has been found on initial examination, nephrotomograms should be done to determine if new stones have formed or existing ones have enlarged. By definition, either of the latter would indicate recurrence of active stone disease, which would in turn be an indication for surgery.

2. Parathyroid surgeon–The most critical consideration in the surgical management of primary hyperparathyroidism is selection of a surgeon with extensive experience in parathyroid surgery and the ability to distinguish between an enlarged or abnormal parathyroid gland or lesion and a normal gland.

3. Surgical procedures–Two different procedures are currently used. The most widely accepted procedure consists of identifying all 4 parathyroid glands (using biopsy if necessary) followed by removal of a single enlarged parathyroid gland or of 3½ glands if multiple glands are involved (Table 11–5). If

Table 11–5. Extent of parathyroidectomy.

Number of Glands Involved	Procedure
All 4	Removal of 3 glands and all but 35–50 mg of the fourth gland; suture tagging of remnant or transplant to forearm.
Two or 3	Removal of all but half of a normal gland; suture tagging of remaining half.
One	Removal of involved gland; identification of remaining glands (often by biopsy); suture tagging of remaining glands.

abnormal parathyroid tissue cannot be identified, hemithyroidectomy should be performed, preferably on the side of a "missing" gland, because an intrathyroidal lesion may be present. All remaining parathyroid glands or remnants are marked with nonabsorbable sutures to facilitate future identification of parathyroid tissue if repeat surgery for recurrent hyperparathyroidism is necessary.

The less commonly used procedure consists of exploring one side of the neck first and removing any single enlarged parathyroid gland. If the second gland on the same side is normal, the other side is not explored. If the second gland is abnormal, it is removed and the other side of the neck is explored and all parathyroid tissue removed except for one-half of a gland. This second approach leaves the unoperated side without scar tissue and makes it easier to explore at some future time for recurrent hyperparathyroidism. However, it fails to establish whether multiple glands are involved, since enlarged glands may be present on the unoperated side.

No matter which approach is taken, it is important to make accurate records of the number and location of glands identified and removed (preferably by detailed diagram). This information is essential in finding the missed glands if hypercalcemia persists or recurs.

4. Parathyroid autotransplantation–Autotransplantation of a portion of an enlarged parathyroid gland to the muscles of the forearm can be beneficial in special circumstances, such as when the last known parathyroid gland is removed because of recurrent primary hyperparathyroidism. Without transplantation, patients of this type may become hypoparathyroid. The functioning of such transplants can be easily assessed by measuring serum iPTH in venous blood from both forearms. A "step-up" in the concentration of serum iPTH in the transplanted forearm in comparison with the nontransplanted one is indicative of a functioning graft. If such patients develop hypercalcemia, portions of the transplanted gland can be removed easily.

5. Ectopic location–About 20% of abnormal parathyroid glands are in the mediastinum. However, 95% of these are in the superior part of the cavity, attached to the thymus or mediastinal fat pad. These abnormal glands are readily identified and removed during routine neck exploration by lifting the contents of the superior mediastinum into the neck incision. The remaining 5% are located elsewhere in the mediastinum and can only be made accessible for excision by splitting the sternum. Before the advent of localization procedures (see above), the success rate in removing abnormal parathyroid tissue from the mediastinum was only 50%. The success rate is markedly improved if mediastinal lesions can be localized, but they are localized less frequently than are neck lesions (approximately 70+%). The decision to perform mediastinal exploration largely depends on the accuracy and completeness of the information obtained during initial neck exploration. If the exploration was inadequate or the records incomplete, repeat neck exploration is probably indicated. A recent study in which patients of this type were explored again showed an 80% success rate in finding missed abnormal parathyroid glands in the neck or superior mediastinum attached to the thymus. In rare cases, a fifth or sixth parathyroid gland may be present and abnormal.

C. Postoperative Care:

1. Hypocalcemia–If surgery is successful, serum calcium concentrations decrease to the normal range or lower within 24–48 hours. It is possible to determine if all abnormal parathyroid tissue has been removed by measuring decreased cAMP in a "spot" urine collection within 2 hours after parathyroidectomy. Patients with significant bony demineralization may develop severe hypocalcemia postoperatively. This is presumably due to the avidity of demineralized bone for extracellular fluid calcium ("hungry bone syndrome"). It can be distinguished from the development of hypoparathyroidism by the absence of hyperphosphatemia and the presence of increased serum iPTH. Treatment may be difficult (see Hypoparathyroidism, above) and requires large quantities of intravenous calcium given continuously by infusion plus calcium carbonate given orally in doses of $1–10$ g/d, depending upon the serum calcium response. Ergocalciferol (vitamin D_2) (usually 50,000–100,000 units daily) is of uncertain value. In the authors' experience, $1,25(OH)_2D_3$ (calcitriol, Rocaltrol) in relatively large doses ($1–2$ μg/d) has been useful.

2. Hypoparathyroidism–Most patients who develop hypocalcemia and mild hyperphosphatemia have temporary hypoparathyroidism, as evidenced by low normal serum levels of iPTH. A few of these patients will develop permanent hypoparathyroidism that requires treatment.

3. Other complications–Worsening of renal function (temporary or permanent), metabolic acidosis, hypomagnesemia, pancreatitis, and gout or pseudogout are other complications that may occur in the postoperative period. The problem of deterioration of renal function should be anticipated in patients who have abnormal renal function before the operation, and prophylactic infusions of mannitol should be given early in the postoperative period to initiate and maintain osmotic diuresis. Likewise, exacerbations of gout or pseudogout should be anticipated in patients with intra-articular calcifications or a history of arthritic attacks.

4. Follow-up–Follow-up is recommended for about 10 years. This is especially important for patients with multiple-gland disease, because of the likelihood of recurrence. Another concern is the rare but real possibility that an excised lesion (in spite of histologic evidence of benignity) may have been malignant. In such cases, early detection of hypercalcemia may permit definitive surgical treatment before the development of local or distant metastases.

SECONDARY HYPERPARATHYROIDISM OF CHRONIC RENAL FAILURE

An increase in PTH secretion that is adaptive and unrelated to intrinsic disease of the parathyroid glands is called secondary hyperparathyroidism. The disorder is associated with prolonged stimulation of the parathyroid glands by chronic decreases in the concentration of ionic calcium in the blood. Several conditions cause chronic hypocalcemia and secondary hyperparathyroidism (Table 11–6). However, except in extreme cases, chronic renal failure is the only one in which secondary hyperparathyroidism produces clinically significant manifestations. Thus, this section will emphasize hyperparathyroidism associated with chronic renal failure.

Interest in the hyperparathyroidism of chronic renal failure and its associated bone disease, **renal osteodystrophy,** is a fairly recent development. Before the advent of hemodialysis, the sequelae of progressive nephron destruction were not studied seriously, because the life expectancy of patients with chronic renal failure was so short. Since these patients are now maintained with dialysis and renal transplantation, the problems of chronic management must be identified and solved.

Table 11–6. Major causes of chronic hypocalcemia other than parathyroprival hypoparathyroidism.

Dietary deficiency of vitamin D or calcium.
Decreased intestinal absorption of vitamin D or calcium due to primary small bowel disease, short bowel syndrome, and post-gastrectomy syndrome.
Drugs that cause rickets or osteomalacia such as phenytoin, phenobarbital, cholestyramine, and laxatives.
States of tissue resistance to vitamin D.
Excessive intake of inorganic phosphate compounds.
Pseudohypoparathyroidism.
Severe hypomagnesemia.
Chronic renal failure.

Pathogenesis of Secondary Hyperparathyroidism in Chronic Renal Failure

Serum iPTH progressively increases in patients with chronic renal failure as glomerular filtration rate (GFR) decreases below 40 mL/min (Fig 11–23). This relationship might have been predicted on the basis of older studies that showed increases in serum phosphorus concentrations at this same level of GFR (40 mL/min). However, it was not until the investigations of Bricker et al that the role of decreased renal filtration of phosphate and subsequent hyperphosphatemia in the genesis of renal hyperparathyroidism was appreciated. According to their hypothesis, each decrement in GFR is accompanied by a transient increase in serum phosphorus, which in turn leads to a transient decrease in serum calcium and a compensatory increase in secretion of PTH. Restoration of serum calcium and serum phosphorus toward normal occurs as a result of the effects of increased serum PTH on mobilization of bone mineral and renal tubular reabsorption of phosphate, respectively. As the cycle is repeated, secondary hyperparathyroidism progressively worsens and parathyroid hyperplasia develops.

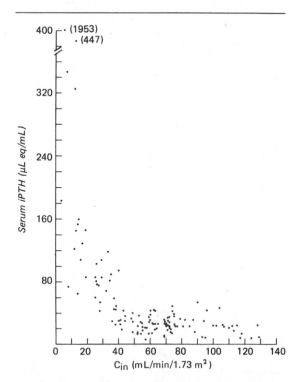

Figure 11–23. Serum iPTH as a function of the renal clearance of inulin in normal subjects and patients with varying degrees of renal failure. The assay used GP1M as the antiserum. (Reproduced, with permission, from Arnaud CD et al: Page 349 in: *Urinary Calculi: Recent Advances in Aetiology, Stone Structure, and Treatment.* International Symposium on Renal Stone Research, 1973.)

The evidence in support of the hypothesis of Bricker et al is impressive, First, a reduction in phosphate intake in proportion to the reduction in GFR prevents renal hyperparathyroidism in dogs that have had progressive renal failure for as long as 1 year. Second, there is a consistent positive correlation between serum concentrations of phosphate and iPTH in patients with chronic renal failure (Fig 11–24). Third, reductions in the serum concentrations of phosphate by dietary restriction and administration of aluminum hydroxide gels in patients with chronic renal failure are associated with increases in serum calcium and decreases in serum iPTH.

The hyperphosphatemia of chronic renal failure may also have a negative influence on the production of $1,25(OH)_2D_3$, even before the destruction of nephrons is so complete that the renal $25OHD_3$-converting enzymes are eliminated. As illustrated in Figure 11–2, such an effect would result in a decrease in the intestinal absorption of calcium—a well-established finding in patients with chronic renal failure. This decrease would contribute further to hypocalcemia and secondary hyperparathyroidism. It is well known that serum concentrations of $1,25(OH)_2D_3$ are low in patients with end-stage renal disease, but there have been no systematic studies of the relation between serum concentrations of this vitamin D metabolite and the degree of chronic renal failure.

The osseous manifestations of progressive increases in PTH secretion and decreases in $1,25(OH)_2D_3$ production by the kidney are evident in patients with chronic renal failure. They include classic osteitis fibrosa cystica similar to that seen in primary hyperparathyroidism (Fig 11–18A and 11–18B) and osteomalacia (Fig 11–34). In addition, osteosclerosis and osteoporosis are often present at the same time. The causes of these 2 disorders are unknown and are probably multiple. It is thought that the osteosclerosis is related to the hyperphosphatemia, and the osteoporosis to diminished sex hormone function and the metabolic acidosis of uremia. Finally, there is evidence that the bones of patients with chronic renal failure are resistant to the calcemic actions of PTH. Although there may be several underlying reasons for such resistance, it is commonly thought that the major factors are the decreased serum concentration of $1,25(OH)_2D_3$ and the dependency of PTH on normal vitamin D metabolism for its action on bone.

The pathogenesis of renal hyperparathyroidism during the progressive destruction of nephrons is illustrated in Figure 11–25. The process schematically described result in the classic biochemical and physiological abnormalities of mineral and bone metabolism observed in patients with chronic renal failure, including hypocalcemia, hyperphosphatemia, decreased intestinal absorption of calcium and negative calcium

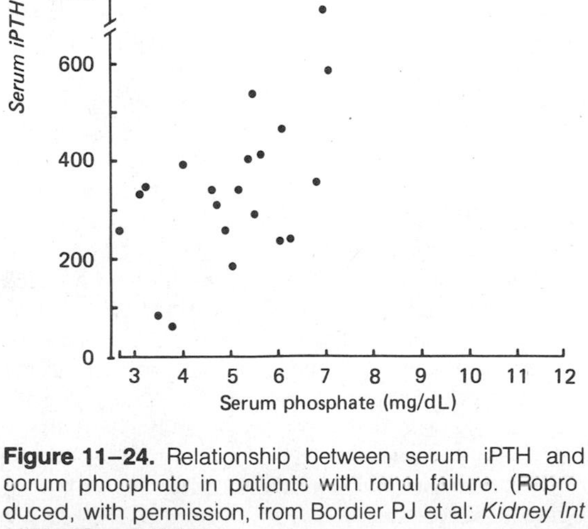

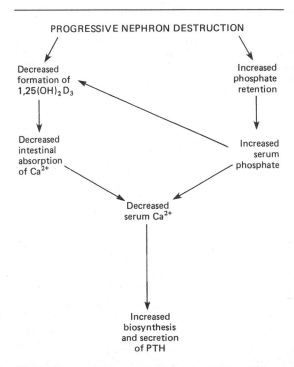

Figure 11–24. Relationship between serum iPTH and serum phosphate in patients with renal failure. (Reproduced, with permission, from Bordier PJ et al: *Kidney Int* 1975;7[Suppl 2]:102.)

Figure 11–25. Pathogenesis of parathyroid hyperplasia during progressive destruction of nephrons. (Reproduced, with permission, from Arnaud CD et al: *Kidney Int* 1973;4:89.)

balance, marked increases in circulating PTH, and the different bone diseases noted above.

Natural History

A. Chronic Renal Failure (Renal Osteodystrophy): The natural history of disorders of mineral and bone metabolism that are associated with chronic renal failure is not well understood. A group of untreated patients with chronic renal failure of varying severity and duration who were not undergoing hemodialysis has been studied in order to provide such information. In spite of the limitations imposed on interpretation of results from a cross-sectional study, it was possible to roughly categorize the development of mineral abnormalities as a function of time and severity (Fig 11–26). The first detectable abnormality appears to be an increase in serum iPTH. This occurs when GFR falls below 40 mL/min and before there are detectable changes in serum phosphate or calcium. This is not unexpected, if increased PTH secretion represents the major mechanism by which the organism adapts to renal phosphate retention. The important question is whether this adaptive mechanism, which appears to be so successful in maintaining extracellular calcium and phosphate homeostasis under physiologic conditions, is in the best interest of the patient with renal failure or whether externally applied therapeutic measures designed to achieve the same purpose might serve such a patient better in the long run.

In the study noted above, all of the patients who had mild to moderate degrees of chronic renal failure

(serum creatinine ≤ 3 mg/dL) had histomorphometric evidence of excess circulating PTH in bone biopsies, and many had subperiosteal bone resorption on hand radiographs (stage I), in spite of normal serum levels of calcium and phosphorus. Thus, it appears that maintenance of normal levels of serum calcium and phosphorus in patients with early renal failure by adaptive increases in PTH secretion occurred as a result of an important trade-off—loss of osseous integrity.

Stage II was marked by the development of hypocalcemia, hyperphosphatemia, and further increases in serum iPTH. A transition to this stage probably reflects the development of severe vitamin D deficiency caused by the hyperphosphatemia and the loss of $1,25(OH)_2D_3$ hydroxylase that occurs with progressive destruction of the kidney. Deficiency of $1,25(OH)_2D_3$ results in superimposition of osteomalacia on osteitis fibrosa cystica, which, having developed during stage I, now becomes worse. It is probably the degree and duration of the hypocalcemia of stage II that determine whether patients enter stages III and IV. These latter stages are characterized by worsening hyperparathyroidism, restoration of the serum calcium first to normal and then to hypercalcemic levels, and development of severe hyperphosphatemia. In fact, it is likely that some time during the transition from stage II to stage III, hyperparathyroidism becomes self-perpetuating and relatively autonomous (referred to by some as "tertiary" hyperparathyroidism). Phosphorus, as well as calcium, is released from bone during the process of PTH-induced bone resorption, and the initial perturbation causing hyperparathyroidism—hyperphosphatemia—is aggravated by the adaptive process originally developed to control it. In this manner, the negative feedback system that operates between bone and parathyroid glands when a normal kidney is present may be transformed into a biologically unstable "positive feedback" system when phosphorus cannot be excreted by a functioning kidney. Evidence of a defect in the ability of hypercalcemia to suppress PTH secretion in stage III and stage IV patients is illustrated in Figure 11–27. Whereas the expected negative correlation between serum iPTH and serum calcium is evident in stage I and stage II patients (lower panel), a positive correlation between these 2 variables exists in stage III and stage IV patients. The determinants of the transformation from stage II to stage III are poorly understood, but they probably include dietary levels of calcium, phosphate, and vitamin D and the rapidity with which the patient loses nephrons. During stages III and IV, osteitis fibrosa cystica and osteomalacia become even more prominent, and, because the product of the serum concentrations of calcium and phosphate increases to levels that favor precipitation, soft tissue calcification ensues.

B. "Aluminum" Osteodystrophy: A newly recognized syndrome of osteodystrophy that does not conform to the bone disease characterizing the 4 stages

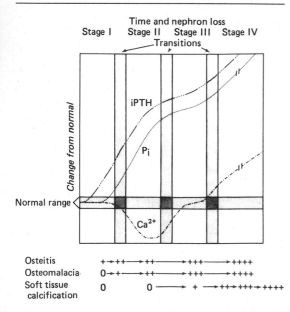

Figure 11–26. Stages of biochemical and osseous abnormalities in renal osteodystrophy as a function of time and nephron loss. (Reproduced, with permission, from Bordier PH et al: *Kidney Int* 1975;**7**[Suppl 2]:102.)

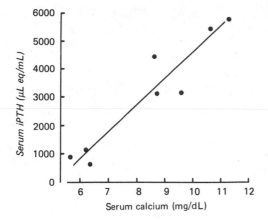

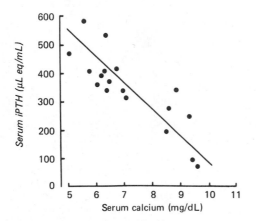

Figure 11–27. Relationship between serum iPTH and serum calcium. *Top:* Stage III and stage IV patients with high iPTH values. *Bottom:* Stage I and stage II patients with relatively low iPTH values. (Reproduced, with permission, from Bordier PJ et al: *Kidney Int* 1975;7[Suppl 2]:102.)

shown in Figure 11–26 has been described in patients with chronic renal failure. This syndrome is present in an increasing number of patients with renal osteodystrophy. Its cause is unknown, although accumulation of aluminum in bone (especially at the calcification front) due to the aluminum contained in dialysis baths or phosphate-binding agents has been recently implicated. Patients with this disorder have bone pain and multiple fractures and tend to develop hypercalcemia. Thus, superficially at least, they resemble patients with stage III or stage IV disease. However, instead of severe degrees of osteitis fibrosa cystica and hyperparathyroidism, these patients have a bone disease characterized by low-turnover osteomalacia and osteoporosis with only small or moderate increases in serum iPTH. Patients who have been subjected to parathyroidectomy have responded poorly or not at all. This is in striking contrast to patients with true stage IV renal hyperparathyroidism and osteodystrophy, who almost always respond favorably as long as they are carefully managed to prevent recrudescence of hyperparathyroidism after subtotal parathyroidectomy. The effectiveness of deferoxamine, a drug that chelates aluminum, is currently being assessed in the treatment of "aluminum" osteodystrophy.

Clinical Features

The clinical manifestations of renal hyperparathyroidism and osteodystrophy are related to hypocalcemia in stage II patients and to soft tissue calcifications, osteodystrophy, and pruritus in stage III and stage IV patients. Although not common, symptoms of neuromuscular irritability and tetany similar to those in hypoparathyroidism may occur. Osteodystrophy may cause bone pain due to either osteitis fibrosa or multiple fractures (frequently of the ribs). Soft tissue calcification of the joints (usually the shoulder) may be evident in rare cases as hard irregular masses over the joints. Pruritus is most debilitating when it occurs, and its cause is poorly understood. However, it routinely abates after successful medical or surgical management of hyperparathyroidism. Radiographs of the skeleton may show the ravages of osteitis fibrosa cystica (Fig 11–18A and 11–18B), osteomalacia (Fig 11–34), and osteosclerosis. This latter condition is classically observed as the "rugger jersey sign" (referring to the striped shirts worn by British rugby teams) and is caused by increased density of the upper and lower margins of vertebral bodies, separated by central horizontal zones of decreased density. Soft tissue calcifications often seen on x-ray in the later stages are most prominent in large vessels and joints but have been observed in extreme cases in lung, stomach, and heart. It is thought that soft tissue calcification of small blood vessels is responsible for the rare development of necrotic skin lesions on legs, abdomen, and fingertips.

Prevention

Little effort has been made to systematically interrupt the adaptive cycle described in the section on pathogenesis and to prevent the development of the pathologic "positive feedback" between bone and parathyroid glands during the course of renal failure. This is probably because patients are generally asymptomatic and reluctant to take medicines early in the course of renal failure. In addition, no long-term prospective studies have been reported showing that appropriate therapy instituted early and directed at preventing the development of positive phosphorus balance, negative calcium balance, and hyperparathyroidism will significantly decrease the incidence or severity of mineral and bone complications that occur in the late stages of renal failure, during hemodialysis, or after kidney transplantation. However, investigations during the past 10 years have shown that restoration of serum calcium and phosphorus levels toward normal by the use of oral phosphate-binding gels and calcium con-

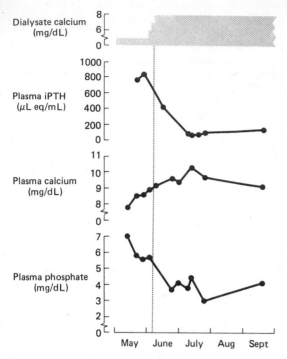

Figure 11–28. Serial values of plasma iPTH, calcium, and phosphate during treatment of a patient with low and then high calcium levels in the dialysate. Plasma phosphate was reduced to 6 mg/dL by oral administration of aluminum hydroxide gel, after which dialysate calcium concentrations were progressively increased to 8 mg/dL. (Reproduced, with permission, from Goldsmith RS et al: *Am J Med* 1971;**50**:692.)

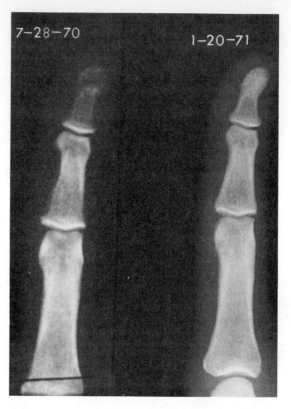

Figure 11–29. X-rays of index finger of a patient before *(left)* and after *(right)* plasma phosphate was reduced to normal with aluminum hydroxide gel and 6 months of dialysis against a bath of 8 mg/dL calcium. (Reproduced, with permission, from Vosik WM et al: *Mayo Clin Proc* 1972:**47**:110.)

centrations of 6–7 mg/dL in the dialysate for patients undergoing hemodialysis decreases serum levels of iPTH (Fig 11–28) and causes improvement in established renal osteodystrophy (Fig 11–29). It is therefore likely that the component of renal osteodystrophy that is due to hyperparathyroidism could be prevented if steps were taken *early* in the course of chronic renal failure to avoid adaptive increases in PTH secretion. Since the stimulus of PTH secretion is hypocalcemia induced by hyperphosphatemia and decreased intestinal absorption of calcium, it is logical to assume that a combination of ingestion of a low-phosphate diet, administration of phosphate-binding gels, and treatment with relatively large doses of absorbable calcium and physiologic doses of $1,25(OH)_2D_3$ (calcitriol) might be successful in restoring extracellular calcium and phosphorus homeostasis and preventing secondary hyperparathyroidism.

Treatment

A. Management of Stage I Renal Osteodystrophy: The major difficulty in this stage is determining when to begin treatment in individual patients, because serum calcium and phosphorus concentrations

are usually within the normal range early in the course of chronic renal failure. In spite of this, serum iPTH is increased during the first stage (Fig 11–26). Unfortunately, this change may be difficult to detect with some radioimmunoassays. Assays specific for the mid or carboxyl region of the PTH molecule show that serum iPTH is increased uniformly in patients with chronic renal failure. Although an increased level of serum iPTH may reflect diminished clearance of carboxyterminal fragments by diseased kidneys, mid- and carboxy-region assays show that institution of the therapy noted below results in a progressive decline in serum iPTH toward the normal range. This result suggests that there is either a decrease in PTH secretion or improved clearance of carboxy-terminal fragments by the kidney. The latter possibility is a remote one, and it is likely that the observed decreases in serum iPTH reflect success in directly interrupting the development of adaptive hyperparathyroidism.

1. Dietary restriction of phosphorus–It appears that the single most important marker for stage I renal osteodystrophy—and the major indication for considering a patient with chronic renal failure for treatment with dietary restriction of phosphate, calcium supplementation, and with vitamin D therapy—is an abnormally high serum iPTH value as measured by a mid- or carboxy-region assay. Although dietary restriction of phosphate may be sufficient for some patients, others may require the addition of phosphate-binding antacids in order to reduce serum iPTH.

2. Removal of phosphate—There are many aluminum-containing phosphate-binding antacids on the market. Alu-Capsules, high-potency liquid Basaljel, and aluminum hydroxide–containing cookies (commercially prepared or baked at home) appear to be the most effective and the best tolerated because of their almost complete absence of aluminum taste. The patient should be offered a variety of preparations and dosage forms and should be allowed to choose an acceptable combination. Dosage must be adjusted for each patient, and prolonged hypophosphatemia should be avoided. The initial dose should be between 0.25 and 0.5 g/d; the dose should be increased if serum phosphate and serum iPTH fail to decrease. For maximal effect on dietary phosphate absorption, antacids should always be taken with meals.

3. Calcium supplementation—Because low-phosphate diets are also low in calcium, it is necessary to provide supplementation with some form of absorbable calcium. Calcium carbonate is preferred because it is cheap and well tolerated, it combats renal acidosis, and it is an effective phosphate-binding agent. Calcium supplementation is necessary even when the patient is on a normal diet, because enteral absorption of calcium is usually decreased in chronic renal failure. Serum calcium should be monitored because a few patients develop hypercalcemia. However, doses as high as 10 g/d may be tolerated well.

4. Vitamin D therapy—It is reasonable to maintain patients with early renal failure on relatively small doses (1000–2000 units/d) of ergocalciferol (vitamin D_2), providing no more than 10 times the daily requirement. Experience with $1,25(OH)_2D_3$ (calcitriol) in patients with stage I disease has not yet been reported.

B. Management of Stage II Renal Osteodystrophy: Most patients with end-stage renal failure present with the mineral and osseous abnormalities found in stage II disease. The hallmarks of this stage are hypocalcemia, hyperphosphatemia, and increases in serum iPTH greater than those in stage I. Generally, serum iPTH measured by a mid- or carboxy-region assay is 10–20 times normal values.

Since stages III and IV tend to be much less reversible by medical means than stage I or stage II, it is important to manage the patient with stage II disease aggressively. In treating such a patient, one must recognize that the hypocalcemia seen in stage II probably reflects a fortuitous protective adaptation of the organism to severe hyperparathyroidism. In other words, the permissive influence of vitamin D on the bone-resorbing action of PTH has been largely removed by

the final destruction of the kidneys, and the devastating effects of enormously high concentrations of circulating PTH have been naturally averted. Thus, it is probably important to delay the introduction of vitamin D or one of its biologically active metabolites or analogues until the hyperparathyroidism has been partially brought under control. This can be done in almost all dialyzed patients by restoring serum calcium and phosphorus to normal levels by the simple manipulation of dietary and dialysate calcium and dietary phosphate described above. Serum phosphate should be reduced to less than 5 mg/dL before attempts to increase serum calcium are made; this prevents increases in the calcium × phosphate product greater than 70 and the tendency to soft tissue calcifications. The regimen is most easily initiated in the hospital and should take no longer than 1 week. After serum iPTH begins to decrease, some form of vitamin D therapy may be introduced. The most effective form of vitamin D therapy has not yet been determined. A combination of metabolites may be necessary to restore both intestinal calcium absorption and bone formation processes to normal. Dihydrotachysterol (0.125 mg twice weekly to 1 mg daily) is used extensively. However, the more expensive $1,25(OH)_2D_3$ (Rocaltrol), at doses of 0.5–2 μg/d, is probably the drug of choice. Equivalent doses of ergocalciferol or any of the available vitamin D metabolites (Table 11–2) may also be used.

C. Management of Patients on Dialysis: Stage I and II Renal Osteodystrophy: When stage I and II patients who are treated as described in the previous section reach the end stage of renal failure and it becomes necessary for them to begin a hemodialysis program, they will have only minor hyperparathyroidism and renal osteodystrophy. These patients should present few problems in continuing prophylaxis. Since a PTH-induced increase in release of phosphate from bone into the circulation has been at least partly averted, dietary phosphate need not be severely restricted, and the dose of phosphate-binding agent needed to maintain serum phosphorus in the normal range should be tolerated by the average patient. Although these patients may require only supplements of vitamin D_2 (ergocalciferol) to avoid development of osteomalacia, one or more active vitamin D metabolites is occasionally necessary.

Dialysis patients with stage II renal osteodystrophy should respond to the treatment outlined for patients in stage II who are not on hemodialysis. The important consideration in patients on hemodialysis is to avoid aggravating negative calcium balance, which occurs when dialysate calcium concentrations are below 5.7 mg/dL. In fact, it is possible and probably desirable to use hemodialysis as a means of producing positive calcium balance by employing calcium concentrations of 6.5–8 mg/dL. However, this should not be attempted until serum phosphate concentrations are below 5 mg/dL, because extraosseous mineralization may be induced when the serum calcium × phosphate product is 70 or more. This therapeutic regimen is illustrated in Figure 11–28, where the reduction of plasma phosphate to 3 mg/dL combined with the gradual introduction of dialysate calcium concentrations of 8 mg/dL resulted in an increase in plasma calcium from 8 to 10 mg/dL and a concomitant and permanent decrease in plasma iPTH from values up to 20 times normal to values just above the upper limits of normal within a period of 2.5 months. Once abnormal mineral metabolism is brought under control, dialysate calcium concentrations should be reduced to about 6.5 mg/dL.

D. Management of Stage III and IV Renal Osteodystrophy: Stage III disease can be identified by the presence of hyperphosphatemia and eucalcemia with serum iPTH values (as measured by mid- or carboxy-region assay) from 50 to 100 times normal levels; in stage IV disease, there is hypercalcemia with elevations of serum iPTH to 200–1000 times normal levels. Whether patients with stage III or IV disease should be treated with the regimen illustrated in Figure 11–28 is controversial. It is clear that with heroic effort, it can be successfully applied to these patients. Figure 11–29 shows improvement in bone disease in one such patient. Ordinarily, patients with stage III or IV renal osteodystrophy should probably be treated initially with subtotal parathyroidectomy in order to decrease the size of the parathyroid gland mass, followed by the regimen described for patients with stage II renal osteodystrophy. This rather radical approach is justified because mineral complications and persistence of hyperparathyroidism after renal transplantation are less severe in patients whose hyperparathyroidism and osteodystrophy were well controlled before transplantation. It generally takes much longer to bring stage III and stage IV patients under control, and success is less common than in patients with stage II disease. Therefore, considering the unpredictable availability of donor kidneys for transplantation and the probable desirability of having hyperparathyroidism and renal osteodystrophy under control prior to transplantation, it is important to decide as soon as possible whether patients have stage III or stage IV renal osteodystrophy. When in doubt, the clinician should institute an intensive regimen of medical treatment, and if marked improvement in hyperparathyroidism and osteodystrophy is not observed within 3–6 months, subtotal parathyroidectomy should be considered.

E. Renal Transplantation: Depending upon the stage of renal hyperparathyroidism and osteodystrophy, successful renal transplantation may reverse the entire course of these complications. Patients who receive transplants during stage I or II achieve normal levels of serum iPTH, calcium, and phosphorus within months. Patients who receive transplants during stage III or IV may never achieve normal levels of serum iPTH and often suffer from hypercalcemia and hypophosphatemia for years, even when the transplanted kidney is functioning normally. Ultimately, some pa-

tients in this latter group require subtotal parathyroidectomy, but the indications for the procedure in such patients are poorly defined.

Prognosis & Future Prospects

It is becoming clear that the outcome of the mineral and osseous complications of end-stage renal failure depends upon early recognition and treatment of these complications, particularly before hemodialysis is started. At present, it is uncertain whether such an approach will succeed in the long-term management of patients, because some elements of the prophylactic regimen described in this section may be unavailable or unacceptable to the patient. The most important of these is an oral phosphate-binding preparation that does not contain aluminum and that will be enthusiastically accepted by patients. Another is a reliable, inexpensive PTH radioimmunoassay, specific for the mid or carboxyl region of the molecule, for patient follow-up. Finally, the underlying cause of the newly described syndrome of low-turnover osteomalacia in patients with end-stage renal failure must be determined (see above). It is possible that this syndrome is related to the widespread use of phosphate-binding agents that contain aluminum; if so, its incidence will increase. This might mean that an entirely new approach to the treatment of renal osteodystrophy would have to be developed.

DISORDERS OF CALCITONIN (CT) SECRETION

No clinical disorder has been reported to date in which hypocalcitoninemia plays a definitive role. However, there are a number of conditions in which hypercalcitoninemia is found—most notably medullary carcinoma of the thyroid gland (see also Chapters 10 and 28).

MEDULLARY CARCINOMA OF THE THYROID GLAND

Medullary carcinoma is a malignant tumor of the parafollicular cells of the thyroid gland. It occurs sporadically but may also be inherited as an autosomal dominant trait as part of the type II multiple endocrine neoplasia (MEN) syndrome. This syndrome includes medullary carcinoma of the thyroid gland and pheochromocytoma. There are 2 variants of the syndrome: type IIa and type IIb. Patients with MEN type IIa have a normal appearance but a high incidence of hyperparathyroidism, most frequently due to enlargement of multiple parathyroid glands. Patients with MEN type

IIb have a striking appearance due to labial and mucosal ganglioneuromas, a marfanoid habitus, and other somatic abnormalities. Hyperparathyroidism is unusual in this variant.

Incidence

Medullary carcinoma constitutes 1–3% of all thyroid cancers. The sex incidence is almost equal (male:female ratio of 1.3:1 in sporadic cases and 1:1 in familial cases). In general, familial cases present at a younger age than do sporadic ones.

Pathology

Medullary carcinoma appears as a solid, often hard mass confined to but not encapsulated in the thyroid gland. It is often unilateral in sporadic cases and bilateral in familial cases. The lesion is composed of sheets of cells with granular cytoplasms and usually contains irregular masses of amyloid and fibrous tissue. Most patients who present with a thyroid mass already have metastases to cervical lymph nodes. Some masses spread to the upper mediastinum. Metastases beyond the mediastinum, usually delayed until late in the natural history of the disease, most commonly occur in lungs, liver, bones, and adrenal glands.

Pathophysiology

Medullary carcinomas secrete large quantities of CT and respond to provocative stimuli such as intravenous pentagastrin or hypercalcemia induced by intravenous calcium. Although CT produces hypocalcemia and hypophosphatemia in experimental animals, these biochemical findings are unusual in patients with medullary carcinoma in spite of extremely high levels of immunoreactive calcitonin (iCT). This paradox is probably due to a combination of factors, including homologous desensitization of tissues that normally respond to the actions of CT.

Medullary carcinomas may secrete many other bioactive substances in addition to CT, each with the potential of causing symptoms. These include biogenic amines, ACTH and corticotropin-releasing hormone, prostaglandins, nerve growth factor, and possibly a prolactin-releasing hormone. Diarrhea is present in about 20% of patients. This symptom relents after surgical excision of the tumor and is therefore thought to be humorally mediated. Cushing's syndrome is present in about 5% of cases, secondary to secretion of excessive ACTH.

Clinical Features

Most patients with sporadic medullary carcinoma present with an asymptomatic thyroid mass. Patients with MEN type IIb may complain of neuromas and their marfanoid appearance. Hypercalcemia may be detected in the course of routine blood screening in patients with MEN type IIa with primary hyperparathyroidism. Most importantly, hypertension in patients with MEN type IIa or IIb may reflect the presence of pheochromocytoma, which may be more immediately life-threatening than medullary carcinoma.

Paraneoplastic syndromes (eg, Cushing's syndrome) as well as intractable diarrhea and flushing should alert the physician to the possible existence of medullary carcinoma. A family history of more than one case of thyroid cancer should certainly raise a suspicion of MEN type IIa in a patient with bizarre symptoms.

Other neural manifestations of MEN type IIb include medullated nerves in the cornea on slit lamp examination of the eye and ganglioneuromas of the gastrointestinal tract. The latter may cause gastrointestinal obstruction as well as megacolon.

Medullary cancers occasionally calcify. Thus, the discovery of a calcified thyroidal mass does not indicate that it is benign; rather, this is probably an indication for measurement of serum iCT (see below).

Diagnosis

The cornerstone of the laboratory investigation of patients suspected of having medullary carcinoma is radioimmunoassay of plasma CT. Although not absolutely specific for the tumor (see below), increased serum levels of iCT in patients with a thyroid mass, a family history of medullary carcinoma, or pheochromocytoma virtually establish the diagnosis. Other conditions in which increased levels of serum iCT have been reported include (1) ectopic secretion by almost any malignant tumor (especially small cell carcinoma of the lung), (2) chronic renal failure, (3) gastrointestinal disorders such as endocrine tumors of the pancreas and pernicious anemia, (4) subacute Hashimoto's thyroiditis, and (5) pregnancy.

The diagnostic accuracy of CT radioimmunoassay is greatly enhanced when combined with provocative tests. As many as 30% of members of a family with MEN type IIa or IIb who harbor small medullary carcinomas will have normal basal levels of plasma iCT. Their neoplastic disease can only be detected by provocative tests with intravenous administration of pentagastrin, 0.5 mg over 5–10 seconds, or calcium chloride, 150 mg over 10 minutes (Fig 11–30). Plasma iCT increases abnormally in most cases within 2–5 minutes. The CT radioimmunoassay used should be sensitive enough to measure plasma iCT in the normal range. Otherwise, the assay is unlikely to detect relatively small increases above the stimulated normal range, thus making the test impossible to interpret.

To rule out familial medullary carcinoma, iCT should be measured during a provocative test in all available first-degree relatives of patients with medullary carcinoma, regardless of the family history. In a few affected patients with minimal parafollicular cell disease, false-negative results may be obtained with any of the tests mentioned. Provocative tests should therefore be performed annually in first-degree relatives who have had negative tests. About half of the

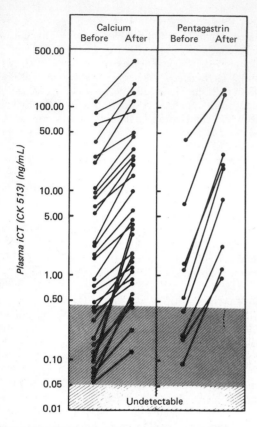

Figure 11–30. Maximal plasma iCT concentrations measured with antiserum CK 513 in patients with histologically proved medullary thyroid carcinoma of C cell hyperplasia before and after administration of calcium (left panel) or pentagastrin (right panel). The upper limit of stimulated plasma iCT concentrations in normal persons (shaded areas) is 0.42 ng/mL. (Reproduced, with permission, from Sizemore GW et al: *Surg Clin North Am* 1977;57:633.)

members of a given family in which one member has MEN type IIa or IIb eventually develop medullary cancer. Early detection will permit definitive surgical treatment.

Treatment

In patients with medullary carcinoma, pheochromocytoma must be excluded or treated first. Medullary carcinoma is then treated by total thyroidectomy. Total thyroidectomy is especially important in patients with MEN type IIa or IIb, because medullary carcinoma is almost always bilateral and polycentric. Lymph nodes in the midline compartment should be removed and those in both internal jugular chains sampled. If jugular lymph nodes are involved, modified neck dissection should be performed. Postoperatively, all patients should be studied with provocative tests to determine if residual tumor is present. They should also be given thyroid hormone replacement. The overall prev-

alence of residual or metastatic medullary cancer after such surgery is about 35%. Most of these patients are older and have had regional metastases at the time of surgery. Long-term follow-up with provocative tests every year is advised for all patients. Although it is usually difficult to determine the location of metastases that are responsible for a positive test, local recurrences can be suspected and dealt with surgically. There is no known effective chemotherapeutic, radiopharmaceutical, or radiation treatment of medullary carcinoma.

Prognosis

Patients with sporadic medullary carcinoma have the least favorable prognosis because metastases are usually present at the time of diagnosis; only 46% of these patients survive for 10 years. Patients with MEN type IIa appear to fare better, with few deaths reported. Conversely, in a Mayo Clinic series of 107 patients with MEN type IIb, 67% have had residual disease after surgery and 18% died of medullary cancer. The reasons for the apparent difference in prognosis between MEN type IIa and MEN type IIb are unknown.

HYPERCALCIURIA

Hypercalciuria is usually detected in the course of evaluation of a patient with renal stone disease. It is variably defined as excretion of more than 300 mg of calcium per 24 hours in men and 250 mg per 24 hours in women. Urinary calcium excretion depends on many factors, but the most important is dietary intake of calcium. It is the *concentration* of calcium in the urine that determines whether calcium will interact with anionic constituents (particularly oxalate) of the urine to form stones. Thus, prevention of calcium-containing stones requires reduction in urinary concentrations of calcium and oxalate. It has been shown that increased excretion of uric acid in the urine is not only responsible for the formation of uric acid stones but may also be important in the formation of calcium oxalate stones. This means that the clinician should pay careful attention to uric acid excretion in patients with calcium oxalate stones and should attempt to reduce it if it is elevated. Likewise, low urinary levels of citrate should be corrected, because this condition contributes to calcium oxalate precipitation.

The present section will concentrate on evaluation of the metabolic causes of hypercalciuria and calcium-containing stones, with the exception of infection, medullary sponge kidney, and renal tubular acidosis. The reader should consult the references at the end of this chapter for excellent reviews on cystine, uric acid, and magnesium ammonium phosphate stones.

Epidemiologic Considerations

Hypercalciuria appears to be common in the general population, but there is little accurate information about its incidence. The true incidence of stone disease is also unknown, although it is likely that 1–3% of people in most industrialized countries have had or will have a renal stone. Geography, race, and occupation probably have some influence on the incidence of stone disease, but the underlying factors are poorly understood. The frequency of calcium phosphate stones is equal in men and women. They occur in patients with sterile alkaline urines—ie, in cases of renal tubular acidosis, protracted use of carbonic anhydrase inhibitors, or primary hyperparathyroidism. Calcium oxalate stones occur more frequently in men (3–8:1) and in patients with idiopathic hypercalciuria.

Biochemical Characteristics of Calcium Stones

The most common anionic constituent of calcium-containing stones is oxalate. Calcium phosphate is also often present (mixed stones). Urinary saturation with calcium phosphate or calcium oxalate correlates roughly with the stone content of either anion. Hypercalciuria is observed in patients who make either mixed or unmixed stones, regardless of whether urinary calcium excretion is expressed as concentration, quantity per unit of time, or as the ratio of calcium to creatinine. Oxalate excretion is increased in patients who form calcium oxalate stones, and urinary pH is increased in those who form mixed stones.

Pathogenesis of Hypercalciuria

The reader is again referred to the "butterfly" diagram (Fig 11–2) while studying the pathogenetic concepts discussed below.

A. Hypercalcemia: In the presence of a normal rate of renal glomerular filtration, hypercalcemia due to any cause (see section on primary hyperparathyroidism), if sufficiently severe, results in hypercalciuria. One exception is benign familial hypercalcemia (familial hypocalciuric hypercalcemia), in which hypocalciuria is the biochemical hallmark of the disease. Another is mild hyperparathyroidism, in which urinary calcium may be normal in spite of hypercalcemia because of the hypocalciuric effects of excess PTH. However, even in such cases of hyperparathyroidism, calcium stones are common and may be due to the presence of other risk factors, such as hyperoxaluria, hyperuricosuria, and increased urine pH. For the most part, renal stone disease occurs primarily in patients who have had chronic hypercalcemia. In fact, this historical information is sometimes important in making the differential diagnosis of hypercalcemia (Table 11–3). Hypercalcemia in patients with documented stone disease is much more likely to be due to primary hyperparathyroidism than to cancer.

B. Diet: High dietary intake of protein causes both increased intestinal absorption and increased urinary excretion of calcium. These effects are poorly understood, but evidence indicates that dietary protein has a greater influence than dietary calcium on urinary calcium when calcium intake is in the range of 800–1400 mg/d. Urolithiasis has been reported in patients who have inordinately high protein intakes.

Increased dietary carbohydrate increases urinary calcium excretion at least in part because it increases the glomerular filtration rate. The calciuric response to a carbohydrate load is greater in stone-formers and their relatives than in normal subjects, but there is no difference between these groups in fractional urinary calcium excretion.

Lactose ingestion also increases urinary excretion of calcium, but lactose appears to act primarily by facilitating intestinal absorption of calcium. Lactose is known to be highly lithogenic in animals, and milk restriction may be important in the management of some patients with calcium stones (see below).

Urinary calcium increases in parallel with dietary intake of elemental calcium. It is presumed that much of the absorbed calcium is transferred from intestine to blood by a passive transport process, because with a high calcium intake, the hormonal mechanisms that regulate active calcium transport across the intestine adapt to decrease active transport (Fig 11–2). Therefore, decreasing the dietary intake of calcium in patients with hypercalciuric stone disease would seem to be appropriate. However, the situation is not so simple. Although calcium restriction reduces urinary calcium excretion, it also increases intestinal absorption and renal excretion of oxalate and, in the long term, results in secondary hyperparathyroidism and possibly osteopenia. Increased calcium intake, on the other hand, decreases intestinal absorption and renal excretion of oxalate by inducing calcium oxalate precipitation in the gut while increasing urinary calcium. Therefore, either of these dietary manipulations could aggravate calcium stone disease in hypercalciuric patients, and the authors cannot recommend them. Instead, a nutritionally adequate intake of calcium (600–800 mg/d) should be maintained in most patients and pharmacologic agents used to lower urinary calcium excretion (see treatment section below).

C. Intestinal Hyperabsorption of Calcium: Most patients with hypercalciuria that is unrelated to chronic states of hypercalcemia, drugs, or diet absorb too much calcium. Many of these patients have decreased serum levels of iPTH and decreased nephrogenous cAMP, presumably reflecting decreased PTH secretion caused by small increases in serum calcium within the normal range. In general, serum phosphorus is below the normal mean; and in one-third of patients, serum levels of $1,25(OH)_2D_3$ are increased. Clearly, in these latter patients, the normal adaptive decrease in $1,25(OH)_2D_3$ production in response to hyperabsorption of calcium and decreased levels of serum PTH fails to occur. It has been suggested that hypophosphatemia due to a renal phosphate leak is responsible (see intestinal loop of Fig 11–2). In this pathogenetic scheme, the renal phosphate leak is postulated to be the primary defect, and hyperabsorption of calcium and hypercalciuria are secondary to the effects of increased serum levels of $1,25(OH)_2D_3$.

The cause of intestinal hyperabsorption of calcium in the remaining two-thirds of patients with hypercalciuria, whose serum concentrations of $1,25(OH)_2D_3$ are normal or low, is unknown. It is possible that endocrine abnormalities not yet identified may be present. On the other hand, these patients may represent a group whose hyperabsorption of calcium is due to an intrinsic defect in the intestine, in which greater than normal quantities of calcium are transported from intestinal lumen to blood.

D. "Renal Leak" of Calcium: It is generally agreed that few patients with hypercalciuria have a true "renal calcium leak." It is possible, however, that some patients with intestinal hyperabsorption of calcium also have a renal tubule defect that permits excessive urinary excretion of calcium. Patients whose hypercalciuria is due solely to a renal leak of calcium have serum concentrations of calcium in the lower range of normal; this results in small increases in serum levels of PTH, which increase bone resorption and the production of $1,25(OH)_2D_3$. The resulting increase in serum levels of $1,25(OH)_2D_3$ causes intestinal hyperabsorption of calcium and produces pathophysiologic changes that superficially resemble hypercalciuria due to "primary" intestinal hyperabsorption of calcium. Thus, only the increased levels of serum iPTH and increased nephrogenous cAMP distinguish patients with hypercalciuria due to renal calcium leak from those with hypercalciuria due to intestinal hyperabsorption of calcium. A sensitive radioimmunoassay of PTH that can measure serum iPTH in the normal range is required for these diagnostic criteria to be applied systematically. Severe, long-standing hypercalciuria may result in increased bone turnover and osteopenia.

Diagnosis

A. Measurement of Urine Calcium: The diagnosis of hypercalciuria is made by measuring the calcium excreted in the urine over a 24-hour period while the patient is ingesting a diet containing normal amounts of calcium (about 800–1000 mg/d). Values greater than 250 mg/24 h in women and 300 mg/24 h in men indicate the presence of hypercalciuria. Patients who present with renal stone disease should undergo a full evaluation, including measurement of the 24-hour urinary excretion of calcium, phosphate, creatinine, oxalate, uric acid, and citrate. If a renal stone is not available, patients should strain their urine. A biochemical and crystallographic analysis of the stone should be made so that the patient can be in-

structed in decreasing the urinary concentrations of the stone's constituents. Particular attention should be paid to excluding other metabolic disorders such as primary hyperparathyroidism, which may be primary or contributing factors. When nephrolithiasis is present, it is important to obtain baseline radiographic studies of the kidneys (intravenous urogram and nephrotomograms and sonograms) to identify the number and size (diameter) of stones present. Similar follow-up studies will give an indication of the activity of the stone disease. (Growth of a stone or appearance of a new stone indicates that stone disease is active.) If a patient is in the inactive phase of nephrolithiasis, specific drug therapy is probably not indicated. If the patient is passing gravel, stone disease is active, and intensive therapy is indicated.

B. History: In seeking the underlying cause of hypercalciuria, a careful history, including diet and drug intake, is important. A history of an extremely high intake of protein, dairy products, or carbohydrates may account for hypercalciuria. Excessive self-medication with calcium-containing antacids, low-phosphate diets, or phosphate-binding antacids can also produce hypercalciuria. The mechanism involved in the latter 2 phenomena is poorly understood. Hypercalciuric patients who are vegetarians may be especially prone to the development of nephrolithiasis, because their diet may be high in oxalate-containing foods or inadequate in phosphate content.

C. Serum iPTH: Although a number of provocative tests of the calciuric and nephrogenous cAMP responses to ingested calcium have been described for distinguishing between intestinal hyperabsorption of calcium and renal leak of calcium, measurement of serum iPTH is the most helpful test available. As noted in the section on pathogenesis, increased serum iPTH in the presence of low normal serum calcium reflects the presence of a renal leak of calcium, whereas normal or decreased serum iPTH in conjunction with high normal serum calcium generally reflects hyperabsorption of calcium. Further study of patients with increased serum iPTH levels may be necessary to distinguish them from patients with primary hyperparathyroidism associated with a renal leak of calcium. For some reason, this latter syndrome occurs most frequently in women, and although unusual, it should be suspected whenever a woman presents with hypercalciuria, because removal of the parathyroid lesion is curative. In most cases, primary hyperparathyroidism can be excluded in patients with increased serum iPTH by determining if serum iPTH decreases during thiazide administration. As will be discussed in the treatment section, thiazide diuretics increase the tubular reabsorption of calcium and thereby increase serum calcium. If serum iPTH decreases with thiazide administration, hyperparathyroidism is probable and occurs secondary to a renal leak of calcium. If serum iPTH fails to decrease with thiazides, the patient probably has associated primary hyperparathyroidism.

Treatment

A. Hypercalciuria Without Nephrolithiasis: Specific drug therapy (see below) should probably be avoided in patients with hypercalciuria without nephrolithiasis. Excessive intake of protein, carbohydrates, dairy products, antacids, and low-phosphate diets should be discontinued or curtailed. Patients should be instructed to avoid foods high in oxalate and to consume at least 2500–3000 mL of water per day.

B. Hypercalciuria With Nephrolithiasis: Surgical treatment of obstructive uropathy caused by nephrolithiasis is always indicated. Medical management is indicated for prevention of calcium stone disease.

1. Hypercalciuria—All of the therapeutic measures mentioned above should be used, except that water intake should be greater (4000 mL/d). The patient should be instructed to drink one or 2 glasses of water in the middle of the night because the concentration of urinary solutes is greatest then. If stones contain oxalate, the patient should be instructed in the preparation and planning of a low-oxalate diet. Some foods to be avoided are listed in Table 11–7.

2. Active nephrolithiasis—If nephrolithiasis is active (see above), one or more of 6 therapeutic agents should be used: (1) thiazide diuretics, (2) orthophosphate, (3) the xanthine oxidase inhibitor allopurinol, and (4) magnesium oxide and pyridoxine, (5) potassium citrate, and (6) cellulose phosphate. Thiazide diuretics and orthophosphate have been reported to reduce the rate of stone recurrence. Thiazide diuretics decrease hypercalciuria by increasing the tubular reabsorption of calcium. Medication should be given at 12-hour intervals—eg, 50 mg of hydrochlorothiazide, twice daily. The only significant complications of thiazide therapy are potassium depletion and annoying polyuria; potassium supplements of 20–40 meq/d should be administered to most patients. The potassium-sparing diuretic, amiloride (Moduril), is an effective substitute, but triamterine should be avoided because it has intrinsic stone-forming potential. Oral supplements of orthophosphate decrease urinary calcium by an unknown mechanism. One to 1.5 g of elemental phosphorus should be administered in 3 divided doses daily as neutral phosphate compounds (eg, K-Phos Neutral, 4–6 tablets/d). Few side effects other than occasional diarrhea have been reported with this therapy, and long-term studies have shown no significant changes in serum iPTH. Orthophosphate therapy is indicated only for patients with sterile urines, because it accelerates stone growth in individuals with ammonium phosphate stones caused by urea-splitting organisms. Magnesium oxide (200 mg/d) plus large doses of pyridoxine (100–150 mg/d) may be of value in the treatment of idiopathic calcium oxalate stones, but systematic studies of the efficacy of this regimen have been meager.

3. Uric acid excretion—Many patients with calcium oxalate stones excrete abnormally large quantities of uric acid. Treatment of these patients with allopurinol (100–200 mg twice daily) reduces the urinary excretion of uric acid and the rate of stone formation when combined with thiazide diuretics. The mechanism of this action of allopurinol is unknown.

4. Potassium citrate—This drug, given in doses of 30–80 meq/kg, is effective in hypocitraturic calcium oxalate nephrolithiasis (eg, renal tubular acidosis, diarrheal states with hyperoxlaluria) and in hyperuricosuria.

5. Cellulose phosphate—This drug has been advocated for severe absorptive hypercalciuria. It is expensive and may lead to magnesium depletion and to oxalate hyperabsorption.

METABOLIC BONE DISEASE

Functions of Bone

Bone has 3 major functions: (1) It provides rigid support to extremities and body cavities containing vital organs. In disease situations in which bone is weak or defective, erect posture may be impossible, and vital organ function may be compromised. (An example is the cardiopulmonary dysfunction that occurs in patients with severe kyphosis due to vertebral collapse.) (2) Bones are crucial to locomotion in that they provide efficient levers and sites of attachment for muscles. With bony deformity, these levers become defective, and severe abnormalities of gait develop. (3) Finally, bone provides a large reservoir of ions, such as calcium, phosphorus, magnesium, and sodium, that are critical for life and can be mobilized when the external environment fails to provide them.

Structure of Bone

As a living tissue, bone is unique in that it is not only rigid and resists forces that would ordinarily break brittle materials but is also light enough to be moved by coordinated muscle contractions. These characteristics are functions of the strategic locations of 2 major types of bone (Fig 11–31). Cortical bone, composed of densely packed, mineralized collagen laid down in layers, provides rigidity and is the major component of

Table 11–7. High-oxalate foods.

Vegetables	Fruits	Miscellaneous
Asparagus	Concord grapes	Almonds
Beans	Cranberries	Cashews
Beets and beet greens	Currants	Cocoa
Brussels sprouts	Oranges	Tea
Potatoes	Pineapple	
Rhubarb	Plums	
Spinach	Strawberries	

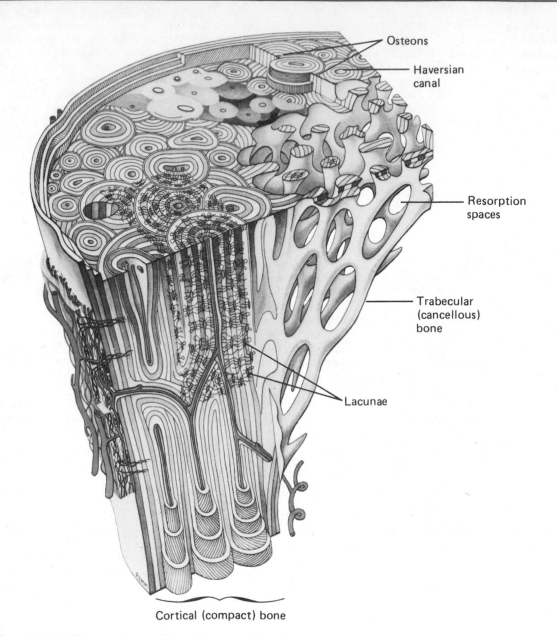

Figure 11–31. Diagram of some of the main features of the microstructure of mature bone seen in both transverse section *(top)* and longitudinal section. Areas of cortical (compact) and trabecular (cancellous) bone are included. The central area in the transverse section simulates a microradiograph, with the variations in density reflecting variations in mineralization. Note the general construction of the osteons, the distribution of the osteocyte lacunae, the haversian canals, resorption spaces, and the different views of the structural basis of bone lamellation. See text for description. (Reproduced, with permission, from page 217 in: *Gray's Anatomy.* 35th ed. Warwick R, Williams PL [editor]. Longman, 1973.)

tubular bones. Trabecular (cancellous) bone is spongy in appearance, provides strength and elasticity, and constitutes the major portion of the axial skeleton. Disorders in which cortical bone is defective or scanty lead to fractures of the long bones, whereas disorders in which trabecular bone is defective or scanty lead to vertebral fractures. Fractures of long bones may also occur because normal trabecular bone reinforcement is lacking.

Two-thirds of the weight of bone is due to mineral; the remainder is due to water and collagen. Minor organic components such as proteoglycans, lipids, noncollagenous proteins, and acidic proteins containing γ-carboxyglutamic acid are probably important, but their functions are poorly understood.

A. Bone Mineral: The mineral of bone is present in 2 forms. The major form consists of hydroxyapatite in crystals of varying maturity. The remainder is amorphous calcium phosphate, which lacks a coherent x-ray diffraction pattern, has a lower calcium-to-phosphate ratio than pure hydroxyapatite, occurs in regions of active bone formation, and is present in larger quantities in young bone.

B. Formation and Resorption of Bone: Bone is resorbed and formed continuously throughout life, and these important processes are dependent upon 3 major types of bone cells, each with different functions (Fig 11–32).

1. Osteoblasts–Osteoblasts form new bone on surfaces of bone previously resorbed by osteoclasts. The osteoblasts are thought to be derived from a population of dividing cells on bone surfaces that arise from mesenchymal cells in bone connective tissue. Osteoblasts are actively involved in the synthesis of matrix components of bone (primarily collagen) and probably facilitate the movement of mineral ions between extracellular fluids and bone surfaces (Figs 11–3 and 11–4). The physiologic importance of such ion transport by osteoblasts—if it occurs at all—is controversial, but there is widespread agreement that osteoblast-mediated deposition of calcium and phosphate is involved in the mineralization of collagen, which in turn is crucial to the formation of bone. In the process of bone formation, osteoblasts gradually become encased in the bone matrix they have produced.

2. Osteocytes–Once osteoblasts are trapped in the mineralized matrix, their functional and morphologic characteristics are changed and they are then called osteocytes. Protein synthetic activity decreases markedly, and the cells develop multiple processes that reach out through lacunae in bone tissue to "communicate" with processes of other osteocytes within a unit of bone (osteon) and also with the cell processes of surface osteoblasts (Figs 11–4, 11–31, and 11–32). The physiologic importance of osteocytes is controversial, but they are believed to act as a cellular syncytium that permits translocation of mineral in and out of regions of bone removed from surfaces.

3. Osteoclasts–The osteoclast is a multinucleated giant cell that is responsible for bone resorption (Figs 11–4 and 11–32). It is probably derived from circulating mononucleated macrophages, which differentiate into the mature osteoclasts by fusion in the bone environment. These cells contain all of the enzymatic components that, when secreted into their environs, are capable of solubilizing matrix and releasing calcium and phosphate. Once released, mineral is transported through the osteoclast into the extracellular fluid and ultimately into blood. Opinion has varied over the years concerning the relative importance of osteoclastic resorption of bone and the translocation of mineral from the surface of bone into the extracellular space by surface osteoblasts in extracellular mineral homeostasis.

C. Structural Features of Bone: Microscopically, there are 2 types of bone structure: woven and lamellar. Both may be found in either cortical or trabecular bone. However, whereas woven bone is a normal constituent of embryonic bone, it usually reflects the presence of disease in adult bone.

Lamellar bone is stronger than woven bone and is formed more slowly. It progressively replaces woven bone as the skeleton develops after birth. Whereas woven bone is characterized by nonparallelism of collagen fibers, with many osteocytes per unit area of matrix and mineral that is poorly incorporated into collagen fibrils, lamellar bone has a parallel arrangement of collagen fibers, few osteocytes per unit area of matrix, and a mineral phase that is within the collagen fibrils. Cortical lamellar bone is present in concentric layers surrounding vascular channels that comprise the haversian systems of cortical bone (osteons) (Fig 11–31). By contrast, the lamellar bone of trabeculae is present in layers and is laid down in long sheaves and sheets.

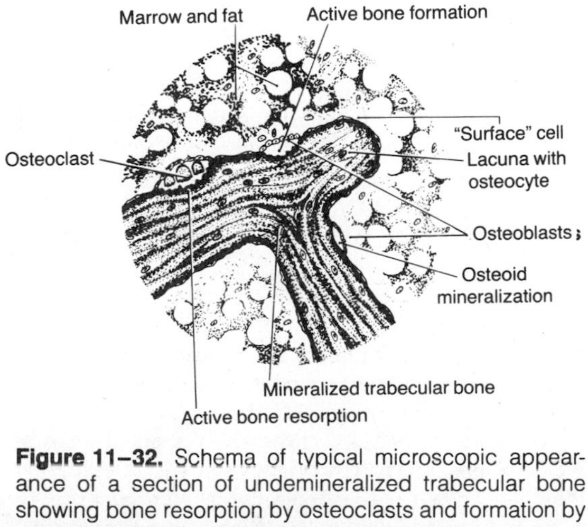

Dynamics of Bone

The term "modeling" as applied to bone denotes processes involved in formation of the macroscopic skeleton. Thus, modeling ceases at maturity (age 18–20). The term "remodeling" denotes those processes occurring at bone surfaces before and after adult development which are required to maintain the structural integrity of bone. Abnormalities of remodeling are responsible for metabolic bone diseases, and these will be discussed in this section. These abnormalities involve alterations in the balance between bone formation and bone resorption that lead to diminished structural integrity of bone and ultimately compromise its functions.

Normally, in spite of continuous bone remodeling, there is no net gain or loss of skeletal mass after longitudinal growth has ceased. This has led to the view that bone resorption and formation are closely "coupled"

Figure 11–32. Schema of typical microscopic appearance of a section of undemineralized trabecular bone showing bone resorption by osteoclasts and formation by osteoblasts. Note layers of lamellar bone.

and that this coupling is the result of the coordinated activity of "packets" of interacting osteoblasts and osteoclasts. These "packets" have been termed "basic multicellular units." The temporal activity of such a unit is characterized by osteoclastic resorption of a defined quantity of bone (on the surface in trabecular bone and by actual excavation in cortical bone), followed by repair of the defect by osteoblasts. Such repair occurs as a result of laying down of collagen (osteoid) and its subsequent mineralization.

By use of sequential, timed labeling of bone with orally administered tetracycline (which binds to recently mineralized collagen) and quantitative histomorphometric analysis of transiliac bone biopsies from normal adult humans, it has been possible to time the activities of a basic multicellular unit. Such estimates indicate that osteoclastic resorption proceeds for about 1 month in a normal 30-year-old adult, and osteoblastic repair takes about 3 months.

The term "sigma" denotes the total duration of activity of a typical basic multicellular unit (ie, 4 months). This concept of "sigma" has added a new dimension to conventional views about the pathogenesis of metabolic bone disease. Thus, not only might alterations in the relative numbers and activities of osteoblasts and osteoclasts be important in production of an imbalance of bone formation and bone resorption, but abnormalities in the relative durations of activities of these 2 cell types could underlie such an imbalance.

Analysis of Bone Biopsy

Presently, quantitative histomorphometric analysis of transiliac bone biopsies has achieved almost the status of a fine art. The procedure is employed in centers established to evaluate metabolic bone disease from both diagnostic and therapeutic points of view. The procedure is most useful (1) in establishing a diagnosis of osteomalacia (see below) and (2) in determining if, in a given patient, diminished bone density is associated with quantitatively significant changes in "sigma" and its bone formation and bone resorption components.

OSTEOMALACIA

Osteomalacia is failure of the organic matrix (osteoid) of bone to mineralize normally. Rickets, which will be only briefly discussed in this chapter, is failure of normal mineralization and maturation of the growth plate at the epiphysis in children.

Etiology & Incidence

A number of factors are critical for normal bone mineralization. An absence or defect of any of them may led to osteomalacia. The most frequent underlying biochemical causes of mineralization defects—individually or in combination—are a decrease in the product of the concentrations of calcium and phosphate in the extracellular fluid such that the supply of minerals to bone-forming surfaces is inadequate; abnormal functioning of bone-forming cells; abnormal or defective collagen production; and a decrease in the pH below 7.6 at sites of mineralization.

Table 11–8 lists the major disorders that can lead to osteomalacia, including those due to vitamin D deficiency, phosphate deficiency, systemic acidosis, drug toxicity, and primary defects of bone. Because of the vague symptomatology of osteomalacia (see below), the disease is often not suspected and is probably much more common than is usually thought.

A. Vitamin D Deficiency: Whereas it was formerly thought that vitamin D deficiency due to inadequate sunlight exposure rarely caused osteomalacia, certain social and environmental developments have almost certainly led to an increased incidence of this problem. This is particularly true in the case of the elderly, who are frequently institutionalized or stay indoors at home and fail to receive either adequate sunlight exposure or dietary supplements of vitamin D.

Although the facts are difficult to document, industrialization without adequate smog control will almost certainly result in an increased incidence of osteomalacia and rickets by filtering out the ultraviolet wavelengths of light from the atmosphere. This can be prevented by systematic supplementation with vitamin D.

With the increase in world population, extreme northern and southern latitudes could become more populated. People living there would be susceptible to osteomalacia and rickets because of the diminished amount of ultraviolet irradiation.

In people who habitually cover their bodies with excessive clothing, the migration from areas of intense ultraviolet exposure to areas of marginal ultraviolet exposure can lead to the development of osteomalacia and rickets. This phenomenon has been reported in Great Britain in immigrants from India, Pakistan, and other Commonwealth countries since the 1950s.

1. Malabsorption–One of the most common causes of osteomalacia due to vitamin D deficiency is gastrointestinal disease associated with malabsorption of vitamin D and calcium. This is particularly true of disorders in which the enterohepatic circulation of vitamin D is interrupted. The biologically active metabolites of vitamin D that are normally secreted into the bile are either diverted (biliary fistula) or not reabsorbed (chronic steatorrhea, gluten-sensitive enteropathy, surgical resection of large parts of the distal jejunum and ileum). In these situations, not only is exogenous vitamin D poorly absorbed, but the body's stores of vitamin D and its metabolites that originate from skin biosynthesis are also depleted by biliary or fecal loss.

2. Impaired renal synthesis–As noted in previous sections, impaired synthesis of $1,25(OH)_2D_3$ by the kidney can lead to osteomalacia. This can occur in chronic kidney disease, in which there is extensive

Table 11–8. Etiology of osteomalacia.

Vitamin D deficiency
Inadequate sunlight exposure without dietary supplementation.
House- or institution-bound people.
Atmospheric smog.
Long-term residence in far northern and far southern latitudes.
Excessive covering of body with clothing.
Gastrointestinal disease that interrupts the normal entero-hepatic recycling of vitamin D and its metabolites, resulting in their fecal loss.
Chronic steatorrhea (pancreatic)
Malabsorption (gluten-sensitive enteropathy).
Surgical resection of large parts of intestine.
Formation of biliary fistulas.
Impaired synthesis of $1,25(OH)_2D_3$ by the kidney.
Nephron loss, as occurs in chronic kidney disease (see section on renal hyperparathyroidism).
Functional impairment of $1,25(OH)_2D_3$ hydroxylase (eg, in hypoparathyroidism).
Congenital absence of $1,25(OH)_2D_3$ hydroxylase (vitamin D-dependency rickets type I).
Suppression of $1,25(OH)_2D_3$ production by endogenously produced substances (cancer).
Target cell resistance to $1,25(OH)_2D_3$—eg, absent or diminished number of $1,25(OH)_2D_3$ receptors, as in vitamin D-dependency rickets type II.

Phosphate deficiency
Dietary.
Low intake of phosphate.
Excessive ingestion of aluminum hydroxide.
Impaired renal tubular reabsorption of phosphate.
X-linked hypophosphatemia.
Adult-onset hypophosphatemia.
Other acquired and hereditary renal tubular disorders associated with renal phosphate loss (Fanconi's syndrome, Wilson's disease).
Tumor-associated hypophosphatemia.

Systemic acidosis
Chronic renal failure.
Distal renal tubular acidosis.
Ureterosigmoidoscopy.
Chronic acetazolamide and ammonium chloride administration.

Drug-induced osteomalacia
Excessive bisphosphonate administration.
Excessive fluoride administration.
Anticonvulsant administration.

Toxin-induced osteomalacia
Aluminum.
Lead.
Cadmium.

Primary mineralization defects
Hypophosphatasia.
Osteopetrosis.
Fibrogenesis imperfecta ossium.

nephron loss, or when other conditions are unfavorable for the synthesis of $1,25(OH)_2D_3$, such as in hypoparathyroidism when serum phosphate is increased and the trophic stimulus of PTH is missing (Fig 11–2).

3. Genetic defects–Two recessively inherited vitamin D deficiency states associated with rickets and osteomalacia are characterized by resistance to treatment with large doses of vitamin D. In one, vitamin D–dependency rickets type I, serum concentrations of $1,25(OH)_2D_3$ are very low. This disease is thought to be due to a defect in $1,25(OH)_2D_3$ hydroxylase in the kidney. In the other, vitamin D-dependency rickets type II, serum concentrations of $1,25(OH)_2D_3$ are high. This disease is thought to be due to target cell resistance to the action of $1,25(OH)_2D_3$. Patients have been described recently whose cultured skin fibroblasts are deficient in receptors for $1,25(OH)_2D_3$.

4. Oncogenic disease–Osteomalacic syndromes have been associated with certain tumors. Although proof is not yet available, recent findings suggest that the underlying cause of the bone disease is a humoral substance secreted by the tumor that suppresses the synthesis of $1,25(OH)_2D_3$.

B. Lowering of Phosphorus: Any sustained lowering of serum phosphorus will ultimately result in rickets and osteomalacia. Phosphate deficiency can occur as a result of failure of intestinal absorption of phosphate (dietary lack of sequestering of phosphate in the intestine by binding of the mineral to aluminum hydroxide in antacids) or excessive renal excretion of phosphate. Vegetarians who do not include diary products in their diets are particularly susceptible to phosphate deficiency, as are elderly or debilitated individuals who are fed a diet low in phosphate. Although it is likely that only excessive use of phosphate-binding antacids will result in a deficiency in phosphate severe enough to produce osteomalacia, the potential for this disorder is great because these drugs are widely available.

The classic example of rickets and osteomalacia due to renal phosphate wasting is the heritable disease X-linked hypophosphatemia, in which a renal phosphate transport defect is manifest. Similar renal phosphate wasting and osteomalacia occur in many patients with Fanconi's syndrome and in patients with adult-onset hypophosphatemia.

Severe phosphate wasting is occasionally associated with benign or malignant lesions, such as sclerosing hemangiomas, angiosarcomas, hemangiopericytomas, and nonossifying fibromas. Some of these involve bone and others soft tissues. Surgical removal of these lesions almost always restores serum phosphate and urinary phosphate excretion to normal and heals the osteomalacia, suggesting that the tumors secrete a humoral substance that either promotes phosphaturia or interferes with vitamin D metabolism.

Aside from chronic renal failure, the disorders listed in Table 11–8 that cause systemic acidosis and osteomalacia are uncommon. The evidence that they produce osteomalacia on the basis of systemic acidosis per se is based only on therapeutic responses achieved when blood pH is restored to normal with bicarbonate therapy. Thus, it is possible that the acidosis acts indirectly, by inducing other systemic abnormalities that then produce osteomalacia.

The mechanisms involved in the development of

osteomalacia due to drugs and the primary mineralization defects listed in Table 11–8 are largely unknown.

Pathology

There is little (if anything) unusual about the gross characteristics of the bones of patients with osteomalacia, except perhaps that they are easier to biopsy because they are soft. Histomorphometrically, however, there are major deviations from normal, primarily related to the thickness and surface coverage of unmineralized osteoid and the degree of mineralization of osteoid. Characteristically, the average thickness of osteoid exceeds 20 μm (normal, 15 ± 2.3 μm), and over 20% of the bone surface is covered by osteoid (normal, $2.1 \pm 1\%$). The "calcification front" at the junction of mineralized bone and osteoid, which is normally marked intensely by tetracycline labels incorporated into bone prior to biopsy, is barely visible. These changes in the quantity of osteoid are due not to increased synthesis of collagen by bone-forming cells but rather to a failure in collagen mineralization. The rate of collagen synthesis may actually be decreased. Because the rate of mineralization is slowed, "sigma" (see above) is prolonged.

Pseudofractures, which are characteristic of osteomalacia, are defects in cortical bone that are bordered by osteoid-encased lamellar bone, with interspersed areas of variably mineralized woven bone.

Depending upon the stage of development of osteomalacia or rickets, bone resorption surfaces may be increased or decreased. After secondary hyperparathyroidism due to hypocalcemia has been established, increased osteoclastic resorption may be observed. Late in the course of development of the disease, when osteoid covers the greater portion of mineralized surfaces, little exposed mineral is available for osteoclastic attack, and bone resorption surfaces are decreased.

Pathophysiology

A. Vitamin D Deficiency: The most useful information about the pathogenesis of osteomalacia and rickets has been provided by studies of the natural history of these diseases. It has not been possible, because of ethical considerations, to conduct longitudinal investigations of the parameters of calcium metabolism in patients with rickets and osteomalacia. However, measurements of these parameters have been reported in individual patients suffering from rickets or osteomalacia of varying degrees of severity. Figure 11–33, which provides an idealized scheme of the results of these studies, depicts 3 stages of development of vitamin D–deficiency rickets or osteomalacia. These stages are characterized by unique changes in the serum concentrations of calcium, phosphate, iPTH, and $25OHD_3$ and the severity of radiographically assessed bone lesions.

B. Stages of Osteomalacia: In the first stage of rickets or osteomalacia, there is mild hypocalcemia,

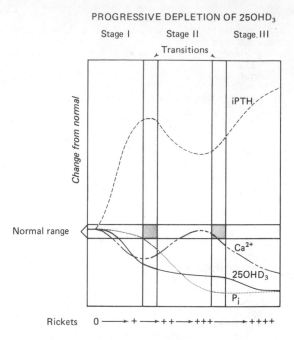

Figure 11–33. Serum biochemical changes and severity of bone disease in the 3 stages of rickets or osteomalacia. See text for description. (Reproduced, with permission, from Arnaud SB et al: *Vitamin D and Problems in Uremic Bone Disease.* Walter de Gruyter, 1975.)

appropriately increased serum iPTH, normal or slightly decreased serum phosphate, and decreased serum $25OHD_3$, which is approximately half the mean value for age-matched normal controls.

In the second stage, serum $25OHD_3$ decreases slightly or not at all. The serum calcium concentration is restored to normal, but paradoxically, there is only a small decrease in serum iPTH. Hypophosphatemia and bone lesions worsen.

In the third stage, when florid rickets or osteomalacia becomes manifest, serum $25OHD_3$ decreases to almost undetectable levels. Hypocalcemia again is apparent and is more severe than in stage I; the degree of hypophosphatemia is the same as for stage II; and serum iPTH increases further and is again appropriate for the degree of hypocalcemia.

The underlying defect leading to these biochemical and osseous changes is the decrease in production of $1,25(OH)_2D_3$, which is due to the diminished availability of the major circulating metabolite of vitamin D, $25OHD_3$. As Figure 11–2 shows, decreased $1,25(OH)_2D_3$ results in decreased intestinal calcium absorption, decreased bone resorption, hypocalcemia, increased PTH secretion, and hypophosphatemia (stage I). The resulting decreased calcium $\times$ phosphate product in serum is insufficient for the normal mineralization of bone, and the osteomalacic process is initiated. The increased PTH secretion and hypophosphatemia represent compensatory phenomena designed to correct the hypocalcemia, but they occur at the expense of osseous demineralization caused by hyperparathyroidism. As stage I shifts to stage II, the severity of the hyperparathyroidism restores serum calcium toward normal. This restoration probably depends upon increased production of $1,25(OH)_2D_3$ from residual stores of $25OHD_3$; this increased production is the result of the stimulation of renal 1α-hydroxylase by increased serum levels of PTH. The mechanism whereby increased PTH secretion is maintained in spite of normocalcemia in this stage is poorly understood. A negative feedback relationship between vitamin D metabolites and PTH secretion may exist, wherein normal levels of vitamin D metabolites are required for physiologic concentrations of serum calcium to suppress parathyroid gland activity. During the transition from stage II to stage III, vitamin D stores are depleted, and in spite of the hyperparathyroidism and hypophosphatemia, $1,25(OH)_2D_3$ production stops because $25OHD_3$, the substrate, is lacking. In stage III, hypocalcemia develops again and is worse than in stage I because of an even greater decrease in intestinal absorption of calcium. PTH secretion increases further in response to hypocalcemia; however, because vitamin D is required for PTH to resorb bone, this compensatory mechanism fails and hypocalcemia persists. In this stage, hypocalcemia and hypophosphatemia become so severe that the serum calcium × phosphate product is too low for normal bond formation, and florid osteomalacia or rickets becomes evident.

C. Phosphate Deficiency: The pathogenesis of the rickets or osteomalacia associated with phosphate deficiency is poorly understood but is presumed to be related to a decrease in the serum calcium × phosphate product below the level required for normal bone formation. Dietary phosphate deficiency is known to be associated with increases in serum concentrations of $1,25(OH)_2D_3$ and calcium and in urinary excretion of calcium. Serum concentrations of iPTH are appropriately decreased, and the PTH-induced demineralization of bone seen in vitamin D deficiency is not observed. Thus, as long as phosphate deficiency is not complicated by deficiencies in vitamin D or calcium, the biochemical changes seen in vitamin D deficiency, rickets, or osteomalacia do not occur.

D. Acidosis: The pathogenesis of the rickets and osteomalacia associated with acidosis is also poorly understood. Possible underlying causes include inhibition of mineralization due to a decrease in pH below 7.6 at calcification sites, acidosis-induced hypophosphatemia, and acidosis-induced resistance to the actions of vitamin D. In addition, the hypercalciuria often observed in acidosis may cause hyperparathyroidism, and the combined effects on bone of the excess PTH and negative calcium balance may be important in the ultimate bone disease associated with acidosis.

Clinical Features

A. Symptoms and Signs: The clinical manifestations of osteomalacia in adults often go unrecognized. This is especially true in patients with osteomalacia due to a vitamin D deficiency caused by disorders of the gastrointestinal tract, because the symptoms of the primary disorder are so prominent. Thus, diffuse skeletal pain and muscular weakness without a specific pattern may be overlooked, and the diagnosis of bone disease may not be suspected until roentgenograms reveal osteomalacia as an incidental finding.

There are few if any characteristic clinical signs of osteomalacia, except for deformities caused by fractures in the ribs, vertebrae, and long bones. Such extensive disease is rare. Classically, patients with osteomalacia have a characteristic waddling gait that is due both to proximal muscular weakness and to pain and discomfort during movement of limbs. Some patients have severe muscular hypotonia and paradoxically brisk deep tendon reflexes. This latter finding is probably due to associated hypocalcemia. In contrast to hypoparathyroidism, osteomalacia is rarely associated with hypocalcemia tetanic manifestations. This difference is probably due to the presence of hyperphosphatemia and lower levels of serum ionized calcium in patients with hypoparathyroidism.

B. Laboratory Findings: The serum biochemistry of osteomalacia and rickets is described above. The values of serum calcium, phosphate, iPTH, and $25OHD_3$ clearly depend upon the stage of the disease at the time the patient is seen (Fig 11–33). Generally, low levels of $25OHD_3$ indicate that osteomalacia is severe, but this is not always true. Increased serum alkaline phosphatase is characteristic. The cause of this abnormality is not well understood; it is probably related to increased but ineffective activity of osteoblasts.

C. X-Ray Findings: The radiologic features of osteomalacia also depend upon the stage of the disease and may be dramatic. There is usually some decrease in bone density. Cortices may be thinned, and roentgenograms of the vertebrae may reveal both loss of trabeculae and blurring of trabecular markings. In stage I and early stage II osteomalacia, radiologic changes may be indistinguishable from those seen in osteoporosis. The most characteristic finding in osteomalacia—and one that is almost pathognomonic—is the radiolucent band termed a **pseudofracture,** a defect in bone that is perpendicular to the bone surface (Fig 11–34A and B). These bands, which may be present at multiple sites, are usually symmetric and bilateral; the characteristic locations include the inner aspects of the femur, the pubic rami, the outer edges of the scapulas, the upper fibula, and the metatarsals. Pseudofractures almost always occur where major arteries cross bones. It is thought that trauma due to arterial pulsation or other factors is responsible for their location and symmetry. Pseudofractures are also termed Looser's zones or Milkman's

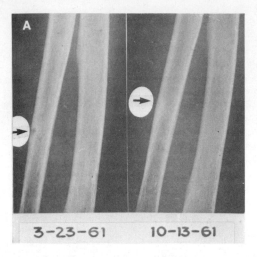 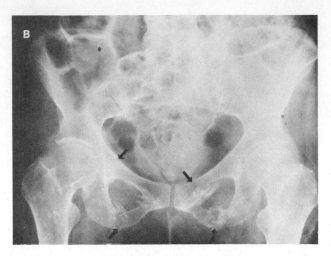

Figure 11–34. *A:* X-rays of the radius and ulna of a patient with severe osteomalacia, showing healing of a pseudofracture (arrows) during 7 months of treatment with ergocalciferol. *B:* X-ray of the pelvis, showing pseudofractures (Looser's zones, or Milkman's fractures) in a woman with severe osteomalacia. (Courtesy of G Gordan.)

fractures, after the individuals who first described them.

Paradoxically, patients with untreated osteomalacia due to specific defects in renal tubular phosphate transport may show increased rather than decreased osseous density and even bony spurs on x-rays. However, such hyperostotic bone is abnormal. It fractures easily and consists of thickened cortices and trabeculae invested in large quantities of thickened osteoid. The cause of this hyperostosis is unknown.

Differential Diagnosis

Osteomalacia and rickets are usually suspected on the basis of the history or the presence of other disorders that frequently cause osteomalacia and rickets. Patients with muscular weakness and skeletal pain should be screened. Children with histories of irritability, poor growth and development, and convulsions should also be investigated. Patients who are taking drugs that have been associated with the development of osteomalacia (Table 11–8) are at risk for this disease and should be evaluated annually for hypocalcemia, hypophosphatemia, and hypocalciuria. Decreased urinary calcium is one of the earliest biochemical signs of osteomalacia and is probably due to increased PTH secretion secondary to mild hypocalcemia. Patients with chronic intestinal disease, particularly those with gluten-sensitive enteropathy or pancreatic insufficiency, should also be considered to have osteomalacia unless this is disproved. Nutritional deprivation and chronic deprivation of sunlight exposure also increase the risk of osteomalacia. Patients with a family history of short stature should be investigated for one of the inherited forms of osteomalacia.

Screening tests for the presence of osteomalacia should include measurements of total serum calcium; serum phosphate, magnesium, iPTH, $25OHD_3$, alkaline phosphatase, and urinary calcium. The presence of hypocalcemia, hyperphosphatemia, increased iPTH, hyper- or hypophosphatasia, or hypocalciuria should prompt further investigations, including x-rays of the skeleton and a radionuclide bone scan (pseudofractures show increased uptake on bone scan). If these latter procedures do not reveal pseudofractures, a transiliac bone biopsy with double tetracycline labeling should be performed. Patients with full-blown osteomalacia due to vitamin D deficiency will have all of the above biochemical findings as well as pseudofractures, and the bone biopsies only offer confirmation. Measurement of 72-hour excretion of fat in the stool is recommended to exclude intestinal malabsorption as a factor in the development of osteomalacia, because this disease is often unaccompanied by overt symptoms. Serum levels of $25OHD_3$ are generally low but may be normal in patients whose diets contain vitamin D at the time of investigation. After restoration of serum $25OHD_3$ concentrations to normal levels, there is a long time lag before the restoration of other important minerals to normal and the healing of bone lesions. Serum concentrations of $1,25(OH)_2D_3$ should be measured in children whose rickets or osteomalacia appears to be resistant to therapeutic doses of vitamin D. Low values will be found in patients with vitamin D–dependency rickets type I and extremely high values in patients with vitamin D–dependency rickets type II.

More often than not, osteomalacia due to mild degrees of vitamin D deficiency is manifested only by small increases in serum iPTH and hypocalciuria. In such cases, only bone biopsy will establish the diagnosis.

A. Hypophosphatemia: Most patients with osteomalacia due to untreated phosphate deficiency

(Table 11–8) have normal serum concentrations of calcium, $25OHD_3$, and iPTH. This distinguishes them from individuals with vitamin D deficiency. However, excessive treatment of these patients with inorganic phosphate frequently produces mild hypocalcemia and increased serum levels of iPTH. Aside from the occasional presence on x-rays of increased bone density in patients with X-linked hypophosphatemic rickets and variable evidence of osteitis fibrosa cystica in patients with vitamin D deficiency, there appears to be no difference between osteomalacic lesions due to vitamin D deficiency and those due to phosphate deficiency.

B. Inherited Osteomalacia: All patients suspected of having an inherited form of osteomalacia should be studied for the presence of renal tubular acidosis using ammonium chloride loading and measurement of urine pH. This is important because successful therapy of renal tubular acidosis depends upon treatment with alkali. Such treatment is not part of the regimen recommended for osteomalacia caused by vitamin D or phosphate deficiencies.

C. Hypoparathyroidism: The differentiation of hypoparathyroidism from osteomalacia is generally not difficult. Patients with hypoparathyroidism usually have hyperphosphatemia (rather than hypophosphatemia) and a history of thyroidectomy. In rare instances, hypoparathyroidism is associated with steatorrhea; in these cases, both hypophosphatemia and osteomalacia may be present, and measurement of serum iPTH may be the key in making the correct diagnosis. Serum concentrations of iPTH are low or undetectable in hypoparathyroidism, but they are generally increased in patients with osteomalacia, unless severe hypomagnesemia is also present.

D. Hypophosphatasia: The finding of a serum alkaline phosphatase at the lower limits of normal should prompt measurement of plasma levels and urinary excretion of phosphorylethanolamine, which are markedly elevated in patients with hypophosphatasia.

E. Tumor: The clinician should search for subcutaneous and bone tumors in all patients with osteomalacia, since such tumors may be the underlying cause of the osteomalacia and their removal may cure the disease.

Treatment

A. Vitamin D: Patients with rickets or osteomalacia due to simple dietary deficiency of vitamin D or lack of exposure to sunlight respond well to small daily supplements of ergocalciferol and calcium or regular periods of exposure to ultraviolet light (artificial or natural). Administration of oral doses of ergocalciferol (0.05 mg [2000 IU] daily) for several months will heal the bone disease and restore serum calcium, phosphate, alkaline phosphatase, and iPTH to normal in most cases. This dose is insufficient to influence the course of rickets or osteomalacia due to any other cause. Although $25OHD_3$ (Calderol) and $1,25(OH)_2D_3$ (calcitriol) have been successful in the treatment of simple rickets and osteomalacia due to inadequate sunlight exposure, dihydrotachysterol has not.

Vitamin D treatment usually results in an increase in serum phosphorus within several days, but serum calcium may not increase for a week or more. In fact, in some patients with severe rickets or osteomalacia, serum calcium may actually decrease for a short period, and in children the development of tetany and convulsions has been described. Phosphate supplements are contraindicated during the early stages of treatment with vitamin D because they may aggravate hypocalcemia. Serum alkaline phosphatase and iPTH decrease slowly over a period of several weeks, but improvement in radiographic abnormalities may not be apparent for several months. The previously absent mineralization front in osteoid that underlies osteoblasts appears rapidly. This occurs even before important changes in the serum concentrations of calcium and phosphate and has been interpreted as evidence that vitamin D affects bone mineralization directly.

B. Calcium: Decreases in serum calcium have been ascribed to rapid movement of calcium from the extracellular fluids into bone as a result of its vitamin D–induced mineralization. For this reason—and to provide adequate calcium for bone mineralization—it is important to administer calcium (2 g of elemental calcium daily for children and 1 g for adults) along with vitamin D.

C. Malabsorption Therapy: Patients with rickets or osteomalacia due to intestinal malabsorption may not respond to treatment with vitamin D compounds because the vitamin is poorly absorbed. Those patients with gluten-sensitive enteropathy respond to ingestion of a gluten-free diet if sunlight exposure is adequate or small doses of oral vitamin D are given. Patients with other forms of malabsorption (Table 11–8) may require up to 5 mg (200,000 IU) per day of oral ergocalciferol, and some may require 40,000–80,000 IU of ergocalciferol (calciferol) given intravenously or intramuscularly. Unfortunately, preparations of vitamin D suitable for parenteral use are not generally available. Oral calcifediol and calcitriol in larger-than-usual doses may also be effective.

D. Long-Term Therapy: Patients with impaired synthesis of $1,25(OH)_2D_3$ or target cell resistance to $1,25(OH)_2D_3$ should be treated with calcitriol (Rocaltrol), although they may respond to large doses of either ergocalciferol or calcifediol. The treatment of patients with renal osteodystrophy or hypoparathyroidism has already been discussed. Patients with vitamin D–dependency rickets types I and II have been treated traditionally with large doses of ergocalciferol. Regimens must be individually tailored and careful lifelong follow-up maintained. Initial doses should be 25 μg (1000 IU) of ergocalciferol per kilogram of body weight per day. After approximately 2 months of treatment, the response to this dose is evaluated with x-rays of bony lesions and measurements of

Table 11–9. High-potency ergocalciferol (vitamin D$_2$) preparations in liquid form.

Ergocalciferol oral solution, 8000 IU vitamin D$_2$ per milliliter. Calciferol, 500,000 IU vitamin D$_2$ per milliliter (should be diluted to 100,000 IU/mL [1:5] with edible vegetable oil before dispensing).

---

serum calcium, phosphate, iPTH, and alkaline phosphatase. If no improvement is observed, the dose of vitamin D is increased by 25%; if signs of healing are observed, the dose is increased by only 15%. Similar evaluations should be made every 2 months, with appropriate increases in vitamin D dose until a satisfactory maintenance dose has been determined. The requirement for ergocalciferol varies among patients but is usually in the range of 40–50 μg/kg/d. Serum calcium should be measured every 3–4 months for life.

The development of hypercalcemia can be avoided by maintaining serum concentrations of calcium in the low normal range. Vitamin D therapy should be discontinued at the earliest sign of hypercalcemia. If detected early, serum calcium returns to the normal range within a week; if it remains normal for 2 weeks, vitamin D therapy can be reinstituted at a dose 15% lower than that which caused the hypercalcemia. Successful therapy is marked by "catch-up" skeletal growth, followed by normal growth.

Liquid forms of vitamin D should be used in patients with vitamin D–dependency rickets, because precise doses can be metered out to the patient with a small, well-calibrated syringe. Table 11–9 lists available liquid preparations of vitamin D$_2$.

Calcifediol (100–900 μg/d) has been used successfully in the treatment of vitamin D–dependency rickets, but it is expensive and offers little advantage over ergocalciferol except that hypercalcemia resolves sooner after calcifediol is discontinued. Calcitriol, on the other hand, provides an important advantage because of its rapid onset and termination of action. Long-term experience in the treatment of patients with vitamin D–dependency rickets with calcitriol has not yet accrued. The doses of dihydrotachysterol required for successful treatment of these patients are large, and this drug offers no special advantage over vitamin D.

E. Hypophosphatemic Rickets: The treatment of X-linked hypophosphatemic rickets is extremely challenging and requires persistence and excellent relationships with family members, so that patients will be compliant in their ingestion of phosphate. Lifelong treatment with orthophosphate supplements by mouth in doses ranging from 1 to 5 g of elemental phosphorus per day in divided doses every 5–6 hours will heal the rickets and osteomalacia of this disease. Phosphate supplements (Table 11–10) may be distasteful and can cause diarrhea initially, but with persistence, serum concentrations of phosphorus are restored toward normal (4 mg/dL), and the side effects generally disappear. The only major complication of phosphate therapy is the development of secondary hyperparathyroidism. The reason for this complication is poorly understood, since normal children who maintain similar levels of serum phosphate do not develop secondary hyperparathyroidism. Secondary hyperparathyroidism can be prevented only by coincident treatment with a vitamin D preparation that prevents decreases in ionized calcium that are ordinarily caused by phosphate therapy. Although ergocalciferol in doses of 0.1–1.25 mg (4000–50,000 IU) daily was used previously, it has recently been determined that calcitriol is equally effective or even more effective. Calcitriol is recommended in the treatment of patients with X-linked hypophosphatemia because hypercalcemia resolves rapidly after its discontinuation and because it may have specific antirachitic effects.

In following patients with X-linked hypophosphatemia who are under treatment with phosphate supplements and vitamin D, procedures similar to those described in the treatment of vitamin D dependency rickets should be used. Serum calcium, phosphate, and iPTH should be measured at intervals of 3–4 months. If hypercalcemia supervenes, vitamin D should be discontinued and then reinstituted at a lower dose when eucalcemia is restored. If serum iPTH increases much above the upper limit of the normal range, orthophosphate should be withheld temporar-

Table 11–10. Phosphate supplements for oral administration in hypophosphatemia.

Acidic phosphate (Joulie's solution)		Dissolve the phosphate salt in about 750 mL of warm water to which the phosphoric acid has been added. Make the solution up to 1L with distilled water. Store at room temperature. The concentration of phosphorus in this solution is 2.76 g/dL; the pH is 4.3.
Dibasic sodium phosphate (Na$_2$HPO$_4$ • 7H$_2$O) (reagent grade)	102	
Phosphoric acid NF (85%)	58.8	
Distilled water, qs ad	1000	
Neutral phosphate solution		Mix the phosphate salts and dispense in dry form as packets. Dissolve the packet of salts in distilled water by gently warming. Store in refrigerator at 4° C. Shake well if precipitate forms. Each batch lasts several days. The concentration of phosphorus in this solution is 2.08 g/dL; the pH is neutral.
NaH$_2$PO$_4$ • H$_2$O (reagent grade)	18.2	
Na$_2$HPO$_4$ • 7H$_2$O (reagent grade)	145	
Distilled water, qs ad	1000	
Neutra-Phos-K, K-Phos Neutral; others		Dissolve capsules in water and take orally. Take tablets orally with water.
Inorganic phosphorus, 250 mg per capsule or tablet		

ily; in some cases, however, it may be necessary to increase the dose of vitamin D. Renal function should be monitored carefully by measuring serum creatinine serially. Twenty-four-hour urinary phosphorus can be monitored to assess patient compliance with the phosphate regimen. Values in excess of 1000–2000 mg/d suggest compliance, but it must be remembered that patients and parents may be interested in pleasing the physician, and patients may take phosphate supplements immediately prior to 24-hour collection of urine but not chronically as prescribed.

F. Renal Tubular Acidosis: Rickets and osteomalacia due to distal renal tubular acidosis are expeditiously treated by correcting the acidosis with sodium bicarbonate, potassium bicarbonate, or potassium citrate. Adults require 5–10 g/d and children 1–5 g/d. Response to therapy should be monitored by measurements of blood pH, with values maintained at nearly physiologic levels. Rickets may heal slowly, and the response may be accelerated by the addition of vitamin D (in relatively high doses) to the treatment regimen. Therapy should be monitored by measuring serum calcium, and the dose of vitamin D should be regulated accordingly. Once rickets has healed, vitamin D therapy is rarely required, but it is probable that lifelong treatment with alkali will be necessary.

G. Rickets Due to Tumor: The response of tumor-associated rickets and osteomalacia to surgical removal of the offending tumor is dramatic. Serum phosphate increases within 1–2 days, and bone lesions heal within 6 months to 1 year.

H. Hypophosphatasia: In treatment of bone lesions associated with hypophosphatasia, use of conventional drugs (eg, vitamin D and calcium) has been unsatisfactory. Recently, increases in alkaline phosphatase and some degree of healing have been observed with doses of fluoride ion in the range of 40 mg/d. Spontaneous remissions have been reported.

OSTEOPOROSIS

Osteoporosis is a generalized disorder of bone characterized by a decrease in the quantity of bone but no change in its quality. The decrease in quantity results in increased bone fragility and fractures following minimal or no trauma.

Etiology & Incidence

Osteoporosis occurs most frequently in postmenopausal women and the aged. It has been estimated that at least 20% of women have suffered one or more fractures (vertebral, wrist, or proximal femur) by age 65 and as many as 40% have fractures thereafter. This enormous increase in fracture rate in comparison to the rate in premenopausal women is directly related to the progressive decrease in bone mass that occurs with aging in women. Osteoporosis is a major source of morbidity in this population. Decreases in bone

mass in men are delayed until after age 60, when fracture rates progressively increase. As many as 5–20% of older patients hospitalized with hip fracture die of cardiopulmonary problems, thus making hip fracture due to osteoporosis one of the more frequent indirect causes of death in North America. As many as 50% of the patients who survive become dependent on nursing home care.

The major types of osteoporosis are listed in Table 11–11 according to frequency of occurrence. The specific cause of the most common form of osteoporosis—that associated with menopause and aging—is unknown, but the major risk and complicating factors are listed in Table 11–12.

Table 11–11. Classification of osteoporosis according to frequency of occurrence.

Frequent	Infrequent
Postmenopausal	Juvenile
Senile	Young adult
Hypogonadism (oophorectomy)	Osteogenesis imperfecta
	Chromosomal abnormalities
Corticosteroid-induced	Migratory
Immobilization	Disappearing bones
Neoplasms (eg, myeloma)	Cushing's syndrome
	Hyperthyroidism
	Iron storage disease

Table 11–12. Risk factors and complicating factors in osteoporosis.

Genetic factors
  Nonblack race
  Northern European stock
  Small bone mass
  Defects in collagen synthesis or structure
Nutritional deficiency
  Calcium and phosphate
  Vitamin D (sunlight deprivation without dietary supplementation)
  Vitamin C
  Protein
Hypogonadism
Drugs
  Alcohol
  Corticosteroids
  Thyroid hormone
  Anticonvulsants
  Cancer chemotherapy
  Heparin
  Caffeine
Smoking
Gastrointestinal disease
  Gastric or intestinal resection
  Malabsorption
  Pancreatic insufficiency
  Hepatic disease
Renal disease
Hyperparathyroidism
Hyperthyroidism
Immobilization and lack of exercise
Excessive exercise leading to weight loss, amenorrhea, or both

A. Estrogen and Calcium Deficiency: There is little question that loss of sex hormone function is of major importance in bone loss associated with aging. Well-controlled trials in several centers have shown that treatment of perimenopausal or oophorectomized women with physiologic doses of estrogen prevents bone loss, in contrast to control subjects given low doses of estrogen or placebo. It has also been established that older persons not only ingest less calcium-containing foods than young men and women but also generally require considerably more calcium in their diets (1400 mg of elemental calcium daily versus 800 mg daily, respectively) to maintain total body calcium balance. Thus, it appears likely that sex hormone deficiency at menopause and calcium deficiency in the aged are the major etiologic factors in the development of osteoporosis.

Although many elderly persons lose bone, not all develop fractures. The absolute quantity of bone present at the time sex hormone and calcium deficiencies develop ultimately determines whether susceptibility to fractures will occur. Hence, if the rate of bone loss is similar among individuals, the critical point of bone "weakness" permitting fracture with minimal trauma will be reached more rapidly in individuals beginning with small amounts of bone than in those beginning with large amounts.

B. Other Factors: Less important risk factors in the development of osteoporosis include alcohol abuse, smoking, immobilization, and lack of exercise. The means by which these factors accelerate bone loss are poorly understood, but they are controllable and should be considered in the treatment of osteoporosis due to any cause. Complicating factors include the conditions that may be associated with vitamin D deficiency, excessive circulating concentrations of PTH, thyroid hormone, or corticosteroids, and a variety of drugs. Particularly important among the latter are corticosteroids, thyroid hormone, and anticonvulsants, which are all commonly used for disorders unrelated to osteoporosis. The true extent and frequency with which osteoporosis is associated with chemotherapy in the treatment of cancer or with heparin therapy are unknown.

C. Juvenile Osteoporosis: Juvenile osteoporosis is rare, and its cause is unknown. It occurs in late childhood and adolescence and is self-limited, lasting about 5 years. Young adult osteoporosis is also rare. It occurs at a later age (20–40), but in contrast to juvenile osteoporosis, it may progress rapidly to an almost total collapse of the axial skeleton and death from respiratory failure. Its cause is also unknown.

D. Osteogenesis Imperfecta: Osteogenesis imperfecta is a relatively common heritable disorder of bone that is probably caused by defects in collagen synthesis or structure. The most severely affected individuals suffer multiple fractures early in life that ultimately produce severe deformity and growth retardation. Other manifestations include bluish-gray scleras

(an inconstant finding), ligamentous laxity, and hearing loss in adults. It has been suggested that some patients who develop osteoporosis in later life may have mild forms of osteogenesis imperfecta.

E. Chromosomal Abnormalities: Although sex hormone deficiency may be responsible in part for the osteoporosis observed in patients with chromosomal abnormalities (eg, Turner's XO and Klinefelter's XXY syndromes), other unknown factors are probably also involved.

F. Immobilization: The osteoporosis of immobilization can be localized (associated with casts for fractures or with painful limbs), generalized (associated with prolonged bed rest or space travel), or neurologic (associated with paraplegia or quadriplegia). The causes are unknown, but absence of stress and muscle pull on bone is an underlying factor in all of these disorders.

G. Vitamin C Deficiency and Hemochromatosis: Osteoporosis may be associated with severe vitamin C deficiency and hemochromatosis. Vitamin C is a cofactor in the enzymatic hydroxylation of proline and lysine in collagen. Because of this, a deficiency in vitamin C is thought to produce abnormalities in collagen biosynthesis and maturation that interfere with bone formation. A similar mechanism may be involved in the osteoporosis of hemochromatosis; the abnormal accumulation of iron may promote oxidation of vitamin C, resulting in its depletion. Hemochromatosis of the testes or of the pituitary, which causes hypogonadism and sex hormone deficiency, is almost certainly an important contributing factor in the production of the osteoporosis of this disorder.

H. Migratory Osteoporosis and Sudeck's Atrophy: There are 2 rare forms of local osteoporosis that appear to be unrelated to immobilization. The first is transitory or regional migratory osteoporosis. It is characterized by painful loss of bone, usually in the upper femoral shafts, which almost always reverses without treatment. The second is the syndrome of "disappearing bones," in which one or more parts of limb bones disappear radiologically and are replaced by fibrous tissue. This disorder probably represents an extreme form of Sudeck's atrophy of bone which occurs after trauma or fracture. It is variably reversible, and no specific treatment is available. The underlying causes of these conditions are unknown.

Anatomic & Chemical Pathology

Osteoporosis can often be detected during transiliac bone biopsy. The biopsy needle saws through the outer table of bone with little difficulty, and extreme care is needed to avoid crushing the specimen. Examination of such a specimen shows that the mass of bone per unit volume of bone tissue is reduced, but its mineral content per unit mass is normal. In contrast, the bone in osteomalacia has a reduced mineral content per unit mass.

Tetracycline labeling of bone in vivo has shown that

bone formation decreases with age and bone resorption remains constant. Microradiographic studies show increases in bone resorption surfaces, probably resulting from the failure of bone formation processes to repair previously resorbed bone. Since it has not yet been possible to investigate the dynamic properties of human bone cells, it is still unknown whether bone cell function in osteoporosis is abnormal.

Pathogenesis

A. Postmenopausal and Senile Osteoporosis: The pathogenesis of postmenopausal and senile osteoporosis is poorly understood, but important observations during the past decade have led to a hypothesis with therapeutic implications. Although evidence is incomplete, it is likely that sex hormones protect bone against the destructive effects of PTH. Thus, the incidence of osteoporosis in postmenopausal women with hypoparathyroidism is decreased, and estrogen treatment in patients with hyperparathyroidism reduces blood calcium levels toward normal. Most importantly, estrogen treatment in patients with postmenopausal osteoporosis causes decreased bone resorption surfaces (as observed in transiliac bone biopsies), small decreases in serum levels of calcium, and appropriate increases in serum levels of iPTH. By inference, therefore, the loss of sex hormone function at the menopause may permit normal levels of circulating PTH to act on bone unopposed, resulting in relatively greater bone resorption in comparison with formation. Negative bone balance ensues, and the resulting increase in the release of calcium from bone causes small increases in the serum levels of calcium, which in turn decreases serum levels of iPTH. The consequences of chronic decreases in PTH secretion are manifest and can be predicted from Fig 11–2. Serum concentrations of phosphate increase because of a decrease in PTH-induced phosphate excretion. The combination of decreased PTH secretion and increased serum phosphate results in diminished $1,25(OH)_2D_3$ production and decreased intestinal calcium absorption. Likewise, urinary calcium excretion is increased as a result of a decrease in PTH-induced renal tubular reabsorption of calcium. These adaptive mechanisms are normally quite effective in preventing increases in serum calcium due to environmental perturbations (eg, increased intestinal absorption of calcium). They can only be considered maladaptive when increases in serum calcium are induced by a primary defect in bone that causes a relative increase in resorption over formation (eg, postmenopausal osteoporosis). Thus, if the sequence of events described above is correct, the decrease in intestinal absorption of calcium and increase in renal excretion of calcium observed in postmenopausal osteoporosis represent epiphenomena of negative bone balance that can only aggravate the primary bone lesions by producing a negative balance in total body calcium.

Serum iPTH has been shown to increase with age in apparently normal subjects. Although this could be due to an intrinsic change in the secretory activity of the parathyroid glands, it is likely that a combination of a dietary deficiency in calcium in the aged, diminished intestinal calcium absorption, and possibly decreased renal function is responsible. Significant increases in serum iPTH above the normal mean value are generally not observed under the age of 60, and they could themselves be responsible for the osteoporosis observed in old people. More intriguing, however, is the possibility that the adverse effects of sex hormone deficiency and secondary hyperparathyroidism due to calcium deficiency merge as age progresses and are responsible for the ultimate clinical picture of advanced osteoporosis in the very old. A working classification of the osteoporosis of aging, based on these 2 pathogenetic schemes, has been proposed: type I denotes osteoporosis due to sex hormone deficiency, and type II denotes that due to secondary hyperparathyroidism.

It has recently been suggested that decreased secretion of calcitonin in women may be an additional etiologic factor.

B. Glucocorticoid-Induced Osteoporosis: Glucocorticoid-induced osteoporosis occurs in patients with Cushing's disease and in other patients treated with glucocorticoids. Diminished bone mass can be observed within months following initiation of high-dose steroid therapy and can result in the rapid compromise of skeletal integrity. Corticosteroids have many effects on extracellular mineral and bone metabolism. They almost certainly interfere with normal production of bone collagen by osteoblasts, and there is evidence in cultured bone cells in vitro that they increase cellular sensitivity to PTH. Corticosteroids also inhibit intestinal absorption of calcium. The mechanism of this action is poorly understood, but it probably does not involve interference with the normal metabolism of vitamin D to its biologically active metabolite $1,25(OH)_2D_3$. It is more likely due to a direct toxic effect on the intestinal calcium transport system. Negative calcium balance due to decreased intestinal absorption and increased renal excretion of calcium is almost always manifest, and the resulting mild hypocalcemia causes appropriate increases in serum concentrations of iPTH. The secondary hyperparathyroidism and possibly the increased sensitivity of bone to PTH are reflected histomorphometrically in an increase in bone resorption surfaces. Thus, the combined effects of diminished bone formation and increased bone resorption result in severe negative bone balance and a rapid decrease in bone mass.

C. Hyperthyroidism: There are dramatic histomorphometric changes in the bones of patients with hyperthyroidism. These are characterized by increased osteoclastic resorption and increased osteoblastic bone formation. Osteoid seams are frequently increased in width owing to accelerated matrix production, and marrow fibrosis may be present. These changes are almost certainly due to the direct effects of thyroid hormones on bone cells and are reflected by increased urinary excretion of hydroxyproline and hydroxylysine and increased serum concentrations of alkaline phosphatase. Alterations in extracellular mineral homeostasis are not always obvious, probably because the increases in bone formation and bone resorption are equivalent. Nevertheless, mild hypercalcemia is occasionally observed and is associated with adaptive decreases in serum iPTH, increases in serum phosphate due to decreased phosphate excretion, marked hypercalciuria, and decreases in intestinal absorption of calcium.

The bone loss that occurs in hyperthyroidism or in patients receiving excessive amounts of thyroid hormone rarely achieves clinical significance in the young but may sufficiently aggravate the bone loss in postmenopausal women or old men to precipitate fractures.

Quantitative Measurement of Bone Mass

There are 3 approaches to quantitative assessment of bone mass. The first uses careful x-rays of the hands and measurements of the periosteal and endosteal diameters of a metacarpal bone (the second, third, or fourth). The thickness of the cortical bone is determined by subtracting the internal diameter from the external diameter. Measurements are best made with a precision caliper. The precision of this measurement is about ±2%.

The second approach uses photon beam absorptiometry, introduced by Cameron and Sorenson. The single-beam method measures the attenuation by bone (usually the radius) of gamma ray emission from isotopes (^{125}I or ^{247}Am). Commercial instruments are now available, and with careful application the precision of measurements is also about ±2%. The disadvantage of this technique is that accessible limb bones have little trabecular bone, and measurements thus reflect chiefly cortical bone. Since most osteoporosis of clinical significance involves principally trabecular bone, there is a large overlap in values for normal subjects and patients with proved osteoporosis.

The recently developed dual-photon absorptiometry (DPA) method can measure mass in almost any bone in the body. Thus, the bones most frequently fractured in patients with osteoporosis (vertebrae and femoral neck) can be assessed directly. The overlap in bone mass values between normal subjects and patients with proved osteoporosis is considerably less than that observed using the single-beam technique.

Another technique, introduced by Genant and Cann, uses quantitative computer-assisted tomography (QCT) to obtain direct measurements of bone mass in the central portion of a given vertebra. This is in contrast with DPA, which measures bone mass in entire vertebrae as well as overlying tissues (eg, calcified aorta). QCT is therefore a more specific mea-

surement of the trabecular bone in the vertebral bodies. The most recent addition to the technology of bone mineral content measurement is dual-energy radiography (DER or DEX), which uses an x-ray source rather than an isotope source to generate photon beams. This method is more rapid, is as accurate and as precise as DPA, and has greater resolution than DPA. It therefore is likely to become the standard for future measurement of bone mineral content. QCT, DPA and DER can provide the clinician with accurate measurements of changes in bone mass during observation or treatment. They should also help in assessing the value of various new treatments for osteoporosis. While there is some controversy as to the cost-effectiveness of bone mineral measurements in patients at risk for the development of osteoporosis, there is little question that they are essential for triaging such patients into groups requiring or not requiring sex hormone prophylaxis against menopausal bone loss.

Clinical Features

A. Symptoms and Signs: Patients with uncomplicated osteoporosis without bone fractures are usually asymptomatic. The first manifestation of reduced bone mass is usually a wrist fracture or a vertebral crush fracture caused by a small amount of force. A fresh vertebral fracture produces severe localized pain in the back that frequently radiates anteriorly into the chest, sometimes resembling the pain of a cardiopulmonary catastrophe. Torso movement aggravates the pain and recumbency relieves it, with improvement occurring within 1–2 months. Subsequent vertebral fractures may occur and may contribute to chronic back pain, but more often the intensity of pain is poorly related to the degree of spinal deformity seen on x-rays. During the acute phase of fracture, spot tenderness occurs over the back, but neurologic signs are rare.

1. Dorsal kyphosis and loss of height—The single most prominent finding in patients with well-established osteoporosis is dorsal kyphosis (so-called dowager's hump) and loss of height. Accurate measurements of height and arm span are most important in assessing the development and progress of osteoporosis in patients who have undergone oophorectomy or orchiectomy or in patients undergoing routine evaluation after the age of 45 years. Normally, total erect height equals arm span but becomes progressively less than arm span with vertebral collapse.

All of the classic signs of hip fracture are present in patients with osteoporosis who are afflicted with this problem, but because most patients are aged, the incidence of fatal complications is increased.

2. Signs of other disorders—Patients with osteoporosis due to causes other than sex hormone deficiency and aging may have symptoms and signs related to the underlying disorder (eg, Cushing's syndrome due to excessive corticosteroids).

B. Laboratory Findings: Serum calcium, phosphate, alkaline phosphatase, and iPTH are within normal ranges in patients with osteoporosis due to sex hormone deficiency and aging. In the acute phase of development, urinary calcium and hydroxyproline may be slightly increased, but these indices have no diagnostic value. Significant abnormalities in serum calcium, phosphate, alkaline phosphatase, iPTH, and serum proteins should be regarded with suspicion, and one or more of the complicating factors listed in Table 11–12 should be sought.

C. X-Ray Findings: X-rays of the skeleton do not show a decrease in osseous density until at least 30% of bone mass has been lost. Although such a decrease in density may be observed in all bones, the most valuable x-rays for diagnostic purposes are those of the lateral lumbar and thoracic spine. One should look for loss of horizontal trabeculae and prominent end plates of the vertebral bodies (Fig 11–35). Intervertebral disks are more prominent than is normal, and mechan-

ical failure of vertebrae is manifested by wedging and protrusion of the disk into the body of the vertebra (Fig 11–35). The latter finding has been termed "codfish spine" because this species has biconcave vertebral bodies.

X-rays of the upper part of the femur that are taken so as to accentuate trabecular patterns may be most helpful in assessing the clinical importance of reduced bone mass (Singh index) (Fig 11–36). Disappearance of the superior trabecular pattern that traverses the greater trochanter (arrow in grade 3 sketch) probably indicates that the osteoporosis is severe enough to increase the risk of hip fracture.

Differential Diagnosis

Without radiographic evidence of vertebral fractures or a history of fracture of other bones with minimal trauma, the detection of significant decreases in bone mass may be difficult. Even with the use of the

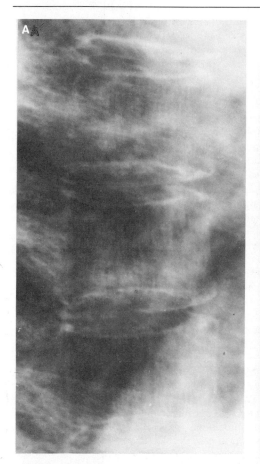
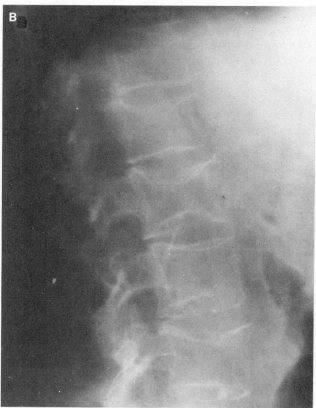

Figure 11–35. *A:* Magnified x-rays of thoracic vertebrae from a woman with osteoporosis. Note the relative prominence of vertical trabeculae and the absence of horizontal trabeculae. *B:* Lateral x-ray of the lumbar spine of a woman with postmenopausal osteoporosis. Note the increased density of the superior and inferior cortical margins of vertebrae, the marked demineralization of vertebral bodies, and the central compression of articular surfaces of vertebral bodies by intervertebral disks. (Courtesy of G Gordan.)

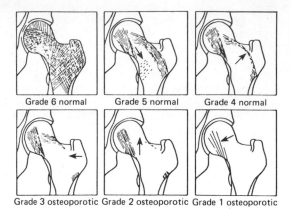

Grade 6 normal   Grade 5 normal   Grade 4 normal

Grade 3 osteoporotic Grade 2 osteoporotic Grade 1 osteoporotic

Figure 11–36. The effects of increasingly severe osteoporosis on the pattern of trabecular bone in the upper end of the femur. Arrows show progressive radiologic disappearance of trabecular groups. (Reproduced, with permission, from Singh M et al: *Ann Intern Med* 1972;**77**:63.)

most sophisticated techniques (see previous section), single values for bone mass may be within the normal range for age after 20% of the skeleton has been lost. Serial measurements showing progressive loss of bone are necessary in order to estimate the original bone mass that might have been present in an individual patient before osseous destruction. The physician should also be aware of conditions and risk factors that may lead to loss of bone mass (Table 11–12). Therapeutic or prophylactic measures should be instituted as rapidly as possible and systematic measurements made at regular intervals to determine the progress of the disease or the effect of treatment.

There are many disorders that mimic or complicate postmenopausal or senile osteoporosis. The routine history and physical examination are very useful in discovering them. The history will reveal drug treatment, gastric or intestinal resections, oophorectomy, sunlight deprivation, and immobilization. Physical examination may reveal the presence of Cushing's syndrome or hyperthyroidism as well as the presence of hepatomegaly or splenomegaly. Liver enlargement suggests liver disease and, in men, the possibility of hemochromatosis. Small, soft testicles should raise suspicions about hypogonadism due to a variety of causes, including Klinefelter's syndrome (see Chapters 16 and 18). Short stature in a woman may be a sign of Turner's syndrome (see Chapters 17 and 18).

Multiple myeloma and diffuse metastasis of malignant tumors to the vertebrae are commonly misdiagnosed as postmenopausal or senile osteoporosis. These conditions should be suspected when the history indicates that the patient may have cancer. In the absence of historical clues, unusually rapid progression of osseous destruction often indicates the presence of cancer. In such cases, bone marrow examination or direct biopsy of lesions may be most helpful.

Total serum calcium, phosphate, magnesium, alkaline phosphatase, albumin and globulin, iPTH, cortisol, and thyroxine should be measured in all patients with osteoporosis. In patients with postmenopausal or senile osteoporosis, the values of all of these indices should be within the normal range. Abnormalities indicate the presence of disorders that mimic or complicate postmenopausal or senile osteoporosis, and a specific diagnosis should be established as soon as possible. Serum $25OHD_3$ should be measured in patients suspected of sunlight deprivation or malabsorption, and in men, measurement of serum testosterone is indicated to exclude hypogonadism.

Treatment

The treatment of osteoporosis depends on establishing its underlying cause to the extent possible. Patients with endocrine abnormalities can usually be treated by either hormone replacement (hypogonadism) or removal of hyperfunctioning endocrine tissue. In most instances, drugs that induce osteoporosis can be discontinued or replaced by other drugs, or the dosage can be reduced. In the case of corticosteroid therapy, measures designed to help prevent osteoporosis should be considered. Alternate-day corticosteroid therapy in conjunction with oral calcium supplements (1–2 g of elemental calcium daily) to decrease PTH secretion may be helpful in this regard. Alternatively, it may be possible in the future to treat patients with corticosteroid preparations that possess anti-inflammatory activity but have little or no adverse effects on bone. Recent studies suggest that a glucocorticoid analogue called deflazacort may be such a compound. It is not yet available in the USA.

Once it has been established that a patient is at risk or has postmenopausal osteoporosis, the risk factors listed in Table 11–12 should be eliminated whenever possible. Small women of northern European ancestry whose Singh index (Fig 11–36) for the upper femoral trabecular pattern is grade 3 or below or whose bone mineral content at the femur is at or below the fracture threshold should be warned that hip fracture is likely to occur with minimal trauma. These patients should eliminate hazards that might cause them to fall (eg, waxed floors and throw rugs).

At first evaluation, baseline measurement of bone mass of the hip and of the lumbar vertebrae should be obtained using one or more of the techniques described above.

A. Calcium: After 24-hour urinary calcium is measured (to rule out idiopathic hypercalciuria), oral calcium supplements of 1–2 g of elemental calcium daily—preferably as calcium carbonate or calcium citrate—are begun. Such therapy increases intestinal absorption of calcium, decreases serum levels of iPTH, and decreases resorption surfaces. If undue hypercalciuria is noted, thiazides are indicated.

B. Estrogens: It has been shown that estrogen prevents bone loss in oophorectomized and perimenopausal women, and a recent study indicates that calcium and estrogen together markedly decrease the fracture rate in osteoporotic women. However, noncyclic estrogen therapy is controversial because some reports indicate that such treatment may increase the incidence of uterine cancer. The conservative approach would be to maintain calcium supplements for a year, at which time bone mass should be measured again and estrogen treatment started if values are significantly below previously obtained baseline values. The more aggressive approach would be to administer cyclic ethinyl estradiol (0.02 mg/d) or conjugated estrogen (0.625 mg/d) for 3 of every 4 weeks. Then progesterone (5–10 mg) should be given during the last week to 10 days that estrogen is administered. In patients with a uterus, menstrual bleeding may be expected during the week off estrogen and progesterone. However, it should be recognized that the possible adverse effects of long-term progesterone therapy have not been fully evaluated. Absolute contraindications to estrogen therapy include a personal or family history of breast or genital cancer or of phlebitis. The transdermal patch, Estraderm (estradiol, 0.05 mg/d or 0.1 mg/d twice weekly) offers an alternative to oral therapy. It is possible that anabolic steroid preparations (eg, stanozolol) may offer another alternative form of therapy to these women.

C. Fluoride: Fluoride ion is the only form of treatment available that has been demonstrated to increase bone mass. Radiographic evidence shows that spinal density increases in patients with osteoporosis who have been given sodium fluoride (50 mg/d), oral calcium (1 g/d), and vitamin D (50,000 IU every 3–5 days). In another study, the combination of fluoride, calcium, and estrogen appeared to decrease fracture rates to a greater extent than did the combination of estrogen and calcium; vitamin D alone had no influence on fracture rates. It is important to recognize that numerous side effects occur with fluoride therapy, including lower extremity pain, joint swelling and gastrointestinal intolerance, all of which may require cessation of therapy. Most importantly, fluoride is at present an investigational drug not approved by the FDA for treatment of osteoporosis.

D. Androgens for Men: Men with osteoporosis should be treated in a manner similar to that described for women, except that androgens should be given instead of estrogens. Unfortunately, androgens may aggravate prostatic hyperplasia. Combined androgen and estrogen therapy (eg, Deladumone) may be of value in this regard.

E. Phosphate: Although phosphate supplements might be expected to increase bone formation, they are associated with development of secondary hyperparathyroidism and apparent worsening of bone disease in patients with osteoporosis. The effect of combining phosphate with other drugs of proved efficacy has yet to be studied extensively.

F. Calcitonin: Calcitonin (Calcimar) was expected to provide the ideal therapy for osteoporosis because of its supposed inhibitory action on bone resorption. However, calcitonin increases serum iPTH and does little to inhibit bone resorption unless calcium supplements are used to prevent hyperparathyroidism. Calcitonin has recently been approved by the FDA for the treatment of osteoporosis in doses of 100 IU/d. It must be given parenterally and is expensive but may be an alternative to estrogen therapy when this drug is contraindicated or not tolerated.

G. Parathyroid Hormone: In an effort to increase bone formation, synthetic human PTH (1–34) has been given to osteoporotic patients in low doses. Early results suggest that such treatment produces positive calcium balance and increases trabecular bone formation. A recent report has described increases in spinal bone mass when PTH treatment is combined with $1,25(OH)_2D_3$ administration.

H. Bisphosphonate Compounds: Bisphosphonate compounds have been shown to decrease bone resorption and therefore might be expected to have a beneficial effect in patients with osteoporosis. Using the only compound currently available in the USA (etidronate disodium), one study has demonstrated a reduction in both bone formation and bone resorption in osteoporotic patients. Although this drug is known to produce osteomalacia when given in high doses, other bisphosphonate compounds do not. It is therefore possible that these latter agents may prove to be of use in the treatment of osteoporosis. A recent report describing the prevention of steroid-induced osteoporosis with the bisphosphonate, 3-amino-1-hydroxy-propylidine-1,1-bisphosphonate (APD), is hopeful in this regard.

I. Life-Style: It is important to encourage osteoporotic patients to take adequate sunlight exposure, increase dietary intake of calcium, decrease intake of alcohol, tobacco, caffeine, and certain drugs (Table 11–12) and make physical exercise a part of their lives. Such measures usually decrease chronic back pain and promote a sense of well-being. Adequate back supports are most important.

PAGET'S DISEASE
(Osteitis Deformans)

Although Paget's disease of bone is a disorder of bone remodeling, it cannot be classified strictly as a metabolic bone disease, because the abnormalities are focal. The disease is characterized by histologic and gross osseous deformities due to local uncontrolled bone resorption, which is caused by excessive numbers of osteoclasts and osteoblasts and ultimately leads to formation of structurally fragile osseous tissue. Any bone of the body may be involved, but the most frequent sites are the femur, tibia, skull, lumbosacral spine, and pelvis. The disease is usually asymptomatic, and except for a similar bone disease in young children called hereditary bone dysplasia with hyperphosphatasia, or "juvenile Paget's disease," patients generally come to medical attention only after age 40.

Paget's disease occurs in a fairly distinct geographic distribution. About 4% of people over 40 years of age in Germany and England have the disease, whereas it is considerably less common in North America and relatively rare in Scandinavia, Africa, and the Near and Far East. It is likely that fewer than 2% of patients with radiographic evidence of Paget's disease are symptomatic. The disease may occur in families and has been reported in identical twins.

Coexistence of primary hyperparathyroidism and Paget's disease has been noted, but this observation must be interpreted cautiously in light of the fact that both disorders are common, and when one is detected, the usual laboratory investigations will almost certainly reveal the other, if present.

Etiology

Recently, the old idea that Paget's disease may be due to some chronic inflammatory process has been revived. Nuclear inclusions resembling virus particles have been observed in the osteoclasts of patients with Paget's disease, suggesting that its underlying cause may be a slow virus.

Pathology

The gross pathologic features of Paget's disease in its full-blown state consist of diffuse bony deformities, including marked enlargement of the skull, expansion and compression of the vertebrae, platybasia with compression of the cerebellum and spinal cord, anterior and lateral bowing of the extremities, and protrusion of the femoral head into the acetabulum as a result of the pelvic involvement. Histologically, all bone cell types are increased in number and apparently in activity. Lamellar bone in the cortex and trabeculae is progressively replaced by woven bone, so that its gross architecture becomes chaotic. As lesions progress, woven bone is replaced by randomly laid lamellar bone; sections thus present a characteristic mosaic structure when observed under polarized light. Osteoid volume is increased but the calcification front is normal, indicating that new bone formation is occurring at a rapid rate. Osteoclasts show great variation in size and may contain up to 100 nuclei. Osteoblasts may be very large, with irregularly shaped nuclei. Osteocytic osteolysis is a prominent finding. Areas of bone that have undergone a full "pagetic cycle" retain architectural abnormalities, but cell numbers and activity are normal.

Pathogenesis

Although bone mineral turnover may be many times greater than normal in Paget's disease, calcium balance is generally maintained because the rates of bone resorption and formation are similar. Only when Paget's disease is complicated by disorders causing further increases in bone resorption (eg, prolonged immobilization or primary hyperparathyroidism) will abnormalities of extracellular mineral metabolism become evident. The hypercalcemia of immobilization may be extremely severe and lead to suppression of PTH secretion, hypercalciuria, decreased intestinal absorption of calcium, and negative calcium balance. If primary hyperparathyroidism is present, hypercalcemia may be more severe than might be predicted by the levels of serum iPTH.

Characteristically, serum alkaline phosphatase levels are markedly increased. These increased levels are probably due to the increased numbers of osteoblasts present in pagetic bone, since serum alkaline phosphatase activity appears to correlate well with histomorphometric values for active bone formation surface. Serum acid phosphatase activity may also be increased in some patients, and this increase is thought to be due to increased numbers of osteoclasts present in lesions.

Urinary excretion of hydroxyproline is increased in most patients, owing to increased rates of synthesis and destruction in bone collagen.

Clinical Features

A. Symptoms and Signs: Relatively few patients with radiologically proved Paget's disease have significant symptoms. The diagnosis is often made as an incidental finding on x-rays taken for other reasons or with the serendipitous finding of an elevated serum alkaline phosphatase value. The chief symptom is bone pain over lesions. Joint symptoms produced by Paget's disease may be difficult to distinguish from those of arthritis. Deafness in patients with Paget's disease of the skull is usually related to bony abnormalities of the internal and external auditory apparatus rather than compression of the eighth nerve by temporal bone enlargement. Vertebral crush fractures occur frequently. In rare cases, there are severe neurologic complications resulting from spinal cord compression and dislocation of cervical vertebrae.

Fractures of long bones may occur. Incomplete ("fissure") fractures, frequently painful, are usually present on the convex surfaces of lower limb bones and may progress to complete fracture with minimal or no trauma. Fractures usually heal rapidly. Redness with increased skin temperature over pagetic bone is a common finding; rarely, bruits may be heard. Increased cardiac output is common in patients with extensive disease. These vascular manifestations are probably due to increased blood flow in involved areas both in bone and in overlying skin. High-output congestive heart failure may occur in patients with underlying heart disease.

The risk of osteogenic sarcoma is greater in patients with Paget's disease than in the population at large. Its major sites are the humerus and skull.

B. Laboratory Findings: Serum calcium, phosphate, magnesium, and iPTH are usually normal. Abnormalities should be taken as evidence of a superimposed condition, such as immobilization or primary hyperparathyroidism. Serum alkaline phosphatase levels are markedly increased, and acid phosphatase levels may also be increased. Urinary hydroxyproline is usually increased except in patients with minimal disease.

C. X-Ray Findings: There is a vast spectrum of characteristic radiologic abnormalities, ranging from pure osteolytic lesions to areas that show both osteolysis and sclerosis. Subperiosteal bone resorption has not been noted in Paget's disease; when present, it suggests associated primary hyperparathyroidism. The classic bony abnormality seen in the extremities is a large, uniform resorption front that appears as a V-shaped wedge on x-ray (Fig 11–37). As the front advances along the shaft, sclerotic bone is laid down behind it, resulting in anterior or lateral bowing. Thick bony trabeculae are common and may fill in the medullary cavity of bones. The skull is often grossly enlarged, and the mixture of sclerotic and lytic areas gives rise to the classic "cotton wool" appearance on x-ray. Initially, the skull may show a purely osteolytic lesion (osteoporosis circumscripta). Thickening of long bones and vertebrae occurs frequently, and crush fractures or "disappearing vertebrae" cause varying degrees of kyphosis.

The development of radionuclide bone scans using 99mTc-labeled bisphosphonate or pyrophosphate and 67gallium citrate has aided greatly in documenting the extent of the disease and revealing lesions that may not be apparent radiologically (Fig 11–38).

Differential Diagnosis

The diagnosis of Paget's disease is relatively straightforward. It is based on the presence of typical bone lesions on x-ray or radionuclide bone scans; normal levels of serum calcium, phosphate, and iPTH; increased serum levels of alkaline phosphatase; and

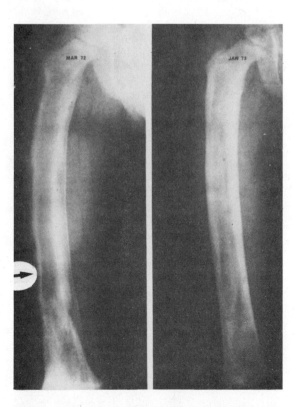

Figure 11–37. X-rays of the right femur in a patient with juvenile Paget's disease before *(left)* and after *(right)* 10 months of treatment with calcitonin. Note the advancing V-shaped resorption front (arrow). A striking improvement in the appearance of diseased bone is seen after treatment. (Reproduced, with permission, from Doyle P et al. *Br J Radiol* 1974;47:9.)

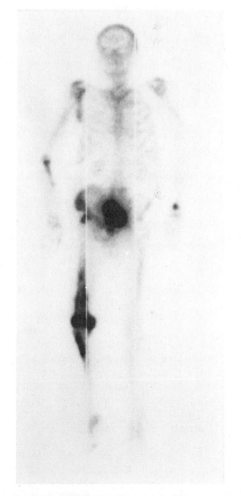

Figure 11–38. Bone scan of patient with severe Paget's disease of the skull, ribs, spine, pelvis, right femur, and acetabulum. Note localization of bone-seeking isotope (99mTc-labeled bisphosphonate) in these areas.

increased excretion of total hydroxyproline in the urine. The only major disorder that mimics Paget's disease is cancer that has metastasized to bone. Osteoblastic metastases such as those from the prostate may be indistinguishable from Paget's lesions on x-ray or radionuclide scanning, and alkaline phosphatase may be increased. The only distinguishing feature may be a marked elevation in the serum level of acid phosphatase in prostatic cancer; this enzyme is only occasionally increased in Paget's disease. In most instances in which metastatic cancer is suspected, confirmation by biopsy either of the primary lesion or of bone metastases is necessary. In contrast, osteolytic lesions such as those that occur in multiple myeloma do not produce markedly abnormal bone scans. Serum alkaline phosphatase may be increased in patients who have metastatic osteolytic lesions due to liver metastases, and fractionation of serum alkaline phosphatase will show that the bulk of the enzyme is not derived from bone. Ultimately, lesions must be biopsied to determine whether bone metastases are present. The development of a sarcoma in association with a pagetic bone lesion is suggested by the appearance of a lytic area within dense bone, a marked increase in pain over the lesion, and a rapid unexplained increase in serum alkaline phosphatase levels.

Treatment

The consensus at present is that only patients with symptoms should be treated. However, the underlying cause of symptoms is sometimes difficult to determine because the pain of degenerative arthritis often mimics that of Paget's disease. When doubt exists, a therapeutic trial of nonsteroidal anti-inflammatory agents should be given before therapy for Paget's disease is initiated. In patients who fail to respond to these agents, one of several courses can be followed; each has its advantages and disadvantages. Before any treatment is started, patients with mild disease and without deformity should be reassured that most patients with the disease do not develop the disfiguring deformities they may have read or heard about.

During the last 5 years, calcitonin, bisphosphonates, and mithramycin have become available for treatment. They all suppress the number and activity of the abnormal bone cells, but they act by different mechanisms. As will be noted below, mithramycin is a toxic drug of last resort. Presently, the choice of calcitonin or bisphosphonate treatment in an individual patient is almost arbitrary, although calcitonin is preferred in primarily lytic bone disease. The advantage of calcitonin is that radiologic evidence of healing has been observed in some patients after treatment. The advantage of bisphosphonates is that they can be administered orally. Osteogenic sarcoma developing in pagetic lesions is virtually unresponsive to any form of therapy.

The treatment of juvenile Paget's disease is similar to the treatment of adult Paget's disease, although calcitonin appears to be the drug of choice.

A. Calcitonin: Synthetic salmon calcitonin (Calcimar) is most commonly used. Synthetic human calcitonin has recently become available. Porcine calcitonin, extracted from pig thyroid glands, was used in the initial pharmacologic studies of treatment of Paget's disease; its availability is limited, and there is no reason to prefer it over salmon or human calcitonin.

The rationale for the use of calcitonin is that it decreases bone resorption. When administered to patients with Paget's disease in doses of about 100 units/d subcutaneously or intramuscularly, it markedly decreases the number of active osteoclasts. Urinary hydroxyproline decreases within 24 hours after the initial injection, but serum alkaline phosphatase does not begin to fall until approximately 2 weeks after treatment is started. Brief but significant hypocalcemia and hypophosphatemia occur shortly after administration, and appropriate increases in serum iPTH in response to the hypocalcemia have been observed. Serum calcium, phosphate, and iPTH return to normal within 4–6 hours and remain so until calcitonin is administered again. Negative calcium balance improves, with decreases in urinary and fecal calcium excretion. Radiologic improvement may not occur for months or years; the criteria for healing are decreased bone volume, increased density of cortices with restoration of a normal corticomedullary junction, and restoration of normal trabecular bone. Histomorphometry of bone biopsy specimens is difficult to evaluate because of the dynamics of untreated pagetic lesions. It has been shown, however, that along with a decrease in osteoclast numbers, there is a decrease in the surface of bone covered by osteoblasts, as well as replacement of woven bone by lamellar bone.

Although it is difficult to evaluate pain objectively, there is apparent relief of pain and bone tenderness within weeks following initiation of therapy. Objective signs of response include a decrease in redness and heat of the skin over involved bones and decreases in cardiac output. Neurologic signs (when present) may improve, but hearing rarely improves. Withdrawal of calcitonin treatment usually results in the return of symptoms and progression of bone lesions.

On the basis of decreases in alkaline phosphatase and urinary excretion of hydroxyproline, it appears that most patients given calcitonin have good long-term responses. However, some patients respond only briefly, with the indices returning to previously high levels in months. Others experience prolonged remissions followed by late recrudescence of the disease. There is no rational explanation for these relapses except in a very few patients who develop high titers of calcitonin antibodies when a nonhuman species of calcitonin is used. In such cases, human calcitonin usually produces a remission.

The ideal dose and schedule for treatment of Paget's disease with calcitonin have not been determined. It is conventional to give 100 Medical Research Council (MRC) units subcutaneously per day, although therapeutic effects have been observed at half this dose. Patients generally administer the drug themselves with a tuberculin syringe after instruction about rotation of injection sites. In patients with Paget's disease who also have hypercalcemia due to immobilization, higher doses (200–400 MRC units) should be given intravenously by slow infusion over 24 hours. A dramatic decrease in serum calcium usually occurs. Treatment is maintained for 2–5 years, depending on the response and on the extent of the disease.

Some patients develop side effects that necessitate discontinuation of treatment. These include flushing, fatigue, nausea, diarrhea, vomiting, pain at the injection site, rash, and a sense of being disconnected from reality. In most cases, these symptoms can be minimized by administering calcitonin at bedtime or lowering the dosage.

Low titers of antibodies to salmon calcitonin develop in about half of patients, but only 10% develop antibody titers high enough to cause relapse. In such cases, human calcitonin should be used, since it has not been shown to produce antibodies.

B. Bisphosphonate: The bisphosphonates are analogues of pyrophosphate, with a P–C–P rather than a P–O–P structure, and are resistant to enzymatic and chemical hydrolysis. They are adsorbed onto the surface of bone mineral and thus inhibit both bone resorption and formation. Evidence indicates that they also are taken up by bone cells and may interfere with bone cell activity.

Currently, only etidronate disodium (Didronel) is available in North America. In doses of 5 mg/kg/d orally, etidronate disodium causes a dramatic decrease in serum alkaline phosphatase and total urinary hydroxyproline excretion, as well as symptomatic improvement in most patients with Paget's disease. Unfortunately, the intestinal absorption of this drug is inconstant, so that it must be given after an overnight fast or 2–3 hours after a meal. Most of the drug accumulates in bone and is not metabolized. It is excreted unchanged in the urine. If it is well absorbed, doses higher than 5 mg/kg/d may cause osteomalacia.

Etidronate is given in courses of about 3–6 months and is reinstituted when serum alkaline phosphatase and total hydroxyproline levels increase after remission. Remissions vary in duration but have lasted as long as 2 years or more. Pagetic lesions have been shown to regress histologically in bone biopsies, but radiographic evidence of healing has rarely been reported.

Etidronate causes few side effects. Diarrhea occurs occasionally but can often be prevented by administering the agent with foods low in calcium content; this decreases absorption to a variable degree, but patients still achieve therapeutic effects. Serum concentrations of phosphate increase within a week after starting treatment, especially with doses larger than 5 mg/kg, but serum concentrations of calcium remain normal, and there is no change in serum iPTH. The effect on serum phosphate is probably related to the drug's effect on renal tubular handling of phosphate.

In patients with very severe disease or in those who fail to respond to either drug, larger doses (eg, 10–15 mg/kg/d of etidronate) or alternating or combination therapy with etidronate and calcitonin may produce a biochemical response. Other bisphosphonates as yet not available in the USA (eg, 3-amino-1-hydroxypropylidine-1,1-bisphosphonate [APD]) have been reported to cause remission in patients resistant to etidronate. Rapid responses of severe Paget's disease to intravenous APD with prolonged remissions have also been observed.

C. Mithramycin (Plicamycin): As noted in the discussion of the treatment of hypercalcemia, mithramycin is a cytotoxic antibiotic that inhibits RNA synthesis. It decreases serum alkaline phosphatase levels and urinary hydroxyproline excretion in patients with Paget's disease. It is given intravenously in doses of about 10–15 μg/kg at weekly intervals until biochemical remission occurs or toxic effects appear. Toxicity may be severe and includes liver dysfunction, renal failure, and suppression of platelet production. For this reason, it should be used only under the most desperate circumstances (eg, spinal cord compression). It is possible to obtain long-lasting remissions when this drug is combined with bisphosphonates.

REFERENCES

EXTRACELLULAR & BONE MINERAL HOMEOSTASIS

Albright F, Reifenstein EC Jr: *The Parathyroid Glands and Metabolic Bone Disease.* Williams & Wilkins, 1948.

Arnaud CD: Calcium homeostasis: Regulatory elements and their integration. *Fed Proc* 1978;**37**:2557.

Arnaud CD: Minerals. Chapter 13 in: *Diet and Health: Implications for Reducing Chronic Disease Risk.* National Academy Press, 1989.

Aurbach GD et al: Parathyroid hormone, calcitonin and the calciferols. Page 1137 in: *Williams Textbook of Endocrinology,* 7th ed. Wilson JD, Foster DW (editors). Saunders, 1985.

Bringhurst FR, Potts JT: Calcium and phosphate distribution, turnover and metabolic actions. Page 805 in: *Endocrinology,* 2nd ed. Vol 2. DeGroot LJ et al (editors). Grune & Stratton, 1989.

Centrella M, Canalis E: Local regulators of skeletal growth: A perspective. *Endocr Rev* 1985;**6**:544.

Martin TJ et al: Calcium regulation and bone metabolism. Page 1 in: *Clinical Endocrinology of Calcium Metabo-*

lism. Martin TJ, Raisz LG (editors). Marcel Dekker, 1987.

Neer RM: Calcium and inorganic phosphate homeostasis. Page 927 in: *Endocrinology,* 2nd ed. Vol 2. DeGroot LJ et al (editors). Grune & Stratton, 1989.

PARATHYROID HORMONE

Structure & Biosynthesis

Cohn DV, Elting JJ: Synthesis and secretion of parathormone and secretory protein I by the parathyroid gland. Page 1 in: *Bone and Mineral Research Annual 2*. Peck WA (editor). Elsevier, 1984.

Habener JF et al: Parathyroid hormone: Biochemical aspects of biosynthesis, secretion, action, and metabolism. *Physiol Rev* 1984;**64**:985.

Rosenblatt M et al: Parathyroid hormone: Physiology, chemistry, biosynthesis, secretion, metabolism, and mode of action. Page 848 in: *Endocrinology,* 2nd ed. Vol 2. DeGroot LJ et al (editors). Grune & Stratton, 1989.

Control of Secretion

Anast CS et al: Evidence for parathyroid failure in magnesium deficiency. *Science* 1972;**177**:606.

Cohn DV, Elting JJ: Synthesis and secretion of parathormone and secretory protein I by the parathyroid gland. Page 1 in: *Bone and Mineral Research Annual 2*. Peck WA (editor). Elsevier, 1984.

Heath H III: Biogenic amines and the secretion of parathyroid hormone and calcitonin. *Endocr Rev* 1980; **1**:319.

Oldham SB et al: Dynamics of parathyroid hormone secretion in vitro. *Am J Med* 1971;**50**:650.

Rosenblatt M et al: Parathyroid hormone: Physiology, chemistry, biosynthesis, secretion, metabolism, and mode of action. Page 848 in: *Endocrinology,* 2nd ed. Vol 2. DeGroot LJ et al (editors). Grune & Stratton, 1989.

Metabolism & Circulating Forms

Berson SA, Yalow RS: Immunochemical heterogeneity of parathyroid hormone in plasma. *J Clin Endocrinol Metab* 1968;**28**:1037.

DiBella F et al: Hyperfunctioning parathyroid glands: Major source of immunoheterogeneity. Proceedings of the Sixth Parathyroid Conference. *Excerpta Medica* 1978;**421**:337.

Fischer JA et al: Calcium-regulated parathyroid hormone peptidase. *Proc Natl Acad Sci USA* 1972;**69**:2341.

Flueck JA et al: Immunoheterogeneity of parathyroid hormone in venous effluent serum from hyperfunctioning parathyroid glands. *J Clin Invest* 1977;**60**:1367.

Goltzman D et al: Studies of the multiple molecular forms of bioactive parathyroid hormone and parathyroid hormonelike substances. *Recent Prog Horm Res* 1986;**42**:665.

Martin KV et al: The peripheral metabolism of parathyroid hormone. *N Engl J Med* 1979;**301**:1092.

Mayer GP et al: Effects of plasma calcium concentrations on the relative proportion of hormone and carboxyl-terminal fragments in parathyroid venous blood. *Endocrinology* 1979;**104**:1778.

Rosenblatt M et al: Parathyroid hormone: Physiology, chemistry, biosynthesis, secretion, metabolism, and

mode of action. Page 848 in: *Endocrinology,* 2nd ed. Vol 2. DeGroot LJ et al (editors). Grune & Stratton, 1989.

Segre GV et al: Parathyroid hormone in human plasma: Immunochemical characterization and biological implications. *J Clin Invest* 1972;**51**:3163.

Silverman R, Yalow RS: Heterogeneity of parathyroid hormone. *J Clin Invest* 1973;**52**:1958.

Actions

Albright F, Reifenstein EC Jr: *The Parathyroid Glands and Metabolic Bone Disease*. Williams & Wilkins, 1948.

Arnaud C, Rasmussen H, Anast C: Further studies on the interrelationship between parathyroid hormone and vitamin D. *J Clin Invest* 1966;**45**:1955.

Bijvoet OLM: Kidney function in calcium and phosphate metabolism. Page 118 in: *Metabolic Bone Disease*. Vol 1. Avioli LV, Krane SM (editors). Academic Press, 1977.

Dennis VW et al: Renal handling of phosphate and calcium. *Annu Rev Physiol* 1979;**41**:257.

Forte LR, Nickols GA, Anast CS: Renal adenylate cyclase and the interrelationship between parathyroid hormone and vitamin D in the regulation of urinary phosphate and adenosine cyclic $3',5'$-monophosphate excretion. *J Clin Invest* 1976;**57**:559.

Klahr S, Hruska KA: Effects of parathyroid hormone on the renal reabsorption of phosphorus and divalent cations. Page 65 in: *Bone and Mineral Research Annual 2*. Peck WA (editor). Elsevier, 1984.

Knox FG et al: Phosphate transport along the nephron. *Am J Physiol* 1977;**233**:261.

Raisz LG: Bone metabolism and calcium regulation. Page 32 in: *Metabolic Bone Disease*. Vol 1. Avioli LV, Krane SM (editors). Academic Press, 1977.

Rosenblatt M et al: Parathyroid hormone: Physiology, chemistry, biosynthesis, secretion, metabolism, and mode of action. Page 848 in: *Endocrinology,* 2nd ed. Vol 2. DeGroot LJ et al (editors). Grune & Stratton, 1989.

Shelling DH: *The Parathyroids in Health and Disease*. Mosby, 1935.

Mechanisms of Action

Donahue HJ et al: Differential effects of parathyroid hormone and its analogues on cytosolic calcium ion and cAMP levels in cultured rat osteoblast-like cells. *J Biol Chem* 1988;**263**:13522.

Karpf DB et al: Structural properties of the renal parathyroid hormone receptor: Hydrodynamic analysis and protease sensitivity. *Endocrinology* 1988;**123**:2611.

Klahr S, Hruska KA: Effects of parathyroid hormone on the renal reabsorption of phosphorus and divalent cations. Page 65 in: *Bone and Mineral Research Annual 2*. Peck WA (editor). Elsevier, 1984.

Nissenson RA, Kleine RF: Parathyroid hormone receptors. Page 481 in: *Peptide Hormone Receptors*. Kalimi MY, Hubbard JR (editors). De Gruyter, 1987.

Nissenson RA et al: Covalent labeling of a high-affinity, guanyl nucleotide sensitive parathyroid hormone receptor in canine renal cortex. *Biochemistry* 1987; **26**:1874.

Pun KK, Arnaud CD, Nissenson RA: Parathyroid hormone receptors in human dermal fibroblasts: structural and functional characterization. *J Bone Miner Res* 1988;**3**:453.

Rasmussen H, Pechet M, Fast D: Effect of dibutyryl cyclic adenosine 3′,5′-monophosphate, theophylline and other nucleotides upon calcium and phosphate metabolism. *J Clin Invest* 1968;**47**:1843.

Reid IR et al: Parathyroid hormone acutely elevates intracellular calcium in osteoblastlike cells. *Am J Physiol* 1987;**253**:E45.

Rosenblatt M et al: Parathyroid hormone: Physiology, chemistry, biosynthesis, secretion, metabolism, and mode of action. Page 848 in: *Endocrinology,* 2nd ed. Vol 2. DeGroot LJ et al (editors). Grune & Stratton, 1989.

Shigeno C et al: Photoaffinity labeling of parathyroid hormone receptors in clonal rat osteosarcoma cells. *J Biol Chem* 1988;**263**:3864.

Silve CM et al: Parathyroid hormone receptor in intact embryonic chicken bone: Characterization and cellular localization. *J Cell Biol* 1982;**94**:379.

Teitelbaum AP et al: Coupling of the canine renal parathyroid hormone receptor to adenylate cyclase: Modulation by guanyl nucleotides and N-ethylmaleimide. *Endocrinology* 1982;**111**:1524.

Yamaguchi DT et al: Parathyroid hormone-activated calcium channels in an osteoblast-like clonal osteosarcoma cell line: cAMP-dependent and cAMP-independent calcium channels. *J Biol Chem* 1987;**262**:7711.

Assay in Biologic Fluids

Arnaud C, Tsao HS, Littledike ET: Radioimmunoassay of human parathyroid hormone in serum. *J Clin Invest* 1971;**50**:21.

Bikle DD (editor): *Assay of Calcium-Regulating Hormones.* Springer-Verlag, 1983.

Blind E et al: Two-site assay of intact parathyroid hormone in the investigation of primary hyperparathyroidism and other disorders of calcium metabolism compared with a midregion assay. *J Clin Endocrinol Metab* 1988;**67**:353.

Brown RC et al: Circulating intact parathyroid hormone measured by a two-site immunochemiluminometric assay. *J Clin Endocrinol Metab* 1987;**65**:407.

Forero MS et al: Effect of age on circulating immunoreactive and bioactive parathyroid hormone levels in women. *J Bone Miner Res* 1987;**2**:363.

Goltzman D et al: Cytochemical bioassay of parathyroid hormone: Characteristics of the assay and analysis of circulating hormonal forms. *J Clin Invest* 1980;**65**:1309.

Mallette LE et al: Radioimmunoassay for the middle region of human parathyroid hormone using an homologous antiserum with a carboxy-terminal fragment of bovine parathyroid hormone as radioligand. *J Clin Endocrinol Metab* 1982;**54**:1017.

Marx SJ et al: Radioimmunoassay for the middle region of human parathyroid hormone: Studies with a radioiodinated synthetic peptide. *J Clin Endocrinol Metab* 1981;**53**:76.

Nissenson RA et al: Endogenous biologically active human parathyroid hormone: Measurement by guanyl nucleotide-amplified renal adenylate cyclase assay. *J Clin Endocrinol Metab* 1981;**52**:840.

Nussbaum SR et al: Highly sensitive two-site immunoradiometric assay of parathyrin, and its clinical utility in evaluating patients with hypercalcemia. *Clin Chem* 1987;**33**:1364.

Segre GV, Potts JT: Differential diagnosis of hypercalcemia: Methods and clinical applications of parathyroid assays. Page 984 in: *Endocrinology,* 2nd ed. Vol 2. DeGroot LJ et al (editors). Grune & Stratton, 1989.

CALCITONIN

Austin LA, Heath HH III: Calcitonin: Physiology and pathophysiology. *N Engl J Med* 1981;**304**:269.

Austin LA et al: Regulation of alcitonin secretion in normal man by changes of serum calcium within the physiologic range. *J Clin Invest* 1979;**64**:1721.

Bikle DD (editor): *Assay of Calcium-Regulating Hormones.* Springer-Verlag, 1983.

Heath HH III, Sizemore GW: Plasma calcitonin in normal man: Differences between men and women. *J Clin Invest* 1977;**60**:1135.

MacIntyre I: Calcitonin: Physiology, biosynthesis secretion, metabolism, and mode of action. Page 892 in: *Endocrinology,* 2nd ed. Vol 2. DeGroot LJ et al (editors). Grune & Stratton, 1989.

Owyang C et al: Comparison of the effects of pentagastrin injection and meal-stimulated gastrin on plasma calcitonin in normal man. *Am J Dig Dis* 1978;**23**:1084.

Talmage RV et al: The physiological significance of calcitonin. Page 74 in: *Bone and Mineral Research Annual I.* Peck WA (editor). Excerpta Medica, 1983.

VITAMIN D

Audran M, Kumar R: The physiology and pathophysiology of vitamin D. *Mayo Clin Proc* 1985;**60**:851.

Bikle DD (editor): *Assay of Calcium-Regulating Hormones.* Springer-Verlag, 1983.

Brommage R, DeLuca HF: Evidence that 1,25-dihydroxyvitamin D_3 is the physiologically active metabolite of vitamin D_3. *Endocr Rev* 1985;**6**:491.

DeLuca HF: The metabolism, physiology and function of vitamin D. Page 1 in: *Vitamin D: Basic and Clinical Aspects.* Kumar R (editor). Martinus Nijhoff, 1984.

DeLuca HF: The vitamin D endocrine system in health and disease. Page 41 in: *Nutrition in the Young and the Elderly.* Haller EW, Cotton GE (editors). Collamore Press, 1983.

Holick MF: Vitamin D: Biosynthesis, metabolism, and mode of action. Page 902 in: *Endocrinology,* 2nd ed. Vol 2. DeGroot LJ et al (editors). Grune & Stratton, 1989.

Norman AW: The vitamin D endocrine system. *Physiologist* 1985;**28**:219.

Parfitt AM et al: Vitamin D and bone health in the elderly. *Am J Clin Nutr* 1982;**36**:1014.

Suda T et al: Modulation of cell differentiation, immune responses and tumor promotion by vitamin D compounds. Page 1 in: *Bone and Mineral Research.* Vol 4. Peck WA (editor). Elsevier, 1986.

DISORDERS OF PARATHYROID FUNCTION

Hypoparathyroidism

Ahn TG et al: Familial isolated hypoparathyroidism: A molecular genetic analysis of 8 families with 23 affected persons. *Medicine* 1986;**65**:73.

Avioli LV: The therapeutic approach to hypoparathyroidism. *Am J Med* 1974;**57**:34.

Nicar MJF, Pak CY: Calcium bioavailability from calcium carbonate and calcium citrate. *J Clin Endocrinol Metab* 1985;**61**:391.

Nusynowitz ML, Frame B, Kolb FO: The spectrum of the hypoparathyroid states. *Medicine* 1976;**55**:105.

Okano K et al: Comparative efficacy of various vitamin D metabolites in the treatment of various types of hypoparathyroidism. *J Clin Endocrinol Metab* 1982;**55**:238.

Palmer RF, Searles HH, Boldrey EB: Papilledema and hypoparathyroidism simulating brain tumor. *J Neurosurg* 1959;**16**:378.

Parfitt AM: The incidence of hypoparathyroid tetany after thyroid operations: Relationship of age, extent of resection and surgical experience. *Med J Aust* 1971;**1**:1103.

Parfitt AM: The spectrum of hypoparathyroidism. *J Clin Endocrinol Metab* 1972;**34**:152.

Parfitt AM: Surgical, idiopathic and other varieties of parathyroid hormone–deficient hypoparathyroidism. Page 1049 in: *Endocrinology,* 2nd ed. Vol 2. DeGroot LJ et al (editors). Grune & Stratton, 1989.

Porter RH et al: Treatment of hypoparathyroid patients with chlorthalidone. *N Engl J Med* 1978;**298**:577.

Rude RK, Oldham SB, Singer FR: Functional hypoparathyroidism and parathyroid hormone end-organ resistance in human magnesium deficiency. *Clin Endocrinol* 1976;**5**:209.

Russell R: Hypoparathyroidism and malabsorption. *Br Med J* 1967;**3**:781.

Spinner MW et al: Familial distribution of organ-specific antibodies in the blood of patients with Addison's disease and hypoparathyroidism and their relatives. *Clin Exp Immunol* 1969;**5**:461.

Suh SM et al: Pathogenesis of hypocalcemia in primary hypomagnesemia: Normal end-organ responsiveness to parathyroid hormone, impaired parathyroid gland function. *J Clin Invest* 1973;**52**:153.

Pseudohypoparathyroidism & Pseudopseudohypoparathyroidism

Albright F et al: Pseudohypoparathyroidism: An example of the "Seabright-bantam syndrome." *Endocrinology* 1942;**20**:922.

Bell NH et al: Effects of dibutyryl cyclic adenosine 3′,5′-monophosphate and parathyroid extract on calcium and phosphorus metabolism in hypoparathyroidism and pseudohypoparathyroidism. *J Clin Invest* 1972;**51**:816.

Chase LR, Melson GL, Aurbach GD: Pseudohypoparathyroidism: Defective excretion of 3′,5′-AMP in response to parathyroid hormone. *J Clin Invest* 1969;**48**:1822.

Downs RW Jr et al: Deficient adenylate cyclase regulatory protein in renal membranes from a patient with pseudohypoparathyroidism. *J Clin Invest* 1983;**71**:231.

Drezner M, Neelon FA, Lebavitz HE: Pseudohypoparathyroidism type II: A possible defect in the reception of the cyclic AMP signal. *N Engl J Med* 1973;**289**:1056.

Farfel Z et al: Defect of receptor-cyclase coupling protein in pseudohypoparathyroidism. *N Engl J Med* 1980;**303**:237.

Farfel Z et al: Pseudohypoparathyroidism: Inheritance of deficient receptor-cyclase coupling activity. *Proc Natl Acad Sci USA* 1981;**78**:3098.

Kolb FO, Steinbach HL: Pseudohypoparathyroidism with secondary hyperparathyroidism and osteitis fibrosa. *J Clin Endocrinol Metab* 1962;**22**:59.

Kooh SW et al: Treatment of hypoparathyroidism and pseudohypoparathyroidism with metabolites of vitamin D to 1,25-dihydroxyvitamin D. *N Engl J Med* 1975;**293**:840.

Levine MA, Aurbach GD: Pseudohypoparathyroidism. Page 1065 in: *Endocrinology,* 2nd ed. Vol 2. DeGroot LJ et al (editors). Grune & Stratton, 1989.

Levine MA et al: Activity of the stimulatory guanine nucleotide-binding protein is reduced in erythrocytes from patients with pseudohypoparathyroidism and pseudopseudohypoparathyroidism: Biochemical, endocrine, and genetic analysis of Albright's hereditary osteodystrophy in six kindreds. *J Clin Endocrinol Metab* 1986;**62**:497.

Levine MA et al: Deficient activity of guanine nucleotide regulatory protein in erythrocytes from patients with pseudohypoparathyroidism. *Biochem Biophys Res Commun* 1980;**94**:1319.

Levine MA et al: Deficient guanine nucleotide regulatory unit activity in cultured fibroblast membranes from patients with pseudohypoparathyroidism type I: A cause of impaired synthesis of 3′,5′-cyclic AMP by intact and broken cells. *J Clin Invest* 1983;**72**:316.

McElduff A et al: A 6-hour human parathyroid hormone (1–34) infusion protocol: Studies in normal and hypoparathyroid subjects. *Calcif Tissue Int* 1987;**41**:267.

Silve C et al: Selective resistance to parathyroid hormone in cultured skin fibroblasts from patients with pseudohypoparathyroidism type Ib. *J Clin Endocrinol Metab* 1986;**62**:640.

Van Dop C, Bourne HR: Pseudohypoparathyroidism. *Annu Rev Med* 1983;**34**:259.

Primary Hyperparathyroidism

Arnaud CD, Tsao HS, Littledike T: Radioimmunoassay of human parathyroid hormone in serum. *J Clin Invest* 1971;**50**:21.

Benson RC et al: Radioimmunoassay of parathyroid hormone in hypercalcemic patients with malignant disease. *Am J Med* 1974;**56**:821.

Bilezikian JP: The medical management of primary hyperparathyroidism. *Ann Intern Med* 1982;**96**:198.

Blind E et al: Two-site assay of intact parathyroid hormone in the investigation of primary hyperparathyroidism and other disorders of calcium metabolism compared with a midregion assay. *J Clin Endocrinol Metab* 1988;**67**:353.

Brandi ML et al: Parathyroid mitogenic activity in plasma from patients with familial multiple endocrine neoplasia type 1. *N Engl J Med* 1986;**314**:1287.

Broadus AE: Nephrogenous cyclic AMP. *Recent Prog Horm Res* 1981;**37**:667.

Canfield RE (editor): Etidronate disodium: A new therapy for hypercalcemia of malignancy. *Am J Med* 1987;**82 (Suppl 2A)**:1. [Entire issue.]

Christianssen T et al: Prevalence of hypercalcemia in health screening in Stockholm. *Acta Med Scand* 1976;**200**:131.

Dauphine RT, Riggs BL, Scholz DA: Back pain and vertebral crush fractures: An unemphasized mode of presentation for primary hyperparathyroidism. *Ann Intern Med* 1975;**83**:365.

Fitzpatrick LA, Bilezikian JP: Acute primary hyperparathyroidism. *Am J Med* 1987;**82**:275.

Foley TP Jr et al: Familial benign hypercalcemia. *J Pediatr* 1972;**81**:1060.

Genant HK et al: Primary hyperparathyroidism: A comprehensive study of clinical, biochemical and radiographic manifestations. *Radiology* 1973;**109**:513.

Goldsmith RE et al: Familial hyperparathyroidism: Description of a large kindred with physiological observations and a review of the literature. *Ann Intern Med* 1976;**94**:36.

Habener JF, Potts JT: Primary hyperparathyroidism: Clinical features. Page 954 in: *Endocrinology,* 2nd ed. Vol 2. DeGroot LJ et al (editors). Grune & Stratton, 1989.

Heath H III, Hodgson SF, Kennedy MA: Primary hyperparathyroidism: Incidence, morbidity, and potential economic impact in a community. *N Engl J Med* 1980;**302**:189.

Heath H III, Purnell DC: Asymptomatic hypercalcemia and primary hyperparathyroidism. Page 189 in: *Calcium Disorders.* Heath DA, Marx SJ (editors). Butterworth, 1982.

Kochersberger G et al: What is the clinical significance of bone loss in primary hyperparathyroidism? *Arch Intern Med* 1987;**147**:1951.

Lambert PW, Heath H III, Sizemore GW: Pre- and postoperative studies of plasma calcitonin in primary hyperparathyroidism. *J Clin Invest* 1979;**63**:602.

Levin KE, Clark OH: Localization of parathyroid glands. *Annu Rev Med* 1988;**39**:29.

Levin KE et al: Localizing studies in patients with persistent or recurrent hyperparathyroidism. *Surgery* 1987;**102**:917.

Marx SJ: Genetic defects in primary hyperparathyroidism. (Editorial.) *N Engl J Med* 1988;**318**:699.

Neer RM, Potts, JT: Medical management of hyperparathyroidism and hypercalcemia. Page 1002 in: *Endocrinology,* 2nd ed. Vol 2. DeGroot LJ et al (editors). Grune & Stratton, 1989.

Norton JA et al: Surgical management of hyperparathyroidism. Page 1013 in: *Endocrinology,* 2nd ed. Vol 2. DeGroot LJ et al (editors). Grune & Stratton, 1989.

Prinz RA et al: Radiation associated hyperparathyroidism: A new syndrome? *Surgery* 1977;**82**:296.

Purnell DC et al: Primary hyperparathyroidism: A prospective clinical study. *Am J Med* 1971;**50**:670.

Purnell DC et al: Treatment of primary hyperparathyroidism. *Am J Med* 1974;**56**:800.

Ralston SH: The pathogenesis of humoral hypercalcemia of malignancy. *Lancet* 1987;**2**:1443.

Richardson ML et al: Bone mineral changes in primary hyperparathyroidism. *Skeletal Radiol* 1986;**15**:85.

Segre GV, Potts JT: Differential diagnosis of hypercalcemia: Methods and clinical applications of parathyroid assays. Page 984 in: *Endocrinology,* 2nd ed. Vol 2. DeGroot LJ et al (editors). Grune & Stratton, 1989.

Scholz DA, Purnell DC: Asymptomatic primary hyperparathyroidism: Ten-year prospective study. *Mayo Clin Proc* 1981;**56**:473.

Sier HC et al: Primary hyperparathyroidism and delirium in the elderly. (Clinical Conference.) *J Am Geriatr Soc* 1988;**36**:157.

Stewart AF, Insogna KF, Broadus AE: Malignancy-associated hypercalcemia. Page 967 in: *Endocrinology,* 2nd ed. Vol 2. DeGroot LJ et al (editors). Grune & Stratton, 1989.

Stewart AF et al: Biochemical evaluation of patients with cancer-associated hypercalcemia: Evidence for humoral and nonhumoral groups. *N Engl J Med* 1980;**30**:1377.

Stewart AF et al: N-terminal amino acid sequence of two novel tumor-derived adenylate cyclase-stimulating proteins: Identification of parathyroid hormone-like and parathyroid hormone-unlike domains. *Biochem Biophys Res Commun* 1987;**146**:672.

Strewler GJ et al: Parathyroid hormonelike protein from human renal carcinoma cells: Structural and functional homology with parathyroid hormone. *J Clin Invest* 1987;**80**:1803.

Suva LJ et al: A parathyroid hormone–related protein implicated in malignant hypercalcemia: Cloning and expression. *Science* 1987;**237**:893.

Wang CA: Surgical management of primary hyperparathyroidism. *Curr Probl Surg* 1985;**22**:1.

Secondary Hyperparathyroidism of Chronic Renal Failure

Arnaud CD: Hyperparathyroidism and renal failure. *Kidney Int* 1973;**4**:80.

Bordier PJ, Marie PJ, Arnaud CD: Evolution of renal osteodystrophy: Correlation of bone histomorphometry and serum mineral and immunoreactive parathyroid hormone values before and after treatment with calcium carbonate or 25-hydroxycholecalciferol. *Kidney Int [Suppl]* 1975;**No. 2**:102.

Bricker NS: On the pathogenesis of the uremic state: An exposition of the "trade-off" hypothesis. *N Engl J Med* 1972;**286**:1093.

Coburn JW, Slatopolsky E: Vitamin D, parathyroid hormone, and renal osteodystrophy. Page 1657 in: *The Kidney,* 3rd ed. Brenner BM, Rector FC Jr (editors). Saunders, 1986.

Coburn JW et al: A skeletal mineralizing defect in dialysis patients: A syndrome resembling osteomalacia but unrelated to vitamin D. *Contrib Nephrol* 1980;**18**:172.

Fournier A et al: Calcium carbonate, an aluminum-free agent for control of hyperphosphatemia, hypocalcemia, and hyperparathyroidism in uremia. *Kidney Int* 1986;**18**:S114.

Fournier AE et al: Etiology of hyperparathyroidism and bone disease during hemodialysis. 2. Factors affecting serum immunoreactive parathyroid hormone. *J Clin Invest* 1971;**50**:599.

Johnson WJ et al: Prevention and reversal of progressive secondary hyperparathyroidism in patients maintained by hemodialysis. *Am J Med* 1974;**56**:827.

Massry SG et al: Skeletal resistance to parathyroid hormone in renal failure. *Ann Intern Med* 1973;**78**:357.

Nebeker HF, Coburn JW: Aluminum and renal osteodystrophy. *Annu Rev Med* 1986;**37**:79.

Parker TF et al: Jejunal absorption and secretion of calcium in patients with chronic renal disease on hemodialysis. *J Clin Invest* 1974;**54**:358.

Portale AA et al: Effect of dietary phosphorus on circulating concentrations of 1,25-dihydroxyvitamin D and immunoreactive parathyroid hormone in children with moderate renal insufficiency. *J Clin Invest* 1984;**73:**1580.

Salusky IB, Coburn JW: The renal osteodystrophies. Page 1032 in: *Endocrinology*, 2nd ed. Vol 2. DeGroot LJ et al (editors). Grune & Stratton, 1989.

Slatopolsky E et al: Calcium carbonate as a phosphate binder in patients with chronic renal failure undergoing dialysis. *N Engl J Med* 1986;**315:**157.

Slatopolsky E et al: Marked suppression of secondary hyperparathyroidism by intravenous administration of 1,25-dihydroxy-cholecalciferol in uremic patients. *J Clin Invest* 1984;**74:**2136.

Slatopolsky E et al: On the pathogenesis of hyperparathyroidism in chronic experimental and renal insufficiency in the dog. *J Clin Invest* 1971;**50:**492.

Slatopolsky E et al: On the prevention of secondary hyperparathyroidism in experimental chronic renal disease using "proportional reduction" of dietary phosphorus intake. *Kidney Int* 1972;**2:**147.

Stanbury SW, Lumb GA: Parathyroid function in chronic renal failure: A statistical survey of the plasma and biochemistry in azotaemic renal osteodystrophy. *Q J Med* 1966;**35:**1.

DISORDERS OF CALCITONIN SECRETION

Austin LA, Heath H III: Calcitonin, physiology and pathophysiology. *N Engl J Med* 1981;**304:**269.

Chong GC et al: Medullary carcinoma of the thyroid gland. *Cancer* 1975;**35:**695.

Graze K et al: Natural history of familial medullary thyroid carcinoma: Effect of a program for early diagnosis. *N Engl J Med* 1978;**299:**980.

Saad MF et al: The prognostic value of calcitonin immunostaining in medullary carcinoma of the thyroid. *J Clin Endocrinol Metab* 1984;**59:**850.

Schwartz KE et al: Calcitonin in nonthyroidal cancer. *J Clin Endocrinol Metab* 1979;**49:**438.

Silva OL et al: Calcitonin as a marker for bronchogenic cancer. *Cancer* 1979;**44:**680.

Sizemore GW et al: Epidemiology of medullary carcinoma of the thyroid gland: A 5 year experience (1971–1976). *Surg Clin North Am* 1977;**57:**633.

Williams ED: Medullary carcinoma of the thyroid. Page 1132 in: *Endocrinology*, 2nd ed. Vol 2. DeGroot LJ et al (editors). Grune & Stratton, 1989.

HYPERCALCIURIA

Chadwick KS et al: Mechanism for hyperoxaluria in patients with ileal dysfunction. *N Engl J Med* 1973;**289:**172.

Coe FL: Treated and untreated recurrent calcium nephrolithiasis in patients with idiopathic hypercalciuria, hyperuricosuria, or no metabolic disorder. *Ann Intern Med* 1977;**87:**404.

Coe FL, Bushinski DA: Pathophysiology of hypercalciuria. *Am J Physiol* 1984;**247:**1.

Coe FL (editor): *Hypercalciuric States: Pathogenesis, Consequences and Treatment*. Grune & Stratton, 1984.

Danielson BG et al: Treatment of idiopathic calcium stone disease. (Editorial.) *Calcif Tissue Int* 1983;**35:**715.

Finlayson B: Calcium stones: Some physical and clinical aspects. Page 337 in: *Calcium Metabolism in Renal Failure and Nephrolithiasis*. David DS (editor). Wiley, 1977.

Frame B, Potts JT (editors): Idiopathic hypercalciuria. Page 401 in: *Clinical Disorders of Bone and Mineral Metabolism*. Section XV. International Congress Series 617. Excerpta Medica, 1983.

Kolb FO: Non-operative management of renal calculi. *J Genitourin Med* (March) 1979;**1:**29.

Pak CY: Pathogenesis of hypercalciuria. Page 303 in: *Bone and Mineral Research*. Vol 4. Peck WA (editor). Elsevier, 1986.

Peacock M, Robertson WG: Urinary calcium stone disease. Page 1111 in: *Endocrinology*, 2nd ed. Vol 2. DeGroot LJ et al (editors). Grune & Stratton, 1989.

Seldin DW, Wilson JD: Renal tubular acidosis. Page 1548 in: *The Metabolic Basis of Inherited Disease*, 4th ed. Stanbury JB et al (editors). McGraw-Hill, 1972.

Shen FH, Baylink DJ: Increased serum 1,25-dihydroxyvitamin D in idiopathic hypercalciuria. *J Lab Clin Med* 1977;**90:**955.

Smith LH et al: Management of cystinuria and cystine-stone disease. *J Urol* 1959;**81:**61.

Smith LH et al: Orthophosphate therapy in calcium renal lithiasis. Page 188 in: *Urinary Calculi*. Delatt LC et al (editors). Karger, 1973.

Yendt ER et al: The use of thiazides in the prevention of renal calculi. *Can Med Assoc J* 1970;**102:**614.

METABOLIC BONE DISEASE

General

Bordier PJ, Tun-Chot S: Quantitative histology of metabolic bone disease. *Clin Endocrinol Metab* 1972;**1:**197.

Frame B, Potts JT (editors): Assessment of trabecular bone status. Page 27 in: *Clinical Disorders of Bone and Mineral Metabolism*. Section II. International Congress Series 617. Excerpta Medica, 1983.

Frost HM: A method of analysis of trabecular bone dynamics. Pages 445–476 in: *Bone Histomorphometry*. Meunier PJ (editor). Armour Montagu, 1977.

Frost, HM: Tetracycline based analysis of bone remodeling. *Calcif Tissue Res* 1969;**3:**211.

Genant HK et al: Quantitative computed tomography in the assessment of osteoporosis. Pages 49–71 in: *Osteoporosis Update 1987*. Genant HK (editor). Univ of California Press, 1987.

Genant HK et al: Quantitative computed tomography of vertebral spongiosa: A sensitive method for detecting early bone loss after oophorectomy. *Ann Intern Med* 1982;**97:**699.

Health and Public Policy Committee, American College of Physicians: Radiologic methods to evaluate bone mineral content. *Ann Intern Med* 1984;**100:**908.

Krane SM, Schiller AL: Metabolic bone disease: Introduction and classification. Page 1511 in: *Endocrinology*, 2nd ed. Vol 2. DeGroot LJ et al (editors). Grune & Stratton, 1989.

Maluche HH, Faugere MC: *Atlas of Mineralized Bone Histology*. Karger, 1986.

Marcus R: Normal and abnormal bone remodeling in man. *Annu Rev Med* 1987;**38:**129.

Mazess RB: The noninvasive measurement of skeletal mass. Page 223 in: *Bone and Mineral Research Annual 1*. Peck WA (editor). Excerpta Medica, 1983.

Mazess RB, Barden HS: Single and dual-photon absorptiometry for bone measurement in osteoporosis. Pages 73–80 in: *Osteoporosis Update 1987*. Genant HK (editor). Univ of California Press, 1987.

Meunier PJ: Histomorphometry of the skeleton. Page 191 in: *Bone and Mineral Research Annual 1*. Peck WA (editor). Excerpta Medica, 1983.

Meunier PJ, Bersot C: Endocrine influences on bone cells and bone remodeling evaluated by clinical histomorphometry. Page 445 in: *Endocrinology of Calcium Metabolism*. Parson JA (editor). Raven Press, 1982.

Ott DM, Kilcoyne RF, Chesnut CH III: Ability of four different techniques of measuring bone mass to diagnose vertebral fractures in postmenopausal women. *J Bone Miner Res* 1987;**2**:201.

Parfitt AM: The cellular basis of bone turnover and bone loss. *Clin Orthop* 1977;**127**:236.

Rasmussen HR, Bordier PJ: *The Physiological and Cellular Basis of Metabolic Bone Disease*. Williams & Wilkins, 1974.

Rodan GA, Martin TJ: Role of osteoblasts in hormonal control of bone resorption: A hypothesis. *Calcif Tissue Int* 1981;**33**:349.

Osteomalacia

Dunningan MG et al: Acquired disorders of vitamin D metabolism. Page 125 in: *Calcium Disorders*. Heath DA, Marx SJ (editors). Butterworth, 1982.

Frame B, Parfitt AM: Osteomalacia: Current concepts. *Ann Intern Med* 1978;**89**:966.

Fraser D et al: Hyperparathyroidism as the cause of hyperaminoaciduria and phosphaturia in human vitamin D deficiency. *Pediatr Res* 1967;**1**:425.

Fraser D et al: Pathogenesis of hereditary vitamin D-dependent rickets: An inborn error of vitamin D metabolism involving defective conversion of 25-hydroxyvitamin D to 1α,25-dihydroxyvitamin D. *N Engl J Med* 1973;**289**:817.

Glorieux FH et al: Use of phosphate and vitamin D to prevent dwarfism and rickets in X-linked hypophosphatemia. *N Engl J Med* 1972;**287**:481.

Goldring SR, Krane SM: Disorders of calcification: Osteomalacia and rickets. Page 1165 in: *Endocrinology*, 2nd ed. Vol 2. DeGroot LJ et al (editors). Grune & Stratton, 1989.

Haddad JG Jr: Serum 25-hydroxycalciferol levels and bone mass in children on anticonvulsant therapy. *N Engl J Med* 1975;**292**:550.

Maclaren NK, Lifshitz F: Vitamin D-dependency rickets in institutionalized, mentally retarded children on long-term anti-convulsant therapy. 2. The response to 25-hydroxycholecalciferol and vitamin D. *Pediatr Res.* 1973;**7**:914.

Marel GM, McKenna MJ, Frame B: Osteomalacia. Page 335 in: *Bone and Mineral Research*. Vol 4. Peck WA (editor). Elsevier, 1986.

Morgan DB et al: The osteomalacia syndrome after stomach operations. *Q J Med* 1970;**39**:395.

Morris RC et al: Renal acidosis. *Kidney Int* 1972;**1**:332.

Nassin JR et al: The effects of vitamin D and gluten-free diet in idiopathic steatorrhea. *Q J Med* 1958;**28**:141.

Ryan EA, Reiss E: Oncogenic osteomalacia. *Am J Med* 1984;**77**:501.

Scriver CR et al: Hereditary rickets. Page 1 in: *Calcium Disorders*. Heath DA, Marx SJ (editors). Butterworth, 1982.

Stamp TCB, Round JM: Seasonal changes in human plasma levels of 25-hydroxyvitamin D. *Nature* 1974;**247**:563.

Steinbach HL, Noetzli M: Roentgen appearance of the skeleton in osteomalacia and rickets. *Am J Roentgenol Radium Ther Nucl Med* 1964;**91**:955.

Twenty-first Nestle Nutrition Workshop: Rickets. Buenos Aires, December 5–8, 1988; Velvy, Switzerland. [In press.]

Osteoporosis

Aloia JF et al: Prevention of involutional bone loss by exercise. *Ann Intern Med* 1978;**89**:356.

Arnaud CD: Osteoporosis. Chapter 23 in: *Diet and Health: Implications for Reducing Chronic Disease Risk*. National Academy Press, 1989.

Arnaud CD et al: On the role of parathyroid hormone in the osteoporosis of aging. Page 215 in: *Osteoporosis: Recent Advances in Pathogenesis and Treatment*. DeLuca HF et al (editors). University Park Press, 1981.

Auwerx J, Bouillon R: Mineral and bone metabolism in thyroid disease: A review. *Q J Med* 1986;**60**:737.

Avioli LV: Osteoporosis. Page 280 in: *Bone and Mineral Research Annual 1*. Peck WA (editor). Excerpta Medica, 1983.

Avioli LV (editor): *The Osteoporotic Syndrome: Detection, Prevention and Treatment*. Grune & Stratton, 1983.

Balsan S et al: Effects of long-term maintenance therapy with a new glucocorticoid, deflazacort, on mineral metabolism and statural growth. *Calcif Tissue Int* 1987;**40**:303.

Cann CE et al: Decreased spinal mineral content in amenorrheic women. *JAMA* 1984;**251**:626.

Christiansen C, Johansen JS, Riis BJ (editors): International symposium on osteoporosis. September 27–October 2, 1987; Aalborg, Denmark. Osteopress Aps, 1987.

Consensus Conference: Osteoporosis. *JAMA* 1984; **252**:799.

Cummings SR et al: Epidemiology of osteoporosis and osteoporotic fractures. *Epidemiol Rev* 1985;**7**:178.

DeLuca HF: The vitamin D endocrine system in health and disease. Page 41 in: *Nutrition in the Young and the Elderly*. Haller EW, Cotton GE (editors). Collamore Press, 1983.

Drinkwater BL et al: Bone mineral content of amenorrheic and eumenorrheic athletes. *N Engl J Med* 1984;**311**:277.

Ettinger B, Genant HK, Cann CE: Long-term estrogen replacement therapy prevents bone loss and fractures. *Ann Intern Med* 1985;**102**:319.

Genant HK (editor): *Osteoporosis Update 1987*. Univ of California Press, 1987.

Gennari C: Glucocorticoids and bone. Page 213 in: *Bone and Mineral Research*. Vol 3. Peck WA (editor). Elsevier, 1985.

Gordon GS, Picchi J, Roof BS: Antifracture efficacy of long-term estrogen for osteoporosis. *Trans Assoc Am Physicians* 1973;**86**:326.

Gruber HE et al: Long-term calcitonin therapy in postmenopausal osteoporosis. *Metabolism* 1984;**33**:295.

Heaney RP: Calcium, bone health and osteoporosis. Page

255 in: *Bone and Mineral Research*. Vol 4. Peck WA (editor). Elsevier, 1986.

Horsman A et al: The effect of estrogen dose on postmenopausal bone loss. *N Engl J Med* 1983;**309:**1405.

Ireland P, Fordtran JS: Effect of dietary calcium and age on jejunal calcium absorption in humans studied by intestinal perfusion. *J Clin Invest* 1973;**52:**2672.

Jee WS, Clark I: Glucocorticoid-induced osteoporosis. Page 331 in: *Osteoporosis: Recent Advances in Pathogenesis and Treatment*. DeLuca HF et al (editors). University Park Press, 1981.

Johnson CC Jr: Studies on prevention of age-related bone loss. Page 233 in: *Bone and Mineral Research*. Vol 3. Peck WA (editor). Elsevier, 1985.

Lindsay R et al: Long-term prevention of postmenopausal osteoporosis by estrogen. *Lancet* 1976;**2:**1038.

MacLaughlin J, Holick MF: Aging decreases the capacity of human skin to produce vitamin D_3. *J Clin Invest* 1985;**76:**1536.

Marcus R et al: Menstrual function and bone mass in elite women distance runners: Endocrine and metabolic features. *Ann Intern Med* 1985;**102:**158.

Nilas L, Christiansen C: Bone mass and its relationship to age and the menopause. *J Clin Endocrinol Metab* 1987;**65:**697.

Odell WD, Swerdloff RS: Male hypogonadism. *West J Med* 1976;**124:**446.

Parfitt AM et al: Vitamin D and bone health in the elderly. *Am J Clin Nutr* 1982;**36:**1014.

Paul TL et al: Long-term L-thyroxine therapy is associated with decreased hip bone density in premenopausal women. *JAMA* 1988;**259:**3137.

Peck WA: Corticosteroids and bone. *Calcif Tissue Int* 1984;**36:**4.

Reid IR et al: Prevention of steroid-induced osteoporosis with (3-amino-1-hydroxypropylidene)-1,1-bisphosphonate (APD). *Lancet* 1988;**1:**143.

Riggs BL: Osteoporosis. Page 1188 in: *Endocrinology*, 2nd ed. Vol 2. DeGroot LJ et al (editors). Grune & Stratton, 1989.

Riggs, BL: Treatment of osteoporosis with sodium fluoride: An appraisal. Page 366 in: *Bone and Mineral Research Annual 2*. Peck WA (editor). Elsevier, 1984.

Riggs BL, Melton LJ III: Evidence for two distinct syndromes of involutional osteoporosis. (Editorial.) *Am J Med* 1983;**75:**899.

Riggs BL, Melton LJ III: Involutional osteoporosis. *N Engl J Med* 1986;**314:**1676.

Riggs BL, Melton LJ III (editors): *Osteoporosis: Etiology, Diagnosis and Management*. Raven Press, 1988.

Riggs BL et al: Effect of the fluoride/calcium regimen on vertebral fracture occurrence in postmenopausal osteoporosis. *N Engl J Med* 1982;**306:**446.

Riggs BL et al: A syndrome of osteoporosis, increased parathyroid hormone and inappropriately low 1,25-dihydroxyvitamin D. *Mayo Clin Proc* 1978;**53:**701.

Rigotti NA et al: Osteoporosis in women with anorexia nervosa. *N Engl J Med* 1984;**311:**1601.

Riis B, Thomsen K, Christianssen C: Does calcium supplementation prevent postmenopausal bone loss? A double-blind, controlled clinical study. *N Engl J Med* 1987;**316:**173.

Seeman E et al: Risk factors for spinal osteoporosis in men. *Am J Med* 1983;**75:**977.

Singh M et al: Femoral trabecular pattern index for evaluation of spinal osteoporosis. *Ann Intern Med* 1972;**77:**63.

Slovik DM et al: Restoration of spinal bone in osteoporotic men by treatment with human parathyroid hormone (1–34) and 1,25-dihydroxyvitamin D. *J Bone Miner Res* **1986;1:**377.

Tsai K-S et al: Impaired vitamin D metabolism with aging in women: Possible role in pathogenesis of senile osteoporosis. *J Clin Invest* 1984;**73:**1668.

Weisman Y et al: Inadequate status and impaired metabolism of vitamin D in the elderly. *Isr J Med Sci* 1981;**17:**19.

Paget's Disease

Altman RD, Collins-Yudiskas B: Synthetic human calcitonin in refractory Paget's disease of bone. *Arch Intern Med* 1987;**147:**1305.

Arnold A: Paget's disease of bone: Pathophysiology and diagnosis. Page 1208 in: *Endocrinology,* 2nd ed. Vol 2. DeGroot LJ et al (editors). Grune & Stratton, 1989.

Avioli LV: Paget's disease: State of the art. *Clin Ther* 1987;**9:**567.

Cawley MI: Complications of Paget's disease of bone. *Gerontology* 1983;**29:**276.

Delmas PD et al: Beneficial effects of aminohexane diphosphonate in patients with Paget's disease of bone resistant to sodium etidronate. *Am J Med* 1987;**83:**276.

Fleish H: Bisphosphonates: Mechanisms of action and clinical applications. Page 319 in: *Bone and Mineral Research Annual 1*. Peck WA (editor). Excerpta Medica, 1983.

Freeman DA: Paget's disease of bone. *Am J Med Sci* 1988;**295:**144.

Huvos AG et al: Osteogenic sarcoma associated with Paget's disease of bone: A clinicopathologic study of 65 patients. *Cancer* 1983;**52:**1489.

Krane SM: Paget's disease of bone. *Calcif Tissue Res* 1986;**38:**309.

Rebel A (editor): Symposium: Paget's disease. *Clin Orthop* (April) 1987;**217:**2. [Entire issue.]

Singer FR: *Paget's Disease of Bone*. Plenum Press, 1977.

Singer FR, Mills BG: Evidence for a viral etiology of Paget's disease of bone. *Clin Orthop* 1983;**178:**245.

Singer FR, Mills BG: Paget's disease of bone: Etiology and therapeutic aspects. Page 394 in: *Bone and Mineral Research Annual 2*. Peck WA (editor). Elsevier, 1984.

Strewler GJ: Paget's disease of bone. *West J Med* 1984;**140:**763.

Wallach S: Treatment of Paget's disease. *Adv Intern Med* 1982;**27:**1.

Glucocorticoids & Adrenal Androgens | 12

J. Blake Tyrrell, MD, David C. Aron, MD, & Peter H. Forsham, MD

The adrenal cortex produces many steroid hormones of which the most important are cortisol, aldosterone, and the adrenal androgens. Disorders of the adrenal glands lead to classic endocrinopathies such as Cushing's syndrome, Addison's disease, hyperaldosteronism, and the syndromes of congenital adrenal hyperplasia. This chapter describes the physiology and disorders of the glucocorticoids and the adrenal androgens. Disorders of aldosterone secretion are discussed in Chapter 13 and congenital defects in adrenal hormone biosynthesis in Chapters 13 and 18.

Advances in diagnostic procedures have simplified the evaluation of adrenocortical disorders; in particular, the assay of plasma glucocorticoids, androgens, and ACTH has allowed more rapid and precise diagnosis. In addition, advances in surgical and medical treatment have improved the outlook for patients with these disorders.

EMBRYOLOGY & ANATOMY

Embryology

The adrenal cortex is of mesodermal origin and is identifiable as a separate organ in the 2-month-old fetus. At 2 months' gestation, the cortex is composed of a **fetal zone** and a **definitive zone** similar to the adult adrenal cortex. The adrenal cortex then increases rapidly in size; at mid gestation, it is considerably larger than the kidney and much larger than the adult gland in relation to total body mass. The fetal zone makes up the bulk of the weight of the adrenal cortex at this time. Factors other than ACTH, such as insulin-like growth factor II, may be involved in the development of the fetal adrenal cortex.

The fetal adrenal is under the control of ACTH by mid pregnancy, but the fetal zone is deficient in the activity of 3β-hydroxysteroid dehydrogenase (see section on biosynthesis of cortisol and adrenal androgens, below) and thus produces mainly dehydroepiandrosterone (DHEA) and DHEA sulfate, which serve as precursors of maternal-placental estrogen production after conversion in the liver to 16α-hydroxylated derivatives. The definitive zone synthesizes a number of steroids and is the major site of fetal cortisol synthesis.

Acronyms Used in This Chapter

ACTH	Adrenocorticotropic hormone
ADH	Antidiuretic hormone (vasopressin)
cAMP	Cyclic adenosine monophosphate
CBG	Corticosteroid-binding globulin
CRH	Corticotropin-releasing hormone
DHEA	Dehydroepiandrosterone
DNA	Deoxyribonucleic acid
DOC	Deoxycorticosterone
GH	Growth hormone
GnRH	Gonadotropin-releasing hormone
HLA	Human leukocyte antigen
LH	Luteinizing hormone
LPH	Lipotropin
mRNA	Messenger ribonucleic acid
NADPH	Dihydronicotinamide adenine dinucleotide phosphate
P-450scc	Side-chain cleavage enzyme
PMN	Polymorphonuclear neutrophil
PRL	Prolactin
PTH	Parathyroid hormone
REM	Rapid eye movement
RNA	Ribonucleic acid
SHBG	Sex hormone-binding globulin
TRH	Thyrotropin-releasing hormone
TSH	Thyroid-stimulating hormone (thyrotropin)

Anatomy

The anatomic relationship of the fetal and definitive zones is maintained until birth, at which time the fetal zone gradually disappears, with a consequent decrease in adrenocortical weight in the 3 months following delivery. During the next 3 years, the adult adrenal cortex develops from cells of the outer layer of the cortex and differentiates into the 3 adult zones: glomerulosa, fasciculata, and reticularis.

The adult adrenal glands, with a combined weight of 8–10 g, lie in the retroperitoneum above or medial to the upper poles of the kidneys (Fig 12–1). A fibrous capsule surrounds the gland; the yellowish outer cortex comprises 90% of the adrenal weight, the inner medulla about 10%.

The adrenal cortex is richly vascularized and receives its main arterial supply from branches of the

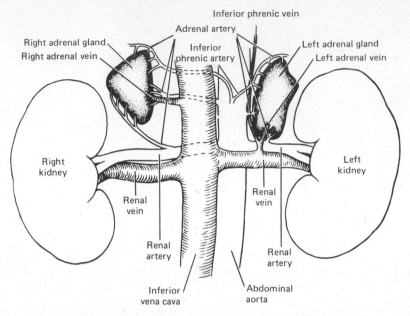

Figure 12–1. Location and blood supply of the adrenal glands (schematic). (Reproduced, with permission, from Baxter JD, Tyrrell JB: The adrenal cortex. In: *Endocrinology and Metabolism*. Felig P et al [editors]. 2nd ed. McGraw-Hill, 1987.)

inferior phrenic artery, the renal arteries, and the aorta. These small arteries form an arterial plexus beneath the capsule and then enter a sinusoidal system that penetrates the cortex and medulla, draining into a single central vein in each gland. The right adrenal vein drains directly into the posterior aspect of the vena cava; the left adrenal vein enters the left renal vein. These anatomic features account for the fact that it is relatively easier to catheterize the left adrenal vein than it is to catheterize the right adrenal vein.

Microscopic Anatomy

Histologically, the adult cortex is composed of 3 zones: an outer zona glomerulosa, a zona fasciculata, and an inner zona reticularis (Fig 12–2). However, the inner 2 zones appear to function as a unit (see below). The **zona glomerulosa,** which produces aldosterone, is deficient in 17α-hydroxylase activity and thus cannot produce cortisol or androgens (see below and Chapter 13). The zona glomerulosa lacks a well-defined structure, and the small lipid-poor cells are scattered beneath the adrenal capsule. The **zona fasciculata** is the thickest layer of the adrenal cortex and produces cortisol and androgens. The cells of the zona fasciculata are larger and contain more lipid and thus are termed "clear cells." These cells extend in columns from the narrow zona reticularis to either the zona glomerulosa or to the capsule. The inner **zona reticularis** surrounds the medulla and also produces cortisol and androgens. The "compact" cells of this narrow zone lack significant lipid content but do contain lipofuscin granules. The zonae fasciculata and re-

ticularis are regulated by ACTH; excess or deficiency of this hormone alters their structure and function. Thus, both zones atrophy when ACTH is deficient; when ACTH is present in excess, hyperplasia and hypertrophy of these zones occur. In addition, chronic stimulation with ACTH leads to a gradual depletion of the lipid from the clear cells of the zona fasciculata at the junction of the 2 zones; these cells thus attain the characteristic appearance of the compact reticularis cells. With chronic excessive stimulation, the compact reticularis cells extend outward and may reach the outer capsule. It is postulated that the zona fasciculata cells can respond acutely to ACTH stimulation with increased cortisol production, whereas the reticularis cells maintain basal glucocorticoid secretion and that induced by prolonged ACTH stimulation.

BIOSYNTHESIS OF CORTISOL & ADRENAL ANDROGENS

Steroidogenesis

The major hormones secreted by the adrenal cortex are cortisol, the androgens, and aldosterone. The carbon atoms in the steroid molecule are numbered as shown in Figure 12–3, and the major biosynthetic pathways and hormonal intermediates are illustrated in Figures 12–4 and 12–5.

The scheme of adrenal steroidogenic synthesis has been clarified by analysis of the steroidogenic enzymes. Most of these enzymes belong to the family of cytochrome P-450 oxygenases. In mitochondria,

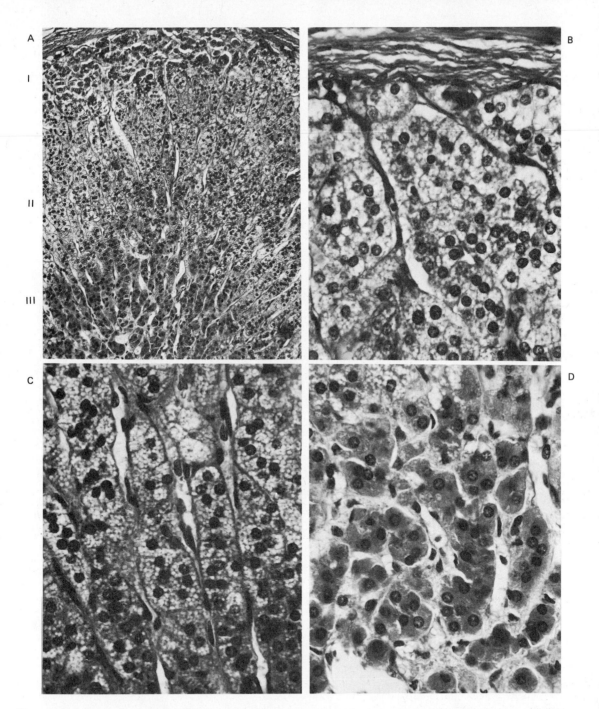

Figure 12–2. Photomicrographs of the adrenal cortex (H&E stain). *A:* A low-power general view. I, the glomerulosa; II, the fasciculata; III, the reticularis. × 80. *B:* The capsule and the zona glomerulosa. × 330. *C:* The zona fasciculata. × 330. *D:* The zona reticularis. × 330. (Reproduced, with permission, from Junqueira LC, Carneiro J: *Basic Histology,* 6th ed. (Appleton & Lange, 1989.)

P-450 is responsible for side-chain cleavage of cholesterol, while the single enzyme, P-450c11 mediates 3 activities: 11 β-hydroxylase, 18-hydroxylase, and 18 methyl-oxidase (aldehyde synthetase). In the endoplasmic reticulum the single enzyme P-450c17 mediates both 17α-hydroxylase activity and 17,20-lyase activity, while P-450c21 mediates the 21-hydroxylation of both progesterone and 17-hydroxyprogesterone. The 3β-hydroxysteroid dehydrogenase and Δ5-Δ4 isomerase enzymes are non-P-450 enzymes.

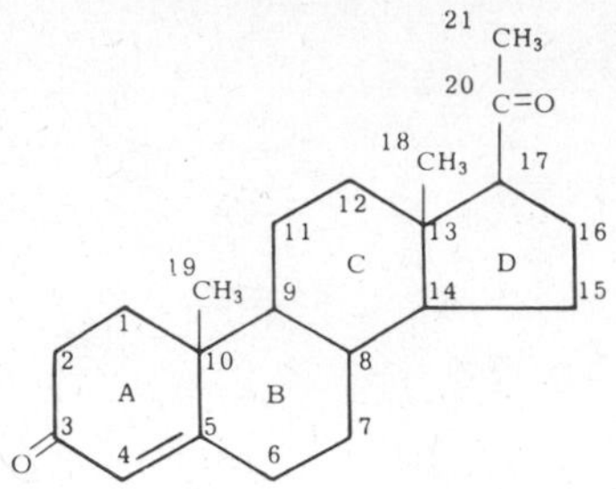

C21 steroid (progesterone)

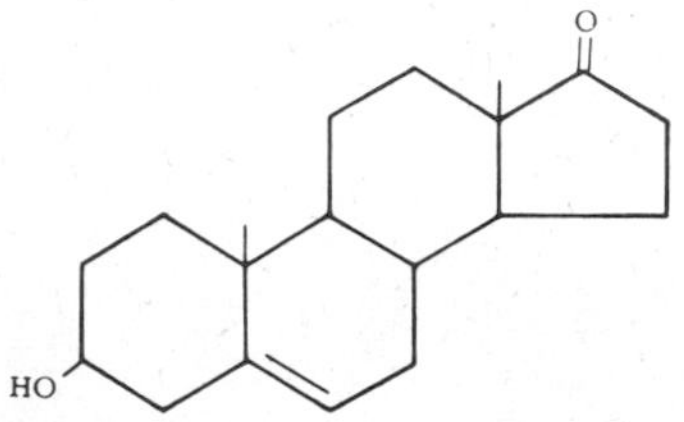

C19 steroid (dehydroepiandrosterone)

Figure 12–3. Structure of adrenocortical steroids. The letters in the formula for progesterone identify the A, B, C, and D rings; the numbers show the positions in the basic C21 steroid structure. The angular methyl groups (positions 18 and 19) are usually indicated simply by straight lines, as in the lower formula. Dehydroepiandrosterone is a "17-ketosteroid" formed by cleavage of the side chain of the C21 steroid 17-hydroxypregnenolone and its replacement by an O atom. (Reproduced, with permission, from Ganong WF: *Review of Medical Physiology,* 14th ed. Appleton & Lange, 1989.)

A. Zones and Steroidogenesis: Because of enzymatic differences between the zona glomerulosa and the inner 2 zones, the adrenal cortex functions as 2 separate units, with differing regulation and secretory products. Thus, the zona glomerulosa, which produces aldosterone, lacks 17α-hydroxylase activity and cannot synthesize 17α-hydroxypregnenolone and 17α-hydroxyprogesterone, which are the precursors of cortisol and the adrenal androgens. The synthesis of aldosterone by this zone is primarily regulated by the renin-angiotensin system and by potassium, as discussed in Chapter 13.

The zona fasciculata and zona reticularis (Fig 12–4) produce cortisol, androgens, and small amounts of estrogens. These zones, primarily regulated by ACTH, do not contain the enzymatic system necessary to dehydrogenate 18-hydroxycorticosterone and thus do not synthesize aldosterone. (See Chapter 13.)

B. Cholesterol Uptake and Synthesis: Synthesis of cortisol and the androgens by the zonae fasciculata and reticularis begins with cholesterol, as does the synthesis of all steroid hormones. Plasma lipoproteins are the major source of adrenal cholesterol, though synthesis within the gland from acetate also

occurs. A small pool of free cholesterol within the adrenal is available for rapid synthesis of steroids when the adrenal is stimulated. When stimulation occurs, there is also increased hydrolysis of stored cholesteryl esters to free cholesterol, increased uptake from plasma lipoproteins, and increased cholesterol synthesis within the gland.

C. Cholesterol Metabolism: The conversion of cholesterol to pregnenolone is the rate-limiting step in adrenal steroidogenesis and the major site of ACTH action on the adrenal. This step occurs in the mitochondria and involves 2 hydroxylations and then the side-chain cleavage of cholesterol. A single enzyme, P-450scc, mediates this process; each step requires molecular oxygen and a pair of electrons. The latter are donated by NADPH to adrenodoxin reductase, a flavoprotein, and then to adrenodoxin, an iron-sulfur protein, and finally to P-450scc. Both adrenodoxin reductase and adrenodoxin are also involved in the action of P-450c11 (see above). Electron transport to microsomal cytochrome P-450 involves P-450 reductase, a flavoprotein distinct from adrenodoxin reductase. Pregnenolone is then transported outside the mitochondria before further steroid synthesis occurs.

D. Synthesis of Cortisol: Cortisol synthesis proceeds by P-450c17 17α-hydroxylation of pregnenolone within the smooth endoplasmic reticulum to form 17α-hydroxypregnenolone. This steroid is then converted to 17α-hydroxyprogesterone after conversion of its 5,6 double bond to a 4,5 double bond by the 3β-hydroxysteroid dehydrogenase Δ^5-Δ^4-oxosteroid isomerase enzyme complex, which is also located within the smooth endoplasmic reticulum. An alternative but apparently less important pathway in the zonae fasciculata and reticularis is from pregnenolone → progesterone → 17α-hydroxyprogesterone (Fig 12–4).

The next step, which is again microsomal, involves the 21-hydroxylation by P-450c21 of 17α-hydroxyprogesterone to form 11-deoxycortisol; this compound is further hydroxylated within mitochondria by 11β-hydroxylation (P-450c11) to form cortisol. The zonae fasciculata and reticularis also produce 11-deoxycorticosterone (DOC), 18-hydroxydeoxycorticosterone, corticosterone, and 18-hydroxycorticosterone. However, as noted above, the absence of mitochondrial 18-hydroxysteroid dehydrogenase prevents production of aldosterone by these zones of the adrenal cortex (Fig 12–5).

E. Synthesis of Androgens: The production of adrenal androgens from pregnenolone and progesterone requires prior 17α-hydroxylation (P-450c17) and thus does not occur in the zona glomerulosa. The major quantitative production of androgens is by conversion of 17α-hydroxypregnenolone to the 19-carbon compounds (C19 steroids) DHEA and its sulfate conjugate DHEA sulfate. Thus, 17α-hydroxypregnenolone undergoes removal of its 2-carbon side chain at the C17 position by micro-

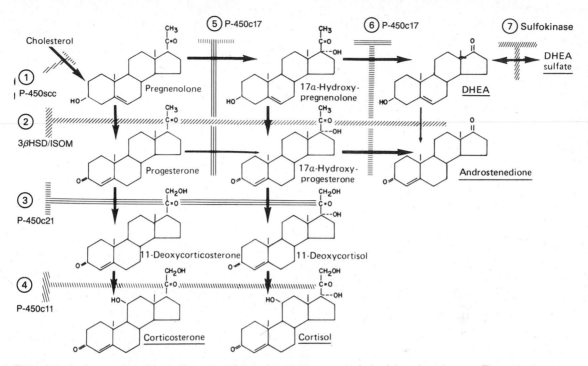

Figure 12–4. Steroid biosynthesis in the zona fasciculata and zona reticularis of the adrenal cortex. The major secretory products are underlined. The enzymes for the reactions are numbered on the left and at the top of the chart, with the steps catalyzed shown by the shaded bars. ① P-450scc = Cholesterol 20,22-hydroxylase:20,22 desmolase activity; ② 3βHSD/ISOM = 3β-hydroxysteroid dehydrogenase: Δ^5-oxosteroid isomerase activity; ③ P-450c21 = 21α-hydroxylase activity; ④ P-450c11 = 11β-hydroxylase activity; ⑤ P-450c17 = 17α-hydroxylase activity; ⑥ P-450c17 = 17,20-lyase/desmolase activity; ⑦ Sulfokinase. (See also Figs 16–2, 18–13, and 18–14.) (Modified and reproduced, with permission, from Ganong, WF: *Review of Medical Physiology,* 14th ed. Appleton & Lange, 1989.)

somal 17,20-desmolase, yielding DHEA with a keto group at C17. DHEA is then converted to DHEA sulfate by a reversible adrenal sulfokinase. The other major adrenal androgen, androstenedione, is produced from 17α-hydroxyprogesterone by 17,20-desmolase and to a lesser extent from DHEA. Androstenedione can be converted to testosterone, though adrenal secretion of this hormone is minimal. The adrenal androgens, DHEA, DHEA sulfate, and androstenedione, have minimal intrinsic androgenic activity, and they contribute to androgenicity by their peripheral conversion to the more potent androgens testosterone and dihydrotestosterone. Although DHEA and DHEA sulfate are secreted in greater quantities, androstenedione is qualitatively more important, since it is more readily converted peripherally to testosterone.

Regulation of Secretion

A. Secretion of CRH and ACTH: ACTH is the trophic hormone of the zonae fasciculata and reticularis and the major regulator of cortisol and androgen production by the adrenal cortex. ACTH in turn is regulated by the hypothalamus and central nervous system via neurotransmitters and corticotropin-releasing hormone (CRH). The neuroendocrine control of

CRH and ACTH secretion is discussed in Chapters 5 and 6 and involves 3 mechanisms to be discussed below.

B. ACTH Effects on the Adrenal Cortex: The delivery of ACTH to the adrenal cortex leads to the rapid synthesis and secretion of steroids; plasma levels of these hormones rise within minutes after ACTH administration. ACTH increases RNA, DNA, and protein synthesis. Chronic stimulation leads to adrenocortical hyperplasia and hypertrophy; conversely, ACTH deficiency results in decreased steroidogenesis and is accompanied by adrenocortical atrophy, decreased gland weight, and decreased protein and nucleic acid content.

C. ACTH and Steroidogenesis: ACTH binds to high-affinity plasma membrane receptors of adrenocortical cells, thereby activating adenylate cyclase and increasing cAMP, which in turn activates intracellular phosphoprotein kinases (Fig 12–6). This process stimulates the rate-limiting step of cholesterol to Δ^5-pregnenolone conversion and initiates steroidogenesis. The exact mechanisms of ACTH stimulation of the side-chain cleavage enzyme (P-450scc) are unknown, as is their relative importance; however, ACTH has a number of effects, including increased free cholesterol formation as a consequence of in-

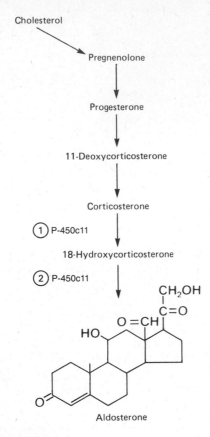

Figure 12–5. Steroid biosynthesis in the zona glomerulosa. The steps from cholesterol to corticosterone are the same as in the zona fasciculata and zona reticularis. However, the zona glomerulosa lacks 17α-hydroxylase activity and only the zona glomerulosa can convert 18-hydroxycorticosterone to aldosterone. ① P-450c11 = Corticosterone methyloxidase I activity; ② P-450c11 = Corticosterone methyloxidase II activity. (See also Figs 16–2, 18–13, and 18–14.) (Modified and reproduced, with permission, from Ganong, WF: *Review of Medical Physiology,* 14th ed. Appleton & Lange, 1989.)

creased cholesterol esterase activity and decreased cholesteryl ester synthetase; increased lipoprotein uptake by the adrenal cortex; increased content of certain phospholipids, which may increase cholesterol side-chain cleavage; and increased binding of cholesterol to the cytochrome P-450scc enzyme in mitochondria.

D. Neuroendocrine Control: Cortisol secretion is closely regulated by ACTH, and plasma cortisol levels parallel those of ACTH (Fig 12–7). There are 3 mechanisms of neuroendocrine control: (1) episodic secretion and the circadian rhythm of ACTH, (2) stress responsiveness of the hypothalamic-pituitary adrenal axis, and (3) feedback inhibition by cortisol of ACTH secretion.

1. Circadian rhythm–Circadian rhythm is superimposed on episodic secretion; it is the result of central nervous system events that regulate both the number

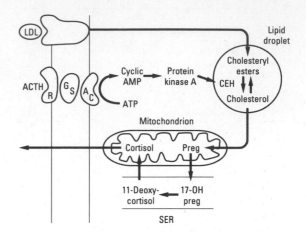

Figure 12–6. Mechanism of action of ACTH on cortisol-secreting cells in the inner 2 zones of the adrenal cortex. When ACTH binds to its receptor (R), adenylate cyclase (AC) is activated via G_s. The resulting increase in cyclic AMP activates protein kinase A, and the kinase phosphorylates cholesterol ester hydrolase (CEH), increasing its activity. Consequently, more free cholesterol is formed and converted to pregnenolone in the mitochondria. Note that in the subsequent steps in steroid biosynthesis, products are shuttled between the mitochondria and the smooth endoplasmic reticulum (SER). (Reproduced, with permission, from Ganong WF: *Review of Medical Physiology,* 14th ed. Appleton & Lange, 1989.)

and magnitude of CRH and ACTH secretory episodes. Cortisol secretion is low in the late evening and continues to decline in the first several hours of sleep, at which time plasma cortisol levels may be undetectable. During the third and fifth hours of sleep, there is an increase in secretion; but the major secretory episodes

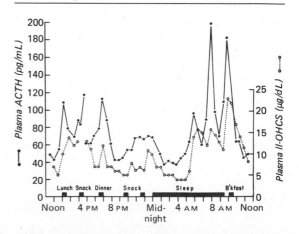

Figure 12–7. Fluctuations in plasma ACTH and glucocorticoids (11-OHCS) throughout the day. Note the greater ACTH and glucocorticoid rises in the morning before awakening. (Reproduced, with permission, from Krieger DT et al: *J Clin Endocrinol Metab* 1971;**32**:266.)

begin in the sixth to eighth hours of sleep (Fig 12–7) and then begin to decline as wakefulness occurs. About half of the total daily cortisol output is secreted during this period. Cortisol secretion then gradually declines during the day, with fewer secretory episodes of decreased magnitude; however, there is increased cortisol secretion in response to eating and exercise.

Although this general pattern is consistent, there is considerable intra- and interindividual variability, and the circadian rhythm may be altered by changes in sleep pattern, light-dark exposure, and feeding times. The rhythm is also changed by (1) physical stresses such as major illness, surgery or trauma, or starvation; (2) psychologic stress, including severe anxiety, endogenous depression, and the manic phase of manic-depressive psychosis; (3) central nervous system and pituitary disorders; (4) Cushing's syndrome; (5) liver disease and other conditions that affect cortisol metabolism; (6) chronic renal failure; and (7) alcoholism. Cyproheptadine inhibits the circadian rhythm, possibly by its antiserotoninergic effects, whereas other drugs usually have no effect.

2. Stress responsiveness–Plasma ACTH and cortisol secretion are also characteristically responsive to physical stress. Thus, plasma ACTH and cortisol are secreted within minutes following the onset of stresses such as surgery and hypoglycemia (Fig 12–8), and these responses abolish circadian periodicity if the stress is prolonged. Stress responses originate in the central nervous system and increase hypothalamic CRH and thus pituitary ACTH secretion. Stress responsiveness of plasma ACTH and cortisol is abolished by prior high-dose glucocorticoid administration and in spontaneous Cushing's syndrome; conversely, the responsiveness of ACTH secretion is enhanced following adrenalectomy.

3. Feedback inhibition–The third major regulator of ACTH and cortisol secretion is that of feedback inhibition by glucocorticoids of CRH, ACTH, and cortisol secretion. Glucocorticoid feedback inhibition occurs at both the pituitary and hypothalamus and involves 2 distinct mechanisms—fast and delayed feedback inhibition (Fig 12–9).

Fast feedback inhibition of ACTH secretion is rate-dependent; ie, it depends on the rate of increase of the glucocorticoid but not the dose administered. This phase is rapid, and basal and stimulated ACTH secretion both diminish within minutes after the plasma glucocorticoid level increases. This fast feedback phase is transient and lasts less than 10 minutes, suggesting that this effect is not mediated via cytosolic glucocorticoid receptors but rather via actions on the cell membrane.

Delayed feedback inhibition after the initial rate-dependent effects of glucocorticoids further suppresses CRH and ACTH secretion by mechanisms that are both time- and dose-dependent. Thus, with continued glucocorticoid administration, ACTH levels continue to decrease and become unresponsive to stimulation. The ultimate effect of prolonged glucocorticoid administration is suppression of CRH and ACTH release and atrophy of the zonae fasciculata and reticularis as a consequence of ACTH deficiency. The suppressed hypothalamic-pituitary-adrenal axis fails to respond to stress and stimulation. Delayed feedback appears to act via the classic glucocorticoid receptor (see below), thus reducing synthesis of the messenger

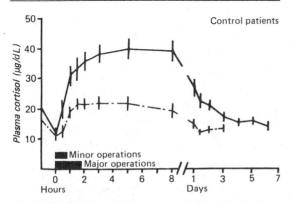

Figure 12–8. Plasma cortisol responses to major surgery (continuous line) and minor surgery (broken line) in normal subjects. Mean values and standard errors for 20 patients are shown in each case. (Reproduced, with permission, from Plumpton FS, Besser GM, Cole PV: *Anaesthesia* 1969;**24**:3).

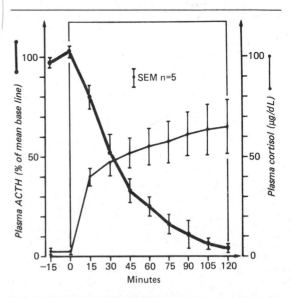

Figure 12–9. Feedback inhibition of plasma ACTH levels during intravenous cortisol infusion at a rate of 50 mg/h in patients with Addison's disease. ACTH values are expressed as percentages of mean basal levels. (Reproduced, with permission, from Fehm HL et al: *J Clin Invest* 1979;**63**:247.)

RNA for pro-opiomelanocortin, the precursor of ACTH.

E. ACTH Effects on Regulation of Androgen Production: Adrenal androgen production in adults is also regulated by ACTH; both DHEA and androstenedione exhibit circadian periodicity in concert with ACTH and cortisol. In addition, plasma concentrations of DHEA and androstenedione increase rapidly with ACTH administration and are suppressed by glucocorticoid administration, confirming the role of endogenous ACTH in their secretion. DHEA sulfate, because of its prolonged metabolic clearance rate, does not exhibit a diurnal rhythm. Thus, adrenal androgen secretion is regulated by ACTH, and, in general, the secretion of these hormones parallels that of cortisol. The existence of a separate anterior pituitary hormone that regulates adrenal androgen secretion has been postulated but not yet proved.

CIRCULATION OF CORTISOL & ADRENAL ANDROGENS

Cortisol and the adrenal androgens circulate bound to plasma proteins. The plasma half-life of cortisol (70–90 minutes) is determined by the extent of plasma binding and by the rate of metabolic inactivation.

Plasma Binding Proteins

Cortisol and adrenal androgens are secreted in an unbound state; however, these hormones bind to plasma proteins upon entering the circulation. Cortisol binds mainly to corticosteroid-binding globulin (CBG, transcortin) and to a lesser extent to albumin, whereas the androgens bind chiefly to albumin. The precise physiologic role of plasma protein binding is unclear, since bound steroids are biologically inactive and the active fraction is that which circulates unbound. Furthermore, CBG is not required for cortisol transport to target tissues or for full biologic activity of the steroid. The plasma proteins may provide a pool of circulating cortisol by delaying metabolic clearance, thus preventing more marked fluctuations of plasma free cortisol levels during episodic secretion by the gland.

Free & Bound Cortisol

In basal conditions, about 10% of the circulating cortisol is free, about 75% is bound to CBG, and the remainder is bound to albumin. The plasma free cortisol level is approximately 1 μg/dL, and it is this biologically active cortisol which is regulated by ACTH.

A. Corticosteroid-Binding Globulin (CBG): CBG has a molecular weight of about 50,000, is produced by the liver, and binds cortisol with high affinity. The CBG in plasma has a cortisol-binding capacity of about 25 μg/dL. When total plasma cortisol concentrations rise above this level, the free concentration rapidly increases and exceeds its usual fraction of 10%

of the total cortisol. Other endogenous steroids do not appreciably affect cortisol binding to CBG under usual circumstances; an exception is in late pregnancy, when progesterone may occupy about 25% of the binding sites on CBG. Synthetic steroids do not bind significantly to CBG—with the exception of prednisolone, which has a high affinity. CBG levels are increased in high-estrogen states (pregnancy; estrogen or oral contraceptive use), hyperthyroidism, diabetes, certain hematologic disorders, and on a genetic basis. CBG concentrations are decreased in familial CBG deficiency, hypothyroidism, and protein deficiency states such as severe liver disease or nephrotic syndrome.

B. Albumin: Albumin has a much greater capacity for cortisol binding but a lower affinity. It normally binds about 15% of the circulating cortisol, and this proportion increases when the total cortisol concentration exceeds the CBG binding capacity. Synthetic glucocorticoids are extensively bound to albumin; eg, 77% of dexamethasone in plasma is bound to albumin.

C. Androgen Binding: Androstenedione, DHEA, and DHEA sulfate circulate weakly bound to albumin. However, testosterone is bound extensively to a specific globulin, sex hormone–binding globulin (SHBG). (See Chapters 16 and 17.)

METABOLISM OF CORTISOL & ADRENAL ANDROGENS

The metabolism of the steroids renders them inactive and increases their water solubility, as does their subsequent conjugation with glucuronide or sulfate groups. These inactive conjugated metabolites are more readily excreted by the kidney. The liver is the major site of steroid catabolism and conjugation, and 90% of these metabolized steroids are excreted by the kidney.

Conversion & Excretion of Cortisol

Cortisol is modified extensively before excretion in urine; less than 1% of secreted cortisol appears in the urine unchanged.

A. Hepatic Conversion: Hepatic metabolism of cortisol involves a number of metabolic conversions of which the most important (quantitatively) is the irreversible inactivation of the steroid by Δ^4-reductases, which reduce the 4,5 double bond of the A ring. Dihydrocortisol, the product of this reaction, is then converted to tetrahydrocortisol by a 3-hydroxysteroid dehydrogenase. Cortisol is also converted extensively to biologically inactive cortisone, which is then metabolized by the enzymes described above to yield tetrahydrocortisone. Tetrahydrocortisol and tetrahydrocortisone can be further altered to form the cortoic acids. These conversions result in the excretion of approximately equal amounts of cortisol and cortisone metabolites. Cortisol and cortisone are also metabo-

lease of glycerol and free fatty acids. This is partially due to direct stimulation of lipolysis by glucocorticoids, but it is also contributed to by decreased glucose uptake and enhancement by glucocorticoids of the effects of lipolytic hormones. Although glucocorticoids are lipolytic, increased fat deposition is a classic manifestation of glucocorticoid excess. This paradox may be explained by the increased appetite caused by high levels of these steroids and by the lipogenic effects of the hyperinsulinemia that occurs in this state. The reason for abnormal fat deposition in states of cortisol excess is unknown. In these instances, fat is classically deposited centrally in the face, cervical area, trunk, and abdomen; the extremities are usually spared.

D. Summary: The effects of the glucocorticoids on intermediary metabolism can be summarized as follows: (1) Effects are minimal in the fed state. However, during fasting, glucocorticoids contribute to the maintenance of plasma glucose levels by increasing gluconeogenesis, glycogen deposition, and the peripheral release of substrate. (2) Hepatic glucose production is enhanced, as is hepatic RNA and protein synthesis. (3) The effects on muscle are catabolic, ie, decreased glucose uptake and metabolism, decreased protein synthesis, and increased release of amino acids. (4) In adipose tissue, lipolysis is stimulated. (5) In glucocorticoid deficiency, hypoglycemia may result, whereas in states of glucocorticoid excess there may be hyperglycemia, hyperinsulinemia, muscle wasting, and weight gain with abnormal fat distribution.

Effects on Other Tissues & Functions

A. Connective Tissue: Glucocorticoids in excess inhibit fibroblasts, lead to loss of collagen and connective tissue, and thus result in thinning of the skin, easy bruising, stria formation, and poor wound healing.

B. Bone: The physiologic role of glucocorticoids in bone metabolism and calcium homeostasis is unknown; however, in excess, they have major deleterious effects. Glucocorticoids directly inhibit bone formation by decreasing cell proliferation and the synthesis of RNA, protein, collagen, and hyaluronate. Glucocorticoids also directly stimulate bone-resorbing cells, leading to osteolysis and increased urinary hydroxyproline excretion. In addition, they potentiate the actions of PTH and 1,25-dihydroxycholecalciferol $(1,25[OH]_2D_3)$ on bone, and this may further contribute to net bone resorption.

C. Calcium Metabolism: Glucocorticoids also have other major effects on mineral homeostasis. They markedly reduce intestinal calcium absorption, which tends to lower serum calcium. This results in a secondary increase in PTH secretion, which maintains serum calcium within the normal range by stimulating bone resorption. In addition, glucocorticoids may directly stimulate PTH release. The mechanism of decreased intestinal calcium absorption is unknown, though recent studies have shown that it is not due to decreased synthesis or decreased serum levels of the active vitamin D metabolites; in fact, $1,25(OH)_2D_3$ levels are normal or even increased in the presence of glucocorticoid excess. Increased $1,25 (OH)_2D_3$ synthesis in this setting may result from decreased serum phosphorus levels (see below), increased PTH levels, and direct stimulation by glucocorticoids of renal 1α-hydroxylase. Glucocorticoids also increase urinary calcium excretion, and hypercalciuria is a consistent feature of cortisol excess. They also reduce the tubular reabsorption of phosphate, leading to phosphaturia and decreased serum phosphorus concentrations.

Thus, glucocorticoids in excess result in negative calcium balance, with decreased absorption and increased urinary excretion. Serum calcium levels are maintained, but at the expense of net bone resorption. Decreased bone formation and increased resorption ultimately result in the disabling osteopenia that is often a major complication of spontaneous and iatrogenic glucocorticoid excess (see Chapter 11).

D. Growth and Development: Glucocorticoids accelerate the development of a number of systems and organs in fetal and differentiating tissues, although the mechanisms are unclear. As discussed above, glucocorticoids are generally inhibitory, and these stimulatory effects may be due to glucocorticoid interactions with other growth factors. Examples of these development-promoting effects are increased surfactant production in the fetal lung and the accelerated development of hepatic and gastrointestinal enzyme systems.

Glucocorticoids in excess inhibit growth in children, and this adverse effect is a major complication of therapy. This may be a direct effect on bone cells, although decreased growth hormone (GH) secretion and somatomedin generation also contribute (see Chapter 8).

E. Blood Cells and Immunologic Function:

1. Erythrocytes–Glucocorticoids have little effect on erythropoiesis and hemoglobin concentration. Although mild polycythemia and anemia may be seen in Cushing's syndrome and Addison's disease, respectively, these alterations are more likely to be secondary to altered androgen metabolism.

2. Leukocytes–Glucocorticoids influence both leukocyte movement and function. Thus, glucocorticoid administration increases the number of intravascular polymorphonuclear leukocytes by increasing PMN release from bone marrow, by increasing the circulating half-life of PMNs, and by decreasing PMN movement out of the vascular compartment. Glucocorticoid administration reduces the number of circulating lymphocytes, monocytes, and eosinophils, mainly by increasing their movement out of the circulation. The converse—ie, neutropenia, lymphocytosis, monocytosis, and eosinophilia—is seen in adrenal insufficiency. Glucocorticoids also decrease the migration of inflammatory cells (PMNs, monocytes, and lymphocytes) to sites of injury, and this is probably a major mechanism of the anti-inflammatory actions and increased susceptibility to infection that occur following chronic administration. Glucocorticoids also decrease lymphocyte production and the mediator and effector functions of these cells.

3. Immunologic effects–Glucocorticoids influence multiple aspects of immunologic and inflammatory responsiveness, including the mobilization and function of leukocytes, as discussed above. They also impair release of effector substances such as the lymphokine interleukin-I, antigen processing, antibody production and clearance, and other specific bone marrow–derived and thymus-derived lymphocyte functions. The immune system, in turn, affects the hypothalamic-pituitary-adrenal axis; interleukin-I stimulates the secretion of CRH and ACTH.

F. Cardiovascular Function: Glucocorticoids may increase cardiac output, and they also increase peripheral vascular tone, possibly by augmenting the effects of other vasoconstrictors, eg, the catecholamines. Thus, refractory shock may occur when the glucocorticoid-deficient individual is subjected to stress. Glucocorticoids in excess may cause hypertension independently of their mineralocorticoid effects; however, the incidence and the precise cause of this problem are unclear.

G. Renal Function: These steroids affect water and electrolyte balance by actions mediated either by mineralocorticoid receptors (sodium and water retention, hypokalemia, and hypertension) or via glucocorticoid receptors (increased glomerular filtration rate due to increased cardiac output or due to a direct renal effect). Thus, corticosteroids such as betamethasone or dexamethasone that have little mineralocorticoid activity increase sodium and water excretion. Glucocorticoid-deficient subjects therefore have decreased glomerular filtration rates and are unable to excrete a water load. This may be contributed to by increased ADH secretion, which may occur in glucocorticoid deficiency.

H. Central Nervous System Function: Glucocorticoids readily enter the brain, and although their physiologic role in central nervous system function is unknown, their excess or deficiency may profoundly alter behavior and cognitive function.

1. Excessive glucocorticoids–In excess, the glucocorticoids initially cause euphoria; however, with prolonged exposure, a variety of psychologic abnormalities occur, including irritability, emotional lability, and depression. Hyperkinetic or manic behavior is less common; overt psychoses occur in a small number of patients. Many patients also note impairment in cognitive functions, most commonly memory and concentration. Other central effects include increased appetite, decreased libido, and insomnia, with decreased REM sleep and increased stage II sleep.

2. Decreased glucocorticoids–Patients with Addison's disease are apathetic and depressed and tend to be irritable, negativistic, and reclusive. They have decreased appetite but increased sensitivity of taste and smell mechanisms.

I. Effects on Other Hormones:

1. Thyroid function–Glucocorticoids in excess affect thyroid function. Although basal TSH levels are usually normal, TSH responsiveness to thyrotropin-releasing hormone (TRH) is frequently subnormal. Serum total thyroxine (T_4) concentrations are usually low normal; however, thyroxine-binding globulin is decreased, and free T_4 levels are normal. Total and free T_3 (triiodothyronine) concentrations may be low, since glucocorticoid excess decreases the conversion of T_4 to T_3 and increases conversion to reverse T_3. Despite these alterations, manifestations of hypothyroidism are not apparent.

2. Gonadal function–Glucocorticoids also affect gonadotropin and gonadal function. In males, they inhibit gonadotropin secretion, as evidenced by decreased responsiveness to administered gonadotropin-releasing hormone (GnRH) and subnormal plasma testosterone concentrations. In females, glucocorticoids also suppress LH responsiveness to GnRH, resulting in suppression of estrogens and progestins with inhibition of ovulation and amenorrhea.

J. Miscellaneous Effects:

1. Peptic ulcer–The role of steroid excess in the production or reactivation of peptic ulcer disease is controversial. Ulcers in spontaneous Cushing's syndrome and with modest exposure to glucocorticoid therapy are unusual, although current data suggest that steroid-treated patients with established ulcers and those on high-dose therapy may be at increased risk.

2. Ophthalmologic effects–Intraocular pressure varies with the level of circulating glucocorticoids and parallels the circadian variation of plasma cortisol levels. In addition, glucocorticoids in excess increase intraocular pressure in patients with open-angle glaucoma. Glucocorticoid therapy may also cause cataract formation.

ADRENAL ANDROGENS

The direct biologic activity of the adrenal androgens (androstenedione, DHEA, and DHEA sulfate) is minimal, and they function primarily as precursors for peripheral conversion to the active androgenic hormones testosterone and dihydrotestosterone. Thus, DHEA sulfate secreted by the adrenal undergoes limited conversion to DHEA; this peripherally converted DHEA and that secreted by the adrenal cortex can be further converted in peripheral tissues to androstenedione, the immediate precursor of the active androgens.

The actions of testosterone and dihydrotestosterone

are described in Chapter 16. This section will deal only with the adrenal contribution to androgenicity.

Effects in Males

In males with normal gonadal function, the conversion of adrenal androstenedione to testosterone accounts for less than 5% of the production rate of this hormone, and thus the physiologic effect is negligible. In adult males, excessive adrenal androgen secretion has no clinical consequences; however, in boys, it causes premature penile enlargement and early development of secondary sexual characteristics.

Effects in Females

In females, ovarian androgen production is low; thus, the adrenal substantially contributes to total androgen production by the peripheral conversion of androstenedione. In the follicular phase of the menstrual cycle, adrenal precursors account for two-thirds of testosterone production and one-half of dihydrotestosterone production. During midcycle, the ovarian contribution increases, and the adrenal precursors account for only 40% of testosterone production.

In females, abnormal adrenal function as seen in Cushing's syndrome, adrenal carcinoma, and congenital adrenal hyperplasia results in excessive secretion of adrenal androgens, and their peripheral conversion results in androgen excess, manifested by acne, ·hirsutism, and virilization.

LABORATORY EVALUATION

Cortisol and the adrenal androgens are measured by specific plasma assays. Certain urinary assays, particularly measurement of 24-hour urine free cortisol, can also be useful. In addition, plasma concentrations of ACTH can be determined. The plasma steroid methods commonly used measure the total hormone concentration and are therefore influenced by alterations in plasma binding proteins. Furthermore, since ACTH and the plasma concentrations of the adrenal hormones fluctuate markedly (Fig 12–7), single plasma measurements are frequently unreliable. Thus, plasma levels must be interpreted cautiously, and more specific diagnostic information is usually obtained by performing appropriate stimulation and suppression tests.

Plasma ACTH

A. Methods of Measurement: Plasma ACTH measurements by radioimmunoassay are extremely useful in the diagnosis of pituitary-adrenal dysfunction; however, they are less commonly available than assays for other polypeptide hormones (see Chapter 6). In general, antisera that react with the biologically active 1–24 sequence of human ACTH are preferable, since they do not detect biologically inactive fragments. The normal range of plasma ACTH is 20–100 pg/mL (4.4–22.2 pmol/L) in the morning, and the

sensitivity of these assays is 5–20 pg/mL (1.1–4.4 pmol/L). ACTH is unstable, and specimens must be handled carefully. They should be collected in heparinized plastic syringes and tubes on ice, centrifuged immediately after collection, and then frozen until assayed.

B. Interpretation: Plasma ACTH levels are most useful in differentiating pituitary causes from adrenal causes of adrenal dysfunction: (1) In **adrenal insufficiency** due to primary adrenal disease, plasma ACTH levels are elevated, usually over 250 pg/mL (55.5 pmol/L). Conversely, in pituitary ACTH deficiency and secondary hypoadrenalism, plasma ACTH levels are less than 50 pg/mL (11 pmol/L) and are usually below the limit of detection even with sensitive assays. (2) In **Cushing's syndrome** due to primary glucocorticoid-secreting adrenal tumors, plasma ACTH is suppressed, and a level less than 20 pg/mL (4.4 pmol/L) is diagnostic. In patients with Cushing's disease (pituitary ACTH hypersecretion), plasma ACTH levels are normal or only modestly elevated (40–200 pg/mL [8.8–44 pmol/L]). Plasma ACTH levels in the ectopic ACTH syndrome range from 100 to several thousand picograms per milliliter (22–666 pmol/L). They are usually markedly elevated; however, overlap occurs with levels seen in Cushing's disease. (3) Plasma ACTH levels are also markedly elevated in patients with the common forms of **congenital adrenal hyperplasia** and are useful in the diagnosis and management of these disorders (see Chapters 13 and 18).

Plasma β-Lipotropin & β-Endorphin

β-Lipotropin (β-LPH) is secreted in equimolar amounts with ACTH and is measured by radioimmunoassay. Because of its greater stability and ease of measurement, it has some advantage over the measurement of ACTH. Alterations in β-LPH levels in disease states parallel those of ACTH as described above. Most assays of β-LPH also measure β-endorphin, and thus separation of these hormones is required for precise measurement of β-endorphin. This can be accomplished by chromatography; however, the clinical utility of β-endorphin measurements has not been established.

Plasma Cortisol

A. Methods of Measurement: Plasma cortisol methods of measurement in current use include radioimmunoassay, high-performance liquid chromatography, competitive protein-binding assay, and fluorimetric assay. These methods measure total cortisol (both bound and free) in plasma. Methods that measure plasma free cortisol—ie, that not bound to CBG—are not yet clinically available.

1. Radioimmunoassays—Radioimmunoassays of plasma cortisol depend on inhibition of binding of radiolabeled cortisol to an antibody by the cortisol present in a plasma sample. Current assays are very sensitive, so that small plasma volumes can be used. In addition, cross-reactivity of current antisera with other endogenous steroids is minimal, and radioimmunoassay thus gives a reliable measurement of total plasma cortisol levels. Cross-reactivity with some synthetic glucocorticoids, eg, prednisone, is variable. Other commonly used drugs and medications do not interfere with this assay.

2. High-performance liquid chromatography– This test also provides a specific method of cortisol determination. Other endogenous steroids are excluded by chromatography, but it is possible that prednisone and prednisolone might interfere. Drug interference does not occur.

3. Competitive protein-binding assay– This method is similar in principle to radioimmunoassay except that CBG is utilized to bind cortisol instead of an antibody. Although other endogenous steroids bind CBG with high affinity, their plasma concentrations are usually much lower than that of cortisol, and they therefore do not cause significant interference. The synthetic glucocorticoids prednisolone and 6α-methylprednisolone bind to CBG in appreciable amounts and may interfere with the assay, although other hormones and medications do not.

4. Fluorimetric assay– This method, which is less commonly used, measures the fluorescence of steroids with 11-hydroxyl groups and thus measures plasma 11-hydroxycorticosteroids. Cortisol is the major hormone measured, but the method also detects corticosterone and 21-deoxycortisol. The latter 2 steroids are usually present in low concentrations and thus do not cause significant interference. Synthetic glucocorticoids do not cross-react in this assay. Since plasma has nonspecific background fluorescence, this method overestimates the plasma cortisol concentration by 2–3 µg/dL (0.06–0.08 µmol/L). Background fluorescence may be increased in the plasma of uremic or jaundiced patients, and spironolactone, quinacrine, quinidine, fusidic acid, niacin, and heparin preparations containing benzyl alcohol interfere with the assay.

B. Interpretation: The diagnostic utility of single plasma cortisol concentrations is limited by the episodic nature of cortisol secretion and its appropriate elevations during stress. As explained below, more information is obtained by dynamic testing of the hypothalamic-pituitary-adrenal axis.

1. Normal values– Normal plasma cortisol levels vary with the method used. With radioimmunoassay and the competitive protein-binding radioassay, levels at 8 AM range from 3 to 20 µg/dL (0.08–0.55 µmol/L) and average 10–12 µg/dL (0.28–0.33 µmol/L). Values obtained later in the day are lower and at 4 PM are approximately half of morning values. At 10 PM to 2 AM, the plasma cortisol concentrations by these methods are usually under 3 µg/dL (0.08 µmol/L).

2. Levels during stress– Cortisol secretion increases in patients who are acutely ill, during surgery, and following trauma. Plasma concentrations may reach 40–60 µg/dL (1.1–1.7 µmol/L).

3. High-estrogen states– The total plasma cortisol concentration is also elevated with increased CBG binding capacity, which occurs most commonly when circulating estrogen levels are high, eg, during pregnancy and when exogenous estrogens or oral contraceptives are being used. In these situations, plasma cortisol may reach levels 2–3 times normal.

4. Other conditions– CBG levels may be increased or decreased in other situations, as discussed above in the sections on circulation and metabolism. Total plasma cortisol concentrations may also be increased in severe anxiety, endogenous depression, starvation, anorexia nervosa, alcoholism, and chronic renal failure.

Urinary Corticosteroids
A. Free Cortisol:

1. Methods of measurement– The assay of unbound cortisol excreted in the urine is an excellent method for the diagnosis of Cushing's syndrome. Normally, less than 1% of the secreted cortisol is excreted unchanged in the urine. However, in states of excess secretion, the binding capacity of CBG is exceeded, and plasma free cortisol therefore increases, as does its urinary excretion. Urine free cortisol is measured in a 24-hour urine collection by radioimmunoassay or competitive protein-binding assay after extraction of the cortisol.

2. Normal values– The normal range of these assays is nil to 110 µg/24 h (0.30 µmol/24 h), and elevated levels are found in over 90% of patients with spontaneous Cushing's syndrome.

3. Diagnostic utility– This method is particularly useful in differentiating simple obesity from Cushing's syndrome, since levels are not elevated in obesity, as are the urinary 17-hydroxycorticosteroids (see below). The levels may be elevated in the same conditions that increase plasma cortisol (see above), including a slight elevation during pregnancy. This test is not useful in adrenal insufficiency, because of the lack of sensitivity of the method at low levels and because low cortisol excretion is often found in normal persons.

B. 17-Hydroxycorticosteroids and 17-Ketogenic Steroids: These urinary steroids are less frequently measured at present, because of the greater utility of plasma cortisol and urine free cortisol measurements. Urinary 17-ketosteroid measurements are discussed in the following section on androgens.

1. 17-Hydroxycorticosteroids–

a. Methods of assay– Urine 17-hydroxycorticosteroids are assayed by the colorimetric Porter-Silber reaction, which detects cortisol and cortisone metabolites.

b. Normal values–Normal values are 3–15 mg/24 h (8.3–41.4 μmol/24 h) or 3–7 mg/g (0.9–2.2 mmol/mol) of urine creatinine.

c. Altered excretion–Total excretion is increased in obesity; however, these values are normal when corrected for creatinine excretion. 17-Hydroxycorticosteroids are increased in hyperthyroidism and decreased in hypothyroidism, starvation, liver disease, renal failure, and pregnancy. Drugs that induce hepatic microsomal enzymes increase cortisol conversion to 6β-hydroxycortisol, which is not measured by the 17-hydroxycorticosteroid method, and therefore reduce 17-hydroxycorticosteroid excretion (see section on metabolism).

d. Drug interference–Direct drug interference with the colorimetric reaction occurs with spironolactone, chlordiazepoxide, hydroxyzine, meprobamate, phenothiazines, and quinine.

2. 17-Ketogenic steroids–The 17-ketogenic steroids include not only the metabolites of cortisol but also those of a number of other steroids, eg, pregnanetriol. The procedure for measurement first converts these steroids to 17-ketosteroids, and they are then measured colorimetrically by the Zimmermann reaction. Normal values are 6–20 mg/24 h (0.016–0.055 mmol/24 h). This is less specific for cortisol metabolites than measurement of 17-hydroxycorticosteroids and is less reliable in the diagnosis of Cushing's syndrome. Values are increased by penicillin G and decreased by glucose, meprobamate, and radiographic contrast agents.

C. Cortisol Secretion Rate: There are several research techniques available to measure the cortisol secretion rate, which normally is 8–25 mg/24 h (0.022–0.07 mmol/24 h). The rate is decreased in adrenal insufficiency and increased in Cushing's syndrome, obesity, hyperthyroidism, and pregnancy. Expression of the secretion rate in terms of creatinine excretion allows differentiation of Cushing's syndrome from exogenous obesity. Thus, in normals and in obese subjects, cortisol secretion is less than 20 mg/24 h/g (0.055 mmol/24 h/g) of urinary creatinine, whereas in patients with Cushing's syndrome values greater than 26 mg/24 h/g (0.07 mmol/24 h/g) of creatinine are obtained. Although useful, these methods are not generally available.

Dexamethasone Suppression Tests

A. Low-Dose Tests: These procedures are used to establish the presence of Cushing's syndrome regardless of its cause. Dexamethasone, a potent glucocorticoid, normally suppresses pituitary ACTH release with a resulting fall in plasma and urine corticosteroids, thus assessing feedback inhibition of the hypothalamic-pituitary-adrenal axis. In Cushing's syndrome, this mechanism is abnormal, and steroid secretion fails to be suppressed in the normal way.

Dexamethasone in the doses used does not interfere with the measurement of plasma and urinary corticosteroids.

1. Overnight 1-mg dexamethasone suppression test–This is a suitable screening test for Cushing's syndrome. Dexamethasone, 1 mg orally, is given as a single dose at 11 PM, and the following morning a plasma sample is obtained for cortisol determination. Cushing's syndrome is excluded if the plasma cortisol level is less than 5 μg/dL (0.137 μmol/L). If the level is greater than 10 μ/dL (0.276 μmol/L)—in the absence of conditions causing false-positive responses—Cushing's syndrome is the probable cause, and the diagnosis should be confirmed with other procedures.

Over 98% of patients with Cushing's syndrome have abnormal responses. Although false-negative results are rare, they may occur in patients in whom dexamethasone metabolism is abnormally slow, since plasma levels of dexamethasone in these patients are higher than normally achieved and result in apparently normal suppression of cortisol. Simultaneous measurement of plasma dexamethasone and cortisol levels will identify these patients; however, dexamethasone measurements are available only on a research basis.

False-positive results occur in 15% of patients with obesity and in 25% of hospitalized and chronically ill patients. Acute illness, depression, anxiety, alcoholism, high-estrogen states, and uremia may also cause false-positive results. Patients taking phenytoin, barbiturates, and other inducers of hepatic microsomal enzymes may have accelerated metabolism of dexamethasone and thus fail to achieve adequate plasma levels to suppress ACTH.

2. Two-day low-dose test–This test is performed by administering dexamethasone, 0.5 mg every 6 hours for 2 days. Twenty-four-hour urine collections are obtained before and on the second day of dexamethasone administration. The test provides the same information as the overnight 1-mg test but is more time-consuming and requires urine collections. However, it is very useful when the results of other tests are equivocal. In response to this procedure, patients *without* Cushing's syndrome suppress urine 17-hydroxycorticosteroids to less than 4 mg/24 h (10.1 μmol/24 h) or to less than 1 mg/g (0.3 mmol/mol) of urinary creatinine on the second day of dexamethasone administration. The response of urine free cortisol is less well standardized; however, a reduction in excretion to less than 25 μg/24 h (0.068 μmol/24 h) appears to exclude Cushing's syndrome. Although the plasma cortisol response has been less extensively studied, a morning cortisol level of less than 5 μg/dL (0.137 μmol/L) (obtained 6 hours after the last dose of dexamethasone has been given) is considered a normal response.

About 95% of patients with Cushing's syndrome have abnormal responses. False-positive results occur rarely in patients with obesity and in high-estrogen states. However, false-positive results do occur with acute and chronic illness, depression, alcoholism, and phenytoin therapy.

B. High-Dose Tests: High-dose dexamethasone tests differentiate Cushing's disease (pituitary ACTH hypersecretion) from the ectopic ACTH syndrome and adrenal tumors, since the hypothalamic-pituitary axis in Cushing's disease is suppressible with supraphysiologic doses of glucocorticoids, whereas cortisol secretion is autonomous in patients with adrenal tumors or ectopic ACTH syndrome and is therefore nonsuppressible. Exceptions to these responses are discussed in the section on diagnosis of Cushing's syndrome.

1. Overnight high-dose dexamethasone suppression test–This test is faster and simpler to perform than the 2-day test described below. After a baseline morning cortisol specimen is obtained, a single dose of dexamethasone, 8 mg orally, is administered at 11 PM, and plasma cortisol is measured at 8 AM the following morning. In Cushing's disease, plasma cortisol levels are reduced to less than 50% of baseline values in 95% of patients, whereas steroid secretion in patients with ectopic ACTH syndrome or cortisol-producing adrenal tumors is not suppressed to this extent and is usually unchanged. This single-dose test is more reliable than the 2-day high-dose test and can be regarded as the procedure of choice.

2. Two-day high-dose test–This test is performed by administering dexamethasone, 2 mg orally every 6 hours for 2 days. Twenty-four-hour urine samples are collected before and on the second day of dexamethasone administration. Patients with Cushing's disease have a reduction in urine 17-hydroxycorticosteroid excretion to less than 50% of baseline values, whereas those with adrenal tumors or the ectopic ACTH syndrome usually have little or no reduction in urinary 17-hydroxycorticosteroids. Urine free cortisol or plasma cortisol appears to give equally adequate responses, and the same criteria apply; the response of urine 17-ketogenic steroids appears to be less reliable. Regardless of the parameter measured, 15–30% of patients with Cushing's disease fail to achieve 50% suppression of corticosteroid levels, thus limiting the reliability of the procedure.

Pituitary-Adrenal Reserve

Determinations of pituitary-adrenal reserve are used to evaluate the patient's adrenal and pituitary reserve and to assess the ability of the hypothalamic-pituitary-adrenal axis to respond to stress. ACTH administration directly stimulates adrenal secretion; metyrapone inhibits cortisol synthesis, thereby stimulating pituitary ACTH secretion; and insulin-induced hypoglycemia stimulates ACTH release by increasing CRH secretion. More recently, CRH has been utilized to directly stimulate pituitary corticotrophs to release ACTH and β-LPH. The relative utility of these procedures is dis-

cussed below in the section on adreno-cortical insufficiency and also in Chapter 6.

A. ACTH Stimulation Testing:

1. Procedure and normal values–The rapid ACTH stimulation test measures the acute adrenal response to ACTH and is used to diagnose both primary and secondary adrenal insufficiency. A synthetic human α^{1-24}-ACTH called tetracosactrin or cosyntropin (Cortrosyn) is used. It has full biologic potency and a lower incidence of allergic reactions than occurred with animal ACTH derivatives. Fasting is not required, and the test may be performed at any time of the day. A baseline cortisol sample is obtained; cosyntropin is administered in a dose of 0.25 mg intramuscularly or intravenously; and additional samples for plasma cortisol are obtained at 30 or 60 minutes following the injection. The normal response is a peak cortisol level greater than 15–18 μg/dL (0.41–0.50 μmol/L), with an increment greater than 5 μg/dL (0.137 μmol/L). If a value of 20 μg/dL (0.55 μmol/L) is obtained, the response is normal regardless of the increment.

2. Subnormal responses–If the cortisol response to the rapid ACTH stimulation test is inadequate, adrenal insufficiency is present. In primary adrenal insufficiency, destruction of cortical cells reduces cortisol secretion and increases pituitary ACTH secretion. Therefore, the adrenal is already maximally stimulated, and there is no further increase in cortisol secretion when exogenous ACTH is given; ie, there is decreased adrenal reserve. In secondary adrenal insufficiency due to ACTH deficiency, there is atrophy of the zonae fasciculata and reticularis, and the adrenal thus is unresponsive to acute stimulation with exogenous ACTH. In either primary or secondary types, a subnormal response to the rapid ACTH stimulation test accurately predicts deficient responsiveness of the axis to insulin hypoglycemia, metyrapone, and surgical stress.

3. Normal responses–A normal response to the rapid ACTH stimulation test excludes both primary adrenal insufficiency (by directly assessing adrenal reserve) and overt secondary adrenal insufficiency with adrenal atrophy. However, a normal response does not rule out partial ACTH deficiency (decreased pituitary reserve) in patients whose basal ACTH secretion is sufficient to prevent adrenocortical atrophy. These patients may be unable to further increase ACTH secretion and thus may have subnormal pituitary ACTH responsiveness to stress or hypoglycemia. In such patients, further testing with metyrapone or hypoglycemia may be indicated. For further discussion, see the section on diagnosis of adrenocortical insufficiency.

4. Aldosterone secretion–The rapid ACTH stimulation test also increases aldosterone secretion and has been used to differentiate primary from secondary adrenocortical insufficiency. In the primary form with destruction of the cortex, both cortisol and aldosterone are unresponsive to exogenous ACTH. However, in secondary adrenal insufficiency, the zona glomerulosa, which is controlled by the renin-angiotensin system, is usually normal. Therefore, the aldosterone response to exogenous ACTH is normal. The normal increment in plasma aldosterone is more than 4 ng/dL (111 pmol/L).

5. Three-day tests–Three-day ACTH stimulation tests are rarely used at present, since the rapid ACTH test and measurements of plasma ACTH are usually sufficient to diagnose and establish the cause of adrenocortical insufficiency.

B. Metyrapone Testing: Metyrapone testing is used to diagnose adrenal insufficiency and to assess pituitary-adrenal reserve. The test procedures are detailed in Chapter 6. Metyrapone blocks cortisol synthesis by inhibiting the 11β-hydroxylase enzyme that converts 11-deoxycortisol to cortisol. This stimulates ACTH secretion, which in turn increases the secretion and plasma levels of 11-deoxycortisol. Urinary 17-hydroxycorticosteroid levels also increase because of increased excretion of the metabolites of 11-deoxycortisol that are measured by this method. The overnight metyrapone test is most commonly used and is best suited to patients with suspected pituitary ACTH deficiency; patients with suspected primary adrenal failure are usually evaluated with the rapid ACTH stimulation test as described above and discussed in the section on diagnosis of adrenocortical insufficiency. The normal response to the overnight metyrapone test is a plasma 11-deoxycortisol level greater than 7 μg/dL (0.19 μmol/L) and indicates both normal ACTH secretion and adrenal function. A subnormal response establishes adrenocortical insufficiency but does not differentiate primary and secondary forms. A normal response to metyrapone accurately predicts normal stress responsiveness of the hypothalamic-pituitary axis and correlates well with responsiveness to insulin-induced hypoglycemia.

C. Insulin-Induced Hypoglycemia Testing: The details of this procedure are described in Chapter 6. Hypoglycemia induces a central nervous system stress response, increases CRH release, and in this way increases ACTH and cortisol secretion. It therefore measures the integrity of the axis and its ability to respond to stress. The normal plasma cortisol response is an increment greater than 8 μg/dL (0.22 μmol/L) and a peak level greater than 18–20 μg/dL (0.50–0.55 μmol/L). The plasma ACTH response to hypoglycemia is not well standardized. A normal plasma cortisol response to hypoglycemia excludes adrenal insufficiency and decreased pituitary reserve. Thus, patients with normal responses do not require cortisol therapy during illness or surgery.

D. CRH Testing: The procedure for CRH testing is described in Chapter 6. ACTH responses are exaggerated in patients with primary adrenal failure and absent in patients with hypopituitarism. Delayed responses may occur in patients with hypothalamic disorders.

Androgens

Androgen excess is usually evaluated by the measurement of basal levels of these hormones, since suppression and stimulation tests are not as useful as in disorders affecting the glucocorticoids.

A. Plasma Levels: Assays are available for total plasma levels of DHEA, DHEA sulfate, androstenedione, testosterone, and dihydrotestosterone; these tests are of greater diagnostic utility than the traditional measurement of urinary androgen metabolites measured as urinary 17-ketosteroids.

Because it is present in greater quantities, DHEA sulfate can be measured directly in unextracted plasma. However, because of their similar structures and lower plasma concentrations, the other androgens require extraction and purification steps prior to assay. This is accomplished by solvent extraction followed by chromatography, and the purified steroids are then measured by radioimmunoassay or competitive protein-binding radioassay. These methods allow measurement of multiple steroids in small volumes of plasma.

B. Free Testosterone: Plasma free testosterone (ie, testosterone not bound to SHBG) can be measured and is a more direct measure of circulating biologically active testosterone than the total plasma level. These methods require separation of the bound and free hormone prior to assay and are technically difficult. The plasma free testosterone concentration in normal women averages 5 pg/mL (17.3 pmol/L), representing approximately 1% of the total testosterone concentration. In hirsute women, average levels are 16 pg/mL (55.4 pmol/L), with a wide range.

C. SHBG Binding Capacity: The binding capacity of SHBG can be measured, although these methods are not in general use. SHBG binding capacity is higher in women; it is increased in pregnancy, in women receiving exogenous estrogens, in hepatic cirrhosis, and in hyperthyroidism and is decreased in hirsute women with increased androgens and in patients with acromegaly.

D. Urinary 17-Ketosteroids: Measurement of urinary androgen metabolites (eg, the 17-ketosteroids) is much less useful in the evaluation of androgen excess than the plasma methods described above. The biologically active androgens testosterone and dihydrotestosterone account for less than 1% of total urinary 17-ketosteroids; the major steroids measured are the metabolites of DHEA and DHEA sulfate. The ketosteroids are separated by solvent extraction and measured colorimetrically by the Zimmermann reaction. Normal values are 5–15 mg/24 h (17–52 nmol/24 h) in women and 9–22 mg/24 h (31–76 nmol/24 h) in men. A number of drugs interfere with this method. Thus, penicillin, spironolactone, chlorpromazine, ethinamate, meprobamate, and nalidixic acid falsely elevate the values, whereas chlordiazepoxide, propoxyphene, progestins, reserpine, and etryptamine acetate reduce them.

DISORDERS OF ADRENOCORTICAL INSUFFICIENCY

Deficient adrenal production of glucocorticoids or mineralocorticoids results in adrenocortical insufficiency, which is either the consequence of destruction or dysfunction of the cortex (primary adrenocortical insufficiency, Addison's disease) or secondary to deficient pituitary ACTH secretion (secondary adrenocortical insufficiency). Secondary adrenocortical insufficiency due to glucocorticoid therapy is the most common cause.

PRIMARY ADRENOCORTICAL INSUFFICIENCY
(Addison's Disease)

Etiology & Pathology

The etiology of primary adrenocortical insufficiency has changed over time. Prior to 1920, tuberculosis was the major cause of adrenocortical insufficiency. Since 1950, autoimmune adrenalitis with adrenal atrophy has accounted for about 80% of cases. It is associated with disordered organ-specific immunity and a high incidence of other immunologic and autoimmune endocrine disorders (see below). Tuberculosis of the adrenal gland is responsible for most of the other cases. Rare causes are listed in Table 12–1. Primary adrenocortical insufficiency, or Addison's disease, is rare, with a reported prevalence of 39 per million population in the United Kingdom and 60 per million in Denmark. It is more common in females, with a female:male ratio of 2.6:1. Tuberculous adrenal destruction is most common in males, giving an overall female:male ratio of 1.25:1. Addison's disease is usually diagnosed in the third to fifth decades; mean ages of 34 and 38 years have been reported for the autoimmune and tuberculous types, respectively. As the number of patients with acquired immunodeficiency syndrome (AIDS) increases, and as patients with malignant disease live longer, more cases of adrenal insufficiency will be seen.

A. Autoimmune Adrenocortical Insufficiency: Lymphocytic infiltration of the adrenal cortex is the characteristic histologic feature. The adrenals are small and atrophic, and the capsule is thickened. The adrenal medulla is preserved, though cortical cells are largely absent, show degenerative changes, and are

Table 12–1. Causes of primary adrenocortical insufficiency.[1]

Major causes
  Autoimmune (about 80%)
  Tuberculosis (about 20%)
Rare causes
  Adrenal hemorrhage and infarction
  Fungal infections
  Metastatic and lymphomatous replacement
  Amyloidosis
  Sarcoidosis
  Hemochromatosis
  Radiation therapy
  Surgical adrenalectomy
  Enzyme inhibitors (metyrapone, aminoglutethimide, trilostane)
  Cytotoxic agents (mitotane; o,p'-DDD)
  Congenital (enzyme defects, hypoplasia, familial glucocorticoid deficiency)

[1]Modified and reproduced, with permission, from Baxter JD, Tyrrell JB, in: *Endocrinology and Metabolism.* Felig P et al (editors). McGraw-Hill, 1981.

surrounded by a fibrous stroma and lymphocytic infiltrates.

Autoimmune Addison's disease is frequently accompanied by other immune disorders. Two distinct polyglandular syndromes involve the adrenal glands: one includes adrenal insufficiency, hypoparathyroidism, and chronic mucocutaneous candidiasis, and the other includes adrenal insufficiency, Hashimoto's thyroiditis, and insulin-dependent diabetes mellitus. Ovarian failure is common in both syndromes. Alopecia, malabsorbtion syndromes, chronic hepatitis, vitiligo, and pernicious anemia are also found in association with autoimmune Addison's disease—one or more of these associated disorders is found in 40–53% of patients. There is an even higher incidence of antibodies to various endocrine organs and other tissues in the absence of overt clinical disease (see Chapter 28).

1. Schmidt's syndrome–The association of Addison's disease with lymphocytic thyroiditis and diabetes mellitus has been termed Schmidt's syndrome, which is a subset of the syndromes of multiglandular failure. Genetic and HLA associations are discussed in Chapter 28. These disorders are not present in Addison's disease due to infection or metastatic malignant tumors.

2. Ovarian failure–This occurs in approximately 25% of female patients and usually presents as secondary amenorrhea. Patients with both ovarian and adrenal failure also have a very high incidence of hypoparathyroidism and thyroid disease. Hypoparathyroidism is most frequent in those with primary amenorrhea.

3. Testicular failure–Testicular failure is uncommon and occurs in fewer than 5% of males with autoimmune Addison's disease.

4. Thyroid disorders–Clinical thyroid disorders occur in 16% of patients. The incidence of subclinical thyroiditis is even higher; about 80% of patients with autoimmune Addison's disease have lymphocytic infiltration of the thyroid, and there is a high incidence of elevated TSH levels. Hyperthyroidism occurs in 7% of patients, of whom the majority are female; clinical hypothyroidism or Hashimoto's thyroiditis with goiter occurs in 9% of patients.

5. Diabetes mellitus—This is present in about 12% of patients with autoimmune Addison's disease and is typically type I (insulin-dependent). The mean age at diagnosis of the 2 disorders is approximately 30 years. Sex distribution is equal, and islet cell autoantibodies are common in these patients.

6. Hypoparathyroidism—Hypoparathyroidism occurs in 6% of patients with autoimmune Addison's disease. These 2 disorders occur at younger ages than the other disorders listed above, with a mean age at diagnosis of 12 years. There is also an increased incidence of early ovarian failure, usually presenting as primary amenorrhea, in patients with autoimmune Addison's disease and hypoparathyroidism.

7. Circulating autoantibodies—The incidence of autoantibodies to adrenal and other tissue antigens is increased in patients with autoimmune Addison's disease (Table 12–2) but not in patients with adrenal failure due to other causes. Circulating adrenal autoantibodies are present in over 60% of patients with autoimmune Addison's disease. Thyroid autoantibodies occur in 45% of patients with autoimmune Addison's disease and are present more frequently (2:1) in female patients. Gastric parietal cell and intrinsic factor autoantibodies are present in 30% and 9%, respectively; parathyroid autoantibodies in 26%; autoantibodies to steroid-producing cells in 17%; and islet cell autoantibodies in 8% of patients with autoimmune Addison's disease.

B. Adrenocortical Insufficiency Due to Invasive and Hemorrhagic Disorders: Invasive or hemorrhagic disorders causing adrenocortical failure result in total or near-total destruction of both glands. With septicemia or hemorrhage, the adrenal is rapidly destroyed, whereas gradual destruction usually occurs in conditions such as tuberculosis.

Table 12–2. Incidence of circulating autoantibodies in autoimmune adrenocortical insufficiency.[1]

	Percent
Adrenal	64
Thyroid	
Cytoplasm	45
Thyroglobulin	22
Stomach	
Parietal cells	30
Intrinsic factor	9
Parathyroid	26
Gonad	17
Islet cell	8

[1]Reproduced, with permission, from Baxter JD, Tyrrell JB, in: *Endocrinology and Metabolism.* Felig P et al (editors). McGraw-Hill, 1981.

1. Adrenal tuberculosis and other destructive causes—Adrenal tuberculosis is due to hematogenous infection of the cortex and usually occurs as a complication of systemic tuberculous infection (lung, gastrointestinal tract, or kidney). The adrenal glands are replaced by caseous necrosis; both cortical and medullary tissue is destroyed. Calcification of the adrenals is frequent and is radiologically demonstrable in about 50% of cases.

2. Bilateral adrenal hemorrhage—Hemorrhage may cause acute adrenal insufficiency. In children, fulminant meningococcemia and *Pseudomonas* septicemia are the most common causes. In adults (mostly > age 50), anticoagulant therapy given for other major illnesses is responsible for one-third of cases. Other causes in adults include septicemia, coagulation disorders, adrenal vein thrombosis, adrenal metastases, trauma, abdominal surgery, and obstetric gestational and postpartum complications.

The adrenal glands are often massively enlarged; there is replacement of the medulla and inner cortex by hemorrhage and ischemic necrosis of the outer cortex, so that only a few subcapsular cortical cells survive. Venous thrombosis frequently accompanies the hemorrhage. In surviving patients, the hematomas may calcify.

3. Adrenal metastases—Although metastases to the adrenals occur frequently with tumors of the lung, breast, stomach, and with melanoma and may occur with many other tumors, frank adrenal insufficiency is relatively uncommon; more than 80–90% of the adrenal must be destroyed before frank insufficiency develops. The adrenals are often massively enlarged, and this may be detected by computed tomography (CT scan). Since the symptoms of adrenal insufficiency may be mistaken for those of the underlying cancer, and since treatment of the adrenal insufficiency may improve the patients' quality of life, a high degree of clinical suspicion should be maintained.

4. Acquired immunodeficiency syndrome (AIDS)—Postmortem examination reveals the adrenal to be the endocrine gland most commonly affected in AIDS, often by opportunistic infection (especially cytomegalovirus) or Kaposi's sarcoma. Although pathologic involvement and subclinical alterations in steroidogenesis are common, clinical adrenal insufficiency is uncommon. Ketoconazole, an antifungal agent frequently used in patients with AIDS, interferes with cytochrome P-450 enzymes in several organs, including the adrenal and the gonads, and result in decreased steroidogenesis. Adrenal insufficiency is usually dose-related and reversible, but it may occur with low doses and it may be persistent.

C. Familial Glucocorticoid Deficiency: Familial glucocorticoid deficiency is a rare disorder in which there is hereditary adrenocortical unresponsiveness to ACTH. This leads to adrenal insufficiency with subnormal glucocorticoid and adrenal androgen secretion and elevated plasma ACTH levels.

In this disorder, cortisol secretion is unresponsive to both endogenous and exogenous ACTH stimulation. However, aldosterone secretion responds to both posture change and sodium deprivation, except in a few subjects who have partial aldosterone deficiency. Presentation is usually in childhood and may be accompanied by achalasia. Histologically, there is preservation of the zona glomerulosa, with degenerative changes in the zonae fasciculata and reticularis. These features and the absence of lymphocytic infiltration of the adrenal cortex differentiate this condition from idiopathic adrenocortical insufficiency.

Pathophysiology

Loss of more than 90% of both adrenal cortices results in the clinical manifestations of adrenocortical insufficiency. Gradual destruction such as occurs in the idiopathic and invasive forms of the disease leads to chronic adrenocortical insufficiency. However, more rapid destruction occurs in many cases; about 25% of patients are in crisis or impending crisis at the time of diagnosis. With gradual adrenocortical destruction, the initial phase is that of decreased adrenal reserve; ie, basal steroid secretion is normal, but secretion does not increase in response to stress. Thus, acute adrenal crisis can be precipitated by the stresses of surgery, trauma, or infection, which require increased corticosteroid secretion. With further loss of cortical tissue, even basal secretion of mineralocorticoids and glucocorticoids becomes deficient, leading to the manifestations of chronic adrenocortical insufficiency. Destruction of the adrenals by hemorrhage results in sudden loss of both glucocorticoid and mineralocorticoid secretion, accompanied by acute adrenal crisis.

With decreasing cortisol secretion, plasma levels of ACTH and β-lipotropin (β-LPH) are increased because of decreased negative-feedback inhibition of their secretion. In chronic states, the elevated ACTH levels cause hyperpigmentation; this is usually absent when adrenal destruction is rapid.

Clinical Features

A. Symptoms and Signs: Cortisol deficiency causes weakness, fatigue, anorexia, nausea and vomiting, hypotension, and hypoglycemia. Mineralocorticoid deficiency produces renal sodium wasting and potassium retention and can lead to severe dehydration, hypotension, hyponatremia, hyperkalemia, and acidosis.

1. Chronic primary adrenocortical insufficiency—The chief symptoms (Table 12–3) are hyperpigmentation, weakness and fatigue, weight loss, anorexia, and gastrointestinal disturbances.

Hyperpigmentation is the classic physical finding, and its presence in association with the above manifestations should suggest primary adrenocortical insufficiency. Generalized hyperpigmentation of the skin and mucous membranes is the earliest manifestation of Addison's disease. It is increased in sun-ex-

Table 12–3. Clinical features of primary adrenocortical insufficiency.[1]

	Percent
Weakness, fatigue, anorexia, weight loss	100
Hyperpigmentation	92
Hypotension	88
Gastrointestinal disturbances	56
Salt craving	19
Postural symptoms	12

[1]Reproduced, with permission, from Baxter JD, Tyrrell JB, in: *Endocrinology and Metabolism.* Felig P et al (editors). McGraw-Hill, 1981.

posed areas and accentuated over pressure areas such as the knuckles, toes, elbows, and knees. It is accompanied by increased numbers of black or dark-brown freckles. The classic hyperpigmentation of the buccal mucosa and gums is preceded by generalized hyperpigmentation of the skin; adrenal insufficiency should also be suspected when there is increased pigmentation of the palmar creases, nail beds, nipples, areolae, and perivaginal and perianal mucosa. Scars that have formed after the onset of ACTH excess become hyperpigmented, whereas older ones do not. Although pigmentation of the buccal mucosa, palmar creases, vulva, and anus is a normal phenomenon in dark-skinned races, patients frequently describe increase in pigmentation of these sites. Pigmentation of the tongue is an abnormal finding in all races.

General weakness, fatigue and malaise, anorexia, and weight loss are invariable features of the disorder. Weight loss may reach 15 kg with progressive adrenal failure. Gastrointestinal disturbances, especially nausea and vomiting, occur in most patients; diarrhea is less frequent. An increase in gastrointestinal symptoms during an acute adrenal crisis may confuse the diagnosis by suggesting a primary intra-abdominal process.

Hypotension is present in about 90% of patients and causes orthostatic symptoms and occasionally syncope. In more severe chronic cases and in acute crises, recumbent hypotension or shock is almost invariably present. Vitiligo occurs in 4–17% of patients with autoimmune Addison's disease but is rare in Addison's disease due to other causes. Salt craving occurs in about 20% of patients.

Severe hypoglycemia may occur in children. This finding is unusual in adults but may be provoked by fasting, fever, infection, or nausea and vomiting, especially in acute adrenal crisis.

Amenorrhea is common in Addison's disease. It may be due to weight loss and chronic illness or to primary ovarian failure. Loss of axillary and pubic hair may occur in women as a result of decreased secretion of adrenal androgens.

2. Acute adrenal crisis—Acute adrenal crisis represents a state of acute adrenocortical insufficiency and occurs in patients with Addison's disease who are ex-

Table 12–4. Clincial features of acute adrenal crisis.

Hypotension and shock
Fever
Dehydration, volume depletion
Nausea, vomiting, anorexia
Weakness, apathy, depressed mentation
Hypoglycemia

posed to the stress of infection, trauma, surgery, or dehydration due to salt deprivation, vomiting, or diarrhea.

The symptoms are listed in Table 12–4. Anorexia and nausea and vomiting increase and worsen the volume depletion and dehydration. Hypovolemic shock may occur, and adrenal insufficiency should be considered in any patient with unexplained vascular collapse. Abdominal pain may occur and mimic an acute abdominal emergency. Weakness, apathy, and confusion are usual. Fever is usual and may be due to infection or to hypoadrenalism per se. Hyperpigmentation is present unless the onset of adrenal insufficiency is rapid and should suggest the diagnosis.

Additional findings that suggest the diagnosis are hyponatremia, hyperkalemia, lymphocytosis, eosinophilia, and hypoglycemia.

Shock and coma may rapidly lead to death in untreated patients.

3. Acute adrenal hemorrhage–(See Table 12–5.) Bilateral adrenal hemorrhage and acute adrenal destruction in an already compromised patient with major medical illness follow a progressively deteriorating course. The usual manifestations are abdominal, flank, or back pain and abdominal tenderness. Abdominal distention, rigidity, and rebound tenderness are less frequent. Hypotension, shock, fever, nausea and vomiting, confusion, and disorientation are common; tachycardia and cyanosis are less frequent.

With progression, severe hypotension, volume depletion, dehydration, hyperpyrexia, cyanosis, coma, and death ensue.

Table 12–5. Clinical features of adrenal hemorrhage.[1]

	Percent
General features	
Hypotension and shock	74
Fever	59
Nausea and vomiting	46
Confusion, disorientation	41
Tachycardia	28
Cyanosis or lividity	28
Local features	
Abdominal, flank, or back pain	77
Abdominal or flank tenderness	38
Abdominal distention	28
Abdominal rigidity	20
Chest pain	13
Rebound tenderness	5

[1]Reproduced, with permission, from Baxter JD, Tyrrell JB, in: *Endocrinology and Metabolism.* Felig P et al (editors). McGraw-Hill, 1981.

The diagnosis of acute adrenal hemorrhage should be considered in the deteriorating patient with unexplained abdominal or flank pain, vascular collapse, hyperpyrexia, or hypoglycemia.

B. Laboratory and Electrocardiographic Findings and Imaging Studies:

1. Gradual adrenal destruction–Hyponatremia and hyperkalemia are classic manifestations of the mineralocorticoid deficiency of primary adrenal insufficiency and should suggest the diagnosis. Hematologic manifestations include normocytic, normochromic anemia, neutropenia, eosinophilia, and a relative lymphocytosis. Azotemia with increased concentrations of blood urea nitrogen and serum creatinine is due to volume depletion and dehydration. Mild acidosis is frequently present. Hypercalcemia of mild to moderate degree occurs in about 6% of patients.

Abdominal radiographs reveal adrenal calcification in half of patients with tuberculous Addison's disease and in some patients with other invasive or hemorrhagic causes of adrenal insufficiency. Computed tomography (CT scan) is a more sensitive detector of adrenal calcification and adrenal enlargement. Bilateral adrenal enlargement in association with adrenal insufficiency may be seen with tuberculosis, fungal infections, cytomegalovirus, malignant and nonmalignant infiltrative diseases, and adrenal hemorrhage.

Electrocardiographic features are low voltage, a vertical QRS axis, and nonspecific ST–T wave abnormalities secondary to abnormal electrolytes.

2. Acute adrenal hemorrhage–Hyponatremia and hyperkalemia occur in only a small number of cases, but azotemia is a usual finding. Increased circulating eosinophils may suggest the diagnosis.

SECONDARY ADRENOCORTICAL INSUFFICIENCY

Etiology

Secondary adrenocortical insufficiency due to ACTH deficiency is most commonly a result of exogenous glucocorticoid therapy. Pituitary or hypothalamic tumors are the most common causes of naturally occurring pituitary ACTH hyposecretion. These and other less common causes are reviewed in Chapter 6.

Pathophysiology

ACTH deficiency is the primary event and leads to decreased cortisol and adrenal androgen secretion. Aldosterone secretion remains normal except in a few cases. In the early stages, basal ACTH and cortisol levels may be normal; however, ACTH reserve is impaired, and ACTH and cortisol responses to stress are therefore subnormal. With further loss of basal ACTH secretion, there is atrophy of the zonae fasciculata and reticularis of the adrenal cortex; and, therefore, basal cortisol secretion is decreased. At this stage, the entire pituitary adrenal axis is impaired; ie, there is not only decreased ACTH responsiveness to stress but also decreased adrenal responsiveness to acute stimulation with exogenous ACTH.

The manifestations of glucocorticoid deficiency are similar to those described for primary adrenocortical insufficiency. However, since aldosterone secretion by the zona glomerulosa is usually preserved, the manifestations of mineralocorticoid deficiency are absent.

Clinical Features

A. Symptoms and Signs: Secondary adrenal insufficiency is usually chronic, and the manifestations may be nonspecific. However, acute crisis can occur in undiagnosed patients or in corticosteroid-treated patients who do not receive increased steroid dosage during periods of stress.

The clinical features of secondary adrenal insufficiency differ from those of primary adrenocortical insufficiency in that pituitary secretion of ACTH and β-LPH is deficient and hyperpigmentation is therefore not present. In addition, mineralocorticoid secretion is usually normal. Thus, the clinical features of ACTH and glucocorticoid deficiency are nonspecific.

Volume depletion, dehydration, and electrolyte abnormalities are usually absent. Hypotension is usually not present except in acute presentations. Hyponatremia may occur as a result of water retention and inability to excrete a water load but is not accompanied by hyperkalemia. Prominent features are weakness, lethargy, easy fatigability, anorexia, nausea, and occasionally vomiting. Arthralgias and myalgias also occur. Hypoglycemia is occasionally the presenting feature. Acute decompensation with severe hypotension or shock unresponsive to vasopressors may occur.

B. Associated Features: Patients with secondary adrenal insufficiency commonly have additional features that suggest the diagnosis. A history of glucocorticoid therapy or, if this is not available, the presence of cushingoid features suggests prior glucocorticoid use. Hypothalamic or pituitary tumors leading to ACTH deficiency usually cause loss of other pituitary hormones (hypogonadism and hypothyroidism). Hypersecretion of GH or prolactin (PRL) from a pituitary adenoma may be present.

C. Laboratory Findings: Findings on routine laboratory examination consist of normochromic, normocytic anemia, neutropenia, lymphocytosis, and eosinophilia. Serum sodium, potassium, creatinine,

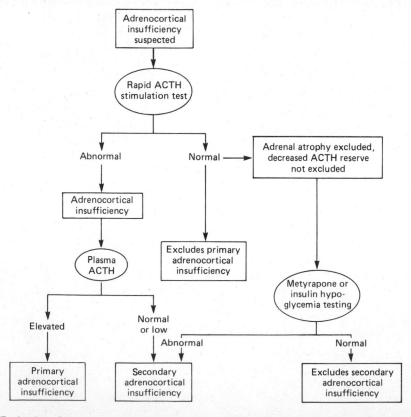

Figure 12–11. Evaluation of suspected primary or secondary adrenocortical insufficiency. Boxes enclose clinical decisions, and circles enclose diagnostic tests. (Redrawn and reproduced, with permission, from Baxter JD, Tyrrell JB: The adrenal cortex. In: *Endocrinology and Metabolism.* Felig P et al [editors]. McGraw-Hill, 1981.)

and bicarbonate and blood urea nitrogen are usually normal; plasma glucose may be low, though severe poglycemia is unusual.

DIAGNOSIS OF ADRENOCORTICAL INSUFFICIENCY

Although the diagnosis of adrenal insufficiency should be confirmed by assessment of the pituitary adrenal axis, therapy should not be delayed nor should the patient be subjected to procedures that may increase volume loss and dehydration and further contribute to hypotension. If the patient is acutely ill, therapy should be instituted and the diagnosis established when the patient is stable.

Diagnostic Tests

Since basal levels of adrenocortical steroids in either urine or plasma may be normal in partial adrenal insufficiency, tests of adrenocortical reserve are necessary to establish the diagnosis (Fig 12–11). These tests are described in the section on laboratory evaluation and in Chapter 6.

Rapid ACTH Stimulation Test

The rapid ACTH stimulation test assesses adrenal reserve and is the initial procedure in the assessment of possible adrenal insufficiency, either primary or secondary.

Subnormal responses to exogenous ACTH administration are an indication of decreased adrenal reserve and establish the diagnosis of adrenocortical insufficiency. Further diagnostic procedures are not required, since subnormal responses to the rapid ACTH stimulation test indicate lack of responsiveness to metyrapone, insulin-induced hypoglycemia, or stress. However, this test does not permit differentiation of primary and secondary causes. This is best accomplished by measurement of basal plasma ACTH levels, as discussed below.

A normal response to the rapid ACTH stimulation test excludes primary adrenal failure, since a normal cortisol response indicates normal cortical function. However, normal responsiveness does not exclude partial secondary adrenocortical insufficiency in those few patients with decreased pituitary reserve and decreased stress responsiveness of the hypothalamic-pituitary-adrenal axis who maintain sufficient basal ACTH secretion to prevent adrenocortical atrophy. If this situation is suspected clinically, pituitary ACTH responsiveness may be tested directly with metyrapone or insulin-induced hypoglycemia. (See section on laboratory evaluation and below.)

Plasma ACTH Levels

If adrenal insufficiency is present, plasma ACTH levels are used to differentiate primary and secondary forms. In patients with primary adrenal insufficiency, plasma ACTH levels are over 250 pg/mL (55.5 pmol/L) and usually range from 400 to 2000 pg/mL (88.8–444 pmol/L). With pituitary ACTH deficiency, plasma ACTH levels range from 0 to 50 pg/mL (0–11 pmol/L) and are usually less than 20 pg/mL (4.4 pmol/L) (Fig 12–12).

Partial ACTH Deficiency

When partial ACTH deficiency and decreased pituitary reserve are suspected despite normal responsiveness to the rapid ACTH stimulation test, the following procedures may be used for more direct assessment of hypothalamic-pituitary function:

A. Methods of Testing: The overnight **metyrapone test** is used in patients with suspected hypothalamic or pituitary disorders when hypoglycemia is contraindicated and in those with prior glucocorticoid therapy. **Insulin-induced hypoglycemia** is used in patients with suspected hypothalamic or pituitary tumors, since both ACTH and GH responsiveness can be assessed (see Chapter 6).

B. Interpretation: A normal response to either metyrapone or hypoglycemia excludes secondary adrenocortical insufficiency. (See section on laboratory evaluation.) Subnormal responses, in the presence of a normal response to ACTH administration, establish the diagnosis of secondary adrenal insufficiency.

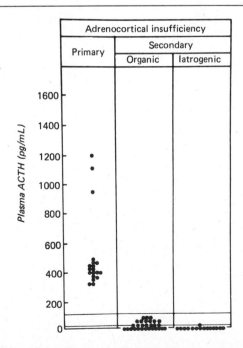

Figure 12–12. Basal plasma ACTH levels in primary and secondary adrenocortical insufficiency. (Reproduced, with permission, from Irvine WJ, Toft AD, Feek CM: Addison's disease. In: *The Adrenal Gland*. James VHT [editor]. Raven Press, 1979.)

TREATMENT OF ADRENOCORTICAL INSUFFICIENCY

The aim of treatment of adrenocortical insufficiency is to produce levels of glucocorticoids and mineralocorticoids equivalent to those achieved in an individual with normal hypothalamic-pituitary-adrenal function under similar circumstances.

Acute Addisonian Crisis (Table 12–6)

Treatment for acute addisonian crisis should be instituted as soon as the diagnosis is suspected. Therapy includes administration of glucocorticoids; correction of dehydration, hypovolemia, and electrolyte abnormalities; general supportive measures; and treatment of coexisting or precipitating disorders.

A. Cortisol (Hydrocortisone): Parenteral cortisol in soluble form (hydrocortisone hemisuccinate or phosphate) is the glucocorticoid preparation most commonly used. This agent has sufficient sodium-retaining potency so that additional mineralocorticoid therapy is not required in patients with primary adrenocortical insufficiency who have deficient secretion of both aldosterone and cortisol.

Cortisol in doses of 100 mg intravenously is given every 6 hours for the first 24 hours. The response to therapy is usually rapid, with improvement occurring within 12 hours or less. If improvement occurs and the patient is stable, 50 mg every 6 hours is given on the second day, and in most patients the dosage may then be gradually reduced to approximately 10 mg 3 times daily by the fourth or fifth day. (See section on maintenance therapy, below.)

1. In severely ill patients, especially in those with additional major complications (eg, sepsis), higher cortisol doses (100 mg intravenously every 6–8 hours) are maintained until the patient is stable.

2. In primary Addison's disease, mineralocorticoid replacement, in the form of fludrocortisone (see below), is added when the total cortisol dosage has been reduced to 50–60 mg/d.

3. In secondary adrenocortical insufficiency with acute crisis, the primary requirement is glucocorticoid replacement and is satisfactorily supplied by the administration of cortisol, as outlined above. If the possibility of excessive fluid and sodium retention in such patients is of concern, equivalent parenteral doses of synthetic steroids such as prednisolone or dexamethasone may be substituted.

4. Intramuscular cortisone acetate is contraindicated in acute adrenal failure for the following reasons: (1) absorption is slow; (2) it requires conversion to cortisol in the liver; (3) adequate plasma levels of cortisol are not obtained; and (4) there is inadequate suppression of plasma ACTH levels, indicating insufficient glucocorticoid activity.

B. Intravenous Fluids: Intravenous glucose and saline are administered to correct volume depletion, hypotension, and hypoglycemia. Volume deficits may be severe in Addison's disease, and hypotension and shock may not respond to vasopressors unless glucocorticoids are administered. Hyperkalemia and acidosis are usually corrected with cortisol and volume replacement; however, an occasional patient may require specific therapy for these abnormalities.

Maintenance Therapy (Table 12–7)

Patients with Addison's disease require lifelong therapy, usually with both glucocorticoids and mineralocorticoids. Cortisol (hydrocortisone) is the glucocorticoid preparation most often used. The total dosage is usually 25–30 mg/d orally, given as 15–20 mg in the morning on arising and 10 mg at 4–5 PM. Other glucocorticoids such as oral cortisone acetate (37.5 mg/d), which is rapidly absorbed and converted to cortisol, or equivalent doses of synthetic steroids (eg, prednisone or prednisolone) may also be used.

Cortisol in twice-daily doses gives satisfactory responses in most patients; however, some patients may require only a single morning dose, and others may require 3 doses per day to maintain well-being and normal energy levels. Insomnia as a side effect of glucocorticoid administration can usually be prevented by administering the last daily dose at 4–5 PM.

Fludrocortisone (9α-fluorocortisol; Florinef) is used for mineralocorticoid therapy; the usual doses are 0.05–0.1 mg/d orally in the morning. Because of the long half-life of this agent, divided doses are not re-

---

Table 12–6. Treatment of acute adrenal crises.

Glucocorticoid replacement
  (1) Administer cortisol (as hydrocortisone phosphate or hemisuccinate), 100 mg intravenously every 6 hours for 24 hours.
  (2) When the patient is stable, reduce the dosage to 50 mg every 6 hours.
  (3) Taper to maintenance therapy by day 4 or 5 and add mineralocorticoid therapy as required.
  (4) Maintain or increase the dose to 200–400 mg/d if complications persist or occur.

General and supportive measures
  (1) Correct volume depletion, dehydration, and hypoglycemia with intravenous saline and glucose.
  (2) Evaluate and correct infection and other precipitating factors.

Table 12–7. Regimen for maintenance therapy of primary adrenocortical insufficiency.[1]

(1) Cortisol, 15–20 mg in AM and 10 mg at 4–5 PM.
(2) Fludrocortisone, 0.05–0.1 mg orally in AM.
(3) Clinical follow-up: Maintenance of normal weight, blood pressure, and electrolytes with regression of clinical features.
(4) Patient education plus identification card or bracelet.
(5) Increased cortisol dosage during "stress."

[1]Reproduced, with permission, from Baxter JD, Tyrrell JB, in: *Endocrinology and Metabolism.* Felig P et al (editors). McGraw-Hill, 1981.

quired. About 10–20% of addisonian patients can be managed with cortisol and adequate dietary sodium intake alone and do not require fludrocortisone.

Secondary adrenocortical insufficiency is treated with the cortisol dosages described above for the primary form. Fludrocortisone is rarely required. The recovery of normal function of the hypothalamic-pituitary-adrenal axis following suppression by exogenous glucocorticoids may take weeks to years, depending on the dose and on the duration of therapy. Consequently, prolonged replacement therapy may be required.

Response to Therapy; Clinical Assessment

There are no currently available biochemical procedures for assessing the response to treatment of adrenocortical insufficiency. Measurement of plasma cortisol and ACTH levels is of no particular value, because of the wide variability in plasma levels in relationship to the timing of the cortisol dose and the time of plasma sampling. Measurement of urine free cortisol levels has been suggested, but a significant advantage has not yet been substantiated.

The adequacy of glucocorticoid and mineralocorticoid replacement is currently best evaluated by the clinical response to therapy. Thus, in appropriately treated patients, there is improvement or resolution of the features of glucocorticoid and mineralocorticoid deficiency, and most patients lead normal lives without significant disability.

A. Cortisol Therapy: Adequate treatment results in the disappearance of weakness, malaise, and fatigue. Anorexia and other gastrointestinal symptoms resolve, and weight returns to normal. The hyperpigmentation invariably improves but may not entirely disappear. Inadequate cortisol administration leads to persistence of these symptoms of adrenal insufficiency, and excessive pigmentation will remain. Greater than physiologic doses of glucocorticoids result in weight gain and may cause cushingoid features.

B. Mineralocorticoid Therapy: This should be monitored by frequent measurement of blood pressure and of serum electrolytes. With adequate treatment, the blood pressure is normal without orthostatic change, and serum sodium and potassium remain within the normal range. Hypertension and hypokalemia result if the fludrocortisone dose is excessive; conversely, undertreatment may lead to fatigue and malaise, orthostatic symptoms, and subnormal supine or upright blood pressure, with hyperkalemia and hyponatremia.

Prevention of Adrenal Crisis

The development of acute adrenal insufficiency in previously diagnosed and treated patients is almost entirely preventable in cooperative individuals. The 2 essential elements are patient education and increased glucocorticoid dosages during illness.

The patient should be informed about the necessity for lifelong therapy, the possible consequences of acute illness, and the necessity for increased therapy and medical assistance during acute illness. An identification card or bracelet should be carried or worn at all times.

The cortisol dose should be increased by the patient to 60–80 mg/d with the development of minor illnesses; the usual maintenance dosage may be resumed in 24–48 hours if improvement occurs. Increased mineralocorticoid therapy is not required.

If symptoms persist or become worse, the patient should continue increased cortisol doses and call the physician.

Vomiting may result in inability to ingest or absorb oral cortisol, and diarrhea in addisonian patients may precipitate a crisis because of rapid fluid and electrolyte losses. Patients must understand that if these symptoms occur, they should seek immediate medical assistance so that parenteral glucocorticoid therapy can be given.

Steroid Coverage for Surgery (Table 12–8)

Patients with primary or secondary adrenocortical insufficiency scheduled for elective surgery require increased glucocorticoid coverage. This problem is most frequently encountered in patients with pituitary-adrenal suppression due to exogenous glucocorticoid therapy. The principles of management are outlined in Table 12–8. *Note:* Intramuscular cortisone acetate should not be used, for the reasons discussed above in the section on treatment of acute addisonian crisis.

PROGNOSIS OF ADRENOCORTICAL INSUFFICIENCY

Before glucocorticoid and mineralocorticoid therapy became available, primary adrenocortical insufficiency was invariably fatal, with death usually occurring within 2 years after onset. Survival now depends upon the underlying cause of the adrenal insufficien-

Table 12–8. Steroid coverage for surgery.[1]

(1) Correct electrolytes, blood pressure, and hydration if necessary.

(2) Give hydrocortisone phosphate or hemisuccinate, 100 mg intramuscularly, on call to operating room.

(3) Give hydrocortisone phosphate or hemisuccinate, 50 mg intramuscularly or intravenously, in the recovery room and every 6 hours for the first 24 hours.

(4) If progress is satisfactory, reduce dosage to 25 mg every 6 hours for 24 hours and then taper to maintenance dosage over 3–5 days. Resume previous fludrocortisone dose when the patient is taking oral medications.

(5) Maintain or increase cortisol dosage to 200–400 mg/d if fever, hypotension, or other complications occur.

[1]Reproduced, with permission, from Baxter JD, Tyrrell JB, in: *Endocrinology and Metabolism.* Felig P et al (editors). McGraw-Hill, 1981.

cy. In patients with autoimmune Addison's disease, survival approaches that of the normal population, and most patients lead normal lives. In general, death from adrenal insufficiency now occurs only in patients with rapid onset of disease who may die before the diagnosis is established and appropriate therapy started.

Secondary adrenal insufficiency has an excellent prognosis with glucocorticoid therapy.

Adrenal insufficiency due to bilateral adrenal hemorrhage is still often fatal, with most cases being recognized only at autopsy.

CUSHING'S SYNDROME

Chronic glucocorticoid excess, whatever its cause, leads to the constellation of symptoms and physical features known as **Cushing's syndrome.** It is most commonly iatrogenic, resulting from chronic glucocorticoid therapy. "Spontaneous" Cushing's syndrome is caused by abnormalities of the pituitary or adrenal or may occur as a consequence of ACTH secretion by nonpituitary tumors (**ectopic ACTH syndrome**). **Cushing's disease** is defined as the specific type of Cushing's syndrome due to excessive pituitary ACTH secretion. This section will review the various types of spontaneous Cushing's syndrome and discuss their diagnosis and therapy. (See also Chapter 6.)

Classification & Incidence

Cushing's syndrome is conveniently classified as either ACTH-dependent or ACTH-independent (Table 12–9).

The ACTH-dependent types of Cushing's syndrome—ectopic ACTH syndrome and Cushing's disease—are characterized by chronic ACTH hypersecretion, which results in hyperplasia of the adrenal zonae fasciculata and reticularis and therefore increased adrenocortical secretion of cortisol, androgens, and DOC.

Table 12–9. Classification and etiology of Cushing's syndrome.[1]

	Percent
ACTH-dependent	
Cushing's disease	68
Ectopic ACTH syndrome	15
ACTH-independent	
Adrenal adenoma	9
Adrenal carcinoma	8
	100

[1]Reproduced, with permission, from Baxter JD, Tyrrell JB, in: *Endocrinology and Metabolism.* Felig P et al (editors). McGraw-Hill, 1981.

ACTH-independent Cushing's syndrome is due to autonomous glucocorticoid-secreting adrenocortical adenomas or carcinomas; in these cases, the resulting cortisol excess suppresses pituitary ACTH secretion.

A. Cushing's Disease: This is the most frequent type of Cushing's syndrome and is responsible for about 70% of reported cases. Cushing's disease is much more common in women than in men (female:male ratio of about 8:1) and the age at diagnosis is usually between 20 and 40 years.

B. Ectopic ACTH Hypersecretion: This disorder is said to account for about 15% of cases of Cushing's syndrome. That figure is probably an underestimate, since it is likely that many patients are not diagnosed because they lack the classic features of hypercortisolism. In addition, severe hypercortisolism and rapid death are common. Ectopic ACTH secretion is most common with small cell carcinoma of the lung; this tumor is responsible for about 50% of cases of the syndrome. Ectopic ACTH hypersecretion is estimated to occur in 0.5–2% of patients with this tumor. Other tumors are discussed below. The ectopic ACTH syndrome is more common in men, presumably because of their higher incidence of small-cell carcinoma. The female:male ratio is 1:3, and the peak incidence is at age 40–60 years.

C. Primary Adrenal Tumors: Primary adrenal tumors cause 17–19% of cases of Cushing's syndrome; adenoma and carcinoma occur with about equal frequency in adults. Glucocorticoid-secreting adrenal adenomas are more common in females. Adrenocortical carcinomas causing cortisol excess are also more common in females; however, if all types (including nonsecreting tumors) are considered, the overall incidence is higher in males. Adrenal carcinoma occurs in about 2 per million population per year; the mean age at diagnosis is 38 years; and 75% of cases occur in adults.

D. Childhood Cushing's Syndrome: Cushing's syndrome in childhood and adolescence is distinctly unusual; however, in contrast to the incidence in adults, adrenal carcinoma is the most frequent cause (51%), and adrenal adenomas are present in 14%. These tumors are more common in girls than in boys, and most occur between the ages of 1 and 8 years. Cushing's disease is more common in the adolescent population and accounts for 35% of cases; most of these patients are over 10 years of age at diagnosis, and the sex incidence is equal.

Pathology

A. Anterior Pituitary Gland:

1. Pituitary adenomas–Pituitary adenomas are present in over 90% of patients with Cushing's disease. These tumors are typically smaller than those secreting GH or PRL; 80–90% are less than 10 mm in diameter. A small group of patients have larger tumors (> 10 mm); these macroadenomas are frequently invasive, leading to extension outside the sella turcica. Malignant pituitary tumors occur rarely.

Microadenomas are located within the anterior pituitary; they are not encapsulated but surrounded by a rim of compressed normal anterior pituitary cells. With routine histologic stains, these tumors are composed of compact sheets of well-granulated basophilic cells in a sinusoidal arrangement. ACTH, β-LPH, and β-endorphin have been demonstrated in these tumor cells by immunocytochemical methods. Larger tumors may appear chromophobic on routine histologic study; however, they also contain ACTH and its related peptides. These ACTH-secreting adenomas typically show Crooke's changes (a zone of perinuclear hyalinization that is the result of chronic exposure of corticotroph cells to hypercortisolism). Electron microscopy demonstrates secretory granules that vary in size from 200 to 700 nm. The number of granules varies in individual cells; they may be dispersed throughout the cytoplasm or concentrated along the cell membrane. A typical feature of these adenomas is the presence of bundles of perinuclear microfilaments (average 7 nm in diameter) surrounding the nucleus; these are responsible for Crooke's hyaline changes visible on light microscopy.

2. Hyperplasia–Diffuse hyperplasia of corticotroph cells has been reported rarely in patients with Cushing's disease. These cases may be the consequence of excessive stimulation of the anterior pituitary by CRH.

3. Other conditions–In patients with adrenal tumors or ectopic ACTH syndrome, the pituitary corticotrophs show prominent Crooke hyaline changes and perinuclear microfilaments. The ACTH content of corticotroph cells is reduced consistent with their suppression by excessive cortisol secretion present in these conditions.

B. Adrenocortical Hyperplasia: Bilateral hyperplasia of the adrenal cortex occurs with chronic ACTH hypersecretion. Three types have been described: simple, that associated with ectopic ACTH syndrome, and bilateral nodular hyperplasia.

1. Simple adrenocortical hyperplasia–This condition is usually due to Cushing's disease. Combined adrenal weight (normal, 8–10 g) is modestly increased, ranging from 12 to 24 g. On histologic study, there is equal hyperplasia of the compact cells of the zona reticularis and the clear cells of the zona fasciculata; consequently, the width of the cortex is increased. Electron microscopy reveals normal ultrastructural features.

2. Ectopic ACTH syndrome–In this disorder, the adrenals are frequently markedly enlarged; combined weights range from 24 g to more than 50 g. The characteristic microscopic feature is marked hyperplasia of the zona reticularis; columns of compact reticularis cells expand throughout the zona fasciculata and into the zona glomerulosa. The zona fasciculata clear cells are markedly reduced.

3. Bilateral nodular hyperplasia–Macronodular hyperplasia occurs in about 20% of cases of adrenocortical hyperplasia. The exact pathogenesis of this lesion is unclear; most cases appear to be secondary to pituitary ACTH excess, but in a minority of cases there may be autonomous function of the adrenals. The adrenals are enlarged; adrenal weight is increased and may be markedly so if large nodules are present. Grossly, there are multiple nodules of various sizes within the adrenal cortices, with widening of the intervening cortex. The nodules are typically yellow and on histologic examination resemble the clear cells of the normal zona fasciculata. The adrenal cortex not involved by the nodules shows the histologic features of simple adrenocortical hyperplasia (see above). Adrenal carcinoma in association with nodular hyperplasia has been described in a few patients. Micronodular hyperplasia occurs less frequently. Both adrenals are involved, and there are multiple small nodules that may be pigmented; the intervening cortex is atrophic. The pathogenesis of this lesion is also unclear, but it appears not to involve ACTH. This disorder presents at a younger age. It may be familial and may also occur in association with cardiac myxomas, spotty pigmented lesions of the skin, and other endocrine disorders such as growth hormone-producing pituitary tumors.

C. Adrenal Tumors: Adrenal tumors causing Cushing's syndrome are independent of ACTH secretion and are either adenomas or carcinomas.

1. Glucocorticoid-secreting adrenal adenomas–These adenomas are encapsulated, weigh 10–70 g, and range in size from 1 to 6 cm. Microscopically, clear cells of the zona fasciculata type predominate, although cells typical of the zona reticularis are also seen.

2. Adrenal carcinomas–Adrenal carcinomas usually weigh over 100 g and may exceed several kilograms. Thus, they are commonly palpable as abdominal masses. Grossly, they are encapsulated and highly vascular; necrosis, hemorrhage, and cystic degeneration are common, and areas of calcification may be present. The histologic appearance of these carcinomas varies considerably; they may appear to be benign or may exhibit considerable pleomorphism. Vascular or capsular invasion is predictive of malignant behavior, as is local extension. These carcinomas invade local structures (kidney, liver, and retroperitoneum) and metastasize hematogenously to liver and lung.

3. Uninvolved adrenal cortex–The cortex contiguous to the tumor and that of the contralateral gland are atrophic in the presence of functioning adrenal adenomas and carcinomas. The cortex is markedly thinned, whereas the capsule is thickened. Histologically, the zona reticularis is virtually absent; the remaining cortex is composed of clear fasciculata cells. The architecture of the zona glomerulosa is normal.

Etiology & Pathogenesis

A. Cushing's Disease: The causes and natural history of Cushing's disease are reviewed in Chapter 6.

Current evidence is consistent with the view that spontaneously arising corticotroph-cell pituitary adenomas are the primary cause and that the consequent ACTH hypersecretion and hypercortisolism lead to the characteristic endocrine abnormalities and hypothalamic dysfunction. This is supported by evidence showing that selective removal of these adenomas by pituitary microsurgery reverses the abnormalities and is followed by return of the hypothalamic-pituitary-adrenal axis to normal.

Although these primary pituitary adenomas are responsible for the great majority of cases, a few patients have been described in whom pituitary disease has been limited to corticotroph-cell hyperplasia; these may be secondary to excessive CRH secretion by rare, benign hypothalamic gangliocytoma.

B. Ectopic ACTH Syndrome: This syndrome arises when nonpituitary tumors synthesize and hypersecrete biologically active ACTH. The related peptides β-LPH and β-endorphin are also synthesized and secreted, as are inactive ACTH fragments. Production of CRH has also been demonstrated in ectopic tumors secreting ACTH, but whether CRH plays a role in pathogenesis is unclear. A few cases in which nonpituitary tumors produced only CRH have been reported.

Ectopic ACTH syndrome occurs predominantly in only a few tumor types (Table 12–10); small-cell carcinoma of the lung causes half of cases. Other tumors causing the syndrome are epithelial thymoma; pancreatic islet cell tumors; carcinoid tumors of lung, gut, pancreas, or ovary; medullary thyroid carcinoma; and pheochromocytoma and related tumors. Other rare miscellaneous tumor types have also been reported (see Chapter 27).

C. Adrenal Tumors: Glucocorticoid-producing adrenal adenomas and carcinomas arise spontaneously. They are not under hypothalamic-pituitary control and autonomously secrete adrenocortical steroids. Rarely, adrenal carcinomas develop in the setting of chronic ACTH hypersecretion in patients with either Cushing's disease and nodular adrenal hyperplasia or congenital adrenal hyperplasia.

Pathophysiology

A. Cushing's Disease: In Cushing's disease, ACTH hypersecretion is random and episodic and causes cortisol hypersecretion with absence of the normal circadian rhythm. Feedback inhibition of ACTH (secreted from the pituitary adenoma) by physiologic levels of glucocorticoids is absent; thus, ACTH hypersecretion persists despite elevated cortisol secretion and results in chronic glucocorticoid excess. The episodic secretion of ACTH and cortisol results in variable plasma levels that may at times be within the normal range. However, measurement of the cortisol production rate, urine free cortisol, or sampling of multiple cortisol levels over 24 hours confirms cortisol hypersecretion (see sections on laboratory evaluation and diagnosis of Cushing's syndrome). In addition, because of the absence of diurnal variability, plasma ACTH and cortisol remain elevated throughout the day and night. This overall increase in glucocorticoid secretion causes the clinical manifestations of Cushing's syndrome; however, ACTH and β-LPH secretion are not usually elevated sufficiently to cause hyperpigmentation.

1. Abnormalities of ACTH secretion–Despite ACTH hypersecretion, stress responsiveness is absent; stimuli such as hypoglycemia or surgery fail to further elevate ACTH and cortisol secretion. This is probably due to suppression of hypothalamic function and CRH secretion by hypercortisolism, resulting in loss of hypothalamic control of ACTH secretion (see Chapter 6).

2. Effect of cortisol excess–Cortisol excess not only inhibits normal pituitary and hypothalamic function, affecting ACTH, thyrotropin, GH, and gonadotropin release, but also results in all the systemic effects of glucocorticoid excess described in previous sections and in the section on clinical features below.

3. Androgen excess–Secretion of adrenal androgens is also increased in Cushing's disease, and the degree of androgen excess parallels that of ACTH and cortisol. Thus, plasma levels of DHEA, DHEA sulfate, and androstenedione may be moderately elevated in Cushing's disease; the peripheral conversion of these hormones to testosterone and dihydrotestosterone leads to androgen excess. In women, this causes hirsutism, acne, and amenorrhea. In men with Cushing's disease, cortisol suppression of LH secretion decreases testosterone secretion by the testis, resulting in decreased libido and impotence. The increased adrenal androgen secretion is insufficient to compensate for the decreased gonadal testosterone production.

B. Ectopic ACTH Syndrome: Hypersecretion of ACTH and cortisol is usually greater in patients with ectopic ACTH syndrome than in those with Cushing's disease. ACTH and cortisol hypersecretion is randomly episodic, and the levels are often greatly elevated. With few exceptions, ACTH secretion by ectopic tumors is not subject to negative-feedback control; ie, secretion of ACTH and cortisol is nonsuppressible with pharmacologic doses of glucocorticoids (see section on diagnosis).

Table 12–10. Tumors causing the ectopic ACTH syndrome.[1]

Small-cell carcinoma of the lung (50% of cases)
Thymoma
Pancreatic islet cell tumors
Carcinoid tumors (lung, gut, pancreas, ovary)
Medullary carcinoma of the thyroid
Pheochromocytoma and related tumors

[1]Modified and reproduced, with permission, from Baxter JD, Tyrrell JB, in: *Endocrinology and Metabolism.* Felig P et al (editors). McGraw-Hill, 1981.

Plasma levels, secretion rates, and urinary excretion of cortisol, the adrenal androgens, and DOC are often markedly elevated; despite this, the typical features of Cushing's syndrome are usually absent, presumably because of rapid onset of hypercortisolism, anorexia, and other manifestations of the associated malignant disease. However, features of mineralocorticoid excess (hypertension and hypokalemia) are frequently due to DOC and the mineralocorticoid effects of cortisol.

C. Adrenal Tumors:

1. Autonomous secretion–Primary adrenal tumors, both adenomas and carcinomas, autonomously hypersecrete cortisol. Circulating plasma ACTH levels are suppressed, resulting in cortical atrophy of the uninvolved adrenal. Secretion is randomly episodic, and these tumors are typically unresponsive to manipulation of the hypothalamic-pituitary axis with pharmacologic agents such as dexamethasone and metyrapone.

2. Adrenal adenomas–Adrenal adenomas causing Cushing's syndrome typically present solely with clinical manifestations of glucocorticoid excess, since they usually secrete only cortisol. Thus, the presence of androgen or mineralocorticoid excess should suggest that the tumor is an adrenocortical carcinoma.

3. Adrenal carcinomas–Adrenal carcinomas frequently hypersecrete multiple adrenocortical steroids and their precursors. Cortisol and androgens are the steroids most frequently secreted in excess; 11-deoxycortisol is often elevated, and there may be increased secretion of DOC, aldosterone, or estrogens. Plasma cortisol, urine free cortisol, and urine 17-hydroxycorticosteroids are often markedly increased; androgen excess is usually even greater than that of cortisol. Thus, high levels of plasma DHEA and DHEA sulfate and of urinary 17-ketosteroids typically accompany the cortisol excess. Clinical manifestations of hypercortisolism are usually severe and rapidly progressive in these patients. In women, features of androgen excess are prominent; virilism may occasionally occur. Hypertension and hypokalemia are frequent and most commonly result from the mineralocorticoid effects of cortisol; less frequently, DOC and aldosterone hypersecretion also contribute.

Clinical Features
(Table 12–11)

A. Symptoms and Signs:

1. Obesity–Obesity is the most common manifestation, and weight gain is usually the initial symptom. It is classically central, affecting mainly the face, neck, trunk, and abdomen, with relative sparing of the extremities. Generalized obesity with central accentuation is equally common, particularly in children.

Accumulation of fat in the face leads to the typical "moon facies," which is present in 75% of cases and is accompanied by facial plethora in most patients. Fat accumulation around the neck is prominent in the su-

Table 12–11. Cinical features of Cushing's syndrome.[1]

	Percent
Obesity	94
Facial plethora	84
Hirsutism	82
Menstrual disorders	76
Hypertension	72
Muscular weakness	58
Back pain	58
Striae	52
Acne	40
Psychologic symptoms	40
Bruising	36
Congestive heart failure	22
Edema	18
Renal calculi	16
Headache	14
Polyuria-polydipsia	10
Hyperpigmentation	6

[1]Reproduced, with permission, from Baxter JD, Tyrrell JB, in: *Endocrinology and Metabolism.* Felig P et al (editors). McGraw-Hill, 1981.

praclavicular and dorsocervical fat pads; the latter is responsible for the "buffalo hump."

Obesity is absent in a handful of patients who do not gain weight; however, they usually have central redistribution of fat and a typical facial appearance.

2. Skin changes–Skin changes are frequent, and their presence should arouse a suspicion of cortisol excess. Atrophy of the epidermis and its underlying connective tissue leads to thinning (a transparent appearance of the skin) and facial plethora. Easy bruisability following minimal trauma is present in about 40%. Striae occur in 50–70%; these are typically red to purple, depressed below the skin surface secondary to loss of underlying connective tissue, and wider (not infrequently 0.5–2 cm) than the pinkish white striae that may occur with pregnancy or rapid weight gain. These striae are most commonly abdominal but may also occur over the breasts, hips, buttocks, thighs, and axillae.

Minor wounds and abrasions may heal slowly, and surgical incisions sometimes undergo dehiscence.

Mucocutaneous fungal infections are frequent, including tinea versicolor, involvement of the nails (onychomycosis), and oral candidiasis.

Hyperpigmentation of the skin is rare in Cushing's disease or adrenal tumors but is common in ectopic ACTH syndrome.

3. Hirsutism–Hirsutism is present in about 80% of female patients owing to hypersecretion of adrenal androgens. Facial hirsutism is most common, but increased hair growth may also occur over the abdomen, breasts, chest, and upper thighs. Acne and seborrhea usually accompany hirsutism. Virilism is unusual except in cases of adrenal carcinoma, in which it occurs in about 20%.

4. Hypertension–Hypertension is a classic feature of spontaneous Cushing's syndrome; it is present in about 75% of cases, and the diastolic blood pressure is greater than 100 mm Hg in over 50%. Hypertension and its complications contribute greatly to the morbidity and mortality rates in spontaneous Cushing's syndrome; in the series of Plotz et al, 40% of those dying with the syndrome did so as a direct result of hypertension or atherosclerosis.

5. Gonadal dysfunction–This is very common as a result of elevated androgens (in females) and cortisol (in males and to a lesser extent in females). Amenorrhea occurs in 75% of premenopausal women and is usually accompanied by infertility. Decreased libido is frequent in males, and some have decreased body hair and soft testes.

6. Psychologic disturbances–Psychologic disturbances occur in about 40% of patients. Mild symptoms consist of emotional lability and increased irritability. Anxiety, depression, poor concentration, and poor memory may also be present. Euphoria is frequent, and occasional patients manifest overtly manic behavior. Sleep disorders are present in most patients, with either insomnia or early morning awakening.

Severe psychologic disorders occur in a few patients and include severe depression, psychosis with delusions or hallucinations, and paranoia. Some patients have committed suicide.

7. Muscle weakness–This occurs in about 60% of cases; it is more often proximal and is usually most prominent in the lower extremities.

8. Osteoporosis–Osteoporosis is present in most patients; back pain is an initial complaint in 58% of cases. Pathologic fractures occur in severe cases involving the ribs and vertebral bodies. Compression fractures of the spine are demonstrable radiographically in 16–22%.

9. Renal calculi–Calculi secondary to glucocorticoid-induced hypercalciuria occur in approximately 15% of patients, and renal colic may occasionally be a presenting complaint.

10. Thirst and polyuria–Thirst and polyuria secondary to overt hyperglycemia and diabetes mellitus occur in about 10% of patients, whereas asymptomatic glucose intolerance is much more frequent. Diabetic ketoacidosis is rare, as are diabetic microvascular complications.

B. Laboratory Findings: Routine laboratory examinations are described here. Specific diagnostic tests to establish the diagnosis of Cushing's syndrome are discussed in the section on diagnosis.

High normal hemoglobin, hematocrit, and red cell counts are usual; polycythemia is rare. The total white count is usually normal; however, both the percentage of lymphocytes and the total lymphocyte count may be subnormal. Eosinophils are also depressed, and a total eosinophil count less than $100/\mu L$ is present in most patients. Serum electrolytes, with rare exceptions, are normal in Cushing's disease; however, hypokalemic alkalosis occurs when there is marked steroid hyper-

secretion with the ectopic ACTH syndrome or adrenocortical carcinoma.

Fasting hyperglycemia or clinical diabetes occurs in only 10–15% of patients; postprandial hyperglycemia is more common. Glycosuria is present in patients with fasting or postprandial hyperglycemia. Most patients have secondary hyperinsulinemia and abnormal glucose tolerance tests.

Serum calcium is normal; serum phosphorus is low normal or slightly depressed. Hypercalciuria is present in 40% of cases.

C. X-Ray Findings: Routine radiographs may reveal cardiomegaly due to hypertensive or atherosclerotic heart disease. Vertebral compression fractures, rib fractures, and renal calculi may be present.

D. Electrocardiographic Findings: Hypertensive, ischemic, and electrolyte-induced changes may be present on the ECG.

Features Suggesting a Specific Cause

A. Cushing's Disease: Cushing's disease typifies the classic clinical picture: female predominance, onset generally between ages 20 and 40, and a slow progression over several years. Hyperpigmentation and hypokalemic alkalosis are rare; androgenic manifestations are limited to acne and hirsutism. Secretion of cortisol and adrenal androgens is only moderately increased.

B. Ectopic ACTH Syndrome (Carcinoma): In contrast, this syndrome occurs predominantly in males, with the highest incidence between ages 40 and 60. The clinical manifestations of hypercortisolism are frequently limited to weakness, hypertension, and glucose intolerance; the primary tumor is usually apparent. Hyperpigmentation, hypokalemia, and alkalosis are common, as are weight loss and anemia. The hypercortisolism is of rapid onset, and steroid hypersecretion is frequently severe, with equally elevated levels of glucocorticoids, androgens, and DOC.

C. Ectopic ACTH Syndrome (Benign Tumor): A minority of patients with ectopic ACTH syndrome due to more "benign" tumors, especially bronchial carcinoids, present a more slowly progressive course, with typical features of Cushing's syndrome. These patients may be clinically identical with those having pituitary-dependent Cushing's disease, and the responsible tumor may not be apparent. Hyperpigmentation, hypokalemic alkalosis, and anemia are variably present. Further confusion may arise, since a number of these patients with occult ectopic tumors may have ACTH and steroid dynamics typical of Cushing's disease (see below).

D. Adrenal Adenomas: The clinical picture in patients with adrenal adenomas is usually that of glucocorticoid excess alone, and androgenic effects such as hirsutism are usually absent. Onset is gradual, and hypercortisolism is mold to moderate. Urinary 17-

ketosteroids and plasma androgens are usually in the low normal or subnormal range.

E. Adrenal Carcinomas: In general, adrenal carcinomas have a rapid onset of the clinical features of excessive glucocorticoid, androgen, and mineralocorticoid secretion and are rapidly progressive. Marked elevations of both cortisol and androgens are usual; hypokalemia is common, as are abdominal pain, palpable masses, and hepatic and pulmonary metastases.

Diagnostic Procedures
(Fig 12–13)

A. Diagnosis of Hypercortisolism (Cushing's Syndrome):

1. Overnight dexamethasone and urine free cortisol—Suspected hypercortisolism is investigated by means of the overnight 1-mg dexamethasone suppression test plus measurement of free cortisol in a 24-hour urine specimen collected on an outpatient basis. If the overnight suppression test is normal (plasma cortisol < 5 μg/dL [0.14 μmol/L]), the diagnosis is very unlikely; if the urine free cortisol is also normal, Cushing's syndrome is excluded.

If these 2 tests are abnormal, hypercortisolism is present and the diagnosis of Cushing's syndrome can be considered established if conditions causing false-positive responses are excluded (see discussion below).

2. Two-day low-dose dexamethasone test—In patients with equivocal or borderline results, a 2-day low-dose dexamethasone suppression test is performed. Normal responses to this test are 17-hydroxycorticosteroid levels less than 4 mg/24 h (11.2 μmol/24 h) (or 1 mg/g of creatinine [0.3 mmol/mol of

creatinine]), free cortisol less than 25 μg/24 h (69 nmol/24 h), and plasma cortisol less than 5 μg/dL (0.14 μmol/L). A normal response excludes Cushing's syndrome, and abnormal suppressibility is consistent with the diagnosis, since the incidence of false-positive responses is negligible.

3. Other tests—Other tests are less reliable in diagnosis and are no longer recommended; these include basal morning cortisol levels, afternoon or early evening cortisol, basal 24-hour urine 17-hydroxysteroids, 17-ketogenic steroids, or 17-ketosteroids, and responsiveness to either ACTH or metyrapone stimulation tests (see Laboratory Evaluation, above).

B. Differential Diagnosis of Hypercortisolism: A number of factors may complicate the diagnosis of Cushing's syndrome. These include both rare false-negative results in patients with Cushing's syndrome and, more commonly, false-positive results in those who do not have the disorder.

1. False-negative responses—False-negative results occur rarely in Cushing's syndrome. In these patients, normal suppression of glucocorticoid secretion with low-dose dexamethasone may be due to delayed clearance of dexamethasone and thus higher than usual plasma levels. However, elevated urine free cortisol will establish the diagnosis. Periodic or episodic hormonogenesis in Cushing's syndrome also makes diagnosis difficult. In these unusual patients, hypercortisolism may be cyclic, with regular periodicity of days to weeks, or irregularly episodic; thus, cortisol secretion may be normal or nearly so between cycles or episodes. With spontaneously varying cortisol secretion, adrenal function may be normal at times, and dexamethasone administration during phases of nor-

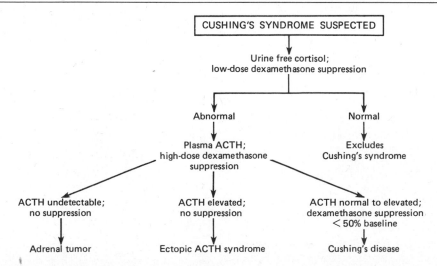

Figure 12–13. Diagnostic evaluation of Cushing's syndrome and procedures for determining the cause. Exceptions and diagnostic difficulties are discussed in the text. (Redrawn and reproduced, with permission, from Baxter JD, Tyrrell JB: The adrenal cortex. In: *Endocrinology and Metabolism.* Felig P et al [editors]. 2nd ed. McGraw-Hill, 1987.)

mal secretion may appear to reveal normal suppressibility. In these patients, repeated evaluation is required to establish the diagnosis.

2. False-positive responses–False-positive results are more common:

a. Acute or chronic illness–Especially in hospitalized patients, acute or chronic illness may appropriately elevate glucocorticoid secretion. Patients may have elevated plasma cortisol and urine free cortisol and are frequently nonsuppressible with the 1-mg overnight dexamethasone test. If Cushing's syndrome is suspected, diagnostic evaluation should be repeated when acute stress has resolved.

b. Obesity–Obesity is the most common differential problem in Cushing's syndrome. Urinary 17-hydroxycorticosteroids and 17-ketogenic steroids are often elevated; furthermore, about 15% of obese patients do not adequately suppress plasma cortisol in response to the 1-mg overnight dexamethasone suppression test. However, urine free cortisol excretion is normal in simple obesity, as is normal suppressibility of urine corticosteroids with the 2-day low-dose suppression test.

c. High-estrogen states–Pregnancy, estrogen therapy, and oral contraceptives increase CBG and thus elevate total plasma cortisol levels to 40–60 μg/dL (1.1–1.7 μmol/L). The overnight 1-mg suppression test may be abnormal; however, urine free cortisol is normal, and there is normal suppressibility of urine steroids with the 2-day low-dose test.

d. Drugs–Various drugs, especially phenytoin, phenobarbital, and primidone, cause false-positive low-dose dexamethasone tests; however, urine free cortisol is normal.

e. Alcoholism–A number of alcoholic patients have both clinical and biochemical features of Cushing's syndrome (alcohol-induced pseudo-Cushing's syndrome) with elevated basal plasma cortisol levels, abnormal diurnal variation, increased cortisol production rate, increased urinary corticosteroid excretion, and abnormal dexamethasone suppressibility. These abnormalities revert to normal following abstinence from alcohol.

f. Depression–Endogenous depression frequently causes increased cortisol secretion with elevated plasma levels, absence of diurnal variation, increased urine free cortisol, increased urine 17-hydroxycorticosteroids, and impaired dexamethasone suppressibility in the overnight dexamethasone test. The abnormal steroid dynamics revert to normal upon psychologic recovery. These patients can be differentiated from those with true Cushing's syndrome, since patients with depression alone maintain normal cortisol responsiveness to insulin-induced hypoglycemia, whereas patients with Cushing's syndrome do not. In addition, depressed patients usually maintain normal responses to the 2-day low-dose dexamethasone test.

C. Differential Diagnosis of Cushing's Syndrome: When Cushing's syndrome is present, pituitary ACTH hypersecretion (Cushing's disease) must be differentiated from ectopic ACTH syndrome and primary adrenal tumors.

1. Procedures–The 2 most specific procedures are measurement of basal plasma ACTH levels and high-dose dexamethasone suppression testing (see Laboratory Evaluation, above). The combined results of these 2 tests will establish the correct diagnosis in most instances.

2. Results–

a. Cushing's disease–Patients with Cushing's disease have normal to modestly elevated plasma ACTH levels (Fig 12–14), and the presence of detectable levels is consistent with bilateral adrenocortical hyperplasia. Plasma ACTH levels in Cushing's disease range from 40 to 200 pg/mL (8.8 to 44.4 pmol/L) (normal, 20–100 pg/mL [4.4–22.2 pmol/L]), and

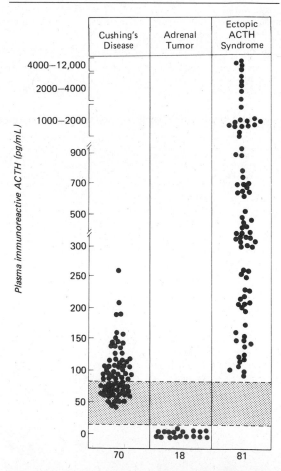

Figure 12–14. Basal plasma ACTH concentrations in patients with spontaneous Cushing's syndrome. (Reproduced, with permission, from Scott AP et al: Pituitary adrenocorticotropin and the melanocyte stimulating hormones. In: *Peptide Hormones.* Parsons JA [editor]. University Park Press, 1979.)

about 50% of patients have values consistently within the normal range. Patients with Cushing's disease characteristically maintain suppressibility of ACTH secretion; ie, cortisol secretion is suppressible to below 50% of basal levels with the high-dose dexamethasone tests.

b. Ectopic ACTH syndrome–In the ectopic ACTH syndrome, plasma ACTH levels are often markedly elevated (500–10,000 pg/mL [111–2222 pmol/L]) and are above 200 pg/mL (44.4 pmol/L) in 65% of patients. However, since at lower levels these overlap with the range seen in Cushing's disease, dexamethasone suppression testing must also be used. Since hypothalamic control of ACTH secretion is absent, cortisol secretion is classically not suppressible with high-dose dexamethasone. In addition, the primary tumor is clinically evident in most patients.

c. Adrenal tumors–Glucocorticoid-secreting adrenal tumors function autonomously, and the resulting suppression of the normal hypothalamic-pituitary axis leads to undetectable plasma ACTH levels ($<$ 20 pg/mL [4.4 pmol/L]) and absent steroid suppression with high-dose dexamethasone.

3. Other tests–CRH testing in Cushing's syndrome reveals that the majority of patients with Cushing's disease respond to CRH, whereas those with ectopic ACTH syndrome do not. However, exceptions have already been reported in both entities, and thus the ultimate clinical utility of this procedure is not yet clear. Metyrapone testing and ACTH stimulation tests do not adequately distinguish the various causes of Cushing's syndrome and are of little diagnostic utility.

D. Problems in Making Etiologic Diagnoses:

1. Episodic hypercortisolism–Problems are encountered in rare patients with periodic, cyclic, or episodic hormonogenesis who may have either Cushing's disease, ectopic ACTH syndrome, or adrenal tumors. Variable responses to high-dose dexamethasone may be observed, and there may be apparent suppressibility if steroid secretion is declining spontaneously at the time of dexamethasone administration. When studied at other times, these patients may be nonsuppressible or even show paradoxic increases during high-dose dexamethasone treatment. Repeated evaluations and use of the localizing procedures described below may be necessary to establish the correct etiologic diagnosis in such patients.

2. Nonsuppressible Cushing's disease and nodular adrenal hyperplasia–About 10–30% of patients with Cushing's disease fail to suppress urinary 17-hydroxycorticosteroids with the standard 2-day high-dose dexamethasone suppression test. This incidence of inadequate suppressibility is less with the overnight 8-mg high-dose dexamethasone suppression test, and the overnight test is therefore preferred. Nonsuppressible Cushing's disease may occur with large pituitary tumors; however, it is also seen in patients with microadenomas and in patients without an obvious pituitary adenoma in whom ACTH is

measurable; these findings falsely suggest the ectopic ACTH syndrome.

In these patients, additional procedures are required. Higher doses of dexamethasone (16 or 32 mg) may be administered, and if steroid suppression is demonstrated, Cushing's disease is suggested. The diagnosis is confirmed by demonstration of the pituitary adenoma using high-resolution CT scanning or the demonstration of pituitary ACTH hypersecretion by selective venous sampling. (See section on tumor localization, below.)

Some of these nonsuppressible patients have macronodular adrenal hyperplasia, which is usually secondary to pituitary ACTH hypersecretion. This disorder frequently causes diagnostic difficulties, since about 75% of these patients are nonsuppressible with the standard 2-day high-dose dexamethasone suppression test. Plasma ACTH levels may be undetectable, normal, or elevated and may vary dramatically in the same patient. These patients should be evaluated with higher doses of dexamethasone (as described above) and pituitary localizing procedures to differentiate them from patients with either the ectopic ACTH syndrome or primary adrenal tumors. In addition, CT scanning of the adrenals may demonstrate nodular hyperplasia.

3. Ectopic ACTH syndrome–Although the ectopic ACTH syndrome is usually easily diagnosed by elevated ACTH levels and nonsuppressible steroid hypersecretion in the presence of an extrapituitary tumor, there are cases in which the tumor is occult, and in these, steroid secretion may be dexamethasone-suppressible and metyrapone-responsive. In addition, the tumor may not make its presence felt for a number of years following the onset of Cushing's syndrome. These occult tumors are usually carcinoids, and the plasma ACTH levels may be in the range of those seen with Cushing's disease. These findings may lead to a mistaken diagnosis of Cushing's disease and inappropriate pituitary therapy. Although it is not possible to make this differentiation with confidence in all cases, certain features should increase the suspicion of ectopic ACTH syndrome: male sex, rapid onset, severe hypercortisolism, hypokalemia, anemia, and weight loss. If ectopic ACTH syndrome is suspected but no tumor is obvious, selective venous ACTH sampling is helpful. Thus, the demonstration of a pituitary ACTH gradient establishes the diagnosis of Cushing's disease. In the absence of a pituitary gradient, ectopic ACTH syndrome is a likely diagnosis, and selective venous sampling may localize the ACTH-secreting ectopic tumor. If localization is not achieved by this method, additional diagnostic and radiologic procedures should be directed to the common sites of ACTH production, ie, the lungs, thymus, pancreas, thyroid, and adrenals.

E. Tumor Localization: The procedures described below are useful in the localization of tumors in Cushing's syndrome, but they should be preceded if possible by a definite biochemical diagnosis, since radiologic procedures may occasionally give misleading results. For example, nodular hyperplasia of the adrenals with a solitary or dominant nodule may be misinterpreted as an autonomous hyperfunctioning adenoma; or enlargement of the sella turcica may be due to the empty sella syndrome rather than to a pituitary tumor.

1. Neuroradiologic studies—In Cushing's disease, neuroradiologic procedures are used to localize the pituitary adenoma and to define sellar size, anatomy, and extrasellar tumor extension. (See also Chapter 6.)

a. Macroadenomas—In patients with larger tumors (macroadenomas) magnetic resonance imaging (MRI) or CT scanning is used to document tumor size, suprasellar extension, lateral expansion, or the presence of a partially empty sella turcica.

b. Microadenomas—The problem of tumor localization in patients with Cushing's disease who have microadenomas has not been solved, necessitating a secure biochemical diagnosis. MRI is the current procedure of choice; however, because of the small size of pituitary adenomas in Cushing's disease, they are detected by current imaging methods in only about 50% of patients. Patients with normal imaging studies should undergo selective venous sampling (see Chapter 6 and below).

2. Selective venous sampling for ACTH determination—This procedure is used when the source of ACTH hypersecretion is in doubt, eg, in patients in whom biochemical data suggest Cushing's disease but MRI does not localize the tumor. This procedure is also very useful in those with suspected dexamethasone-nonsuppressible Cushing's disease, nodular adrenal hyperplasia, or an occult ectopic ACTH-secreting tumor, as discussed above. In these circumstances, venous sampling may establish the pituitary as the source of ACTH and in some cases will localize an ectopic tumor. ACTH samples are obtained from the inferior petrosal sinuses (a major site of venous drainage of the anterior pituitary), from the jugular venous bulb, and from other sites and are compared with simultaneous peripheral vein samples. In patients with Cushing's disease, ACTH levels are higher in the inferior petrosal sinus samples than in the peripheral vein samples (ratios usually $> 2:1$). In patients with ectopic ACTH syndrome, no inferior petrosal-to-peripheral ACTH gradient is demonstrable, but selective venous sampling may localize the ectopic tumor.

3. Adrenal localizing procedures—CT scan (Fig 12–15), MRI, ultrasonography, and isotope scanning with iodocholesterol are used to define adrenal lesions. In patients with ACTH hypersecretion, these procedures exclude an adrenal tumor and confirm bilateral adrenal hyperplasia or nodular adrenal hyperplasia. These procedures also effectively localize adrenal tumors, since these tumors are usually over 2 cm in diameter. Invasive procedures such as arteriography and venography are rarely required.

Treatment

A. Cushing's Disease: The aim of treatment of Cushing's syndrome is to remove or destroy the basic lesion and thus correct hypersecretion of adrenal hormones without inducing pituitary or adrenal damage, which requires permanent replacement therapy for hormone deficiencies.

Treatment of Cushing's disease is currently directed at the pituitary to control ACTH hypersecretion; available methods include microsurgery, various forms of radiation therapy, and pharmacologic inhibition of ACTH secretion. Treatment of hypercortisolism per se by surgical or medical adrenalectomy is less commonly used. These methods are discussed in Chapter 6.

B. Ectopic ACTH Syndrome: Cure of ectopic ACTH syndrome is usually possible only in cases involving the more "benign" tumors such as thymomas, bronchial carcinoids, or pheochromocytomas. Treatment is made difficult by the presence of metastatic malignant tumors and accompanying severe hypercortisolism. Therapy directed to the primary tumor is usually unsuccessful, and other means must be used to correct the steroid-excess state.

Severe hypokalemia may require potassium replacement in large doses and spironolactone to block mineralocorticoid effects.

Drugs that block steroid synthesis (ketoconazole, metyrapone, and aminoglutethimide) are useful, but they may produce hypoadrenalism, and steroid secretion must be monitored and replacement steroids given if necessary. The dosage of ketoconazole is 400–800 mg/d in divided doses and is usually well tolerated.

Because of its slow onset of action and its side effects, mitotane (o,p'-DDD) is less useful, and several weeks of therapy may be required to control cortisol secretion (see below).

Bilateral adrenalectomy is rarely required, but it may be necessary if hypercortisolism cannot otherwise be controlled.

C. Adrenal Tumors:

1. Adrenal adenomas—Patients with adrenal adenomas are successfully treated by unilateral adrenalectomy, and the outlook is excellent. Since the hypothalamic-pituitary axis and the contralateral adrenal are suppressed by prolonged cortisol secretion, these patients have postoperative adrenal insufficiency and require glucocorticoid therapy both during and following surgery until the remaining adrenal recovers.

2. Adrenal carcinomas—Therapy in cases of adrenocortical carcinoma is less satisfactory, since the tumor has frequently already metastasized (usually to the retroperitoneum, liver, and lungs) by the time the diagnosis is made.

a. Operative treatment—Surgical cure is rare, but excision serves to reduce the tumor mass and the de-

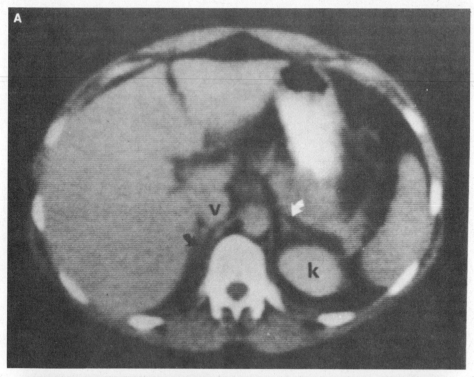

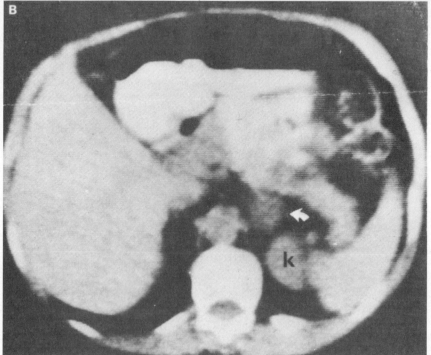

Figure 12–15. Adrenal CT scans in Cushing's syndrome. *A:* Patient with ACTH-dependent Cushing's syndrome. The adrenal glands are not detectably abnormal by this procedure. The curvilinear right adrenal (black arrow) is shown posterior to the inferior vena cava (V) between the right lobe of the liver and the right crus of the diaphragm. The left adrenal (white arrow) has an inverted Y appearance anteromedial to the left kidney (K). *B:* A 3-cm left adrenal adenoma (white arrow) is shown anteromedial to the left kidney (K). (Reproduced, with permission, from Korobkin MT et al: *Am J Roentgenol* 1979;**132:**231.)

gree of steroid hypersecretion. Persisting nonsuppressible steroid secretion in the immediate postoperative period indicates residual or metastatic tumor.

b. Medical treatment–Mitotane (Lysodren; *o,p'*-DDD) is the drug of choice. The dosage is 6–12 g/d orally in 3 or 4 divided doses. The dose must often be reduced because of side effects in 80% of patients (diarrhea, nausea and vomiting, depression, somnolence). About 70% of patients achieve a reduction of steroid secretion, but only 35% achieve a reduction in tumor size. Since mitotane reduces urinary 17-hydroxycorticosteroid excretion by altering the hepatic metabolism of cortisol, these patients require follow-up by plasma cortisol or urine free cortisol assays.

Ketoconazole, metyrapone, or aminoglutethimide (singly or in combination) are useful in controlling steroid hypersecretion in patients who do not respond to mitotane.

Radiotherapy and conventional chemotherapy have not been useful in this disease.

D. Nodular Adrenal Hyperplasia: When pituitary ACTH dependency can be demonstrated, macronodular hyperplasia may be treated like other cases of Cushing's disease. When ACTH dependency is not present, as in micronodular hyperplasia and in some cases of macronodular hyperplasia, bilateral adrenalectomy is appropriate.

Prognosis

A. Cushing's Syndrome: Untreated Cushing's syndrome is frequently fatal, and death may be due to the underlying tumor itself, as in the ectopic ACTH syndrome and adrenal carcinoma. However, in many cases, death is the consequence of sustained hypercortisolism and its complications, including hypertension, cardiovascular disease, stroke, thromboembolism, and susceptibility to infection. In older series, 50% of patients died within 5 years after onset.

B. Cushing's Disease: With current refinements in pituitary microsurgery and heavy particle irradiation, the great majority of patients with Cushing's disease can be treated successfully, and the operative mortality and morbidity rates that attended bilateral adrenalectomy are no longer a feature of the natural history of this disease. Survival in these patients is considerably longer than in older series. However, survival is still less than that of age-matched controls; the increased mortality rate is due to cardiovascular causes. Patients with Cushing's disease who have large pituitary tumors at the time of diagnosis have a much less satisfactory prognosis and may die as a consequence of tumor invasion or persisting hypercortisolism.

C. Adrenal Tumors: The prognosis in adrenal adenomas is excellent, although the mortality and morbidity rates associated with adrenalectomy must be considered in these patients. In adrenal carcinoma, the prognosis is almost universally poor, and the median survival from the date of onset of symptoms is about 4 years.

D. Ectopic ACTH Syndrome: Prognosis is also poor in patients with ectopic ACTH syndrome due to malignant tumors, and in these patients with severe hypercortisolism, survival is frequently only days to weeks. Some patients respond to tumor resection or chemotherapy. The prognosis is better in patients with benign tumors producing the ectopic ACTH syndrome.

HIRSUTISM & VIRILISM

Excessive adrenal or ovarian secretion of androgens or excessive conversion of androgens in peripheral tissues leads to hirsutism and virilism. As previously discussed, the adrenal secretory products DHEA, DHEA sulfate, and androstenedione are weak androgens; however, the peripheral conversion to testosterone and dihydrotestosterone can result in a state of androgen excess. In most patients with hirsutism and in virtually all with virilism, plasma androgen concentrations are increased; a few have normal androgen and plasma concentrations but increased peripheral conversion or sensitivity.

Androgen excess in men may cause testicular atrophy but does not cause other manifestations. The clinical consequences of androgen excess in children are described in Chapter 19. In women, hirsutism is the usual clinical syndrome, and virilism due to markedly excessive androgen production is rare. Hirsutism in women is defined as excessive growth of hair in androgen-sensitive areas, most commonly resulting in increased facial hair. The severity ranges from a mild increase in the amount of hair on the upper lip and chin and at the sideburn areas to heavy facial growth requiring daily shaving. There may also be excessive hair in the pubic area, upper thighs, and lower abdomen (male pattern of hair growth) and on the lower back, chest, and breasts. These patients frequently have oily skin, acne, and menstrual irregularity or amenorrhea. Virilism results from marked androgen excess; in addition to hirsutism, these women have temporal recession of the hairline, male pattern baldness, clitoral enlargement, and masculine features, including increased muscle bulk, a male habitus, deepening of the voice, and amenorrhea. (See Chapter 17.)

Excessive androgen production is seen in both adrenal and ovarian disorders. Adrenal causes include Cushing's syndrome, adrenal carcinoma, and congenital adrenal hyperplasia (see previous sections and Chapter 18). Mild adult-onset cases of congenital adrenal enzyme deficiencies have been described; these appear to be relatively uncommon. Ovarian causes include the polycystic ovary syndrome and, rarely, androgen-secreting tumors or stromal hyperthecosis (see Chapter 17). Polycystic ovary syndrome is the most common of these causes, and milder variants of this syndrome may be responsible for many cases of idiopathic hirsutism not accompanied by ovarian enlargement or menstrual irregularity. Idiopathic hirsutism is also common, and although most patients have demonstrable androgen hypersecretion, the site of abnormal androgen production is unclear. Thus, the ovary, adrenal, or both glands may contribute; current suppression and stimulation tests and even venous catheterization of the adrenals and ovaries have failed to resolve this controversy.

In children, androgen excess is usually due to congenital adrenal hyperplasia or adrenal carcinoma. In women, hirsutism accompanied by amenorrhea, infertility, ovarian enlargement, and elevated plasma LH levels is typical of the polycystic ovary syndrome, whereas in Cushing's syndrome hirsutism is accompanied by features of cortisol excess. Late-onset 21-hydroxylase deficiency is accompanied by elevated levels of plasma 17-hydroxyprogesterone. Virilism and severe androgen excess in adults are usually due to androgen-secreting adrenal or ovarian tumors; virilism is unusual in the polycystic ovary syndrome and rare in Cushing's disease. In the absence of these syndromes, hirsutism in women is usually idiopathic or due to milder forms of polycystic ovary syndrome.

Evaluation of possible androgen excess requires measurement of plasma androgens; one or more of these hormones are elevated in 85% of women with hirsutism. Urinary 17-ketosteroids are elevated in fewer than 20% of such patients. Although plasma assays are useful, certain guidelines are necessary in their use. First, androgen secretion is episodic and varies both with the circadian rhythm of ACTH and with the menstrual cycle. Thus, single plasma samples may not be diagnostic, and more reliable information is obtained by taking multiple samples that may be pooled before assay. Second, measurement of total plasma levels may not accurately reflect the biologically active free hormone concentration. This is of particular importance in states of androgen excess in which the circulating androgens reduce SHBG levels and binding capacity. Thus, in hirsutism, testosterone production, metabolic clearance, and free

plasma testosterone concentration are usually increased; however, total plasma testosterone concentration is frequently normal. Therefore, measurement of the plasma free testosterone concentration, if available, is the most useful single measurement in these patients; it is elevated in 85% of patients. If free testosterone is normal or the test is not available, several measurements of the total androgen level should be done, since at least one of them will be elevated in almost every patient with hirsutism. The frequency of abnormal values is as follows: dihydrotestosterone, 75%; DHEA sulfate, 66%; testosterone, 60%; androstenedione, 45%; and DHEA, 45%. Androstanediol and its glucuronide, which are metabolic products of dihydrotestosterone, are elevated more frequently and are thus useful markers of androgen excess.

In the presence of excess androgens, the diagnosis of idiopathic hirsutism depends on exclusion of the other causes discussed above.

The therapy of hirsutism is discussed in Chapter 17.

INCIDENTALLY DISCOVERED ADRENAL MASSES

Unsuspected adrenal masses have been identified in 0.6–1.3% of abdominal CT scans. These tumors, "incidentalomas," vary in diameter from 0.5 cm to more than 6 cm. Unilateral masses may represent adrenal cortical neoplasms (benign or malignant), metastases, cysts, pheochromocytomas, or myelolipomas. Since benign clinically silent adrenocortical adrenomas are found frequently at autopsy and occult adrenocortical carcinoma is rare, the approach to "incidentalomas" is controversial. Screening tests should be performed to determine whether the lesions produce glucocorticoids, mineralocorticoids, sex steroids, or catecholamines. Most authors recommend removal of all functional (eg, hormone-producing) lesions and all masses greater than 3–6 cm in diameter. For nonfunctional lesions smaller than 3 cm (and for some between 3 and 6 cm), follow-up with serial CT scanning and needle puncture of cysts is appropriate.

REFERENCES

General

Baxter JD, Tyrrell JB: The adrenal cortex. In: *Endocrinology and Metabolism,* 2nd ed. Felig P et al (editors). McGraw-Hill, 1987.

Besser GM, Rees LH: The pituitary-adrenocortical axis. *Clin Endocrinol Metab* 1985;**14**:765.

Frohman LA: Diseases of the anterior pituitary. In: *Endocrinology and Metabolism,* 2nd ed. Felig P et al (editors). McGraw-Hill, 1987.

Norman AW, Litwack G: *Hormones.* Academic Press, 1987. [See Chapters 2, 5, 10, and 12.]

Embryology & Anatomy

Neville AM, O'Hare MJ: Aspects of structure, function and pathology. In: *The Adrenal Gland.* James VHT (editor). Raven Press, 1979.

Neville AM, O'Hare MJ: Histopathology of the human adrenal cortex. *Clin Endocrinol Metab* 1985;**14**:791.

Voutilainen R, Miller WL: Developmental and hormonal regulation of mRNAs for insulin-like growth factor II and steroidogenic enzymes in human fetal adrenals and gonads. *DNA* 1988;**7:**9.

Biosynthesis of Cortisol & Adrenal Androgens

Fehm HL et al: Differential and integral corticosteroid effects on ACTH secretion in hypoadrenocorticism. *J Clin Invest* 1979;**63:**247.

Gill GN: ACTH regulation of the adrenal cortex. In: *Pharmacology of Adrenal Cortical Hormones.* Gill GN (editor). Pergamon, 1979.

Hale AC, Rees LH: ACTH and related peptides. In: *Endocrinology,* 2nd ed. DeGroot LJ et al (editors). Saunders, 1989.

Jones MT: Control of adrenocortical hormone secretion. In: *The Adrenal Gland.* James VHT (editor). Raven Press, 1979.

Keller-Wood ME, Dallman MF: Corticosteroid inhibition of ACTH secretion. *Endocr Rev* 1984;**5:**1.

Miller, WL: Molecular biology of steroid hormone synthesis. *Endocr Rev* 1988;**9:**295.

Miller WL, Levine LS: Molecular and clinical advances in congenital adrenal hyperplasia. *J Pediatr* 1987; **111:**1.

Plumpton FS, Besser GM, Cole PV: Corticosteroid treatment and surgery. *Anaesthesia* 1969;**24:**3.

Sapolsky R et al: Interleukin 1 stimulates the secretion of hypothalamic corticotropin-releasing factor. *Science* 1987;**238:**522.

Taylor, AL, Fishman LM: Corticotropin-releasing hormone. *N Engl J Med* 1988;**319:**213.

Vale W et al: Characterization of a 41-residue ovine hypothalamic peptide that stimulates secretion of corticotropin and β-endorphin. *Science* 1981;**213:**1394.

White PC, New MI, Dupont B: Congenital adrenal hyperplasia. *N Engl J Med* 1987;**316:**1519, 1580.

Circulation & Metabolism of Cortisol & Adrenal Androgens

Abraham GE: Ovarian and adrenal contribution to peripheral androgens during the menstrual cycle. *J Clin Endocrinol Metab* 1974;**39:**340.

Ballard PL: Delivery and transport of glucocorticoids to target cells. In: *Glucocorticoid Hormone Action.* Baxter JD, Rousseau GG (editors). Springer-Verlag, 1979.

Brooks RV: Biosynthesis and metabolism of adrenocortical steroids. In: *The Adrenal Gland.* James VHT (editor). Raven Press, 1979.

Brown MS et al: Receptor-mediated uptake of lipoprotein-cholesterol and its utilization for steroid synthesis in the adrenal cortex. *Recent Prog Horm Res* 1979;**35:**215.

Finkelstein M, Shaefer JM: Inborn errors of steroid biosynthesis. *Physiol Rev* 1979;**59:**353.

Gill GN: Biosynthesis, secretion and metabolism of hormones. In: *Endocrinology and Metabolism,* 2nd ed. Felig P et al (editors). McGraw-Hill, 1987.

Grant JK: An introductory review of adrenocortical steroid biosynthesis. In: *The Endocrine Function of the Human Adrenal Cortex.* James VHT et al (editors). Academic Press, 1978.

Migeon CJ: Adrenal androgens in man. *Am J Med* 1972;**53:**606.

Biologic Effects

Adams EF et al: Effect of nizoral on ACTH secretion by human pituitary corticotrophic tumours in cell culture. *Clin Endocrinol* 1985;**22:**631.

Baxter JD: Mechanisms of glucocorticoid inhibition of growth. *Kidney Int* 1978;**14:**330.

Baxter JD, Rousseau GG (editors): *Glucocorticoid Hormone Action.* Springer-Verlag, 1979.

Baylink DJ: Glucocorticoid-induced osteoporosis. *N Engl J Med* 1983;**309:**306.

Bertagna X et al: Peripheral antiglucocorticoid action of RU486 in man. *Clin Endocrinol* 1988;**28:**537.

Blalock JE: New concepts in endocrinology: Neuroendocrine and immune system interactions. Pages 15–28 in: *Yearbook of Endocrinology.* Yearbook, 1987.

Chrousos GP et al: Primary cortisol resistance in man: A glucocorticoid receptor–mediated disease. *J Clin Invest* 1982;**69:**1261.

Craddock CG: Corticosteroid-induced lymphopenia, immunosuppression and body defense. *Ann Intern Med* 1978;**88:**564.

Evans RM: The steroid and thyroid hormone receptor superfamily. *Science* 1988;**240:**889.

Fauci AS, Dale DC, Balow JE: Glucocorticoid therapy: Mechanisms of action and clinical considerations. *Ann Intern Med* 1976;**84:**304.

Findling JW et al: Vitamin D metabolites and parathyroid hormone in Cushing's syndrome: Relationship to calcium and phosphorus homeostasis. *J Clin Endocrinol Metab* 1982;**54:**1039.

Gaillard GC et al: RU486 inhibits peripheral effects of glucocorticoids in humans. *J Clin Endocrinol Metab* 1985;**61:**1009.

Hyams JS, Carey DE: Corticosteroids and growth. *J Pediatr* 1988;**133:**249.

Katt KJ: Molecular mechanisms of hormone action: Control of target-cell function by peptide, thyroid and steroid hormones. In: *Endocrinology and Metabolism,* 2nd ed. Felig P et al (editors). McGraw-Hill, 1987.

Malerbi D et al: Glucocorticoids and glucose metabolism: Hepatic glucose production in untreated Addisonian patients and on two different levels of glucocorticoid administration. *Clin Endocrinol* 1988;**28:**415.

Munch A, Guyre PM, Holbrook NJ: Physiologic functions of glucocorticoids in stress and their relation to pharmacological actions. *Endocr Rev* 1984; **5:**25.

Oikarinen AI, Vitto J, Oikarinen J: Glucocorticoid action on connective tissue: From molecular mechanisms to clinical practice. *Med Biol* 1986;**64:**221.

Parillo JE, Fauci AS: Mechanisms of glucocorticoid action on immune processes. *Annu Rev Pharmacol Toxicol* 1979;**19:**179.

Tyrrell JB, Baxter JD: Glucocorticoid therapy. In: *Endocrinology and Metabolism,* 2nd ed. Felig P et al (editors). McGraw-Hill, 1987.

Walters MR: Steroid hormone receptors and the nucleus. *Endocr Rev* 1985;**6:**512.

Whitworth JA: Mechanisms of glucocorticoid-induced hypertension. *Kidney Int* 1987;**31:**1213.

Laboratory Evaluation

APA Task Force on Laboratory Tests in Psychiatry: The dexamethasone suppression test: An overview of its current status in psychiatry. *Am J Psychiatry* 1987;**144:**1253.

Abraham GE, Chakmakjian ZH: Plasma steroids in hirsutism. *Obstet Gynecol* 1974;**44**:171.

Borst GC, Michenfelder HJ, O'Brian JT: Discordant cortisol response to exogenous ACTH and insulin-induced hypoglycemia in patients with pituitary disease. *N Engl J Med* 1982;**306**:1462.

Chrousos GP et al: The corticotropin-releasing factor stimulation test: An aid in the evaluation of patients with Cushing's syndrome. *N Engl J Med* 1984;**310**:622.

Crapo L: Cushing's syndrome: A review of diagnostic tests. *Metabolism* 1979;**28**:955.

Cunningham SK, Moore A, Mckenna TJ: Normal cortisol response to corticotropin in patients with secondary adrenal failure. *Arch Intern Med* 1982;**143**:2276.

Givens JR: Normal and abnormal androgen metabolism. *Clin Obstet Gynecol* 1978;**21**:115.

Liddle GW: Tests of pituitary adrenal suppressibility in the diagnosis of Cushing's syndrome. *J Clin Endocrinol Metab* 1960;**12**:1539.

Lindholm J, Kehlet H: Re-evaluation of the clinical value of the 30 min ACTH test in assessing the hypothalamic-pituitary-adrenocortical function. *Clin Endocrinol* 1987;**26**:53.

Maroulis GB, Manlimos FS, Abraham GE: Comparison between urinary 17-ketosteroids and plasma androgens in hirsute patients. *Obstet Gynecol* 1977;**49**:454.

May ME, Carey RM: Rapid adrenocorticotrophic hormone test in practice: Retrospective review. *Am J Med* 1985;**79**:679.

Nelson JC, Tindall DJ: A comparison of of the adrenal responses to hypoglycemia, metyrapone and ACTH. *Am J Med Sci* 1978;**275**:165.

Paulsen JD et al: Free testosterone concentrations in serum: Elevation is the hallmark of hirsutism. *Am J Obstet Gynecol* 1977;**128**:851.

Rosenfield RL: Plasma free androgen patterns in hirsute women and their diagnostic implications. *Am J Med* 1979;**66**:417.

Scott AP et al: Pituitary adrenocorticotrophin and the melanocyte stimulating hormones. In: *Peptide Hormones*. Parsons JA (editor). University Park Press, 1979.

Spiger M et al: Single dose metyrapone test: Review of a four-year experience. *Arch Intern Med* 1975;**135**:698.

Streeten DHP et al: Normal and abnormal function of the hypothalamic-pituitary-adrenocortical system in man. *Endocr Rev* 1984;**5**:371.

Vermeulen A: Adrenal virilism. In: *The Adrenal Gland*. James VHT (editor). Raven Press, 1979.

Vermeulen A, Ando S: Metabolic clearance rate and interconversion of androgens and the influence of the free androgen fraction. *J Clin Endocrinol Metab* 1979;**48**:320.

Wade CE et al: Upon admission adrenal steroidogenesis is adapted to the degree of illness in intensive care unit patients. *J Clin Endocrinol Metab* 1988;**67**:223.

Disorders of Adrenocortical Insufficiency

Best TR et al: Persistent adrenal insufficiency secondary to low dose ketoconazole therapy. *Am J Med* 1987;**82**:676.

Burke CW: Adrenocortical insufficiency. *Clin Endocrinol Metab* 1985;**14**:947.

Byyny RL: Withdrawal from glucocorticoid therapy. *N Engl J Med* 1976;**295**:30.

Glasgow BJ et al: Adrenal pathology in the acquired immune deficiency syndrome. *Am J Clin Pathol* 1985;**84**:594.

Green LW et al: Adrenal insufficiency as a complication of the acquired immunodeficiency syndrome. *Ann Intern Med* 1984;**101**:497.

Irvine WJ, Toft AD, Feek CM: Addison's disease. In: *The Adrenal Gland*. James VHT (editor). Raven Press, 1979.

Leshin M: Polyglandular autoimmune syndromes. *Am J Med Sci* 1985;**290**:77.

Membreno L et al: Adrenocortical function in acquired immunodeficiency syndrome. *J Clin Endocrinol Metab* 1987;**65**:482.

Nerup J: Addison's disease: Clinical studies. A report of 108 cases. *Acta Endocrinol* 1974;**76**:127.

Nerup J: Addison's disease: A review of some clinical, pathological and immunological features. *Dan Med Bull* 1974;**21**:201.

Neufeld M, Maclaren NK, Blizzard RM: Two types of autoimmune Addison's disease associated with different polyglandular autoimmune (PGA) syndromes. *Medicine* 1981;**60**:355.

Plumpton FS, Besser GM, Cole PV: Corticosteroid treatment and surgery. 2. The management of steroid cover. *Anaesthesia* 1969;**24**:12.

Redman BG et al: Prospective evaluation of adrenal insufficiency in patients with adrenal metastasis. *Cancer* 1987;**60**:103.

Schulte HM et al: The corticotropin-releasing hormone stimulation test: A possible aid in the evaluation of patients with adrenal insufficiency. *J Clin Endocrinol Metab* 1984;**58**:1064.

Shibutani Y: Prolactin dynamics in a patient with isolated ACTH deficiency accompanied by hyperprolactinemia. *Am J Med Sci* 1988;**295**:140.

Stacpoole PW et al: Isolated ACTH deficiency: A heterogeneous disorder. *Medicine* 1982;**61**:13.

Thompson DG, Mason AS, Goodwin FJ: Mineralocorticoid replacement in Addison's disease. *Clin Endocrinol* 1979;**10**:499.

Vita JA et al: Clinical clues to the cause of Addison's disease. *Am J Med* 1985;**78**:461.

Watson CA, Rosenfeld RL, Fang VS: Recovery from glucocorticoid inhibition of the responses to corticotrophin-releasing hormone. *Clin Endocrinol* 1988;**28**:471.

Xarli VP et al: Adrenal hemorrhage in the adult. *Medicine* 1978;**57**:211.

Cushing's Syndrome

Aron DC et al: Cushing's syndrome: Problems in diagnosis. *Medicine* 1981;**60**:25.

Aron DC et al: Cushing's syndrome: Problems in management. *Endocr Rev* 1982;**3**:229.

Aron DC, Findling JW, Tyrrell JB: Cushing's disease. *Endocrinol Metab Clin North Am* 1987;**16**:705.

Asa SL et al: Cushing's disease associated with an intrasellar ganglicocytoma producing corticotrophin-releasing factor. *Ann Intern Med* 1984;**101**:789.

Besky JL et al: Cushing's syndrome due to ectopic production of corticotropin-releasing factor. *J Clin Endocrinol Metab* 1985;**60**:496.

Carney JA et al: The complex of myxomas, spotty pigmentation, and endocrine overactivity. *Medicine* 1985;**64**:270.

Dwyer AJ et al: Pituitary adenomas in patients with Cushing's disease: Initial experience with Gd-DTPA-enhanced MR imaging. *Radiology* 1987;**163:**421.

Findling JW, Tyrrell JB: Occult ectopic secretion of corticotropin. *Arch Intern Med* 1986;**146:**929.

Findling JW et al: Selective venous sampling for ACTH in Cushing's syndrome. *Ann Intern Med* 1981;**94:**647.

Fitzgerald PA et al: Cushing's disease: Transient secondary adrenal insufficiency after selective removal of pituitary microadenomas: Evidence for a pituitary origin. *J Clin Endocrinol Metab* 1982;**54:**413.

Howlett TA, Rees LH, Besser GM: Cushing's syndrome. *Clin Endocrinol Metab* 1985;**14:**911.

Howlett TA et al: Diagnosis and management of ACTH-dependent Cushing's syndrome: Comparison of the features in ectopic and pituitary ACTH production. *Clin Endocrinol* 1986;**24:**699.

Hutter AM, Kayhoe DE: Adrenal cortical carcinoma: Clinical features of 138 patients. *Am J Med* 1966;**41:**572.

Jex RK et al: Ectopic ACTH syndrome: Diagnostic and therapeutic aspects. *Am J Surg* 1985;**149:**276.

Larsen JL, Cathey WJ, O'Dell WD: Primary adrenocortical nodular dysplasia: A distinct subtype of Cushing's syndrome. *Am J Med* 1986;**80:**976.

Mampalam TJ, Tyrrell JB, Wilson CB: Transsphenoidal microsurgery for Cushing's disease. *Ann Intern Med* 1988;**109:**487.

Marcovitz S et al: The diagnostic accuracy of preoperative CT scanning in the evaluation of pituitary ACTH-secreting adenomas. *Am J Roentgenol* 1987;**149:**803.

McNicol AM, Teasdale GM, Beastall GH: A study of corticotroph adenomas in Cushing's disease: No evidence of intermediate lobe origin. *Clin Endocrinol* 1986;**24:**715.

Pojunas KW et al: Pituitary and adrenal CT of Cushing's syndrome. *Am J Roentgenol* 1986;**146:**1235.

Ross, EJ, Linch DC: The clinical response to treatment in adult Cushing's syndrome following remission of hypercortisolaemia. *Postgrad Med J* 1985;**61:**205.

Sheeler LR: Cushing's syndrome 1988. *Cleve Clin J Med* 1988;**55:**329.

Sonino N et al: Prolonged treatment of Cushing's disease by ketoconazole. *J Clin Endocrinol Metab* 1985;**61:**718.

Styne DM et al: Treatment of Cushing's disease in childhood and adolescence by transsphenoidal microadenomectomy. *N Engl J Med* 1984;**310:**889.

Tyrrell JB: Diagnosis of Cushing's disease. In: *Secretory Tumors of the Pituitary Gland.* Black PM et al (editors). Raven Press, 1984.

Tyrrell JB et al: Cushing's disease: Selective transsphenoidal resection of pituitary adenomas. *N Engl J Med* 1978;**298:**753.

Tyrrell JB et al: An overnight high-dose dexamethasone suppression test: Rapid differential diagnosis of Cushing's syndrome. *Ann Intern Med* 1986;**104:**180.

Watson RGK et al: Results of adrenal surgery for Cushing's syndrome: 10 years' experience. *World J Surg* 1986;**10:**531.

Hirsutism & Virilism

Baskin HJ: Screening for late-onset congenital adrenal hyperplasia in hirsutism or amenorrhea. *Arch Intern Med* 1987;**147:**847.

Biffignandi P, Massucchetti C, Molinatti GM: Female hirsutism: Pathophysiological considerations and therapeutic implications. *Endocr Rev* 1984;**5:**498.

Chetkowski RJ et al: The incidence of late-onset congenital adrenal hyperplasia due to 21-hydroxlase deficiency among hirsute women. *J Clin Endocrinol Metab* 1984;**58:**595.

Cumming DC et al: Treatment of hirsutism with spironolactone. *JAMA* 1982;**247:**1295.

Gabrilove JL et al: Virilizing adrenal adenoma with studies on the steroid content of adrenal venous effluent and a review of the literature. *Endocr Rev* 1981;**2:**462.

Hatch R et al: Hirsutism: Implications, etiology and management. *Am J Obstet Gynecol* 1981;**140:**815.

Horton R, Hawks D, Lobo R: $3\alpha,17\beta$-Adrostanediol glucuronide in plasma: A marker of androgen action in idiopathic hirsutism. *J Clin Invest* 1982;**69:**1203.

Lackelin GCL et al: Long term effects of nightly dexamethasone administration in patients with polycystic ovarian disease. *J Clin Endocrinol Metab* 1982;**55:**768.

Longcope C: Adrenal and gonadal androgen secretion in normal females. *Clin Endocrinol Metab* 1986;**15:**213.

Maroulis GB: Evaluation of hirsutism and hyperandrogenemia. *Fertil Steril* 1981;**36:**273.

McKenna TJ: Pathogenesis and treatment of polycystic ovary syndrome. *N Engl J Med* 1988;**318:**558.

Moltz L, Schwartz U: Gonadal and adrenal androgen secretion in hirsute females. *Clin Endocrinol Metab* 1986;**15:**229.

Rittmaster RS, Loriaux DL: Hirsutism. *Ann Intern Med* 1987;**106:**95.

Incidentally Discovered Adrenal Masses

Copeland PM: The incidentally discovered adrenal mass. *Ann Intern Med* 1983;**98:**940.

Reinig JW et al: Adrenal masses differentiated by MR. *Radiology* 1986;**158:**81.

Thompson NW, Cheung PSY: Diagnosis and treatment of functioning and nonfunctioning adrenocortical neoplasms including incidentalomas. *Surg Clin North Am* 1987;**67:**423.

Mineralocorticoids

13

Edward G. Biglieri, MD, & Claudio E. Kater, MD

The biosynthetic pathways of the mineralocorticoid hormones are shown in Fig 13–1 (see also Figs 12–4 and 12–5). The principal mineralocorticoid hormone is aldosterone. It is produced in the zona glomerulosa exclusively and is primarily controlled by the renin-angiotensin system. Other regulators include sodium and potassium levels, ACTH, and neural components of the adrenergic and dopaminergic systems. The precursors of aldosterone in this pathway normally contribute little to their peripheral concentrations—except for 18-hydroxycorticosterone. In the zona fasciculata, there are 2 steroid pathways—the glucocorticoid (17-hydroxy) and mineralocorticoid (17-deoxy) pathways—both under control of ACTH. The glucocorticoid pathway results in the formation of cortisol. The major mineralocorticoid hormone of the zona fasciculata is deoxycorticosterone (DOC), but corticosterone and 18-hydroxydeoxycorticosterone are also produced in substantial amounts. The bulk of the circulating levels of DOC, 18-hydroxydeoxycorticosterone, and corticosterone originates from the zona fasciculata.

Activity of Aldosterone

The principal effects of aldosterone are on maintenance of normal sodium and potassium concentrations and extracellular volume. Aldosterone combines with an intracellular cytosol mineralocorticoid receptor. The active steroid-receptor complex moves into the nucleus of the target cell, where it initiates the transcription of RNA and subsequently induces a new protein providing the energy required for movement of sodium from the cell via the sodium pump. The major effect of this action quantitatively is to increase the difference in potential across the renal tubule. The increased luminal negativity effects tubular secretion of potassium and hydrogen (Fig 13–2). Tubular sodium, via the sodium pump, enters the extracellular fluid and helps maintain its normal composition and volume. All of these events occur in other secretory systems and can be measured in saliva, sweat, and feces. It is of interest that the increased difference in potential or increased luminal negativity noted in the kidney is also present in the gastrointestinal tract, and its measurement may be used to quantitate mineralocorticoid ac-

Acronyms Used in This Chapter

ACTH	Adrenocorticotropic hormone
CMO	Corticosterone methyloxidase
DHEA	Dehydroepiandrosterone
DOC	Deoxycorticosterone
DOCA	Deoxycorticosterone acetate
MCH	Mineralocorticoid hormone
RNA	Ribonucleic acid

tivity, eg, decreased stool sodium with increased stool potassium.

Although renin and aldosterone move in concert in most situations, aldosterone is also influenced by ACTH, potassium balance and concentration, and probably other factors to maintain volume and electrolyte homeostasis. In the virtual absence of renin, as in patients with primary aldosteronism, circulating levels of aldosterone are modulated by variations in ACTH rhythm. Free aldosterone comprises 30–40% of its total concentration, whereas the free fractions of the steroids of the zona fasciculata comprise 5–10% of their total concentration. Aldosterone is *loosely* bound to corticosteroid-binding globulin, in contrast to the zona fasciculata steroids. Because it is the free hormone that combines with the mineralocorticoid receptor to initiate subsequent mineralocorticoid action, extremely high levels of DOC must be achieved to produce a mineralocorticoid effect.

Interactions of Hormones

The interactions of all circulating steroid hormones, the distribution between their free and bound forms, the influence of peptide hormones, and receptor availability and affinity determine their effectiveness as mineralocorticoids. For example, numerically normal levels of mineralocorticoid hormones can induce a state of hypermineralocorticoidism in situations in which synergistic or "facilitating" substances (enhancers) are also present that increase the receptor affinity for aldosterone. Cortisol itself, in high concentrations, can act as a mineralocorticoid in the presence of normal or even low levels of aldosterone or DOC.

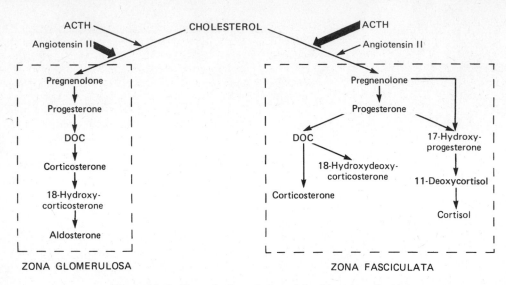

Figure 13–1. Biosynthetic pathways of the mineralocorticoids.

Definition of Terms

Mineralocorticoid and **glucocorticoid hormones** have mineral- and carbohydrate-regulating activity, respectively. A mineralocorticoid is an adrenocortical steroid whose principal action is electrolyte regulation; it is not necessarily produced in the aldosterone biosynthetic pathway or even in the zona glomerulosa. A glucocorticoid hormone is an adrenocortical steroid whose predominant action is related to carbohydrate regulation, protein catabolism, ACTH suppression, and the immune system. Although some glucocorticoid activity can be produced in the zona glomerulosa, it is mainly formed in the zona fasciculata.

The terms **mineralocorticoid excess** and **mineralocorticoid deficiency** denote an absolute elevation and an absolute diminution, respectively, of the endogenous hormones as reflected by their plasma or urine levels. However, this is not necessarily related to the clinical manifestations of mineralocorticoid activity.

A condition characterized by presumed increased mineralocorticoid activity, with salt retention, hypertension, hypokalemia, and metabolic alkalosis, is more appropriately called **hypermineralocorticoidism.** It can occur in the absence of any mineralocorticoid production, eg, in Liddle's syndrome or chronic

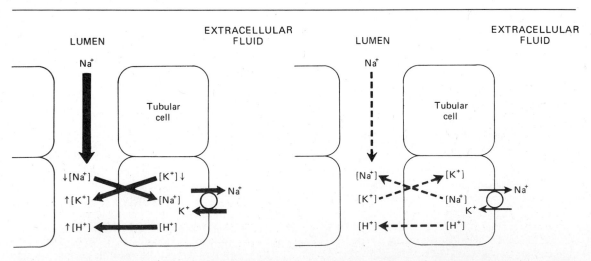

Figure 13–2. Mineralocorticoid action. On the left, high sodium intakes and high tubular sodium with increased mineralocorticoid action lead to K^+ and H^+ secretion and Na^+ movement into extracellular fluid. Similar amounts of mineralocorticoid are ineffective when tubular sodium is reduced (eg, by dietary sodium restriction).

ingestion of licorice. In contrast, in the mineralocorticoid resistance syndromes (receptor deficiency, pseudohypoaldosteronism), an excess of circulating mineralocorticoid cannot express its peripheral action and results in a clinical state of **hypomineralocorticoidism,** presenting with sodium loss, hypotension, hyperkalemia, and metabolic acidosis.

PRIMARY MINERALOCORTICOID EXCESS (Table 13–1)

Disorders in this category are manifested by hypertension, hypokalemia, suppression of the renin system, and normal or low cortisol production. Although technically the mineralocorticoid hormones produced in the 11β- and 17α-hydroxylase deficiency disorders are secondary to ACTH excess, their biochemical findings are those of primary mineralocorticoid excess.

PRIMARY ALDOSTERONISM

1. RECOGNITION & INITIAL DIAGNOSIS

The increased production of aldosterone by abnormal zona glomerulosa tissue (adenoma or hyperplasia) initiates a series of events that result in the clinical abnormality known as primary aldosteronism. Aldosterone excess leads to increased sodium retention, expansion of the extracellular fluid volume, and increased total body sodium content. Although the effects on the kidney are greatest quantitatively, the other secretory tissues also participate in this event. Fecal excretion of sodium, for example, can be decreased to almost nil. The expanded extracellular fluid and plasma volumes are registered by stretch receptors at the juxtaglomerular apparatus and sodium flux at the macula densa, with resultant suppression of renin secretion, measured as suppressed plasma renin activity. These effects of aldosterone are further manifested by normal or elevated serum sodium concentration and reduced hematocrit. With primary (autonomous) increases in aldosterone production, the renin system is greatly suppressed. This is the hallmark of the disorder.

In addition to sodium retention, potassium depletion develops, decreasing the total body and plasma concentration of potassium and producing alkalosis. The extrusion of potassium from its intracellular reservoir is followed by the intracellular movement of hydrogen ion, and along with increased renal secretion of hydrogen ion, alkalosis ensues. With moderate potassium depletion, decreased carbohydrate tolerance (shown by an abnormal glucose tolerance test) and resistance to antidiuretic hormone (vasopressin) occur. Severe potassium depletion blunts baroreceptor function, occasionally producing postural hypotension.

Because aldosterone biosynthesis is intensified, the entire biosynthetic pathway becomes activated. Precursor steroids such as DOC, corticosterone, and 18-hydroxycorticosterone are present in increased amounts in the blood of persons with an aldosterone-producing adenoma (Fig 13–1). Primary aldosteronism is a disease of the zona glomerulosa. Cells of this zone do not have the capacity to make cortisol. There are no abnormalities in cortisol production, plasma cortisol level, or cortisol metabolism.

Table 13–1. Biochemical findings in primary hypermineralocorticoidism.

	Plasma		Aldosterone	Other MCHs	Renin	Cortisol	ACTH	Hct	BUN/ Creatinine
	Na+	K+							
Aldosterone-producing adenoma	N or ↑	↓	↑↑	↑	↓↓	N	N	↓	N
Aldosterone-producing carcinoma	↑	↓	↑↑	↑↑	↓↓	N or ↑	N or ↓	↓	N
Hyperplasia Idiopathic hyperaldosteronism	N	↓	↑	N	↓	N	N	N or ↓	N
Indeterminate hyperaldosteronism	N	N or ↓	↑	N	↓	N	N	N or ↓	N
Glucocorticoid-remediable hyperaldosteronism	N	↓	↑	N	↓	N	N	N or ↓	N
"Primary hyperplasia"	N or ↑	↓	↑↑	↑	↓↓	N	N	↓	N
11β-Hydroxylase deficiency	N	N or ↓	↓	↑	N or ↓	N or ↓	↑	N or ↓	N
17α-Hydroxylase deficiency	N or ↑	↓	↓	↑↑	↓↓	↓	↑	N or ↓	N
11β-Hydroxysteroid dehydrogenase deficiency	N	↓	↓	N	↓	N	N	N	N

BUN, blood urea nitrogen; Hct, hematocrit; MCH, mineralocorticoid hormone; N, normal; ↑, increased; ↓, decreased; ↑↑, ↓↓, markedly increased, decreased.

History & Physical Findings

Patients usually come to medical attention because of symptoms of hypokalemia or detection of previously unsuspected hypertension during the course of physical examination. The medical history reveals no characteristic symptoms—often only nonspecific complaints of tiredness, loss of stamina, weakness, nocturia, and lassitude—all symptoms of potassium depletion. If potassium depletion is more severe, with alkalosis, then increased thirst, polyuria (especially nocturnal), and paresthesias may be present. Headache is a frequent incidental complaint.

Excessive production of mineralocorticoids produces no characteristic physical findings. Blood pressure in patients with primary aldosteronism can range from borderline to severe hypertensive levels. The mean ± SEM blood pressure in the 136 patients reported by the Glasgow unit was 205 ± 21/123 ± 18 mm Hg, with no significant difference between the group with adenoma and that with hyperplasia. Accelerated (malignant) hypertension is extremely rare in patients with primary aldosteronism. Retinopathy is mild, and hemorrhages are rarely (if ever) present. Postural falls in blood pressure without reflex tachycardia are observed in the severely potassium-depleted patient because of blunting of the baroreceptors. Clinical edema is quite rare. A positive Trousseau or Chvostek sign may be suggestive of alkalosis accompanying severe potassium depletion. The heart is usually only mildly enlarged if at all, and electrocardiographic changes are usually those of modest left ventricular hypertrophy and potassium depletion.

Initial Diagnosis
(Fig 13–3)

A. Hypokalemia: Determination of the presence or absence of hypokalemia is the most important initial screening procedure in patients with hypertension. Care must be taken to assess the state of sodium intake or balance in the patient before serum electrolytes are obtained. Serum potassium concentration is closely related to and determined to a great extent by sodium chloride intake. A low-sodium diet, by sparing potassium loss, can correct serum potassium abnormalities, thus masking total potassium depletion; as the amount of sodium ion available for reabsorption is reduced, potassium secretion is retarded in the distal tubule.

In some series, up to 20% of patients with primary aldosteronism have had normal serum potassium concentrations, depending on criteria of dietary sodium and laboratory variability. In the presence of normal renal function and aldosterone excess, salt loading will unmask hypokalemia as a manifestation of potassium depletion. Normokalemic hyperaldosteronism under these conditions has been reported but is probably rare.

B. Salt Intake: In the USA, Japan, and many European countries, the average person consumes more than 110–120 meq of sodium per day—enough to allow hypokalemia to become manifest. If a dietary history of high salt intake is obtained and potassium concentrations are normal, there is no need for further tests. A useful way to demonstrate hypokalemia is to have the patient ingest an unrestricted diet plus 1 g of sodium chloride (as a 1-g sodium chloride USP tablet, ⅕ tsp of table salt, or packets containing 1 g of salt) with each meal for 4 days; blood samples for fasting electrolyte determinations should be obtained on day 5. The finding of a low serum potassium concentration warrants further study (Fig 13–3).

C. Diuretic Therapy: Previous diuretic therapy always poses a problem in interpreting serum potassium concentrations and is the most common cause of hypokalemia in hypertension. The patient should discontinue use of diuretics for at least 3 weeks before potassium levels are measured.

In the absence of previous diuretic therapy, sodium concentrations less than 139 meq/L are rare in patients with primary aldosteronism, but they are common with diuretic therapy. Thus, any lower concentration should suggest secondary hyperaldosteronism. A high serum sodium concentration (140–152 meq/L) in the presence of a reduced hematocrit (due to increased extracellular fluid and plasma volume from sodium retention) is presumptive evidence of mineralocorticoid excess. Additional clues to potassium depletion are failure to concentrate urine (nephrogenic diabetes insipidus), an abnormal glucose tolerance test, and alkalosis.

If hypokalemia is documented, the renin-angiotensin system must be assessed. This is accomplished by a random plasma renin activity measurement. If plasma renin activity is normal or high in a patient who has been off diuretic therapy for 3 weeks, it is very unlikely that primary aldosteronism is present. If the random plasma renin activity is suppressed, primary aldosteronism is a likely diagnosis.

Measurement of Aldosterone
& Other Steroids
(Table 13–2)

Assessment of aldosterone production can best be accomplished by measurement of urinary aldosterone excretion over a 24-hour period under the same conditions of sodium intake described for potassium measurement. Measurement of either the 18-glucuronide or the tetrahydroaldosterone metabolite is sufficient to assess the rate of total production. Blood samples must be obtained under proper conditions in order to yield reliable diagnostic information. Although the value obtained for plasma aldosterone concentration is the aldosterone level only at a given moment, in the properly prepared patient it can provide an excellent assessment of mineralocorticoid production. Both plasma and urinary aldosterone measurements should be performed while the patient is taking a high-salt diet with sodium chloride supplementation, as previously described. This is crucial, because with any diminution

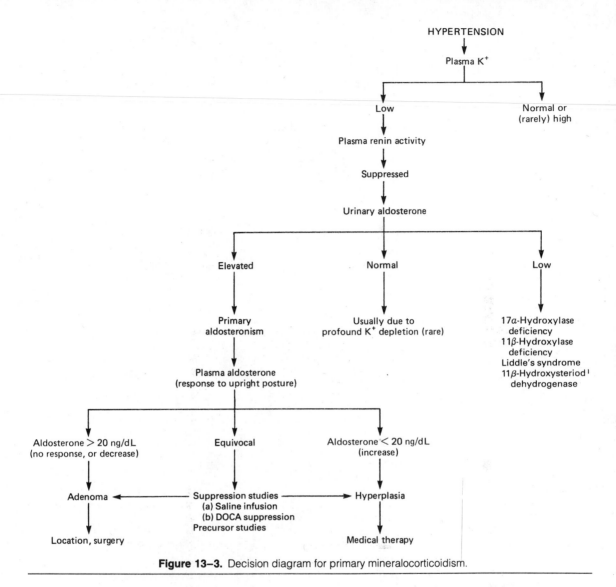

Figure 13–3. Decision diagram for primary mineralocorticoidism.

of salt intake, plasma aldosterone concentration and aldosterone production normally increase. The plasma aldosterone concentration in a group of 47 patients with adenoma was over 20 ng/dL (555 pmol/L) (61.8 ± 10.9 ng/dL [1714 ± 302 pmol/L]); in 19 patients with idiopathic hyperaldosteronism (hyperplasia), it was less than 20 ng/dL (555 pmol/L) (15.2 ± 1.2 ng/dL [422 ± 33 pmol/L]). The normal urinary aldosterone values are 5–20 μg/24 h (13–55.5 nmol/24 h). In one series, there were mean values for adenoma and hyperplasia of 37.6 ± 3 μg/24 h (104 ± 8 nmol/24 h) and 22.5 ± 1.5 μg/24 h (62.4 ± 4.2 nmol/24 h) respectively. Although urinary measurements have been adequate for detecting abnormal production of aldosterone (and in fact superior to plasma aldosterone concentration measurement), it has not been possible to use daily excretion of aldosterone to discriminate between adenoma and hyperplasia.

2. DIFFERENTIAL DIAGNOSIS

Differentiation Between Aldosterone-Producing Adenoma & Adrenocortical Hyperplasia

It is important to distinguish between adenoma and hyperplasia, because surgery is indicated in the former but not in the latter.

A. Measurement of Plasma Aldosterone, Deoxycorticosterone, Corticosterone, & 18-Hydroxycorticosterone Concentrations (Table 13–2): The plasma aldosterone concentration provides not only diagnostic information about hyperaldosteronism but also differential diagnostic information about the pathologic process. After at least 4 days of sodium intake exceeding 120 meq daily and after overnight (at least 6 hours) recumbency, the 8 AM plasma aldosterone concentration can be used to distinguish pa-

Table 13–2. Simultaneous measurements (±SE) of plasma aldosterone, 18-hydroxycorticosterone, and plasma renin concentration in normal subjects and in primary aldosteronism during postural stimulation.[1,2]

	Normal Subjects (n = 14)			Aldosterone-Producing Adenoma (n = 15)			Idiopathic Hyperaldosteronism (n = 14)		
	Aldosterone ng/dL (pmol/L)	18-Hydroxy-corticos-terone ng/dL (pmol/L)	Plasma Renin Concen-tration ng/mL/h (ng/Ls)	Aldosterone ng/dL (pmol/L)	18-Hydroxy-corticos-terone ng/dL (pmol/L)	Plasma Renin Concen-tration ng/mL/h (ng/Ls)	Aldosterone ng/dL (pmol/L)	18-Hydroxy-corticos-terone ng/dL (pmol/L)	Plasma Renin Concen-tration ng/mL/h (ng/Ls)
8 AM recum-bent	8.2 ± 0.6 (228 ± 16.6)	23.5 ± 2.4 (647 ± 66)	3.4 ± 0.7 (0.97 ± .19)	54.7 ± 9.5 (1517 ± 263)	160.0 ± 29.9 (4401 ± 822)	0.49 ± 0.11 (0.14 ± .03)	13.2 ± 1.2 (366 ± 33.3)	24.2 ± 3.7 (666 ± 102)	0.52 ± .08 (0.14 ± .02)
12 noon up-right	22.2 ± 2.3 (616 ± 63.8)	48.6 ± 4.9 (1337 ± 134.8)	8.8 ± 1.7 (2.44 ± .47)	49.8 ± 5.8 (1381 ± 161)	136.9 ± 31.8 (3766 ± 875)	0.61 ± .21 (0.17 ± .06)	32.5 ± 4.9 (902 ± 136)	49.0 ± 9.4 (1348 ± 259)	1.13 ± 0.2 (0.31 ± 0.06)

[1](SI units)

[2]SI unit conversion factors: Aldosterone ng/dL × 27.74 = pmol/L; 18-hydroxycorticosterone ng/dL × 27.51 = pmol/L; plasma renin concentration ng/mL/h × 0.2778 = ng/(L.s).

tients with adenoma from those with hyperplasia. A plasma aldosterone concentration greater than 20 ng/dL (555 pmol/L) indicates adenoma, and less than 20 ng/dL (555 pmol/L) usually indicates hyperplasia. After 2 or 4 hours in the upright posture (which normally activates the renin system, with a rise in plasma aldosterone), plasma aldosterone concentration shows no significant change or diminution in 90% of patients with adenoma, but it almost always increases in patients with adrenocortical hyperplasia (Table 13–2). This important differential maneuver is extremely accurate in identifying the pathogenetic mechanism. The difference is due to the profound suppression of the renin system by excessive aldosterone production caused by adenoma. In addition, the number and affinity of angiotensin II receptors decreases in the tumor; the influence of ACTH also decreases from 8 AM to 12 noon. In contrast, in patients with adrenocortical hyperplasia, increased sensitivity of the hyperplastic gland to minute but measurable increases in renin that occur with assumption of the upright posture leads to an increased aldosterone level. The effectiveness of this maneuver depends on attention to the details of preparation described above.

Additional simultaneous measurements can be made of other precursor steroids and add significantly to the precision of diagnosis. Plasma DOC and corticosterone are frequently increased at 8 AM in patients with adenoma, whereas they are rarely if ever elevated in patients with hyperplasia. 18-Hydroxycorticosterone is invariably increased in patients with adenoma to levels greater than 85 ng/dL (2338 pmol/L) and shows no overlap with the normal or slightly high values of this steroid in patients with hyperplasia.

The procedures just discussed can identify primary aldosteronism and differentiate adenoma from hyperplasia in most cases; when uncertainty remains, 2 other tests, the deoxycorticosterone acetate (DOCA) maneuver and the saline infusion test, can be of further help. They can also be useful in further defining the type of hyperplasia.

B. Deoxycorticosterone Acetate (DOCA) Maneuver: Patients should be hospitalized for the DOCA suppression maneuver, which consists of administration of 10 mg of DOCA intramuscularly every 12 hours for 3 consecutive days accompanied by a salt intake of at least 7 g (120 meq/d). Fludrocortisone, 0.2 mg twice daily orally for 3–4 days, can be used with outpatients. On the third day of this regimen, either plasma aldosterone concentration or urinary aldosterone excretion is compared with pretreatment values. Aldosterone is suppressed minimally or not at all by DOCA in patients with adenoma.

The lack of suppression of the 8 AM recumbent plasma aldosterone concentration or the urinary aldosterone excretion on the third day generally indicates the idiopathic hyperaldosteronism form of hyperplasia or adenoma, whereas suppression of either plasma aldosterone concentration or urinary aldosterone excre-

tion establishes a second subset of hyperplasia patients, those with indeterminate hyperaldosteronism. Patients in the latter group present with milder degrees of hypokalemia, modest elevations of aldosterone production, and suppressed plasma renin concentration. Patients with adenoma do not respond by suppression of the already low plasma renin concentration.

C. Saline Infusion Test: Saline loading establishes aldosterone unresponsiveness to volume expansion and thereby identifies autonomy in patients with aldosterone-producing adenomas. As a rule, 2 L of isotonic saline is administered over a period of 2–4 hours, and blood samples are then obtained. This expansion of the extracellular fluid volume reduces plasma aldosterone concentration promptly in patients with "essential" hypertension but fails to suppress plasma aldosterone concentration into the normal range in patients with adenoma or idiopathic hyperplasia. However, the plasma aldosterone concentration is suppressed in the group with indeterminate hyperplasia.

The saline infusion test and the DOCA or fludrocortisone maneuver clearly distinguish hyperaldosteronism from essential hypertension. Response to upright posture identifies adenoma or hyperplasia. Suppression studies help determine the type of hyperplasia.

Identification of Other Types of Aldosteronism

A. Glucocorticoid-Responsive Aldosteronism: The glucocorticoid-remediable form of hyperaldosteronism is rare, occurs primarily in young men, and is familial. It constitutes a remarkable subset of hyperaldosteronemic patients with hyperplasia in whom all of the biochemical abnormalities can be reversed after 2–3 weeks with the use of ACTH-suppressive doses of glucocorticoids (1–2 mg of dexamethasone daily). Patients with glucocorticoid-remediable hyperaldosteronism will maintain a normal blood pressure, plasma aldosterone, and other biochemical indices as long as the dexamethasone or other ACTH suppressant is administered. Plasma aldosterone concentration is moderately elevated in these patients due to the increased sensitivity of the aldosterone biosynthetic pathway to normal ACTH levels.

B. Aldosteronism Due to Adrenocortical Carcinoma: Malignant tumors producing only aldosterone are extremely rare. The few patients reported have had large tumors with abundant precursor steroids and an absence of circadian rhythm.

Summary of Differential Diagnosis

The most important disorder of the mineralocorticoid hormones is primary aldosteronism due to a solitary adenoma. As diagnostic precision increases, many cases of hypertension and hypokalemia with modest increases of aldosterone production have been identified and characterized as hyperaldosteronism due to hyperplasia. Whether this is a primary adrenal disorder or not is far from clear, but the weight of evidence suggests that it is not. During the course of diagnostic workups of patients with suspected adenoma, conditions involving other mineralocorticoid abnormalities have been found.

Defining the growing numbers of patients with adrenal hyperplasia and hyperaldosteronism is not as important clinically as identifying those patients with adenoma who can be cured by surgery. Hypokalemia in a hypertensive patient means hypermineralocorticoidism. The subsequent suppressed plasma renin activity confirms this.

The high urinary aldosterone level identifies the adrenal as the source of the disorder. If the urinary aldosterone level is low, another adrenal mineralocorticoid hormone is operative. Measurement of plasma aldosterone is perhaps the best means of discriminating between adenoma and hyperplasia by both the degree of elevation and the response to postural change.

Suppression studies in patients with increased aldosterone production help define the type of hyperplasia and autonomy of adenomas. Precursor steroids may be even more important in distinguishing hyperplasia from adenoma, because they are invariably normal in hyperplasia and elevated in adenoma. (18-Hydroxycorticosterone is almost always elevated, and DOC and corticosterone are elevated over half of the time.)

4. MANAGEMENT OF ALDOSTERONE-PRODUCING ADENOMAS

Location of Adenoma

Once the biochemical diagnosis is secure, lateralization procedures in patients with adenoma become extremely important in determining the surgical approach. A number of techniques have been developed: adrenal venography, ^{131}I iodocholesterol scanning, adrenal vein catheterization and bilateral sampling, CT scanning, and, more recently, magnetic resonance imaging (MRI).

Adrenal venography was one of the first techniques used to locate tumors. However, a number of problems occurred, such as extravasation of dye, hemorrhage, and adrenal infarction, making this a potentially traumatic procedure. Tumors smaller than 7 mm cannot be located by this technique, and the success rate in identifying adrenal tumors has varied from 60 to 70%.

Scanning using intravenously administered ^{131}I iodocholesterol has located tumors in about 80% of patients. Again, size of tumor may be a limiting factor, because if tumors are less than 1 cm in diameter, the success rate drops considerably. The procedure is tedious and takes several weeks to accomplish. The use of 6β-iodomethyl-19-norcholesterol (NP59) reduces

the interval between injection and scintiscanning to about 24 hours.

CT scanning, which is as effective as iodocholesterol scanning in locating adenomas, has proved to be even more useful, because it requires considerably less radiation than iodocholesterol scanning, and the diagnostic information is more readily available. Experience with MRI is still limited, but for small adrenal tumors its level of resolution is equal to or slightly better than that of CT scanning.

Adrenal vein catheterization to measure bilateral aldosterone levels continues to be useful in lateralizing tumors only after other lateralizing techniques fail and biochemical evidence still supports the diagnosis of adenoma.

Treatment

Treatment depends for the most part on the precision of diagnosis. In patients with an aldosterone-producing adenoma and no contraindication to operation, unilateral adrenalectomy is recommended. The degree of reduction of blood pressure and correction of hypokalemia achieved with spironolactone provides a surprisingly close approximation to the actual response to surgery; in fact, greater reduction often occurs postoperatively, presumably because of a greater reduction of extracellular fluid. The surgical cure rate of hypertension associated with adenoma is excellent—over 50% in several series—with reduction of hypertension in the remainder.

Preoperative Preparation

Patients should be treated preoperatively with spironolactone, 200–400 mg/d, until the blood pressure and serum potassium are entirely normal; this may take 1–3 months. This drug is particularly beneficial because of its unique mechanism of action as an antagonist—ie, it blocks steroid binding at the mineralocorticoid receptor level. Once both blood pressure and serum potassium levels are normal, the dose can be reduced gradually to a maintenance dose of approximately 100–150 mg of spironolactone per day until the time of surgery. Spironolactone reduces the volume of the expanded extracellular fluid toward normal, promotes potassium retention, and restores normal serum potassium concentration. It often has the additional desirable effect of activating (after 1 or 2 months) the suppressed renin-angiotensin system. This will stimulate the suppressed zona glomerulosa of the nonadenomatous adrenal gland, so that postoperative hypoaldosteronism with hyperkalemia will be less likely, and the preoperative restoration of normal blood pressure is sustained. Preoperative treatment will also permit reversal to some extent of some of the changes in target organs that were produced by the hypertensive and hypokalemic states. Spironolactone is usually well tolerated; the side effects of rashes, gynecomastia, impotence, and epigastric discomfort are rare under the treatment program suggested.

Surgical & Medical Treatment Periods

When the diagnosis and lateralization are certain, surgical removal of the adenoma is recommended. The transperitoneal (anterior) approach has been employed successfully for many years. However, if preoperative lateralization techniques identify the site of tumor, a unilateral posterior approach can be used with considerably less postoperative morbidity.

If the tumor is identified at surgery, exploration of the contralateral adrenal is not indicated. If surgery is contraindicated or refused, indefinite treatment with spironolactone can be effective. The initial dose of 200–400 mg of spironolactone per day must be continued for 4–6 weeks before the full effect on blood pressure is realized. With prolonged treatment, aldosterone production does not increase even though potassium replenishment, decreased sodium and volume spaces, and activation of the renin-angiotensin system occur. In addition, spironolactone directly inhibits aldosterone synthesis by adenomas.

Subtotal adrenalectomy will correct hypokalemia in patients with hyperplasia, but the blood pressure remains elevated. In some cases, removal of adrenal mass ameliorates the hyperaldosterone-dependent hypertensive state. Preoperative identification of these cases is difficult. Primary adrenal hyperplasia appears to be a subtype of hyperaldosteronism (Table 13–1), which accounts for cures following reduction of adrenal tissue mass. Biochemically, patients in this group are indistinguishable from those with tumor, but no lateralization of aldosterone production can be demonstrated. Therefore, other antihypertensive measures (which should include spironolactone) must be used to control hypertension in patients with hyperplasia.

In patients with aldosteronism of indeterminate type, spironolactone alone is usually effective in controlling both the hypertension and the potassium-depleted state. Because of the effectiveness of spironolactone in these patients, other antihypertensive medications can often be discontinued.

Amiloride, a potassium-sparing diuretic, can also be used, in doses of 20–40 mg/d, to manage primary aldosteronism.

Pathologic Findings

Over 50% of patients with primary aldosteronism who have undergone surgery have had unilateral adenoma. Bilateral tumors are rare. The characteristic adenoma is readily identified by its golden-yellow color. In addition, small satellite adenomas are often found, and distinction from micro- or macronodular hyperplasia is frequently difficult. In patients with adenoma, the contiguous adrenal gland can show hyperplasia throughout the gland. Hyperplasia is also present in the contralateral adrenal gland but is not associated with aldosterone abnormalities after removal of the primary adenoma.

DEOXYCORTICOSTERONE EXCESS SYNDROMES

Diagnosis

A. 11β-Hydroxylase Deficiency: 11β-Hydroxylase deficiency syndrome is usually recognized in infants and children because of virilization and the frequent presence of both hypertension and hypokalemia. Plasma 11-deoxycortisol (compound S), 17α-hydroxyprogesterone, urinary 17-ketosteroids, and 17-hydroxycorticosteroids are increased.

The defect is usually partial, so that some cortisol is produced, but it does not increase with further stimulation by ACTH. Blood levels and production rates of cortisol are usually within normal limits. A partial defect of 11β-hydroxylation results in increased production and blood levels of DOC, 11-deoxycortisol, and androgens (see Fig 12–4). Hypertension results from excessive production of DOC by mechanisms previously described for aldosterone.

The blood levels and production rates of aldosterone are normal or reduced. Two mechanisms are proposed. One is that there is only partial inhibition of 11β-hydroxylation in the zona glomerulosa, which is a required biosynthetic step for aldosterone synthesis. The constancy of this block is supported by the fact that after normalization of DOC production and correction of the hypertension (by ACTH suppression), aldosterone production remains reduced and is not increased by sodium restriction. In fact, a sodium-losing state may be provoked by initial treatment. The other mechanism could be that suppression of renin by increased production of DOC might suppress the normal production of aldosterone in the zona glomerulosa. This notion is supported by the increase in renin and aldosterone production after suppression of ACTH and reduction of DOC production. It is still controversial whether the 11β-hydroxylating enzyme in the glomerulosa is the same as that of the fasciculata. The reduced levels of 18-hydroxydeoxycorticosterone (a zona fasciculata steroid) observed in this condition suggest that the 11β- and 18-hydroxylating enzymes may be similar.

B. 17α-Hydroxylase Deficiency: 17α-Hydroxylase deficiency syndrome is usually recognized at the time of puberty in young adults by the presence of hypertension, hypokalemia, and primary amenorrhea in the female or pseudohermaphroditism in the male. These features become more evident at this time because of the lack of increased sex steroid production associated with puberty. In contrast to the 11β-hydroxylation defect, there is no virilization or restricted growth. Patients often present with eunuchoid proportions and appearance. The virtual absence of 17α-hydroxyprogesterone, pregnanetriol, and ketosteroids is diagnostic of this type of hydroxylase deficiency (see Fig 12–4).

The key location of the 17α-hydroxylating system in the steroid biosynthetic pathway prevents normal production of androgens and estrogens. There has been no instance in which the adrenal defect has appeared without a concomitant gonadal defect. The defect seems to be in a single gene coding for the enzyme or in the expression of the gene. The diminution of cortisol production with this deficiency syndrome induces increased production of ACTH. Initially, the entire biosynthetic pathway of mineralocorticoids must be increased—namely, progesterone, DOC, corticosterone, 18-hydroxydeoxycorticosterone, and aldosterone.

Progressive overproduction of the mineralocorticoids in both the zona glomerulosa and zona fasciculata pathways results in expansion of extracellular fluid and blood volumes, hypertension, and subsequent reduction and obliteration, in most cases, of plasma renin activity. Subsequent to this reduction, the plasma aldosterone concentration is virtually absent in most patients. Thus, the principal mineralocorticoid hormones present in great quantities are corticosterone, DOC, 18-hydroxycorticosterone, and 18-hydroxydeoxycorticosterone—all of them ACTH-dependent steroids of the zona fasciculata.

Treatment

Treatment of both of these disorders—11β-hydroxylase deficiency syndrome and 17α-hydroxylase deficiency syndrome—is similar to that of all non-sodium-losing forms of congenital adrenal hyperplasia. Treatment with replacement doses of glucocorticoid, such as hydrocortisone or dexamethasone, restores blood pressure to normal levels, corrects potassium depletion, reduces excessive DOC and corticosterone production in 17α-hydroxylase deficiency syndrome, and reduces DOC and 11-deoxycortisol production in 11β-hydroxylase deficiency syndrome. In 17α-hydroxylase deficiency syndrome, restoration of normal levels of DOC results in a return of plasma renin activity and aldosterone to normal values. A delay in return of the suppressed renin-aldosterone system toward normal can result in hypovolemic crises with the initial natriuresis and diuresis. It may take several years before the aldosterone and renin systems become normal. The amount of glucocorticoid administered must be carefully determined because of apparently exquisite tissue sensitivity to glucocorticoid hormones.

ABNORMALITY OF TERMINAL STEROID METABOLISM (APPARENT MINERALOCORTICOID EXCESS SYNDROME)

An interesting subgroup of patients with hypertension, hypokalemia, and suppressed renin and aldosterone production has been described primarily in children. There is strong evidence that an unknown mineralocorticoid is active, although one has not been identified. Such a steroid responds to ACTH and inten-

sifies the abnormalities. The hypertension is sodium-dependent and responds to treatment with spironolactone. The hallmark of this disorder is the reduced peripheral metabolism of cortisol. There is reduced production of tetrahydrocortisone relative to tetrahydrocortisol owing to reduced activity of 11β-hydroxysteroid dehydrogenase. This abnormality in metabolism of cortisol appears to be primarily a peripheral marker of the disorder. The enzyme deficiency increases cortisol levels in the kidney to make it the causative mineralocorticoid.

SECONDARY MINERALOCORTICOID EXCESS (Table 13–3)

Activation of the zona glomerulosa by the renin-angiotensin system can lead to a variety of conditions in which increased aldosterone production occurs. Activation of the renin system can be accomplished by abnormalities such as sodium-wasting disease, laxative or diuretic abuse, decrease in intravascular volume, and direct overproduction of renin, such as in renovascular hypertension and renin-secreting tumors. This group can be subdivided into disorders with or without hypertension.

SECONDARY MINERALOCORTICOID EXCESS WITH HYPERTENSION

The following hypertensive disorders are for the most part renin-mediated, with hyperaldosteronism and hypokalemia as sequelae.

Renovascular Disease

Renovascular hypertension represents the most common cause of surgically reversible hypertension. It can be due to either atherosclerosis or fibromuscular hyperplasia. Other anatomic lesions may cause hypertension as well: renal infarction, solitary cysts, hydronephrosis, and other parenchymal lesions. Plasma renin activity in peripheral blood vessels is within normal limits in half of the patients with renovascular hypertension. Hyperaldosteronism is not always apparent in these patients; it manifests itself when renin levels are elevated. It is important to appreciate that even though renin levels are within normal limits in the peripheral circulation, they may be inappropriate for the degree of sodium retention that may have occurred during the development of this hypertensive state.

Renin-Secreting Tumors

Renin-secreting tumors are extremely rare and can be mistaken for primary aldosteronism. This is be-

Table 13–3. Biochemical findings in secondary hypermineralocorticoidism.

	Plasma		Aldos-terone	Other MCHs	Renin	Cortisol	ACTH	Hct	BUN/Creatinine
	Na+	K+							
With hypertension									
Renovascular hypertension	N or ↑	N or ↓	↑	N	↑	N	N	↑	N or ↑
Renin-secreting tumor	N or ↑	↓	↑↑	N	↑↑	N	N	↑	N
Accelerated hypertension	N	N or ↓	↑	N	↑	N	N	N or ↑	N or ↑
Estrogen therapy	N	N or ↓	↑	N	N or ↑	N or ↑	N	N or ↓	N
Cushing's disease	N	N or ↓	N or ↓	↑	N	↑	N or ↑	N	N
Without hypertension									
Sodium-wasting nephropathy	↓	↑ or ↓	↑↑	N or ↑	↑↑	N or ↑	N or ↑	↑	N or ↑
Bartter's syndrome	N	↓	↑	N	↑↑	N	N	N	N
Pseudohypoaldosteronism	N or ↓	↑	↑↑	N or ↑	↑↑	N	N	↑	N
Renal tubular acidosis	N	N or ↑	↑	N	↑	N	N	N or ↑	N
Diuretic/laxative abusers	N or ↓	↓	↑↑	N	↑↑	N	N	↑	N

BUN, blood urea nitrogen; Hct, hematocrit; MCH, mineralocorticoid hormone; N, normal; ↑, increased; ↓, decreased; ↑↑, ↓↓, markedly increased, decreased.

cause patients have high plasma levels of aldosterone, marked hypokalemia, and hypertension. The tumors are usually hemangiopericytomas containing elements of the juxtaglomerular cells. They are located by renal vein catheterization. Other tumors (Wilms' tumors, ectopic tumors) that secrete renin have been reported, including a pulmonary tumor that secreted excessive amounts of renin, producing hypertension and hypokalemia with secondary aldosteronism.

Accelerated Hypertension

Accelerated hypertension is characterized by marked elevations of diastolic blood pressure that can be abrupt in onset. This disorder is associated with progressive arteriosclerosis. The plasma levels of aldosterone may be extremely high. It is believed that the intense vasospastic events that occur and the excessive renal cortical nephrosclerosis lead to hyperreninemia and accelerate the hypertensive process. Vigorous antihypertensive therapy usually mitigates the hyperaldosteronism.

Estrogen Therapy

Aldosterone levels are increased during replacement estrogen therapy or use of oral contraceptives. This is due to increases in plasma renin substrate and plasma renin activity. Angiotensin II levels are increased and thus stimulate aldosterone production. However, hypokalemia rarely occurs during estrogen administration. Plasma cortisol levels may be increased due to estrogen-induced increases in CBG concentration.

Cushing's Disease

ACTH-dependent hypercortisolism (Cushing's disease and ectopic ACTH production) is frequently accompanied by increased levels of other ACTH-dependent steroids, especially DOC and corticosterone. Elevated DOC and cortisol levels produce hypertension, occasionally with hypokalemia. Plasma renin activity is normal due to increased production of renin substrate. Levels of aldosterone and 18-hydroxycorticosterone are consistently in or below the low normal range. (See Chapter 12 for a discussion of Cushing's syndrome.)

SECONDARY MINERALOCORTICOID EXCESS WITHOUT HYPERTENSION

Sodium-Wasting Syndromes

In the preceding section we described primary renin overproduction due to direct and local diminution of volume to renin-secreting areas. The abnormalities discussed in this group of disorders are more systemic, resulting in major changes in extracellular fluid volume and affecting renin and aldosterone production accordingly. In patients with severe chronic renal insufficiency, sodium wasting can become a permanent effect, resulting in secondary hyperaldosteronism with hypo- or hypertension, hyponatremia, and hyper- or hypokalemia. Modest renal sodium wasting in patients with renal tubular acidosis may increase renin secretion and result in aldosterone excess, potassium depletion, and hypokalemia. Pseudohypoaldosteronism is a rare genetic disorder in which tubular resistance to mineralocorticoid hormones is present, presumably due to a deficiency of mineralocorticoid hormone receptors. Renal sodium wasting, volume depletion, and shock can occur; hyperkalemia is invariably present.

Diuretic abuse causes renal sodium wasting and thus secondary hyperaldosteronism by activation of the renin system. Similarly, surreptitious vomiting and laxative abuse can cause secondary aldosteronism and increase in renin secretion by depleting extracellular fluid volume via the gastrointestinal tract. Urinary chloride levels are low in this condition.

Edematous States

The classic edematous states associated with secondary aldosteronism are those of cirrhosis with ascites, nephrosis, and congestive heart failure. Activation of the renin system in patients with these diseases most likely results from changes in renal hemodynamics and redistribution of volume into extravascular tissues, so that the increase in the renin-aldosterone system may be looked upon as a homeostatic adjustment. Although presumably a homeostatic mechanism, the hyperaldosteronism can further contribute to the edema. Hypokalemia is not a frequent finding in these patients unless intake of potassium is extremely low, because reabsorption of sodium in proximal nephron sites makes excessive potassium loss in the distal nephron and the collecting tubules less likely.

Bartter's Syndrome

Bartter's syndrome is a disorder characterized by hypokalemia, alkalosis, hyperreninemia, secondary hyperaldosteronism, increased renal prostaglandins, increased urinary levels of kallikreins, and resistance to pressor effects of angiotensin II. The defect seems to be primarily renal. Although its immediate cause has not been clearly identified, an initiating event may be the defect in chloride reabsorption in the ascending limb of Henle's loop (see Chapter 4).

PRIMARY MINERALOCORTICOID DEFICIENCY
(Table 13–4)

Disorders of primary mineralocorticoid deficiency consist of a group of adrenal diseases in which mineralocorticoid hormone production is subnormal or inadequate owing to a decrease in the mass of adrenocortical tissue or defective synthesis. As a consequence, variable degrees of sodium loss ensue, with hyponatremia, diminished effective blood volume, and hypotension. Potassium and hydrogen ion secretion are impaired in the renal tubule, resulting in hyperkalemia and metabolic acidosis. Renin activity, as a reliable index of sodium loss, is typically increased (Table 13–4).

Acute and chronic adrenocortical insufficiencies are discussed in Chapter 12. Some problems relative to mineralocorticoids are reviewed here.

UNILATERAL ADRENALECTOMY

Patients who have had unilateral adrenalectomy for removal of an aldosterone-producing tumor usually have a transient period of relative hypomineralocorticoidism with negative sodium balance, potassium retention, and mild acidosis. Full recovery of the chronically unstimulated, contralateral zona glomerulosa usually takes place in 4–6 months following surgery, but sometimes it takes as long as 18–24 months, particularly in those patients prepared for surgery less than optimally with spironolactone. Restitution of the suppressed renin-angiotensin system to normal function usually precedes a completely normal adrenocortical response similar to the recovery of the pituitary-adrenal axis after removal of cortisol-producing adenoma (Cushing's syndrome). No specific treatment is necessary beyond adequate fluid intake and sodium supplementation, except when renal disease is present. A small percentage of patients (1%) do not have normal recovery of their renin-angiotensin-aldosterone system and require mineralocorticoid replacement therapy for life. Preexisting renal disease usually identifies this group.

CONGENITAL ADRENAL HYPOPLASIA & RELATED METABOLIC DISORDERS

Genetic disorders or congenital anomalies involving the adrenal glands have been reported rarely. Congenital adrenal hypoplasia, alone or in association with pituitary hypoplasia, was found at autopsy in a number of newborns who failed to thrive because of sodium loss and complications of hyperkalemia. Other infrequent metabolic disorders that usually involve the adrenal glands are Wolman's disease, cholesteryl ester storage disease, and adrenoleukodystrophy (X-linked Schilder's disease). Mineralocorticoid production is clearly deficient in patients with these diseases.

CONGENITAL ADRENAL HYPERPLASIA WITH RENAL SODIUM LOSS

In variants of congenital adrenal hyperplasia, cortisol synthesis is always impaired. ACTH is accordingly elevated, producing adrenal hyperplasia and stimulating ACTH-dependent steroid precursors.

The steroid biosynthetic pathways, both in the adrenal glands and the gonads, produce specific steroid hormones: cortisol, aldosterone, and testosterone or estradiol. These terminal products come from a single precursor, cholesterol, via a series of enzymatic reactions that introduce hydroxyl groups at specific sites (Fig 13–1). Recessive autosomal inheritance is re-

Table 13–4. Biochemical findings in primary mineralocorticoid deficiency.

	Plasma		Aldos-terone	Other MCHs	Renin	Cortisol	ACTH	Hct	BUN/Creatinine
	Na+	K+							
Chronic adrenocortical insufficiency	N or ↓	↑	↓	N or ↓	↑	↓	↑	↑	N or ↑
After unilateral adrenalectomy for aldosterone-producing tumor	N or ↓	N or ↑	↓	↓	↓ ↑	N	N	N or ↑	N
21-Hydroxylase deficiency (sodium-losing type)	↓	↑	↓	↓	↑	↓	↑	↑	N
Cholesterol desmolase deficiency	↓	↑	↓	↓	↑	↓	↑	↑	N
3β-Hydroxysteroid dehydrogenase deficiency	↓	↑	↓	↓	↑	↓	↑	↑	N
18-Hydroxylase (CMO type I) deficiency	↓	↑	↓	↑	↑	N	N	↑	N or ↑
18-Hydroxysteroid dehydrogenase (CMO type II) deficiency	↓	↑	↓	↑	↑	N	N	↑	N or ↑

BUN, blood urea nitrogen; Hct, hematocrit; MCH, mineralocorticoid hormone; N, normal; ↑, increased; ↓, decreased; ↑ ↑, ↓ ↓, markedly increased, decreased.

sponsible for deficiencies in each of the enzymatic steps and results in several forms of the syndrome of deficient steroid production known generically as congenital adrenal hyperplasia. Synthesis of cortisol, aldosterone, and sex steroids is therefore involved in many different ways and combinations. The forms discussed here are those in which production of mineralocorticoid hormones is limited.

1. 21-HYDROXYLASE DEFICIENCY

The most common (95%) of the enzymatic abnormalities in steroid biosynthesis that cause congenital adrenal hyperplasia is due to a deficiency or defect in the enzymatic system responsible for 21-hydroxylation of steroids (see Fig 12–4).

The incidence of this particular form of congenital adrenal hyperplasia in the USA is believed to be approximately 1:5000 live births. In about half of these patients, sodium loss is not apparent, and aldosterone secretion or excretion is actually increased. The presence of elevated levels of progesterone, 17-hydroxyprogesterone, and probably other precursor steroids resulting from uninhibited ACTH stimulation of the adrenal cortex up to the level of the 21-hydroxylation block is probably responsible for the renin-mediated increase in aldosterone production, because these precursor steroids act as aldosterone antagonists at the distal tubule in the nephron and promote mild sodium loss. The ability to conserve sodium during periods of low-sodium intake in these patients is dependent, therefore, on how much aldosterone can be generated in the zona glomerulosa to counteract aldosterone antagonists. Because mild to moderate sodium loss can sometimes be demonstrated in the presence of increased aldosterone production, one has to assume that the high aldosterone levels are inadequate to promote sodium conservation. A wide range of clinical manifestations can be observed. The more severely affected patients, who represent approximately one-third of the whole group, have unquestionable deficiency in aldosterone production, with the 21-hydroxylation block unequivocally involving the zona glomerulosa biosynthetic pathway.

Diagnosis

Because 21-hydroxylase deficiency is an inborn error of steroid metabolism, clinical manifestations are likely to occur early in infancy. The disorder should be suspected in any infant or child who has frequent and usually refractory episodes of dehydration and whose genitalia are ambiguous. Diagnosis can be confirmed by laboratory findings of electrolyte disturbance, low levels of urinary metabolites or plasma concentrations of cortisol and aldosterone, and elevated levels of steroid precursors such as 17-hydroxyprogesterone and its urinary metabolite pregnanetriol.

Treatment

Treatment must be instituted promptly, because the sodium and fluid losses result in severe dehydration, shock, and hyperkalemia and thus in usually fatal cardiac arrhythmias. Parenteral isotonic or even hypertonic saline and glucocorticoids (hydrocortisone, 25–50 mg intravenously, and DOCA, 2–5 mg intramuscularly) as required are lifesaving. Cationic resins (eg, sodium polystyrene sulfonate [Kayexalate]) may be used to lower extremely high potassium levels refractory to other treatment. Chronic treatment requires mineralocorticoid replacement and sodium chloride supplementation. In addition, patients achieve improvement in linear growth and experience decreased need for glucocorticoid hormones to suppress ACTH when small supplements of mineralocorticoids are given. For reasons not understood, sodium-retaining ability may improve with age, so that some patients are able to discontinue mineralocorticoid replacement, usually after puberty.

Patients with the "simple virilizing," non-sodium-losing type of 21-hydroxylase deficiency also have been shown to have elevated plasma renin levels. This elevation is presumably due to the increased production of precursor steroids with aldosterone-antagonistic properties, leading to higher plasma aldosterone levels. The level of plasma renin activity is accordingly an index for substitution therapy with added salt or fludrocortisone to correct this abnormality. These observations led some investigators to postulate that even in the non–sodium-losing type of 21-hydroxylase deficiency, a mild degree of sodium loss, usually manifested during stressful situations or low sodium intake, occurs as a consequence of inadequate aldosterone production even though the plasma concentration or urinary level of aldosterone may be elevated. Accordingly, the 21-hydroxylase deficiency should be considered as a single disorder with a wide spectrum of clinical manifestations related to sodium conservation instead of 2 separate disorders—the sodium-losing and non–sodium-losing forms.

2. CHOLESTEROL DESMOLASE DEFICIENCY

Prader in 1955 described a syndrome of sodium loss in which no steroid could be found in the urine. Histologic and postmortem examination of patients showed a "lipoid" hyperplasia of adrenocortical tissue containing a high concentration of cholesterol-laden cells. A defect in cholesterol desmolase, the earliest step in steroid biosynthesis, that impeded the conversion of cholesterol to Δ^5-pregnenolone was proposed as the mechanism. Patients with this uncommon disorder cannot produce steroids from any source and present with a female phenotype and severe sodium loss; they frequently die in the first weeks of life, although a few survive with early recognition and treatment.

3. 3β-HYDROXYSTEROID DEHYDROGENASE & $\Delta^{4,5}$ ISOMERASE DEFICIENCIES

3β-Hydroxysteroid dehydrogenase deficiency is a rare life-threatening form of congenital adrenal hyperplasia that was described by Bongiovanni in 1962. Pregnenolone (Δ^5) can be synthesized but not Δ^4 steroids derived from it, eg, progesterone (see Fig 12–4). The concomitant involvement of the gonads precludes production of sex steroids. Incomplete sexual differentiation is seen in males, whereas mild virilization is seen in females from weaker androgenic steroids derived from pregnenolone, ie, dehydro-

epiandrosterone (DHEA). Aldosterone, which is also derived from the Δ^4 steroid lineage, cannot be produced in adequate amounts, and sodium conservation is therefore poor. Recently, a mild or incomplete defect in this enzymatic step was reported in adults. Analysis of steroid metabolites in the urine or of plasma concentrations of steroids establishes the diagnosis, and treatment should consist of replacement of glucocorticoids, mineralocorticoids, and sex hormones.

4. DISORDERS OF TERMINAL ALDOSTERONE BIOSYNTHESIS

In contrast to congenital adrenal hyperplasia, specific enzymatic deficiencies can result in a syndrome of isolated mineralocorticoid deficiency. Two clinically similar sodium-losing syndromes have been described that present almost exclusively with sodium loss and some degree of growth retardation. The production of aldosterone from corticosterone is a 2-step reaction in which 18-hydroxycorticosterone is presumably formed as an intermediate precursor. However, Ulick proposed that aldosterone and 18-hydroxycorticosterone are both end products of the zona glomerulosa, being synthesized from corticosterone through a mixed function oxidation system. In so-called corticosterone methyloxidase (CMO) type I deficiency (18-hydroxylase deficiency), formation of aldosterone and 18-hydroxycorticosterone is blocked after corticosterone formation. The salt loss and increased renin secretion stimulate the zona glomerulosa pathway and increase production of the 18-hydroxycorticosterone and aldosterone precursors corticosterone and DOC. In the second variant, corticosterone methyloxidase (CMO) type II deficiency (18-hydroxysteroid dehydrogenase deficiency), corticosterone and 18-hydroxycorticosterone are produced in increased amounts in the presence of reduced production of aldosterone. The accumulation of precursors in each case, however, is not sufficient to prevent sodium loss, hyperkalemia, and increased renin production. Both of these uncommon diseases are manifested early in infancy and have a tendency to improve with age. Early detection and treatment with mineralocorticoid and sodium supplements result in an excellent prognosis.

SECONDARY MINERALOCORTICOID DEFICIENCY (Table 13–5)

SECONDARY MINERALOCORTICOID DEFICIENCY WITH HYPERTENSION

Secondary mineralocorticoid deficiency comprises a heterogeneous group of disorders in which endoge-

Table 13–5. Biochemical findings in secondary mineralocorticoid deficiency.

	Plasma		Aldos-terone	Other MCHs	Renin	Cortisol	ACTH	Hct	BUN/Creatinine
	Na+	K+							
With hypertension									
Pseudohyperaldosteronism (Liddle's syndrome)	N or ↑	↓	↓	N or ↓	↓	N	N	↓	N
Arnold-Healy-Gordon syndrome	N or ↑	↑	↓	N or ↓	↓	N	N	N or ↓	N
Synthetic MCH administration	N or ↑	↓	↓	↓²	↓	N	N	↓	N
Chronic ingestion of MCH-like substances	N or ↑	↓	↓	↓²	↓	N	N	↓	N
Without hypertension									
Heparin and heparinoids	N or ↓	N or ↑	N or ↓	N or ↓	N or ↑	N	N	N or ↑	N
Hyporeninemic hypoaldosteronism	N or ↓	↑	↓	N or ↓	↓	N	N	N or ↑	↑
Autonomic insufficiency	N or ↓	N or ↑	↓	N or ↓	↓	N	N	N	N
Renin blockers/angiotensin-converting enzyme inhibitors	N or ↓	N or ↑	↓	N or ↓	↓(↑)¹	N	N	N	N or ↑

[1] Angiotensin II or III is decreased; renin activity or concentration is increased by an artifact.
[2] Endogenous production of mineralocorticoid is decreased; high mineralocorticoid hormone activity results from exogenous administration.
BUN, blood urea nitrogen; Hct, hematocrit; MCH, mineralocorticoid hormone; N, normal; ↑, increased; ↓, decreased; ↑↑, ↓↓, markedly increased, decreased.

nous mineralocorticoid secretion is abnormally low owing to suppressed or insufficient renin production. In the former situation, renin is suppressed by increased sodium retention and volume expansion resulting either from the presence of exogenous mineralocorticoids or mineralocorticoidlike substances or from a renal tubular defect. Hypertension, hypokalemia, and metabolic alkalosis are the usual manifestations. When renin production is insufficient to stimulate mineralocorticoid production, sodium loss, hyperkalemia, and metabolic acidosis occur.

Pseudohyperaldosteronism (Liddle's Syndrome)

In 1963, Liddle et al studied a family in which the affected members had clinical manifestations resembling those of classic primary aldosteronism: hypertension, hypokalemia with renal potassium wasting, metabolic alkalosis, and suppressed plasma renin activity. However, aldosterone production was negligible. This unusual isolated finding suggested the possibility of excessive production of another unidentified mineralocorticoid hormone to explain the clinical manifestations. However, administration of spironolactone, a mineralocorticoid antagonist at the distal tubular receptor level, did not correct either the hypertension or the hypokalemia. Furthermore, the adrenocortical synthesis-blocking agent metyrapone, which inhibits 11β- and 18-hydroxylation of aldosterone precursors, also had no effect. In contrast, administration of triamterene, a diuretic agent with potassium-sparing activity acting at a proximal site in the nephron independently of mineralocorticoid hor-

mones, was effective in correcting the abnormalities. The investigators proposed that a primary defect in sodium-potassium transport across membranes in the renal tubule was responsible for the syndrome, although the precise mechanism remains unclear. The defect is probably generalized, since hyperactivity of Na^+ - K^+ ATPase (the sodium-potassium pump) has also been demonstrated in red blood cells.

Arnold-Healy-Gordon Syndrome

Several patients have been reported in whom hypertension is present in association with hyperkalemia, impairment of potassium excretion, and hyperchloremic metabolic acidosis. A state of hyporeninemic hypoaldosteronism is well documented in the presence of normal renal function. The aldosterone response to stimulatory maneuvers appears to be adequate. Administration of large amounts of mineralocorticoids fails to produce a kaliuretic response and thus correct the hyperkalemia, suggesting a mineralocorticoid-resistant state. Impairment in renal potassium excretion was initially proposed as the primary defect. However, when patients were given a sodium bicarbonate or sulfate load, the increased distal delivery of sodium greatly facilitated potassium excretion and hyperkalemia was virtually corrected, suggesting that the proposed defect in potassium excretion was only secondary. The defect caused increases in chloride reabsorption proximal to the sodium- and mineralocorticoid-dependent driving forces for potassium secretion, resulting in hyperkalemia. By increasing proximal sodium reabsorption with consequent volume expansion, hypertension and suppression of renin and aldosterone production occurred. Abnormalities can be corrected in this syndrome by adding supplementary amounts of sodium bicarbonate, sulfate, or furosemide.

Administration of Synthetic Mineralocorticoid Hormones

In several of the mineralocorticoid deficiency syndromes, the appropriate therapy is mineralocorticoid replacement. The most commonly used synthetic mineralocorticoid is the 9α-fluoro derivative of hydrocortisone, 9α-fluorohydrocortisone (fludrocortisone acetate). Its potent mineralocorticoid activity, which is similar to that of aldosterone, permits it to be used in amounts as small as 0.1 mg daily or every other day. Alternatively, DOCA in a long-acting preparation can be used intramuscularly. Because individual sensitivity to these preparations varies, blood pressure and plasma electrolyte panels should be monitored closely. When used in inappropriately high dosage or in the presence of increased sodium intake or inadequate metabolism, increased mineralocorticoid activity will occur and result in sodium retention, expansion of extracellular fluid volume, hypertension, and hypokalemia. Adjustment of the dosage easily controls undesirable side effects.

Chronic Ingestion of Mineralocorticoidlike Substances

Chronic ingestion of large amounts of substances containing mineralocorticoidlike activity—eg, certain candies, infusions, and some chewing tobaccos containing licorice—results in a syndrome of hypertension, hypokalemia, renal sodium retention, volume expansion, suppressed plasma renin activity, and metabolic alkalosis that is almost indistinguishable from primary hyperaldosteronism. Aldosterone secretion or excretion is, however, low or undetectable, as are other mineralocorticoid precursors in the aldosterone pathway. The responsible agents for this syndrome are certain substances, especially glycyrrhizic acid and its metabolite glycyrrhetimic acid, that are present in certain commercially available products. They inhibit 11β-hydroxydehydrogenase in the kidney which increases free cortisol locally to act as the mineralocorticoid. Hypermineralocorticoidism can be induced by licorice and its derivatives—carbenoxolone (an anti-gastric ulcer drug), sodium hemisuccinate of 18β-glycyrrhetimic acid—and by other fluorinated steroids with powerful mineralocorticoidlike activity contained in some topical preparations such as nasal sprays and dermatologic creams. Electrolyte abnormalities and hypertension disappear within a few days or weeks upon discontinuation of licorice ingestion or carbenoxolone withdrawal.

SECONDARY MINERALOCORTICOID DEFICIENCY WITHOUT HYPERTENSION

Heparin & Heparinoids

Chronic administration of heparin and related compounds, either to humans or to experimental animals, is reportedly associated with decreased aldosterone production in some cases. The mechanism for impaired aldosterone synthesis is not clearly understood, although decreased sensitivity of the zona glomerulosa to renin-angiotensin stimulation is suspected. No evidence of any enzymatic defect induced by heparin has been demonstrated by measuring aldosterone precursors. Anatomic changes in the zona glomerulosa are nonspecific and seem to be reversible after heparin treatment is discontinued.

Hyporeninemic Hypoaldosteronism

An increasing number of patients have recently been reported in whom hyperkalemia and acidosis are present in association with variable degrees of renal failure in the course of diseases such as pyelonephritis, diabetes mellitus, and gout. The patients, usually men in the fifth to seventh decades of life, have an average decrease of 60% in renal function as evaluated by creatinine clearance, and the chronic renal insufficiency per se usually cannot account for the degree of hyperkalemia. Plasma sodium concentration is normal, but sodium conservation is frequently deficient. Plasma concentrations and urinary excretion of aldosterone are low and unresponsive to such stimulatory maneuvers as prolonged ACTH administration, upright posture, dietary sodium deprivation, furosemide administration, and angiotensin III ([des-Asp[1]] angiotensin II) infusion. Plasma renin activity and concentration are consistently low and also unresponsive to stimulation. Cortisol- and ACTH-dependent steroids are normal and increase adequately in response to appropriate stimuli. The cause of the hyporeninemic state is presumably associated with chronic impairment of the juxtaglomerular apparatus. Potassium restriction, furosemide, alkali, and small doses of fludrocortisone (Florinef) (0.05 mg/d), singly or in combination, may be required to correct the acidosis and hyperkalemia.

Autonomic Insufficiency

This subset of hyporeninemic hypoaldosteronism can be further characterized by defective baroreceptor function, vasopressor sensitivity to vasopressin and norepinephrine, and mild sodium wasting.

Progressive degeneration and destruction of sympathetic nerve terminations leading to the juxtaglomerular apparatus and deficient neurotransmission in the afferent or efferent fibers associated with the synthesis and storage of renin granules are potential causes of secondary aldosterone deficiency. Stimuli such as upright posture or acute volume depletion, mediated by baroreceptors, do not effect normal responses in renin. Even stimuli mediated by the sodium concentration in the macula densa (ie, chemoreceptors) fail to initiate a renin-aldosterone response. Aldosterone levels are low normal and subnormally responsive to sodium restriction in this condition. The classic manifestation of this disease is a moderate to sever postural fall in blood pressure. The impaired potassium excretion associated with the hypoaldosteronism can be further aggravated by the diminished renal blood flow, resulting in alarmingly high plasma levels of potassium. Doses of fludrocortisone (Florinef) in the range of 0.1–0.4 mg/d are usually necessary to maintain adequate blood volume, to ensure appropriate accommodation to postural changes, and to prevent potassium retention.

Prolonged Use of Renin Blockers or Angiotensin-Converting Enzyme Inhibitors

Several hypertensive states, especially those associated with high renin levels (angiotensinogenic hypertension)—eg, high-renin essential hypertension, renovascular hypertension, and accelerated hypertension—have been managed either by renin secretion inhibitors such as the beta-receptor blockers or converting enzyme inhibitors of angiotensin II formation such as captopril or enalapril. Although hormonal responses during treatment must be monitored, one can assume that chronic suppression of renin formation or release or continuous inhibition of the renin-angiotensin system cascade may induce varying degrees of aldosterone deficiency, especially in patients with decreased renal function. Prostaglandin synthetase inhibitors (nonsteroidal anti-inflammatory agents) can reduce renin and aldosterone levels, and their use in a patient with impaired renal function may result in hyperkalemia.

REFERENCES

Arteaga E et al: Aldosterone-producing adrenocortical carcinoma: Preoperative recognition and course in three cases. *Ann Intern Med* 1984;**101**:316.

Baxter JD et al: The endocrinology of hypertension. Chapter 14 in: *Endocrinology and Metabolism,* 2nd ed. Felig P et al (editors). McGraw-Hill, 1987.

Biglieri EG: Rare causes of adrenocortical hypertension. *Cardiology* 1985;**72(Suppl 1)**:70.

Biglieri EG, Kater CE: Adrenal enzymatic defects. Chapter 58 in: *Hypertension: Physiopathology and Treatment,* 2nd ed. Genest J, Kuchel O (editors). McGraw-Hill, 1983.

Biglieri EG, Kater CE: Disorders of the adrenal cortex. In: *Internal Medicine.* Stein JH (editor). Little, Brown, 1986.

Blachley JD, Knochel JP: Tobacco chewer's hypokalemia: Licorice revisited. *N Engl J Med* 1980;**302**:784.

Bravo EL et al: The changing clinical spectrum of primary aldosteronism. *Am J Med* 1983;**74**:641.

Carey RM et al: Idiopathic hyperaldosteronism: A possible role for aldosterone-stimulating factor. *N Engl J Med* 1984;**311**:94.

Carey RM, Sen S: Recent progress in the control of aldosterone secretion. *Recent Prog Horm Res* 1986;**42**:251.

Dunnick NR et al: Localization of functional adrenal tumors by computed tomography and venous sampling. *Radiology* 1982;**142**:429.

Dzau VJ, Gibbons GH, Levin DC: Renovascular hypertension: An update on pathophysiology, diagnosis and treatment. *Am J Nephrol* 1983;**3**:172.

Falke TH et al: MR imaging of the adrenals: Correlation with computed tomography. *J Comput Assist Tomogr* 1986;**10**:242.

Gill JR Jr: Bartter's syndrome. *Annu Rev Med* 1980;**31**:405.

Gordon RD: Syndrome of hypertension and hyperkalemia with normal glomerular filtration rate. *Hypertension* 1986;**8**:93.

Griffing GT, Melby JC: Adrenocortical factors in hypertension. *J Clin Pharmacol* 1985;**25**:318.

Hunt TK, Biglieri EG, Tyrrell JB: Adrenals. Chap 35, pp 661–673, in: *Current Surgical Diagnosis & Treatment,* 8th ed. Way LW (editor). Appleton & Lange, 1988.

Irvine WJ, Toft AD, Feek CM: Addison's disease. Pages 131–164 in: *The Adrenal Gland.* James VH (editor). Raven Press, 1979.

Lee PD et al: Biochemical diagnosis and management of corticosterone methyl oxidase type II deficiency. *J Clin Endocrinol Metab* 1986;**62**:225.

Melby JC: Primary aldosteronism. (Clinical conference.) *Kidney Int* 1984;**26**:769.

New MI (editor): Congenital adrenal hyperplasia. *Ann NY Acad Sci* 1985;**458**:1. [Entire issue.]

New MI, Oberfield SE, Levine LS: Hypertension in children. Chapter 54 in: *Hypertension: Physiopathology and Treatment,* 2nd ed. Genest J, Kuchel O (editors). McGraw-Hill, 1983.

Oberfield SE et al: Metabolic and blood pressure responses to hydrocortisone in the syndrome of apparent mineralocorticoid excess. *J Clin Endocrinol Metab* 1983;**56**:332.

Schalekamp MA, Wenting GJ, Man in't Veld AJ: Pathogenesis of mineralocorticoid hypertension. *Clin Endocrinol Metab* 1981;**10**:397.

Schambelan M, Sebastian A, Biglieri EG: Prevalence, pathogenesis, and functional significance of aldosterone deficiency in hyperkalemic patients with chronic renal insufficiency. *Kidney Int* 1980;**17**:89.

Thompson DG, Mason AS, Goodwin FJ: Mineralocorticoid replacement in Addison's disease. *Clin Endocrinol* 1979;**10**:499.

Williams GH: Hyporeninemic hypoaldosteronism. (Editorial.) *N Engl J Med* 1986;**314**:1041.

Young WF, Klee GG: Primary aldosteronism: Diagnostic evaluation. *Endocrinol Metab Clin North Am* 1988;**17**:367.

14

Adrenal Medulla

Alan Goldfien, MD

The adrenal medulla was first distinguished from the adrenal cortex at the beginning of the 19th century. Its major secretory product, **epinephrine,** was isolated, purified, and synthesized a century later. **Norepinephrine** was synthesized in 1904, but not until 1946 was it recognized as a secretory product of the adrenal medulla and as the major neurotransmitter of the postganglionic sympathetic nerves. The adrenal medulla, a highly specialized part of the sympathetic nervous system, functions under stress or whenever marked deviations from normal homeostasis occur—in contrast to the rest of the sympathetic nervous system, which is involved in the minute-to-minute fine regulation of most physiologic processes.

Acronyms Used in This Chapter

ACTH	Adrenocorticotropic hormone
ATP	Adenosine triphosphate
cAMP	Cyclic adenosine monophosphate
COMT	Catechol-O-methyltransferase
DOMA	Dihydroxymandelic acid
DOPA	Dihydroxyphenylalanine
DOPEG	Dihydroxyphenylglycol
IP$_3$	Inositol trisphosphate
MAO	Monoamine oxidase
MEN	Multiple endocrine neoplasia
MIBG	[^{131}I] Metaiodobenzylguanidine
PGE	Prostaglandin E
PNMT	Phenylethanolamine-N-methyltransferase
VIP	Vasoactive intestinal peptide
VMA	Vanillylmandelic acid (3-methoxy-4-hydroxymandelic acid)

ANATOMY

Embryology
(Fig 14–1)

The sympathetic nervous system arises in the fetus from the primitive cells of the neural crest (sympathogonia). At about the fifth week of gestation, these cells migrate from the primitive spinal ganglia in the thoracic region to form the sympathetic chain posterior to the dorsal aorta. They then begin to migrate anteriorly to form the remaining ganglia.

At 6 weeks, groups of these primitive cells migrate along the central vein and enter the fetal adrenal cortex to form the adrenal medulla, which is detectable by the eighth week. The adrenal medulla at this time is composed of sympathogonia and pheochromoblasts, which then mature into pheochromocytes. The cells appear in rosettelike structures, with the more primitive cells occupying a central position. Storage granules can be found in these cells by electron microscopy at 12 weeks. Pheochromoblasts and pheochromocytes also collect on both sides of the aorta to form the paraganglia. The principal collection of these cells is found at the level of the inferior mesenteric artery. They fuse anteriorly to form the organ of Zuckerkandl, which is quite prominent in fetal life. This organ is thought to be a major source of catecholamines during the first year of life, after which it begins to atrophy. Pheochromocytes (chromaffin cells) also are found scattered throughout the abdominal sympathetic plexuses as well as in other parts of the sympathetic nervous system.

Gross Structure

The anatomic relationships between the adrenal medulla and the adrenal cortex are different in different species. These organs are completely separate structures in the shark. They remain separate but in close contact in amphibians, and there is some intermingling in birds. In mammals, the medulla is surrounded by the adrenal cortex. In humans, the adrenal medulla occupies a central position in the widest part of the gland, with only small portions extending into the narrower parts. It constitutes approximately one-tenth of the weight of the gland, although the proportions vary from individual to individual. There is no clear demarcation between cortex and medulla. The central vein is usually surrounded by a cuff of adrenal cortical cells, and there may be islands of cortex elsewhere in the medulla.

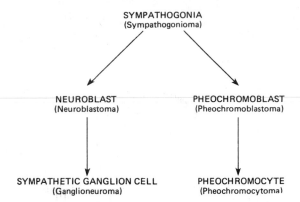

SYMPATHOGONIA
(Sympathogonioma)

NEUROBLAST
(Neuroblastoma)

PHEOCHROMOBLAST
(Pheochromoblastoma)

SYMPATHETIC GANGLION CELL
(Ganglioneuroma)

PHEOCHROMOCYTE
(Pheochromocytoma)

Figure 14–1. The embryonic development of adrenergic cells and tumors that develop from them. Sympathogonia are primitive cells derived from the neural crest. Neuroblasts are also called sympathoblasts; ganglion cells are the same as sympathocytes; and pheochromocytes are mature chromaffin cells.

Microscopic Structure

The **chromaffin cells,** or **pheochromocytes,** of the adrenal medulla are large ovoid columnar cells arranged in clumps or cords around blood vessels. They derive their name from the observation that their granules turn brown (*pheo-*) when stained with chromic acid. The color is due to the oxidation of epinephrine and norepinephrine to melanin. These cells have large nuclei and a well-developed Golgi apparatus. They contain large numbers of vesicles or granules containing catecholamines. Vesicles containing norepinephrine are darker than those containing epinephrine.

The pheochromocytes may be arranged in nests, alveoli, or cords and are surrounded by a rich network of capillaries and sinusoids. The adrenal medulla also contains some sympathetic ganglion cells, singly or in groups. Ganglion cells are also found in association with the viscera, the carotid body, the glomus jugulare, and the cervical and thoracic ganglia.

Nerve Supply

The cells of the adrenal medulla are innervated by preganglionic fibers of the sympathetic nervous system, which release acetylcholine and enkephalins at the synapses. Most of these fibers arise from a plexus in the capsule of the posterior surface of the gland and enter the adrenal glands in bundles of 30–50 fibers without synapsing. They follow the course of the blood vessels into the medulla without branching into the adrenal cortex. Some reach the wall of the central vein, where they synapse with small autonomic ganglia. However, most fibers end in relationship to the pheochromocytes.

Blood Supply

The human adrenal gland derives blood from the superior, middle, and inferior adrenal branches of the inferior phrenic artery, directly from the aorta and from the renal arteries. Upon reaching the adrenal gland, these arteries branch to form a plexus under the capsule supplying the adrenal cortex. A few of these vessels, however, penetrate the cortex, passing directly to the medulla. The medulla is also nourished by branches of the arteries supplying the central vein and cuff of cortical tissue around the central vein. Capillary loops passing from the subcapsular plexus of the cortex also supply blood as they drain into the central vein. It would appear, then, that most of the blood supply to the medullary cells is via a portal vascular system arising from the capillaries in the cortex. There is also a capillary network of lymphatics that drain into a plexus around the central vein.

In mammals, the enzyme that catalyzes the conversion of norepinephrine to epinephrine (phenylethanolamine-N-methyltransferase, PNMT) is induced by cortisol. The chromaffin cells containing epinephrine therefore receive most of their blood supply from the capillaries draining the cortical cells, whereas cells containing predominantly norepinephrine are supplied by the arteries that directly supply the medulla. (See Biosynthesis, below.)

On the right side, the central vein is short and drains directly into the vena cava, although some branches go to the surface of the gland and reach the azygos system. On the left, the vein is somewhat longer and drains into the renal vein.

HORMONES OF THE ADRENAL MEDULLA

CATECHOLAMINES

Biosynthesis
(Fig 14–2)

Catecholamines are widely distributed in plants and animals. In mammals, **epinephrine** is synthesized mainly in the adrenal medulla, whereas **norepinephrine** is found not only in the adrenal medulla but also in the central nervous system and in the peripheral sympathetic nerves. **Dopamine,** the precursor of norepinephrine, is found in the adrenal medulla and in noradrenergic neurons. It is present in high concentrations in the brain, in specialized interneurons in the sympathetic ganglia, and in the carotid body, where it serves as a neurotransmitter. Dopamine is also found in specialized mast cells and in enterochromaffin cells.

The proportions of epinephrine and norepinephrine found in the adrenal medulla vary with the species (Table 14–1). In humans, the adrenal contains 15–20% norepinephrine.

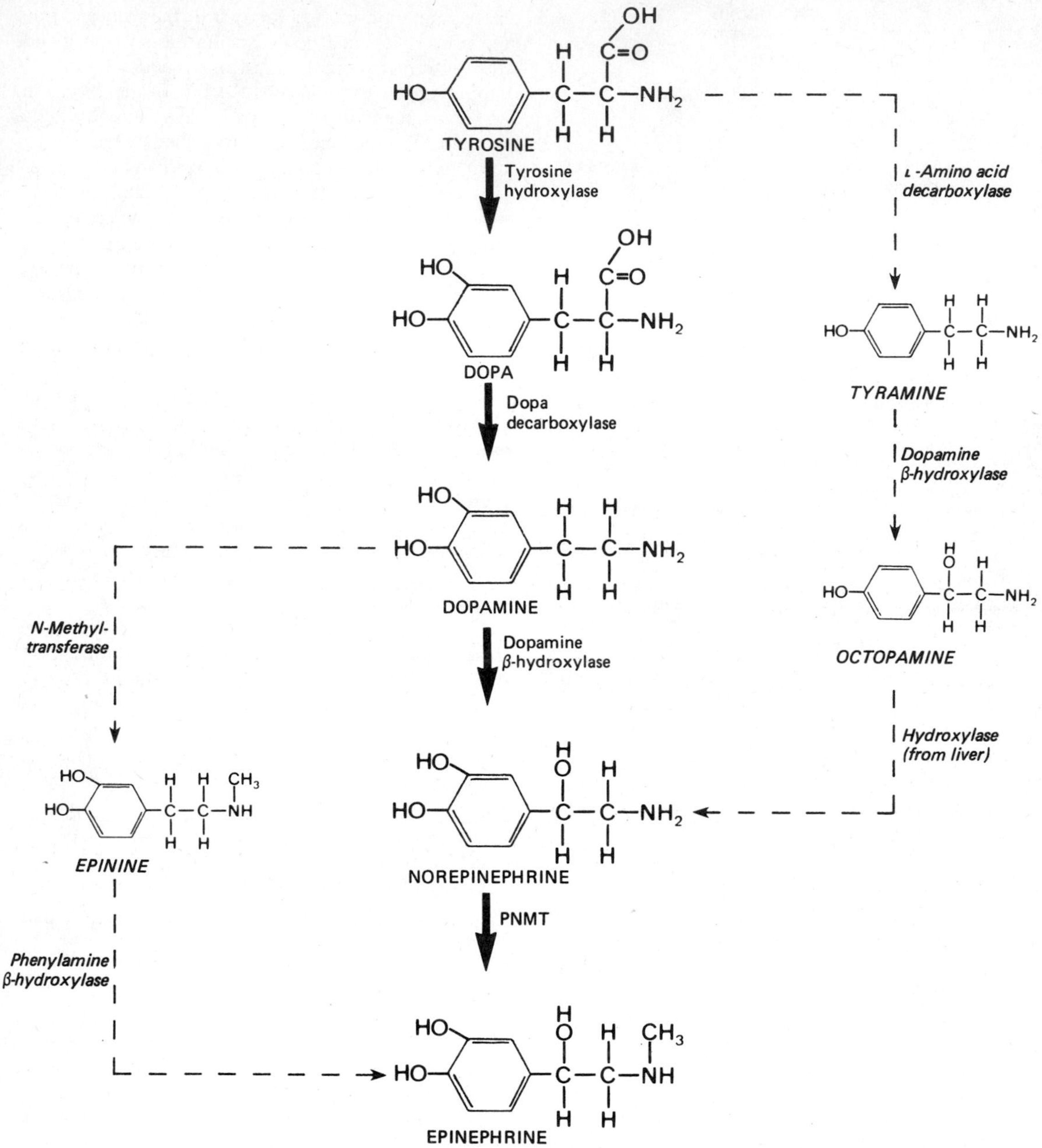

Figure 14–2. Biosynthesis of catecholamines. The alternative pathways shown by the dashed arrows have not been found to be of physiologic significance in humans. PNMT, phenylethanolamine-N-methyltransferase.

A. Conversion of Tyrosine to Dopa: The catecholamines are synthesized from **tyrosine,** which may be derived from ingested food or synthesized from phenylalanine in the liver. Tyrosine circulates at a concentration of 1–1.5 mg/dL of blood. It enters neurons and chromaffin cells by an active transport mechanism and is converted to **dihydroxyphenylalanine (dopa)**. The reaction is catalyzed by **tyrosine hydroxylase,** which is transported via axonal flow to the nerve termi-

nal. Tyrosine hydroxylase activity may be inhibited by a variety of compounds. Alpha-methylmetatyrosine is effective and is sometimes used in the therapy of malignant pheochromocytomas (see p. 383). Substances that chelate iron or compete for the pteridine cofactor also inhibit the enzyme but are not useful clinically. Activity of this enzyme is a reliable marker of intact sympathetic nerve tissue and neurotransmitter synthesis.

Table 14–1. Approximate percentages of total adrenal medullary catecholamines present as norepinephrine in various species.

Whale	70	Horse	25
Chicken	70	Squirrel	25
Lion	55	Cow	25
Frog	50	Human	20
Pig	45	Guinea pig	15
Cat	40	Rat	15
Gazelle	35	Zebra	13
Sheep	35	Rabbit	5
Goat	35	Baboon	0
Dog	30		

B. Conversion of Dopa to Dopamine: Dopa is converted to dopamine by the enzyme aromatic L-amino acid decarboxylase (dopa decarboxylase). This enzyme is found in all tissues, with the highest concentrations in liver, kidney, brain, and vas deferens. The various enzymes have different substrate specificities depending upon the tissue source. Competitive inhibitors of dopa decarboxylase such as methyldopa are converted to substances (an example is α-methylnorepinephrine) that are then stored in granules in the nerve cell and released in place of norepinephrine. These products (false transmitters) were thought to mediate the antihypertensive action of drugs at peripheral sympathetic synapses but are now believed to stimulate the alpha receptors of the inhibitory corticobulbar system, reducing sympathetic discharge peripherally.

C. Conversion of Dopamine to Norepinephrine: The conversion of dopamine to norepinephrine is catalyzed by dopamine β-hydroxylase, a mixed-function oxidase requiring oxygen and an external electron donor. The enzyme does not occur in tissues outside the neuron. Part of the biologic specificity of dopamine β-hydroxylase may result from its compartmentalization. Newly synthesized dopamine β-hydroxylase is incorporated directly into storage vesicles that take up, synthesize, and store the catecholamines. The membranes of these vesicles contain dopamine β-hydroxylase, ATPase, cytochrome P-561, and cytochrome P-561:NADH reductase. Dopamine β-hydroxylase is also found within the granule and is released with norepinephrine during secretion. Inhibitors of the enzyme, such as disulfuramic and picolinic acid, have no clinical importance.

D. Conversion of Norepinephrine to Epinephrine: PNMT catalyzes the N-methylation of norepinephrine to epinephrine, using S-adenosylmethionine as a methyl donor. It is found only in the adrenal medulla and in a few neurons in the central nervous system. The enzyme is found in the cytosol. Norepinephrine leaves the granule and after methylation reenters different granules. This enzyme is induced by the high levels of glucocorticoids (100 times the systemic concentration) found in the adrenal medulla.

The conversion of dopamine to **epinine** is catalyzed by a nonspecific N-methyltransferase.

Catecholamine biosynthesis is coupled to secretion, so that the stores of norepinephrine at the nerve endings remain relatively unchanged even in the presence of marked nerve activity. In the adrenal medulla, it is possible to deplete stores with prolonged hypoglycemia. Biosynthesis appears to be increased during nerve stimulation by activation of tyrosine hydroxylase. Prolonged stimulation leads to the induction of increased amounts of this enzyme.

Storage

The catecholamines are found in the adrenal medulla and various sympathetically innervated organs, and their concentration reflects the density of sympathetic neurons. The adrenal medulla contains about 0.5 mg/g; the spleen, vas deferens, brain, spinal cord, and heart contain 1–5 μg/g; liver, gut, and skeletal muscle contain 0.1–0.5 μg/g. The catecholamines are stored in electron-dense granules approximately 1 μm in diameter that contain catecholamines and ATP in a 4:1 molar ratio, several neuropeptides, calcium, magnesium, and water-soluble proteins called **chromogranins.** The ratio of catecholamines to ATP is much higher in granules isolated from pheochromocytomas. The interior surface of the membrane contains dopamine β-hydroxylase and ATPase. The Mg^{2+}-dependent ATPase facilitates the uptake and inhibits the release of catecholamines by the granules. This activity is inhibited by reserpine. Adrenal medullary granules appear to contain and release a number of active peptides including ACTH, vasoactive intestinal peptide (VIP), chromogranins, and enkephalins. The peptides derived from the chromogranins are physiologically active and may modulate catecholamine release.

Secretion

Adrenal medullary catecholamine secretion is increased by exercise, angina pectoris, myocardial infarction, hemorrhage, ether anesthesia, surgery, hypoglycemia, anoxia and asphyxia, and many other stressful stimuli. The rate of secretion of epinephrine increases more than that of norepinephrine in the presence of hypoglycemia and most other stimuli (Fig 14–3). However, anoxia and asphyxia produce a greater increase in adrenal medullary release of norepinephrine than is observed with other stimuli (Fig 14–4).

Secretion of the adrenal medullary hormones is mediated by the release of acetylcholine from the terminals of preganglionic fibers. The resulting depolarization of the axonal membrane triggers an influx of calcium ion. The contents of the storage vesicles, including the chromogranins and soluble dopamine β-hydroxylase, are released by exocytosis by the calcium ion increase. Membrane-bound dopamine β-hydroxylase is not released. **Tyramine,** however, releases norepinephrine primarily from the free store in the

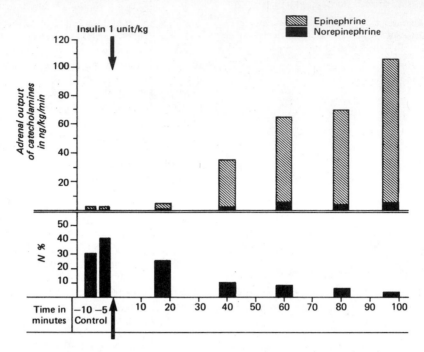

Figure 14–3. Rate of secretion of amines from one adrenal following injection of insulin. The percentage of the total released as norepinephrine is shown below.

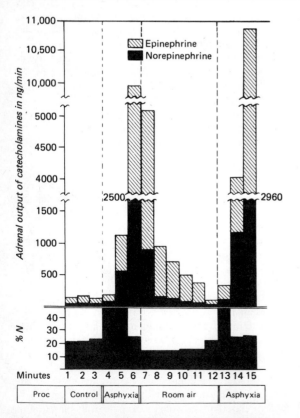

Figure 14–4. Rate of secretion of amines from one adrenal during asphyxia. The percentage of the total released as norepinephrine is shown below.

cytosol. Cocaine and monoamine oxidase inhibitors inhibit the effect of tyramine but do not affect the release of catecholamines by nervous stimulation. The rate of release in response to nerve stimulation is increased or decreased by a wide variety of neurotransmitters acting at specific receptors on the presynaptic neuron. Norepinephrine has an important role in modulating its own release by activating the alpha receptors on the presynaptic membrane. Alpha receptor antagonists inhibit this reaction. Conversely, presynaptic beta receptors enhance norepinephrine release, whereas beta receptor blockers increase it. The effect of such substances are shown in Table 14–2. The accumulation of excess catecholamines that are not in the storage granules is prevented by the presence of intraneuronal monoamine oxidase.

Transport

When released into the circulation, the amines are bound to albumin or a closely associated protein with low affinity and high capacity (K_d 10^{-7}).

Metabolism & Inactivation

The actions of catecholamines are terminated rapidly. Compared to hormones with a more prolonged action they have a relatively low affinity for their receptor and rapidly dissociate from it. The free hormone is removed by several mechanisms. These include reuptake by the sympathetic nerve ending, metabolism by the enzymes catechol-O-methyltransferase (COMT)

Table 14–2. Substances altering the release of norepinephrine at nerve endings by binding to specific presynaptic membrane receptors.

Increase	Decrease
Norepinephrine (beta receptor)	[1]Norepinephrine (alpha receptor)
Angiotensin	Serotonin
Epinephrine	Dopamine
	PGE$_2$
	Purines
	Metenkephalin
	Substance P
	Acetylcholine

[1]The alpha receptor–mediated inhibition of norepinephrine release is the dominant effect.

and monoamine oxidase (Fig 14–5), conjugation with sulfate ion, and direct excretion by the kidney. Estimates of the metabolic clearance rates for epinephrine and norepinephrine are 4000–5000 L/d.

Uptake

A. Neuronal (Uptake 1): A large proportion (85–90%) of the amines released at the synapse are taken up locally by the nerve endings from which they are released (uptake 1). Circulating amines can also be taken up by this mechanism. However, this mecha- nism plays a less important role in the inactivation of circulating catecholamines. The axonal membrane uptake process is energy-requiring, saturable, ster- eoselective, and sodium-dependent. It is blocked by cocaine, other sympathomimetic amines such as meta- raminol and amphetamine, and agents such as tricyclic antidepressants and phenothiazines. Neither calcium nor magnesium ion has any effect on uptake 1. There is also an uptake process for dopamine in neurons of the central nervous system, but this process is not inhibited by tricyclic antidepressants. After being taken up by the neuron, the amines are reutilized or deaminated by monoamine oxidase and the metabolites are released (Fig 14–6). The intraneuronal monoamine oxidase is a flavoprotein and is localized to the outer mitochondrial membrane. Its substrate specificity favors norepi- nephrine, which it oxidizes to dihydroxyphenylglycol (DOPEG) or dihydroxymandelic acid (DOMA). The major functions of monoamine oxidase are (1) to regu- late dopamine and norepinephrine content of the neu- rons; (2) to destroy ingested amines; and (3) to metabo- lize the circulating catecholamines and their O-methyl metabolites. Progesterone increases the level of mono- amine oxidase in women, whereas estrogens inhibit the enzyme.

B. Extraneuronal (Uptake 2): Extraneuronal tissues also take up catecholamines. This process, up-

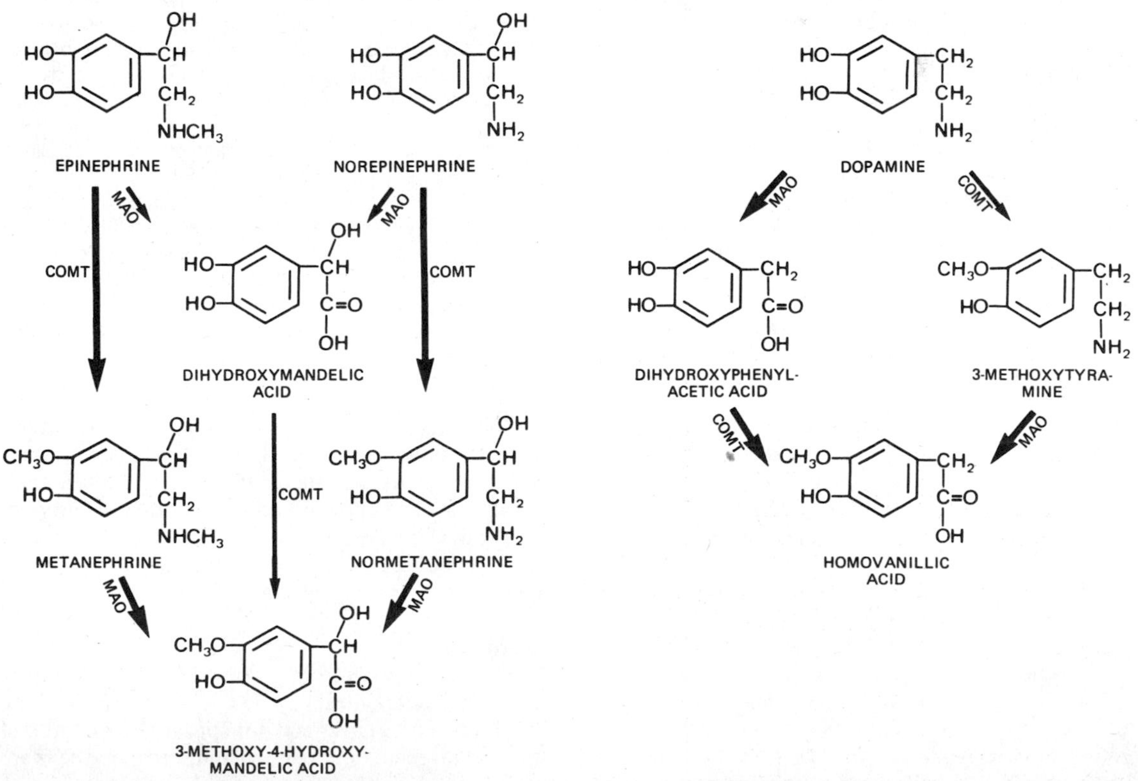

Figure 14–5. Metabolism of catecholamines by catechol-O-methyltransferase (COMT) and monoamine oxidase (MAO).

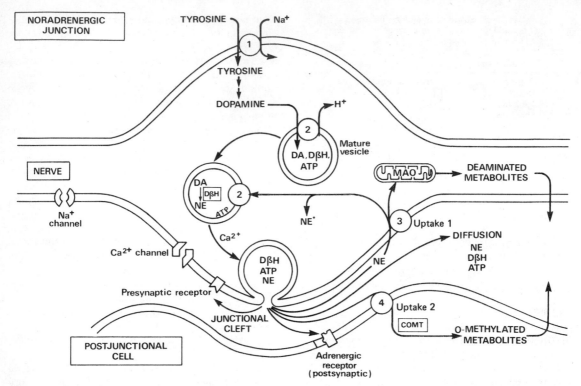

Figure 14–6. Schematic diagram of the neuroeffector junction of the peripheral sympathetic nervous system. The nerves terminate in complex networks with varicosities or enlargements that form synaptic junctions with effector cells. The neurotransmitter at these junctions is norepinephrine, which is synthesized from tyrosine. Tyrosine uptake (①) is linked to sodium uptake and transport into the varicosity where the secretory vesicles form. Tyrosine is hydroxylated by tyrosine hydroxylase to dopa, which is then decarboxylated by dopa decarboxylate to dopamine in the cytoplasm. Dopamine (DA) is transported into the vesicle by a carrier mechanism (②) that can be blocked by reserpine. The same carrier transports norepinephrine (NE) and several other amines into these granules. Dopamine is converted to norepinephrine through the catalytic action of dopamine β-hydroxylase (DβH). ATP is also present in high concentration in the vesicle. Release of transmitter occurs when an action potential is conducted to the varicosity by the action of voltage-sensitive sodium channels. Depolarization of the varicosity membrane opens voltage-sensitive calcium channels and results in an increase in intracellular calcium. The elevated calcium facilitates exocytotic fusion of vesicles with the surface membrane and expulsion of norepinephrine, ATP, and some of the dopamine β-hydroxylase. Release is blocked by drugs such as guanethidine and bretylium. Norepinephrine reaching either pre- or postsynaptic receptors modifies the function of the corresponding cells. Norepinephrine also diffuses out of the cleft, or it may be transported into the cytoplasm of the varicosity (uptake 1, blocked by cocaine, tricyclic antidepressants) (③) or into the postjunctional cell (uptake 2) (④). (Reproduced, with permission, from Katzung BG [editor]: *Basic & Clinical Pharmacology,* 4th ed. Appleton & Lange, 1989.)

take 2, is saturable, is not specific for catecholamines, and is inhibited by various steroids, phenoxybenzamine, and normetanephrine but not by cocaine and other drugs that inhibit neuronal uptake.

At uptake 2, the catecholamines are metabolized to their O-methyl derivatives by COMT (Fig 14–6). This enzyme is found mainly in the soluble fraction of tissue homogenates, with the highest levels in the liver and kidney. S-Adenosylmethionine is the methyl donor, and divalent ions are required for the reaction. It is predominantly an extraneuronal enzyme and acts on circulating catecholamines as well as on the locally released norepinephrine. It is the most important enzyme in the metabolism of circulating amines. Ap-

proximately 70% of circulating epinephrine in humans is methoxylated, and about 24% is also deaminated. These enzymes also metabolize dopamine to homovanillic acid. Although normetanephrine is fairly active at the alpha receptor of the nictitating membrane, the metabolites of the catecholamines are generally devoid of biologic or physiologic activity.

Conjugation

The phenolic hydroxyl group of the catecholamines and their metabolites may be conjugated with sulfate or glucuronide. Liver and gut appear to be important sites of this reaction, and circulating red blood cells are also a significant site of sulfation in humans.

Connective tissue binds catecholamines by a process that is inhibited by oxytetracycline. The significance of this binding is unknown.

Receptors

The catecholamines exert their physiologic effects by binding to receptor molecules on the surfaces of target cells. The mechanism whereby binding of the hormone to the receptor activates the physiologic response is discussed in Chapter 1. Early studies of sympathetic activation suggested that there were 2 classes of responses designated as inhibitory or excitatory. Cannon and his colleagues in the 1930s postulated that this difference was produced by the release of different neurotransmitters: sympathin I and sympathin E. The discovery by von Euler and others that norepinephrine was the neurotransmitter released by peripheral sympathetic nerve endings and was responsible for both types of responses led to the proposal by Ahlquist in 1948 that there were 2 types of receptors that he designated alpha and beta, based on the relative potencies of a series of adrenergic agonists. The subsequent development of relatively specific antagonists confirmed this hypothesis and allowed the development of binding assays for the alpha, beta, and dopaminergic receptors. Subsequent pharmacologic and biochemical studies indicate that alpha, beta, and dopaminergic receptors can be further divided into subtypes. The characteristic interactions of these receptors with various agonists and antagonists are shown in Table 14–3.

A. Types of Receptors: The physiologic effects mediated by the alpha-adrenergic receptor are summarized in Table 14–4. Two subtypes of this receptor have been identified and designated α_1 and α_2. It was initially thought that the α_2 receptor was limited to the

Table 14–3. Characteristic interactions of agonists and antagonists at the adrenergic receptors.

Receptor	Agonist Potency[1]	Antagonist Potency	Agonist Effect on Adenylate Cyclase Activity
Alpha$_1$	Same for α_1 and α_2.	Prazosin > phentolamine > yohimbine.	None
Alpha$_2$	Epinephrine slightly > norepinephrine >> isoproterenol.	Phentolamine slightly > yohimbine >> prazosin.	Decrease
Beta$_1$	Isoproterenol > epinephrine ≅ norepinephrine.	Metoprolol > butoxamine.	Increase
Beta$_2$	Isoproterenol > epinephrine >> norepinephrine.	Butoxamine > metoprolol.	Increase

[1] These potencies are defined by studies of binding competition and pharmacologic response.

Table 14–4. Adrenergic responses of selected tissues.

Organ or Tissue	Receptor	Effect
Heart (myocardium)	β_1	Increased force of contraction Increased rate of contraction
Blood vessels	α	Vasoconstriction
	β_2	Vasodilatation
Kidney	β	Increased renin release
Gut	α, β	Decreased motility and increased sphincter tone
Pancreas	α	Decreased insulin release Decreased glucagon release
	β	Increased insulin release Increased glucagon release
Liver	α, β	Increased glycogenolysis
Adipose tissue	β	Increased lipolysis
Most tissues	β	Increased calorigenesis
Skin (apocrine glands on hands, axillae, etc)	α	Increased sweating
Bronchioles	β_2	Dilatation
Uterus	α	Contraction
	β_2	Relaxation

presynaptic nerve ending and, when activated, served to inhibit the release of norepinephrine. However, these receptors have been found in platelets and postsynaptically in the nervous system, adipose tissue, and smooth muscle.

The adrenergic receptors are transmembrane proteins with an extracellular amino terminus and an intracellular carboxy terminus. Each of their 7 hydrophobic regions spans the cell membrane. Although these regions of the adrenergic receptor subtypes exhibit significant amino acid homology, differences in the fifth and sixth segments determine the specificity of agonist binding. Differences in the fifth and seventh segments determine whether the receptor is coupled to the stimulatory (G_s) or inhibitory (G_i) guanyl nucleotide binding proteins.

The effects of agonist binding to the α_1 receptor are mediated by the activation of phospholipase C, which catalyzes the breakdown of phosphorylated phosphatidylinositol, forming inositol trisphosphate (IP_3). IP_3 releases calcium ion from intracellular stores to initiate a physiologic response. Diacylglycerol remains after the removal of inositol trisphosphate: it activates kinase C, which sustains the physiologic effect. The details of these interactions are discussed in Chapter 1. Agonists binding to the α_2 receptor inhibit the activity of adenylate cyclase, reducing the amount of cyclic AMP formed. Selective α_1 and α_2 antagonists are shown in Table 14–3.

Two subtypes of the beta receptor, β_1 and β_2, have been identified. Beta$_1$ receptors appear to mediate the inotropic and chronotropic effects on cardiac muscle, whereas β_2 receptors mediate smooth muscle relaxation in the bronchi and vascular smooth muscle as well as the uterus and adipose tissue. Norepinephrine is a powerful agonist at the β_1 receptor but weak at the β_2 receptor, compared to epinephrine or isoproterenol. Relatively selective beta agonists have also been developed, as shown in Table 14–3. The role of cAMP as a second messenger of the beta-adrenergic response is discussed in Chapter 1.

Dopaminergic receptors are found in the central nervous system, presynaptic adrenergic nerve terminals, pituitary, heart, renal and mesenteric vascular beds, and other sites. Two subtypes of the dopaminergic receptor, D_1 and D_2, have been identified. The binding affinity of the D_1 receptor is greater for dopamine than for haloperidol; the reverse is true for the D_2 receptor. The effects of the D_1 receptor are mediated by stimulation of the adenylate cyclase system and are found postsynaptically in the brain. Those in the pituitary are D_2 receptors that inhibit the formation of cAMP.

B. Receptors as Regulatory Sites: The receptor also serves as a site of regulation of adrenergic activity. As noted above, presynaptically, norepinephrine released during nerve stimulation binds to alpha receptors and reduces the amount of norepinephrine released. Nerve endings have also been found to have receptors for many other agents presynaptically (Table 14–2).

The number of receptors on the effector cell surface can be reduced by binding of agonist to receptor (antagonists do not have the same effect). This reduction is called "down-regulation." Thyroid hormone, however, has been shown to increase the number of beta receptors in the myocardium. Estrogen, which increases the number of alpha receptors in the myometrium, increases the affinity of some vascular alpha receptors for norepinephrine.

Although the receptors and areas of postreceptor events serve as sites of fine regulation, the major physiologic control is exerted by alterations in activity of the nervous system. The discovery of cAMP and elucidation of its role in controlling physiologic processes—and the finding that most cells in the body have adrenergic receptors—have led to an appreciation of the important regulatory role of the peripheral sympathetic nervous system. In contrast, the effects of the adrenal medulla are mediated via the circulating amines and, therefore, are much more generalized in nature. Furthermore, adrenal medullary secretion increases significantly only in the presence of stress or marked deviation from homeostatic or resting conditions. For example, a minor reduction in the available glucose leads to sympathetic activation of fat mobilization from adipose tissue, whereas the adrenal medulla may not release large amounts of epinephrine until the blood sugar falls to 40–50 mg/dL (3 mmol/L) in normal individuals. A summary of physiologic effects of the catecholamines in various tissues is presented in Table 14–4.

Physiologic Effects

A. Cardiovascular Effects: Catecholamines increase the rate and frequency of contraction and increase the irritability of the myocardium by activating myocardial β_1 receptors. The contractile effects of the catecholamines on vascular smooth muscle are mediated via alpha receptors. Although beta receptors are present and cause dilatation, other mechanisms of vascular dilatation are probably more important. The release or injection of catecholamines can therefore be expected to increase heart rate and cardiac output and cause peripheral vasoconstriction—all leading to an increase in blood pressure. These events are modulated by reflex mechanisms, so that, as the blood pressure increases, reflex stimulation may slow the heart rate and tend to reduce cardiac output. Although norepinephrine in the usual doses will have these effects, the effect of epinephrine may vary depending on the smooth muscle tone of the vascular system at the time. For example, in an individual with increased vascular tone, the net effect of small amounts of epinephrine may be to reduce the mean blood pressure while increasing the heart rate and cardiac output. In an individual with a reduction in vascular tone, the mean blood pressure would be expected to increase. In addition to the reflex mechanisms, vascular output is integrated by the central nervous system, so that, under appropriate circumstances, one vascular bed may be dilated while others remain unchanged. The central organization of the sympathetic nervous system is such that its ordinary regulatory effects are quite discrete—in contrast to periods of stress, when stimulation may be rather generalized and accompanied by release of catecholamines into the circulation. The infusion of catecholamines leads to a rapid reduction in plasma volume, presumably to accommodate to the reduced volume of the arterial and venous beds (Fig 14–7).

B. Effects on Extravascular Smooth Muscle: The catecholamines also regulate the activity of smooth muscle in tissues other than blood vessels. These effects include relaxation and contraction of uterine myometrium, relaxation of intestinal and bladder smooth muscle, contraction of the smooth muscle in the bladder and intestinal sphincters, and relaxation of tracheal smooth muscle and pupillary dilatation.

C. Metabolic Effects: The catecholamines increase oxygen consumption and heat production. Although the effects appear to be mediated by the beta receptor, the mechanism is unknown. The catecholamines also regulate glucose and fat mobilization from storage depots. Glycogenolysis in heart muscle

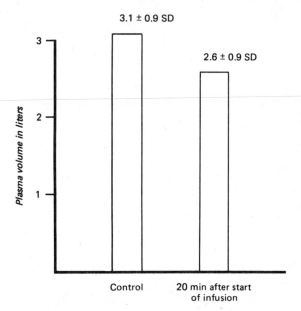

Figure 14–7. Changes in plasma volume produced by infusion of norepinephrine for 20 minutes in a dose sufficient to increase mean arterial pressure from 96 ± 10 mm Hg to 150 ± 16 mm Hg. (Data from Finnerty FA Jr, Buchholz JH, Guillaudeu RL: *J Clin Invest* 1958;**37**:425.)

and in liver leads to an increase in available carbohydrate for utilization. Stimulation of adipose tissue leads to lipolysis and the release of free fatty acids and glycerol into the circulation for utilization at other sites. In humans, these effects are mediated by the beta receptor.

The plasma levels of catecholamines required to produce some cardiovascular and metabolic effects in humans are shown in Table 14–5.

The catecholamines have effects on water, sodium, potassium, calcium, and phosphate excretion in the kidney. However, the mechanisms and the significance of these changes are not clear.

Table 14–5. Approximate circulating plasma levels of epinephrine and norepinephrine required to produce hemodynamic and metabolic changes during infusions of epinephrine and norepinephrine[1]. Values are pg/mL and (nmol/L).

	Norepinephrine	Epinephrine
Systolic blood pressure	Increased at 2500 (15)	Increased at 500 (3)
Diastolic blood pressure	Increased at 2500 (15)	Decreased at 500 (3)
Pulse	Decreased at 2500 (15)	Increased at 250 (1.5)
Plasma glucose	Increased at 2500 (15)	Increased at 250–500 (1.5–3)

[1]Data from Silverberg AB et al: *Am J Physiol* 1978;**234**:E252; and from Clutter WE et al: *J Clin Invest* 1980;**66**:94.

The Regulatory Role of Catecholamines in Hormone Secretion

The sympathetic nervous system plays an important role in the regulation and integration of hormone secretion at 2 levels. Centrally, norepinephrine and dopamine play important roles in the regulation of secretion of the anterior pituitary hormones. Dopamine, for example, has been identified as the prolactin-inhibiting hormone, and the hypothalamic releasing hormones appear to be under sympathetic nervous system control. Peripherally, the secretion of renin by the juxtaglomerular cells of the kidney is regulated by the sympathetic nervous system via the renal nerves and circulating catecholamines. The catecholamines release renin via a beta receptor mechanism. The B cell of the pancreatic islets is stimulated by activation of the beta receptors in the presence of alpha-adrenergic blockade. However, the dominant effect of norepinephrine or epinephrine is inhibition of insulin secretion, which is mediated by the alpha receptor. Similar effects have been observed in the secretion of glucagon by pancreatic A cells. The catecholamines have also been found to increase the release of thyroxine, calcitonin, parathyroid hormone, and gastrin by a beta receptor–mediated mechanism.

OTHER HORMONES

In addition to the catecholamines, the chromaffin cells of the adrenal medulla and peripheral sympathetic neurons synthesize and secrete opiatelike peptides, including met- and leu-enkephalin (see Chapter 6). They are stored in the large, dense-cored vesicles with the catecholamines in the adrenal medulla and at sympathetic nerve endings. These peptides are also found in the terminals of the splanchnic fibers that innervate the adrenal medulla. The observation that naloxone increases plasma catecholamine levels suggests that these peptides may inhibit sympathetic activity.

DISORDERS OF ADRENAL MEDULLARY FUNCTION

HYPOFUNCTION

Hypofunction of the adrenal medulla alone probably occurs only in individuals receiving adrenocortical steroid replacement therapy following adrenalectomy. Such individuals with otherwise intact sympathetic nervous systems suffer no clinically significant disability. Patients with autonomic insufficiency, which

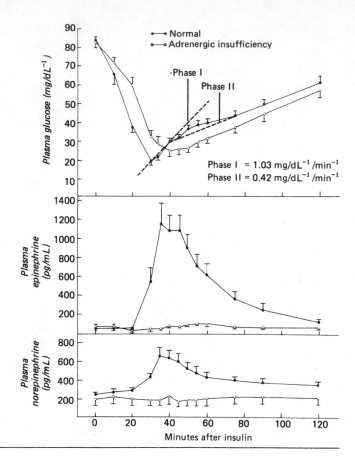

Figure 14–8. Plasma glucose, epinephrine, and norepinephrine levels after insulin administration in 14 normal subjects (●–●) and 7 patients with idiopathic orthostatic hypotension (○–○) with low or absent epinephrine responses. Results are expressed as mean ± SEM. (Reproduced, with permission, from Polonsky RJ et al: *J Clin Endocrinol Metab* 1980;51:1404.)

includes deficiency of adrenal medullary epinephrine secretion, can be demonstrated to have minor defects in recovery from insulin-induced hypoglycemia (Fig 14–8). Patients with generalized autonomic insufficiency usually have orthostatic hypotension. The causes of disorders associated with autonomic insufficiency are listed in Table 14–6.

When a normal individual stands, a series of physiologic adjustments occur that maintain blood pressure and ensure adequate circulation to the brain. The initial lowering of the blood pressure stimulates the baroreceptors, which then activate central reflex mechanisms that cause arterial and venous constriction, increase cardiac output, and activate the release of renin and vasopressin. Interruption of afferent, central, or efferent components of this autonomic reflex results in autonomic insufficiency.

The treatment of symptomatic orthostatic hypotension is dependent upon maintenance of an adequate blood volume. If physical measures such as raising the head of the bed at night and using support garments do not alleviate the condition, pharmacologic measures may be used. Although agents producing constriction of the vascular bed, including ephedrine, phenylephrine, metaraminol, monoamine oxidase inhibitors, levodopa, propranolol, and indomethacin, have been used, volume expansion with fludrocortisone is the most effective treatment.

HYPERFUNCTION

The adrenal medulla is not known to play a significant role in essential hypertension. However, the role of the sympathetic nervous system in the regulation of blood flow and blood pressure has led to extensive investigations of its role in various types of hypertension. Some of the abnormalities observed, such as a resetting of baroreceptor activity, are thought to be

Table 14–6. Disorders associated with autonomic insufficiency.

Familial dysautonomia
Shy-Drager syndrome
Parkinson's disease
Tabes dorsalis
Syringomyelia
Cerebrovascular disease
Peripheral neuropathy due to diabetes
Idiopathic orthostatic hypotension
Sympathectomy
Drugs: antihypertensives, antidepressants

secondary to the change in blood pressure. Others, such as the increased cardiac output found in early essential hypertension, have been thought by some investigators to play a primary role.

Catecholamines can increase blood pressure by increasing cardiac output, by increasing peripheral resistance through their vasoconstrictive action on the arteriole, and by increasing renin release from the kidney, leading to increased circulating levels of angiotensin II. Although many studies show an increase in circulating free catecholamine levels, evidence of increased sympathetic activity has not been a uniform finding in patients with essential hypertension.

PHEOCHROMOCYTOMA

Pheochromocytomas are tumors arising from chromaffin cells in the sympathetic nervous system. They release epinephrine or norepinephrine (or both)—and in some cases dopamine—into the circulation, causing hypertension and other signs and symptoms.

It is estimated that 0.1% of patients with diastolic hypertension have pheochromocytomas. These tumors are found at all ages and in both sexes and are most commonly diagnosed in the fourth or fifth decades. An analysis of data from the National Cancer Registry in Sweden indicates an incidence of about 2 per million in that population.

Although uncommon, this disorder is important to diagnose, because undiagnosed it may be fatal in pregnant women during delivery or in patients undergoing surgery for other disorders. However, with early diagnosis and proper management, almost all patients with benign tumors recover completely.

Clinical Manifestations

A. Symptoms and Signs: Although most patients with functioning tumors have symptoms most of the time, these vary in intensity and are perceived to be mainly episodic or paroxysmal by about half of the patients. Most patients with persistent hypertension also have superimposed paroxysms. A few patients are entirely free of symptoms and hypertension between attacks and give no evidence of excessive catecholamine release during these intervals. In some instances, these tumors occur with minimal clinical manifestations and are only found incidentally on CT or MRI scan. Commonly reported symptoms and signs are listed in Table 14–7.

B. Description of an Attack: In patients with paroxysmal release of catecholamines, the symptoms resemble those produced by injections of epinephrine or norepinephrine, and the symptom complex is far more consistent than is suggested by the variability of pa-

Table 14–7. Common symptoms in patients with hypertension due to pheochromocytoma.

Symptoms during or following paroxysms
Headache
Sweating
Forceful heartbeat with or without tachycardia
Anxiety or fear of impending death
Tremor
Fatigue or exhaustion
Nausea and vomiting
Abdominal or chest pain
Visual disturbances
Symptoms between paroxysms
Increased sweating
Cold hands and feet
Weight loss
Constipation

tients' complaints. An episode usually begins with a sensation of something happening deep inside the chest, and a stimulus to deeper breathing is noted. The patient then becomes aware of a pounding or forceful heartbeat, caused by the β_1 receptor-mediated increase in cardiac output. This throbbing spreads to the rest of the trunk and head, causing headache or a pounding sensation in the head. The intense alpha receptor–mediated peripheral vasoconstriction causes cool, moist hands and feet and facial pallor. The combination of increased cardiac output and vasoconstriction causes marked elevation of the blood pressure when large amounts of catecholamines are released. The decreased heat loss and increased metabolism may cause a rise in temperature or flushing and lead to reflex sweating, which may be profuse and usually follows the cardiovascular effects that begin in the first few seconds after onset of an attack. The increased glycolysis and alpha receptor–mediated inhibition of insulin release cause an increase in blood sugar levels. Patients experience marked anxiety during all but the mildest attacks, and when episodes are prolonged or severe, there may be nausea, vomiting, visual disturbances, chest or abdominal pain, paresthesias, or seizures. A feeling of fatigue or exhaustion usually follows these episodes unless they are very mild or of short duration.

C. Frequency of Attacks: In patients with paroxysmal symptoms, attacks usually occur several times a week or oftener and last for 15 minutes or less though they may occur at intervals of months or as often as 25 times daily and may last from minutes to days. As time passes, the attacks usually increase in frequency but do not change much in character. They are frequently precipitated by activities that compress the tumor (eg, changes in position, exercise, lifting, defecation, or eating) and by emotional distress or anxiety.

D. Variability of Manifestations: Although the pattern of the manifestations described above can be elicited in almost all patients capable of clear communication, the variability of presenting complaints may be confusing and is sometimes misleading. Women whose episodes are first noted around the time of menopause may be thought to be experiencing "hot flushes." The diagnosis may only be made when hormonal therapy has failed to alleviate the "hot flush" or the episode is observed and the blood pressure taken during an attack. When a pheochromocytoma causes hypertension late in pregnancy, it may be confused with preeclampsia. Other causes of increased sympathetic activity must be distinguished from pheochromocytomas (see below) (Table 14–9).

E. Chronic Symptoms: Patients with persistently secreting tumors and chronic symptoms usually experience the symptom complex described above in response to transient increases in the release of catecholamines. In addition, in these patients the increased metabolic rate usually causes heat intolerance, increased sweating, and weight loss or (in children) lack of weight gain. The effects on glycogenolysis and insulin release can produce hyperglycemia and glucose intolerance, and patients may present with diabetes mellitus. Hypertension is usually present. Wide fluctuations of blood pressure are characteristic, and marked increases may be followed by hypotension and syncope. When pressure is elevated, postural hypotension is present. Typically, the hypertension does not respond to commonly used antihypertensive regimens, and such drugs as guanethidine and ganglionic blockers can induce paradoxic pressor responses. On examination, these patients, usually thin, have a forceful heartbeat that is often visible and easily palpable. They feel warm, may have pallor of the face and chest, perspire, have cool and moist hands and feet, and prefer a cool room. A mass may be palpable in the abdomen or neck, and deep palpation of the abdomen may produce a typical paroxysm. Chronic constriction of the arterial and venous beds leads to a reduction in plasma volume in most of these patients. The inability to further constrict these vessels upon arising causes the postural hypotension that is characteristically observed.

Familial Syndromes & Other Tumors

Pheochromocytoma may also occur as a heritable disorder, either alone or more commonly in association with other endocrine tumors. In one syndrome, multiple endocrine neoplasia (MEN) type IIa (Sipple's syndrome), the patient may also have a calcitonin-producing adenoma of the thyroid, a parathyroid hormone-producing adenoma of the parathyroid, or a pituitary adenoma. In the other group (MEN type IIb), pheochromocytomas occur in association with mucosal neuromas, which are numerous and small and are found around the mouth. Transmission of these disorders follows the pattern of an autosomal dominant gene with incomplete penetrance. (See Chapter 28.)

Pheochromocytomas occurring as part of the familial syndromes appear to be the expression of an as yet unidentified stimulus to tumor formation in patients with genetic abnormalities that predispose them to re-

spond with tumor formation. An abnormal gene on chromosome 10 has been reported in some families. In MEN type IIa, bilateral adrenal tumors, frequently producing epinephrine, are common and may develop from hyperplasia of the adrenal medulla. Medullary carcinoma of the thyroid in these patients is commonly bilateral and associated with parafollicular or "C" cell hyperplasia. Multicentric tumors of the parathyroid gland are also quite typical and are found predominantly in patients with MEN type IIa and rarely in those with MEN type IIb. The thyroid tumors have been reported to secrete ACTH, serotonin, prostaglandins, and kallikreins, which may contribute to the clinical manifestations in these patients. Usually, the thyroid tumor (medullary carcinoma) is diagnosed by finding an elevated serum calcitonin level under basal conditions or after provocative testing with stimuli such as calcium or pentagastrin (see Chapters 10 and 11).

Pathology

A. Location of Tumor: Pheochromocytomas occur wherever chromaffin tissue is found (Fig 14–9). The adrenal medulla contains the largest collection of chromaffin cells. They are found in the organ of Zuckerkandl, which is very large in the fetus but is gradually replaced by fibrous tissue after delivery and is small in the adult. Chromaffin cells are also found in

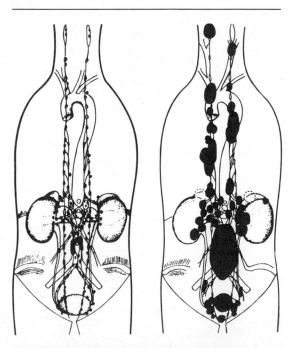

Figure 14–9. *Left:* Anatomic distribution of extra-adrenal chromaffin tissue in the newborn. *Right:* Locations of extra-adrenal pheochromocytomas reported before 1965. (Reproduced, with permission, from Coupland R: *The Natural History of the Chromaffin Cell.* Longmans, Green, 1965.)

association with sympathetic ganglia, nerve plexuses, and nerves.

Over 95% of pheochromocytomas are found in the abdomen, and 85% of these are in the adrenal. Common extra-adrenal sites are near the kidney and in the organ of Zuckerkandl. Those found in the chest are in the heart or the posterior mediastinal area. The intracranial lesions reported are thought to be metastatic in origin. The tumors may be multicentric in origin, particularly when they are familial or part of the syndromes of multiple endocrine neoplasia and when they are seen in children. Although fewer than 10% of adults have multiple tumors, they are found in about one-third of affected children.

B. Size of Tumor: Pheochromocytomas vary in size from less than 1 g to several kilograms. However, they are usually small, most weighing under 100 g. They are vascular tumors and commonly contain cystic or hemorrhagic areas. The cells tend to be large and contain typical catecholamine storage granules similar to those in the adrenal medulla. Multinucleated cells, pleomorphic nuclei, mitoses, and extension into the capsule and vessels are sometimes seen but do not indicate that the tumor is malignant. Fewer than 10% of pheochromocytomas are malignant, and these can be recognized either during surgery, by the finding of extensive local infiltration or metastases, or later, because of postsurgical local recurrence or metastases.

C. Adrenal Medullary Hyperplasia: This has also been described as the cause of an indistinguishable clinical picture and is found in the syndrome of multiple endocrine neoplasia (see Chapter 28).

Complications

Patients with persistent symptoms and hypertension may develop hypertensive retinopathy or nephropathy. Postmortem studies indicate that there are a significant number of patients with pheochromocytomas who have myocarditis characterized by focal degeneration and necrosis of myocardial fibers with infiltration of histiocytes, plasma cells, and other signs of inflammation. Platelet aggregates and fibrin deposition are found in pulmonary arterioles. These changes may be associated with abnormal findings on the ECG but may not become apparent until the patient is exposed to marked cardiovascular stress and heart failure results. In patients harboring pheochromocytomas for long periods, the serious sequelae of hypertension are observed. Cerebrovascular accidents, congestive heart failure, and myocardial infarction have been observed. Some of the causes of death in unoperated patients are shown in Table 14–8.

Differential Diagnosis

The diagnosis of pheochromocytoma should be considered in all patients with paroxysmal symptoms; in children with hypertension; in adults with severe hypertension not responding to therapy; in hypertensive patients with diabetes or hypermetabolism; in patients

Table 14–8. Causes of death in patients with unsuspected pheochromocytomas.

Myocardial infarction
Cerebrovascular accident
Arrhythmias
Irreversible shock
Renal failure
Dissecting aortic aneurysm

with hypertension in whom symptoms resemble those described above or can be evoked by exercise, position change, emotional distress, or antihypertensive drugs such as guanethidine and ganglionic blockers; and in patients who become severely hypertensive or go into shock during anesthesia, surgery, or obstetric delivery. Patients who have disorders sometimes associated with pheochromocytomas (neurofibromatosis, mucosal adenomas, von Hippel's disease, medullary carcinoma of the thyroid) and those with first-degree relatives who have pheochromocytoma or other manifestations of MEN should be investigated. Other disorders associated with marked sympathetic stimulation are listed in Table 14–9. Plasma catecholamine levels at rest and with exercise and various disorders are shown in Table 14–10.

In these and other disorders in which elevated plasma catecholamine levels are under sympathetic nervous system control, it may be possible to reduce catecholamine release by autonomic blockade or sympathetic suppression. Pentolinium and clonidine have been used for this purpose. The reliability and safety of such procedures have not been established.

Ganglioneuromas (which are usually small, well-differentiated tumors arising from ganglion cells) and neuroblastomas (which are highly malignant tumors arising from more primitive sympathoblastic cells) can produce catecholamines and present a similar clinical picture. Dopamine is usually the major active catecholamine produced, and its production leads to elevated concentrations of homovanillic acid in urine.

Diagnostic Tests & Procedures

Assay of catecholamines and their metabolites has markedly simplified the diagnosis of this disorder. Op-

Table 14–9. Disorders presenting with features of sympathetic discharge or hypermetabolism.

Angina due to coronary vasospasm
Severe anxiety states
Hypertension
Hypertensive crises associated with—
  Paraplegia
  Tabes dorsalis
  Lead poisoning
  Acute porphyria
Menopausal hot flushes
Autonomic epilepsy
Thyrotoxicosis
Hyperdynamic beta-adrenergic states

Table 14–10. Range of plasma catecholamine levels observed in healthy subjects and patients.

	Norepinephrine pg/mL (nmol/L)	Epinephrine pg/mL (nmol/L)
Healthy subjects		
Basal	150–400 (0.9–2.4)	25–100 (0.1–0.6)
Ambulatory	200–800 (1.2–4.8)	30–100 (0.1–1)
Exercise	800–4000 (4.8–24)	100–1000 (0.5–5)
Symptomatic hypoglycemia	200–1000 (1.2–6)	1000–5000 (5–25)
Patients		
Hypertension	200–500 (1.2–3)	20–100 (0.1–0.6)
Surgery	500–2000 (3–12)	100–500 (0.5–3)
Myocardial infarction	1000–2000 (6–12)	800–5000 (4–25)

erative exploration for pheochromocytoma should not be done in the absence of chemical confirmation of the diagnosis. With currently available methods, it is possible to avoid unnecessary surgery and to successfully locate a tumor in almost all patients.

A. Hormone Assay: In patients with continuous hypertension or symptoms, levels of plasma or urine catecholamines and their metabolites are usually clearly increased. Therefore, in the selection of a particular assay, it is more important that the test be performed well by the laboratory than that a particular substance be measured. A reliable assay of the catecholamines, metanephrines, or vanillylmandelic acid (VMA) is usually sufficient to confirm the diagnosis. Patients with large tumors may excrete disproportionately greater amounts of catecholamine metabolites, because the amines can be metabolized by enzymes in the tumor cells prior to their release. Malignant tumors may release large amounts of dopamine, leading to the excretion of large amounts of homovanillic acid in the urine. It is important that the appropriate assay procedure be chosen to avoid misleading results and that drugs and foods that interfere with these assays be eliminated (Table 14–11).

In patients having brief and infrequent paroxysms with symptom-free intervals, confirmation of the diagnosis may be more difficult. Although large amounts of catecholamines are produced during the brief episode, the total amount excreted during the 24-hour urine collection period may not be clearly abnormal—in contrast to patients whose tumors secrete continuously. The latter group will accumulate larger amounts of catecholamines and metabolites in the urine even though secretion rates are lower and symptoms are less severe. Therefore, sampling of blood or timed urine collections during a carefully observed episode may be necessary to confirm the diagnosis.

B. Glucagon Test: In patients with infrequent episodes, glucagon can be used to induce a paroxysm. This is rarely necessary and should not be done in patients who have angina, visual changes, or other severe symptoms during spontaneous attacks. Phentolamine should be available to terminate the induced episode. Injection of 1 mg of glucagon intravenously

will induce an attack in more than 90% of patients with pheochromocytoma. A typical response in such a patient is shown in Figure 14–10. In those instances in which glucagon has failed to evoke a paroxysm and the clinical suspicion is very strong, histamine given intravenously in doses of 25–50 μg may also be tried. However, histamine injection is associated with flushing and a brief but severe episode of headache. In general, the provoked episodes are no more severe than those occurring spontaneously. Provocative tests should be reserved for patients in whom it is necessary to rule out the presence of pheochromocytoma when they are seen (eg, prior to surgery or obstetric delivery). At all other times, a timed urine collection during an episode can provide the same information.

C. Clonidine Suppression Test: In patients whose catecholamine levels are elevated because of neurogenic stimulation rather than release of cate-

Table 14–11. Maximal normal concentrations of the catecholamines and their metabolites in urine.[1] Substances interfering with their measurement are listed.

Compound	Excreted mg/24 h (nmol/24 h)	Interfering Substances
Epinephrine Norepinephrine Dopamine	0.02 (0.1) 0.08 (0.5) 0.4 (2.5)	May be increased by highly fluorescent compounds such as tetracyclines and quinidine; by foods[2] and drugs containing catecholamines; and by levodopa, methyldopa, and ethanol.
Metanephrine Normetanephrine	0.4 (2.5) 0.9 (5)	Increased by catecholamines, monoamine oxidase inhibitors, and others, depending on the method.
Vanillylmandelic acid (VMA) Homovanillic acid	8 (47) 7 (45)	Increased by catecholamines, by foods containing vanillin, or by levodopa. Decreased by clofibrate, disulfiram, and monoamine oxidase inhibitors.

[1]Values may be higher under unusual stress, illness, or strenuous activity.
[2]For example, bananas contain significant amounts of norepinephrine.

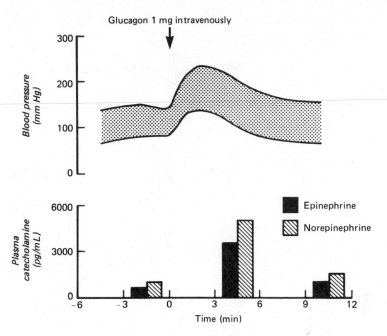

Figure 14–10. Blood pressure and plasma catecholamine levels following glucagon injection in a patient with a paroxysmally secreting pheochromocytoma. The blood sugar at 12 minutes was 180 mg/dL.

cholamine from a tumor, the administration of 0.3 mg of clonidine 2–3 hours before sampling of blood may be useful in reducing plasma norepinephrine levels. This procedure can be used during an office visit or whenever it is not possible to obtain blood under resting conditions.

D. Trial of Phenoxybenzamine: In the occasional patient in whom the chemical tests are inconclusive, it may be useful or convenient to institute therapy with phenoxybenzamine over a period of 1–2 months to observe effects both on the nature and frequency of attacks and on the blood pressure. A salutary effect will sometimes be observed for a few weeks but seldom longer than that in the absence of pheochromocytoma. A good response indicates the need for reappraisal of the patient.

Screening for Pheochromocytoma

In addition to screening patients with typical clinical manifestations, assays for catecholamines and their metabolites can be used to screen other patients at high risk. The indications for screening are listed in Table 14–12. When the presence of an undetected pheochromocytoma is particularly dangerous, as in pregnancy or prior to surgery, screening should be considered even when clinical manifestations are less typical.

Localization of Tumors

When the diagnosis has been established, the tumor must be located in order to facilitate its surgical removal. CT and MR scanning have given excellent results (Fig 14–11). Only the smallest tumors or those

shielded by clips and other metal objects from previous surgery have been elusive.

Analysis of blood samples obtained via percutaneous venous catheterization can be of great value in locating small tumors in unusual locations. An example of the use of this technique is shown in Figure 14–12. Because of a small risk of complications and the discomfort and cost of this procedure, it should be used only after simpler methods fail.

Table 14–12. Patients to be screened for pheochromocytoma.

Young hypertensives
Hypertensive patients with:
  Symptoms listed in Table 14–8
  Weight loss
  Seizures
  Orthostatic hypotension
  Unexplained shock
  Family history of pheochromocytoma or medullary carcinoma
    of thyroid
  Neurofibromatosis and other neurocutaneous syndromes
  Mucosal neuromas
  Hyperglycemia
  Cardiomyopathy
Marked lability of blood pressure
Family history of pheochromocytoma
Shock or severe pressor responses with:
  Induction of anesthesia
  Parturition
  Surgery
  Invasive procedures
  Antihypertensive drugs
Radiologic evidence of adrenal mass

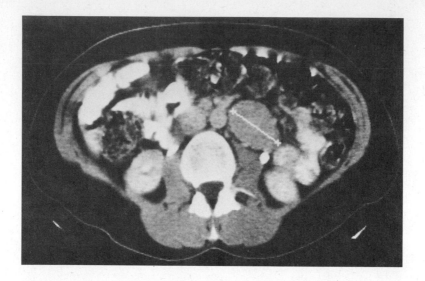

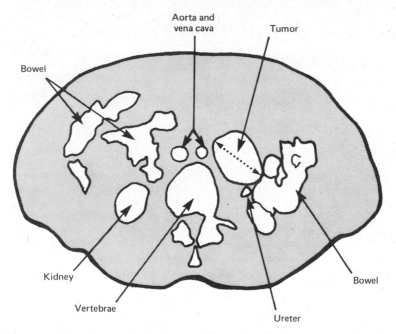

Figure 14–11. Left infrarenal pheochromocytoma shown by CT scanning. The lower diagram identifies many of the visible structures.

A scintigraphic procedure for the localization of pheochromocytomas has been described. [131I]Met-aiodobenzylguanidine (MIBG) is injected into the patient, resulting in detectable images 24–72 hours later. Very small tumors can be safely and conveniently located by this method. Although not all pheochromocytomas will produce detectable images, the specificity of the method seems high, and it has been possible to locate tumors not shown by CT scanning. MIBG is also taken up by some neuroblastomas.

Management

Optimal management of patients with pheochromocytomas requires an understanding of the pathophysiology produced by excessive catecholamines and an acquaintance with the action of adrenergic antagonists and other drugs used in the treatment of these patients.

A. Treatment With Adrenergic Antagonists: As soon as the diagnosis has been confirmed, therapy with adrenergic antagonists should be instituted. Treatment

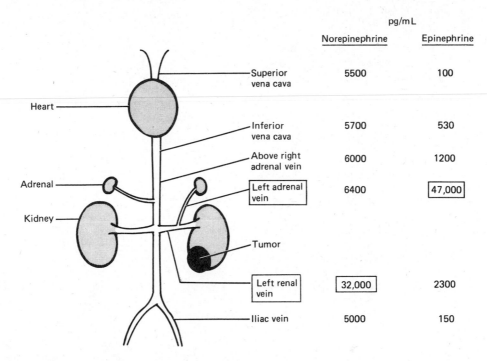

	pg/mL	
	Norepinephrine	Epinephrine
Superior vena cava	5500	100
Inferior vena cava	5700	530
Above right adrenal vein	6000	1200
Left adrenal vein	6400	47,000
Left renal vein	32,000	2300
Iliac vein	5000	150

Figure 14–12. Plasma norepinephrine and epinephrine levels in samples of blood obtained from the vena cava. Note that the level of epinephrine is very high in the left adrenal vein sample, distinguishing it from the drainage of the tumor, which secretes mainly norepinephrine. Note the relatively normal peripheral levels of epinephrine (as seen in the iliac vein or the superior vena cava).

is directed toward reduction of symptoms, lowering of blood pressure, and amelioration of paroxysms occurring spontaneously or induced by studies undertaken to localize the tumors. Such treatment will allow expansion of the vascular bed and plasma volume and will reduce the amount of transfused blood required for maintenance of blood pressure during surgery.

Although only a few days of therapy are required for preoperative study and preparation of most patients for surgery, prolonged medical therapy is advantageous in patients who have had recent myocardial infarctions, those with electrocardiographic or clinical evidence of catecholamine cardiomyopathy, or those in the last trimester of pregnancy. They can be maintained on this regimen until the infant is delivered or the complication resolved, at which time the tumor can be removed.

Agents commonly used in therapy include phentolamine, prazosin, and phenoxybenzamine. Propranolol is occasionally helpful to control marked tachycardia and arrhythmias, but it should not be given until alpha receptor blockade is established.

In patients with persistent hypertension or frequent paroxysms, **phenoxybenzamine** (Dibenzyline), a noncompetitive alpha-adrenergic antagonist with a prolonged effect, is indicated. Treatment is begun with doses of 20–40 mg/d orally and can be increased by 10–20 mg every 1–2 days until the desired effect is achieved. Postural hypotension may be marked at the beginning of therapy, and care should be taken to prevent syncope. However, postural hypotension usually disappears when adequate blockade is achieved. Completely normal blood pressures (<140/90 mm Hg) may not be achieved and are not required. A dose of 60–80 mg daily is usually adequate, but 2–3 times that amount may be necessary. When marked tachycardia or arrhythmias occur prior to or during surgery, small doses of **propranolol** may be required. Patients with infrequent paroxysms and an absence of interval manifestations can be treated in a similar manner.

Rapid titration of the dose may be difficult using phenoxybenzamine, because of its long half-life (36 hours). However, **prazosin** (Minipress), an alpha antagonist with a shorter duration of activity has been found to be useful. Prazosin is predominantly an α_1 antagonist and has not been found to be effective in all patients.

B. Preparation for Surgery: Preparation of the patient as described above minimizes the hazards of anesthesia and surgery. The patient's blood pressure and electrocardiographic patterns should be continuously monitored, and phentolamine and particularly sodium nitroprusside are useful to reduce blood pressure if necessary. Suspected intra-abdominal tumors are usually approached through a transabdominal incision, since this allows exploration of the adrenals, sympathetic ganglia, bladder, and other pelvic structures. However, posterior and flank incisions are preferred by some surgeons for removal of larger tumors. When bilateral adrenal tumors are found and the adrenals removed, adrenocortical steroid replacement is required (see Chapter 12).

C. Postoperative Care: When the tumor is removed, the blood pressure usually falls to about 90/60 mm Hg. Persistence of low blood pressures or poor peripheral perfusion may require blood volume expansion with whole blood, plasma, or other fluids as indicated. Pressor therapy is not usually required and should not be substituted for volume expansion.

Lack of a fall in pressure at the time of tumor removal (even in the presence of adrenergic blockade) indicates the presence of additional tumor tissue.

In patients with tumors producing persistent hypertension, the initial fall in blood pressure may be followed by an elevation of blood pressure in the postoperative period. However, the accompanying symptoms of sympathetic stimulation are gone, and the pressure returns to normal over the next few weeks. If the blood pressure remains elevated but the patient is otherwise asymptomatic, another cause for the elevated blood pressure should be considered. Essential hypertension and renal vascular hypertension have been reported in several patients harboring pheochromocytomas. In patients whose tumors secrete little or no excess of catecholamines and who are free of signs and symptoms other than fixed hypertension, tumor removal will not usually eliminate the elevated blood pressure.

D. Treatment of Malignant Tumors: Patients with nonresectable malignant tumors or metastases or

Table 14–13. Distribution of metastases in 41 cases of malignant pheochromocytoma.[1]

	Autopsy Cases (n = 26)	Nonautopsy Cases (n = 15)	Percentage
Skeleton	12	6	44
Liver	12	3	37
Lymph node	11	4	37
Lungs	9	2	27
Central nervous system	4	0	10
Pleura	4	0	10
Kidneys	2	0	5
Pancreas	1	0	2
Omentum	1	0	2

[1]Reproduced, with permission, from Schönebeck J: *Scand J Urol Nephrol* 1969;**3**:66.

those who for other reasons are not amenable to successful surgical treatment can be managed medically for prolonged periods. Phenoxybenzamine and perhaps prazosin can be used chronically as described above. Patients with malignant tumors have also benefited symptomatically from treatment with α-methylmetatyrosine, an inhibitor of tyrosine hydroxylase, the rate-limiting enzyme in the biosynthetic process. Although some patients with malignant pheochromocytomas die early because of disseminated disease, there are long-term survivors. Sites of metastases are shown in Table 14–13. The most common site of metastases is the skeleton, and bone lesions tend to respond well to radiation therapy. The use of combinations of chemotherapeutic agents such as cyclophosphamide, vincristine, and dacarbazine is effective in controlling soft tissue lesions in some patients.

REFERENCES

General

Coupland RE: *The Natural History of the Chromaffin Cell.* Longmans, Green, 1965.

Cryer PE: Physiology and pathophysiology of the human sympathoadrenal neuroendocrine system. *N Engl J Med* 1980;**303**:436.

Malmejhac J: Activity of the adrenal medulla and its regulation. *Physiol Rev* 1964;**44**:186.

Hormones of the Adrenal Medulla

Ahlquist RP: A study of the adrenotropic receptors. *Am J Physiol* 1948;**153**:586.

Axelrod J: The metabolism, storage and release of catecholamines. *Recent Prog Horm Res* 1965;**21**:597.

Bleasdale J, Eichberg J, Havser G (editors): *Inositol and Phosphoinositides.* Humana Press, 1985.

Brown MR, Fisher LA: Brain peptide regulation of adrenal epinephrine secretion. *Am J Physiol* 1984;**247**:E41.

Clutter WE et al: Epinephrine plasma metabolic clearance rates and physiologic thresholds for metabolic and hemodynamic actions in man. *J Clin Invest* 1980;**66**:94.

Eiden LE: Is chromogranin a prohormone? *Nature* 1987;**325**:301.

Ganong WF, Reid IA: Role of the sympathetic nervous system and central alpha- and beta-adrenergic receptors in regulation of renin activity. *Am J Physiol* 1976;**230**:1733.

Goldfien A: Effects of glucose deprivation on the sympathetic outflow to the adrenal medulla and adipose tissue. *Pharmacol Rev* 1966;**18**:303.

Goldstein DS, Eisenhofer G: Plasma catechols: What do they mean? *News Physiol Sci* 1988;**3**:139.

Iversen LL: Uptake processes for biogenic amines. Pages 381–442 in: *Handbook of Psychopharmacology.* Section 1, Vol. 3. Plenum Press, 1975.

Mannelli M et al: Endogenous dopamine (DA) and DA2 receptors: A mechanism limiting excessive sympathetic-adrenal discharge in humans. *J Clin Endocrinol Metab* 1988;**66**:626.

Murray E et al: Determination of norepinephrine apparent release rate and clearance in humans. *Life Sci* 1979;**25**:1461.

Raum WJ: Methods of plasma catecholamine measurement including radioimmunoassay. *Am J Physiol* 1984;**247**:E4.

Robertson D et al: Use of alpha$_2$ adrenoceptor agonists and antagonists in the functional assessment of the sympathetic nervous system. *J Clin Invest* 1986;**78**:576.

Seeman P: Dopamine receptors. *Pharmacol Rev* 1980;**32**:230.

Silverberg AB et al: Norepinephrine: Hormone and neurotransmitter in man. *Am J Physiol* 1978;**234**:252.

Simon JP, Bader MF, Aunis D: Secretion from chromaffin cells is controlled by chromogranin A-derived peptides. *Proc Natl Acad Sci USA* 1988;**85**:1712.

Trendelenburg U, Weiner N (editors): *Catecholamines*. Vol 90 of *Handbook of Experimental Pharmacology*. Springer-Verlag, 1988.

Weiner N: Regulation of norepinephrine biosynthesis. *Annu Rev Pharmacol* 1970;**10**:273.

Woods SC, Porte D Jr: Neural control of the endocrine pancreas. *Physiol Rev* 1974;**54**:596.

Disorders of Adrenal Medullary Function; Pheochromocytoma

Averbuch SD et al: Malignant pheochromocytoma: Effective treatment with a combination of cyclophosphamide, vincristine, and dacarbazine. *Ann Intern Med* 1988;**109**:267.

Bravo E, Gifford RW Jr: Pheochromocytoma: Diagnosis, localization and management. *N Engl J Med* 1984;**311**:1298.

Engelman K, Sjoerdsma A: Chronic medical therapy for pheochromocytoma. *Ann Intern Med* 1964;**61**:229.

Frohlich ED: The adrenergic nervous system and hypertension: State of the art. Second Pan American Symposium on Hypertension, Part 2. *Mayo Clin Proc* 1977;**52**:361.

Gagel RF et al: The clinical outcome of prospective screening for multiple endocrine neoplasia type 2a: An 18-year experience. *N Engl J Med* 1988;**318**:478.

Goldfien A: Pheochromocytoma: Diagnosis and anesthetic and surgical management. *Anesthesiology* 1963;**24**:462.

Goldstein DS: Plasma norepinephrine in essential hypertension. *Hypertension* 1981;**3**:48.

Hume DM: Pheochromocytoma in the adult and in the child. *Am J Surg* 1960;**99**:458.

Keiser HR et al: Treatment of malignant pheochromocytoma with combination chemotherapy. *Hypertension* 1985;**7(No. 3–Part 2)**:118.

Landsberg L: Catecholamines and hyperthyroidism. *Clin Endocrinol Metab* 1977;**6**:697.

Manger WM: Pheochromocytoma. (Editorial.) *West J Med* 1986;**145**:382.

Manger WM, Gifford RW: *Pheochromocytoma*. Springer, 1977.

Mathew CG et al: A linked genetic marker for multiple endocrine neoplasia type 2A on chromosome 10. *Nature* 1987;**328**:527.

Modlin IM et al: Pheochromocytomas in 72 patients: Clinical and diagnostic features, treatment and long-term results. *Br J Surg* 1979;**66**:456.

Ponder BA, Jackson CE (editors): The second international workshop on multiple endocrine neoplasia type 2 syndromes. *Henry Ford Hosp Med J* 1987;**35**:1. [Entire 2 issues.]

Proye C et al: Dopamine-secreting pheochromocytoma: An unrecognized entity. Classification of pheochromocytomas according to their type of secretion. *Surgery* 1986;**100**:1154.

Schenker JG, Chowers U: Pheochromocytoma and pregnancy: Review of 89 cases. *Obstet Gynecol Surv* 1971;**26**:739.

Schimke NR et al: Syndrome of bilateral pheochromocytoma, medullary thyroid carcinoma and multiple neuromas: A possible regulatory defect in the differentiation of chromaffin tissue. *N Engl J Med* 1968;**279**:1.

Simpson NE et al: Assignment of multiple endocrine neoplasia type 2A to chromosome 10 by linkage. *Nature* 1987;**328**:528.

Sisson JC, Wieland DM: Radiolabeled metaiodobenzylguanidine: Pharmacology and clinical studies. *Am J Physiol Imaging* 1986;**1**:96.

Sizemore GW, Heath H, Carney JA: Multiple endocrine neoplasia type 2. *Clin Endocrinol Metab* 1980;**9**:299.

Sjoerdsma A: Chronic medical therapy for pheochromocytoma. *Ann Intern Med* 1964;**61**:229.

Stenström G, Svärdsudd K: Pheochromocytoma in Sweden 1958–1981: An analysis of the National Cancer Registry data. *Acta Med Scand* 1986;**220**:225.

Visser J, Axt R: Bilateral adrenal medullary hyperplasia: A clinicopathological entity. *J Clin Pathol* 1975;**28**:298.

Yanese T et al: Studies on adrenorphin in pheochromocytoma. *J Clin Endocrinol Metab* 1987;**64**:692.

Robertson D et al: Autonomic insufficiency Isolated failure of autonomic noradrenergic neurotransmission: Evidence for impaired β-hydroxylation of dopamine. *N Engl J Med* 1986;**314**:1494.

Schatz IJ: Orthostatic hypotension. *Arch Intern Med* 1984;**144**:733.

Renal Hormones & Endocrine Hypertension

David J. Ramsay, DM, DPhil

The kidney is involved in 3 major hormonal systems in the body. First, it secretes **renin,** a proteolytic enzyme that initiates a chain of events leading to the production of the circulating peptide **angiotensin II,** which plays an important role in the regulation of salt and water metabolism and of blood pressure. Second, the kidney secretes **erythropoietin,** a glycoprotein that helps to control red cell production. Third, the final step in **activation of vitamin D** occurs in the kidney. The kidney takes up 25-hydroxycholecalciferol from the bloodstream and hydroxylates it to **1,25-dihydroxycholecalciferol.** This agent increases plasma calcium concentration by increasing its intestinal absorption and renal tubular reabsorption and by stimulating bone resorption. In addition, kidney disease and renal hormones are frequently involved in the pathogenesis of human hypertension (Chapter 11).

RENIN & THE RENIN-ANGIOTENSIN SYSTEM

In 1947, Goldblatt noted that reducing the flow of blood to the kidney in experimental animals was followed by an increase in blood pressure. This simple experiment, which implicated the kidney in the pathogenesis of hypertension, stimulated much of the research that led to elucidation of the **renin-angiotensin system** as we know it today.

As the afferent arteriole enters the glomerulus (Fig 15–1), the smooth muscle cells become modified to perform a secretory function. These cells, the **juxtaglomerular cells,** produce and secrete renin. Renin is a proteolytic enzyme with a molecular weight of approximately 40,000. It is derived from the proteolysis of its precursor, **prorenin.** The human kidney secretes both prorenin and renin into the bloodstream.

Prorenin, which has a slightly higher molecular weight than renin, appears to be identical to the molecule previously termed inactive renin and can be present in the circulation at levels as high as or higher than those of renin. Prorenin can be converted into renin in vitro by a number of methods, but it is not known whether significant extrarenal conversion of prorenin occurs. Renin reaches the bloodstream, where it acts upon its only known substrate, **angiotensinogen,** to form a decapeptide, **angiotensin I** (Fig 15–2). Angiotensin I, which is physiologically inert, is converted to **angiotensin II,** an octapeptide, by the action of **converting enzyme.** Angiotensin II accounts for the biologic activity. The half-life of angiotensin II in plasma is less than 1 minute as a result of the action of multiple angiotensinases located in most tissues of the body.

Angiotensinogen

Angiotensinogen (renin substrate) is an α_2-globulin secreted by the liver. It has a molecular weight of approximately 60,000 and is usually present in human plasma at a constant concentration of 1 μmol/L. Although the rate of production of angiotensin II is normally determined by changes in plasma renin concentration, the concentration of angiotensinogen is below the V_{max} for the reaction. Thus, if angiotensinogen concentration increases, the amount of angiotensin produced at the same plasma renin concentration will increase. Hepatic production of angiotensinogen is increased by glucocorticoids and by estrogens. Stimulation of angiotensinogen production by estrogen-containing contraceptive pills may contribute to some of the hypertension encountered as a side effect of this treatment.

In situations such as sodium depletion, where there is a sustained high level of circulating angiotensin II, the rate of breakdown of substrate by renin in the plasma is greatly increased. Because the plasma concentration of angiotensinogen remains constant in these situations, hepatic production must increase to match the increased rate of breakdown. The mechanism of this increase is not clear, although angiotensin II itself is a stimulus to substrate production.

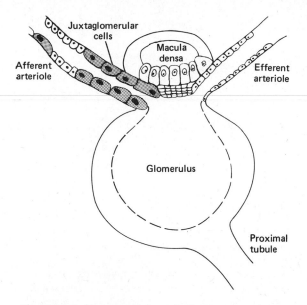

Figure 15–1. Diagram of glomerulus, showing juxtaglomerular apparatus and macula densa.

Converting Enzyme

Converting enzyme is found in most tissues in the body and circulates in plasma. Thus, theoretically, the conversion of angiotensin I to angiotensin II could take place anywhere in the circulatory system. However, there are particularly high activities of the enzyme in the lung such that on a single passage, 70–80% of angiotensin I is converted to angiotensin II. In the whole body, therefore, the lung is quantitatively the most important site of formation of circulating angiotensin II.

Converting enzyme is a dipeptidyl carboxypeptidase, a glycoprotein of MW 130,000–160,000 that cleaves dipeptides from a number of substrates. In addition to angiotensin I, these include bradykinin, enkephalins, and substance P. Potent inhibitors of converting enzyme are available that prevent the formation of angiotensin II in the circulation and thus

block its biologic effects (Fig 15–2). Captopril and enalapril are particularly important converting enzyme inhibitors because they are active when taken by mouth (see below). Because of the participation of converting enzyme in a number of peptide systems, blockade of the enzyme may not always exert its effects solely via the renin-angiotensin system.

EFFECTS OF ANGIOTENSIN II

Peripheral Effects

Angiotensin II is a very potent pressor agent. It exerts its effects on peripheral arterioles to cause vasoconstriction and thus increases total peripheral resistance. Vasoconstriction occurs in all tissue beds, including the kidney, and has been implicated in the phenomenon of renal autoregulation. Angiotensin may also affect the heart, causing increases in rate and strength of contraction, although this is less clear. The possible role of increased circulating levels of angiotensin II in the pathogenesis of hypertension is discussed below.

Angiotensin II acts directly on the adrenal cortex to stimulate aldosterone secretion. In fact, in many situations, angiotensin is the most important regulator of aldosterone secretion and thus plays a central role in the regulation of sodium balance. For example, during dietary sodium depletion, extracellular fluid volume is reduced due to osmotic transfer of water to the intracellular fluid compartment. Subsequent stimulation of the renin-angiotensin system is important in 2 ways. The vasoconstrictor action of angiotensin helps to maintain blood pressure in the face of reduced extracellular fluid volume, whereas the action of angiotensin to stimulate aldosterone secretion and thus sodium retention allows volume to be conserved.

The intrarenal actions of angiotensin II also help to promote sodium retention. Angiotensin II preferentially constricts efferent arterioles, thus maintaining glomerular filtration rate during hypovolemia and arterial hypotension. The subsequent fall in peritubular

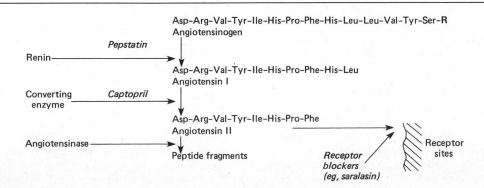

Figure 15–2. Sequence of formation of angiotensin II. Drugs that can be used to block various steps are shown in italics.

capillary hydrostatic pressure aids proximal tubule reabsorption of sodium and water. In addition, angiotensin II itself stimulates proximal tubule sodium reabsorption. Reduced loop of Henle flow—due to reduced glomerular filtration rate and increased proximal reabsorption—and reduced vasa recta flow aid countercurrent multiplication and urinary concentration mechanisms.

Angiotensin II modulates activity at sympathetic nerve endings in peripheral blood vessels and in the heart. It increases sympathetic activity partly by facilitating adrenergic transmitter release and partly by increasing the responsiveness of smooth muscle to norepinephrine. Angiotensin II also stimulates the release of catecholamines from the adrenal medulla.

Blockade of the peripheral effects of angiotensin II is useful therapeutically. For example, in low-output congestive cardiac failure, plasma levels of angiotensin II are high. These high circulating levels promote salt and water retention and—by constricting arterioles—raise peripheral vascular resistance, thus increasing cardiac afterload. Treatment with converting enzyme inhibitors such as captopril results in peripheral vasodilation, thereby improving tissue perfusion and cardiac performance as well as aiding renal elimination of salt and water. The use of converting enzyme inhibitors in the treatment of hypertension is discussed below.

Brain & Central Nervous System Effects

In recent years, many actions of angiotensin on the central nervous system have been described. Angiotensin II is a polar peptide that does not cross the blood-brain barrier. Circulating angiotensin II, however, may affect the brain by acting through one or more of the circumventricular organs (see Chapter 5). These specialized regions within the brain lack a blood-brain barrier, so that receptive cells in these areas are sensitive to plasma composition. Of particular significance to the actions of angiotensin are the subfornical organ, the organum vasculosum of the lamina terminalis, and the area postrema.

Many tissues in the body, including the brain, heart, ovary, adrenal testis, and peripheral blood vessels, contain the components of the renin-angiotensin system. In some of these tissues, there is evidence that angiotensin can be formed locally and that such formation may have physiologic functions. For example, production of angiotensin II in the brain has been implicated in several models of hypertension.

The major actions of angiotensin II on the brain are listed in Table 15–1. Angiotensin II is a potent dipsogen when injected directly into the brain or administered systemically. The major receptors for the dipsogenic action of circulating angiotensin II are located in the subfornical organ. Angiotensin II also stimulates vasopressin secretion, particularly in association with raised plasma osmolality. As such, the renin-angioten-

Table 15–1. Actions of angiotensin on the brain.

Stimulates drinking.
Increases vasopressin secretion.
Stimulates ACTH secretion.
Raises blood pressure.
Increases salt appetite.

sin system may have an important part to play in the control of water balance, particularly during hypovolemia.

Angiotensin also acts on the brain to increase blood pressure, although its effects at this site seem to be less potent than those exerted directly in the systemic circulation. In most animals, the receptors are located in the area postrema.

Other central actions of angiotensin II include stimulation of adrenocorticotropic hormone (ACTH) secretion, suppression of plasma renin activity, and stimulation of sodium appetite, particularly in association with raised mineralocorticoid levels. The full implications of these (and other) central actions of angiotensin remain to be elucidated.

CONTROL OF RENIN SECRETION

The original experimental work that heralded the discovery of renin showed that a reduction of blood pressure to the kidney increases renin secretion. This led to the view that blood pressure is the major renin secretion control mechanism. However, the mechanism of the inverse relationship between blood pressure and renin secretion is not clear. There are 2 main theories. The **baroreceptor theory** argues that the juxtaglomerular cells act as their own baroreceptors. Thus, if blood pressure increases, baroreceptors in the juxtaglomerular cells will be stretched, leading to a decrease in renin output. The second theory is that the **macula densa cells** contain different receptors sensitive to the sodium chloride load of the distal tubular fluid. The macula densa cells are in close contact with juxtaglomerular cells, so that a fall in sodium chloride load passing these cells in the distal tubule will be perceived by the macula densa cells and result in increased renin secretion. A third important stimulus to renin secretion is increased beta-adrenergic stimulation mediated through renal sympathetic nerves.

In general, the important whole body stimulus that leads to renin secretion is **hypovolemia.** Hypovolemia causes a fall in blood pressure and thus, according to the baroreceptor theory, an increase in renin output. A fall in blood pressure will also reduce glomerular filtration rate and distal sodium and chloride load and thus, by the macula densa theory, stimulate renin secretion. Hypovolemic stimulation of renin secretion is enhanced by renal sympathetic nerves. Decreased discharge in atrial and pulmonary stretch receptors, as well as reduced arterial baroreceptor discharge, leads to reflex augmentation of renin release via the renal nerves. The sympathetic nerves act directly on the juxtaglomerular cells as well as indirectly, by reducing blood flow through the kidney.

The significance of other effects on renin secretion is less well understood. Both vasopressin and angiotensin II decrease renin secretion, probably acting at the juxtaglomerular cells. These peptides have actions on renin secretion that can occur with variations of their plasma concentrations over the physiologic range, but the importance of their roles remains to be elucidated.

RENIN & HYPERTENSION

Since the original observation that impaired renal perfusion leads to secretion of renin and an increase in blood pressure, renin has been implicated in the etiology of hypertension. For many years, the evidence linking renin to hypertension was inconclusive, and many investigators discounted the participation of the renin-angiotensin system in all but a few forms of hypertension. For example, rare renin-producing tumors can result in severe hypertension. Renal artery stenosis and coarctation of the aorta above the origin of the renal arteries are associated with renin-dependent hypertension. Similarly, malignant hypertension in endstage renal disease is associated with increased plasma renin levels.

Renovascular Hypertension

The most common known cause of renin-dependent hypertension is renovascular hypertension. Various studies have reported it to be present in 1–4% of patients with hypertension. Renovascular hypertension is usually due to either atherosclerosis or fibromuscular hyperplasia of the renal arteries. These result in decreased perfusion in the renal segment distal to the obstructed vessel, which causes increased renin release from this segment and so increased angiotensin II production. This results in an increase in blood pressure and fluid volume that suppresses renin release from the contralateral kidney and from those segments of the ipsilateral kidney that are unaffected by the stenosis. The increases in angiotensin II, blood pressure and fluid also suppress to some extent the abnormal renin release from the affected kidney segments. Consequently, the total plasma renin activity may be only slightly elevated or even normal.

A single, 100% reliable, and simple screening test for renovascular hypertension is unavailable. Because of this and the low incidence of the disorder, screening all hypertensives for renovascular hypertension is generally not recommended. Instead, most physicians look for indications that the hypertension is inappropriate before deciding to evaluate the patient for renovascular hypertension. As a general guideline, any combination of severe hypertension, accelerated hypertension, onset of hypertension before age 20 or after age 50, the presence of abdominal bruit, or hypokalemia in a patient without a family history of hypertension should lead to evaluation for this disorder. Although hypertension in general is more common in blacks, renovascular hypertension is more common in whites.

Renovascular hypertension is diagnosed by tests that demonstrate the anatomic defect and by functional studies that document the abnormal renin release. There is no general agreement on which of the available tests should be performed or on the order they should be performed in. Although the rapid sequence hypertensive intravenous urogram or pyelogram (IVP) and radionucleotide renal imaging have been traditionally used for screening, these tests are no longer frequently used due to their low sensitivity (around 80%) and specificity (around 80%). The best technique to define the renal artery lesion is renal arteriography, which can define the anatomic constriction and also provide some indication of whether it can be relieved through transluminal angioplasty or other means.

The 2 most popular means for documenting the abnormal renin release are selective sampling from the renal veins by renal vein catheterization (selective venous sampling) and blocking angiotensin II production by converting enzyme administration (captopril test). Basal plasma renin levels by themselves do not indicate the diagnosis unless they are extremely low (arguing against the diagnosis), since normal plasma renin levels can be present in renovascular hypertension and elevated levels are present in a significant number of patients with essential hypertension (discussed below) and other forms of renal disease. In selective venous sampling, plasma samples are taken of the venous effluent from the affected portion of the kidney and from the contralateral kidney. The renin level is ordinarily significantly higher in the sample from the affected kidney than in that from the contralateral kidney. When the value for the affected kidney sample is divided by the value for the unaffected sample, a ratio of greater than 1.5 generally indicates a functional abnormality, although a lower ratio does not exclude the diagnosis. In some centers, the results are analyzed by subtracting the arterial value from the venous value and dividing the result by the arterial plasma renin values. The captopril test involves administering captopril to the patient (on a high- or normal-sodium diet) and measuring the plasma renin levels before and 1 hour after the administration. Captopril induces a reactive hyperreninemia by blocking the negative feedback exerted by intrarenal angiotensin II. This feedback is less pronounced in patients with essential hypertension.

Anatomic correction is the preferred therapy for renovascular hypertension when it is possible and the patient is considered able to tolerate the procedure. Recent advances in transluminal angioplasty have made this the procedure of choice. In special situations, other surgical approaches such as endarterectomy are used. However, renovascular hypertension can be treated medically; this treatment is used when the patient is considered unable to tolerate a surgical procedure or the diagnosis is uncertain. The converting enzyme inhibitors captopril and enalapril are particularly effective, although these agents can lower intrarenal efferent arteriolar resistance and so decrease renal function in patients with bilateral renal artery stenosis. Renovascular hypertension may also respond to beta-adrenergic and calcium channel blockers.

Renin & Essential Hypertension

Most patients with hypertension have essential hypertension, meaning that its cause is unknown. The connection between renin and hypertension has been rationalized largely by the fact that hypertension represents a mixture of clinical entities (Table 15–2). At one end of the spectrum lie various causes of hypertension that have in common intense peripheral vasoconstriction. Thus, increased activity of any **vasoconstrictor agent**—eg, angiotensin in renal vascular hypertension or catecholamines in pheochromocytomas—will cause arteriolar vasoconstriction and an increase in total peripheral resistance and thus an increase in blood pressure. At the other end of the spectrum are increases in blood pressure due to expansion of **extracellular fluid volume.** Thus, any situation that leads to sodium or water retention can lead to an increase in blood pressure.

Much effort has been expended in defining a normal range for plasma renin activity. It is not easy to assess the state of the renin-angiotensin system from a single blood sample drawn for analysis of plasma renin activity, since the secretion rate may be affected by so many factors. Furthermore, assay methodology varies between laboratories in such important aspects as the pH of the incubation step. Of particular importance is the sodium content of the diet. Other factors that affect the interpretation of results include sex, age, race, position (supine, upright, etc.), physical activity, severity of hypertension, concurrent medication such as birth control pills and antihypertensive drugs, and illnesses such as diabetes mellitus, congestive heart

Table 15–2. Contribution of excessive arterial vasoconstriction and excessive blood volume in different types of hypertension. The diseases at the top show the greatest degree of vasoconstriction compared with volume excess; those at the bottom show the greatest degree of volume excess compared with arterial vasoconstriction.

Malignant hypertension.
Pheochromocytoma.
Unilateral renovascular hypertension.
High-renin essential hypertension.
Low-renin essential hypertension unresponsive to diuretics.
Normal-renin essential hypertension.
Bilateral renovascular hypertension.
Low-renin essential hypertension responsive to diuretics.
Primary aldosteronism.

failure, and cirrhosis. Diuretic therapy is especially important to consider, because it can lead to sodium depletion and elevated plasma renin levels.

Several protocols have been used to standardize the plasma renin activity measurements. These include measurements after normal and low sodium diets, pretreatment with a diuretic, overnight recumbency, and four hours of ambulation. Another approach to this problem has been to correlate plasma renin activity with the sodium content of the diet as judged by 24-hour urine collection (Fig 15–3). Investigation of normal subjects has shown that in general, the higher the sodium content of the diet, the lower the plasma renin activity will be. For instance, when standardized with the latter approach, plasma renin activity in patients with essential hypertension varies considerably. Around 5% of such patients have high levels and around 30% have low levels of plasma renin activity. The significance of these differences is not known. In general, the blood pressure of patients with low plasma renin levels responds better to calcium channel blockers and diuretics and that of patients with higher renin levels responds better to converting enzyme inhibitors and beta-adrenergic blockers. However, even patients with normal plasma renin levels exhibit considerable heterogeneity in response to therapy. Thus, despite the logic in the use of "renin profiling" to decide on an appropriate therapeutic agent, this method has not come into general usage.

Measurement of plasma renin activity is useful in helping to diagnose renin-secreting tumors. Although

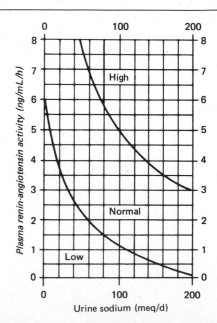

Figure 15–3. Correlation of plasma renin activity with 24-hour sodium excretion in human subjects. (Reproduced, with permission, from Laragh JH, Sealey JE: *Cardiovasc Med* 1977;2:1053.)

these are rare, it is important to spot them, since early detection is likely to improve the chances of surgical cure (see Chapter 13).

ERYTHROPOIETIN

It has long been realized that hypoxia is a potent stimulus to red cell production. Within a few hours after exposure of human subjects to hypoxia, there is an increase in reticulocyte count—denoting the presence of new red blood cells in the circulation—followed by an increase in circulating red cell mass. This is due to the increased production of a glycoprotein, erythropoietin. The kidney is the major source of this hormone, but it is also produced in the liver, particularly in fetuses. Day-to-day production of erythropoietin depends on the Po_2 of blood perfusing the kidneys.

The target cells for erythropoietin are the colony forming units—erythroid (CFU-E) cells in the bone marrow. Erythropoietin reacts with receptors on CFU-E cells, which leads to increased production of proerythroblasts and release of more erythrocytes into the circulation. Human erythropoietin cDNA has been cloned and recombinant erythropoietin is available for therapeutic use.

There is continuous secretion of erythropoietin even in the adult. Anephric patients generally have very low hematocrits, largely as a result of the absence of circulating erythropoietin in the plasma. The suppressed rate of formation of red blood cells due to lack of renal production of erythropoietin is a major problem in the treatment of patients with severe renal failure. Renal transplantation not only restores renal function to the anephric patient but also restores normal erythropoiesis.

Hypoxia is the most important stimulus to erythropoietin production. A number of pathologic conditions affecting the kidney, particularly those that reduce renal blood flow, may increase the rate of release of erythropoietin and inevitably increase red blood cell production. A few cases of erythropoietin-releasing tumors have been described in patients with very high hematocrits and hypertension resulting from the increased peripheral vascular resistance caused by high blood viscosity.

Kallikrein-Kinin System

The kidney contains all the elements of the kallikrein-kinin system. Renal kallikrein is a serine protease that is synthesized in distal tubule cells and is distinct from plasma kallikrein. Kallikrein is secreted into distal tubular fluid where it reacts with filtered hepatic kininogen to form kinin. There are kinin receptors in the cortical and medullary collecting tubules on both the luminal and peritubular surfaces. Kinins ap-

pear to increase the salt and water excretion-inhibiting effects of aldosterone and vasopressin on the collecting tubule epithelium. The physiologic significance of the kallikrein-kinin system is not yet clear.

ATRIAL NATRIURETIC PEPTIDE

Extracts of atrial—but not ventricular—tissue cause marked natriuresis when injected into rats. The material is contained in densely staining granules in the atria of most mammalian species. A number of laboratories have sequenced and synthesized several natriuretic peptides containing between 22 and 28 amino acids, and rat and human atrial cDNA clones that encode atrial natriuretic peptides have been isolated and characterized. The 28-amino-acid peptide is probably normally secreted into the bloodstream. Several terms are used to describe these peptides, including atriopeptin, auriculin, cardionatrin, and atrial natriuretic factor. The major effects of administration of atrial natriuretic peptide are natriuresis and a fall in blood pressure. Although the peptide can cause relaxation of smooth muscle, the fall in blood pressure is due to reduction of venous return and depression of cardiac output in intact animals. The natriuresis is associated with a marked increase in filtration fraction without a sustained increase in renal blood flow, which suggests that the peptide may cause efferent arteriolar constriction. There is some evidence that glomerular membrane permeability may be increased and that tubular reabsorption may be reduced. Atrial natriuretic peptide also inhibits secretion of renin and aldosterone. There is also evidence that baroreflex stimulation of heart rate as well as vasopressin and ACTH secretion is inhibited.

Recently, a number of radioimmunoassays for atrial natriuretic peptide have been developed. Although there are still questions concerning the specificity of these assays, it is clear that there are measurable levels of the material in normal plasma. Maneuvers that expand plasma volume and experiments that increase atrial pressure are associated with increased levels of radioimmunoassayable peptide in plasma. Situations such as congestive heart failure that are associated with chronically raised atrial pressures show raised plasma levels of the peptide. Thus, atrial natriuretic peptide may be involved in the control of sodium balance. When blood volume increases, the associated increase in atrial pressure and atrial stretch may trigger secretion of the peptide and lead to natriuresis and blood pressure reduction. However, the precise role that atrial natriuretic peptide plays in the control of sodium balance and blood volume under physiologic conditions is not clear.

REFERENCES

Baxter JD et al: The endocrinology of hypertension. Chapter 14 in: *Endocrinology and Metabolism,* 2nd ed. Felig P et al (editors). McGraw-Hill, 1987.

Currie MG et al: Purification and sequence analysis of bioactive atrial peptides (atriopeptins). *Science* 1984;**223:**67.

Davis JO, Freeman RH: Mechanisms regulating renin release. *Physiol Rev* 1976;**56:**1.

Dzau VJ, Burt DW, Pratt RE: Molecular biology of the renin-angiotensin system. *Am J Physiol* 1988;**255:**F563.

Fried W, Morley C: Update on erythropoietin. *Int J Artif Organs* 1985;**8:**79.

Genest J, Cantin M: The atrial natriuretic factor: Its physiology and biochemistry. *Rev Physiol Biochem Pharm* 1988;**110:**1.

Hardman JA et al: Primary structure of the human renin gene. *DNA* 1984;**6:**457.

Huang CL et al: Renal mechanism of action of rat atrial natriuretic factor. *J Clin Invest* 1985;**75:**769.

Huang SL: Cloning and expression of human erythropoietic DNA in *Escherichia coli. Proc Natl Acad Sci USA* 1984;**81:**2708.

Laragh JH: Atrial natriuretic hormone, the renin-aldosterone axis, and blood pressure: Electrolyte homeostasis. *N Engl J Med* 1985;**313:**1330.

Laragh JH, Bühler FR, Seldin DW (editors): *Frontiers in Hypertension Research.* Springer-Verlag, 1981.

Laragh JH, Letcher RL, Pickering TG: Renin profiling for diagnosis and treatment of hypertension. *JAMA* 1979;**241:**151.

Levinsky NG, Lieberthal W, Vasilevsky ML: Role of the kallikrein-kinin system in volume homeostasis. In: *Body Fluid Homeostasis.* Brenner BM, Stein JH (editors). Churchill Livingstone, 1986.

Maack T et al: Atrial natriuretic factor: Structure and functional properties. *Kidney Int* 1985;**27:**607.

Oikawa S et al: Cloning and sequence analysis of cDNA encoding a precursor for human atrial polypeptide. *Nature* 1984;**309:**724.

Ramsay DJ: The effects of circulating angiotensin II on the brain. Page 263 in: *Frontiers in Neuroendocrinology.* Vol 7. Ganong WF, Martini L (editors). Raven Press, 1982.

Reid IA, Morris BJ, Ganong WF: The renin-angiotensin system. *Annu Rev Physiol* 1978;**40:**377.

Seidah NG et al: Amino-acid sequence of homologous rat atrial peptides: Natriuretic activity of native and synthetic forms. *Proc Natl Acad Sci USA* 1984;**81:**2640.

Symposium: Biochemistry of the renin-angiotensin system. *Fed Proc* 1983;**42:**2272.

Yamanaka M et al: Clonic and sequence analysis of the cDNA for the rat atrial natriuretic factor precursor. *Nature* 1984;**309:**719.

Testes

16

Glenn D. Braunstein, MD

The testes contain 2 major components, which are structurally separate and serve different functions. The **Leydig cells,** or **interstitial cells,** comprise the major endocrine component. The primary secretory product of these cells, testosterone, is responsible either directly or indirectly for embryonic differentiation along male lines of the external and internal genitalia, male secondary sexual development at puberty, and maintenance of libido and potency in the adult male. The **seminiferous tubules** comprise the bulk of the testes and are responsible for the production of approximately 30 million spermatozoa per day during male reproductive life (puberty to death).

Both of these testicular components are interrelated, and both require an intact hypothalamic-pituitary axis for initiation and maintenance of their function. In addition, several accessory genital structures are required for the functional maturation and transport of spermatozoa. Thus, disorders of the testes, hypothalamus, pituitary, or accessory structures may result in abnormalities of androgen or gamete production, infertility, or a combination of these problems.

ANATOMY & STRUCTURE-FUNCTION RELATIONSHIPS (Fig 16–1)

TESTES

The adult testis is a spheroid with a mean volume of 18.6 ± 4.8 mL (SD). The average length is 4.6 cm (range, 3.6–5.5 cm), and the average width is 2.6 cm (range, 2.1–3.2 cm). The testes are located within the scrotum, which not only serves as a protective envelope but also helps to maintain the testicular temperature approximately 2 °C below abdominal temperature. Three layers of membranes—visceral tunica vaginalis, tunica albuginea, and tunica vasculosa—comprise the testicular capsule. Extensions of the tunica albuginea into the testicle as fibrous septa result in the formation of approximately 250 pyramidal lob-

Acronyms Used in This Chapter	
ACTH	Adrenocorticotropic hormone
cAMP	Cyclic adenosine monophosphate
DHEA	Dehydroepiandrosterone
FSH	Follicle-stimulating hormone
GnRH	Gonadotropin-releasing hormone
hCG	Human chorionic gonadotropin
LH	Luteinizing hormone
mRNA	Messenter ribonucleic acid
PRL	Prolactin
SHBG	Sex hormone-binding globulin

ules each of which contains coiled seminiferous tubules. Within each testis there are almost 200 m of seminiferous tubules, and these structures account for 80–90% of the testicular mass. The approximately 350 million androgen-producing Leydig cells, as well as the blood and lymphatic vessels, nerves, and fibroblasts, are interspersed between the seminiferous tubules.

The blood supply to the testes is derived chiefly from the testicular arteries, which are branches of the internal spermatic arteries. After traversing a complicated capillary network, blood enters multiple testicular veins that form an anastomotic network, the pampiniform plexus. The pampiniform plexuses coalesce to form the internal spermatic veins. The right spermatic vein drains directly into the vena cava; the left enters the renal vein.

The seminiferous tubules in the adult average 165 μm in diameter and are composed of Sertoli cells and germinal cells. The Sertoli cells line the basement membrane and form tight junctions with other Sertoli cells. These tight junctions prevent the passage of proteins from the interstitial space into the lumen of the seminiferous tubules, thus establishing a "blood-testis barrier." Through extension of cytoplasmic processes, the Sertoli cells surround developing germ cells and provide an environment essential for germ cell differentiation. In addition, these cells have been shown to be responsible for the movement of germ cells from the base of the tubule toward the lumen and for the release of mature sperm into the lumen. These cells also actively phagocytose damaged germ cells and residual

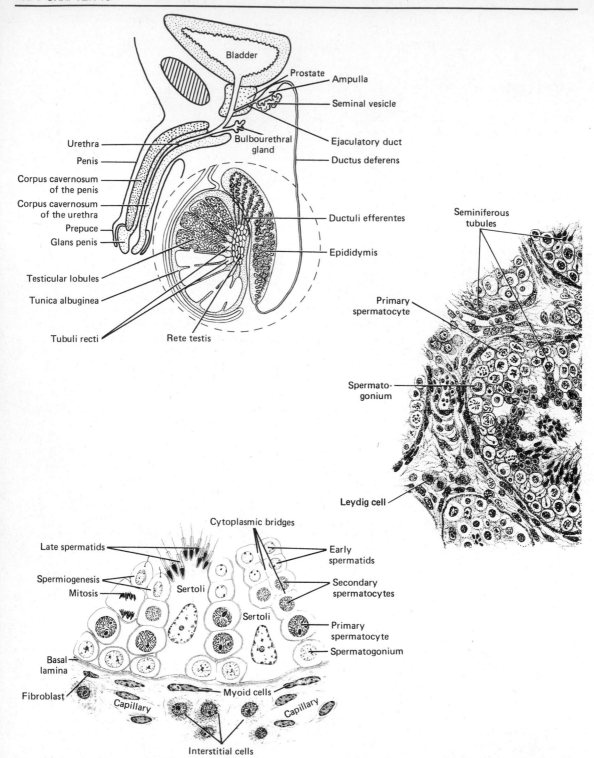

Figure 16–1. Male genital system. *Top:* The testis and the epididymis are in different scales from the other parts of the reproductive system. Observe the communication between the testicular lobules. *Bottom:* Structural organization of the human seminiferous tubule and interstitial tissue. This figure does not show the lymphatic vessels frequently found in the connective tissue. (Both illustrations reproduced, with permission, from Junqueira LC, Carneiro J, Kelley RO: *Basic Histology,* 6th ed. Appleton & Lange, 1989.) *At right:* Section of human testis. (Reproduced, with permission, from Ganong WF: *Review of Medical Physiology,* 14th ed. Appleton & Lange, 1989.)

bodies, which are portions of the germ cell cytoplasm not used in the formation of spermatozoa. Finally, in response to follicle-stimulating hormone (FSH) or testosterone, the Sertoli cells secrete androgen-binding protein, a molecule with high affinity for androgens. This substance, which enters the tubular lumen, provides a high concentration of testosterone to the developing germinal cells during the process of spermatogenesis.

More than a dozen different types of germ cells have been described in males. Broadly, they can be classified as spermatogonia, primary spermatocytes, secondary spermatocytes, spermatids, and spermatozoa. Spermatogenesis occurs in an orderly fashion, with the spermatocytes being derived from the spermatogonia via mitotic division. Through meiotic (or reduction) division, the spermatids are formed; they contain a haploid number of chromosomes (23). The interval from the beginning of spermatogenesis to release of mature spermatozoa into the tubular lumen is approximately 74 days. Although there is little variation in the duration of the spermatogenic cycle, a cross section of a seminiferous tubule will demonstrate several stages of germ cell development.

ACCESSORY STRUCTURES

The seminiferous tubules empty into a highly convoluted anastomotic network of ducts called the rete testis. Spermatozoa are then transported through efferent ductules and into a single duct, the epididymis, by testicular fluid pressure, ciliary motion, and contraction of the efferent ductules. During the approximately 12 days required for transit through the epididymis, spermatozoa undergo morphologic and functional changes essential to confer upon the gametes the capacity for fertilizing an ovum. The epididymis also serves as a reservoir for sperm. Spermatozoa stored in the epididymis enter the vas deferens, a muscular duct 35–50 cm long that propels its contents by peristaltic motion into the ejaculatory duct.

In addition to the spermatozoa and the secretory products of the testes, retia testis, and epididymides, the ejaculatory ducts receive fluid from the seminal vesicles. These paired structures, 10–20 cm long, are composed of alveolar glands, connective tissue, and muscle. They are the source of seminal plasma fructose, which provides nourishment to the spermatozoa. In addition, the seminal vesicles secrete phosphorylcholine, ergothioneine, ascorbic acid, flavins, and prostaglandins. About 60% of the total volume of seminal fluid is derived from the seminal vesicles.

The ejaculatory ducts terminate in the prostatic urethra. There additional fluid (approximately 20% of total volume) is added by the prostate, a tubuloalveolar gland with a fibromuscular stroma that weighs about 20 g and measures 4 × 2 × 3 cm. The constituents of the prostate fluid include spermine, citric acid, cholesterol, phospholipids, fibrinolysin, fibrinogenase, zinc, and acid phosphatase. Fluid is also added to the seminal plasma by the bulbourethral (Cowper) glands and urethral (Littre) glands during its transit through the penile urethra.

PHYSIOLOGY OF THE MALE REPRODUCTIVE SYSTEM

GONADAL STEROIDS (Fig 16–2)

The 3 steroids of primary importance in male reproductive function are testosterone, dihydrotestosterone, and estradiol. From a quantitative standpoint, the most important androgen is testosterone. Over 95% of the testosterone is secreted by the testicular Leydig cells; the remainder is derived from the adrenals. In addition to testosterone, the testes secrete small amounts of the potent androgen dihydrotestosterone and the weak androgens dehydroepiandrosterone (DHEA) and androstenedione. The Leydig cells also secrete small quantities of estradiol, estrone, pregnenolone, progesterone, 17α-hydroxypregnenolone, and 17α-hydroxyprogesterone. The steps in testicular androgen biosynthesis are illustrated in Figure 16–2.

Dihydrotestosterone and estradiol are derived not only by direct secretion from the testes but also by conversion in peripheral tissues of androgen and estrogen precursors secreted by both the testes and the adrenals. Thus, about 80% of the circulating concentrations of these 2 steroids is derived from such peripheral conversion. Table 16–1 summarizes the approximate contributions of the testes, adrenals, and peripheral tissues to the circulating levels of several sex steroid hormones in men.

In the blood, androgens and estrogens exist in either a free (unbound) state or bound to serum proteins. Although about 38% of testosterone is bound to albumin, the major binding protein is sex hormone–binding globulin (SHBG), which binds 60% of the testosterone. This protein is distinct from the androgen-binding protein secreted by the Sertoli cells and is synthesized in the liver. The serum concentrations of this protein are increased by estrogen or thyroid hormone administration, hyperthyroidism, and cirrhosis and are decreased by exogenous androgens or growth hormone, hypothyroidism, acromegaly, and obesity. About 2% of the circulating testosterone is not bound to serum proteins and is able to enter cells and exert its metabolic effects. In addition, some of the protein-bound testosterone may dissociate from the protein and enter target tissues; thus, the amount of

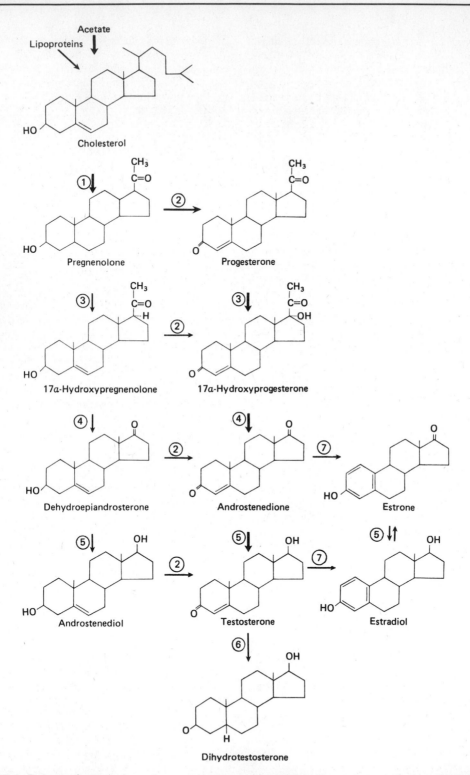

Figure 16–2. Pathways for testicular androgen and estrogen biosynthesis. Heavy arrows indicate major pathways. Circled numbers represent enzymes as follows: ① = 20,22-desmolase (P-450scc); ② = 3β-hydroxysteroid dehydrogenase and Δ⁵,Δ⁴-isomerase; ③ = 17-hydroxylase (P-450scc); ④ = 17,20-desmolase (P-450c17); ⑤ = 17-ketoreductase (P-450c17); ⑥ = 5α-reductase; ⑦ = aromatase. (See also Figs 12–4, 18–13, and 18–14.)

Table 16–1. Relative contributions (approximate percentages) of the testes, adrenals, and peripheral tissues to circulating levels of sex steroids in men.

	Testicular Secretion	Adrenal Secretion	Peripheral Conversion of Precursors
Testosterone	95	<1	<5
Dihydrotestosterone	20	<1	80
Estradiol	20	<1	80
Estrone	2	<1	98
DHEA sulfate	<10	90	. . .

bioavailable testosterone may be greater than just the amount of non–protein-bound testosterone.

As noted below, testosterone may be converted to dihydrotestosterone within specific androgen target tissues. Most circulating testosterone is converted primarily by the liver into various metabolites such as androsterone and etiocholanolone, which, after conjugation with glucuronic or sulfuric acid, are excreted in the urine as 17-ketosteroids. However, it should be noted that only 20–30% of the urinary 17-keto-steroids are derived from testosterone metabolism. The majority of the 17-ketosteroids are formed from the metabolism of adrenal steroids. Therefore, 17-ketosteroid determinations do not reliably reflect testicular steroid secretion.

Testosterone leaves the circulation and rapidly traverses the cell membrane (Fig 16–3). In most androgen target cells, testosterone is enzymatically converted to the more potent androgen dihydrotestosterone by the microsomal enzyme 5α-reductase. Dihydrotestosterone as well as testosterone then binds to the same specific intracytoplasmic receptor protein (R_c in Fig 16–3) that is distinct from both androgen-binding protein and SHBG. The genes that code for this protein are located on the X chromosome. After binding, the dihydrotestosterone- or testosterone-receptor complex is translocated into the nucleus, where it undergoes transformation (to R_n in Fig 16–3), allowing it to bind to the nuclear chromatin. The interaction of the androgen-receptor complex with the chromatin results in the synthesis of messenger RNA (mRNA), which is eventually transported to the cytoplasm, where it directs the transcription of new protein synthesis and other changes that together constitute androgen action.

A variety of biologic effects of androgens have been defined in males. As discussed in Chapter 18, they are essential for appropriate differentiation of the internal and external male genital system during fetal development. During puberty, androgen-mediated growth of the scrotum, epididymis, vas deferens, seminal vesicles, prostate, and penis occurs. The functional integrity of these organs requires androgens. Androgens stimulate skeletal muscle growth and growth of the

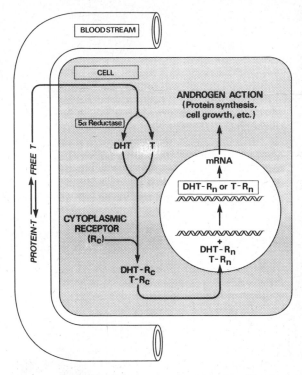

Figure 16–3. Mechanisms of androgen action. T = testosterone; DHT = dihydrotestosterone; R_n = nuclear receptor; mRNA = messenger RNA; R_c = cytoplasmic receptor.

larynx, which results in deepening of the voice; and of the epiphyseal cartilaginous plates, which results in the pubertal growth spurt. Both ambisexual (pubic and axillary) hair growth and sexual (beard, mustache, chest, abdomen, and back) hair growth are stimulated, as is sebaceous gland activity. Other effects include stimulation of erythropoiesis and social behavioral changes.

CONTROL OF TESTICULAR FUNCTION

Hypothalamic-Pituitary-Leydig Cell Axis (Fig 16–4)

The hypothalamus synthesizes a decapeptide, gonadotropin-releasing hormone (GnRH), and secretes it in pulses every 90–120 minutes into the hypothalamohypophyseal portal blood. After reaching the anterior pituitary, GnRH binds to the gonadotropes and stimulates the release of both luteinizing hormone (LH) and, to a lesser extent, FSH into the general circulation. LH is taken up by the Leydig cells, where it binds to specific membrane receptors. This leads to activation of adenylate cyclase and generation of

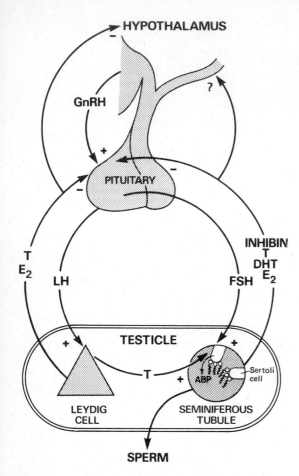

Figure 16–4. Hypothalamic-pituitary-testicular axis. GnRH = gonadotropin-releasing hormone; LH = luteinizing hormone; FSH = follicle-stimulating hormone; T = testosterone; DHT = dihydrotestosterone; ABP = androgen-binding protein; E_2 = estradiol; + = positive influence; − = negative influence.

cAMP and other messengers that ultimately result in the secretion of androgens. In turn, the elevation of androgens inhibits the secretion of LH from the anterior pituitary through a direct action on the pituitary and an inhibitory effect at the hypothalamic level. Both the hypothalamus and the pituitary have androgen and estrogen receptors. Experimentally, pure androgens such as dihydrotestosterone (DHT) reduce LH pulse frequency, while estradiol reduces LH pulse amplitude. However, the major inhibitory effect of androgen on the hypothalamus appears to be mediated principally by estradiol, which may be derived locally through the aromatization of testosterone. Leydig cells also secrete small quantities of oxytocin, lipotropin, β-endorphin, dynorphin, angiotensin, and prostaglandins, which may be important for the paracrine regulation of testicular function.

Hypothalamic-Pituitary-Seminiferous Tubular Axis (Fig 16–4)

After stimulation by GnRH, the gonadotropes secrete FSH into the systemic circulation. This glycoprotein hormone binds to specific receptors in the Sertoli cells and stimulates the production of androgen-binding protein. FSH is necessary for the initiation of spermatogenesis. However, full maturation of the spermatozoa appears to require not only an FSH effect but also testosterone. Indeed, the major action of FSH on spermatogenesis may be via the stimulation of androgen-binding protein production, which allows a high intratubular concentration of testosterone to be maintained.

In addition to androgen-binding protein, the Sertoli cell secretes several other substances including GnRH-like peptide, transferrin, plasmogen activator, ceruloplasmin, müllerian duct inhibitory factor, H-Y antigen, and inhibin. At least 3 genes have been found to direct inhibin synthesis. Two forms of inhibin have been identified, inhibin A and inhibin B. Both are 32,000-dalton proteins composed of the same alpha subunit cross-linked with different beta subunits, and each can selectively inhibit FSH release from the pituitary without affecting LH release. FSH directly stimulates the Sertoli cells to secrete inhibin, and therefore inhibin is probably a physiologic regulator of pituitary FSH secretion, possibly together with the gonadal steroids.

Two additional inhibin-related proteins that have been identified in porcine follicular fluid may also be present in the testes. These factors, designated follicle regulatory protein and activin, are composed of inhibin beta subunit dimers and can selectively stimulate pituitary secretion in vitro. They are structurally similar to transforming growth factor-β, which can also stimulate pituitary FSH release. The physiologic role, if any, that follicle regulatory protein, activin, and transforming growth factor-β have in the regulation of FSH secretion is unknown.

ERECTION & EJACULATION

The male sexual response may be divided into 4 distinct stages: excitement, plateau, orgasm, and resolution. Erotic stimuli result in increased blood pressure, increased cutaneous blood flow, and erection during the excitement stage. Penile erection occurs when blood flow to the penile erectile tissue (corpora cavernosa and spongiosum) increases as a result of dilatation of the urethral artery, the artery of the bulb of the penis, the deep artery of the penis, and the dorsal artery of the penis. Concurrent contraction of the ischiocavernosus muscle leads to compression of the veins draining the corpora cavernosa and spongiosum. This combination results in the distention, engorgement, and rigidity of the penis that constitute erection. Erection is an involuntary reflex that may occur via 2 different mechanisms. Psychogenic stimuli transmitted to the limbic system stimulate the thoracolumbar (T12–L2) parasympathetic nerves, and this in turn results in dilatation of the arteriolar vessels that supply the corpora cavernosa and spongiosum. In addition to the thoracolumbar center, sacral parasympathetic (S2–4) nerves may be activated by direct genital stimuli. The afferent limb for the spinal reflex arc is located within the pudendal nerves.

The plateau phase is the period between the initiation of erection and ejaculation. The duration of this phase is variable. While it lasts, mucus is secreted by Cowper's and Littre's glands.

Orgasm occurs in 2 stages. The first stage consists of reflex activity of the thoracolumbar sympathetic nerves, resulting in rhythmic contractions of the vas deferens, prostate, and seminal vesicles. These contractions propel sperm and seminal fluid into the posterior portion of the urethra (emission). Simultaneously, the bladder neck contracts by closure of the internal sphincter. The presence of semen in the urethral bulb leads to a feeling of impending or inevitable ejaculation. The second stage of the orgasmic phase is the ejaculatory reflex. Ejaculation is mediated through the pudendal nerves, which induce rhythmic contractions—at intervals of 0.8 second—of the bulbocavernosus and ischiocavernosus muscles. These contractions force semen out of the penis. During ejaculation, impulses are transmitted through the anterolateral tracts of the spinal cord to the cerebral cortex, where orgasm is perceived.

Following orgasm, the blood in the corpora cavernosa and spongiosum rapidly leaves the penis, resulting in a return to the flaccid state (resolution phase). A variable interval must elapse following the resolution phase before the sequence can be repeated (refractory period).

EVALUATION OF MALE GONADAL FUNCTION

CLINICAL EVALUATION

Clinical Presentation

The clinical presentation of patients with deficient testosterone production or action depends upon the age at onset of hypogonadism. Androgen deficiency during the second to third months of fetal development results in varying degrees of ambiguity of the genitalia and male pseudohermaphroditism. These topics are covered in Chapters 18 and 19.

Prepubertal androgen deficiency leads to poor secondary sexual development and eunuchoid skeletal proportions (Table 16–2). The penis fails to enlarge, the testes remain small, and the scrotum does not develop the marked rugae characteristic of puberty. The voice remains high-pitched and the muscle mass does not develop fully, resulting in less than normal strength and endurance. The lack of appropriate stimulation of sexual hair growth results in sparse axillary and pubic hair (which receive some stimulation from adrenal androgens) and absent or very sparse facial, chest, upper abdominal, and back hair. Although the androgen-mediated pubertal growth spurt will fail to take place, the epiphyseal plates of the long bones will continue to grow under the influence of somatomedins and other growth factors. Thus, the long bones of the upper and lower extremities will grow out of proportion to the axial skeleton. Healthy white men have an average upper segment (crown to pubis) to lower segment (pubis to floor) ratio of >1, whereas prepubertal hypogonadism results in a ratio of <1. Similarly, the ratio of total arm span to total height averages 0.96 in white men. Because of the relatively greater growth in the upper extremities, the arm span of eunuchoid individuals exceeds height by 5 cm or more.

If testosterone deficiency develops after puberty, the patient may complain of decreased libido, impotence, and low energy. Patients with mild androgen deficiency or androgen deficiency of recent onset may not note a decrease in facial or body hair growth; it appears that although adult androgen levels must be achieved to *stimulate* male sexual hair growth, relatively low levels of androgens are required to *maintain* sexual hair growth. With long-standing hypogonadism, the growth of facial hair will diminish, and the frequency of shaving may also decrease (Fig 16–5). In addition, fine wrinkles may appear in the corners of the mouth and eyes and, together with the sparse beard growth, result in the classic hypogonadal facies.

Genital Examination

Adequate assessment of the genitalia is essential in the evaluation of male hypogonadism. The examina-

Table 16–2. Clinical findings in eunuchoidism.

Symptoms
Deficient growth of axillary, pubic, facial, and body hair.
Low or absent libido, erections, potency.
Diminished strength and endurance compared with age mates.

Signs
Failure to manifest pubertal growth spurt.
Eunuchoid skeletal proportions (upper/lower segment ratio <1; arm span/height ratio >1).
Sparse axillary, pubic, facial, and body hair.
Poor muscle development.
High-pitched (childish) voice.
Small penis, testes, scrotum, and prostate.
Osteoporosis with long-standing hypogonadism.

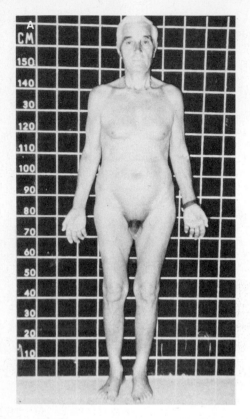
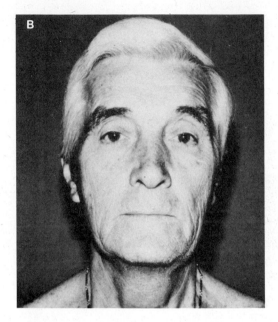

Figure 16–5. *A:* Hypogonadal habitus. Note absence of body and facial hair as well as feminine body distribution. *B.* Hypogonadal facies. Note absence of facial hair and fine wrinkles around the corners of the eyes and lips.

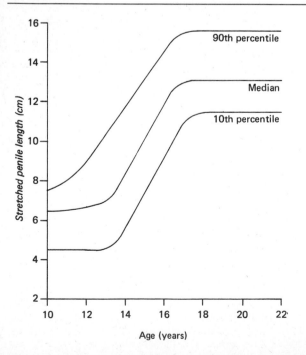
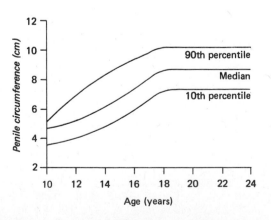

Figure 16–6. Penile length and circumference at various ages. *Left:* Normal values for stretched penile length. *Right:* Normal values for penile circumference. (Both redrawn and reproduced, with permission, from Schonfeld WA: *Am J Dis Child* 1943;**65**:535. Copyright © 1943 by the American Medical Association.)

tion should be performed in a warm room in order to relax the dartos muscle of the scrotum. The penis should be examined for the presence of hypospadias, epispadias, and chordee (abnormal angulation of the penis due to a fibrotic plaque), which may interfere with fertility. The fully stretched dorsal penile length should be measured in the flaccid state from the pubopenile skin junction to the tip of the glans. Penile circumference may also be measured in the flaccid state. Both of these measurements may be compared to normal values (Fig 16–6).

Assessment of testicular volume is also vital to the evaluation of hypogonadism. Careful measurement of the longitudinal and transverse axes of the testes may be made and testicular volume (V) calculated from the formula for a prolate spheriod: $V = 0.52 \times \text{length} \times \text{width}^2$. The mean volume for an adult testis is 18.6 ± 4.8 (SD) mL. The normal ranges for pre- and postpubertal individuals are shown in Figure 16–7. Alternatively, volume may be estimated with the Prader orchidometer, which consists of a series of plastic ellipsoids ranging in volume from 1 to 25 mL (Fig 16–8). Each testis is compared to the appropriate ellipsoid. Adults normally have volumes greater than 15 mL by this method.

Since 80–90% of testicular volume is composed of seminiferous tubules, decrease in volume indicates lack of tubular development or regression of tubular size. The consistency of the testicle should be noted. Small, firm testes are characteristic of hyalinization or fibrosis, as may occur in Klinefelter's syndrome. Small, rubbery testes are normally found in prepubertal males; in an adult, they are indicative of deficient gonadotropin stimulation. Testes with a mushy or soft consistency are characteristically found in individuals with postpubertal testicular atrophy.

The epididymis and vas deferens should also be examined. One of the most important parts of the exam-

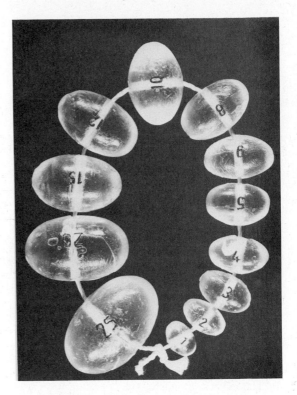

Figure 16–8. Prader orchidometer.

ination is evaluation of the presence of varicocele resulting from incompetence of the internal spermatic vein. As will be discussed later, this is an important and potentially correctable form of male infertility. The patient should be examined in the upright position while performing the Valsalva maneuver. The examiner should carefully palpate the spermatic cords above the testes. A varicocele can be felt as an impulse along the posterior portion of the cord. About 85% of varicoceles are located on the left side, and 15% are bilateral. A unilateral varicocele is rare.

LABORATORY TESTS OF TESTICULAR FUNCTION

Semen Analysis

With some exceptions, a normal semen analysis excludes gonadal dysfunction. However, a single abnormal semen analysis is not a sufficient basis for a diagnosis of disturbance of testicular function, since marked variations in several of the parameters may be seen in normal individuals: At least 3 semen samples must be examined over a 2- to 3-month interval in order to evaluate this facet of male gonadal function. As noted above, approximately 3 months are required for completion of the spermatogenic cycle and movement of the mature spermatozoa through the ductal system. Therefore, when an abnormal semen sample is

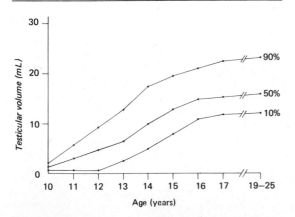

Figure 16–7. Normal values for testicular volume in relation to age. (Redrawn and reproduced, with permission, from Zachmann M et al: *Helv Paediatr Acta* 1974;**29**:61.)

produced, one must question the patient about prior fever, trauma, drug exposure, and other factors that may temporarily damage spermatogenesis.

The semen should be collected by masturbation after 1–3 days of sexual abstinence. If the patient will not masturbate, a specially designed plastic condom (Mylex Corporation, Chicago) can be used during intercourse. Ordinary condoms cannot be used for this purpose, since they contain spermicidal chemicals. If neither of these methods is satisfactory, coitus interruptus may be used as long as the complete ejaculate is collected. It should be stressed to the patient that the greatest concentration of spermatozoa is in the first portion of the ejaculate and that this is the portion most often lost during coitus interruptus.

The specimen should be examined by an experienced technologist within 2 hours after collection. Normal values for semen analysis are given in Table 16–3.

Steroid Measurements

Each of the gonadal steroids may be measured by radioimmunoassay. Although single determinations may distinguish between normal individuals and patients with severe hypogonadism, mild defects in androgen production may be missed. In normal individuals, there are frequent, rapid pulsatile changes in serum testosterone concentration as well as a slight nocturnal elevation. Therefore, at least 3 separate blood samples should be collected at 20- to 40-minute intervals during the morning for testosterone measurement. The testosterone may be measured in each of the serum samples, or equal aliquots of each of the 3 serum samples may be combined, mixed, and subjected to testosterone analysis. The latter procedure provides a savings in cost as well as a mean serum testosterone concentration that takes into account the pulsatile release of testosterone.

Androgen and estrogen radioimmunoassays measure total serum steroid concentrations. This is the sum of the free, biologically active hormone and the protein-bound moiety. Although in most circumstances it is not necessary to determine the actual quantity of free steroid hormones, in some situations alterations in the

Table 16–4. Normal ranges for gonadal steroids, pituitary gonadotropins, and prolactin in men. SI units are shown in parentheses.

Testosterone	300–1100	ng/dL	(10.4–38.2	nmol/L)
Free testos-terone	50–210	pg/mL	(1.7–7.28	pmol/L)
Dihydrotestos-terone	25–75	ng/dL	(0.9–2.6	nmol/L)
Androstenedione	50–200	ng/dL	(1.7–6.9	nmol/L)
Estradiol	15–40	pg/mL	(55–150	pmol/L)
Estrone	15–65	pg/mL	(55.5–240	pmol/L)
FSH	2–15	mIU/mL	(2–15	IU/L)
LH	2–15	mIU/mL	(2–15	IU/L)
PRL	4–18	ng/mL	(4–18	μg/L)

binding protein concentration may occur. Lowered concentrations of SHBG are seen in patients with hypothyroidism, obesity, and acromegaly. In these circumstances, the free testosterone concentration should be directly measured, since it may be normal when the total serum testosterone level is decreased. The normal male serum concentrations of gonadal steroids collected in the basal state are given in Table 16–4.

Gonadotropin & Prolactin Measurements

LH and, to a lesser extent, FSH are released in pulsatile fashion throughout the day. Therefore, as with testosterone, at least 3 blood samples should be obtained at 20- to 40-minute intervals during the day. FSH and LH may be measured in each of the samples or in a single pooled specimen. Although many laboratories give a numerical value for the lower limits of normal for gonadotropins, some normal males have concentrations of FSH and LH undetectable by presently available radioimmunoassay techniques. Furthermore, the concentrations of gonadotropins measured in one laboratory may not be directly comparable to those measured in another because of differences in the reference preparations used. The primary use of basal FSH and LH concentrations is to distinguish between hypergonadotropic hypogonadism, in which either or both of the gonadotropins are elevated, and hypogonadotropic hypogonadism, in which the gonadotropins are low or inappropriately normal in the presence of decreased androgen production.

Elevations of serum prolactin (PRL) inhibit the normal release of pituitary gonadotropins (shown by a reduced LH pulse frequency), probably through an effect on the hypothalamus. Thus, serum PRL measurements should be performed in any patient with hypogonadotropic hypogonadism. Serum PRL concentrations are generally stable throughout the day; therefore, measurement of this hormone in a single sample is usually sufficient. However, the patient should abstain from eating for 3 hours before the blood sample is obtained, since a protein meal may acutely stimulate the release of PRL from the pituitary. The

Table 16–3. Normal values for semen analysis.

Liquefaction time: 3–25 minutes[1]
Volume: 1–6 mL
Concentration of sperm: ≥20 × 10⁶/mL; ≥60 × 10⁶ in total ejaculate
Motility of sperm: ≥2+ on a scale of 1–4+
Morphology: ≥60% normal or oval

[1]Following ejaculation, the semen forms a coagulum that is liquefied by proteolytic enzymes from the prostate.

0 = no motility; 1+ = sperm motile without forward progression; 2+ = sperm motile with slow forward progression; 3+ = sperm motile with forward progression at moderate to good rate of speed; 4+ = sperm motile, moving at high speed and in a straight line.

normal ranges for serum PRL and gonadotropins are shown in Table 16–4.

Dynamic Tests

A. Chorionic Gonadotropin Stimulation Test: (Fig 16–9.) Human chorionic gonadotropin (hCG) is a glycoprotein hormone with biologic actions similar to those of LH. Following an injection of chorionic gonadotropin, this hormone binds to the LH receptors on the Leydig cells and stimulates the synthesis and secretion of testicular steroids. Therefore, the Leydig cells may be directly assessed by the intramuscular injection of 4000 IU of chorionic gonadotropin daily for 4 days. A normal response is a doubling of the testosterone level following the last injection. Alternatively, a single intramuscular dose of chorionic gonadotropin (5000 IU/1.7 m² in adults or 100 IU/kg in children) may be given, with blood samples taken for testosterone measurements 72 and 96 hours later. Patients with primary gonadal disease will have a diminished response following administration of chorionic gonadotropin, while patients with Leydig cell failure secondary to pituitary or hypothalamic disease will have a qualitatively normal response.

B. Clomiphene Citrate Stimulation Test: (Fig 16–10.) Clomiphene citrate (Clomid) is a nonsteroid compound with weak estrogenic activity. It binds to estrogen receptors in various tissues, including the hypothalamus. By preventing the more potent estrogen

estradiol from occupying these receptors, the hypothalamus in effect "sees" less estradiol. As noted above, most if not all of the hypothalamic-pituitary feedback control by testicular androgens is mediated by estradiol, which is derived from the peripheral conversion of androgens. The apparent estradiol deficiency leads to an increase of GnRH release the net result of which is stimulation of the gonadotropes to secrete increased quantities of LH and FSH.

The test is performed by giving clomiphene citrate, 100 mg orally twice daily for 10 days. Three blood samples are collected at 20-minute intervals (see comments above, under Steroid Measurements) 1 day before the drug is administered and again on days 9 and 10 of drug administration. LH, FSH, and testosterone should be measured in pooled aliquots from each of these samples. Healthy men have a 50–250% increase in LH, a 30–200% increase in FSH, and a 30–220% increase in testosterone on day 10 of the test. Patients with pituitary or hypothalamic disease do not show a normal increment in LH or FSH.

C. Gonadotropin-Releasing Hormone Test: (Fig 16–11). The decapeptide GnRH (gonadorelin; Factrel) directly stimulates the gonadotropes of the anterior pituitary to secrete LH and FSH. It was expected that measurement of LH and FSH following the administration of GnRH would be useful in distinguishing between hypothalamic and pituitary lesions, but this has not proved to be the case. Patients

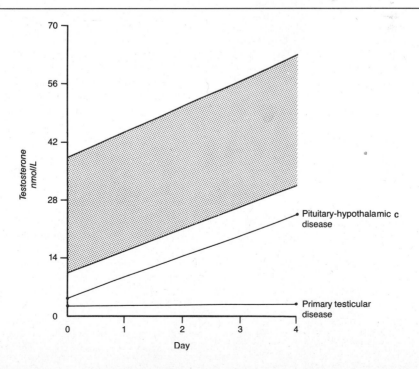

Figure 16–9. Testosterone response following stimulation with chorionic gonadotropin, 4000 IU/d intramuscularly, in normal males (shaded area) and in patients with primary and secondary hypogonadism.

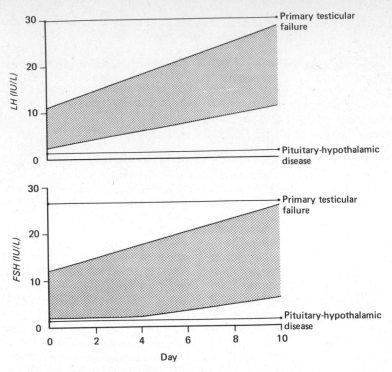

Figure 16–10. LH and FSH response following 10 days of clomiphene citrate, 200 mg/d, in normal males (shaded areas) and in patients with primary and secondary hypogonadism.

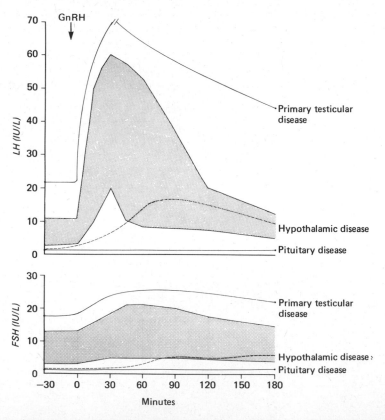

Figure 16–11. LH and FSH responses following a bolus injection of GnRH (gonadorelin; Factrel) in normal males (shaded areas) and in patients with primary testicular, hypothalamic, or pituitary disease. Note that patients with hypothalamic disorders may have a quantitatively normal but delayed rise. Some patients with hypothalamic disease show no response, while some patients with pituitary disease demonstrate a normal response.

with destructive lesions of the pituitary and those with long-standing hypogonadism due to hypothalamic disorders may not show a response to a GnRH test. However, if the releasing factor is administered by repeated injections every 60–120 minutes or by a programmable pulsatile infusion pump for 7–14 days, patients with hypothalamic lesions may have their pituitary responsiveness to GnRH restored, whereas patients with pituitary insufficiency do not. Conversely, a normal LH and FSH response to GnRH in a hypogonadal male does not eliminate hypopituitarism as the cause of the gonadal failure, since patients with mild hypogonadotropic hypogonadism may demonstrate a normal response.

The test is performed by administering 100 μg of gonadorelin by rapid intravenous bolus. Blood is drawn at −15, 0, 15, 30, 45, 60, 90, 120, and 180 minutes for LH and FSH measurements. Normal adult males have a 2- to 5-fold increase in LH over baseline concentrations and an approximately 2-fold rise of FSH. However, some normal males fail to have an increase in FSH following GnRH. Patients with primary testicular disease may respond with exaggerated increases in LH and FSH. If seminiferous tubule damage alone is present, abnormal FSH rise and normal LH response may be seen.

Testicular Biopsy

Testicular biopsy in hypogonadal men is primarily indicated in patients with normal-sized testes and azoospermia in order to distinguish spermatogenic failure and ductal obstruction. Although germinal aplasia, hypoplasia, maturation arrest, and other abnormalities of spermatogenesis may be diagnosed by examination of testicular tissue in oligospermic males, knowledge of the type of defect does not alter therapy. Therefore, testicular biopsy is not usually indicted for evaluation of mild to moderate oligospermia.

Evaluation for Male Hypogonadism

Figure 16–12 outlines an approach to the diagnosis of male gonadal disorders. Semen analysis and determination of the basal concentrations of testosterone, FSH, and LH allow the clinician to distinguish patients with primary gonadal failure who have poor semen characteristics, low or normal testosterone, and elevated FSH or LH from those with secondary gonadal failure and abnormal semen analysis, decreased testosterone, and low or inappropriately normal gonadotropins.

In patients with elevations of gonadotropins resulting from primary testicular disease, chromosomal analysis will help to differentiate between genetic abnormalities and acquired testicular defects. Since no therapy exists that will restore spermatogenesis in an individual with severe testicular damage, androgen replacement is the treatment of choice. Patients with isolated seminiferous tubule failure may have normal or elevated FSH concentrations in association with normal LH and testosterone levels and usually severe oligospermia. Patients with azoospermia require evaluation for the possible presence of ductal obstruction, since this defect may be surgically correctable. Fruc-

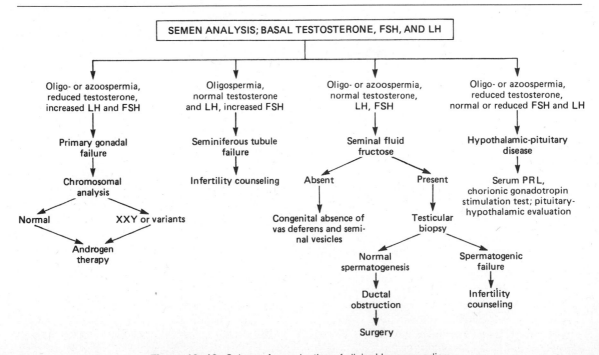

Figure 16–12. Scheme for evaluation of clinical hypogonadism.

tose is added to seminal plasma by the seminal vesicles, and an absence of fructose indicates that the seminal vesicles are absent or bilaterally obstructed. The combination of a poor semen analysis with low testosterone, FSH, and LH is indicative of a hypothalamic or pituitary defect. Such patients need further evaluation of anterior and posterior pituitary gland function with appropriate pituitary function tests, as well as neuroradiologic and neuro-ophthalmologic studies (see Chapter 6).

PHARMACOLOGY OF DRUGS USED TO TREAT MALE GONADAL DISORDERS

ANDROGENS

A variety of drugs are available for the treatment of androgen deficiency. Preparations for sublingual or oral administration such as methyltestosterone, oxymetholone, and fluoxymesterone have the advantage of ease of administration but the disadvantage of erratic absorption, potential for cholestatic jaundice, and decreased effectiveness when compared to the intramuscular preparations. Testosterone propionate is a short-acting androgen. Its main use is in initiating therapy in older men, whose prostate glands may be exquisitely sensitive to testosterone. A dose of 50 mg 2–3 times per week is adequate. Obstructive symptoms due to benign prostatic hypertrophy following therapy with this androgen usually resolve rapidly because of its short duration of action.

Androgen deficiency is currently best treated with testosterone enanthate or cyclopentylpropionate (cypionate) given intramuscularly. The duration of action of these preparations is usually 2 weeks, although some patients note an effect for up to 4 weeks. Unlike the oral androgen preparations, both of these agents are capable of completely virilizing the patients. Therapy may be initiated with 200 mg intramuscularly every 1–2 weeks for 1–2 years. After adequate virilization has been achieved, the androgen effect may be maintained by doses of 100–200 mg every 2–3 weeks. Testosterone pellets may be implanted subcutaneously for a longer duration of effect. However, this therapy has not enjoyed much popularity. Transdermal delivery via a polyethylene-derived membrane impregnated with testosterone is a new method of replacement therapy that should be available soon. The patches must be placed on the scrotum, since this site allows the greatest degree of androgen adsorption through the skin (40 times greater than adsorption through forearm skin). The patches, which must be replaced daily, provide physiologic levels of testosterone that closely mimic the normal diurnal testosterone fluctuation. Elevated serum concentrations of di-

Table 16–5. Adverse effects of androgen therapy.

Prostatic hypertrophy
Cholestatic jaundice (methyltestosterone, fluoxymesterone)
Hepatoma (methyltestosterone, fluoxymesterone)
Premature epiphyseal fusion
Water retention with hypertension
Erythrocytosis
Inhibition of spermatogenesis
Gynecomastia
Priapism
Acne
Aggressive behavior
Alterations of thyroid and adrenal function tests

hydrotestosterone—a finding of unknown clinical significance—have been noted in patients using these patches.

Androgen therapy is contraindicated in patients with known prostatic carcinoma. The adverse reactions that may occur during therapy are listed in Table 16–5. About 1–2% of patients receiving methyltestosterone and fluoxymesterone develop intrahepatic cholestaic jaundice that resolves when the drug is discontinued. Rarely, these methylated or halogenated androgens have been associated with benign and malignant hepatocellular tumors.

Androgen therapy may also cause premature fusion of the epiphyses in an adolescent, and this may result in some loss of potential height. Therefore, androgen therapy is usually withheld until a hypogonadal male reaches 13 years of age. Water retention may be associated with hypertension or congestive heart failure in susceptible individuals. Since androgens stimulate erythropoietin production, erythrocytosis may occur during therapy. This is not usually clinically significant. Inhibition of spermatogenesis is mediated through suppression of gonadotropins by the androgens. Gynecomastia may develop during initiation of androgen therapy but usually resolves with continued administration of the drug. Priapism, acne, and aggressive behavior are dose-related adverse effects and generally disappear after reduction of dosage. Androgens decrease the production of thyroxine-binding globulin and corticosteroid-binding globulin by the liver. Therefore, total serum thyroxine and cortisone concentrations may be decreased though the free hormone concentrations remain normal.

GONADOTROPINS

In patients with hypogonadism due to inadequate gonadotropin secretion, spermatogenesis and virilization may be induced by exogenous gonadotropin injections. Since the gonadotropins are proteins with short half-lives, they must be administered parenterally 2–3 times a week.

The expense and inconvenience of this type of therapy preclude its routine use for the treatment of androgen deficiency. The 2 major indications for exogenous gonadotropins are treatment of cryptorchidism (see below) and induction of spermatogenesis in hypogonadal males who wish to father children.

To induce spermatogenesis, 2000 IU of chorionic gonadotropin may be given intramuscularly 3 times a week for 12–18 months. In some individuals with partial gonadotropin deficiencies, this may induce adequate spermatogenesis. In patients with more severe deficiencies, menotropins (Pergonal), available in bottles containing 75 IU each of FSH and LH, is added to chorionic gonadotropin therapy after 12–18 months and is administered in a dosage of one vial intramuscularly 3 times a week.

Adverse reactions with such therapy are minimal. Acne, gynecomastia, or prostatic enlargement may be noted due to excessive Leydig cell stimulation. Reduction of the chorionic gonadotropin dosage or a decrease in the frequency of chorionic gonadotropin injections generally result in resolution of the problem.

GONADOTROPIN-RELEASING HORMONE

GnRH (gonadorelin, Factrel), administered in pulses every 60–120 minutes by portable infusion pumps, effectively stimulates the endogenous release of LH and FSH in hypogonadotropic hypogonadal patients. This therapy does not currently appear to offer any major advantage over the use of exogenous gonadotropins for induction of spermatogenesis or the use of testosterone enanthate or cypioante for virilization. A long-acting analogue of GnRH, leuprolide acetate (Leupron), is available for the treatment of prostatic carcinoma. Daily subcutaneous administration of 1 mg of leuprolide or monthly intramuscular injections of 7.5 mg of a Depot preparation (Lupron) results in desensitization of the pituitary GnRH receptors, which reduces LH and FSH levels and so ultimately testosterone concentrations. With this therapy, initial remission rates for prostatic carcinoma are similar to those found with orchiectomy or treatment with diethylstilbestrol (about 70%). In patients with benign prostatic hypertrophy, prostate size has been reduced with this therapy. Long-acting GnRH agonists combined with testosterone have been studied as a possible male contraceptive, but they do not uniformly induce azoospermia.

CLINICAL MALE GONADAL DISORDERS

Hypogonadism may be subdivided into 3 general categories (Table 16–6). A thorough discussion of the hypothalamic-pituitary disorders that cause hypogonadism is presented in Chapters 6 and 19. The de-

Table 16–6. Classification of male hypogonadism.

Hypothalamic-pituitary disorders
  Panhypopituitarism
  Isolated LH deficiency (fertile eunuch)
  LH and FSH deficiency
    a. With normal sense of smell
    b. With hyposmia or anosmia (Kallmann's syndrome)
  Prader-Willi syndrome
  Laurence-Moon-Biedl syndrome
  Cerebellar ataxia
  Biologically inactive LH
Gonadal abnormalities
  Klinefelter's syndrome
  Other chromosomal defects (XX male, XY/XXY, XX/XXY, XXXY, XXXXY, XXYY, XYY)
  Bilateral anorchia (vanishing testes syndrome)
  Leydig cell aplasia
  Cryptorchidism
  Noonan's syndrome
  Myotonic dystrophy
  Adult seminiferous tubule failure
  Adult Leydig cell failure
  Defects in androgen biosynthesis
Defects in androgen action
  Complete androgen insensitivity (testicular feminization)
  Incomplete androgen insensitivity
    a. Type I
    b. Type II (5α-reductase deficiency)

fects in androgen biosynthesis and androgen action are described in Chapter 18. The following section emphasizes the primary gonadal abnormalities.

KLINEFELTER'S SYNDROME (XXY Seminiferous Tubule Dysgenesis)

Klinefelter's syndrome is the most common cause of male hypogonadism. An extra X chromosome is present in about 0.2% of live-born males. Sex chromosome surveys of mentally retarded males have revealed an extra X chromosome in 0.45–2.5% of such individuals. Patients with an XXY genotype have classic Klinefelter's syndrome; those with an XXXY, XXXXY, or XXYY genotype or with XXY/chromosomal mosaicism are considered to have variant forms of the syndrome (see below).

Etiology & Pathophysiology
The XXY genotype is usually due to maternal meiotic nondisjunction, which results in an egg with two X chromosomes. Meiotic nondisjunction during spermatogenesis has also been documented. Both observations correlate positively with the epidemiologic findings that both the mother and the father tend to be older than average at the time of the patient's birth.

At birth there are generally no physical stigmas of Klinefelter's syndrome, and during childhood there are no specific signs or symptoms. The chromosomal defect is expressed chiefly during puberty. As the gonadotropins increase, the seminiferous tubules do not enlarge but rather undergo fibrosis and hyalinization, which results in small, firm testes. Obliteration of the seminiferous tubules results in azoospermia.

In addition to dysgenesis of the seminiferous tubules, the Leydig cells are also abnormal. They are present in clumps and appear to be hyperplastic upon initial examination of a testicular biopsy. However, the Leydig cell mass is not increased, and the apparent hyperplasia is actually due to the marked reduction in tubular volume. Despite the normal mass of tissue, the Leydig cells are functionally abnormal. The testosterone production rate is reduced, and there is a compensatory elevation in serum LH. Stimulation of the Leydig cells with exogenous chorionic gonadotropin results in a subnormal rise in testosterone. The clinical manifestations of androgen deficiency vary considerably from patient to patient. Thus, some individuals have virtually no secondary sexual developmental changes, whereas other are indistinguishable from healthy individuals.

The elevated LH concentrations also stimulate the Leydig cells to secrete increased quantities of estradiol and estradiol precursors. The relatively high estradiol:testosterone ratio is responsible for the variable degrees of feminization and gynecomastia seen in these patients. The elevated estradiol also stimulates the liver to produce SHBG. This may result in total serum testosterone concentrations that are within the low normal range for adult males. However, the free testosterone level may be lower than normal.

The pathogenesis of the eunuchoid proportions, personality, and intellectual deficits and associated medical disorders is presently unclear.

Testicular Pathology

Most of the seminiferous tubules are fibrotic and hyalinized, although occasional Sertoli cells and spermatogonia may be present in some sections. Absence of elastic fibers in the tunica propria is indicative of the dysgenetic nature of the tubules. The Leydig cells are arranged in clumps and appear hyperplastic, although the total mass is normal.

Clinical Features
(Fig 16–13)

A. Symptoms and Signs: There are usually no symptoms before puberty other than poor school performance in some affected individuals. Puberty may be delayed, but not usually by more than 1–2 years. During puberty, the penis and scrotum undergo varying degrees of development, with some individuals appearing normal. Most patients (80%) have diminished facial and torso hair growth. The major complaint is often persistent gynecomastia, which is clinically present in over half of patients. The testes are uniformly small (<2 cm in longest axis) and firm as a result of fibrosis and hyalinization. Other complaints include infertility or insufficient libido and potency. The patient may have difficulty putting into words his embarrassment in situations where he must disrobe in

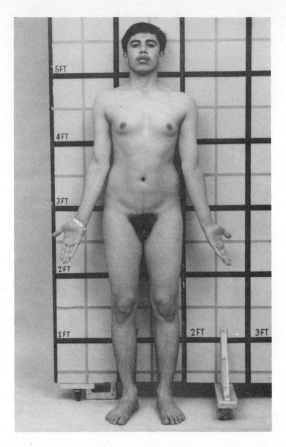

Figure 16–13. Klinefelter's syndrome in a 20-year-old man. Note relatively increased lower/upper body segment ratio, gynecomastia, small penis, and sparse body hair with a female public hair pattern.

the presence of other men, and the subnormal development of the external genitalia along with gynecomastia may lead to feelings of inadequacy that may be partly responsible for the dyssocial behavior some patients exhibit. Osteopenia may be severe in patients with long-standing androgen deficiencies.

Patients with Klinefelter's syndrome have abnormal skeletal proportions that are not truly eunuchoid. Growth of the lower extremities is relatively greater than that of the trunk and upper extremities; therefore, pubis-to-floor height is greater than crown-to-pubis height, and span is less than total height. Thus, the abnormal skeletal proportions are not the result of androgen deficiency per se (which results in span greater than height).

Intellectual impairment is noted in many patients with Klinefelter's syndrome, but the true proportion of affected individuals with subnormal intelligence is not known. Dyssocial behavior is common (see above). Patients generally show want of ambition, difficulties in maintaining permanent employment, and a tendency to ramble in conversations.

Medical disorders found to be associated with Klinefelter's syndrome with greater than chance frequency include chronic pulmonary disease (emphysema, chronic bronchitis), varicose veins, glucose intolerance, primary hypothyroidism, and breast cancer.

B. Laboratory Findings: Serum testosterone is low or normal; FSH and LH concentrations are elevated. Azoospermia is present. The buccal smear is chromatin-positive (>20% of cells having a Barr body), and chromosomal analysis reveals a 47,XXY karyotype.

Differential Diagnosis

Klinefelter's syndrome should be distinguished from other causes of hypogonadism. Small, firm testes should suggest Klinefelter's syndrome. Hypothalamic-pituitary hypogonadism may be associated with small, rubbery testes if puberty has not occurred or atrophic testes if normal puberty has occurred. The consistency of the testes in Klinefelter's syndrome is also different from that noted in acquired forms of adult seminiferous tubular damage. The elevated gonadotropins place the site of the lesion at the testicular level, and chromosomal analysis confirms the diagnosis. Chromosomal analysis is also required to differentiate classic Klinefelter's syndrome from the variant forms.

Treatment

A. Medical: Androgen deficiency should be treated with testosterone replacement. Patients with personality defects should be virilized gradually to decrease the risk of aggressive behavior. Testosterone enanthate or cypionate, 100 mg intramuscularly, may be given every 2–4 weeks initially and increased to 200 mg every 2 weeks if well tolerated. Patients with low normal androgen levels may not require androgen replacement therapy.

B. Surgical: If gynecomastia presents a cosmetic problem, mastectomy may be performed.

Course & Prognosis

Patients generally feel better after androgen replacement therapy has begun. However, the personality defects do not improve, and these patients often require long-term psychiatric counseling. Life expectancy is not affected.

VARIANT KLINEFELTER'S SYNDROME & OTHER CHROMOSOMAL ABNORMALITIES

Several clinical and genotypic variants of Klinefelter's syndrome have been described. The salient clinical features are listed in Table 16–7. In addition to small testes with seminiferous tubular hyalinization, azoospermia, deficient secondary sexual development, and elevated gonadotropins, patients with 3 or more X chromosomes uniformly have severe mental retardation. The presence of more than one Y chromosome tends to be associated with aggressive antisocial behavior and macronodular acne. Skeletal deformities such as radioulnar synostoses, flexion deformities of the elbows, and clinodactyly also are more commonly

Table 16–7. Comparison of classic and variant forms of Klinefelter's syndrome. (Approximate frequencies shown in parentheses if known.) (0 = absent; 1+ = <25%; 2+ = 25–50%; 3+ = 50–75%; 4+ = >75%)

	Klinefelter's (47,XXY) (1:500)	XX Male[1] (1:9000)	XY/XXY[2] (1:1700)	XX/XXY	XXXY[3]	XXXXY[4]	XXYY[5] (1:9000)	XYY[6] (1:1000)
Small testes	4+	4+	3+	4+	4+	4+	4+	0
Azoospermia	4+	4+	3+	4+	4+	4+	4+	0
Deficient secondary sexual development	4+	4+	3+	4+	4+	4+	3+	0
Gynecomastia	2+	2+	2+	2+	3+	0	3+	0
Skeletal deformities	1+	0	1+	0	1+	4+	1+	1+
Mental retardation	1+	0	1+	1+	4+	4+	4+	1+
Cryptorchidism	1+	1+	0	1+	0	2+	1+	0
Increased gonadotropin levels	4+	4+	3+	4+	4+	4+	3+	1+

Other features:
[1] Normal skeletal proportions. Taller than XX female, shorter than XY male.
[2] May be fertile if gonads have XY; testes may have germinal aplasia.
[3] Epicanthal folds, wide mouth.
[4] Peculiar facies, hypoplastic genitalia, congenital heart disease.
[5] Aggressive behavior; tall; varicose veins; acromegalic features.
[6] Antisocial behavior; macronodular acne; tall; electroencephalographic abnormalities; oligospermia.

seen in Klinefelter variants. Patients with sex chromosome mosaicism (XX/XXY) may have only a few of the Klinefelter stigmas. These patients may have normal testicular size and may be fertile if their testes contain the XY genotype.

Phenotypic males with an XY chromosome composition have clinical features similar to those of Klinefelter's syndrome but tend to be shorter and maintain more normal skeletal proportions than patients with the classic syndrome. Mental retardation and behavioral abnormalities also are found less frequently in these patients. Although a Y chromosome is not evident in the karyotype of these patients, their cells do express the H-Y antigen, indicating that X-Y interchange occurs during paternal meiosis or that a Y chromosome-containing cell line was at one time present but was eliminated during development.

Patients with the XXXXY genotype have, in addition to small testes and hypogonadism, severe mental retardation, peculiar facies, and a variety of skeletal deformities. These include epicanthal folds, strabismus, hypertelorism, a broad, flat nose, a large mouth with prognathism, webbing of the neck, and large ears. Patients with the XXXY genotype have clinical features that are intermediate between those with XXXXY and typical Klinefelter's syndrome.

One of the most frequent sex chromosomal abnormalities in phenotypic males is the XYY genotype. In population surveys, this karyotype is found in approximately 1:1000 live male births. However, in penal institutions, the prevalence is 4 times greater; and in combined penal-mental institutions, the frequency is 20 times greater than in the general population. These patients are generally tall, and approximately half have macronodular acne. The aggressive social behavior noted in many of these individuals may in part represent a selection bias, since many of the subjects are identified in prisons. Although some individuals are clearly retarded, mental retardation is seen less frequently than in typical Klinefelter's syndrome. Testicular size is generally normal, and spermatogenesis may be normal or abnormal. Serum testosterone and gonadotropin levels are normal in most patients, although mild elevations of FSH have been noted in patients with the more severe degrees of spermatogenic maturation arrest.

BILATERAL ANORCHIA
(Vanishing Testes Syndrome)

Approximately 3% of phenotypic boys undergoing surgery to correct unilateral or bilateral cryptorchidism are found to have absence of one testis, and in about 1% of cryptorchid males both testes are absent. Thus, bilateral anorchia is found in approximately one out of every 20,000 males.

Etiology & Pathophysiology
(See also Chapters 18 and 19.)

Functional testicular tissue must be present during the first 14–16 weeks of embryonic development in order for wolffian duct growth and müllerian duct regression to occur and for the external genitalia to differentiate along male lines. Absence of testicular function before this time will result in varying degrees of male pseudohermaphroditism with ambiguous genitalia. Prenatal testicular injury occurring after 16 weeks of gestation as a result of trauma, vascular insufficiency, infection, or other mechanisms may result in loss of testicular tissue in an otherwise normal phenotypic male; hence the term "vanishing testes syndrome."

Testicular Pathology

In most instances, no recognizable testicular tissue has been identified despite extensive dissections. Wolffian duct structures are generally normal, and the vas deferens and testicular vessels may terminate blindly or in a mass of connective tissues in the inguinal canal or scrotum.

Clinical Features

A. Symptoms and Signs: At birth, patients appear to be normal phenotypic males with bilateral cryptorchidism. Growth and development are normal until secondary sexual development fails to occur at puberty. The penis remains small; pubic and axillary hair does not fully develop despite the presence of adrenal androgens; and the scrotum remains empty. If the patient does not receive androgens, eunuchoid proportions develop. Gynecomastia does not occur.

An occasional patient will undergo partial spontaneous virilization at puberty. Although anatomically no testicular tissue has been identified in such patients, catheterization studies have demonstrated higher testosterone concentrations in venous blood obtained from the spermatic veins than in the peripheral venous circulation. This suggests that functional Leydig cells are present in some patients, although they are not associated with testicular germinal epithelium or stroma

B. Laboratory Findings: Serum testosterone concentrations are generally quite low, and both LH and FSH are markedly elevated. Serum testosterone concentrations do not rise following a chorionic gonadotropin stimulation test. Chromosomal analysis discloses a 46,XY karyotype.

C. X-Ray Findings: Testicular artery arteriograms and spermatic venograms show vessels that taper and end in the inguinal canal or scrotum without an associated gonad.

D. Special Examinations: Thorough inguinal, abdominal, and retroperitoneal exploration may locate the testes. If testicular vessels and the vas deferens are identified and found to terminate blindly together, it may be assumed that the testis is absent.

Differential Diagnosis

Bilateral cryptorchidism must be differentiated from congenital bilateral anorchia. A normal serum testosterone concentration that rises following stimulation with chorionic gonadotropin is indicative of functional Leydig cells and probable bilateral cryptorchidism. Elevated serum LH and FSH and a low testosterone that fails to rise after administration of exogenous chorionic gonadotropin indicate bilateral absence of functional testicular tissue.

Treatment

Androgen replacement therapy is discussed in the section of pharmacology (see Androgens, above).

Implantation of testicular prostheses for cosmetic purposes may be beneficial after the scrotum has enlarged in response to androgen therapy.

LEYDIG CELL APLASIA

Defective development of testicular Leydig cells is a rare cause of male pseudohermaphroditism with ambiguous genitalia.

Etiology & Pathophysiology

Testes are present in the inguinal canal and contain prepubertal-appearing tubules with Sertoli cells and spermatogonia without germinal cell maturation. The interstitial tissue has a loose myxoid appearance with an absence of Leydig cells. The binding of hCG or LH to testicular extracts from these patients is absent. It is not known whether this represents a primary defect in Leydig cell development due to an abnormality in the Leydig cell precursor cells or is the result of a deficiency of Leydig cell receptors for gonadotropins that may be responsible for inducing Leydig cell differentiation. The presence of a vas deferens and epididymis in these patients indicates that the local concentration of testosterone was high enough during embryogenesis to result in differentiation of the wolffian duct structures. However, the ambiguity of the genitalia indicates that the androgen concentration in these patients was insufficient to bring about full virilization of the external genitalia. The absence of müllerian duct structures is compatible with normal fetal secretion of müllerian duct inhibitory factor from the Sertoli cells.

Clinical Features

A. Symptoms and Signs: These patients may present in infancy with variable degrees of genital ambiguity, including a bifid scrotum, clitoral phallus, urogenital sinus, and blind vaginal pouch. Alternatively, they may appear as normal phenotypic females and escape detection until adolescence, when they present with primary amenorrhea, with or without normal breast development. The gonads are generally located in the inguinal canal. Axillary and pubic hair, although present, may be sparse.

B. Laboratory Findings: Serum gonadotropins are elevated, and testosterone levels are below normal limits for a male and within the low normal range for females. There is no increase in testosterone following chorionic gonadotropin administration.

Differential Diagnosis

Leydig cell aplasia should be differentiated from the vanishing testes syndrome, from testosterone biosynthetic defects, from disorders of androgen action, and from 5α-reductase deficiency. The differential diagnostic features of these disorders are discussed in Chapter 18.

Treatment

Patients with Leydig cell aplasia respond well to the exogenous administration of testosterone, and it would be anticipated that they would be fully virilized and even develop some degree of spermatogenesis with exogenous testosterone administration. However, since the few patients that have been reported have been discovered either late in childhood or as adolescents, it would be inappropriate to attempt a gender reversal at such a late period. Removal of the cryptorchid testes and feminization with exogenous estrogens would appear to be the most prudent course of therapy.

CRYPTORCHIDISM

Cryptorchidism is unilateral or bilateral absence of the testes from the scrotum because of failure of normal testicular descent from the genital ridge through the external inguinal ring. About 3% of full-term male infants have cryptorchidism. In most cases of cryptorchidism noted at birth, spontaneous testicular descent occurs during the first year of life, reducing the incidence to 0.2–0.8% by 1 year of age. Approximately 0.75% of adult males are cryptorchid. Unilateral cryptorchidism is 5–10 times more common than bilateral cryptorchidism.

Almost 50% of cryptorchid testes are located at the external inguinal ring or in a high scrotal position; 19% lie within the inguinal canal between the internal and external inguinal rings (canalicular); 9% are intra-abdominal; and 23% are ectopic, ie, located away from the normal pathway of descent from the abdominal cavity to the scrotum. Most ectopic testes are found in a superficial inguinal pouch above the external inguinal ring.

Etiology & Pathophysiology

Testicular descent usually occurs between the twelfth week of fetal development and birth. Both mechanical and hormonal factors appear to be important for this process: Cryptorchidism is common in patients with congenital defects in androgen synthesis or action and in patients with congenital gonadotropin deficiency, and experimental studies have demonstrated that dihydrotestosterone is required for normal testicular descent. These observations suggest that prenatal androgen deficiency may be of etiologic importance in the development of cryptorchidism.

It is not known whether pathologic changes in the testes are due to the effects of cryptorchidism or to intrinsic abnormalities in the gonad. Experimental studies in animals have shown that an increase in the temperature of the testes by 1.5–2 °C (the temperature differential between the abdomen and scrotum) results in depression of spermatogenesis. Serial testicular biopsies in cryptorchid patients have demonstrated partial reversal of the histologic abnormalities following surgical correction, suggesting that the extrascrotal environment is responsible for the observed pathologic abnormalities.

An intrinsic abnormality in the testes in patients with unilateral cryptorchidism is suggested by the observation that such patients are at increased risk for development of germ cell neoplasms in the scrotal testis. Similarly, the observation that adults with unilateral cryptorchidism surgically corrected before puberty had low sperm counts, high basal serum LH and FSH concentrations, and an exaggerated FSH response to GnRH suggests either that both testes are intrinsically abnormal or that the cryptorchid gonad somehow suppresses the function of the scrotal testis.

Pathology

Histologic studies on cryptorchid testes have demonstrated a decrease in the size of the seminiferous tubules and number of spermatogonia and an increase in peritubular tissue. The Leydig cells usually appear normal. It is unclear at what age these changes first appear. Abnormalities have been detected as early as 18 months to 2 years. It is well established that the longer a testis remains cryptorchid, the more likely it is to show pathologic changes. More severe changes are generally found in intra-abdominal testes than in canalicular testes.

Clinical Features

A. Symptoms and Signs: There are usually no symptoms unless a complication such as testicular torsion, trauma, or malignant degeneration occurs. School-age children may have gender identity problems. Adults may complain of infertility, especially if they have a history of bilateral cryptorchidism.

Absence of one or both testes is the cardinal clinical finding. This may be associated with a small scrotum (bilateral cryptorchidism) or hemiscrotum (unilateral cryptorchidism). Signs of androgen deficiency are not present.

B. Laboratory Findings: Basal or stimulated serum FSH, LH, and testosterone concentrations are not helpful in evaluating prepubertal unilaterally cryptorchid males. However, serum FSH and LH concentrations and the testosterone response to exogenous chorionic gonadotropin are useful in differentiating cryptorchid patients from those with congenital anorchia. The latter have high basal gonadotropins, low serum testosterone, and absent or diminished testosterone rise following chorionic gonadotropin stimulation.

Postpubertal adults may have oligospermia, elevated basal serum FSH and LH concentrations, and an exaggerated FSH increase following GnRH stimulation. Such abnormalities are more prevalent in patients with a history of bilateral cryptorchidism than with unilateral cryptorchidism.

C. X-Ray Findings: Intravenous urography will disclose an associated abnormality of the upper urinary tract in 10% of cases—horseshoe kidney, renal hypoplasia, ureteral duplication, hydroureter, and hydronephrosis.

Differential Diagnosis

Retractile testis (pseudocryptorchidism) is due to a hyperactive cremasteric reflex, which draws the testicle into the inguinal canal. Cold temperature, fear, and genital manipulation commonly activate the reflex, which is most prominent between the ages of 5 and 6 years. The child should be examined with warm hands in a warm room. The testis can usually be "milked" into the scrotum with gentle pressure over the lower abdomen in the direction of the inguinal canal.

Bilateral anorchia is associated with elevated gonadotropins, decreased testosterone, and an absent or subnormal response to stimulation with chorionic gonadotropin.

The virilizing forms of congenital adrenal hyperplasia may result in prenatal fusion of the labial-scrotal folds and clitoral hypertrophy (see Chapter 18). Severely affected females have the appearance of phenotypic males with bilateral cryptorchidism. Because of the potentially disastrous consequences (acute adrenal insufficiency) if this diagnosis is missed, a buccal smear should be performed on bilaterally cryptorchid phenotypic male infants.

Complications & Sequelae

A. Hernia: Approximately 90% of cryptorchid males have associated ipsilateral inguinal hernia resulting from failure of the processus vaginalis to close. This is rarely symptomatic.

B. Torsion: Because of the abnormal connection between the cryptorchid testis and its supporting tissues, torsion may occur. This should be suspected in any patient with abdominal or pelvic pain and an ipsilateral empty scrotum.

C. Trauma: Testes that lie above the pubic tubercle are particularly susceptible to traumatic injury.

D. Neoplasms: A cryptorchid testis is 20–40 times more likely to undergo malignant degeneration than are normal testes. The incidence of such tumors is greater in patients with intra-abdominal testes than in patients with canalicular testes. Seminomas are the neoplasms most commonly associated with maldescended testes. Because of the increased risk of neoplasia, many urologists recommend orchiectomy for a unilaterally undescended testicle in a patient first seen during or after puberty. Patients who present with bilateral cryptorchidism after puberty should have bilateral orchiopexy and testicular biopsies to preserve testicular endocrine function and to make palpation for detection of neoplasia easier.

E. Infertility: Over 90% of untreated bilaterally cryptorchid males are infertile. About 30–50% of bilaterally cryptorchid patients who undergo prepubertal orchiopexy have been found to be fertile. About half of patients with untreated unilateral cryptorchidism are infertile, whereas infertility is found in less than one-fourth of such patients whose cryptorchidism is surgically repaired before puberty.

Prevention

Although cryptorchidism cannot be prevented, the complications can. It is clear that the adverse changes that take place in the testes are related in part to the location of the maldescended testis and the duration of the cryptorchidism. Most testes that are undescended at birth enter the scrotum during the first year of life. However, it is rare for a cryptorchid testis to descend spontaneously after the age of 1 year. Since adverse histologic changes have been noted around the age of 2 years, hormonal or surgical correction should be undertaken at or before that time.

Treatment
A. Medical:
1. Intramuscular chorionic gonadotropin therapy—Because growth of the vas deferens and testicular descent are at least partially dependent upon androgens, stimulation of endogenous testosterone secretion by chorionic gonadotropin may correct the cryptorchidism. Cryptorchidism is corrected in less than 25% of patients treated with a course of chorionic gonadotropin, and recent studies suggest that patients with conditions that respond to hormonal therapy may actually have retractile testes rather than true cryptorchidism. Nevertheless, this therapy should be tried prior to orchiopexy, since it is innocuous and may avoid the need for surgery. For bilateral cryptorchidism, give a short course of chorionic gonadotropin consisting of 3300 units intramuscularly every other day over a 5-day period (3 injections). For unilateral cryptorchidism, give 500 units intramuscularly 3 times a week for 6½ weeks (20 injections).

2. Intranasal GNRH therapy—Recently, GnRH given 3 times a day for 28 days by nasal spray (Cryptolin) has been shown to be as effective as chorionic gonadotropin injections in correcting cryptorchidism in some patients. This preparation of GnRH has not yet been released for clinical use in the USA.

B. Surgical: Several procedures have been devised to place the maldescended testis into the scrotum (orchiopexy). The operation may be performed in one or 2 stages. Inguinal hernia should be repaired if present.

NOONAN'S SYNDROME
(Male Turner's Syndrome)

Phenotypic and genotypic males with many of the physical stigmas of classic Turner's syndrome have been described under a variety of names, including Noonan's syndrome, male Turner's syndrome, pseudo-Turner's syndrome, and Ullrich-Turner syndrome. The incidence and cause of this syndrome are unknown. It may occur sporadically or may be familial, inherited in an autosomal dominant fashion with variable penetrance. A number of pathologic features have been noted, including reduced seminiferous tubular size with or without sclerosis, diminished or absent germ cells, and Leydig cell hyperplasia.

Clinical Features
A. Symptoms and Signs: (Fig 16–14.) The most common clinical features are short stature, webbed neck, and cubitus valgus. Other somatic defects variably observed in these patients are listed in Table 16–8. Congenital cardiac anomalies are common and involve primarily the right side of the heart—in contrast to patients with XO gonadal dysgenesis.

Cryptorchidism is frequently present. Although some affected individuals are fertile, with normal testes, most have small testes and mild to moderate hypogonadism.

B. Laboratory Findings: Serum testosterone concentrations are usually low or low normal, and serum gonadotropins are high. The karyotype is 46,XY.

Differential Diagnosis
The clinical features of Noonan's syndrome are sufficiently distinct so that confusion with other causes of hypogonadism is usually not a problem. However, a rare individual with XY/XO mosaicism may have similar somatic anomalies requiring chromosomal analysis for differentiation.

Treatment
If the patient is hypogonadal, androgen replacement therapy is indicated.

MYOTONIC DYSTROPHY

Myotonic dystrophy is one of the familial forms of muscular dystrophy. About 80% of affected males have some degree of primary testicular failure.

The disorder is transmitted in an autosomal domi-

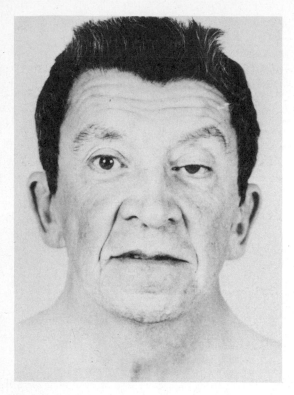

Figure 16–14. Noonan's syndrome. Note ptosis and webbed neck. (Reproduced, with permission, from Bolton MR et al: *Ann Intern Med* 1974;**80**:626.)

Table 16–8. Clinical features of Noonan's syndrome.

Skin
Hyperelasticity
Dermatoglyphic abnormalities
Webbed neck
Nevi
Lymphedema
Low-set posterior hairline
Facial
Hypertelorism
Ptosis
Antimongoloid slant
Low-set ears
Misshapen auricles
Skeletal
Short stature
Short neck
Cubitus valgus
Pectus excavatum
Brachydactyly
High-arched palate
Dental malocclusion
Pes planus
Abnormal vertebrae
Cardiovascular
Pulmonary stenosis
Supravalvular pulmonary artery stenosis
Atrial septal defect
Coarctation of the aorta
Genitourinary
Cryptorchidism
Small testes
Horseshoe kidney
Miscellaneous
Mental retardation
Gynecomastia
Wide-spaced nipples

nant fashion, with marked variability in expression. The underlying cause is unknown, and no chromosomal abnormalities have been described.

Testicular histology varies from moderate derangement of spermatogenesis with germinal cell arrest to regional hyalinization and fibrosis of the seminiferous tubules. The Leydig cells are usually preserved and may appear in clumps.

The testes are normal in affected prepubertal individuals, and puberty generally proceeds normally. Testosterone secretion is normal, and secondary sexual characteristics develop. After puberty, seminiferous tubular atrophy results in a decrease in testicular size and change of consistency from firm to soft or mushy. Infertility is a consequence of disrupted spermatogenesis. If testicular hyalinization and fibrosis are extensive, Leydig cell function may also be impaired.

Clinical Features

A. Symptoms and Signs: (Fig 16–15.) The disease usually becomes apparent in adulthood. Progressive weakness and atrophy of the facial, neck, hand, and lower extremity muscles is commonly observed. Severe atrophy of the temporalis muscles, ptosis due to weakness of the levator muscles of the eye with compensatory wrinkling of the forehead muscles, and frontal baldness comprise the myopathic facies characteristic of the disorder. Myotonia is present in several muscle groups an is characterized by inability to relax the muscle normally after a strong contraction.

Testicular atrophy is not noted until adulthood, and most patients develop and maintain normal facial and body hair growth and libido. Gynecomastia is usually not present.

Associated features include mental retardation cataracts, cranial hyperostosis, diabetes mellitus, and primary hypothyroidism.

B. Laboratory Findings: Serum testosterone is normal to slightly decreased. FSH is uniformly elevated in patients with atrophic testes. LH is also frequently elevated, even in patients with normal serum testosterone levels. Leydig cell reserve is generally diminished, with subnormal increases in serum testosterone following stimulation with chorionic gonadotropin. An excessive rise in FSH and, to a lesser extent, LH is found following GnRH stimulation.

Differential Diagnosis

Myotonic dystrophy should be distinguished from forms of muscular dystrophy not associated with hypogonadism.

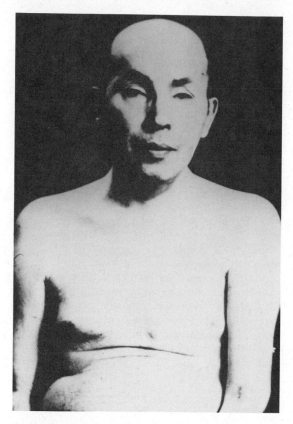

Figure 16–15. Myotonic dystrophy. Note myotonic facies with temporal baldness, ptosis, and wasting of the temporal and sternocleidomastoid muscles. (Reproduced, with permission, from Rimoin DL, Schimke RN: *Genetic Disorders of the Endocrine Glands.* Mosby, 1971.)

Treatment

There is no therapy that will prevent progressive muscular atrophy in this disorder. Testosterone replacement therapy is not indicated unless the serum testosterone levels are subnormal.

ADULT SEMINIFEROUS TUBULE FAILURE

Adult seminiferous tubule failure encompasses a spectrum of pathologic alterations of the seminiferous tubules that results in hypospermatogenesis, germinal cell arrest, germinal cell aplasia, and tubular hyalinization. Almost half of infertile males exhibit some degree of isolated seminiferous tubule failure.

Etiology, Pathology, & Pathophysiology

Etiologic factors in seminiferous tubule failure include mumps or gonococcal orchitis, leprosy, cryptorchidism, irradiation, uremia, alcoholism, para-

plegia, lead poisoning, and therapy with antineoplastic agents such as cyclophosphamide, chlorambucil, vincristine, methotrexate, and procarbazine. Vascular insufficiency resulting from spermatic artery damage during herniorrhaphy, testicular torsion, or sickle cell anemia may also selectively damage the tubules. Similar pathologic changes may be found in oligospermic patients with varicoceles. In many patients, no etiologic factors can be identified, and the condition is referred to as "idiopathic."

The rapidly dividing germinal epithelium is more susceptible to injury than are the Sertoli or Leydig cells. Thus, pressure necrosis (eg, mumps or gonococcal orchitis), increased testicular temperature (eg, cryptorchidism and perhaps varicocele and paraplegia), and the direct cytotoxic effects of irradiation, alcohol, lead, and chemotherapeutic agents primarily injure the germ cells. Although the Sertoli and Leydig cells appear to be morphologically normal, severe testicular injury may result in functional alterations in these cells.

Several different lesions may be found in testicular biopsy specimens. The pathologic process may involve the entire testes or may appear in patches. The least severe lesion is hypospermatogenesis, in which all stages of spermatogenesis are present but there is a decrease in the number of germinal epithelial cells. Some degree of peritubular fibrosis may be present. Cessation of development at the primary spermatocyte or spermatogonial stage of the spermatogenic cycle is classified as germinal cell arrest. More severely affected testes may demonstrate a complete absence of germ cells with maintenance or morphologically normal Sertoli cells (Sertoli cell only syndrome). The most severe lesion is fibrosis or hyalinization of the tubules. This latter pattern may be indistinguishable from that seen in Klinefelter's syndrome.

Irrespective of the etiologic factors involved in damage to the germinal epithelium, the alterations in spermatogenesis result in oligospermia. If the damage is severe, as in the Sertoli cell only syndrome or tubular hyalinization, azoospermia may be present. Since testicular volume consists chiefly of tubules, some degree of testicular atrophy is often present in these patients. Some patients have elevations in basal serum FSH concentrations and demonstrate a hyperresponsive FSH rise following GnRH, suggesting that the Sertoli cells are functionally abnormal despite their normal histologic appearance.

Clinical Features

A. Symptoms and Signs: Infertility is usually the only complaint. Mild to moderate testicular atrophy may be present. Careful examination should be made for the presence of varicocele by palpating the spermatic cord during Valsalva's maneuver with the patient in the upright position. The patients are fully virilized, and gynecomastia is not present.

B. Laboratory Findings: Semen analysis shows oligospermia or azoospermia, and serum testosterone and LH concentrations are normal. Basal serum FSH levels may be normal or high, and an excessive FSH rise following GnRH may be present.

Differential Diagnosis

Patients with hypothalamic or pituitary disorders may have oligospermia or azoospermia and testicular atrophy. The serum FSH and LH concentrations are often in the low normal range, and the testosterone level is usually (not always) diminished. The presence of neurologic and ophthalmologic abnormalities, diabetes insipidus, anterior pituitary trophic hormone deficiencies, or an elevated serum PRL concentration distinguishes these patients from those with primary seminiferous tubule failure. Other causes of primary testicular failure are associated either with clinical signs and symptoms of androgen deficiency or with enough somatic abnormalities to allow differentiation from isolated seminiferous tubule failure.

Prevention

In many instances, damage to the seminiferous tubules cannot be prevented. Early correction of cryptorchidism, adequate shielding of the testes during diagnostic radiologic procedures or radiotherapy, and limitation of the total dose of chemotherapeutic agents may prevent or ameliorate the adverse effects.

Treatment

A. Medical: Attempts to treat oligospermia and infertility medically have included testosterone rebound therapy, low-dose testosterone, exogenous gonadotropins, thyroid hormone therapy, vitamins, and clomiphene citrate. None of these agents have been found to be uniformly beneficial, and several may actually lead to a decrease in the sperm count.

B. Surgical: Some of the pathologic changes in the testes have been reversed by early orchiopexy in cryptorchid individuals. If a varicocele is found in an oligospermic, infertile male, it should be ligated.

Course & Prognosis

Patients who have received up to 300 rads of testicular irradiation may show partial or full recovery of spermatogenesis months to years following exposure. The prognosis for recovery is better for individuals who receive the irradiation over a short interval than for those who are exposed over several weeks.

Recovery of spermatogenesis may also occur months to years following administration of chemotherapeutic agents. The most important factor determining prognosis is the total dose of chemotherapy administered.

Improvement in the quality of the semen is found in 60–80% of patients following successful repair of varicocele. Restoration of fertility has been reported in about half of such patients.

The prognosis for spontaneous improvement of idiopathic oligospermia due to infection or infarction is poor.

ADULT LEYDIG CELL FAILURE
(Male Climacteric Syndrome)

In contrast to the menopause in women, men do not experience an abrupt decline or cessation of gonadal function. However, a gradual diminution of testicular function does occur in many men as part of the aging process (see Chapter 29). It is not known how many men develop symptoms directly attributable to this phenomenon.

Etiology, Pathology, & Pathophysiology

There have been many studies of the relationships between age and testicular function, often with conflicting results. Several investigators have found that after age 50, there is a gradual decrease in the total serum testosterone concentration, although the actual values remain within the normal range. The levels of free testosterone decrease to a greater extent because of an increase in SHBG. The testosterone production rate declines, and Leydig cell responsiveness to hCG also decreases. A gradual compensatory increase in serum LH levels has also been noted. However, some studies on elderly men selected on the basis of their being in excellent physical health have shown no statistical changes in the basal levels of androgens and gonadotropins in comparison to younger healthy males.

Histologic studies of the aging testes have shown patchy degenerative changes in the seminiferous tubules with morphologically normal Leydig cells. The pathologic changes are first noted in the regions most remote from the arterial blood supply. Thus, microvascular insufficiency may be the etiologic basis for the histologic tubular changes and the decrease in Leydig cell function noted with aging. In addition, virtually all of the conditions that cause adult seminiferous tubule failure may lead to Leydig cell dysfunction if testicular injury is severe enough.

Clinical Features

A. Symptoms and Signs: A great many symptoms have been attributed to the male climacteric, including decreased libido and potency, emotional instability, fatigue, decreased concentrating ability, vasomotor instability (palpitations, hot flushes, diaphoresis), and a variety of diffuse aches and pains. There are usually no associated signs unless the testicular injury is severe. In such patients, a decrease in testicular volume and consistency may be present.

B. Laboratory Findings: Serum testosterone may be low or low normal; serum LH concentration is usually high normal or slightly high. Oligospermia is usually present.

C. Special Examinations: Because many men with complaints compatible with Leydig cell failure have testosterone and LH concentrations within the normal adult range, a diagnostic trial of testosterone therapy may be attempted. The test is best performed double-blind over an 8-week period. During the first or last 4 weeks, the patient receives testosterone enanthate, 200 mg intramuscularly per week; during the other 4-week period, placebo injections are administered. The patient is interviewed by the physician 2 weeks after the last course of injections. After the interview, the code is broken; if the patient notes amelioration of symptoms during the period of androgen administration but not during the placebo period, the diagnosis of adult Leydig cell failure is substantiated. If the patient experiences no subjective improvement following testosterone, of if improvement is noted following both placebo and testosterone injections, Leydig cell failure is effectively ruled out.

Differential Diagnosis

Impotence from vascular, neurologic, or psychologic causes must be distinguished from Leydig cell failure. A therapeutic trial of androgen therapy will not help impotence that is not due to androgen deficiency.

Treatment

Androgen replacement therapy is the treatment of choice for symptomatic Leydig cell failure.

IMPOTENCE

Impotence implies erectile dysfunction with or without associated disturbances of libido or ejaculatory ability. The overall prevalence of impotence in the general population is unknown, although it is likely that most men experience occasional episodes of impotence at some time during their lives.

Etiology & Pathophysiology

The physiology of erection and ejaculation is discussed in an earlier section of this chapter. Broadly speaking, erectile dysfunction may be divided into psychogenic and organic causes. Table 16–9 lists various pathologic conditions and drugs that may be associated with impotence. In many patients, however, impotence has a psychogenic basis. Fear, depression, anger, guilt, anxiety, and problems with interpersonal relationships may decrease libido and interfere with the ability to become sexually aroused or the ability to achieve and maintain an erection. Inhibition of sexual function is mediated through the central nervous system by poorly understood mechanisms.

Most organic causes of impotence result from disturbances in the neurologic pathways essential for the initiation and maintenance of erection (temporal lobe,

Table 16–9. Organic causes of impotence.

Neurologic
Anterior temporal lobe lesions
Spinal cord lesions
Autonomic neuropathy
Vascular
Leriche's syndrome
Pelvic vascular insufficiency
Sickle cell disease
Aging (?)
Endocrine
Diabetes mellitus
Hypogonadism
Hyperprolactinemia
Adrenal insufficiency
Feminizing tumors
Hypothyroidism
Hyperthyroidism
Urogenital
Trauma
Castration
Priapism
Systemic illness
Cardiac insufficiency
Cirrhosis
Uremia
Respiratory insufficiency
Lead poisoning
Postoperative
Aortoiliac or aortofemoral reconstruction
Lumbar sympathectomy
Perineal prostatectomy
Retroperitoneal dissection
Drugs
Alcohol
Barbiturates
Spironolactone
Anticholinergics
Estrogens
Guanethidine
Reserpine
Methyldopa
Ketoconazole
Phenothiazines
Butyrophenones
Thiothixenes
Tricyclic antidepressants
Monoamine oxidase inhibitors
Heroin
Methadone
Morphine
Cocaine
Amphetamines
Diuretics
Antiandrogens

spinal cord, peripheral and autonomic nerves) or in the blood supply to the penis (occlusion of the aortic bifurcation [Leriche's syndrome], pelvic vascular insufficiency, sickle cell disease, or microvascular insufficiency). Many of the endocrine disorders, systemic illnesses, and drugs associated with impotence affect libido, the autonomic pathways essential for erection, or the blood flow to the penis. Local urogenital disorders such as Peyronie's disease (idiopathic fibrosis of the covering sheath of the corpus cavernosum) may mechanically interfere with erection. In some patients, the cause of impotence is multifactorial. For example, some degree of erectile dysfunction is reported by over 50% of men with diabetes mellitus. The basis of the impotence is usually autonomic neuropathy. However, vascular insufficiency, antihypertensive medication, uremia, and depression may also cause or contribute to the problem in diabetics.

Clinical Features

A. Symptoms and Signs: Patients may complain of constant or episodic inability to initiate or maintain an erection, decreased penile turgidity, decreased libido, or a combination of these difficulties. Besides the specific sexual dysfunction symptoms, symptoms and signs of a more pervasive emotional or psychiatric problem may be elicited. If an underlying neurologic, vascular, or systemic disorder is the cause of impotence, additional symptoms and signs referable to the anatomic or metabolic disturbances may be present. A history of claudication of the buttocks or lower extremities should direct attention toward arteriovascular insufficiency.

The differentiation between psychogenic and organic impotence can usually be made on the basis of the history. Even though the patient may be selectively unable to obtain or maintain a satisfactory erection to complete sexual intercourse, a history of repeated normal erections at other times is indicative of psychogenic impotence. Thus, a history of erections that occur nocturnally, during masturbation, or during foreplay or with other sexual partners eliminates significant neurologic, vascular, or endocrine causes of impotence. Patients with psychogenic impotence often note a sudden onset of sexual dysfunction concurrently with a significant event in their lives such as loss of a friend or relative, an extramarital affair, or the loss of a job.

Patients with organic impotence generally note a more gradual and global loss of potency. Initially, such individuals may be able to achieve erections with strong sexual stimuli, but ultimately they may be unable to achieve a fully turgid erection under any circumstances. In contrast to patients with psychogenic impotence, patients with organic impotence generally maintain a normal libido. However, patients with systemic illness may have a concurrent diminution of libido and potency. Hypogonadism should be suspected in a patient who has never had an erection (primary impotence).

B. Laboratory Findings and Special Examinations: The integrity of the neurologic pathways and the ability of the blood vessels to deliver a sufficient amount of blood to the penis for erection to occur may be objectively examined by placement of a strain gauge behind the glans penis and at the base of the penis at the time the patient retires for sleep. The occurrence of nocturnal penile tumescence can thus be recorded. Healthy men and those with psychogenic impotence have 3–5 erections a night associated with rapid eye movement (REM) sleep. Absence or reduced frequency of nocturnal tumescence indicates an organic lesion. Penile rigidity as well as tumescence can be evaluated with an ambulatory monitor called RigiScan (Dacomed Corporation, Minneapolis, MN 55420). A less cumbersome screening test can be carried out with a Snap-Gauge (also from Dacomed Corporation), which consists of Velcro straps with 3 plastic connectors, each of which breaks at a defined tensile pressure.

Penile arterial blood pressure may be measured with a small pneumatic cuff wrapped around the base of the penis and connected to a manometer. Penile blood flow is monitored during inflation and deflation of the cuff by a Doppler ultrasound device. Comparison of the ratio of the penile systolic blood pressure with the brachial systolic blood pressure at rest and following exercise of the lower extremities is a useful technique for unmasking pelvic vascular insufficiency.

Neural innervation of the penis may be assessed by measurement of the bulbocavernosus reflex response latency period. This procedure is performed by electrical stimulation of the dorsal nerve to the penis, which evokes contraction of the bulbocavernosus muscle with a normal latency of 30–50 ms. Alternatively, since the autonomic pathways involved in erection and urination are the same, cystometrography with measurement of bladder capacity and residual urine may be used as an indirect measurement of penile innervation.

Serum PRL should be measured in all patients with cryptogenic organic impotence, since hyperprolactinemia, whether drug-induced or due to a pituitary or hypothalamic lesion, appears to inhibit the peripheral effects of androgens. In addition, testosterone measurements may uncover a mild and otherwise asymptomatic androgen deficiency. Because diabetes mellitus is a relatively common cause of impotence and impotence may be the presenting symptom of diabetes, fasting and 2-hour postprandial blood glucose measurements should be ordered. The choice of other laboratory tests depends upon associated organic symptoms or signs.

Treatment

A. Psychogenic Impotence: Simple reassurance and explanation, formal psychotherapy, and various forms of behavioral therapy have a reported 40–70% success rate. Androgen therapy should not be used in patients with psychogenic impotence, since androgens exert no more than a placebo effect and may focus the patient's attention on a nonexistent organic problem.

B. Organic Impotence: Discontinuation of an offending drug usually results in a return of potency. Similarly, effective therapy of an underlying systemic or endocrine disorder may cure the erectile dysfunction.

Patients with permanent impotence due to organic lesions that cannot be corrected should be counseled in noncoital sensate focus techniques. Some patients respond to intracavernous injections of the vasoactive drugs papaverine hydrochloride and phentolamine mesylate, although priapism, infection, and bleeding can complicate this type of therapy. Recently, a device has been developed that uses suction to induce penile engorgement and constrictive bands to maintain the ensuing erection (ErecAid System, Osbon Medical Systems, Augusta, GA). Patients appear to be quite satisfied with this nonsurgical therapy. Alternatively, a penile prosthesis may be surgically implanted. Two major types of such prostheses have been developed. These include semirigid silicone rubber rods that are implanted in the corpora (eg, Small-Carrion and Jonas prostheses) or inflatable penile prostheses that allow the penis to remain flaccid until erection is desired. Both types of prostheses have given satisfactory results in 85–90% of cases.

MALE INFERTILITY

About 15% of married couples are unable to produce offspring. Male factors are responsible in about 40% of cases, female factors in about 40%, and couple factors in 20%.

Etiology & Pathophysiology

In order for conception to occur, spermatogenesis must be normal, the sperm must complete its maturation during transport through patent ducts, adequate amounts of seminal plasma must be added to provide volume and nutritional elements, and the male must be able to deposit the semen near the female's cervix. Any defect in this pathway can result in infertility due to a male factor problem. The spermatozoa must also be able to penetrate the cervical mucus and reach the uterine tubes, where conception takes place. These latter events may fail to occur if there are female reproductive tract disorders or abnormalities of sperm motility or fertilizing capacity.

Table 16–10 lists the identified causes of male infertility. Disturbances in the function of the hypothalamus, pituitary, adrenals, or thyroid are found in approximately 4% of males evaluated for infertility. Sex chromosome abnormalities, cryptorchidism, adult seminiferous tubule failure, and other forms of primary testicular failure are found in 15% of infertile males. Congenital or acquired ductal problems are found in approximately 6% of such patients, and poor coital technique, sexual dysfunction, ejaculatory disturbances, and anatomic abnormalities such as hypospadias are causative factors in 4–5% of patients evaluated for infertility. Idiopathic infertility, in which no cause can be identified with certainty, accounts for approximately 35% of patients. Autoimmune disturbances that lead to sperm agglutination and immobilization causes infertility in only a small fraction of patients. Varicoceles are found in 25–40% of patients classified as having idiopathic infertility. The signifi-

Table 16–10. Causes of male infertility.

Endocrine
  Hypothalamic-pituitary disorders
  Testicular disorders
  Defects of androgen action
  Hyperthyroidism
  Hypothyroidism
  Adrenal insufficiency
  Congenital adrenal hyperplasia
Systemic illness
Defects in spermatogenesis
  Immotile cilia syndrome
  Drug-induced
  Adult seminiferous tubule failure
Ductal obstruction
  Congenital
  Acquired
Seminal vesicle disease
Prostatic disease
Varicocele
Retrograde ejaculation
Antibodies to sperm or seminal plasma
Anatomic defects of the penis
Poor coital technique
Sexual dysfunction
Idiopathic

cance of this finding is uncertain, since 8–20% of males in the general population have varicoceles.

Clinical Features

A. Symptoms and Signs: The clinical features of the hypothalamic-pituitary, thyroid, adrenal, testicular, and sexual dysfunctional disorders have been discussed in preceding sections of this chapter. Evaluation for the presence of varicocele has also been described.

Patients with immotile cilia syndrome have associated mucociliary transport defects in the lower airways that result in chronic pulmonary obstructive disease. Some patients with this disorder also have Kartagener's syndrome, with sinusitis, bronchiectasis, and situs inversus. Infections of the epididymis or vas deferens may be asymptomatic or associated with scrotal pain that may radiate to the flank, fever, epididymal swelling and tenderness, and urethral discharge. The presence of thickened, enlarged epididymis and vas is indicative of chronic epididymitis. Chronic prostatitis is usually asymptomatic, although a perineal aching sensation or low back pain may be described. A boggy or indurated prostate may be found on rectal palpation. A careful examination for the presence of penile anatomic abnormalities such as chordee, hypospadias, or epispadias should be made, since these defects may prevent the deposit of sperm in the vagina.

B. Laboratory Findings: A carefully collected and performed semen analysis is mandatory. A normal report indicates normal endocrine function and spermatogenesis and an intact transport system. Semen analysis should be followed by a postcoital test, which consists of examining a cervical mucus sample obtained within 2 hours after intercourse. The presence of large numbers of motile spermatozoa in mucus obtained from the internal os of the cervix rules out the male factor as a cause of infertility. If a postcoital test reveals necrospermia (dead sperm), asthenospermia (slow-moving sperm), or agglutination of sperm, examination of the female partner for the presence of sperm-immobilizing antibodies or cervical mucus abnormalities should be carried out.

If semen analysis shows abnormalities, at least 2 more specimens should be obtained at monthly intervals. Persistent oligospermia or azoospermia should be evaluated by studies outlined in Figure 16–12.

The female partner should be thoroughly examined to verify patency of the uterus and uterine tubes, normal ovulation, and normal cervical mucus. This examination must be done even in the presence of a male factor abnormality, since infertility is due to a combination of male and female factors in about 20% of cases.

Treatment

A. Endocrine Disorders: Correction of hyperthyroidism, hypothyroidism, adrenal insufficiency, and congenital adrenal hyperplasia generally restores fertility. Patients with hypogonadotropic hypogonadism may have spermatogenesis initiated with gonadotropin therapy. Chorionic gonadotropin (2000 units given intramuscularly 3 times per week) with menotropins (75 units given intramuscularly 3 times per week) added after 12–18 months if sperm do not appear in the ejaculate, will restore spermatogenesis in most hypogonadotropic men. The sperm count following such therapy usually does not exceed 10 million/mL but may still allow impregnation. Patients with isolated deficiency of LH may respond to chorionic gonadotropin alone. There is no effective therapy for adult seminiferous tubule failure not associated with varicocele or cryptorchidism. However, if the oligospermia is mild (10–20 million/mL), cup insemination of the female partner with concentrates of semen may be tried. In vitro fertilization techniques are increasingly being utilized as a method for achieving pregnancy in couples in which the male is oligospermic.

B. Defects of Spermatogenesis: There is no treatment for immotile cilia syndrome or for chromosomal abnormalities associated with defective spermatogenesis. Drugs that interfere with spermatogenesis should be discontinued. These include the antimetabolites, phenytoin, marijuana, alcohol, monoamine oxidase inhibitors, and nitrofurantoin. Discontinuing use of these agents may be accompanied by restoration of normal sperm density.

C. Ductal Obstruction: Localized obstruction of the vas deferens may be treated by vasovasotomy. Sperms are detected in the ejaculate of 60–80% of patients following this procedure. However, the subsequent fertility rate is only 30–35%; the presence of antisperm antibodies that agglutinate or immobilize sperm probably accounts for the high failure rate.

Epididymovasostomy may be performed for epididymal obstruction. Sperm in the postoperative ejaculate have been found in approximately half of patients treated with this procedure, but subsequent fertility has been demonstrated in only 20% of cases.

D. Genital Tract Infections: Acute prostatitis may be treated with daily sitz baths, prostatic massage, and antibiotics. A combination of trimethoprim (400 mg) and sulfamethoxazole (2000 mg), twice a day for 10 days followed by the same dosage once a day for another 20 days, has been used with some success. Acute epididymitis may respond to injections of local anesthetic into the spermatic cord just above the testicle. Appropriate antibiotic therapy should also be given. The prognosis for fertility following severe bilateral chronic epididymitis or extensive scarring from acute epididymitis is poor.

E. Varicocele: The presence of varicocele in an infertile male with oligospermia is an indication for surgical ligation of the incompetent spermatic veins. Improvement in the semen is noted in 60–80% of treated patients, and about half are subsequently fertile.

F. Retrograde Ejaculation: Ejaculation of semen into the urinary bladder may occur following disruption of the internal bladder sphincter or with neuropathic disorders such as diabetic autonomic neuropathy. Normal ejaculation has been restored in a few patients with the latter problem following administration of phenylpropanolamine, 15 mg orally twice daily in timed-release capsules. Sperm can also be recovered from the bladder following masturbation for the purpose of direct insemination of the female partner.

G. Antibodies to Sperm or Seminal Plasma: Antibodies in the female genital tract that agglutinate or immobilize sperm may be difficult to treat. Older methods such as condom therapy or administration of glucocorticoids have not been uniformly successful. Currently, intrauterine insemination with washed spermatozoa, in vitro fertilization, and gamete intrafallopian transfer are considered the most effective treatments.

H. Anatomic Defects of the Penis: Patients with hypospadias, epispadias, or severe chordee may collect semen by masturbation for use in insemination.

I. Poor Coital Technique: Couples should be counseled not to use vaginal lubricants or postcoital douches. In order to maximize the sperm count in cases of borderline oligospermia, intercourse should not be more frequent than every other day. Exposure of the cervix to the seminal plasma is increased by having the woman lie supine with her knees bent up for 20 minutes after intercourse.

Course & Prognosis

The prognosis for fertility depends upon the underlying cause. It is good for patients with nontesticular endocrine abnormalities, varicoceles, retrograde ejaculation, and anatomic defects of the penis. If fertility cannot be restored, the couple should be counseled regarding artificial donor insemination, in vitro fertilization, or adoption.

GYNECOMASTIA

Gynecomastia is common during the neonatal period and is present in about 70% of pubertal males. Clinically apparent gynecomastia has been noted at autopsy in almost 1% of adult males, and 40% of autopsied males have histologic evidence of gynecomastia.

Etiology & Pathophysiology

The causes of gynecomastia are listed in Table 16–11. Several mechanisms have been proposed to account for this disorder. All involve a relative imbalance between estrogen and androgen concentrations or action at the mammary gland level. Decrease in free testosterone may be due to primary gonadal disease or an increase in SHBG as is found in hyperthyroidism and some forms of liver disease (eg, alcoholic cirrhosis). Acute or chronic excessive stimulation of the Leydig cells by pituitary gonadotropins alters the

Table 16–11. Causes of gynecomastia.

Physiologic
  Neonatal
  Pubertal
Drug-induced
  Amphetamines
  Androgens
  Chorionic gonadotropin
  Cimetidine
  Digitalis
  Estrogens
  Hydroxyzine
  Isoniazid
  Marijuana
  Meprobamate
  Methadone
  Methyldopa
  Phenothiazines
  Reserpine
  Spironolactone
Endocrine
  Primary hypogonadism with Leydig cell damage
  Hyperprolactinemia
  Hyperthyroidism
  Hypothyroidism
Systemic diseases
  Hepatic cirrhosis
  Uremia
  Recovery from malnourishment
Neoplasms
  Testicular germ cell or Leydig cell tumors
  Feminizing adrenocortical adenoma or carcinoma
  hCG-secreting nontrophoblastic neoplasms
Familial
Idiopathic

steroidogenic pathways and favors excessive estrogen and estrogen precursor secretion relative to testosterone production. This mechanism may be responsible for the gynecomastia found with hypergonadotropic states such as Klinefelter's syndrome and adult Leydig cell failure. The rise of gonadotropins during puberty may lead to an estrogen-androgen imbalance by similar mechanisms. Patients who are malnourished or have systemic illness may develop gynecomastia during refeeding or treatment of the underlying disorder. Malnourishment and chronic illness are accompanied by a reduction in gonadotropin secretion, and during recovery the gonadotropins rise and may stimulate excessive Leydig cell production of estrogens relative to testosterone.

Excessive stimulation of Leydig cells may also occur in patients with hCG-producing trophoblastic or nontrophoblastic tumors. In addition, some of these tumors are able to convert estrogen precursors into estradiol. Feminizing adrenocortical and Leydig cell neoplasms may directly secrete excessive quantities of estrogens. The mechanisms by which PRL-secreting pituitary tumors and hyperprolactinemia produce gynecomastia are unclear. PRL may directly stimulate breast glandular development through its mammotropic action. Elevated serum PRL levels may also diminish the peripheral actions of testosterone, which may result in an excessive estrogen effect on the breast that is not counteracted by androgens.

Drugs such as phenothiazines, methyldopa, and reserpine may induce gynecomastia through elevations of PRL. Other drugs may reduce androgen production (eg, spironolactone), peripherally antagonize androgen action (spironolactone, cimetidine), or interact with breast estrogen receptors (spironolactone, digitalis, phytoestrogens in marijuana).

Finally, it has been proposed that patients with idiopathic and familial gynecomastia have breast glandular tissue that is inordinately sensitive to normal circulating levels of estrogen or excessively converts estrogen precursors to estrogens.

Pathology

Three histologic patterns of gynecomastia have been recognized. The florid pattern consists of an increase in the number of budding ducts, proliferation of the ductal epithelium, periductal edema, and a cellular fibroblastic stroma. The fibrous type has dilated ducts, minimal duct epithelial proliferation, no periductal edema, and a virtually acellular fibrous stroma. An intermediate pattern contains features of both types.

Although it has been proposed that different causes of gynecomastia are associated with either the florid or the fibrous pattern, it appears that the duration of gynecomastia is the most important factor in determining the pathologic picture. Approximately 75% of patients with gynecomastia of 4 months' duration or less exhibit the florid pattern, while 90% of patients with gynecomastia lasting a year or more have the fibrous type. Between 4 months and 1 year, 60% of patients have the intermediate pattern.

Clinical Features

A. Symptoms and Signs: The principal complaint is unilateral or bilateral concentric enlargement of breast glandular tissue. Nipple or breast pain is present in one-fourth of patients and objective tenderness in about 40%. A complaint of nipple discharge can be elicited in 4% of cases. Histologic examination has demonstrated that gynecomastia is almost always bilateral, although grossly it may be detected only on one side. The patient will often complain of discomfort in one breast despite obvious bilateral gynecomastia. Breast or nipple discomfort generally lasts less than 1 year. Chronic gynecomastia is usually asymptomatic, with the major complaint being the cosmetic one.

Symptoms and signs of underlying disorders may be present. Gynecomastia may be the earliest manifestation of an hCG-secreting testicular tumor; therefore, it is mandatory that careful examination of the testes be performed in any patient with gynecomastia. Enlargement, asymmetry, and induration of a testis may be noted in such patients.

B. Laboratory Findings: Serum hCG by the beta subunit radioimmunoassay method is the most sensitive test for detection of hCG-secreting neoplasms. Feminizing tumors of the adrenals or Leydig cells are associated with marked elevations of serum estradiol. However, most patients with gynecomastia not associated with these neoplasms have total serum estradiol levels within the normal range. Serum PRL and thyroid hormones should be measured to detect hyperprolactinemia and hyper- or hypothyroidism. If hyperprolactinemia is found in a patient who has been taking phenothiazines or other drugs that enhance PRL secretion, the drug should be withdrawn and the PRL concentration measured in 2–3 months.

C. X-Ray Findings: Chest x-ray may detect metastatic disease or an hCG-secreting primary lung neoplasm. CT scans of the pituitary-hypothalamic region should be performed if hyperprolactinemia is present. If gynecomastia is unilateral and especially if the "glandular" tissue is eccentric, mammograms should be taken to exclude breast carcinoma, which accounts for about 0.2% of all cancers in males.

D. Special Examinations: If small testes are found on physical examination, buccal smear or chromosomal analysis should be done, since Klinefelter's syndrome is one of the more common causes of persistent pubertal gynecomastia.

Differential Diagnosis

Gynecomastia should be differentiated from lipomas, neurofibromas, carcinoma of the breast, and obesity. Breast lipomas, neurofibromas, and carcinoma are usually unilateral, painless, and eccentric, whereas gynecomastia characteristically begins in the subareolar areas and enlarges concentrically. The differentiation between gynecomastia and enlarged breasts due to obesity may be difficult. The patient should be supine. Examination is performed by spreading the thumb and index fingers and gently palpating the breasts during slow apposition of the fingers toward the nipple. In this manner, a concentric ridge of tissue can be felt in patients with gynecomastia but not in obese patients without glandular tissue enlargement. The examination may be facilitated by applying soap and water to the breasts.

Complications & Sequelae

There are no complications other than possible psychologic damage from the cosmetic defect. Patients with gynecomastia may have a slightly increased risk of development of breast carcinoma.

Treatment

A. Medical: The underlying disease should be corrected if possible, and offending drugs should be discontinued. Antiestrogens such as tamoxifen and clomiphene citrate have been found useful for relieving pain and reversing gynecomastia in a few patients. Whether this therapy will be useful in most patients with gynecomastia remains to be seen.

B. Surgical: Reduction mammoplasty should be considered for cosmetic reasons in any patient with long-standing gynecomastia that is in the fibrotic stage.

C. Radiologic: Patients with prostatic carcinoma may receive low-dose radiation therapy (900 rads or less) to the breasts before initiation of estrogen therapy. This may prevent or diminish the gynecomastia that usually results from such therapy. Radiotherapy should not be given to other patients with gynecomastia.

Course & Prognosis

Pubertal gynecomastia usually regresses spontaneously over 1–2 years. Patients who develop drug-induced gynecomastia generally have complete or near-complete regression of the breast changes if the drug is discontinued during the early florid stage. Once gynecomastia from any cause has reached the fibrotic stage, little or no spontaneous regression occurs.

TESTICULAR TUMORS

Testicular neoplasms account for 1–2% of all male-related malignant neoplasms and 4–10% of all genitourinary neoplasms. They are the second most frequent type of cancer in men between 20 and 34 years of age. The incidence is 2–3 per 100,000 men in the USA and 4–6 per 100,000 men in Denmark. The incidence is lower in nonwhite than in white populations. Ninety-five percent of testicular tumors are of germ cell origin; 5% are composed of stromal or Leydig cell neoplasms.

Etiology & Pathophysiology

The cause of testicular tumors is not known. Predisposing factors include testicular maldescent and dysgenesis. About 4–12% of testicular tumors are found in association with cryptorchidism, and such a testicle has a 20- to 40-fold greater risk of developing a neoplasm than does a normally descended one. Almost 20% of testicular tumors associated with cryptorchidism arise in the contralateral scrotal testis, suggesting that testicular dysgenesis may be of etiologic importance in the development of germ cell neoplasms. Although trauma is frequently cited as an etiologic factor in testicular tumors, no causal relationship has been established. What is more likely is that testicular trauma serves to call the patient's attention to the presence of a testicular mass.

Bilateral gynecomastia is uncommon in patients who present with testicular cancer. It is generally associated with production of hCG by the trophoblastic elements in the tumor. The hCG stimulates the Leydig cells to produce excessive estrogens relative to androgen production, resulting in estrogen-androgen imbalance and gynecomastia. In addition, the trophoblastic tissue in some of the tumors may convert estrogen precursors to estrogens.

Pathology

A. Germ Cell Tumors: Seminomas account for 33–50% of all germ cell tumors. They are composed of round cells with abundant cytoplasm, prominent nuclei, and large nucleoli. The cells are arranged in cords and nests and have a thin delicate network of stromal connective tissue. Embryonal cell neoplasms comprise 20–33% of germ cell tumors. These tumors have multiple histologic patterns composed of cuboidal pleomorphic cells. One distinct pattern of cellular arrangement is the endodermal sinus tumor (yolk sac tumor), the most frequent germ cell neoplasm found in infants. Immunohistochemical techniques have localized alpha-fetoprotein to the embryonal cells. About 10% of germ cell tumors are teratomas, which are composed of well-differentiated cells derived from all 3 germ layers. When one or more of the teratoid elements are malignant or are mixed with embryonal carcinoma cells, the term teratocarcinoma is applied. These tumors account for one-tenth to one-third of germ cell neoplasms. Choriocarcinoma is the rarest form of germ cell tumor (2%) and is composed of masses of large, polymorphic, multinucleated syncytiotrophoblastic cells. Although pure choriocarcinoma is rare, many testicular tumors contain an occasional trophoblastic giant cell. Immunohistochemical techniques have shown that these cells are the source of hCG in such tumors.

B. Leydig Cell Tumors: Leydig cell (interstitial cell) tumors are rare. Most are benign and are composed of sheets of oval to polygonal cells arranged in lobules separated from one another by thin strands of connective tissue. Malignant Leydig cell tumor disseminates by both lymphatic and venous channels, with initial metastatic deposits being found in the regional lymph nodes, followed by metastases to liver, lung, and bone.

Clinical Features

A. Symptoms and Signs:

1. Germ cell tumors–Testicular tumors usually present as painless enlargement of a testicle with an associated feeling of fullness or heaviness in the scrotum. Thus, about 80% of patients note a testicular swelling or mass, whereas only 25% complain of testicular pain or tenderness. About 6–25% of patients give a history of testicular trauma that brought the testicular mass to their attention. Gynecomastia may be present initially in 2–4% of patients and develops subsequently in another 10%. About 5–10% of patients present with symptoms of distant metastatic disease, including backache, skeletal pains, gastrointestinal and abdominal pains, inguinal adenopathy, and neurologic dysfunction.

A testicular mass or generalized enlargement of the testis is often present on examination. In 5–10% of patients, a coexisting hydrocele may be present. In the presence of metastatic disease, supraclavicular and retroperitoneal lymph node enlargement may be present.

2. Leydig cell tumors–In children, Leydig cell tumors of the testes may produce sexual precocity, with rapid skeletal growth and development of secondary sexual characteristics. Adults with such tumors usually present with a testicular mass and occasionally gynecomastia. Decreased libido may also be present in such patients.

B. Laboratory Findings:

1. Germ cell tumors–The tumor markers hCG and alpha-fetoprotein should be measured in every male presenting with a testicular mass. hCG is found in the sera of 5–10% of males with seminoma, over half of patients with teratocarcinoma or embryonal cell carcinoma, and all patients with choriocarcinoma. hCG should be measured by the beta subunit or other hCG-specific radioimmunoassay method. Elevated serum immunoreactive alpha-fetoprotein concentrations are found in almost 70% of patients with nonseminomatous forms of germ cell neoplasms. Both markers are elevated in over 50% of patients with nonseminomatous germ cell tumors, and at least one of the markers is elevated in 85% of such patients. These markers can also be used to monitor the results of therapy.

2. Leydig cell tumors–Urinary 17-ketosteroids and serum DHEA sulfate concentrations are increased. Both urinary and serum estrogen levels may also be increased. Serum testosterone concentrations tend to be low or within the normal adult range.

C. X-Ray Findings: Staging of testicular tumors requires several radiologic procedures, including chest tomograms, intravenous urograms, liver scans, gallium scans, and bipedal lymphangiography. CT scans of the abdomen and retroperitoneum have replaced lymphangiograms in many institutions.

Differential Diagnosis

Testicular tumors are sometimes misdiagnosed as epididymitis or epididymo-orchitis. An inflammatory reaction of the epididymis often involves the vas deferens. Therefore, both the vas and the epididymis will be thickened and tender on examination during the acute disease. Pyuria and fever also help to differentiate between epididymitis and testicular tumor. Because hydrocele may coexist with testicular tumor, the testes should be carefully examined following aspiration of the hydrocele.

Other conditions that can cause confusion with testicular tumors include inguinal hernia, hematocele, hematoma, torsion, spermatocele, varicocele, and (rarely) sarcoidosis, tuberculosis, and syphilitic gumma. Ultrasonic examination of the scrotum may help distinguish between testicular tumors and extratesticular disease such as acute or chronic epididymitis, spermatocele, or hydrocele.

Benign Leydig cell tumors of the testes must be differentiated from adrenal rest tumors in patients with congenital adrenal hyperplasia. Since the testes and the adrenals are derived from the same embryologic source, ectopic adrenal tissue may be found to migrate with the testes. This tissue can enlarge under the influence of ACTH in patients with congenital adrenal hyperplasia or Cushing's disease. Adrenal rest tumors tend to be bilateral, whereas patients with Leydig cell tumors generally have unilateral disease. Both may be associated with elevated urine 17-ketosteroids and elevated serum DHEA sulfate concentrations. Elevated serum and urinary estrogen concentrations are found with both disorders. However, patients with congenital adrenal hyperplasia or Cushing's disease will have a decrease in 17-ketasteroids, DHEA sulfate, and estrogen concentrations, as well as a decrease in tumor size, following administration of dexamethasone.

Treatment

A. Germ Cell Tumors: Seminomas are quite radiosensitive, and disease localized to the testes is usually treated with orchiectomy and 2000–4000 rads of conventional radiotherapy delivered to the ipsilateral inguinal-iliac and bilateral para-aortic lymph nodes to the level of the diaphragm. For disease that has spread to the lymph nodes below the diaphragm, additional whole abdominal radiotherapy and prophylactic mediastinal and supraclavicular lymph node irradiation are usually given. Widely disseminated disease is generally treated with a combination of radiotherapy and chemotherapy, especially with alkylating agents.

Nonseminomatous tumors are treated with orchiectomy, retroperitoneal lymph node dissection, and, if necessary, radiotherapy or chemotherapy (or both). Although many chemotherapeutic agents have been used, combinations of vinblastine, bleomycin, and cisplatin currently appear to produce the best overall results. Patients with nonseminomatous tumors treated by these means should be monitored with serial measurements of serum hCG and alpha-fetoprotein.

B. Leydig Cell Tumors: Benign Leydig cell tumors of the testes are treated by unilateral orchiectomy. Objective remissions of malignant Leydig cell tumors have been noted following treatment with mitotane.

Course & Prognosis

A. Germ Cell Tumors: In patients with seminoma confined to the testicle, the 5-year survival rates after orchiectomy and radiotherapy are 98–100%. Disease in the lymph nodes below the diaphragm also has an excellent prognosis, with 5-year survival rates of 80–85%. Disease above the diaphragm and disseminated disease have 5-year survival rates as low as 18%.

In patients with nonseminomatous germ cell tumors, aggressive surgery and combination chemotherapy have raised the 5-year survival rates from less than 20% to 60–90%.

B. Leydig Cell Tumors: Removal of a benign Leydig cell tumor is accompanied by regression of precocious puberty in children or feminization in adults. The prognosis for malignant Leydig cell tumor is poor, with most patients surviving less than 2 years from the time of diagnosis.

REFERENCES

Anatomy & Structure-Function Relationships

Fawcett DW: The cell biology of gametogenesis in the male. *Perspect Biol Med* 1979;**2**:S56.

Hafez ESE: *Human Semen and Fertility Regulation in Men*. Mosby, 1976.

Lipshultz LI, Howards SS (editors): *Infertility in the Male*. Churchill Livingstone, 1983.

Physiology

Berkovitz GD, Brown TR, Migeon CJ: Androgen receptors. *Clin Endocrinol Metab* 1983;**12**:155.

Brooks RV: Androgens. *Clin Endocrinol Metab* 1975;**4**:503.

deGroat WC, Booth AM: Physiology of male sexual function. *Ann Intern Med* 1980;**92**:329.

Jeffcoate SL: The control of testicular function in the adult. *Clin Endocrinol Metab* 1975;**4**:521.

Mooradian AD, Morley JE, Korenman SG: Biological actions of androgens. *Endocr Rev* 1987;**8**:1.

Newman HF, Reiss H, Northup JD: Physical basis of emission, ejaculation, and orgasm in the male. *Urology* 1982;**19**:341.

Odell WD, Swerdloff RS: Abnormalities of gonadal function in men. *Clin Endocrinol* 1978;**8**:149.

Sharpe RM: Paracrine control of the testis. *Clin Endocrinol Metab* 1986;**15**:185.

Steinberger E: Hormonal regulation of the seminiferous tubule function. *Curr Top Mol Endocrinol* 1975;**2**:337.

Steinberger E: Hormonal regulation of the seminiferous tubule function. *Curr Top Mol Endocrinol* 1975;**2**:337.

Tsonis CG, Sharpe RM: Dual gonadal control of follicle-stimulating hormone. *Nature* 1986;**321**:724.

Weiss HD: The physiology of human penile erection. *Ann Intern Med* 1972;**76**:793.

Evaluation of Male Gonadal Function

Baker HW, Hudson B: Male gonadal dysfunction. *Clin Endocrinol Metab* 1974;**3**:507.

Blasco L: Clinical tests of sperm fertilizing ability. *Fertil Steril* 1984;**41**:177.

Forest MG: How should we perform the human chorionic gonadotropin (hCG) stimulation test? *Int J Androl* 1983;**6**:1.

Goldzieher JW et al: Improving the diagnostic reliability of rapidly fluctuating plasma hormone levels by optimized multiple-sampling techniques. *J Clin Endocrinol Metab* 1976;**43**:824.

Marshall JC: Investigating procedures. *Clin Endocrinol Metab* 1975;**4**:545.

Nieschlag E: Hormone diagnosis in male hypogonadism and infertility. *Horm Res* 1978;**9**:394.

Penny R: The testis. *Pediatr Clin North Am* 1979;**26**:107.

Santen RJ, Swerdloff RS (editors): *Male Reproductive Dysfunction: Diagnosis and Management of Hypogonadism, Infertility, and Impotence.* Marcel Dekker, 1986.

Schonfeld WA: Primary and secondary sexual characteristics: Study of their development in males from birth through maturity, with biometric study of penis and testes. *Am J Dis Child* 1943;**65**:535.

Wu FC: Male hypogonadism: Current concepts and trends. *Clin Obstet Gynaecol* 1985;**12**:531.

Zachmann M et al: Testicular volume during adolescence: Cross-sectional and longitudinal studies. *Helv Paediatr Acta* 1974;**29**:61.

Pharmacology of Drugs Used in Treatment

Clayton RN: Gonadotropin-releasing hormone: From physiology to pharmacology. *Clin Endocrinol* 1987;**26**:361.

Cutler GB et al: Therapeutic applications of luteinizing hormone-releasing hormone and its analogs. *Ann Intern Med* 1985;**102**:643.

Davidson JM, Camargo CA, Smith ER: Effects of androgen on sexual behavior in hypogonadal men. *J Clin Endocrinol Metab* 1979;**48**:955.

Garcia CR et al (editors): *Current Therapy of Infertility,* 3rd Ed. BC Decker, 1987.

Korenman SG et al: Androgen therapy of hypogonadal men with transscrotal testosterone systems. *Am J Med* 1987;**83**:471.

London DR: Medical aspects of hypogonadism. *Clin Endocrinol Metab* 1975;**4**:597.

O'Carroll R, Shapiro C, Bancroft J: Androgens, behaviour and nocturnal erection in hypogonadal men: The effects of varying the replacement dose. *Clin Endocrinol* 1985;**23**:527.

Santoro N, Filicori M, Crowley WF Jr: Hypogonadotropic disorders in men and women: Diagnosis and therapy with pulsatile gonadotropin-releasing hormone. *Endocr Rev* 1986;**7**:11.

Schally AV, Comaru-Schally AM: Use of luteinizing hormone-releasing hormone analogs in the treatment of hormone-dependent tumors. *Semin Reprod Endocrinol* 1987;**5**:389.

Snyder PJ: Clinical use of androgens. *Annu Rev Med* 1984;**35**:207.

Klinefelter's Syndrome & Variants

Baghdassarian A et al: Testicular function in XXY men. *Johns Hopkins Med J* 1975;**136**:15.

de la Chapelle A: Analytic review: Nature and origin of males with XX sex chromosomes. *Am J Hum Genet* 1972;**24**:71.

Federman DD: *Abnormal Sexual Development: A Genetic and Endocrine Approach to Differential Diagnosis.* Saunders, 1968.

Ferguson-Smith MA: Sex chromatin, Klinefelter's syndrome and mental deficiency. Page 280 in: *The Sex Chromatin.* Moor KL (editor). Saunders, 1966.

Ishida H et al: Studies on pituitary-gonadal endocrine function in XYY men. *J Urol* 1979;**121**:190.

Klinefelter HF: Klinefelter's syndrome: Historical background and development. *South Med J* 1986;**79**:1089.

Ratcliffe SG: The sexual development of boys with the chromosome constitution 47,XXY (Klinefelter's syndrome). *Clin Endocrinol Metab* 1982;**11**:703.

Rimoin DL, Schimke RN: *Genetic Disorders of the Endocrine Glands.* Mosby, 1971.

Schiavi RC et al: Pituitary-gonadal function in XYY and XXY men identified in a population survey. *Clin Endocrinol* 1978;**9**:233.

Walzer S, Gerald PS, Shah SA: The XYY genotype. *Annu Rev Med* 1978;**29**:563.

Zuppinger K et al: Klinefelter's syndrome: A clinical and cytogenetic study in 24 cases. *Acta Endocrinol* 1967;**54(Suppl 113)**:5.

Anorchia

Abeyaratne MR, Aherne WA, Scott JE: The vanishing testis. *Lancet* 1969;**2**:822.

Kirschner MA, Jacobs JB, Fraley EE: Bilateral anorchia with persistent testosterone production. *N Engl J Med* 1970;**282**:240.

Tosi SE, Morin LJ: The vanishing testis syndrome: Indications for conservative therapy. *J Urol* 1976;**115**:758.

Leydig Cell Aplasia

Lee PA et al: Leydig cell hypofunction resulting in male pseudohermaphroditism. *Fertil Steril* 1982;**37**:675.

Cryptorchidism

Lipshultz LI: Cryptorchidism in the subfertile male. *Fertil Steril* 1976;**27:**609.

Rajfer J (editor): Cryptorchidism. *Urol Clin North Am* 1982;**9:**315.

Rafjer J et al: Hormonal therapy of cryptorchidism: A randomized, double-blind study comparing human chorionic gonadotropin and gonadotropin-releasing hormone. *N Engl J Med* 1986;**314:**466.

Noonan's Syndrome

Collins E, Turner G: The Noonan syndrome: A review of the clinical and genetic features of 27 cases. *J Pediatr* 1973;**83:**941.

Schoen E: Diminished testicular function in "male Turner's syndrome." *J Clin Endocrinol Metab* 1965;**25:**101.

Myotonic Dystrophy

Febres F et al: Hypothalamic-pituitary-gonadal function in patients with myotonic dystrophy. *J Clin Endocrinol Metab* 1975;**41:**833.

Takeda R, Ueda M: Pituitary-gonadal function in male patients with myotonic dystrophy: Serum luteinizing hormone, follicle stimulating hormone, and testosterone levels and histological damage of the testis. *Acta Endocrinol* 1977;**84:**382.

Adult Seminiferous Tubule Failure

Abbasi AA et al: Gonadal function abnormalities in sickle cell anemia. *Ann Intern Med* 1976;**85:**601.

Ash PA: The influence of radiation on fertility in man. *Br J Radiol* 1980;**53:**271.

Braunstein GD, Dahlgren J, Loriaux DL: Hypogonadism in chronically lead-poisoned men. *Infertility* 1978;**1:**33.

de Kretser DM: The effects of systemic disease on the function of the testis. *Clin Endocrinol Metab* 1979;**8:**487.

Holdsworth S et al: The pituitary-testicular axis in men with chronic renal failure. *N Engl J Med* 1977;**296:**1245.

Johnsen SG, Agger P: Quantitative evaluation of testicular biopsies before and after operation for varicocele. *Fertil Steril* 1978;**29:**58.

Kikuchi TA et al: The pituitary-gonadal axis in spinal cord injury. *Fertil Steril* 1976;**27:**1142.

Morley JE, Melmed S: Gonadal dysfunction in systemic disorders. *Metabolism* 1979;**28:**1051.

Schilsky RL et al: Gonadal dysfunction in patients receiving chemotherapy for cancer. *Ann Intern Med* 1980;**93:**109.

Van Thiel DH, Lester R: The effect of chronic alcohol abuse on sexual function. *Clin Endocrinol Metab* 1979;**8:**499.

Adult Leydig Cell Failure

Baker HW et al: Changes in the pituitary-testicular system with age. *Clin Endocrinol* 1976;**5:**349.

Hallberg MC et al: Impaired Leydig cell reserve and altered serum androgen binding in the aging male. *Fertil Steril* 1976;**27:**812.

Tsitouras PD: Effects of age on testicular function. *Endocrinol Metab Clin North Am* 1987;**16:**1045.

Werner AA: The male climacteric: Report of 273 cases. *JAMA* 1946;**132:**188.

Impotence

Bodner DR: Impotence: Evaluation and treatment. *Prim Care* 1985;**12:**719.

Buvat J et al: Is intracavernous injection of papaverine a reliable screening test for vascular impotence? *J Urol* 1986;**135:**476.

Krane RJ, Siroky MB, Goldstein I (editors): *Male Sexual Dysfunction.* Little, Brown, 1983.

Morley JE: Impotence. *Am J Med* 1986;**80:**897.

Nelson RP: Male sexual dysfunction: Evaluation and treatment. *South Med J* 1987;**80:**69.

Padma-Nathan H, Goldstein I, Krane RJ: Evaluation of the impotent patient. *Semin Urol* 1986;**4:**225.

Sacks SA: Evaluation of impotence: Comprehensive, compassionate approach. *Postgrad Med* (Oct) 1983;**74:**182.

Schiavi RC: Male erectile disorders. *Annu Rev Med* 1981;**32:**509.

Schurmeyer TH, Nieschlag E: Effect of ketoconazole and other imidazole fungicides on testosterone biosynthesis. *Acta Endocrinol* 1984;**105:**275.

Scott FB, Fishman IJ, Light JK: An inflatable penile prosthesis for treatment of diabetic impotence. *Ann Intern Med* 1980;**92:**340.

Wiles PG: Successful noninvasive management of erectile impotence in diabetic men. *Br Med J* 1988;**296:**161.

Male Infertility

Dubin L, Amelar RD: Etiologic factors in 1294 consecutive cases of male infertility. *Fertil Steril* 1971;**22:**469.

Eliasson R et al: The immotile-cilia syndrome: A congenital ciliary abnormality as an etiologic factor in chronic airway infections and male sterility. *N Engl J Med* 1977;**297:**1.

Hudson RW: The endocrinology of varicoceles. *Fertil Steril* 1988;**49:**199.

Jones WR: Immunologic infertility: Fact or fiction? *Fertil Steril* 1980;**33:**577.

Ross LS: Diagnosis and treatment of infertile men: A clinical perspective. *J Urol* 1983;**130:**847.

Santen RJ, Swerdloff RS (editors): *Male Reproductive Dysfunction: Diagnosis and Management of Hypogonadism, Infertility, and Impotence.* Marcel Dekker, 1986.

Wong TW et al: Pathological aspects of the infertile testis. *Urol Clin North Am* 1978;**5:**503.

Gynecomastia

Bannayan GA, Hajdu SI: Gynecomastia: Clinicopathologic study of 351 cases. *Am J Clin Pathol* 1972;**57:**431.

Carlson HE: Gynecomastia. *N Engl J Med* 1980;**303:**795.

Chopra IJ et al: Alterations in circulating estradiol-17β in male patients with Graves' disease. *N Engl J Med* 1972;**286:**124.

Cook S, Rodriguez-Antunez A: Pre-estrogen irradiation of the breast to prevent gynecomastia. *Am J Roentgenol Radium Ther Nucl Med* 1973;**117:**662.

Nicolis SL, Modlinger RS, Gabrilove JL: A study of the

histopathology of human gynecomastia. *J Clin Endocrinol Metab* 1971;**32:**173.

Niewoehner CB, Nuttall FQ: Gynecomastia in a hospitalized male population. *Am J Med* 1984;**77:**633.

Parker LN et al: Treatment of gynecomastia with tamoxifen: A double-blind crossover study. *Metabolism* 1986;**35:**705.

Williams MJ: Gynecomastia: Its incidence, recognition and host characterization in 447 autopsy cases. *Am J Med* 1963;**34:**103.

Wilson JD, Aiman J, McDonald PC: The pathogenesis of gynecomastia. *Adv Intern Med* 1980;**25:**1.

Testicular Tumors

Azer PC, Braunstein GD: Malignant Leydig cell tumor: Objective tumor response to *o,p'*-DDD. *Cancer* 1981;**47:**1251.

Braunstein GD et al: Germ cell tumors of the testes. *West J Med* 1977;**126:**362.

Catalona WJ: Current management of testicular tumors. *Surg Clin North Am* 1982;**62:**1119.

Einhorn LH, Williams SD: Chemotherapy of disseminated testicular cancer: A random prospective study. *Cancer* 1980;**46:**1339.

Hajdu SI: Pathology of germ cell tumors of the testis. *Semin Oncol* 1979;**6:**14.

Javadpour N (editor): *Principles and Management of Testicular Cancer*. Thieme, 1985.

Sample WF et al: Gray scale ultrasound of the scrotum. *Radiology* 1978;**127:**225.

Scardino PT et al: The value of serum tumor markers in the staging and prognosis of germ cell tumors of the testis. *J Urol* 1977;**118:**994.

17

Ovaries

Alan Goldfien, MD, & Scott E. Monroe, MD

ANATOMY OF THE OVARIES

The mature ovaries are paired nodular structures 2.5–5 × 2 × 1 cm, weighing from 4 to 8 g, the weight varying during the menstrual cycle. They are situated behind the peritoneum attached to the posterior surface of the broad ligament by a fold of the peritoneum called the mesovarium, which contains the blood vessels and nerves leading to the hilum. The ovaries are attached to the uterus by the ovarian ligament and lie in close association with the uterine tubes (oviducts, fallopian tubes) (Fig 17–1).

The ovaries develop from the genital ridges situated between the base of the dorsal mesentery and the mesonephros on either side of the coelomic cavity. The primordial germ cells that originate in the endoderm of the yolk sac at the third week begin to migrate through the hindgut to invade the genital ridges at about the sixth week. These primary oocytes are surrounded by a layer of epithelium and mesenchymal cells that give rise to the primordial follicles. About 1700 germ cells are present before migration to the genital ridge begins; however, these multiply during the process of migration and within the genital ridge, reaching a peak of 7 million oocytes at mid gestation. The primordial germ cells increase in size early in their development and become oogonia. At mid gestation they begin the first meiotic division, becoming primary oocytes. This prophase lasts until just before ovulation, which may occur 12–40 or more years later. In this state, they are no longer capable of multiplication and in fact steadily decline in number (Fig 17–2). About 400 ova are lost through the process of ovulation during a woman's lifetime. The remainder undergo degeneration so that, by the time of the menopause, few are present.

Blood Supply

The arterial vessels supplying the ovary are derived from branches of the ovarian and uterine arteries that enter through the mesovarium and divide into branches leading into the stroma of the medulla and then to the cortex. The small arteries of the ovary are charac-

Acronyms Used in This Chapter

ACTH	Adrenocorticotropic hormone
BSP	Bromsulphalein
CBG	Corticosteroid-binding globulin
DHEA	Dehydroepiandrosterone
EI	Eosinophilic index
FSH	Follicle-stimulating hormone
GH	Growth hormone
GnRH	Gonadotropin-releasing hormone
hCG	Human chorionic gonadotropin
HDL	High-density lipoprotein(s)
KPI	Karyopyknotic index
LDL	Low-density lipoprotein(s)
LH	Luteinizing hormone
MCR	Metabolic clearance rate
MI	Maturation index
mRNA	Messenger ribonucleic acid
PMN	Polymorphonuclear neutrophil
PMS	Premenstrual syndrome
PRL	Prolactin
PTH	Parathyroid hormone
RNA	Ribonucleic acid
SGPT	Serum glutamic-pyruvic transaminase
SHBG	Sex hormone–binding globulin
TBG	Thyroid hormone–binding globulin
TSH	Thyroid-stimulating hormone (thyrotropin)
VLDL	Very low density lipoprotein(s)

teristically spiral. The capillary blood gathers in veins that form a large, thin-walled plexus of vessels called the pampiniform plexus, leaving the ovary by way of the ovarian vein at the hilum. Lymphatics arise in the outer or cortical portion of the ovary and anastomose centrally, leaving through the hilum. Although the lymphatic channels are numerous in the theca externa, corpora lutea, and corpora albicantia, they are not seen in the theca interna, granulosa, or tunica albuginea.

Nerve Supply

The ovary has a rich autonomic innervation arising from the intermesenteric nerves and renal plexus; from the superior hypogastric plexus or presacral nerve and the hypogastric nerve; and from the inferior hypogastric plexus or pelvic plexus. The nerves appear to be mainly sympathetic in origin.

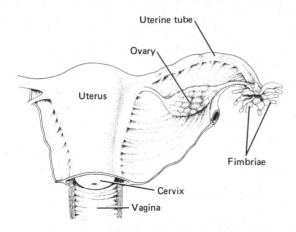

Figure 17–1. Internal organs of the female reproductive system: ovary, fimbriae of infundibulum, uterine tube, uterus, cervix, and vagina. (Reproduced, with permission, from Junqueira LC, Carneiro J, Kelley RO: *Basic Histology,* 6th ed. Appleton & Lange, 1989.)

Microscopic Anatomy

As shown in Figure 17–3, the ovary consists of many different structures. The mature ovary is covered by a layer of columnar cells that constitute the **germinal epithelium.** The dense layer of connective tissue under the epithelium is called the tunica albuginea. The remainder of the organ is divided into outer cortical and inner medullary portions, of which the cortex is the larger. The cortex contains follicular structures in all stages of development, surrounded by the connective tissue elements of the stroma and the

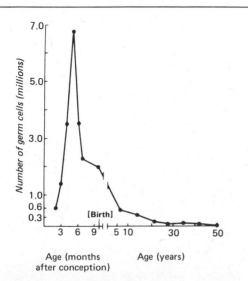

Figure 17–2. Total number of germ cells in the human ovary at different ages. (Reproduced, with permission, from Baker TG: *Reproduction in Mammals.* Austin CR, Short RV [editors]. Cambridge Univ Press, 1972.)

hilar cells, a group of steroid-secreting cells that histologically resemble the Leydig, or interstitial, cells of the testes. The medulla consists of a connective tissue stroma containing elastic fibers, blood vessels, nerves, lymphatics, and smooth muscle fibers.

The follicular complex contains the ova as well as the cells responsible for production of the ovarian hormones and their precursors. Structural changes and hormonal activity that occur throughout the menstrual cycle are discussed below.

HORMONES OF THE OVARY

The mature ovary actively synthesizes and secretes a variety of hormones. Among these are the sex steroids, which include estrogens, progesterone, androgens, and their precursors. In addition, the ovary produces relaxin, inhibin, prostaglandins, and other substances.

STEROID HORMONES

The ovary is normally the major source of estrogens, although the conversion of androgen precursors in other tissues is clinically important after the menopause and in some women with disorders of ovarian function. The ovary also produces and secretes large amounts of progesterone during the luteal phase of the cycle. It is also the source of small amounts of testosterone and other androgens that serve not only as precursors to estrogen synthesis but also are released into the circulation to act on peripheral tissues.

Biosynthesis of Steroid Hormones

The biochemical pathways, including the major enzymes and their intracellular localizations, are similar in the ovary, testis, and adrenal. The process in the ovary is outlined in Figure 17–4. The steroid hormones are synthesized from cholesterol, which is present in the gland both free and esterified to fatty acids (cholesteryl esters). Cholesterol derived either from circulating lipoproteins or from cholesteryl esters in the gland is converted to pregnenolone by removal of a 6-carbon fragment, isocaproic acid. This reaction or group of reactions is the rate-limiting step in the biosynthetic process and is controlled by luteinizing hormone (LH) from the anterior pituitary.

Pregnenolone formed by this reaction may be converted either to progesterone or to 17α-hydroxypregnenolone. The conversion to progesterone requires the action of 3β-hydroxysteroid dehydrogenase and $\Delta^{5,4}$-ketosteroid isomerase, which shifts the double bond from the Δ^5 to the Δ^4 position. Progesterone is secreted

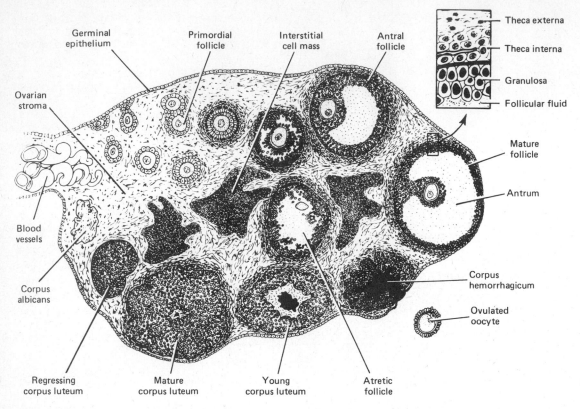

Figure 17–3. Diagram of a mammalian ovary, showing the sequential development of a follicle, formation of a corpus luteum, and, in the center, follicular atresia. A section of the wall of a mature follicle is enlarged at the upper right. The interstitial cell mass is not prominent in primates. (After Patten & Eakin. Reproduced, with permission, from Katzung BG [editor]: *Basic & Clinical Pharmacology,* 3rd ed. Appleton & Lange, 1987.)

by the corpus luteum in large amounts following ovulation (see below). However, it also serves as a precursor for androgen and estrogen, since it is a substrate for P-450c17 (17α-hydroxylase), which converts it to 17α-hydroxyprogesterone in the endoplasmic reticulum. Following 17α-hydroxylation, the 2-carbon (20–21) side chain may be cleaved by the P-450c17 (C17,20-lyase) enzyme to form androgens (see Fig 17–4).

17α-Hydroxypregnenolone is converted by the P-450c17 (lyase) enzyme to dehydroepiandrosterone (DHEA). This compound can then be converted to androstenedione. The relative importance of these pathways to androgen production is not clear. Androstenedione is the major androgen secreted by the ovary, but small amounts of DHEA and testosterone are also released.

Estradiol, the most active estrogen produced by the ovary, is synthesized from androgens by a group of enzymes known as the aromatase complex or system. The process involves 3 steps: hydroxylation of the methyl group at carbon 19, oxidation of this group, and hydroxylation at the 3α position. These steps are thought to occur in the microsomal fraction.

During the menstrual cycle, regulation of biosynthesis and release is controlled by the gonadotropins as well as by local factors.

Secretion of Steroid Hormones

The secretory activity of the steroid-producing granulosa and theca cells is closely coupled to their biosynthetic activity, since little hormone is stored in the cells. Direct measures of secretion rates in humans are difficult to obtain, because they require an accurate measure of the concentration of the hormone in the effluent blood from the gland and a measure of blood flow through the gland. Such samples and measurements are difficult to obtain without interfering with blood flow and normal gland activity. Therefore, indirect measures have been widely used. Some of the most useful information has been obtained by measuring the metabolic clearance rate (MCR) with an in vivo isotope dilution technique. Multiplying MCR by the concentration of the hormone in blood provides a total production rate for the hormone. However, the production rate also includes production of the hormone at other sites from circulating precursors, and it may therefore be greater than the amount secreted by the

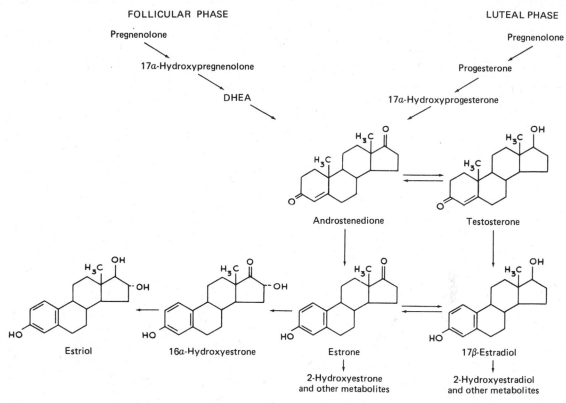

Figure 17–4. Biosynthesis and metabolism of estrogens. (Reproduced, with permission, from Katzung BG [editor]: *Basic & Clinical Pharmacology,* 4th ed. Appleton & Lange, 1989.)

gland. The production rates, plasma levels, and MCRs of various ovarian steroids are shown in Table 17–1.

During pregnancy, the fetal-placental unit produces a large amount of steroid hormone. The placenta produces progesterone, which is released into the maternal circulation, and large amounts of pregnenolone, which is released into the fetal circulation. Enzymatic conversion of pregnenolone by the fetal adrenal and liver produces steroids, including 16-hydroxydehydroepiandrosterone sulfate, which are subsequently converted to estriol and other estrogens in the placenta and released into the maternal circulation (see Chapter 20).

Transport of Steroid Hormones

When released into the circulation, the gonadal steroids bind to plasma proteins. Estradiol binds avidly to a transport globulin called sex hormone–binding globulin (SHBG) and binds with less affinity to albumin. Progesterone binds strongly to corticosteroid-binding globulin (CBG) and weakly to albumin. The percentages of various steroids that bind to these carrier proteins are listed in Table 17–2. The concentration of these binding proteins is increased by estrogen and thyroxine and decreased by androgens and progestins. SHBG is synthesized in the liver, and because

its synthesis is stimulated by estrogens and inhibited by androgen, levels are twice as high in women as in men. The proportions of free and bound estradiol do not vary significantly during the menstrual cycle. However, differences in binding may assume clinical importance after the menopause or in women with abnormal ovarian function associated with excess androgens.

Metabolism of Steroid Hormones

A. Estrogens: Circulating estradiol is rapidly converted in the liver to estrone by 17β-hydroxysteroid dehydrogenase (Fig. 17–5). Some of the estrone reenters the circulation; however, most of it is further metabolized to 16α-hydroxyestrone (which is then converted to estriol) or to 2-hydroxyestrone, a catechol estrogen. Much of the remaining estrone is conjugated to form estrone sulfate. Estriol is converted largely to estriol 3-sulfate-16-glucuronide before excretion by the kidney.

B. Progesterone: Progesterone is rapidly cleared from the circulation, having an initial half-life of about 5 minutes. As indicated by its high clearance rate (Table 17–1), it is rapidly converted to pregnanediol and conjugated to glucuronic acid in the liver. Pregnanediol glucuronide is excreted in the urine and may

Table 17–1. Approximate concentrations, metabolic clearance rates (MCR), production rates, and ovarian secretion rates of steroids in blood.[1]

	MCR (L/d)	Phase of Menstrual Cycle	Plasma Concentration		Production Rate		Secretion Rate (Both Ovaries)	
			(μg/dL)	(nmol/L)	(mg/d)	(μmol/d)	(mg/d)	(μmol/d)
Estradiol	1350	Early follicular	0.006	(0.22)	0.081	(0.3)	0.07	(0.26)
		Late follicular	0.033–0.07	(1.21–2.57)	0.445–0.945	(1.63–3.47)	0.4–0.8	(1.63–2.93)
		Midluteal	0.02	(0.73)	0.27	(1)	0.25	(0.92)
Estrone	2210	Early follicular	0.005	(0.18)	0.11	(0.41)	0.08	(0.3)
		Late follicular	0.015–0.03	(0.55–1.11)	0.331–0.662	(0.86–2.45)	0.25–0.5	(0.92–1.85)
		Midluteal	0.011	(0.41)	0.243	(0.9)	0.16	(0.59)
Progesterone	2200	Late follicular	0.095	(3.02)	2.1	(6.68)	1.5	(4.77)
		Luteal	1.13	(35.9)	25	(79.5)	24	(76.3)
Androstenedione	2010	⋯	0.159	(5.1)	3.2	(11.1)	0.8–1.6	(2.77–5.55)
Testosterone	690	⋯	0.038	(1.32)	0.26	(0.9)	⋯	⋯
Dehydroepiandrosterone	1640	⋯	0.49	(16.8)	8	(27.5)	0.3–3	(1.03–10.3)
Dihydrotestosterone	400	⋯	0.02	(0.69)	0.05	(0.17)	0.01–0.02	(0.03–0.06)

[1]Modified from Lipsett, MB: Steroid hormones. Page 84 in: *Reproductive Endocrinology*. Yen SSC, Jaffe RB (editors). Saunders, 1978.

Table 17–2. Total plasma concentration and percentage of steroid hormone that is free or bound to plasma transport proteins in healthy women in the early follicular phase. During the luteal phase, the total concentrations of estradiol (0.72 nmol/L) and progesterone (38 nmol/L) are higher, but the distribution is the same.[1]

	Total Plasma Concentration (nmol/L)	Percentage Distribution of Steroid			
		Free	SHBG	CBG	Albumin
Estradiol	0.29	1.8	37.3	0.1	60.8
Estrone	0.23	3.6	16.3	0.1	80.1
Progesterone	0.65	2.4	0.6	17.7	79.3
Testosterone	1.3	1.4	66	2.3	30.4
Dihydrotestosterone	0.65	0.5	78.4	0.1	21
Androstenedione	5.4	7.5	6.6	1.4	84.5
Cortisol	400	3.8	0.2	89.7	6.3

[1]Data from Dunn JF, Nisula BC, Rodbard D: *J Clin Endocrinol Metab* 1981;**53**:58.

be used as an index of progesterone production. In addition, small amounts of 20α-hydroxyprogesterone are formed (Fig 17–5). This compound has one-fifth the activity of progesterone.

Physiologic Effects of Steroid Hormones

The biologic effects of the ovarian steroids are mediated by specific hormone receptors (see Chapter 1). The steroids enter cells by passive diffusion but only bind to specific receptor proteins in their target cells. These receptors, upon binding to the hormone, undergo transformation, and the complexes bind to specific sites on the chromosome. The hormone dissociates slowly from this binding site. This interaction with the gene leads to the synthesis of specific messenger RNA (mRNA).

There are estimated to be between 5000 and 20,000 receptor molecules per cell. These receptors also serve as sites for regulation of hormonal activity. For example, estrogens induce development of increased numbers of estrogen receptors in some tissues and also stimulate the synthesis of progesterone receptors. By contrast, progesterone may cause a reduction in the number of estrogen and progesterone receptors.

Although it is clear that these intracellular receptors mediate many of the important effects of steroid hormones, some effects, such as the anesthetic effect of progesterone and the stimulatory effect of estrogens on uterine blood flow, suggest that these steroids also act at the cell membrane.

A. Estrogens: Estrogens are required for the normal maturation of the female. They stimulate the maturation of the vagina, uterus, and uterine tubes at puberty as well as the secondary sex characteristics. They stimulate stromal development and ductal growth in the breast and are responsible for the accelerated growth phase and the closing of the epiphyses of the long bones that occurs at puberty. They alter the distribution of body fat so as to produce typical female body contours, including some accumulation of body fat around the hips and breasts. Larger quantities also stimulate development of pigmentation in the skin, most prominently in the region of the nipples and areolae and in the genital region.

In addition to its effects on growth of uterine muscle, estrogen also plays an important role in development of the endometrial lining. Continuous exposure to estrogens for prolonged periods leads to an abnormal hyperplasia of the endometrium that is usually associated with abnormal bleeding patterns. When estrogen production is properly coordinated with the production of progesterone during the normal human menstrual cycle, regular periodic bleeding and shedding of the endometrial lining occur.

Estrogens have a number of important metabolic effects. They seem to be partially responsible for maintenance of the normal structure of the skin and blood vessels in women. Estrogens decrease the rate of resorption of bone by antagonizing the effect of parathyroid hormone (PTH) on bone; they do not stimulate bone formation. Estrogens may have important effects on intestinal absorption, because they reduce the motility of bowel. In addition to stimulating the synthesis of enzymes leading to uterine growth, they alter the production and activity of many other enzymes in the body. In the liver, there is an increase in the synthesis of binding or transport proteins, including those for estrogen, testosterone, and thyroxine.

Estrogens enhance the coagulability of blood. Many changes in factors influencing coagulation have been reported, including increased circulating levels of factors II, VII, IX, and X. Increased plasminogen levels and decreased platelet adhesiveness have been reported.

Alterations in the composition of the plasma lipids caused by estrogens include an increase in high-density lipoproteins (HDL), a slight reduction in low-density lipoproteins (LDL), and a reduction in plasma cholesterol levels. Plasma triglyceride levels are increased.

Estrogens have many other effects. They are respon-

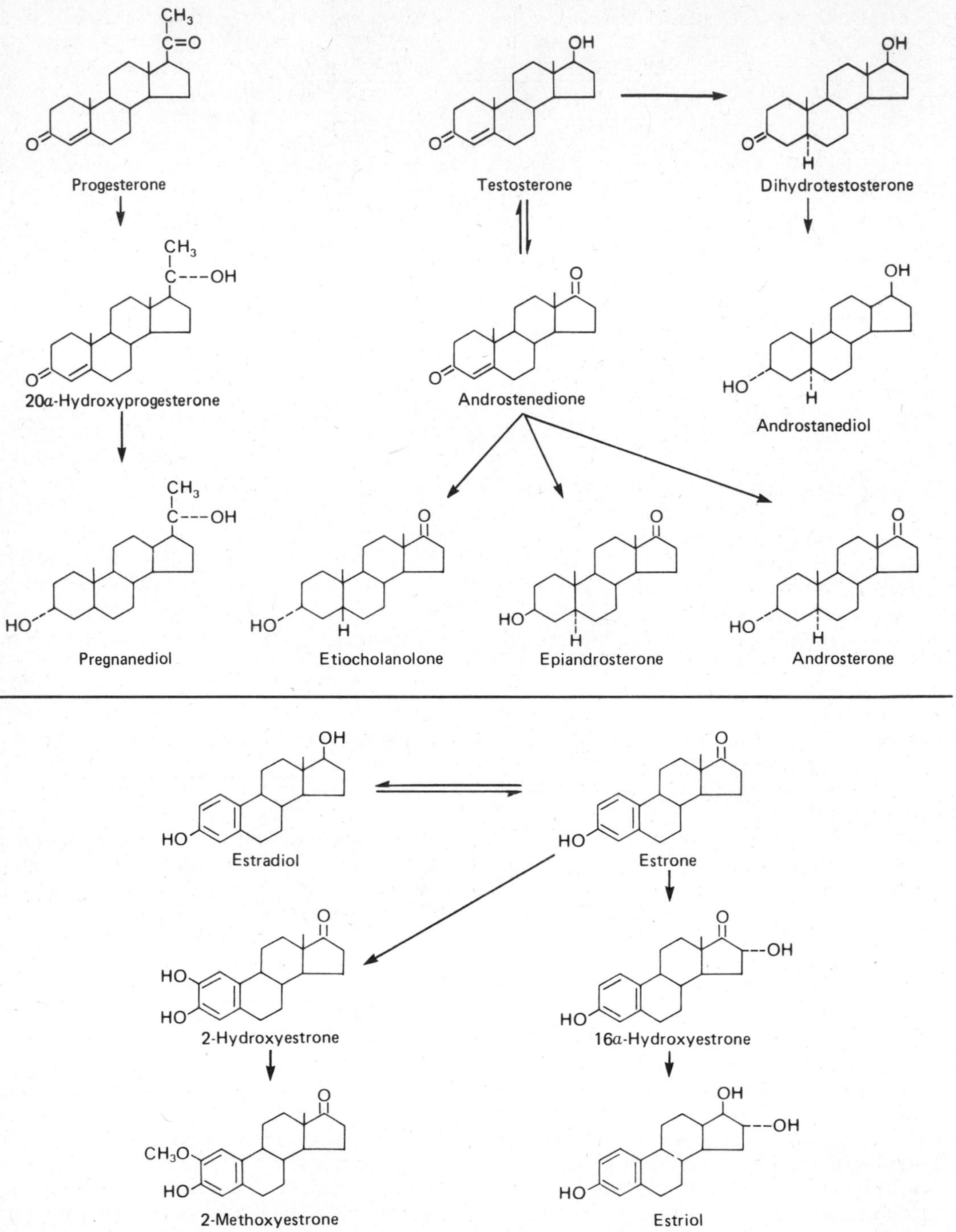

Figure 17–5. Metabolism of ovarian steroid hormones.

sible for estrous behavior in animals and influence libido in humans. They facilitate the loss of intravascular fluid into the extracellular space, producing edema. The resulting decrease in plasma volume causes a compensatory retention of sodium and water

by the kidney. Estrogens also modulate sympathetic nervous system control of smooth muscle function.

B. Progesterone: The effects of progesterone on reproductive organs include the glandular development of the breasts and the cyclic glandular development of the endometrium described below (see Menstrual Cycle) and are critical for successful reproduction. However, progesterone exhibits important metabolic effects in other organs and tissues, producing changes in carbohydrate, protein, and lipid metabolism.

A dose of 50 mg of progesterone intramuscularly daily can lead to increased insulin levels and decreased response of blood glucose levels to insulin as observed in normal pregnancy.

Progesterone can compete with aldosterone at the renal tubule, causing a decrease in Na^+ reabsorption. This leads to an increased secretion of aldosterone by the adrenal cortex—eg, in pregnancy. Progesterone increases the body temperature in humans. The mechanism of this effect is not known, but an alteration of the temperature-regulating centers in the hypothalamus has been suggested. Progesterone also alters the function of the respiratory centers. The ventilatory response to CO_2 is increased, leading to a measurable reduction in arterial and alveolar P_{CO_2} during pregnancy and in the luteal phase of the menstrual cycle. Synthetic progestins with an ethinyl group do not have these respiratory effects. Progesterone and related steroids also have hypnotic effects on the brain.

C. Androgens: The normal ovary produces potent androgens, including testosterone and dihydrotestosterone, as well as androstenedione, Δ^5-androstenediol, and DHEA. Only testosterone and dihydrotestosterone have significant androgenic activity, although androstenedione is converted to testosterone in peripheral tissues. The healthy woman produces less than 300 μg of testosterone in 24 hours, and about one-fourth of this is probably formed in the ovary directly. The physiologic significance of these small amounts of androgens is not established, but they may be partly responsible for normal hair growth at puberty and may have other important metabolic effects. Androgen production by the ovary may be markedly increased in some abnormal states (usually in association with amenorrhea), and less active precursors (eg, androstenedione) may be converted to more active hormones in target tissues such as the hair follicle and sebaceous glands.

RELAXIN

Relaxin is a polypeptide that has been extracted from the ovary. In certain animal species, it appears to play an important role at the time of parturition, causing relaxation of the pelvic ligaments and softening of the uterine cervix. The 3-dimensional structure of relaxin is similar to that of insulin and related growth-promoting polypeptides, although the amino acid sequences are different. It consists of 2 chains linked by disulfide bonds, cleaved from a prohormone. It is found in the ovary, placenta, and uterus and in the blood. Relaxin synthesis has been demonstrated in luteinized granulosa cells of the corpus luteum. In addition to changing the mechanical properties of tissues such as the cervix and pubic ligaments, it increases glycogen synthesis and water uptake by the myometrium and decreases its contractility. It may also have mammotropic effects.

In women, relaxin has been measured by immunoassay. During the menstrual cycle, levels were highest immediately after the LH surge and during menstruation. Circulating levels of relaxin are reported to be 25% higher by the end of the first trimester than during the second and third trimesters.

OTHER OVARIAN HORMONES & REGULATORY SUBSTANCES

Several nonsteroidal substances that may be important in the regulation of both intra- and extraovarian processes have been found in follicular fluid. These substances include factors that can decrease (eg, inhibin or folliculostatin) or increase (eg, activin) FSH secretion, modulate steroid secretion from granulosa cells, and delay the maturation of the oocyte in the developing preovulatory follicle (oocyte maturation inhibitor).

THE MENSTRUAL CYCLE

The female reproductive system undergoes a series of regular cyclic changes termed the menstrual cycle. The most obvious of these changes is periodic vaginal bleeding, resulting from shedding of the endometrial lining of the uterus. Normal menstrual function results from the interaction of the hypothalamus, pituitary, and ovaries and associated changes in the target tissues of the reproductive tract. Although each component is essential for normal reproductive function, the ovary plays a central role in this process, since it appears to be responsible for regulating both the cyclic changes and the length of the menstrual cycle. In most women in the middle reproductive years, menstrual bleeding recurs every 25–35 days, with a median cycle length of 28 days (Fig 17–6). In women with ovulatory cycles, the interval from the onset of menses to ovulation—the follicular (proliferative) phase—is variable in duration and accounts for the range of cycle lengths observed in ovulating women. The interval from ovulation to the onset of menstrual bleeding—the luteal (secretory) phase—is relatively constant and averages 14 ± 2 days in most women. The greatest variability in cycle length is found in the first few years after menarche and the years immediately preceding the menopause. There is a high incidence of anovulatory vaginal bleeding at these times.

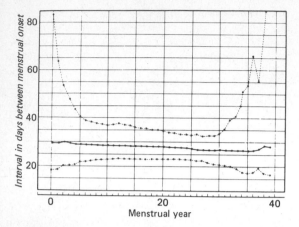

Figure 17–6. Median lengths of menstrual cycles (solid line) throughout reproductive life in women from menarche (year 0) to menopause (year 40). Ninety percent of all cycles fall within the upper and lower dotted lines. (After Treolar AE et al. Reproduced, with permission, from Yen SSC, Jaffe RB [editors]: *Reproductive Endocrinology.* Saunders, 1978.)

HORMONAL PROFILES DURING THE MENSTRUAL CYCLE

Pituitary Gonadotropins

Luteinizing hormone (LH) and follicle-stimulating hormone (FSH) are glycoproteins with molecular weights of about 28,000 and 33,000, respectively. Each hormone is composed of an alpha subunit and a beta subunit. The alpha subunits have essentially the same amino acid sequences. The beta subunits, however, are unique and are responsible for the characteristic biologic activities of each hormone. The initial plasma half-life of LH is approximately 30 minutes, whereas the half-life of FSH is 3 hours. The profiles of LH and FSH throughout the menstrual cycle are illustrated in Figure 17–7. Because of the diversity of standards used to quantitate gonadotropins, the LH and FSH values for the same serum sample reported by different laboratories may vary 2- or 3-fold. The clinician must therefore be aware of the laboratory's upper and lower limits of normal. Serum FSH levels persistently greater than 40 mIU/mL (milli-International Units of the Second International Reference Preparation of Human Menopausal Gonadotropin; mIU-2nd IRP-HMG) usually indicate declining or absent ovarian follicular activity.

In the normal menstrual cycle, serum concentrations of both LH and FSH begin to increase a few days prior to menses. FSH concentrations initially increase more rapidly than those of LH and attain maximum levels during the first half of the follicular phase. FSH levels gradually decline in the latter half of the follicular phase and, with the exception of a brief peak at

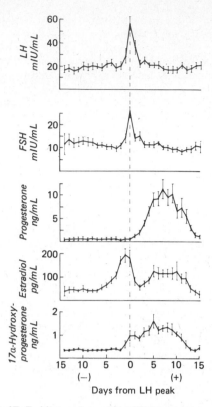

Figure 17–7. Mean values of LH, FSH, progesterone, estradiol, and 17α-hydroxyprogesterone in daily serum samples from 9 women during ovulatory menstrual cycles. Data from different cycles have been combined using the day of the midcycle LH peak as the reference day (day 0). The vertical bars represent one standard error of the mean. (Reproduced, with permission, from Thorneycroft IH et al: *Am J Obstet Gynecol* 1971; **111:**947).

midcycle, continue to fall until the lowest concentrations in the cycle are reached during the second half of the luteal phase. The preovulatory decline in serum concentrations of FSH is a consequence of the rising concentration of estradiol in this period. LH levels increase gradually throughout the follicular phase. At midcycle, there is a large peak in serum concentration of LH (midcycle LH surge) lasting 1–3 days. Subsequently, LH levels gradually decline, also reaching their lowest concentrations late in the luteal phase (Fig 17–7). Frequent measurements of serum gonadotropin levels in individual women indicate that gonadotropin secretion—particularly LH—is pulsatile. These pulses of gonadotropins are dependent upon the pulsatile secretion of gonadotropin-releasing hormone (GnRH) from the hypothalamus. During the follicular phase, pulses of LH occur approximately every hour. During the luteal phase, these pulses gradually decrease in frequency, occurring as infrequently as once every 4–8 hours. The decrease in frequency is secondary to rising levels of progesterone, which slow down the hypothalamic GnRH pulse generator.

Prolactin (PRL)

In contrast to LH and FSH profiles, there are no consistent cyclic changes in individual PRL profiles during the normal menstrual cycle. In studies of large numbers of women, however, mean PRL levels in the preovulatory and luteal phases of the menstrual cycle may be slightly higher than in the follicular phase. There is also a significant diurnal variation in plasma concentrations of PRL, with peak levels during the night and early morning hours. Laboratories vary in their reporting of PRL levels (as they do also in reporting gonadotropin levels) because of the use of standards with different biologic and immunologic potencies. The upper limit of normal may thus vary from 15 ng/mL to 30 ng/mL (0.68–1.4 nmol/L), depending upon the laboratory.

Ovarian Steroids

The ovary secretes progestins, androgens, and estrogens. Many of these steroids are also secreted by the adrenal gland or can be formed by peripheral conversion of other steroid precursors; consequently, plasma concentrations of these hormones may not directly reflect ovarian steroidogenic activity. Table 17–1 summarizes the plasma concentrations, metabolic clearance rates, and production rates of the major steroids secreted by the ovary in normal women.

A. Estrogens: Estradiol (E_2) is perhaps the most important secretory product of the ovary, because of its biologic potency and diverse physiologic effects on peripheral target tissues. Plasma concentrations of estradiol during the first half of the follicular phase are low, generally less than 50 pg/mL (0.18 nmol/L) (Fig 17–7). About 1 week prior to the midcycle gonadotropin surge, estradiol concentrations begin to increase rapidly, and peak levels of approximately 200–300 pg/mL (0.73–1.1 nmol/L) are attained on the day preceding—or, less commonly, the day of—the LH surge. The rise in plasma estradiol levels correlates closely with the increase in size of the preovulatory follicle. After the LH surge, serum estradiol levels fall rapidly for several days. There is a secondary increase in plasma estradiol levels that reaches a peak in the midportion of the luteal phase, reflecting estrogen secretion by the corpus luteum. Plasma patterns of estrone during the menstrual cycle are similar to those of estradiol, but the changes in concentrations are less than those of estradiol; thus, the ratio of estrone to estradiol varies throughout the cycle. The ratio is highest at the time of menses, when estradiol secretion is minimal, and lowest in the preovulatory period, when estradiol secretion is maximal. While most of the estradiol in the peripheral circulation results from direct ovarian secretion, a significant fraction of the circulating estrone arises from estradiol and the peripheral

conversion of androstenedione. Catheterization studies have shown that increased plasma concentrations of estradiol in the preovulatory and midluteal phases of the cycle principally reflect secretion from the ovary containing the dominant or preovulatory follicle, which later becomes the corpus luteum.

B. Progesterone: Throughout the follicular phase, serum concentrations of progesterone are low—less than 1 ng/mL (3.18 nmol/L). At the time of the LH surge, there is a small increase in plasma concentrations of progesterone, followed by a rise over the next 4–5 days (Fig 17–7). Progesterone levels reach a plateau at concentrations between 10 and 20 ng/mL (32–64 nmol/L) during the midportion of the luteal phase. Thereafter, progesterone levels decline rapidly, reaching concentrations of about 1 ng/mL (3.18 nmol/L) by the first day of menses. Although catheterization studies have shown that progesterone is secreted by both ovaries during the first half of the follicular phase, most of the circulating progesterone at this time appears to be derived from the extraglandular conversion of the adrenal steroids, pregnenolone and pregnenolone sulfate, and from the direct secretion of small amounts of progesterone by the adrenal glands.

During the luteal phase of the cycle, virtually all of the circulating progesterone arises by direct secretion from the corpus luteum. Measurement of plasma concentrations of progesterone is widely used to monitor ovulation. Concentrations greater than 4 or 5 ng/mL (12.7–15.9 nmol/L) suggest that ovulation has occurred.

C. Androgens: In healthy women, circulating androgens can be derived from secretion by the ovaries and the adrenal glands and also by peripheral conversion of steroid precursors of ovarian and adrenal origin. In healthy women, testosterone is secreted in small quantities by the ovaries and adrenal glands. About 50–70% of the circulating testosterone, however, arises primarily from the peripheral conversion of androstenedione. Mean plasma concentrations of testosterone range from 0.2 ng/mL to 0.4 ng/mL (0.69–1.39 nmol/L) during most of the follicular and luteal phases and increase slightly in the preovulatory phase. Androstenedione arises primarily from direct secretion by the ovaries and adrenal glands. Only a small percentage (about 10%) is formed by peripheral conversion. Secretion of androstenedione by the adrenal does not vary significantly during different phases of the menstrual cycle, although there is a diurnal variation in adrenal secretion of androstenedione similar to that of cortisol. Ovarian secretion of androstenedione, however, fluctuates throughout the menstrual cycle, and the pattern of secretion resembles that of estradiol. Serum concentrations of androstenedione increase in the late follicular phase of the cycle and are maximal at the time of the midcycle gonadotropin surge. There is a small secondary peak of androstenedione during the midluteal phase. Plasma concentrations of both DHEA and DHEA sulfate vary independently of the phase of the menstrual cycle. Both hormones are secreted primarily by the adrenal gland.

THE OVARIAN CYCLE

Ovarian Structure

Throughout adult reproductive years, the structural composition and hormonal activity of the ovary are continually changing (Figs 17–3 and 17–8). These changes in composition and activity are responsible for many of the physiologic events in the normal menstrual cycle. The 2 major functions of the adult ovary—the synthesis and secretion of sex steroids and the release of a mature ovum every 28–30 days—normally progress in concert with one another and are closely interrelated. The basic reproductive unit of the ovary is the small **primordial follicle,** consisting of (1) a small oocyte (<25 μm in diameter) arrested in the diplotene stage of meiotic prophase; (2) a few, or a complete ring of, poorly differentiated granulosa cells; and (3) a basement membrane that surrounds the granulosa cells, separating them from the adjacent ovarian stroma. Primordial follicles are found principally in the outer cortex just beneath the fibrous capsule of the ovary. These primordial follicles constitute an inactive or resting pool from which all ovulatory follicles will eventually develop. During late fetal life and throughout the prepubertal years, a small percentage of these small, inactive follicles are continually resuming growth. At an early stage of development and prior to antrum formation, however, growth is arrested and the follicles undergo atresia. Although ovulation does not occur, the continual process of limited growth and atresia in the prepubertal ovary depletes a large portion of the small primordial follicles, so that only about 400,000 primordial follicles remain at puberty (Fig 17–2). Of these follicles, only about 400 will reach full development and release an oocyte during ovulation in the adult.

The earliest morphologic change indicating that the primordial follicle has left the pool of resting follicles and resumed the process of growth is an increase in size of the oocyte. As the oocyte enlarges, the zona pellucida, a membrane that will eventually surround the oocyte, begins to form. The flat, poorly differentiated granulosa cells, which form a single layer, assume a cuboid shape as the oocyte approaches its maximum size of 80–100 μm. At this stage of development, the follicular unit is known as a **primary follicle.** Subsequently, the granulosa cells rapidly proliferate, forming a multilayered covering around the oocyte. Small patches of fluid form between the granulosa cells. Blood vessels, however, do not penetrate the basement membrane surrounding the granulosa cells, and the granulosa layer remains avascular until after ovulation has occurred. As the follicle continues to enlarge, cells that are indistinguishable from mesenchymal fibroblasts align themselves concentrically outside the basement membrane. These cells form the thecal layer and complete the formation of the **secondary follicle (preantral follicle).** As the granulosa cells continue to multiply, there is further production and accumulation of fluid within the granulosa cell layer, leading to the formation of a follicular cavity, or **antrum.** The oocyte and a portion of the surrounding granulosa cells (cumulus cells) are gradually displaced to one side of the follicular cavity, and a **tertiary follicle (antral follicle)** is formed. There is both a rapid accumulation of follicular fluid and additional growth of granulosa cells, causing further enlargement of the **preovulatory (graafian) follicle.** The follicle reaches a diameter of 2–2.5 cm shortly before ovulation. Following ovulation, the antrum fills with blood and lymph fluid (Fig 17–3). The wall of the follicle collapses and becomes convoluted, and vessels from the thecal layer invade the granulosa layer. The appearance of the granulosa cells changes markedly after ovulation, and they become luteinized. In conjunction with the contiguous thecal layer or adjacent stromal cells, the luteinized granulosa layer forms the **corpus luteum.** If pregnancy does not follow ovulation, the corpus luteum lasts about 14 days and is gradually replaced by fibrous tissue, forming a **corpus albicans.** The mechanisms responsible for regression (luteolysis) of the corpus

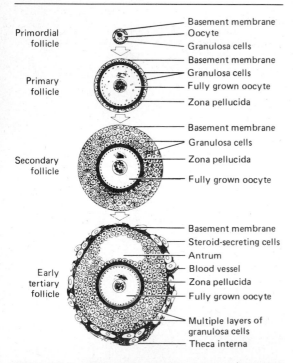

Figure 17–8. Morphologic changes that occur in ovarian follicles during growth and development. (Reproduced, with permission, from Erickson GF: Follicular growth and development. Chapter 12 in: *Gynecology and Obstetrics.* Vol 5. Sciarra JJ [editor]. Harper & Row, 1981.)

luteum after 14 days in humans are incompletely understood. In nonprimates, prostaglandins appear to play an important role in luteolysis.

Control of Growth & Steroidogenesis in Ovarian Follicles

The factors that stimulate resting primordial follicles to resume growth and development are unknown. Pituitary gonadotropins, however, are not involved in initiating these events. Cohorts of primordial follicles in prepubertal girls—in whom LH and FSH levels are undetectable—and in hypophysectomized laboratory animals are continually leaving the large pool of inactive primordial follicles and resuming growth. Development beyond the preantral or early antral stage, however, depends upon the interaction of pituitary gonadotropins, ovarian steroids, and other local factors within the follicle.

Receptors for FSH have been found only in granulosa cells. Each cell is estimated to contain about 1000 receptors. The binding of FSH to its receptor stimulates the synthesis of enzymes which have aromatase activity and which convert androgen precursors to estrogens. Estradiol, in turn, plays a critical role in follicular growth and development both by a local effect on granulosa cells and via positive and negative feedback regulation of FSH and LH secretion (see below). In small follicles, estradiol induces the proliferation of granulosa cells. In the absence of FSH, estradiol per se can stimulate follicular growth to the

preantral stage, but further development is dependent upon gonadotropin stimulation. FSH and estradiol, working in concert, also induce the formation of LH receptors in granulosa cells. In contrast to FSH receptors, which are restricted to granulosa cells, LH receptors also have been found in theca, interstitial, and luteal cells.

The cellular origin of estradiol in large ovarian follicles in primates remains controversial. In the rat, granulosa cells lack the enzymes 17α-hydroxylase and C17,20 lyase and thus are unable to directly synthesize androgens or estrogens from C21 precursors—eg, progesterone or pregnenolone. Therefore, estradiol production by granulosa cells is dependent upon the availability of C19 androgenic precursors (testosterone and androstenedione), which can be aromatized to estrogens. These observations have led to the formation of the "2-cell theory" to explain estradiol formation within the follicular complex (Fig 17–9). According to this hypothesis, LH stimulates the synthesis of androgenic precursors, primarily androstenedione and to a lesser extent testosterone, by the theca cells. The androgens diffuse across the basement membrane that separates the theca and granulosa cells. Some of the androstenedione and testosterone enters the antral fluid, while the remainder is converted to estradiol by the granulosa cells. Studies in primates, however, have shown that both the thecal layer and the granulosa cells of antral follicles are able to synthesize estradiol; consequently, it is unclear whether it is the theca cells or the granulosa cells that are the principal site of es-

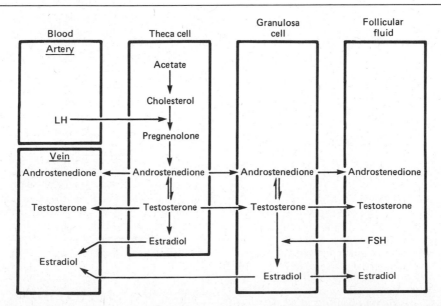

Figure 17–9. Pathways involved in the synthesis and secretion of androgens and estradiol by the preovulatory follicle. In primates, it is not known if the theca cells or granulosa cells are the major source for estradiol in plasma. (Reproduced, with permission, from Peters H, McNatty KP: *The Ovary: A Correlation of Structure and Function in Mammals.* Granada Publishing, 1980.)

tradiol synthesis in the mid and late follicular phases of the menstrual cycle. A study in the rhesus monkey suggested that most of the estradiol production in the preovulatory period was of theca cell—not granulosa cell—origin. It is possible that most of the estradiol produced by the granulosa cells remains within the follicular fluid, while estradiol in the serum arises primarily from the thecal layer.

In the normal ovary, androgens produced by the thecal layer—particularly androstenedione—serve, in part, as precursors of estrogen synthesis by granulosa cells. Androgens utilized in this fashion thus indirectly facilitate follicular growth via estradiol stimulation. However, high concentrations of testosterone or dihydrotestosterone—or increased ratios of androgen to estrogen—have been found in follicles undergoing atresia, and this suggests an inhibitory action of androgens on follicular development. This could explain, in part, the lack of normal follicular development in polycystic ovary syndrome. In this disorder, high levels of LH may promote excessive androgen production by the thecal layer. Since FSH levels are low, granulosa cells may have a reduced capacity to convert these androgens to estrogens.

All of the developing follicles within the ovary are initially exposed to similar concentrations of FSH and LH. Since fewer than 1% of these follicles will eventually reach full maturity and ovulate, local factors must play a critical role in selection of the dominant preovulatory follicle. There are significant differences in the concentrations of protein and steroid hormones in the antral fluid of follicles of differing sizes and at differing stages of the menstrual cycle. The presence of this fluid-filled cavity provides a mechanism by which the granulosa cells and oocyte of one developing follicle can be exposed to a unique microenvironment that differs from that of the other developing follicles within the ovary. Studies have shown that it is the concentrations of pituitary gonadotropins and ovarian steroids within the follicular fluid rather than the serum concentrations of these hormones that correlate most closely with both the mitotic and synthetic activity of the granulosa cells as well as with the future viability of the oocyte. The highest concentrations of FSH and LH in antral fluid are found in the largest follicles during the late follicular phase of the menstrual cycle. Prolactin (PRL) levels, in contrast, are highest in small follicles and lower in large follicles in the late follicular phase. The concentrations of LH and FSH in follicular fluid are generally lower than corresponding serum levels, but the concentrations of ovarian steroids—androstenedione, testosterone, dihydrotestosterone, and estradiol—may be 10–40,000 times greater than their serum levels. Although androgen concentrations do not differ greatly in follicular fluid from either small or large follicles, mean estradiol concentrations in antral fluid increase markedly, reaching levels in excess of 1500 ng/mL (5507 nmol/L) in large follicles in the late follicular phase of

the menstrual cycle. It is not known at present whether these increases in the absolute concentration of estradiol and the ratio of estradiol to androgen in antral fluid are a consequence of follicular growth and development or play an important role in the process that leads to selection of a single preovulatory follicle.

Nonsteroidal Ovarian Regulatory Factors

Several proteins that can alter the secretion of FSH and/or modify estradiol secretion by granulosa cells have been identified in ovarian follicular fluid. The best characterized of these are the inhibins A and B, which are glycoprotein heterodimers with 2 subunits. Both inhibins have a common alpha subunit but somewhat different beta subunits, called β_a and β_b. Inhibin preferentially inhibits the secretion of FSH; it is thought to be produced by ovarian granulosa cells. If the beta subunits of inhibin are combined, forming a dimer without the usual alpha subunit, the resultant proteins, known as activins, can stimulate the secretion of FSH. The exact physiologic roles of inhibins and activins during the menstrual cycle remain to be elucidated.

HORMONE INTERACTION & REGULATION DURING THE MENSTRUAL CYCLE

Gonadotropin-Releasing Hormone (GnRH)

GnRH (also referred to as luteinizing hormone–releasing hormone [LHRH]; luteotropin-releasing hormone [LRH]; and luteotropin-releasing factor [LRF]) is a decapeptide synthesized by neurosecretory cells located primarily within the hypothalamus. It regulates the secretion of LH and FSH and is essential for their synthesis and release. LH and FSH cannot be detected in serum from peripheral blood of women with congenital absence of hypothalamic GnRH. Ovarian sex steroids are not essential for the synthesis of LH and FSH, but they modulate release of these hormones by altering either gonadotrope response to GnRH or secretion of hypothalamic GnRH. Concentrations of GnRH in serum from peripheral blood are very low, and the pattern of GnRH secretion throughout the menstrual cycle in humans has not been well characterized. However, studies in humans suggest that GnRH secretion may be increased in the preovulatory period. GnRH has been measured in the pituitary portal blood of rhesus monkeys. In these nonhuman primates, GnRH is secreted in pulses every 1–3 hours. Concentrations of GnRH in the portal blood of nonhuman primates during the follicular phase of the menstrual cycle range from less than 10 pg/mL (which is undetectable) to 200 pg/mL. Studies in sheep have shown that each episode of LH release is triggered by a pulse of GnRH from the hypothalamus. Continuous infusions of GnRH initially increase the secretion of LH and FSH. After several hours or days of continuous infusion, desensitization and receptor "down-regulation" occur, and the pituitary gonadotropes become refractory to further stimulation by GnRH.

Regulation of GnRH Secretion

In both rhesus monkeys and humans, intermittent pulses of GnRH every 60–90 minutes stimulate indefinitely the release of LH and FSH. In rhesus monkeys, changes in the frequency of the GnRH pulses can selectively increase or decrease the serum concentration of either LH or FSH. This observation suggests a mechanism by which a single releasing hormone, GnRH, can alter the ratio of LH to FSH in serum and further supports the concept that GnRH is the only hypothalamic hormone required for the regulation of both LH and FSH secretion.

Effects of Ovarian Steroids & Peptides on Gonadotropin Secretion

A. Negative Feedback: Under most conditions, ovarian steroids limit or reduce the secretion of pituitary gonadotropins. Serum concentrations of both FSH and LH increase markedly following ovariectomy or menopause, whereas the administration of estrogen (or estrogen and progesterone) lowers serum gonadotropin levels. Throughout most of the normal menstrual cycle, the negative feedback effects of ovarian steroids predominate and plasma gonadotropin concentrations remain below 25 mIU/ mL. The physiologic importance of inhibin and other inhibitory peptides of ovarian origin during the normal menstrual cycle has not yet been determined.

B. Positive Feedback: Estradiol and progesterone, under certain conditions, can induce the release of LH and FSH. During the menstrual cycle, rising concentrations of estradiol in the latter part of the follicular phase initiate the preovulatory surge of LH via this mechanism. This increase in LH secretion in turn stimulates a small but significant increase in the secretion of progesterone that further augments the LH surge and, coupled with estradiol, initiates the midcycle surge of FSH. Although the negative feedback action of ovarian steroids may become apparent within a few hours, positive feedback develops more slowly, and 48–72 hours of sustained estrogen stimulation is generally required before an increase in LH secretion is observed. It is probable that the negative and positive feedback actions of ovarian sex steroids result from both (1) a direct effect of the steroids on the pituitary gonadotropes that alters their sensitivity to GnRH and (2) modulation of the frequency and magnitude of the pulses of hypothalamic GnRH.

Neural Regulation of the Menstrual Cycle

In nonhuman primates—and perhaps in humans as well—the neural components that control both the

tonic and surge secretion of gonadotropins are located within the medial basal hypothalamus. When the medial basal hypothalamus, which includes the median eminence, the arcuate nucleus, and portions of the ventromedial nucleus, was surgically isolated from the remainder of the brain without disrupting the hypothalamic-pituitary-portal vasculature, gonadotropin secretion in rhesus monkeys was not significantly altered. Both the negative and positive feedback actions of estradiol remained intact, and many monkeys continued to have spontaneous ovulatory menstrual cycles. It is probable, however, that other neural areas outside the hypothalamus (eg, limbic structures) normally modify gonadotropin secretion.

GnRH plays a permissive, though still essential, role in the regulation of LH and FSH secretion throughout the menstrual cycle. Pulsatile administration of exogenous GnRH every 60–90 minutes induced ovulatory menstrual cycles in monkeys with hypothalamic lesions or in humans with congenital absence of hypothalamic GnRH. In these cycles, the serum profiles of pituitary gonadotropins and ovarian steroids were within normal limits. These observations suggest that the cyclic nature of the menstrual cycle in primates is regulated by the ovary and not by the brain. The length of the menstrual cycle thus is determined by both the time required for development of a mature follicle and by the functional life span of the corpus luteum. Following luteolysis, follicular development resumes, and a new menstrual cycle begins. The major hypothalamic-pituitary-gonadal interactions that regulate the menstrual cycle are summarized in Figure 17–10.

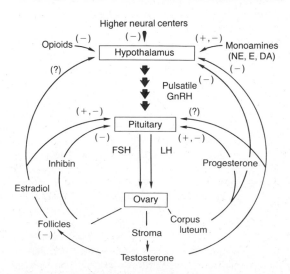

Figure 17–10. The major hypothalamic-pituitary-gonadal interactions thought to regulate the menstrual cycle. Ovarian sex steroids and neural monoamines may exert stimulatory (+) or inhibitory (−) (or both) effects on the secretion of GnRH or pituitary gonadotropins (or both).

CYCLIC CHANGES IN THE FEMALE REPRODUCTIVE TRACT

As a consequence of the changing rates of secretion of estrogen and progesterone throughout the menstrual cycle, the female reproductive tract undergoes a series of regular and cyclic changes. These changes can be recognized by histologic study of the endometrium, the composition and appearance of the cervical mucus, and the cytologic features of the vaginal epithelium. The end of each cycle is marked by uterine bleeding that continues for 3–7 days.

HISTOLOGY OF THE ENDOMETRIUM THROUGHOUT THE MENSTRUAL CYCLE

The endometrium consists of 2 distinct layers or zones differing in both histologic appearance and functional responsiveness to hormonal stimulation: a **basal layer** and a **functional layer.** The basal layer is in direct contact with the myometrium, undergoes little change throughout the menstrual cycle, and is not sloughed during menses. The functional layer arises from the basal layer and eventually surrounds the entire lumen of the uterine cavity. The functional layer can be subdivided further into 2 components: a thin superficial **compact layer** and a deeper **spongiosa layer,** of which most of the secretory or fully developed endometrium is composed. The blood supply of the endometrium consists of a highly specialized network of arterial and venous channels. The **spiral arteries** arise within the myometrium from branches of the uterine artery, pass through the basal endometrial layer, and extend into the functional zone. The proximal portion of the spiral artery, the **straight artery,** distributes blood to tissues of the basal layer and is not influenced by changes in estrogen and progesterone secretion. The spiral arteries, however, undergo cyclic regeneration and degeneration during each menstrual cycle in response to hormonal changes.

The endometrial cycle can be subdivided into 3 major phases: proliferative, secretory, and menstrual. The morphologic changes of the endometrium that occur during the normal menstrual cycle have been described in great detail and are summarized in Figure 17–11. For convenience, the changes described in this figure and the following discussion are based on a hypothetical menstrual cycle of 28 days, in which the follicular and luteal phases are each approximately 14 days in length.

Proliferative Phase

When menstrual flow ceases, a thin layer of basal endometrial tissue remains. This tissue, consisting of the remnants of glands and stroma, grows rapidly. Epithelial cells from the glands proliferate and cover the raw stromal surfaces with a layer of simple columnar epithelium. In the early proliferative phase, most of the glands are straight, short, and narrow. The glandular epithelium exhibits increasing mitotic activity. Throughout the proliferative phase, there is continued and rapid growth of both the epithelial and stromal components of the endometrium. By the late proliferative phase of the menstrual cycle, the surface of the endometrium is somewhat undulant. The glands are becoming tortuous and are lined by tall columnar cells with basal nuclei. Pseudostratification of nuclei is prominent. The stroma at this time is moderately dense, with many mitotic figures.

Secretory Phase

During the secretory phase, histologic changes occur very rapidly. During the first half of this phase, the appearance of the glandular epithelium is most useful in precise dating of the endometrium, whereas in the second half, accurate dating depends largely on the characteristics of the stroma. On the 16th day of the cycle (second postovulatory day), subnuclear glycogen-rich vacuoles become prominent in the glandular epithelium. The vacuoles push the epithelial cell nuclei into a central position within the cells. By the 19th day (fifth postovulatory day), few vacuoles remain within the cells. Acidophilic intraluminal glandular secretory material is most apparent on day 21. Stromal edema, which is variable during the proliferative phase, also becomes prominent at this time and peaks on day 22. By day 24, pseudodecidual or predecidual changes begin to appear within the stroma. These changes are initially most apparent near the spiral arteries and eventually encompass large areas of the stroma. Lymphocytic infiltration of the stroma increases markedly in conjunction with the appearance of pseudodecidual changes, and by day 26, PMN invasion also is apparent.

If the blastocyst implants successfully, serum concentrations of hCG and, secondarily, progesterone begin to increase 7–10 days after ovulation (ie, days 21–24 of the menstrual cycle). The rising levels of progesterone produce a type of endometrial change known as decidualization. The decidua of pregnancy consists primarily of plump, eosinophilic stromal cells that have a pavementlike appearance. In the early stages of pregnancy, the cells of the glandular epithelium become distended with clear cytoplasm and possibly with enlarged and hyperchromatic nuclei, a feature called the Arias-Stella phenomenon. With advancing pregnancy, the endometrial glands gradually atrophy.

Menstrual Phase

In the absence of pregnancy, changes in the endometrium secondary to declining hormone production by the corpus luteum can be observed by day 24. The functional layer of the stroma begins to shrink, and the endometrial glands become more tortuous and saw-

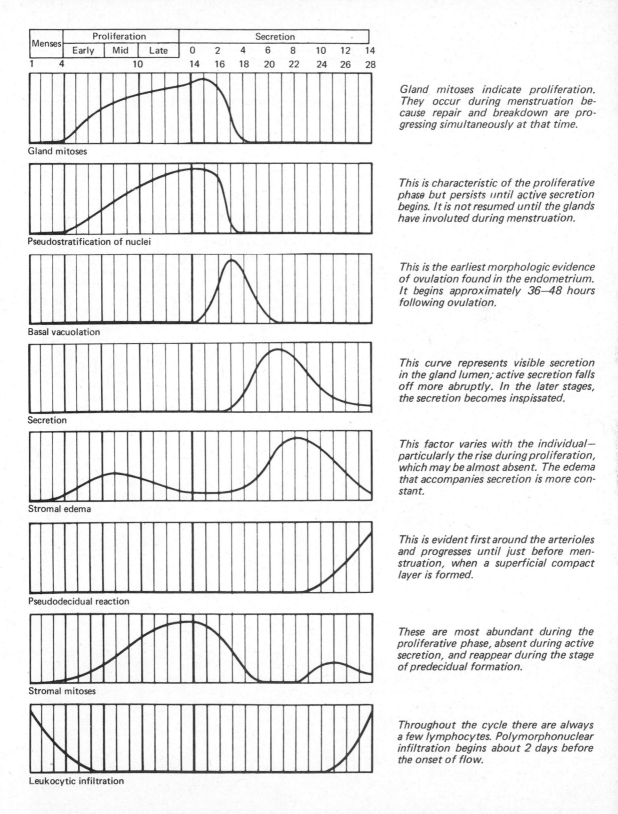

Figure 17–11. Morphologic changes in the endometrium that are useful in determining the stage of the menstrual cycle. (After Noyes, Hertig, & Rock. Reproduced, with permission, from Benson RC [editor]: *Current Obstetric & Gynecologic Diagnosis & Treatment,* 5th ed. Lange, 1984.)

toothed in appearance. Intermittent constriction of the spiral arteries leads to stasis within the capillaries of the functional layer, tissue ischemia, and extravasation of blood into the stroma with formation of small hematomas. Eventually, desquamation and sloughing of the entire functional layer of the endometrium occurs.

Endometrial biopsy has been used extensively in the past to assess progesterone secretion in women with menstrual dysfunction and infertility. With the widespread availability of reliable radioimmunoassays to measure serum concentrations of progesterone, the need for endometrial biopsy is limited; it should be used primarily to assess the response of the endometrium to hormonal stimulation. Endometrial biopsy is most informative when performed a few days before the anticipated menstrual period. Although biopsy late in the luteal phase may potentially interrupt a pregnancy if conception has occurred, the risk is minimal.

CERVICAL MUCUS

Cervical mucus is a complex secretion produced by the glands of the endocervix. It is composed of 92–98% water and approximately 1% inorganic salts, of which NaCl is the main constituent. The mucus also contains free simple sugars, polysaccharides, proteins, and glycoproteins. Its pH is usually alkaline and ranges from 6.5 to 9.0. Several physical charac-teristics of cervical mucus can be evaluated readily by the clinician. Since these characteristics are influenced by serum estrogen and progesterone levels, it is often possible to gain an approximate assessment of the hormonal status of a patient by examination of cervical mucus. Estrogen stimulates the production of copious amounts (up to 700 mg/d) of clear, watery mucus through which sperm can penetrate most readily. Progesterone, however, even in the presence of high plasma levels of estrogen, reduces the secretion of mucus. Both during the luteal phase of the menstrual cycle and during pregnancy, the mucus is scant, viscous, and cellular. During most of the menstrual cycle, 20–60 mg of mucus is produced each day.

Figure 17–12 summarizes those characteristics of cervical mucus that the clinician can readily determine and correlates them with the day of the menstrual cycle.

Spinnbarkeit is the property that allows cervical mucus to be stretched or drawn into a thread. Spinnbarkeit can be estimated by stretching a sample of mucus between 2 glass slides and measuring the maximum length of the thread before it breaks. At midcycle, spinnbarkeit usually exceeds 10 cm. **Ferning,** or **arborization,** refers to the characteristic microscopic pattern cervical mucus forms when dried on a slide (Fig 17–13). Ferning results from the crystallization of inorganic salts around small and optimal amounts of organic material present in cervical mucus. As serum

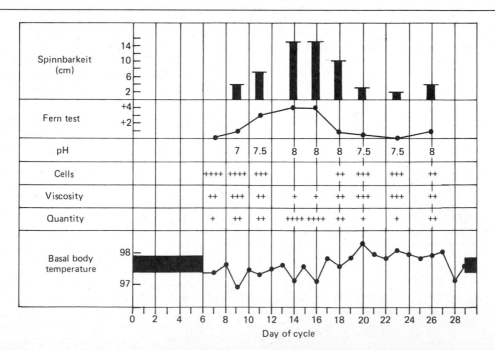

Figure 17–12. Changes in the composition and properties of cervical mucus throughout the menstrual cycle. (Modified and reproduced, with permission, from Moghissi KS: Composition and function of cervical secretion. Chapter 31 in: *Handbook of Physiology,* Section 7: Endocrinology, Vol 2, Part 2. Greep RO [editor]. American Physiological Society, 1973.)

Normal cycle, 14th day

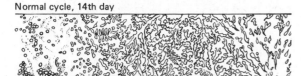

Midluteal phase, normal cycle

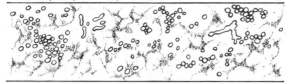

Anovulatory cycle with estrogen present

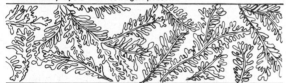

Figure 17–13. Patterns formed when cervical mucus is smeared on a slide, permitted to dry, and examined under the microscope. Progesterone makes the mucus thick and cellular. In the smear from a patient who failed to ovulate (*bottom*), there is no progesterone to inhibit the estrogen-induced fern pattern. (Reproduced, with permission, from Ganong WF: *Review of Medical Physiology,* 14th ed. Appleton & Lange, 1989.)

concentrations of estradiol increase, the composition of cervical mucus changes, so that dried mucus begins to demonstrate ferning in the latter part of the follicular phase. In the periovulatory interval, when estradiol levels are maximal and prior to significant progesterone secretion, ferning is most prominent and the mucus is thin, watery, and contains few cells. As serum progesterone concentrations increase following ovulation, the quality of the mucus changes and ferning disappears. The absence of ferning can reflect either inadequate stimulation of endocervical glands by estrogen or inhibition by increased secretion of progesterone. Persistent ferning throughout the menstrual cycle suggests anovulatory cycles or insufficient progesterone secretion.

VAGINAL EPITHELIUM

The vaginal mucosa is composed of a stratified squamous epithelium and does not contain glands. Cells in the outer layer during the reproductive years are flattened and may contain keratohyaline granules, but true cornification does not normally occur. The epithelial cells of the vagina, like other tissues of the female reproductive tract, respond to changing levels of ovarian sex steroids. Estrogen stimulates the proliferation and maturation of the epithelial cells, resulting in a thickening of the vaginal mucosa and increased glycogen content of the epithelial cells. This glycogen is fermented to lactic acid by the normal bacterial flora of the vagina, thus accounting for the mildly acid pH of vaginal fluid. The histologic and cytologic changes of the vaginal epithelium of women during the normal menstrual cycle are less marked than those occurring in the estrous cycle of rodents.

Cytologists describe 3 types of exfoliated vaginal epithelial cells—superficial, intermediate, and basal-parabasal—which do not refer to the locations of the cells within the epithelium but to their degree of cellular maturity or differentiation. Exfoliated cells, obtained by light scrapings from the midportion of the lateral vaginal wall, are most useful for cytohormonal assessment.

Superficial cells are mature, flat, usually polygonal, squamous epithelial cells with pyknotic, hyperchromatic nuclei. These cells develop in response to high levels of unopposed estrogen stimulation.

Intermediate cells are relatively mature squamous epithelial cells with eosinophilic or cyanophilic cytoplasm and a vesicular, nonpyknotic nucleus. The appearance of the nucleus is the critical factor in differentiating intermediate cells from superficial cells. Intermediate cells predominate in endocrinologic states in which progesterone levels are high, such as in pregnancy or in the midluteal phase of the menstrual cycle.

Basal-parabasal cells are thick, small, oval or round, immature cells with large vesicular nuclei and cyanophilic cytoplasm. Parabasal cells usually indicate estrogen deficiency and are the predominant cell type in the prepubertal and postmenopausal periods.

Among the various indices that describe the ratio or percentage of superficial, intermediate, and basal-parabasal cells are (1) the karyopyknotic index (KPI), the ratio of superficial cells to intermediate cells; (2) the eosinophilic index (EI), the ratio of mature eosinophilic cells to mature cyanophilic cells; and (3) the maturation index (MI), the percentage of parabasal, intermediate, and superficial cells present, in that order. Since only MI includes as a factor the presence of all 3 cell types, it may provide more information than the other 2 indices.

In general, only 2 diagnostic patterns of vaginal epithelial cells are clinically useful. When the vaginal epithelium has been stimulated by estrogen, MI may range from (0/40/60) at midcycle, when estradiol concentrations are highest, to (0/70/30) late in the luteal phase, when progesterone effects are most prominent. A finding of parabasal cells with a few intermediate cells and no superficial cells indicates that the vaginal epithelium has received little or no estrogen stimulation. The MI in this instance may be (100/0/0) or (80/20/0). The vaginal smear can be used to provide a qualitative assessment of estrogen production in women with amenorrhea.

EXTRAGENITAL SYMPTOMS ASSOCIATED WITH NORMAL MENSTRUAL FUNCTION

PREMENSTRUAL SYNDROME

The premenstrual syndrome (PMS) designates a wide variety of symptoms commonly associated with the normal menstrual cycle. Common symptoms are described below, but the particular pattern of symptoms varies in different women. They are severe enough to be noticeable in about 50% of women, although many of those not consciously aware of symptoms are able to recognize that their menses are about to begin before the bleeding starts. In rare instances, the symptoms may be completely disabling and even require hospitalization. The symptoms usually begin a few days to a week before the onset of menses and cease abruptly or are markedly ameliorated with the onset of menstrual flow. However, patterns vary greatly, and in some women symptoms may be more severe during the first few days of bleeding.

The transitory increase in water content of body tissues contributes to weight gain, edema, bloating, and breast tenderness. These appear to be predominantly the result of estrogen secretion, which facilitates the loss of electrolytes and fluid into the extravascular tissues. The resulting hypovolemia causes a secondary increase in aldosterone and antidiuretic hormone release, resulting in retention of sodium and water by the kidney. These symptoms frequently respond to diuretic therapy.

Neurologic and behavioral symptoms are often the most difficult to manage. Women may become nervous, irritable, agitated, and depressed. In severe cases, these disturbances frequently disrupt family and other personal relationships. The cause of the symptoms is unknown but is probably related to the central nervous system effects of the hormones as well as social, cultural, and psychologic factors.

Diagnosis & Treatment

The physician must be informed and willing to listen carefully to the woman describe her symptoms. Some of these symptoms will probably be related to the cycle and therefore will be facilitated or triggered by the chemical changes that occur. Adoption of a life-style that includes regular hours, a healthy diet, and exercise is a good place to start in the treatment of this syndrome.

The patient's major complaints should be identified and dealt with pragmatically. Empiric treatment of symptoms may be helpful (eg, using diuretics for breast swelling and prostaglandin synthetase inhibitors for cramps and mastodynia). Changes in behavior,

anxiety, depression, agitation, and irritability are usually more difficult to treat, but severe symptoms may respond to anxiolytics and antidepressants.

If the patient does not want children, suppressing ovulation with oral contraceptives will often effectively abolish these symptoms. Danazol (in low doses), clonidine, naltrexone, alprazolam, and GnRH agonists have also been found to effectively alleviate these symptoms in placebo-controlled double-blind studies. Many other agents and hormones, including vitamin B_6, progesterone, and thyroxine, have been reported to be of value in treating PMS. However, careful studies have not found these agents to be more effective than a placebo. Hysterectomy that preserves the ovaries does not eliminate the behavioral symptoms.

DYSMENORRHEA

Dysmenorrhea unrelated to any identifiable disorder almost always begins before age 20 but seldom within the first year or so after menarche. It is one of the most important causes of lost working hours and failure to attend school. The pain is colicky in nature and thought to be related to uterine contractions caused by prostaglandins released at the time of endometrial breakdown. When severe, the pain may radiate from the pelvic region to the back and thighs and is frequently accompanied by nausea and in some women vomiting and diarrhea. Treatment with aspirin before the onset of pain is effective in milder cases; however, the nonsteroidal anti-inflammatory compounds that are active inhibitors of prostaglandin synthesis are more effective when the pain is severe. Naproxen (Naprosyn), 250 mg twice daily, and ibuprofen (Motrin), 400 mg 3 times daily, are useful for this purpose, as is indomethacin (Indocin), 25 mg 3–4 times daily, or mefenamic acid (Ponstel), 250 mg 4 times daily. These compounds are often more effective if started before the pain begins. Since dysmenorrhea rarely accompanies bleeding in the absence of ovulation, suppression of ovulation with oral contraceptives is also effective treatment.

DISORDERS OF OVARIAN & MENSTRUAL FUNCTION

Abnormal ovarian endocrine function is manifested by (1) evidence of inappropriate estrogen secretion (eg, precocious puberty); (2) deficient estrogen secretion (eg, delayed puberty); (3) disturbances or alterations of the menstrual cycle in mature women; or (4) evidence of excessive androgen production. In this chapter, emphasis will be placed on disorders occurring in postpubertal adults, since these comprise the vast majority of disorders encountered and because disorders of development and differentiation are described in Chapters 8 and 18 and pituitary disorders in Chapter 6.

The pattern of menstrual bleeding with regard to the frequency, duration, and amount of flow tends to be fairly consistent in most healthy women. Periodic, regular menstrual cycles are usually ovulatory. However, there are a wide variety of organic and functional disturbances of menstrual flow. In general, when the basic pattern of bleeding is undisturbed and there are superimposed episodes of spotting or bleeding, the cause is likely to be a local organic lesion or hematologic disorder. When the basic pattern of bleeding is changed, it is more often due to lack of ovulation and disturbances in the pattern of hormone secretion. Table 17–3 sets forth the terms frequently used to describe abnormalities of menses, their definitions, and some common causes.

The great majority of disorders of ovarian function causing amenorrhea occur without known or identifiable structural changes in the components of the complex system required for normal ovulatory cycles. They can result from abnormalities in function of the central mechanism that regulates the pulsatile secretion of GnRH; from abnormalities in feedback; or from changes in intraovarian regulatory mechanisms. Environmental changes, physical and emotional stress,

Table 17–3. Types of abnormal vaginal bleeding.

	Definition	Causes
Hypermenorrhea (menorrhagia)	Cyclic bleeding in excessive amount.	Uterine myomas and endometrial polyps, hyperplasia, adenomyosis, endometritis, von Willebrand's disease.
Hypomenorrhea	Cyclic bleeding in abnormally small amount	Cervical obstruction, synechia of endometrium, tuberculosis of endometrium.
Polymenorrhea	Frequent periods (cycle length of <21 days).	Shortening of follicular phase, luteal insufficiency, frequent anovulatory bleeding.
Oligomenorrhea	Infrequent periods (cycle length of >35 days).	Anovulation, systemic disturbances.
Amenorrhea	More than 6 months since last menstrual period.	Anovulation or outflow tract disorder.
Metrorrhagia	Bleeding between normal cycles.	Except for ovulatory bleeding or spotting, this symptom usually indicates disease of the vagina, cervix, or uterus.

extreme weight loss, and drugs seem to be able to interfere with the functioning of the hypothalamic centers and their control of GnRH secretion. In such cases, a variety of hormonal abnormalities may be identified. In some patients, follicle stimulation by FSH is insufficient to produce adequate growth and maturation of ovarian follicles, with a resulting decrease in ovarian estradiol secretion. Failure of the preovulatory LH surge to occur even though follicles have developed and produced estrogen will also disrupt normal ovarian and menstrual function. However, the continuous secretion of increased amounts of LH in the absence of normally developing follicles may result in overproduction of androgens and lead to amenorrhea and hirsutism (eg, polycystic ovary syndrome). The role of estrogens, androgens, and other local hormones in the ovary is not presently well delineated, but these hormones may be responsible for abnormalities in ovarian function in some patients. Abnormalities of gonadotropin secretion leading to anovulation are sometimes associated with the release of increased amounts of PRL in the absence of any demonstrable lesion of the pituitary. In such patients, amenorrhea may be associated with galactorrhea.

Treatment of these disorders depends to some extent on their causes and manifestations. However, the desired outcome is the critical consideration. It would be fruitless, for example, to treat hirsutism secondary to excess production of ovarian androgens by suppressing the ovary with oral contraceptives in a patient whose main objective was to achieve a pregnancy.

In considering the possible causes of amenorrhea in a given patient, it is useful to review the requirements for normal cyclic ovarian function: (1) a normal outflow tract, (2) normal ovaries, (3) a normal pituitary gland, and (4) a normal central nervous system. Each of these systems can be examined by means of the history, direct observation, and appropriate laboratory tests or procedures. The problem may be more complex in young women with primary amenorrhea and no evidence of sexual maturation. In women with secondary amenorrhea, however, the process may require very few laboratory tests. By the time one has begun to speak to the patient, one has already observed her approximate age, appearance, stature, and extent of sexual development; this information provides some direction for taking her history and doing the physical examination.

AMENORRHEA IN THE ABSENCE OF SEXUAL MATURATION

The diagnostic considerations for a young, immature woman are quite different from those for a mature woman with secondary amenorrhea. In the otherwise healthy but sexually immature patient over 16 years of age, the first question to resolve is whether normal puberty is merely delayed. This question can sometimes be answered by finding a normal level of gonadotropins and a history of late puberty in the family. No conclusion can be drawn if the levels of gonadotropins are low. In these patients, LH and FSH responses to testing with GnRH or a GnRH agonist analogue may help to differentiate delayed puberty from a more serious disorder.

Elevated concentrations of FSH and LH indicate unresponsiveness or absence of functioning ovarian tissue. If the patient is short in stature and has obvious stigmas of Turner's syndrome (gonadal dysgenesis), gonadotropins will be elevated. Chromosomal analysis will confirm the diagnosis, determine the genotype, and indicate the need for gonadectomy if a Y chromosome mosaicism is found. If the patient is of normal height or has relatively longer arms and legs compared with the length of the trunk (eunuchoid proportions), gonadal absence or agenesis must be differentiated from selective hypogonadotropism. FSH will be elevated in the former and low in the latter. If height and stature are normal and gonadotropins are low, one must also consider a central nervous system defect such as Kallmann's syndrome. These patients also have anosmia, which can be determined by the history or by testing the ability to smell.

Patients with amenorrhea and hypogonadism in whom the levels of gonadotropins are normal or lower than normal may be experiencing a delay in onset of puberty. However, after age 16, this is sufficiently unusual to warrant further investigation. When the cause is craniopharyngioma or pituitary tumor, there is commonly an interference with growth secondary to deficient GH secretion. Clinical or laboratory evidence of thyroid or adrenal insufficiency or decreased reserve also may be present. These and other pituitary disorders causing amenorrhea and conditions of abnormal pubertal development are discussed in Chapters 6 and 19.

Primary Ovarian Disorders

A. Gonadal Agenesis: Hypogonadism may result from absent or incomplete development of the ovary. This abnormality could result from environmentally induced abnormalities in development early in pregnancy (see Chapter 18).

B. Turner's Syndrome (Gonadal Dysgenesis): Turner's syndrome and related variants of gonadal dysgenesis are the most common cause of congenital hypogonadism. The karyotype in affected patients is most frequently 45,X, showing an absence of the second X chromosome. Clinical features, in addition to the lack of sexual maturation, include short stature, webbed neck, shield chest, and valgus deformity of the elbow. This syndrome and its variants are described in detail in Chapter 18. Gonadal dysgenesis may also occur in the presence of multiple cell lines with varying chromosomal composition. This is called "mosaicism." Many patients with mosaicism have typical phenotypic characteristics of Turner's syndrome, and

the diagnosis may be made before puberty. A karyotype should be performed on all of these patients to determine whether or not a Y chromosome is present. Patients having Y chromosomes require laparotomy and excision of the gonadal area to prevent development of gonadoblastomas. It should also be noted that patients having an XX constituent to their mosaicism may have functional ovarian tissue. In some of these, normal puberty (including menses) occurs, and they are able to reproduce. These individuals frequently experience premature menopause.

C. 17α-Hydroxylase (P-450c17) Deficiency: Hypogonadism and elevated levels of gonadotropin can be found in patients with 17α-hydroxylase deficiency, a rare form of congenital adrenal hyperplasia in which there is impaired conversion of pregnenolone and progesterone to cortisol and to androgens and estrogens. The impairment leads to increased production of deoxycorticosterone and corticosterone, resulting in hypokalemia and hypertension (see Chapter 13).

Disorders Due to Central Nervous System Disease

A. Hypogonadotropism and Anosmia: This syndrome, similar to Kallmann's syndrome in the male, is a rare cause of amenorrhea. Patients fail to mature at the expected time for puberty and are found to have low gonadotropins, normal stature, anosmia, and a female karyotype. The disorder is believed to involve failure of development of the olfactory lobe and a deficiency of GnRH. Ovulation can be induced by injection of menopausal gonadotropins and by pulsatile injection of GnRH.

B. Prepubertal Pituitary-CNS Tumors: Pituitary and central nervous system disorders which interfere with ovarian function, or tumors such as craniopharyngeomas and pituitary adenomas are discussed in Chapters 6 and 19.

AMENORRHEA IN PATIENTS WITH NORMAL SECONDARY SEX CHARACTERISTICS

The evaluation of women with amenorrhea but otherwise normal sexual development begins with the history and physical examination plus a few laboratory tests (Fig 17–14). This initial evaluation will localize the underlying cause of the amenorrhea to dysfunction of either the outflow tract, the ovary, or the hypothalamic-pituitary complex. In most cases, further diagnostic procedures will not be required. The medical history should include a complete description of prior menstrual patterns, the presence or absence of breast discharge, and any changes that might suggest increased androgen secretion. The possibility of pregnancy should always be considered.

The initial evaluation consists of a qualitative assessment of the patient's endogenous estrogen level

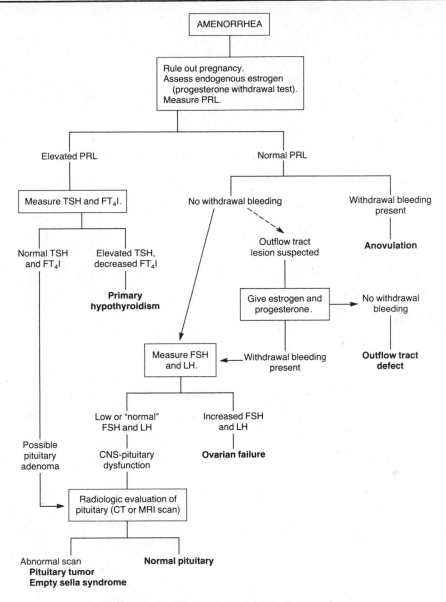

Figure 17–14. Diagnostic evaluation of amenorrhea.

and determination of the serum PRL concentration. The presence of endogenous estrogens can be established by attempting to induce withdrawal uterine bleeding by administering progesterone. An oral progestin with no estrogenic activity—eg, medroxyprogesterone, 10 mg daily for 5–7 days—or a single intramuscular injection of 200 mg of progesterone in oil may be used. The presence of vaginal bleeding within 7 days after conclusion of the progesterone treatment indicates that the outflow tract is intact and that the patient is producing sufficient estrogen to stimulate endometrial growth. If the serum PRL concentration is also within normal limits, a pituitary tumor is very unlikely. These patients can be considered to be anovulatory, and in most cases no further evaluation is

required. The choice of treatment, if any, will depend upon the objectives of the patient.

Failure to induce menstrual bleeding by exogenous progestin indicates either a defect of the outflow tract with normal estrogen production (an infrequent cause of secondary amenorrhea) or insufficient estrogen production secondary to hypothalamic-pituitary-ovarian dysfunction. To differentiate between these possibilities in women with normal PRL levels, gonadotropin levels are obtained to differentiate between ovarian failure and hypothalamic-pituitary dysfunction. If an abnormality of the outflow tract is suspected, its integrity can be assessed by administering oral estrogen (1.25–2.5 mg of conjugated estrogens [Premarin, etc] or 50 μg of ethinyl estradiol per day) for 21 days. A progestin should be added during the last 5 days of treatment. Lack of withdrawal bleeding following treatment usually indicates an abnormality of the outflow tract. In most instances, however, bleeding will occur and the outflow tract is found to be normal.

To differentiate between ovarian failure and hypothalamic-pituitary dysfunction, gonadotropin levels are obtained. If ovarian failure is the primary cause of amenorrhea, serum FSH and LH levels will be elevated because of the loss of negative feedback by ovarian sex steroids. If serum concentrations of FSH and LH are low or low normal or if prolactin levels are elevated, radiologic or magnetic resonance examination of the pituitary gland is indicated to rule out a pituitary tumor. Therapy for these disorders is discussed below.

Abnormalities of the Outflow Tract

Patients with amenorrhea in whom gonadal tissue is presumed to be present because they have undergone normal sexual maturation may have abnormalities of the outflow tract. Patients who cannot be induced to bleed by treatment with a progestational agent and who fail to bleed following administration of estrogens in conjunction with a progestational agent after several attempts can be presumed to have an abnormality of the outflow tract. In these patients, the presence or absence of ovulation can be determined by following the basal body temperature over a month or more or by measuring serum progesterone levels once a week for several weeks.

A. Müllerian Defects: In women with no history of vaginal bleeding, developmental abnormalities of the müllerian tube must be considered. These abnormalities range from the presence of an imperforate hymen to the total absence of müllerian structures. In the presence of a uterus lined with endometrium, interruption of the outflow tract by an abnormal cervix, interruptions of the vaginal canal, or imperforate hymen may be accompanied by collection of the menstruum proximal to the point of obstruction. This leads to pain and distention of the proximal structures or accumulation of blood in the peritoneal cavity. **Absence of the vagina,** with varying degrees of uterine development associated with normal ovarian function, is one of the more common abnormalities of müllerian development (Mayer-Rokitansky-Küster-Hauser syndrome). Affected patients commonly have developmental abnormalities of the urinary and skeletal systems. Surgical creation of an artificial vagina is indicated when there is evidence that a functioning uterus exists and that fertility might be restored. Otherwise, progressive dilation by the use of vaginal dilators can be used to form a functional vagina.

B. Asherman's Syndrome (Uterine Synechia): In women in whom menses have once been established, destruction of the endometrial cavity by chronic infections such as tuberculosis or destruction of the endometrium by curettage can lead to amenorrhea.

Such scarring (Asherman's syndrome) is uncommon and can be treated by careful dilatation under hysteroscopic view, followed by insertion of a small Foley catheter or other device to prevent adhesions from recurring. Treatment should include the use of broad-spectrum antibiotics for 10 days following the procedure and cyclic stimulation of endometrial development with large doses of estrogen plus a progestin.

Primary Gonadal Disorders

In patients with amenorrhea and a normal outflow tract, abnormal ovarian function may result from disorders of the ovary itself or disorders of the controlling mechanisms. A plasma FSH of more than 40 mIU/mL accompanied by high levels of LH is evidence of failure of ovarian hormone production. This is a very serious diagnosis, not only because of the hormone deficiency, which is correctable, but also—and more importantly from the patient's point of view—because lack of a functioning follicular apparatus results in sterility. For this reason, it is worth repeating the test to be sure there is no error. In women near menopause, elevated gonadotropin levels are sometimes found in the presence of ovulatory cycles. However, a misdiagnosis in this group of patients is rarely clinically important unless the patient is pregnant.

A. Premature Ovarian Failure: Ovarian failure occasionally occurs in women under the age of 35 following spontaneous sexual maturation. In some patients, ovarian failure is associated with ovarian autoantibodies and is probably due to autoimmune destruction of the ovary. It is frequently associated with autoantibodies to other glands such as the thyroid and adrenal (Schmidt's syndrome) (see Chapters 10, 12, and 28). In other patients, the ovaries show a few primordial follicles, and in some they resemble menopausal ovaries.

B. Testicular Feminization: This disorder in its classic form is characterized by primary amenorrhea, an absent uterus, and the absence of pubic and axillary hair. Affected patients are male pseudohermaphrodites with testes and an XY karyotype. Incomplete forms of this disorder have also been described. They are discussed in detail in Chapter 18.

C. Resistant Ovary Syndrome: Rarely, women exhibit amenorrhea and elevated gonadotropin levels in the presence of potentially functional ovarian follicles. It may be possible to induce follicular growth and estrogen secretion in these patients by administration of large amounts of exogenous gonadotropins. However, it is usually difficult or impossible to induce ovulation and subsequent pregnancy in these patients. Although this disorder can only be diagnosed with certainty by ovarian biopsy, the infrequency of the disorder and the poor prognosis dictate that ovarian biopsy be performed only rarely in patients with high gonadotropins and normal karyotype.

D. Functioning Ovarian Tumors: Hormone-producing tumors of the ovary presenting clinically as endocrine disorders are uncommon. Classification of these tumors is made difficult by the uncertainty of embryonic origin in some and the lack of correlation between the functional and morphologic characteristics. However, it is convenient to divide them into broad morphologic categories, keeping in mind that the diagnostic approach will be based on the clinical presentation. Detection of androgen-producing tumors is considered in the section on amenorrhea with excess androgen production (see below). The estrogen-producing tumors cause amenorrhea or anovulatory bleeding in premenopausal women, irregular bleeding after the menopause, and precocious puberty in children. A classification of these tumors is presented in Table 17–4.

1. Germ cell tumors–

a. Germinomas (dysgerminoma, seminoma, gonocytoma, embryonal carcinoma)–These tumors of the ovary are usually found on routine examination in young women. They are generally small and asymptomatic unless associated with teratomatous elements that produce hCG. When hCG is produced, the patient will develop amenorrhea and other signs and symptoms of early pregnancy.

b. Teratomas–Teratomas arising in gonadal tissue are common. Although rarely active hormonally, they may contain hormone-secreting elements. Tumors containing thyroid tissue (struma ovarii) can release thyroxine. Carcinoid tumors producing serotonin have also been reported.

Choriocarcinoma of the ovary is usually secondary to uterine choriocarcinoma and very rarely arises within the ovary. It is composed of trophoblastic tissue, usually with extensive hemorrhage and necrosis. These tumors produce large amounts of hCG. The elevated plasma levels of this hormone are useful in diagnosing the tumor and in monitoring treatment. Treatment is similar to that of tumors of trophoblastic origin in the uterus. However, the prognosis is less favorable.

c. Gonadoblastomas–These rare tumors arise in dysgenetic gonads. They are typically seen in phenotypic females with a Y chromosome. They are morphologically similar to germinomas but also have cells of mesenchymal or sex cord origin. The latter may differentiate into Leydig or granulosa cells and secrete androgens or estrogens. Prophylactic removal of the dysgenetic gonads is recommended in patients with a Y chromosome (see Chapter 18).

2. Sex cord–mesenchymal tumors–

a. Granulosa–theca cell tumors–These tumors constitute 5–10% of ovarian neoplasms. They are usually associated with some clinical or pathologic evidence of estrogen secretion. Androgen-producing tumors of this type have been reported but are rare. Granulosa cell tumors are unilateral in 90% of patients. They are usually solid and vary in appearance from mature granulosa cells arranged in circumferential rows around spaces ("Call-Exner bodies") to immature cells with a sarcomatous appearance. The cells may take on the polyhedral appearance of the luteinized granulosa cells of the corpus luteum. Although the prognosis following removal of these tumors is better than for ovarian carcinomas, about 20% recur in 5 years and about 40% in 10 years. The recurrences may be circumscribed and can be quite sensitive to radiation.

b. Sertoli–Leydig cell tumors (arrhenoblastoma, androblastoma)–This group of tumors, as noted above, may cause feminization. They more commonly produce virilization and under these circumstances are commonly called arrhenoblastomas or androblastomas. They are not common, accounting for fewer than 5% of ovarian tumors. They vary in size and, although usually small, may become large. The histologic pattern varies from that of well-differentiated testicular tubules (Pick's adenoma) to an undifferentiated sarcomatous appearance and mixtures of both.

Typically, the first manifestation of an androgen-producing tumor is amenorrhea, followed by hirsutism, acne, and breast atrophy; clitoral hypertrophy, balding, and deepening of the voice occur later. Plasma androgen levels are usually in the normal male range and cannot be suppressed by administration of estrogens or estrogen-containing oral contraceptives. Removal of the tumor is followed by a return of menses and partial or complete loss of abnormal hair. The tumors are seldom bilateral and usually benign.

Table 17–4. Classification and clinical features of functioning ovarian tumors.

	Hormones[1]	Usual Age at Onset	Percent Palpable	Percent Bilateral	Percent Malignant
Germ cell tumors					
Germinomas-teratomas					
Struma ovarii	Thyroxine	10–40	90	10	Rare
Carcinoid tumors	Serotonin	10–40	90	10	Rare
Choriocarcinomas	Chorionic gonadotropin	6–15	100	Rare	100
Gonadoblastomas	Androgens, estrogens	10–30		40	50
Sex cord–mesenchymal tumors					
Granulosa–theca cell tumors	Estrogens, androgens, progestins	30–70	90	10	20
Sertoli–Leydig cell tumors (arrhenoblastomas)	Androgens, estrogens	20–50	80	Rare	20
Hilar cell tumors	Androgens, estrogens	45–75	50	Rare	Rare

[1]Steroid-producing tumors may produce estrogens or androgens. The usual hormone released is listed first.

3. Hilar cell (lipoid cell) tumors—These androgen-producing tumors usually occur in older patients and cause severe masculinization, including hirsutism, balding, clitoral enlargement, and deepening of the voice. They are usually small and less likely to be palpated than other ovarian tumors. Histologically, they are typical steroid-producing cells and contain Reinke crystalloids, which are characteristically found in the interstitial cells of the testis. They are almost always benign and are treated by extirpation, which reverses the hirsutism, baldness, and metabolic changes, though clitoral enlargement and voice changes persist.

Disorders of the Pituitary

The anterior pituitary gland plays a key role in normal ovarian function. In adults, the loss of pituitary gonadotropic activity is usually noted before the loss of other pituitary trophic functions when the organ is damaged by vascular, inflammatory, or neoplastic processes.

A. Pituitary Tumors: Most patients with amenorrhea and low gonadotropin levels have decreased or altered secretion of GnRH secondary to altered hypothalamic or central nervous system activity. However, the presence of a pituitary tumor must be considered and excluded. Amenorrhea may be the only clue to a nonfunctioning tumor. Most commonly, however, pituitary tumors in young women with amenorrhea cause hyperprolactinemia, and galactorrhea is found in more than 50% of patients with PRL-secreting adenomas (see Chapter 6). In contrast, GH-secreting tumors are associated with clinical signs of acromegaly. Although this is an unusual cause of amenorrhea, it is important to consider the diagnosis in appropriate clinical circumstances, since early diagnosis and treatment can prevent the permanently disfiguring effects of excessive GH. Amenorrhea may also be the presenting symptom in patients with Cushing's syndrome due to a pituitary tumor (Cushing's disease).

B. Empty Sella Syndrome: Amenorrhea and galactorrhea may occur in the presence of the empty sella syndrome (see Chapter 6). In this condition, there appears to be an extension of the subarachnoid space into the pituitary fossa, which leads to flattening of pituitary tissue against the wall of the sella and may lead to its enlargement. The disorder is found in 5% of patients at autopsy. It is benign and requires no treatment unless associated abnormalities of pituitary function are present. This condition can be differentiated from tumor by CT or MRI scanning.

Disorders Due to Central Nervous System Abnormalities of Regulation of Gonadotropin Secretion

A. Hypothalamic Amenorrhea: This term is used to described amenorrhea due to functional abnormalities in the neural mechanisms that regulate the pulsatile secretion of GnRH. Young women commonly fail to ovulate at times of increased stress such as may be occasioned by academic or career pressures, disruption of personal life-styles, change in residences, or illness. These events may mark the onset of periods of amenorrhea.

In most instances, the period of amenorrhea is self-limited and ovulatory menstrual function returns spontaneously. If this does not occur, treatment is dependent upon the expectations of the patient. If she wishes to become pregnant, induction of ovulation by clomiphene would be the initial treatment. If this does not induce ovulation, treatment with clomiphene plus chorionic gonadotropin, with menotropins (Pergonal), or with pulsatile administration of GnRH will be required. If the patient does not want to become pregnant, her estrogenic status will help to determine treatment. Most of these women will have a positive progesterone challenge test (withdrawal bleeding) and either normal or only moderately reduced levels of estrogen. Cyclic treatment with a progestational agent will prevent endometrial hyperplasia in these women. Rarely, these women will have a negative progesterone challenge test (no withdrawal bleeding) and may have significant loss of calcium with the eventual development of osteoporosis secondary to low levels of estrogen. In these patients, preventative treatment with estrogen and a cyclic progestin should be considered.

B. Amenorrhea in Athletes: Menstrual abnormalities are sufficiently common in female athletes to suggest a causal relationship between vigorous physical effort and amenorrhea. About one-third of long-distance runners experience amenorrhea or oligomenorrhea. The incidence appears to vary with the degree of stress and effort in other activities. The incidence of amenorrhea correlates directly with the amount of weight lost and inversely with the percentage of body weight as fat. It is less frequent in multiparous women. No consistent changes in plasma estradiol, testosterone, or gonadotropin levels have been reported. In general, these menstrual abnormalities disappear with a reduction of physical activity and a return to the individual's natural weight and proportion of body weight as fat. Some of these women with prolonged amenorrhea show excessive bone loss in spite of their intense physical activity, and appropriate hormone replacement therapy should be instituted.

C. Anorexia: Anorexia nervosa in its classic form is a serious but uncommon disorder characterized by extreme malnutrition and hypogonadotropism. It is considered to be a severe behavioral disorder, with endocrine changes secondary to both psychologic and nutritional disturbances. Amenorrhea may precede weight loss. Milder forms of malnutrition and amenorrhea are more commonly seen in formerly overweight women with an abnormal fear of regaining weight lost by dieting. These patients may respond to psychotherapy and antidepressant drug therapy. Malnutrition may result from refusal to eat, induced vomiting (bulimia), and excessive use of laxatives. Psychiatric treatment is required, and hospitalization may be necessary to prevent death from starvation, suicide, or intercurrent illnesses.

D. Post-Pill Amenorrhea: Although it has not been possible to clearly demonstrate an increase in prolactinomas or a reduction in the fertility rate of women following the use of oral contraceptives, studies are available that show a moderate increase in the incidence of amenorrhea in such women. Furthermore, the syndrome of amenorrhea with galactorrhea (see below) is more common in women treated with oral contraceptives. Although the nature of this relationship is not established, it is clear that most women who develop amenorrhea following the use of contraceptive pills would probably have developed amenorrhea without them, and the disorder must be investigated as in other women.

Amenorrhea with Galactorrhea

Galactorrhea may be induced by a wide variety of stimuli ranging from local irritation or stimulation of the chest wall to ingestion of drugs that interfere with the hypothalamic release of dopamine or its binding to the pituitary lactotrophs (see Chapter 6). The expression of even 1 drop of fluid from the nipple is clinically significant and is rarely seen in healthy women who have not taken oral contraceptives or who have not been recently pregnant or exposed to drugs such as phenothiazines (which cause galactorrhea) or to excessive breast stimulation. In women with amenorrhea, an attempt should be made to elicit such a secretion by gentle manual pressure at the base of the breast, working toward the nipple. The secretion may be present in only one breast at any given time.

Whether or not galactorrhea is present, however, prolactin levels should be measured in patients with persistent amenorrhea (Fig 17–14). When a detectable tumor is present, prolactin levels are usually elevated. In the presence of nonsecreting tumors impinging on the pituitary stalk, prolactin levels may be only minimally elevated. It is advisable to obtain CT or MRI studies of the pituitary in most patients with galactorrhea or elevated prolactin levels. Studies of pituitary function, including the gonadotropin response to GnRH and the effect of levodopa and other drugs on PRL secretion, do not reliably identify patients with pituitary tumors. However, these and other tests of pituitary function are useful in assessing residual pituitary function. CT scanning will detect microadenomas as small as 3–5 mm in size. Bulging and demineralization of the sella turcica usually occur when the tumor exceeds 1 cm in diameter, and larger tumors are usually found in patients presenting with visual field defects.

Criteria for the selection of patients with tumors for surgical treatment or medical treatment with bromocriptine have not been firmly established and may be expected to change over the next few years. About 10–20% of women examined at autopsy show small pituitary adenomas. The natural history of the disorder is not well understood.

Although clomiphene or gonadotropins may induce ovulation in these patients, bromocriptine is more effective. Bromocriptine mesylate (Parlodel) is an ergot alkaloid that acts by binding to the dopaminergic receptors in the pituitary, resulting in inhibition of PRL secretion. In 90% or more of these patients, treatment leads to the onset of menses in 3–5 weeks. The usual dose is 2.5 mg 2 or 3 times a day. Since there are side effects of nausea and mild dizziness, it is useful to start with a small dose, such as 2.5 mg daily—or half that amount given at bedtime in sensitive patients—and increase to 2.5 mg twice daily. PRL levels should be depressed to normal if treatment is adequate.

The long-term use of bromocriptine to induce regression of pituitary tumors is under study. Preliminary results indicate that at least in some patients tumors can be shown to regress. Even incomplete regression may be useful in patients whose tumors are too large to favor the transsphenoidal approach to the removal of the tumor. As noted above, the indications for surgery in patients with small tumors have not been established. Transsphenoidal tumor removal will restore normal gonadal function and normal PRL levels in the large majority of these patients. However, others have been followed for many years without evidence of tumor enlargement. In any case, patients must be followed carefully with PRL levels. Patients with tumors require radiologic reevaluation of the sella every 1–2 years. (See Chapter 6.)

Amenorrhea with Androgen Excess

The presence of excessive amounts of androgen is usually associated with oligomenorrhea or amenorrhea. Causes of androgen excess are shown in Table 17–5.

A. Polycystic Ovary Syndrome: Polycystic ovary (Stein-Leventhal) syndrome is a complex of varying symptoms ranging from amenorrhea to anovulatory

Table 17–5. Causes of increased androgen production, hirsutism, or both.

Ovarian causes
  Polycystic ovary syndrome
  Hyperthecosis
  Androgen-producing tumors
  Virilization of pregnancy (luteoma)
Adrenal causes
  Congenital or adult-onset adrenal hyperplasia
  Androgen-producing tumors
Combined ovarian-adrenal dysfunction: polycystic ovary syndrome
Cushing's syndrome
Obesity
Idiopathic or familial hirsutism
Postmenopausal state
Incomplete testicular feminization
Iatrogenic (eg, phenytoin, diazoxide, danazol, minoxidil)

bleeding often associated with obesity and hirsutism. The term has been used to describe such a variety of symptom complexes (Table 17–6) that it is almost a barrier to communication. In the most characteristic form of the disorder, the term denotes an absence of ovulation in association with continuous stimulation of the ovary by disproportionately high levels of LH. The chronic stimulation leads to increased ovarian androgen secretion and characteristic morphologic changes in the ovaries. The ovaries are usually (not always) enlarged and may reach several times their normal size; one ovary may be significantly larger than the other. The ovaries typically appear glistening white because of a thickened capsule and show many small follicles in various stages of development and atresia at the surface. The theca cells are often hyperplastic and luteinized. The syndrome is also associated with changes in adrenal androgen production in some patients. Estrogen production in these patients is usually a result of the peripheral conversion of androgens to estrogens, predominantly androstenedione to estrone. This can produce endometrial hyperplasia and eventually lead to adenocarcinoma of the endometrium, since the estrogen action is unopposed by progesterone.

1. Etiology–The cause of this syndrome is unknown, and it is possible that there are several causes. Each of the functional changes that occur tends to maintain the cycle of functional abnormalities as shown in Figure 17–15. It has been suggested that in some patients this disorder may be initiated by excessive adrenal androgen production at the time of puberty or by a stress-induced increase in adrenal androgen secretion. The peripheral conversion of androgen to estrogen could facilitate the secretion of increased

Table 17–6. Incidence of various clinical findings in women with polycystic ovary syndrome. Data are derived from 187 references comprising a total of 1079 cases.[1]

	Incidence (%)	
	Mean	**Range**
Infertility	74	35–94
Hirsutism	69	17–83
Amenorrhea	51	15–77
Obesity	41	16–49
Functional bleeding	29	6–65
Dysmenorrhea	23	
Corpus luteum at surgery	22	0–71
Virilization	21	0–28
Biphasic basal body temperature	15	12–40
Cyclic menses	12	7–28

[1]Reproduced, with permission, from Goldzieher JW: Polycystic ovarian disease. In: *Progress in Infertility*, 2nd ed. Behrman SH, Kistner RW (editors). Little, Brown, 1975.

amounts of LH, leading to increased ovarian androgen production and impaired follicular maturation. In some patients, there is a strong family history, and the pattern of inheritance suggests that the trait is dominant and may be linked to the X chromosome. A group of patients have also been found in whom amenorrhea and androgen excess are associated with acanthosis nigricans and insulin resistance.

This syndrome could also result from central nervous system abnormalities, leading to inappropriate secretion of hypothalamic GnRH. This, in turn, could increase the secretion of LH and reduce the secretion of FSH. High levels of LH may promote excessive androgen production by the thecal layer. Since FSH levels also are low, granulosa cells may have a reduced capaci-

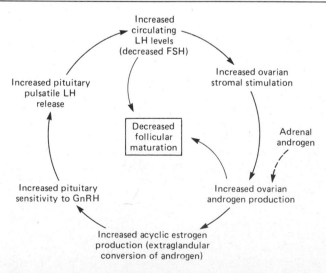

Figure 17–15. Pathophysiology of chronic anovulation in women with polycystic ovary syndrome. (Reproduced, with permission, from Yen SSC, Jaffe RB [editors]: *Reproductive Endocrinology.* Saunders, 1978.)

ty to convert these androgens to estrogens. High local levels of androstenedione and testosterone in the polycystic ovary may impede normal follicular growth and increase the rate of atresia, resulting in the formation of numerous small cystic follicles. Serum levels of estrone and free estradiol are elevated secondarily to increased peripheral aromatization of the ovarian androgens. The elevated levels of estrogen, in turn, may further sensitize the pituitary gland to hypothalamic GnRH, sustaining the abnormality.

Although androgen production is quite variable, it seldom reaches the levels seen in the presence of androgen-producing ovarian tumors. As a result, the vast majority of women show hirsutism and increased activity of the sebaceous glands often associated with acne. Signs of more severe virilization, such as male pattern (bitemporal) balding, clitoral hypertrophy, and voice changes, are rare. In general, there is a good correlation between levels of free testosterone and clinical evidence of androgen excess.

2. Management–The major manifestations of polycystic ovary syndrome are hirsutism secondary to androgen excess and failure of ovulation causing amenorrhea and infertility. The goals of therapy in the individual patient are of prime importance in determining the appropriate therapeutic program.

Induction of ovulation is required for anovulatory patients who wish to conceive. Most women ovulate in response to clomiphene citrate (see Ovulation Induction, below). In women whose ovaries fail to respond, combined therapy consisting of adrenal suppression and clomiphene may be more successful. The use of pulsatile GnRH to induce ovulation has generally not been effective. Wedge resection of the ovaries is rarely employed today.

In patients who have amenorrhea but do not wish to become pregnant, treatment may not be required. Some obese patients have been reported to resume ovulation and reduce androgen secretion on a program of weight reduction alone. In patients producing moderate to large amounts of estrogen continuously, endometrial hyperplasia with consequent bleeding and even endometrial carcinoma may develop. In such patients, the cyclic administration of a progestational agent may be required (see Anovulatory Bleeding, below). Hirsutism can be treated by suppression of ovarian androgen production or by antiandrogen therapy, as discussed in the Treatment of Hirsutism section, below.

B. Other Causes of Androgen Excess: Excessive production of androgens is more commonly of ovarian than adrenal origin. The exact cause needs to be established to rule out androgen-producing adrenal and ovarian tumors, Cushing's syndrome, and mild forms of congenital adrenal hyperplasia. Other causes of androgen excess are shown in Table 17–5. The general clinical approach to the evaluation of patients with excess androgen production is discussed below and summarized in Figure 17–16.

HIRSUTISM

Hair can be classified as either vellus or terminal. Vellus hairs are fine, soft, and nonpigmented. They are found over most of the body and predominate prior to puberty. They are often so fine that they are barely visible. Terminal hairs are coarse and pigmented. Before puberty, terminal hairs normally are found only on the scalp and eyebrows. Under the influence of increasing levels of androgen at puberty, vellus hairs are transformed into terminal hairs. In women, this conversion to terminal hairs involves principally the axillary and pubic regions and to a lesser extent the extremities. Under conditions of excessive androgen production or increased 5α-reductase activity (which increases conversion of testosterone to dihydrotestosterone), there is increased conversion of vellus to terminal hairs. Terminal hairs may thus develop in body regions where such hair growth is normally considered to be a male secondary sex characteristic. The presence of increasing numbers of terminal hairs on the face, chest, back, lower abdomen, and inner thighs is referred to as hirsutism. In many women, hirsutism is accompanied by menstrual dysfunction (usually oligomenorrhea but sometimes amenorrhea). Rarely, abnormal androgen production increases to levels normally found only in men. In such instances, the high circulating levels of androgen also produce somatic changes referred to as virilization. These changes include frontal balding, deepening of the voice, breast atrophy, clitoral enlargement, increased muscle mass, and loss of normal female body contours. The clinical assessment and treatment of women with mild to moderate hirsutism may be complicated by the difficulty in determining if the pattern of hair growth is secondary to an increase in androgen production or utilization or is merely a normal familial trait. The availability of specific and sensitive radioimmunoassays to estimate androgen production, however, may facilitate this difficult differential diagnosis.

Production & Metabolism of Serum Androgens

The major circulating androgens in women are testosterone, dihydrotestosterone, androstenedione, dehydroepiandrosterone (DHEA), and DHEA sulfate. The relative androgenic activity, serum concentrations, and sources of these androgens are summarized in Table 17–7. Testosterone is the principal circulating androgen in normal women. Both the ovaries and the adrenals normally secrete testosterone. Approximately 50% of the testosterone in serum, however, is derived from the peripheral conversion of steroid precursors, principally androstenedione and to a lesser extent DHEA. In many androgen-sensitive tissues, such as hair follicles, the enzyme 5α-reductase converts testosterone to dihydrotestosterone. It is believed that dihydrotestosterone per se (and not testosterone) is mainly responsible for stimulating hair growth in many areas

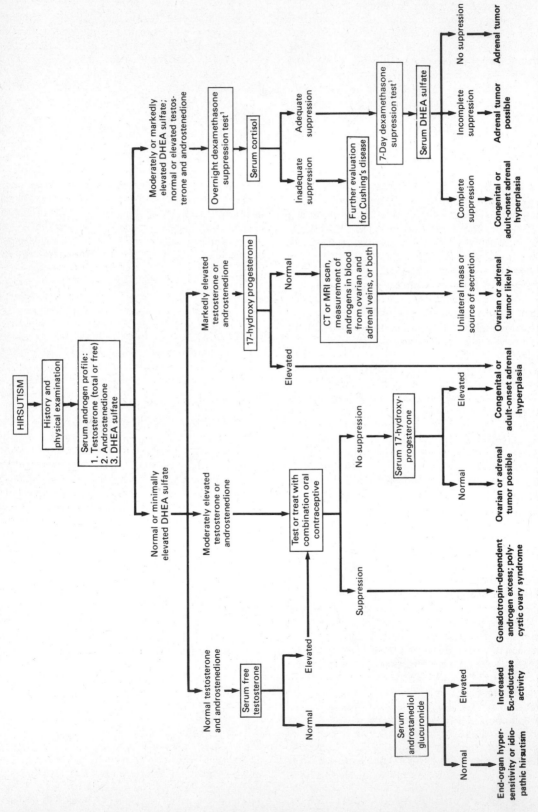

Figure 17–16. A guide to the use of hormone measurements in the evaluation of hirsutism. [1] See text for discussion of dexamethasone suppression tests.

Table 17–7. Circulating androgens and their relative androgenic activity, serum concentration, and site of formation in women.

Hormone	Relative Androgenic Activity[1]	Serum Concentration[2]		Source of Circulating Hormone (Percentage of Total)		
		(ng/mL)	(nmol/L)	Adrenal	Ovary	Peripheral Conversion
Testosterone	100	0.2–0.7	(0.69–2.43)	5–25	5–25	50–70
Dihydrotestosterone	250	0.05–0.3	(0.17–1.03)	. . .	. . .	100
Androstenedione	10–20	0.5–2.5	(1.72–8.6)	30–45	45–60	10
DHEA	5	1.3–9.8	(4.5–34)	80	20	. . .
DHEA sulfate	Minimal	400–3200	(790–6318)	>95	<5	. . .

[1]Testosterone has been assigned a potency of 100. Values are approximate and may vary depending upon the biologic system in which the hormones are evaluated.
[2]Normal ranges will vary in different laboratories.

of the body. Virtually all of the dihydrotestosterone in the circulation is formed in androgen-dependent peripheral tissues by 5α-reductase conversion of testosterone. Most of the dihydrotestosterone formed in these target tissues is metabolized further to androstanediols. Circulating androstenedione, in contrast to testosterone and dihydrotestosterone, is derived primarily from direct secretion by the ovaries and adrenals. Although androstenedione is a relatively weak androgen, possessing only 10–20% of the biologic activity of testosterone, it can be converted to testosterone in androgen-sensitive target tissues. Increased production and secretion of androstenedione thus may play a role in promoting the development of hirsutism in many women. DHEA is a very weak androgen with little biologic activity. DHEA sulfate has little or no androgenic activity. Virtually all of the DHEA sulfate in the serum is derived from the adrenal glands. Measurement of serum DHEA sulfate is useful in assessing adrenal androgen production.

Pathophysiology of Hirsutism

A. Increased Androgen Production: Studies in which women with mild to moderate hirsutism have been evaluated with sensitive and specific laboratory techniques have shown that most women with excessive hair growth have increased serum androgen levels (ie, increased concentrations of free testosterone) or increased 5α-reductase activity. Thus, fewer women are currently classified as having "idiopathic" hirsutism. The source (adrenal, ovarian, or both) of the increased production of androgens in women with mild to moderate hirsutism is sometimes difficult to establish. Many published reports support a combined adrenal-ovarian source for the increased serum levels of androgens, with the ovary as the major contributor in most instances. Approximately 1–5% of women with mild hirsutism have elevated serum levels of 17-hydroxyprogesterone and are thought to have increased androgen production secondary to adult-onset adrenal hyperplasia.

B. Serum Binding Proteins and the Serum Transport of Androgens: As reviewed earlier (Table 17–2), circulating steroid hormones are bound, to varying degrees, to plasma proteins, eg., albumin and specific transport proteins. In normal women, approx-

imately 65% of the circulating testosterone is tightly bound to SHBG, while most of the remaining hormone is loosely bound to albumin. Only 1–2% of the total testosterone is free (not bound to protein). It is generally thought that testosterone bound to SHBG is not readily available to intracellular androgen receptors at target tissues and therefore has little biologic activity. Factors that can alter the serum concentration of SHBG are shown in Table 17–8. Hirsute women often have reduced serum concentrations of SHBG. Thus, a small increase in total testosterone, accompanied by a decrease in the concentration of SHBG, may result in a significant increase in biologically active hormone. The measurement of free, or non-SHBG bound, testosterone levels in serum is a more sensitive indicator of androgen activity. A greater proportion of women with mild to moderate hirsutism have elevated concentrations of free—as compared to total—plasma testosterone.

C. Androgen Metabolism in Skin and Hair Follicles: Factors that alter the activity of 5α-reductase can influence the androgenic activity of testosterone. In vitro studies utilizing skin biopsies from hair-bearing regions have demonstrated increased 5α-reductase activity in hirsute women; thus, many women presently thought to have idiopathic hirsutism may actually have increased formation of dihydrotestosterone in hair follicles. This mechanism also is suggested by the relatively high percentage of women with hirsutism and normal levels of testosterone who have been found to have increased serum levels of androstanediol

Table 17–8. Conditions affecting SHBG synthesis and therefore the percentage of plasma testosterone that is free.

	SHBG Synthesis
Hypothyroidism Androgen therapy Corticosteroid therapy Obesity Acromegaly	Decreased
Hyperthyroidism Pregnancy Estrogen therapy Cirrhosis	Increased

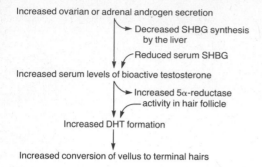

Increased ovarian or adrenal androgen secretion

→ Decreased SHBG synthesis
by the liver

↙ Reduced serum SHBG

Increased serum levels of bioactive testosterone

→ Increased 5α-reductase
↙ activity in hair follicle

Increased DHT formation

Increased conversion of vellus to terminal hairs

Figure 17–17. Development factors of androgen-dependent hirsutism.

glucuronide, a major metabolite of dihydrotestosterone. The factors responsible for the development of androgen-dependent hirsutism are summarized in Figure 17–17.

Evaluation of Women with Hirsutism

The common causes of increased androgen production and hirsutism are listed in Table 17–5. The initial assessment of hirsute women should include a thorough history and physical examination. Hirsutism is usually secondary to a mild increase in androgen activity. The increase in body hair occurs gradually and may be accompanied by other symptoms of mild androgen excess such as acne, oily skin, and oligomenorrhea or amenorrhea. The sudden appearance of rapid hair growth and amenorrhea associated with virilization, however, suggests an ovarian or adrenal androgen-producing tumor (see Chapter 12 and Table 17–4). The physical examination should detect signs of associated endocrine dysfunction, such as Cushing's syndrome or virilization. The degree and extent of growth of terminal hairs should be carefully recorded. This will help the physician decide if further endocrine investigation is warranted and help assess the effects of any future therapy. A pelvic examination also should be included in the initial evaluation of the patient, especially if she has oligomenorrhea or amenorrhea.

The laboratory evaluation of women with hirsutism is important for ruling out a serious underlying disease process such as an ovarian or adrenal androgen-producing tumor, steroid enzymatic defect (eg, partial 21-hydroxylase deficiency), or Cushing's syndrome. Once therapy has been initiated, measurement of serum androgen levels also can be used to determine if androgen secretion has been reduced. Suppression of androgen production or action at the hair follicle will, in most women, reduce the extent of excessive hair growth.

A general approach to the hormonal evaluation of women with hirsutism is shown in Figure 17–16. The rate of ovarian and adrenal androgen secretion can be estimated initially by measuring the serum concentrations of testosterone (total or free), androstenedione, and DHEA sulfate. In many women with hirsutism, serum testosterone or androstenedione will be somewhat elevated. Patients with raised levels of these hormones and normal or minimally increased levels of DHEA sulfate can be evaluated further by administering a combination oral contraceptive to suppress pituitary LH and FSH secretion. If the excess production of androgen is gonadotropin-dependent and of ovarian origin (eg, as in polycystic ovary syndrome), serum androgen levels (especially free testosterone levels) also will be suppressed after a 1-month trial of oral contraceptives. Treatment may be continued in those women with LH-dependent androgen secretion. Failure of serum androgens to suppress indicates that the excessive production is either of adrenal origin (eg, a tumor or enzyme defect) or secondary to an ovarian neoplasm. Women with adult-onset adrenal hyperplasia secondary to a 21-hydroxylase deficiency will have elevated serum levels of 17-hydroxyprogesterone, which are readily suppressed by dexamethasone.

Women with initially normal serum levels of total testosterone and androstenedione can be evaluated further by measuring free testosterone. If free testosterone levels also are within normal limits, 5α-reductase activity in the hair follicles can be estimated by measuring serum levels of androstenediol glucuronide (measurement of serum androstenediol glucuronide is rarely justified for clinical management). Only a small percentage of hirsute women eventually will be found to have both normal androgen production and 5α-reductase activity. These women can be diagnosed as having idiopathic hirsutism.

Women with signs or symptoms of virilization generally will have greatly elevated testosterone levels (> 3 ng/mL [10.4 nmol/L]), androstenedione levels above 5 ng/mL (17.3 nmol/L), or both. These women are most likely to have an androgen-producing *ovarian* tumor if DHEA sulfate levels are normal or an androgen-producing *adrenal* tumor if DHEA sulfate levels are elevated. Rarely, an androgen-secreting adrenal tumor can be found in the presence of normal serum DHEA sulfate levels. Women with 21-hydroxylase deficiencies may also have normal or minimally elevated levels of DHEA sulfate. Further evaluation of women with virilization should include suppression tests (dexamethasone for adrenal suppression and an oral contraceptive for ovarian suppression) as well as CT or MRI scans of the adrenals and ovaries. If the androgens are not suppressible, surgical exploration is required. A few patients have been found to have tumors with LH-dependent androgen secretion.

Moderately to markedly elevated serum levels of DHEA sulfate indicate increased adrenal androgen secretion resulting from excessive stimulation (eg, Cushing's disease) or indicate adrenal hyperplasia secondary to an enzyme defect, stress, or a tumor. In these cases, serum testosterone and androstenedione levels may vary from minimally to markedly elevated. Initially, women in this group should be evaluated by an overnight dexamethasone suppression test (1 mg of dexamethasone given at bedtime, and serum cortisol levels measured in the morning) to rule out Cushing's syndrome. Suppression of serum cortisol levels to less than 5 μg/dL (138 nmol/L) excludes this disorder. If suppression to this level is not achieved, further assessment of adrenal function, as described in Chapter 12, is required. An overnight dexamethasone suppression test, however, is inadequate to assess adrenal androgen production as reflected by levels of DHEA sulfate, since this hormone has a long plasma half-life. In women who have elevated levels of DHEA sulfate but in whom Cushing's syndrome has been excluded, dexamethasone (2 mg/d) given for 4–7 days will differentiate an adrenal tumor (no suppression) from other causes of increased adrenal androgen production.

Treatment of Hirsutism

Medical therapies directed at reducing the production of ovarian or adrenal androgens are effective primarily in reducing or preventing the formation of new hair growth. For the most part, such treatment has limited effect on terminal hairs previously formed, since the cycle of hair growth ordinarily occurs only every 6 months to 2 years. Consequently, an effective approach to the management of hirsutism usually consists of both medical and cosmetic treatment.

A. Suppression of Androgen Production: The reduction of serum levels of androgens by trials with combination oral contraceptives, progestins, or glucocorticoids should provide a rational basis for choosing one or another of these various forms of therapy. However, most women with hirsutism have only slightly increased androgen production, and its precise source or sources cannot be identified readily. In these patients, estrogen-containing oral contraceptives are generally more effective and are most often the initial form of treatment.

1. Oral contraceptives or progestins–Oral contraceptives containing both an estrogen and a progestin suppress the secretion of LH and FSH and reduce LH-dependent ovarian androgen production. The progestin component also increases the metabolic clearance rate of testosterone, while the estrogen component stimulates the production of SHBG. Although treatment with a progestin alone (ie, oral or injectable medroxyprogesterone acetate) suppresses the secretion of LH and increases the metabolic clearance rate of androgens, there is no concomitant increase in SHBG levels. Progestins are therefore generally less effective than combination oral contraceptives. They may be useful when estrogens are contraindicated.

The available combination oral contraceptives are listed in Table 17–11. In selecting a particular contraceptive for the treatment of hirsutism, the physician

should avoid compounds containing the more androgenic progestins, particularly norgestrel. Contraceptives containing a minimum of 35–50 μg of ethinyl estradiol may increase serum concentrations of SHBG and reduce the levels of both total and free testosterone in most patients. If significant clinical improvement—eg, a decrease in acne, skin oiliness, and rate of hair growth—is not apparent after 3 months of treatment, serum androgen levels should be reevaluated to make certain that adequate suppression of ovarian function has occurred. Treatment with oral contraceptives is discussed in a subsequent section of this chapter.

2. Glucocorticoids–If increased androgen production is predominantly or entirely of adrenal origin—such as occurs in adult-onset adrenal hyperplasia—treatment with glucocorticoids is indicated. In these cases, dexamethasone, 0.5–0.75 mg/d, or prednisone, 5–7.5 mg/d, has been used to reduce the production of adrenal androgens. In most women with hirsutism, however, excess androgen secretion is generally of ovarian origin, and glucocorticoids are not effective.

3. Gonadotropin-releasing hormone analogues–GnRH analogues are also effective in the management of hirsutism due to excessive ovarian androgens. They inhibit pituitary FSH and LH secretion and thus decrease ovarian androgen production. Since ovarian estradiol production will also be reduced, treatment with GnRH analogues will produce symptoms and other changes of estrogen deficiency. These can be prevented by concurrent low-dose estrogen replacement.

B. Antiandrogens–Cyproterone acetate was the first antiandrogen to be employed extensively for the treatment of hirsutism. Clinical studies with this drug in Europe have resulted in a high rate of improvement. Cyproterone acetate is a derivative of the progestin chlormadinone acetate and possesses both progestational and antiandrogenic activity. It suppresses the secretion of LH, with a subsequent decrease in ovarian androgen production, and blocks the binding of androgens to receptors in the hair follicles. Estrogen is usually administered concurrently, since endogenous estrogen production also is reduced during treatment. Although few serious side effects have been reported, cyproterone acetate is not available in the USA. A commonly used dosage is 2 mg of cyproterone acetate plus 50 μg of ethinyl estradiol daily on days 5–20 of each menstrual cycle.

Spironolactone, a competitive inhibitor of aldosterone, has been shown to possess antiandrogenic properties and competes with dihydrotestosterone for androgenic receptors in target tissues. It also decreases 17α-hydroxylase activity and thus reduces serum levels of testosterone and androstenedione. Doses ranging from 50 to 200 mg/d have been used to treat hirsutism. Spironolactone is especially useful for therapy in women in whom oral contraceptives are contraindicated or ineffective. Irregular uterine bleeding is a common side effect of treatment with spironolactone.

C. Cosmetic Therapy: The initial response to medical treatment is generally slow, and 3–6 months of therapy may be required before there is noticeable improvement in hirsutism. During the initial period of treatment, the patient can either continue with or start a simple and inexpensive method for the temporary removal of hair, eg, shaving or use of a depilatory or hot wax. After several months of medical treatment, the rate of formation of new terminal hairs will be reduced markedly, and permanent hair removal by electrolysis can be initiated, if desired. If permanent hair removal is tried prior to adequate medical treatment, the results will be transient, since new terminal hairs will continue to be formed.

ANOVULATORY BLEEDING

In the absence of ovulatory cycles, the pattern of bleeding (Table 17–3) is dependent upon the amount and timing of estrogen secretion, since the bleeding is due to estrogen stimulation of the endometrium. When estrogen secretion is low, there is usually no bleeding. However, the heaviest bleeding is observed in association with continuous secretion of substantial amounts of estrogen. In these instances, the estrogen produces proliferation of the endometrium, leading to hyperplasia or adenomatous hyperplasia. In some of these women, endometrial carcinoma will develop over long periods.

When the level of estrogen fluctuates, bleeding will occur during periods of reduced secretion. However, when the secretion is continuous and maturation is not synchronized by progesterone, the tissue is subject to spontaneous breakdown and bleeding of differing portions of the endometrium at different times. Furthermore, local factors such as the coiling and contraction of the spiral vessels do not contribute to the hemostasis, and bleeding may be severe. Such bleeding is more common in postpubertal teenagers and in the premenopausal period in older women. It is also seen in some patients in association with polycystic ovary syndrome and in women receiving estrogen therapy.

OVULATION INDUCTION

CLOMIPHENE CITRATE

Clomiphene citrate (Clomid) is a weak estrogen that effectively inhibits the action of stronger estrogens and stimulates the secretion of gonadotropins; it is used for the treatment of anovulatory patients in whom ovulation is desired. In general, a single ovulation is induced by a single course of therapy, and the patient must be treated repeatedly until pregnancy is achieved. The compound is of no use in the treatment of ovarian or pituitary failure.

The recommended initial dose of clomiphene citrate is 50 mg/d for 5 days. If ovulation occurs, this same course may be repeated until pregnancy is achieved. If ovulation does not occur, the dose is doubled to 100 mg/d for 5 days. If ovulation and menses occur, the next course can be started on the fifth day of the cycle. About 80% of patients with anovulatory disorders or amenorrhea can be expected to respond to this treatment by having ovulatory cycles. Approximately half of these patients will become pregnant. In patients in whom pregnancy is achieved, the incidence of early abortion seems to be slightly increased, as is the occurrence of multiple pregnancy (10%). Although a variety of congenital defects have been described in the offspring of these pregnancies, the incidence does not appear to be greater than that of the general population. Ovulation can be induced in some of the patients not responding to 50 or 100 mg of clomiphene daily for 5 days by using larger doses (up to 200 mg/d) for longer periods or by injecting 5000 units of chorionic gonadotropin at the time of expected ovulation. The combination of clomiphene and bromocriptine has also been reported to be successful in some patients with normal PRL levels. Clomiphene has also been used in combination with menotropins to reduce the amount of the latter required to induce ovulation.

The effective use of clomiphene is associated with some stimulation of the ovaries and usually with ovarian enlargement. The degree of enlargement tends to be greater and its incidence higher in patients who have enlarged ovaries at the beginning of therapy.

The most common side effects in patients treated with this drug are hot flushes, which resemble those experienced by menopausal patients. These tend to be mild and disappear when the drug is discontinued. There have been occasional reports of visual disturbances consisting of intensification and prolongation of afterimages. These are generally of short duration. Headache, constipation, allergic skin reactions, and reversible hair loss have been reported occasionally.

HUMAN MENOPAUSAL GONADOTROPINS (Menotropins)

Human menopausal gonadotropins, or menotropins (Pergonal), in conjunction with chorionic gonadotropin, are used to stimulate ovulation in anovulatory patients who have potentially functional ovarian tissue. Patients with ovarian failure should not be considered for therapy. Menotropins are generally used only after less complicated therapies, such as clomiphene citrate or bromocriptine, have been unsuccessful. Since therapy is difficult and expensive, it is also important to exclude other factors that might preclude pregnancy (eg, obstruction of the uterine tubes or abnormalities in sperm production by the husband) prior to initiating treatment. The possibility of multiple births must be acceptable to the patient. This treatment has induced ovulation in patients with hypopituitarism and other defects of gonadotropin secretion and in patients with amenorrhea or anovulatory cycles in whom ovulatory disturbances are associated with galactorrhea or hirsutism. In patients undergoing in vitro fertilization, menotropins are used to stimulate the development of multiple large follicles to increase the number of available ova.

Contraindications & Cautions

The most common problem encountered is excessive ovarian stimulation. Ovarian enlargement is common. When marked, as in the ovarian hyperstimulation syndrome, it may be accompanied by pain, ascites, and pleural effusion. A few patients experience fever and swelling along with discomfort at the injection site. Undesirable results of therapy include a high incidence of multiple pregnancy and abortion. The frequency of birth defects has not been increased in the offspring of patients who have succeeded in carrying their pregnancies to term.

The typical outcome of therapy in properly selected patients treated by experienced physicians is shown in Table 17–9. Menotropins are potentially dangerous and should be administered by physicians with experience in endocrine disturbances and problems of reproductive function. This mode of therapy is complicated, time-consuming, and expensive and should not be undertaken unless simpler therapeutic measures have failed.

Dosages

Human menopausal gonadotropins (menotropins, Pergonal) are supplied in lyophilized form in ampules containing 75 units each of FSH and LH and 10 mg of lactose. The usual dosage is one or more ampules intramuscularly daily until estrogen production is optimal—ie, plasma levels of 600–1000 pg/mL (2.2–3.7 nmol/L). Growth of ovarian follicles should also be monitored by ultrasonography to assist in determining the optimal dosage and duration of treatment. Chorionic gonadotropin (see Chapter 20) in doses of 5000–10,000 units intramuscularly is then adminis-

tered once to induce ovulation from the mature follicle and then several times after ovulation to support corpus luteum function. If estrogen production becomes excessive during the preovulatory treatment phase, chorionic gonadotropin should be withheld to avoid the ovarian hyperstimulation syndrome. Patients must be examined frequently (daily or on alternate days) for 2 weeks following the last injection to detect signs of overstimulation and should be advised to have intercourse at least every other day near the time of expected ovulation.

GONADOTROPIN-RELEASING HORMONE

The pulsatile administration of GnRH in doses of 1–10 μg per pulse at 60- to 120-minute intervals will induce ovulation in most patients with amenorrhea due to hypothalamic dysfunction associated with decreased secretion of endogenous GnRH. GnRH can be given intravenously or subcutaneously using a peristaltic pump. Although the method is somewhat cumbersome, less frequent monitoring of the patient is required and ovarian hyperstimulation is less likely to occur.

BROMOCRIPTINE

Although bromocriptine is occasionally effective in treating patients with amenorrhea in the absence of elevated serum levels of PRL, its use is generally reserved for patients with hyperprolactinemia or galactorrhea. Its use in such patients is described elsewhere in this chapter.

THERAPEUTIC USE OF OVARIAN HORMONES & THEIR SYNTHETIC ANALOGUES

Estrogens are used in combination with progestins by more than 40 million women for contraception and are widely used after the menopause. Estrogens are also used to limit the height of tall girls and to replace absent or deficient endogenous hormone in patients with hypogonadism or after gonadectomy. It is therefore important to understand the effects of these agents and problems engendered by their use.

TREATMENT OF PRIMARY HYPOGONADISM

Treatment of primary hypogonadism is usually begun at 11–13 years of age in order to stimulate the development of secondary sex characteristics and

Table 17–9. Results of treatment with menotropins.

Pregnancy achieved: 25–40%
Multiple births
Twins, 10–20%
Triplets, etc, 5–10%
Abortions, 20%
Hyperstimulation syndrome: 0.5–1.5%

menses and to promote optimal growth. Treatment consists mainly of the administration of estrogens and progestins. Androgens and anabolic agents have also been used in these patients to stimulate growth, but no further increase in final height was achieved. Furthermore, acne, hirsutism, clitorimegaly, and premature closure of the epiphyses have occurred as unwanted effects of androgens and anabolic agents. Progestins are advisable in conjunction with estrogens, because long-term replacement therapy, even when used cyclically in modest doses, has been associated with an increase in the incidence of endometrial hyperplasia and endometrial carcinoma. Oral contraceptives have also been used for replacement therapy.

OVARIAN SUPPRESSION

Estrogen-progestin combinations (oral contraceptives) are used to suppress ovarian function in patients with LH-dependent excess androgen production or endometriosis and are discussed elsewhere in this chapter.

Progestational hormones alone are used to produce long-term ovarian suppression when estrogens are contraindicated. When used parenterally in large doses—eg, medroxyprogesterone acetate, 150 mg intramuscularly every 90 days—prolonged anovulation and amenorrhea are produced. This procedure has been employed in the treatment of dysmenorrhea, endometriosis, hirsutism, and bleeding disorders. The major problem encountered with this regimen is the prolonged time required for ovulatory function to return after cessation of therapy in some patients. Irregular spotting also occurs. This treatment should not be used for patients planning a pregnancy in the near future.

THREATENED ABORTION

Progestins do not appear to have any place in the therapy of threatened or habitual abortion. Early reports of the usefulness of these agents were based on the unwarranted assumption that after several abortions the likelihood of repeated abortions was over 90%. When progestational agents were administered to patients with previous abortions, a salvage rate of 80% was achieved. It is now recognized that similar patients abort only 20% of the time even when untreated.

In some patients with "threatened" abortion, progesterone production is decreased. It is likely that the decrease in progesterone reflects damage to the placenta or fetus and is a result of events leading to abortion rather than a cause of the abortion. Administration of progesterone in these circumstances, especially in the presence of declining serum levels of hCG, does not appear to be useful and may allow retention of the dead fetus, thus delaying recognition of an abortion that has occurred. Prolonged postpartum bleeding has also been reported in some patients treated with repository medroxyprogesterone or hydroxyprogesterone caproate.

INADEQUATE LUTEAL PHASE

Progesterone and medroxyprogesterone have been used in the treatment of women who have difficulty in conceiving and who demonstrate a slow rise in basal body temperature. Some investigators believe that these patients suffer from a relative luteal insufficiency, and progesterone or related compounds are given to replace the deficiency. There is no convincing evidence that this treatment is effective. In the absence of satisfactory controls, the successes reported are impossible to distinguish from placebo effects.

DIAGNOSTIC USES

Progesterone is also used as a test of estrogen secretion. A single intramuscular injection of 200 mg of progesterone in oil or a course of medroxyprogesterone, 10 mg/d for 5–7 days, is followed by withdrawal bleeding in amenorrheic patients only when the endometrium has been stimulated by estrogens. In the absence of withdrawal bleeding, a combination of estrogen and progestin can be given to test the responsiveness of the endometrium in patients with amenorrhea.

INHIBITORS OF OVARIAN FUNCTION

GONADOTROPIN-RELEASING HORMONE ANALOGUES

As noted above, GnRH administered in a pulsatile manner will induce ovulation in patients with amenorrhea. However, when large amounts are administered continuously, inhibition of gonadotropin release occurs. This property has been exploited by the development of highly potent agonist analogues, such as leuprolide, buserelin, and nafarelin. These analogues can be administered subcutaneously or intranasally. In sufficient doses, they can inhibit ovarian function, both reducing the secretion of sex steroids and inhibiting ovulation. GnRH analogues have been used to treat patients with sex hormone-dependent disorders such as precocious puberty, endometriosis, uterine fibroids, and hirsutism secondary to excess ovarian androgen production.

TAMOXIFEN

Tamoxifen is a nonsteroidal competitive inhibitor of estradiol at its receptor. It can be given orally and is being used in the palliative treatment of advanced breast cancer in postmenopausal women (see Chapter 26). Peak plasma levels are reached in a few hours. It has an initial half-life of 7–14 hours in the circulation and is predominantly excreted by the liver. It is dispensed as the citrate in the form of tablets (Nolvadex) containing the equivalent of 10 mg of tamoxifen. It is used in doses of 10–20 mg twice daily. Hot flushes and nausea and vomiting occur in 25% of patients, and many other adverse effects have been reported.

DANAZOL

Danazol (Danocrine), an isoxazole derivative of ethisterone (17α-ethinyl testosterone) with weak progestational and androgenic activities, is used to suppress ovarian function. It inhibits the midcycle surge of LH and FSH and can prevent the compensatory increase in LH and FSH following castration in animals, but it does not significantly lower or suppress basal LH or FSH levels in healthy humans. Danazol binds to androgen, progesterone, and glucocorticoid receptors and can initiate androgen-specific RNA synthesis. It does not bind to intracellular estrogen receptors, but it does bind to SHBG and CBG. It inhibits the cholesterol-cleaving enzyme, 3α-hydroxysteroid dehydrogenase, 17α-hydroxysteroid dehydrogenase, 17,21-lyase, 17α-hydroxylase, 11α-hydroxylase, and 21-hydroxylase, but it does not inhibit aromatase. It increases the mean clearance rate of progesterone, probably by competition for binding to CBG, and may have similar effects on other active steroid hormones. Ethisterone, a major metabolite, has both progestational and mild androgenic effects.

Danazol has been employed as an inhibitor of gonadal function and has found its major use in the treatment of endometriosis. For this purpose, it is usually administered at a starting dose of 400 mg/d, and in patients who do not respond, the dose can be increased to 600 or 800 mg/d. In most patients requiring the larger doses, the dosage can be reduced after several months of therapy without a return of symptoms. Danazol has also been used to treat fibrocystic breast disease and several hematologic disorders.

The major side effects are weight gain, edema, decreased breast size, acne and oily skin, mild hirsutism, deepening of the voice, headache, hot flushes, changes in libido, and muscle cramps. Although these side effects do not present any health risks, many women discontinue treatment because of them.

Danazol should be used with great caution in patients with hepatic dysfunction, since it has been reported to produce mild to moderate hepatocellular damage in some patients, as evidenced by enzyme changes. Danazol treatment also markedly decreases the HDL:LDL ratio in most women. It is contraindicated during pregnancy and breast-feeding, as it can produce urogenital abnormalities in the offspring.

ANTIPROGESTINS

Mifepristone (17β-hydroxy-11β(4-dimethylaminophenyl)-17α(1-propynyl)estra-4,9-diene-3-one, RU-486), a 19 norsteroid, binds strongly to the progesterone receptor (in addition to binding to the glucocorticoid receptor) and inhibits the binding and activity of progesterone. Preliminary studies indicate that it has luteolytic properties in many women when given in the midluteal period. The mechanism of this effect is unknown. These luteolytic properties could make mifepristone useful as a contraceptive. However, its long half-life and large dose requirement may prolong the follicular phase of the subsequent cycle and make it difficult to use for this purpose. This drug has been used for the termination of early pregnancy. Doses of 400–600 mg/d for 4 days or 800 mg/d for 2 days successfully terminated pregnancy in 85% of the women studied. The major side effect was prolonged bleeding that did not require treatment.

Preliminary studies have found that epostane, a 3β-hydroxysteroid dehydrogenase inhibitor, decreases the synthesis of progesterone and can terminate early pregnancy.

ANTIANDROGENS

The possibility of using antiandrogens to treat hirsutism and other disorders due to excessive amounts of testosterone has led to a search for effective drugs via 2 approaches that have met with limited success experimentally. Several compounds have been developed that inhibit the 17-hydroxylation of progesterone or pregnenolone, thereby preventing the action of the side chain-splitting enzyme and the further transformation of these steroid precursors to active androgens. A few of these compounds have been tested clinically but have been too toxic for prolonged use. Another approach has been the development of steroids that are chemically similar and act as competitive inhibitors. A few of them have been tried in patients on a limited basis.

Cyproterone and **cyproterone acetate** are effective antiandrogens that inhibit the action of the androgens at the target organ. The acetate form has a marked progestational effect that suppresses LH and FSH, thus leading to a more effective antiandrogen effect. These compounds have been used to decrease excessive sexual drive in disturbed individuals and are being studied in other conditions in which reduction of androgenic effects would be useful. In Europe, they are used in the treatment of hirsutism (see page 473). They are not available in the USA.

Ketoconazole, an inhibitor of glucocorticoid and androgen synthesis in the adrenal, has also been shown to inhibit human ovarian 17-hydroxylase and 3β-hydroxysteroid dehydrogenase. It does not affect ovarian aromatase, but reduces human placental aromatase activity. The drug has been used experimentally to treat hirsutism in women and prostate cancer in men. Men treated with ketoconazole have increased estradiol:testosterone ratios, which may cause the gynecomastia seen during therapy. Ketoconazole does not appear to be clinically useful in women.

MENOPAUSE

Menopause begins with the last episode of menstrual bleeding induced by the cyclic endogenous secretion of ovarian hormones. It normally occurs between the ages of 42 and 60 years. It occurs prematurely as a result of surgical removal, irradiation, or abnormalities of the ovaries.

HORMONAL CHANGES

The changes in endocrine function are not abrupt in women undergoing spontaneous menopause. The circulating levels of gonadotropins begin to increase several years before ovulation ceases. Production of estrogen and progesterone decreases, and irregular cycles and anovulatory bleeding are not uncommon (Table 17–10). The increase in FSH is greater than that of LH and reflects the lack of feedback inhibition by estrogen or inhibin, or both. The stromal cells of the ovary respond to increased LH stimulation by producing more androstenedione but only tiny amounts of estrogen.

The average production rate of estradiol falls to 12 μg/24 h (44 nmol/24 h), and the clearance rate is reduced. Since very little estradiol is found in ovarian or adrenal veins, most of the circulating estradiol is derived from estrone, which in itself is produced by the peripheral conversion of androstenedione. The average production rate for estrone is 55 μg/24 h (202 nmol/24 h), and there is a 20% reduction in its clearance.

Progesterone levels are approximately 30% of the concentration seen in young women during the follicular phase. The source of this progesterone appears to be the adrenal.

Androgen levels are also reduced postmenopausally. Androstenedione falls to about half of the concentration found in young women, and most of that apparently comes from the adrenal, as suggested by its peak concentrations at 8 AM and nadir concentrations at 3–4 PM. The clearance rate does not change. The average production rate is about 1.5 mg/24 h (5200 nmol/24 h). About 20% of it is thought to come from the ovary. Testosterone production rates are approximately 150 μg/24 h (520 nmol/24 h), as compared to about 200 μg/24 h (693 nmol/24 h) in younger women. This fall is less than that seen after ovariectomy, indicating that testosterone is produced by conversion of androstenedione as well as being secreted by the adrenal and ovary. It is of interest that DHEA and DHEA sulfate also fall with age, although almost all of these steroids come from the adrenal gland.

CLINICAL MANIFESTATIONS OF MENOPAUSE

Menstrual Changes

The interval prior to the menopause is usually characterized sequentially by cycles with a shortening of the follicular phase, an interval of very irregular cycles, and an interval of anovulatory bleeding. Fertility is usually very low during this time. Although menses may cease abruptly, usually there is a gradual diminution in the amount of menstrual flow as well as its duration. However, if secretion of estrogen is prolonged in the absence of ovulation, endometrial hyperplasia may occur and cause heavy bleeding. It is some-

Table 17–10. Serum concentrations (mean ± SEM) of steroids in premenopausal and postmenopausal women.[1]

Steroid	Premenopausal[2]		Postmenopausal	
	(ng/mL)	(nmol/L)	(ng/mL)	(nmol/L)
Progesterone	0.47 ± 0.03	(1.49 ± 0.1)	0.17 ± 0.02	(0.54 ± 0.06)
DHEA	4.2 ± 0.5	(14.5 ± 1.7)	1.8 ± 0.2	(6.2 ± 0.69)
DHEA sulfate	1600 ± 350	(3159 ± 691)	300 ± 70	(592 ± 138)
Androstenedione	1.5 ± 0.1	(5.2 ± 0.35)	0.6 ± 0.01	(2.08 ± 0.03)
Testosterone	0.32 ± 0.02	(1.11 ± 0.07)	0.25 ± 0.03	(0.87 ± 0.1)
Estrone	0.08 ± 0.01	(0.29 ± 0.04)	0.029 ± 0.002	(0.11 ± 0.01)
Estradiol	0.05 ± 0.005	(0.18 ± 0.02)	0.013 ± 0.001	(0.05 ± 0.004)

[1]Reproduced, with permission, from Pernoll ML, Benson RC (editor): *Current Obstetric & Gynecologic Diagnosis & Treatment,* 6th ed. Appleton & Lange, 1987.
[2]Follicular phase concentrations.

times difficult to clinically distinguish this type of bleeding from that produced by organic diseases, including endometrial carcinoma. Any bleeding that occurs more than a year after the last previous period is likely to be an indication of organic disease.

Vasomotor Symptoms

The most common menopausal complaint is hot flushes, which occur in 75% of women at the menopause. They are due to declining estrogen levels. Women with estrogen deficiency from childhood do not develop hot flushes unless they have been treated with exogenous estrogens and treatment is interrupted. Episodes of flushing are associated with periodic increases in core temperature, causing reflex peripheral vasodilatation, a small increase in pulse rate, and sweating. They are synchronous with the pulsatile release of LH but are not caused by increased secretion of gonadotropins. Rather, they appear to be linked to the central mechanism controlling the release of GnRH. These symptoms occur most frequently in a warm environment and are common at night, contributing to insomnia.

The hot flush often starts with a sensation of pressure in the head, followed by a feeling of warmth in the head and neck and upper thorax. It may be associated with palpitations and gradually spreading waves of heat over the entire body. The feeling of warmth and flushing is quickly followed by sweating. The sweating and vasodilatation lead to heat loss and a decrease in core temperature of approximately 0.2 °C. These episodes last 10–20 minutes.

In 20% of patients, hot flushes are a transient phenomenon lasting for less than 1 year, but 25–50% of women experience them for more than 5 years. Estrogen therapy is remarkably effective in controlling hot flushes in over 90% of patients.

Atrophic Changes in the Genitourinary System

The decline in estrogen production results in reduction in mucus secretion and gradual atrophy of the vaginal and urethral epithelium. The rugae progressively disappear with thinning of the epithelium. The surface may appear vascular at first but then becomes pale. These changes lead to itching, dyspareunia, and burning. Similar changes in the urinary tract may give rise to atrophic cystitis, with symptoms of urgency, incontinence, and frequency. The cervix decreases in size, and the mucus secretion diminishes. The endometrium and myometrium also undergo atrophy. Myomas become smaller and endometriosis less symptomatic. The adverse symptoms can be treated by administration of estrogens locally as well as systemically (see below).

Osteoporosis

Osteoporosis results from a combination of increased bone resorption and decreased bone formation. In its early stages, it is predominantly a disease of trabecular bone. Affected patients show increased calcium loss from bone, which could account for the slight elevation of plasma Ca^{2+}, reduction of $1,25(OH)_2D_3$, and reduction in the intestinal absorption of Ca^{2+} found in this disorder. The problem is enhanced in winter months because of decreased activity and decreased exposure to sunlight and by the difficulty of maintaining calcium balance at normal levels of intake (see Chapters 11 and 29).

During the first few years following menopause, women lose an average of about 1% of their metacarpal cortical bone mass per year (Fig 17–18). The initial rapid bone loss is inhibited by estrogen. Loss of bone mass leads to reduced skeletal strength and susceptibility to fractures. There is, for example, a 10-fold increase in the incidence of Colles' fractures in women between the ages of 35 and 55, although a similar increase is not seen in men (Fig 17–19). Hip fractures, which are ultimately fatal in about one-third of patients and disable others for life, also occur more frequently.

The availability of methods for assessing bone density has led to a better understanding of the disorder and its response to therapy. Studies indicate that bone density decreases in women as the years advance. However, the loss is accelerated at menopause. Other studies indicate that estrogen therapy started at that time can prevent the loss (Fig 17–18). If estrogens are administered subsequently, the process can be arrested. However, when treatment is delayed for 5–6 years, little effect is noted. Treatment with estrogen decreases plasma Ca^{2+} and increases plasma PTH and $1,25(OH)_2D_3$, which, in turn, increases calcium absorption. The risk for osteoporosis is highest in smokers who are thin, Caucasian, inactive, and have a low calcium intake and a strong family history of osteoporosis. (See also Chapter 11.)

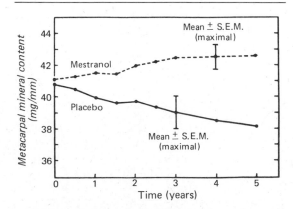

Figure 17–18. Metacarpal mineral content in postmenopausal women treated with mestranol or placebo for 5 years. Note loss of bone density in placebo but not mestranol treatment group. (Reproduced, with permission, from Lindsay R et al: Long-term prevention of postmenopausal osteoporosis by oestrogen. *Lancet* 1976; **1:**1038.)

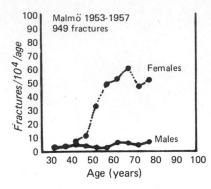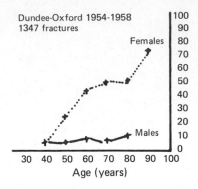

Figure 17–19. Indices of Colles' fracture in relation to age in Malmö and Dundee-Oxford. (Reproduced, with permission, from Cope E: Physical changes associated with post-menopausal years. Page 4 in: *Management of the Menopause and Post-Menopause Years.* Campbell S [editor]. MTP Press Ltd, 1976.)

Skin & Hair Changes

At the time of the menopause, changes in the skin due to aging are noticeable. There is some thinning and wrinkling. Although estrogen creams are widely used cosmetically, it is not clear that they have any effects other than enhancement of the dermal water content. Changes in hair include loss of some underarm and pubic hair and occasionally replacement of vellus hair on the chin and upper lip by terminal hairs.

Emotional Changes

Anxiety, depression, and irritability are commonly reported around the time of the menopause. There is no good evidence that these symptoms are directly related to estrogen deficiency. However, sleep disturbances caused by hot flushes may contribute to the irritability. The majority of women treated with estrogens report some improvement in their sense of well-being and relief of insomnia and other symptoms produced by estrogen deficiency.

MANAGEMENT OF MENOPAUSE

Hormonal Therapy

The major indications for hormonal therapy in menopausal patients are the treatment of hot flushes and atrophic vaginitis and the prevention of osteoporosis in patients at high risk for development of that disorder. Estrogens should be used in the smallest dose consistent with relief of symptoms. In women with a uterus, estrogen therapy should be given for the first 21–25 days of each month and a progestational agent administered during the last 10–14 days of estrogen administration. The recommended daily dosage of estrogen is 0.3–1.25 mg of conjugated estrogens or 0.01–0.02 mg of ethinyl estradiol. Doses in the middle of these ranges have been shown to be maximally effective in preventing the decrease in bone density occurring at the menopause. In order to prevent osteoporosis, it is important to begin therapy as soon as possible after the menopause. Studies indicate that addition of 10 mg medroxyprogesterone acetate orally daily for the last 10–14 days of estrogen therapy markedly reduces the risk of endometrial carcinoma.

Some women are reluctant to accept the periodic vaginal bleeding associated with cyclic estrogen-progestin therapy despite its benefits. Preliminary studies indicate that continuous daily administration of 0.625 mg of conjugated equine estrogens and 2.5 mg of medroxyprogesterone will eliminate cyclic bleeding in most patients while providing relief from vasomotor symptoms and genital atrophy and protection from endometrial hyperplasia. About half of these patients will experience breakthrough bleeding in the first few months. Further studies will be required to determine the long-term effects on cardiovascular risk factors.

Patients at low risk for development of osteoporosis with only mild atrophic vaginitis can be treated with local vaginal preparations. This route of application is also useful in treatment of urinary tract symptoms. It is important to realize, however, that locally administered estrogens are almost completely absorbed into the circulation and should be used intermittently.

Although the estrogens share most, if not all, of their hormonal effects, their relative potencies vary depending on the agent and the route of administration. As noted above, estradiol is the most active endogenous estrogen and has the highest affinity for the estrogen receptor. However, its metabolites estrone and estriol have weak uterotropic effects. 2-Hydroxyestrone, another important metabolite, possesses neurotransmitter activity in the brain. It also competes with catecholamines for catechol-O-methyltransferase and inhibits tyrosine hydroxylase. For a given level of gonadotropin suppression, oral compounds have a greater effect on the circulating levels of corticosteroid and sex hormone-binding proteins. This effect, which is thought to be due to larger concentrations of hormone reaching the liver by this route, has led to the development of transdermal preparations. When administered transdermally, 50–100 μg of estradiol had effects similar to those of 0.625–1.25 mg conjugated oral estrogens on gonadotropin levels, endometrium, and vaginal epithelium. However, only the oral estrogen increased levels of renin substrate, CBG, and TBG, while the higher dose of conjugated estrogens had favorable effects on high- and low-density lipoprotein levels.

In patients in whom estrogen replacement therapy is contraindicated (eg, those with estrogen-sensitive tumors), relief of vasomotor symptoms may be obtained by the use of progestational agents. Medroxyprogesterone acetate, 150 mg intramuscularly once a month, norgestrel, 250 μg orally daily, or medroxyprogesterone, 10 mg orally daily, can be useful. Mild tranquilizers and clonidine are also effective in some patients, as are atropine-barbiturate mixtures. Calcium carbonate supplements (eg, Os-Cal) are useful in bringing the total daily calcium intake up to 1500 mg. Vitamin D therapy may be useful when calcium intake is less than optimal. Preliminary studies show that fluoride in adequate amounts can increase bone density, but the effects on bone strength have not been assessed.

Adverse Effects of Therapy

Therapeutic use of estrogens is accompanied by adverse effects of varying degrees of severity (see Hormonal Contraception, below).

Estrogen therapy has now become the major cause of postmenopausal bleeding. Unfortunately, vaginal bleeding at this time of life may be due to carcinoma of the endometrium, and many women are being subjected to dilatation and curettage of the uterus unnecessarily. In order to avoid this complication, patients should be treated with the smallest effective amount of estrogen, given cyclically, with addition of a progestational agent in the last 10 days of estrogen in each cycle. This will usually produce regular and predictable withdrawal bleeding.

Nausea and breast tenderness are common and can be minimized by using the smallest effective dose. These symptoms may be more marked at the beginning of therapy. The presence of cystic mastitis or fibroids that increase in size during treatment may also interfere with the use of estrogen. Hyperpigmentation also occurs. Estrogen therapy is associated with an increase in frequency of migraine headaches as well as cholestasis, hypertension, and gallbladder disease.

The relationship of estrogen therapy to cancer continues to be the subject of active investigation. It has not been possible to establish whether or not there is an increased risk in the incidence of breast cancer. Nor is it clear that it is safe to use estrogen in patients at high risk for development of this tumor. The risk of endometrial carcinoma is increased in patients taking estrogens without adjunct progestins and varies with the dose and duration of treatment. It increases 15 times in patients taking large doses of estrogen for 5 or more years but only 2–4 times in patients receiving lower doses for 2 years. The concomitant use of a progestin

not only prevents this increased risk but actually reduces the incidence of endometrial cancer below that in the general population.

HORMONAL CONTRACEPTION (Oral Contraceptives)

A large number of oral contraceptives containing estrogens or progestins (or both) are now available for clinical use (Table 17–11). These preparations vary in chemical composition and, as might be expected, have many properties in common, but there are also differences. Two types of preparations are used for oral contraception: (1) monophasic, biphasic, and triphasic combinations of estrogens and progestins; and (2) progestins without concomitant administration of estrogens.

PHARMACOLOGIC EFFECTS OF ESTROGENS & SYNTHETIC PROGESTINS

Mechanisms of Contraceptive Action

Estrogens and progestin combinations inhibit gonadotropin secretion, which prevents ovulation. They also change the cervical mucus, the endometrium, and tubal motility and secretion, all of which decrease the likelihood of conception and implantation. Continuous use of progestins alone does not inhibit ovulation, and the other effects play a major role in prevention of pregnancy when these agents are used.

Genital Effects of Oral Contraceptives

Chronic use of estrogen-progestin combinations depresses ovarian function. The ovary shows minimal follicular development and an absence of corpora lutea, larger follicles, stromal edema, and other morphologic features normally seen in ovulating women. Estrogen production is decreased, and progesterone secretion is minimal. Although cystic follicles have been described in patients taking oral contraceptives, the ovaries usually become smaller even when previously enlarged.

Cytologic findings on vaginal smears vary depending on the preparation used. However, with almost all of the combined drugs, a midzone maturation index is found because of the presence of progestational agents.

Effects on the uterus include hypertrophy of the cervix and polyp formation after prolonged use. The cervical mucus becomes thick and less copious and contains much cellular debris. Initially, there may be some

Table 17–11. Oral contraceptive agents in use. The estrogen-containing compounds are arranged in order of increasing content of estrogen (ethinyl estradiol and mestranol have similar potencies). The relative progestational potencies are shown in the last column.[1]

	Estrogen (mg)		Progestin (mg)		pp[2]
Monophasic combination tablets					
Loestrin 1/20	Ethinyl estradiol	0.02	Norethindrone acetate	1.0	4
Loestrin 1.5/30	Ethinyl estradiol	0.03	Norethindrone acetate	1.5	6
Lo/Ovral	Ethinyl estradiol	0.03	dl-Norgestrel	0.3	18
Nordette	Ethinyl estradiol	0.03	L-Norgestrel	0.15	18
Brevicon Modicon	Ethinyl estradiol	0.035	Norethindrone	0.5	1
Demulen 1/35	Ethinyl estradiol	0.035	Ethynodiol diacetate	1.0	30
Norinyl 1/35 Ortho-Novum 1/35	Ethinyl estradiol	0.035	Norethindrone	1.0	2
Ovcon 35	Ethinyl estradiol	0.035	Norethindrone	0.4	0.8
Demulen 1/50	Ethinyl estradiol	0.05	Ethynodiol diacetate	1.0	30
Norlestrin 1/50	Ethinyl estradiol	0.05	Norethindrone acetate	1.0	4
Norlestrin 2.5/50	Ethinyl estradiol	0.05	Norethindrone acetate	2.5	10
Ovcon 50	Ethinyl estradiol	0.05	Norethindrone	1.0	2
Ovral	Ethinyl estradiol	0.05	dl-Norgestrel	0.5	30
Norinyl 1/50 Ortho-Novum 1/50	Mestranol	0.05	Norethindrone	1.0	2
Enovid 5	Mestranol	0.075	Norethynodrel	5.0	11
Norinyl 1/80 Ortho-Novum 1/80	Mestranol	0.08	Norethindrone	1.0	2
Enovid E	Mestranol	0.1	Norethynodrel	2.5	6
Norinyl-2 Ortho-Novum-2	Mestranol	0.1	Norethindrone	2.0	4
Ovulen	Mestranol	0.1	Ethynodiol diacetate	1.0	30
Biphasic combination tablets Ortho-Novum 10/11					
Days 1–10	Ethinyl estradiol	0.035	Norethindrone	0.5	1
Days 11–21	Ethinyl estradiol	0.035	Norethindrone	1.0	2
Triphasic combination tablets Triphasil					
Days 1–6	Ethinyl estradiol	0.03	L-Norgestrel	0.05	2
Days 7–11	Ethinyl estradiol	0.04	L-Norgestrel	0.075	3
Days 12–21	Ethinyl estradiol	0.03	L-Norgestrel	0.125	5
Ortho-Novum 7/7/7					
Days 1–7	Ethinyl estradiol	0.035	Norethindrone	0.5	1
Days 8–14	Ethinyl estradiol	0.035	Norethindrone	0.75	1.5
Days 15–21	Ethinyl estradiol	0.035	Norethindrone	1.0	2
Tri-Norinyl					
Days 1–7	Ethinyl estradiol	0.035	Norethindrone	0.5	1
Days 8–16	Ethinyl estradiol	0.035	Norethindrone	1.0	2
Days 17–21	Ethinyl estradiol	0.035	Norethindrone	0.5	1
Daily progestin tablets					
Micronor	. . .		Norethindrone	0.35	0.7
Nor-QD	. . .		Norethindrone	0.35	0.7
Ovrette	. . .		dl-Norgestrel	0.075	3

[1]Modified and reproduced, with permission, from Katzung BG (editor): *Basic & Clinical Pharmacology,* 4th ed. Appleton & Lange, 1989.
[2]Progestational potency.

stimulation of the uterine muscle, resulting in softening. Stromal deciduation occurs toward the end of the
cycle. The agents containing 19-nortestosterone derivatives combined with smaller amounts of estrogen tend
to produce more glandular atrophy and less bleeding
than agents containing progestins that stimulate glandular development.

Although studies in humans are not available, experiments in animals indicate that alterations in the
transport of the gamete through the uterine tube are
produced by estrogens and progestins. The effect on
germ cell transport is thought by some to be an important mechanism for the impairment of fertility, particularly with the use of low-dosage continuous progestin
therapy.

Stimulation of the breasts occurs in most patients
receiving estrogen-containing agents. Some enlargement is generally noted. These agents tend to suppress
lactation, but when the doses are small, the effects on
breast feeding are not appreciable. Preliminary studies
of transport of oral contraceptives into the breast milk
suggest that only small amounts of these compounds
are found and they have not been considered to be of
importance.

Extragenital Effects of Oral Contraceptives

It is important to understand the extragenital effects
of oral contraceptives, because of the large and growing number of normal individuals using them.

A. Central Nervous System Effects: The effects
of the oral contraceptives on the central nervous system have not been well studied in humans. In animals,
estrogens tend to lower the threshold of excitability in
the brain, whereas progesterone tends to increase it. In
addition, the increased respiration and thermogenic
actions of progesterone and some of the synthetic progestins are thought to be due to effects on the central
nervous system. The suppression of ovarian function
results in part from inhibition of GnRH secretion by
the hypothalamus.

It is very difficult to evaluate any behavioral or emotional effects of these compounds. Although there is a
low incidence of pronounced changes in mood, affect,
and behavior in most studies, milder changes are
common.

B. Endocrinologic Effects: The combined agents
inhibit the secretion of pituitary gonadotropins, as
mentioned above. Estrogens increase the plasma concentration of CBG. This increases plasma cortisol concentrations but does not lead to chronic alteration in the
rate of cortisol secretion. It has also been observed that
the ACTH response to the administration of
metyrapone is attenuated by estrogens and the oral
contraceptives.

These preparations alter the angiotensin-aldoster-
one system, increasing plasma renin activity and therefore aldosterone secretion. The relationship between

these alterations and the hypertension that occurs in
some patients taking oral contraceptives is not clear.

TBG is increased, resulting in higher circulating
thyroxine levels. However, the free thyroxine level in
these patients is normal.

C. Hematologic Effects: Serious thromboembolic
phenomena occurring in women taking oral contraceptives have stimulated a great many studies of their
effects on blood coagulation. A clear picture of such
effects has not yet emerged. The oral contraceptives do
not consistently alter bleeding or clotting times. Conflicting information has arisen from studies of effects
of these agents on the clotting factors. However, in
general they indicate that the changes observed are
similar to those reported in pregnancy and include an
increase in factors VII, VIII, IX, and X. Increased
amounts of coumarin derivatives are required to prolong prothrombin time in patients taking oral contraceptives. The platelet aggregation response to catecholamines is also increased.

Significant alterations in the cellular components of
blood have not been reported with any consistency.
Oral contraceptives inhibit the conversion of poly-
glutamic folate found in food to the monoglutamic
folate that is absorbed in the gastrointestinal tract,
thereby causing folic acid–deficiency anemias, which
can be reversed by folic acid supplementation or by
discontinuing oral contraceptives.

D. Hepatic Effects: The liver plays an important
role in the metabolism of the estrogens and progestins
used in oral contraceptives. These hormones also affect liver function. (See Adverse Effects of Oral Contraceptives, below.)

Estrogens increase the synthesis of the various
transport globulins and fibrinogen and decrease the
synthesis of serum haptoglobins.

Important alterations in drug excretion and metabolism also occur in the liver. Estrogens in the amounts
present during pregnancy or ingested in oral contraceptive agents delay the clearance of sulfobromoph-
thalein (Bromsulphalein, BSP) and reduce bile flow.

Oral contraceptives increase the saturation of cholesterol in bile, and the ratio of cholic acid to chenodeoxycholic acid is increased. These changes may
cause the observed increase in cholelithiasis associated
with use of these agents.

E. Effects on Lipid Metabolism: Estrogens increase plasma high-density lipoproteins (HDL) and
very low density lipoproteins (VLDL) while lowering
low-density lipoproteins (LDL). In young women with
normal lipids, this results in higher circulating triglyceride and free and esterified cholesterol levels. In older
women with higher cholesterol levels, a reduction is
usually observed because of the reduction of LDL.
Phospholipid levels are increased. Although the effects are marked with doses of 100 μg of mestranol or
ethinyl estradiol, doses of 50 μg or less have minimal
effects. The progestins—particularly the 19-nor-

testosterone derivatives—tend to antagonize the effects of estrogen. Preparations containing small amounts of estrogen and a progestin may slightly decrease triglycerides and high-density lipoproteins.

F. Effects on Carbohydrate Metabolism: The administration of oral contraceptives produces alterations in carbohydrate metabolism similar to those observed in pregnancy (see Chapter 20). There is a reduction in the rate of absorption of carbohydrates from the gastrointestinal tract. These agents antagonize the effects of insulin, causing decreases in glucose tolerance or increased secretion of insulin following administration of glucose. Studies in experimental animals indicate that estrogens enhance islet cell function, whereas progesterone interferes with insulin action. The changes in glucose tolerance are reversible on discontinuing medication.

G. Cardiovascular Effects: These agents cause small increases in cardiac output associated with slightly higher systolic and diastolic blood pressure and heart rate. Pathologic increases in blood pressure occur in a small number of patients, in whom the pressure slowly returns to normal when treatment is terminated. It is important that blood pressure be followed in each patient.

Venous engorgement has been reported. Changes in connective tissue in the arteries of rodents have been reported, but their significance is not known. Plasma from women taking oral contraceptives stimulates growth of arterial smooth muscle in tissue culture, and it is postulated that this effect could enhance the atherosclerotic process.

H. Dermatologic Effects: Oral contraceptives have been noted to increase pigmentation of the skin (chloasma). This effect seems to be enhanced in women with dark complexions and by exposure to ultraviolet light. Agents with larger amounts of androgenic progestins may increase the production of sebum and cause acne. However, estrogen-dominant oral contraceptive preparations usually decrease sebum production by suppressing the ovarian production of androgens.

CLINICAL USES OF ORAL CONTRACEPTIVES

The most important use of the estrogen and progestin compounds is for prevention of pregnancy. Many preparations are available, and they are packaged to provide for ease of administration. When these agents are taken according to directions, the risk of conception is estimated to be about 0.5–1 per 100 woman years.

These compounds are also used in the treatment of endometriosis. When severe dysmenorrhea is the major symptom of this disorder, suppression of ovulation with estrogen may be followed by painless periods. In some patients, long-term continuous administration of large doses of progestins or estrogen-progestin combinations

to prevent cyclic breakdown of the endometrial tissue leads to endometrial fibrosis and prevents the reactivation of implants for prolonged periods.

As is true with most hormonal preparations, many of the adverse effects are physiologic or pharmacologic effects of the drug that are objectionable only because they are not pertinent to the situation for which they are being used. Therefore, the product containing the smallest amounts of hormones should be selected for use.

The differences between preparations can be used to advantage for individualized treatment. These preparations differ in amounts and types of estrogen and progestin (Table 17–11). Preparations containing larger amounts of estrogen tend to produce more withdrawal bleeding, nausea, and mastalgia. Preparations containing 19-nortestosterone derivatives tend to reduce the amount of withdrawal bleeding and have more anabolic or androgenic effects.

ADVERSE EFFECTS OF ORAL CONTRACEPTIVES

The incidence of serious adverse effects associated with the use of these drugs is low. There are a number of reversible changes in intermediary metabolism. However, the long-term effects of the metabolic alterations are not well understood. Minor adverse effects are frequent but transient and may respond to simple changes in pill formulation. Although it is not often necessary to discontinue taking the pills because of these adverse effects, one-third of patients started on oral contraception discontinue therapy for reasons other than a desire to become pregnant.

Mild Adverse Effects

Breakthrough bleeding is the most common problem in use of progestational agents alone for contraception, occurring in as many as 25% of patients. It also occurs in patients taking combined agents and is more common with preparations containing less than 50 μg of ethinyl estradiol (or equivalent). The newer biphasic and triphasic formulations containing 35 μg of ethinyl estradiol and varying doses of progestin (Table 17–11) reduce breakthrough bleeding without increasing the total amount of hormone administered during a cycle.

Nausea, mastalgia, excessive withdrawal bleeding, and edema are more common with larger amounts of estrogen and can often be alleviated by a shift to a preparation containing smaller amounts of estrogen or more potent progestational compounds.

Psychologic changes are often transient and are not predictable with any of the preparations. In general, most patients "feel better" because they are relieved of anxiety about becoming pregnant. Some patients experience symptoms of irritability and depression throughout the cycle. Depression and fatigue may respond to a reduction in progestin content.

Withdrawal bleeding sometimes fails to occur and may cause confusion with regard to pregnancy. If this is disturbing to the patient, a preparation with higher estrogenic or lower progestational potency may be tried or another method of contraception used. Increased estrogen potency can also reduce early and midcycle spotting.

Moderately Severe Adverse Effects

Any of the following may require discontinuation of oral contraceptives:

Mild and transient headaches may occur. Migraine is often made worse and is associated with an increased frequency of cerebrovascular accidents. Therefore, when migraine becomes more severe or has its onset during therapy with these agents, treatment should be discontinued.

Weight gain is more common with the combination agents containing more potent progestins. It can usually be controlled by shifting to preparations with less progestin effect or by dieting.

Increased skin pigmentation occurs in 5% of women at the end of the first year and about 40% after 8 years. It is thought to be exacerbated by vitamin B deficiency. The condition improves upon discontinuance of medication, but pigmentation may disappear very slowly.

Acne may be exacerbated by agents containing androgenic progestins, whereas agents containing larger amounts of estrogen frequently cause marked improvement in acne in women with androgen excess.

Hirsutism may be aggravated by the 19-nortestosterone derivatives. This effect is seldom seen, because the suppression of ovarian androgens usually causes a net reduction in androgen effect.

Ureteral dilatation similar to that observed in pregnancy has been reported, and bacteriuria is more frequent.

Vaginal infections are more common and more difficult to treat in patients who are receiving oral contraceptives.

When therapy is terminated, the great majority of patients return to normal menstrual patterns. About 75% will ovulate in the first posttreatment cycle and 97% by the third posttreatment cycle. Patients with a history of irregular cycles more commonly develop amenorrhea following cessation of therapy.

About 2% of patients remain amenorrheic for up to several years after stopping the pills, and the prevalence of amenorrhea, often with galactorrhea, is higher in women who have used this form of contraception.

Severe Adverse Effects

A. Vascular Disorders: Thromboembolism was one of the earliest of the serious unanticipated effects to be reported and has been the most thoroughly studied. Studies were devised to determine whether the case reports represented coincidental occurrences or an increased risk due to treatment with these preparations. By use of case control and cohort studies, it has

been possible in most cases to determine the incidence of a disorder in oral contraceptive users compared to that in nonusers and in some instances to determine whether this disorder occurs rarely or commonly. It should be kept in mind that almost all of these studies have been conducted in Great Britain, the USA, and Scandinavia and that effects in other populations might be somewhat different. During the past 15 years, the amounts of estrogen used in these preparations have been reduced, and this decline has been associated with a reduction in frequency of many of these effects. The most important adverse effect of the oral contraceptives is the increased risk of cardiovascular disease, including venous thromboembolism, myocardial infarction, and stroke.

1. Venous thromboembolic disease–Epidemiologic studies indicate that about one woman per 1000 woman years not using oral contraceptives will develop superficial or deep thromboembolic disease. The overall incidence of these disorders in patients taking oral contraceptives is about 3 per 1000 woman years. Data obtained by studying changes in plasma fibrinogen or by ^{125}I fibrinogen uptake studies suggest that subclinical thrombosis occurs much more frequently than overt disease. An incidence of one episode per person per year lasting about 1 month is found in healthy nonpregnant women of reproductive age; in patients using oral contraceptives who are otherwise comparable, it is approximately 3 per year. The risk for this disorder is increased during the first month of contraceptive use and remains constant for several years or more. The risk returns to normal within a month when treatment is discontinued. The risk of venous thrombosis or pulmonary embolism among women with predisposing conditions may be higher than that in healthy women.

The incidence of this complication is related to the estrogen content of oral contraceptives. A reduction from 100–150 μg to 50–80 μg reduced the incidence of pulmonary embolism by 50% or more. The most recent studies employing contraceptives containing 30 μg of estrogen indicate that the risk of death from pulmonary embolism is even lower. There is no clear relationship between progestin content and the incidence of this complication. The risk of superficial or deep thromboembolic disease in patients treated with oral contraceptives is not related to age, parity, mild obesity, or cigarette smoking. However, the risk of idiopathic deep venous thromboembolic disease in women with blood types A, B, or AB is twice as great as in those with blood type O who are not taking contraceptives and 3 times as great in type O women using these compounds. These studies indicate a genetic susceptibility to this disorder and suggest that oral contraceptives magnify the effect. Decreased venous blood flow, endothelial proliferation in veins and arteries, and increased coagulability of blood due to changes in platelet coagulation and fibrinolytic systems contribute to the increased incidence of thrombosis. In general, these changes are similar to those seen in pregnancy. It has been proposed that the main factor responsible is a decrease in the ability to halt the progression of intravenous coagulation and inhibition of fibrin clot dissolution. The major plasma inhibitor of thrombin is antithrombin 3, which is substantially decreased during oral contraceptive use. This change occurs in the first month of treatment and lasts as long as treatment persists.

Current information, therefore, suggests that oral contraceptives increase both the risk of overt venous thromboembolic disease and the occurrence of subclinical venous thromboembolic disease, primarily by increasing the size of the intravenous clots formed in response to endothelial injury or other stimuli that lead to thrombin formation. This effect appears to be primarily due to the estrogenic component of the oral contraceptives and appears to involve decreased antithrombin 3 activity.

2. Myocardial infarction—Myocardial infarction occurs more frequently in oral contraceptive users but is unrelated to the duration of use. The attributable risk of myocardial infarction is about 5–7 per 100,000 current user years at age 30–39, rising to approximately 60 at age 40–44. The risk is related to the dose of estrogen and is significantly lower in women using low-dose estrogen compounds. There are also data indicating that the risk is increased in women using oral contraceptives containing 3–4 mg, as compared to 1 or 2 mg, of the progestin norethindrone acetate.

The use of oral contraceptives is associated with a higher risk of myocardial infarction in women who smoke 15 or more cigarettes a day, who have a history of preeclampsia or hypertension, or who have type II hyperlipoproteinemia or diabetes. The risk attributable to oral contraceptives in women 30–39 years of age who do not smoke is about 4 cases per 100,000 users per year, as compared to 185 cases per 100,000 among women 40–44 who smoke heavily. The pathogenesis of myocardial infarction is thought to be related to acceleration of atherogenesis, decreased levels of HDL, and increased platelet aggregation. However, the facilitation of coronary arterial spasm may play a role in some of these patients. The progestational component of oral contraceptives decreases HDL cholesterol, whereas the estrogenic component increases it. The net difference, therefore, will depend entirely on the specific composition of the pill used and the patient's susceptibility to the particular effects. Preparations containing norgestrel, 0.5 mg, or norethindrone acetate, 2.5 mg, have been reported to have strong antiestrogenic effects and to decrease HDL cholesterol, while some of the others have no effect.

3. Cerebrovascular disease—The risk of stroke is concentrated in women over 35. It is increased in current users but not in past users. However, the incidence of subarachnoid hemorrhage is increased among both current and past users and may increase with time. The risk of thrombotic or hemorrhagic stroke attributable to oral contraceptives is about 37 cases per 100,000 users per year. Ten percent of these strokes are fatal, and most of them are due to subarachnoid hemorrhage. Insufficient data are available on which to base an assessment of the effects of smoking and other risk factors.

Elevations in blood pressure may also increase the risk, since there is a 3- to 6-fold increase in the incidence of overt hypertension in women taking oral contraceptives.

In summary, the information available indicates that oral contraceptives increase the risk of various cardiovascular disorders at all ages and among both smokers and nonsmokers. *However, this risk appears to be concentrated in women 35 years of age or older who are heavy smokers. The presence of these risk factors must be considered in each individual patient for whom oral contraceptives are considered.*

B. Gastrointestinal Disorders: Many cases of cholestatic jaundice have been reported in patients taking progestin-containing drugs. The differences in incidence of these disorders from one population to another suggest that genetic factors are involved. The jaundice caused by these agents is similar to that produced by other 17-alkyl–substituted steroids. It is most often observed in the first 3 cycles and is particularly common in women with a history of cholestatic jaundice during pregnancy. Liver biopsies from such women show bile thrombi in the canaliculi and occasional areas of focal necrosis. Serum alkaline phosphatase and SGPT are increased. The BSP retention and serum enzyme changes observed in some patients may indicate liver damage. Jaundice and pruritus disappear 1–8 weeks after the drug is discontinued.

These agents have also been found to increase the incidence of symptomatic gallbladder disease, including cholecystitis and cholangitis. This is probably the result of alterations in bile secretion and content.

It also appears that the incidence of hepatic adenomas is increased in women taking oral contraceptives. Ischemic bowel disease secondary to thrombosis of celiac and superior and inferior mesenteric arteries and veins has also been reported in women using these drugs.

C. Depression: Depression severe enough to require stopping the pills occurs in about 6% of patients taking some preparations.

D. Other Disorders: In addition to the above effects, a number of other adverse reactions have been reported for which a causal relationship has not been established. These include alopecia, erythema multiforme, erythema nodosum, and other skin disorders.

NONCONTRACEPTIVE ADVANTAGES OF HORMONAL CONTRACEPTION

The advent of oral contraceptives with low hormone content has significantly reduced the incidence of serious adverse effects. Furthermore, it has become apparent that their use is associated with important health benefits such as less risk of developing endometrial cancer, iron deficiency anemia, benign breast disease, functional ovarian cysts, premenstrual tension syndrome, and dysmenorrhea.

These and other benefits make hormonal contraception with low-dose, low-potency combination pills an excellent contraceptive method for younger women who do not smoke.

CONTRAINDICATIONS & CAUTIONS

Oral contraceptives are contraindicated in patients with thrombophlebitis, thromboembolic phenomena, and cerebrovascular disorders or a past history of these conditions. They should not be used to treat vaginal bleeding when the cause is unknown. They should be avoided in patients known or suspected to have a tumor of the breast or other estrogen-dependent neoplasm. They are contraindicated in adolescents in whom epiphyseal closure has not yet been completed, because they may prevent attainment of normal adult height.

Since these preparations have caused aggravation of preexisting disorders, they should be avoided or used with caution in patients with liver disease, hypertriglyceridemia, asthma, eczema, migraine, diabetes, hypertension, congestive heart failure, optic neuritis, retrobulbar neuritis, or convulsive disorders.

Estrogens may increase the rate of growth of fibroids. Therefore, for women with these tumors, agents with the smallest amounts of estrogen and the most potent progestins should be selected. The use of progestational agents alone for contraception might be especially useful in such patients (see below).

CONTRACEPTION WITH PROGESTINS

Small doses of progestins administered orally can be used for contraception (Table 17–11). They are particularly suited for patients who should not take estrogens. They are about as effective as intrauterine devices or combination pills containing 20–30 μg of ethinyl estradiol. There is a high incidence of abnormal bleeding. Giving infrequent injections of long-acting progestins such as medroxyprogesterone acetate has also found limited usefulness. Progestins have also been incorporated into an intrauterine device's and implanted under the skin.

POSTCOITAL CONTRACEPTIVES

Pregnancy can be prevented following coitus by the administration of estrogens alone or in combination with progestins. Insertion of an intrauterine device within 5 days has also been effective.

A variety of schedules have been tested and found

Table 17–12. Schedules for use of postcoital contraceptives.

Conjugated estrogens: 10 mg 3 times daily for 5 days
Ethinyl estradiol: 2.5 mg twice daily for 5 days
Diethylstilbestrol: 50 mg daily for 5 days
Norgestrel, 0.5 mg, with ethinyl estradiol, 0.05 mg: 2 tablets and 2 in 12 hours

effective, and these are shown in Table 17–12. When treatment is begun within 72 hours, the failure rate is less than 1%. Since 40% of patients treated experience nausea or vomiting, antiemetics are recommended. Headache, dizziness, breast tenderness, and abdominal and leg cramps have also been reported as adverse effects. Because these compounds have serious teratogenic effects early in pregnancy and because vaginal adenosis and cancer, cervical abnormalities, and impairment of reproductive function have been found in the offspring of women treated with diethylstilbestrol during gestation, voluntary termination of pregnancy is advised when conception occurs in these patients.

Mifepristone (see above), when given in the midluteal phase or at intervals during the menstrual cycle, can also prevent pregnancy. Its use for this purpose is under study.

INFERTILITY

Infertility is usually defined as failure of conception by a couple who have been having regular intercourse for 1 year or more without contraception. The intensity of the patients' concern varies, and a physician may be consulted after only a few months or many years of trying to become pregnant. Semen abnormalities are responsible for infertility in about half of cases. Some of the more common problems encountered are listed in Table 17–13.

SEMEN ABNORMALITIES

Semen analysis is usually obtained early in the investigation of infertile couples, because male factors are a common cause of infertility and because the test is relatively simple and inexpensive; furthermore, sperm abnormalities may compound the problem in women who fail to ovulate or have other problems reducing fertility. The characteristics of normal semen and sperm are discussed in Chapter 16. Male infertility is commonly attributed to varicocele of the left internal spermatic vein. Although this hypothesis is controversial, surgical correction of this disorder usually results in marked improvement in sperm motility, and even when lower than normal sperm counts remain, preg-

Table 17–13. Causes of infertility.

Male (40–50%)	Female (50–60%)

Abnormalities of sperm
  Infection (mumps)
  Failure to liquefy
  Agglutination
  Chronic infection (epididymitis,
    prostatitis)
High scrotal temperature
  Varicocele
  Baths
  Jockey shorts
  Prolonged sitting
Radiation exposure
**Drugs (cimetidine, sulfasalazine,
  nitrofurantoin, etc)**
Retrograde ejaculation
Severe allergic reactions (rare)
Endocrine disorders
Immunologic abnormalities[1]
	Tubal disease (20%)
	Anovulation (15%)
	Cervical factors (5%)
	Unknown (10–20%)
	Immunologic abnor-
	  malities[1]

[1]Failure of conception correlates best with agglutinating antibodies to sperm in the male and with agglutinating and immobilizing antibodies in the female.

nancy is achieved about half the time. The quality and concentration of sperm can also be improved in some men by the use of split ejaculates. In about 90% of men, the first few drops of semen contain a higher concentration of sperm with better motility than the remainder of the ejaculate. The combination of this technique with artificial insemination increases the chances of pregnancy in some couples.

OVULATORY DISORDERS

Absent or infrequent ovulation accounts for about 15% of infertility problems. Whether ovulation is completely absent or occurs infrequently, the opportunity for conception is diminished, and the patient should be treated by ovulation induction. (see page 474)

Women who have menstrual bleeding at regular intervals preceded by recognizable symptoms or who have dysmenorrhea almost always ovulate regularly. The occurrence of ovulation can be confirmed by the finding of a progesterone level greater than 4 ng/mL. However, it is useful to obtain daily basal body temperatures in order to determine the length of the luteal phase and to find out whether coitus has occurred at the time of ovulation. The timing of coitus is important, since the egg is fertilizable for only 12–24 hours, and sperm retain their ability to fertilize for 24–48 hours. Ideally, coitus should occur every other day for the 3 days preceding and following ovulation.

INFERTILITY IN THE PRESENCE OF OVULATION

When conception has not occurred in spite of a normal sperm analysis in the man and regular ovulation in

the woman, a postcoital test of cervical mucus should be done near the time of expected ovulation as indicated by basal body temperature charts, length of cycle, or the patient's observation of increased amounts of clear mucus at an appropriate time of the cycle. The cervical mucus at this time is under the influence of high estrogen levels and is clear and abundant. It can be stretched between a slide and cover slip as much as 10 cm at this time ("spinnbarkeit"). When the mucus is dried on the slide, the interaction of the electrolytes and protein results in a crystalline pattern called "ferning" (Fig 17–13). This mucus contains chains of glycoproteins that form channels through which the sperm can migrate. In order to perform the test, mucus is obtained from the cervix following intercourse, preferably within 8 hours. If the mucus is thick and cloudy, the specimen may have been obtained too late in the cycle, and the test should be repeated. Absence of spermatozoa in the specimen indicates the need for a more careful study of the semen specimen, as does the presence of dead sperm cells without motility. The presence of 20 or more motile sperm per high dry field is associated with a higher fertility rate than when few sperm are found. However, pregnancies occur even when no motile sperm cells are found in this test. The finding of dead cells suggests the use of spermicidal lubricants or may indicate the need for sperm antibody testing.

Tests of Tubal Patency

When there is a history of pelvic infection or pelvic surgery, tubal patency should be examined by hysterosalpingography or at the time of diagnostic laparoscopy. Such examinations are also indicated in patients in whom other factors have not been identified that might explain the infertility. Hysterosalpingography is best performed a few days following cessation of menstrual flow, thus avoiding the disruption of an early pregnancy. It is contraindicated in the presence of active pelvic inflammatory disease, as indicated by the presence of pelvic masses, tenderness, or an elevated sedimentation rate. Radiation should be minimized by the use of image intensification fluoroscopy and by taking the minimum number of films. An increased number of conceptions has been reported following this procedure when oil-based dye is used. The increase has been attributed to various mechanical and chemical effects of lavage with an iodine-containing and possibly bacteriostatic substance.

When semen analysis and the above tests are found to be normal in the infertile couple, the possibility of endometriosis should be considered even in the absence of typical signs and symptoms such as severe dysmenorrhea, dyspareunia, thickening of the broad ligament, nodularity and tenderness, or fixation of the uterus on pelvic examination. In these instances, laparoscopy may detect the presence and indicate the extent of any intrapelvic disease. Surgical treatment of minimal endometriosis established in this manner is followed by conception in half of women so treated. Hormonal treatment (eg, danazol or GnRH analogues) also may be effective in some patients.

IN VITRO FERTILIZATION

In vitro fertilization and transfer of the fertilized ovum into the uterus is now a therapeutic option to achieve pregnancy. After thorough fertility evaluation and study of the patient's menstrual cycles, the patient is given clomiphene citrate, menotropins, or both to increase the number of large mature follicles. Just be-fore ovulation, several ova are obtained by laparo-scopy or percutaneously under ultrasound guidance. The ova are incubated for several hours, and washed sperm are added to the culture medium. After 2–3 days of incubation, several 4- to 6-cell conceptuses are transferred to the uterus via the cervix.

Seventy to 80% of mature ova obtained can be fertil-ized. Early abortion is frequent, and the overall suc-cess rate is less than 30% even in experienced hands. The process is very expensive, lengthy, and time-con-suming. However, the risks of fetal abnormalities and maternal complications are low.

REFERENCES

General

Hodgen GD: The dominant ovarian follicle. *Fertil Steril* 1982;**38**:281.

Hseuh AJ et al: Hormonal regulation of the differentiation of cultured ovarian granulosa cells. *Endocr Rev* 1984;**5**:76.

Peters H, McNatty KP: *The Ovary: A Correlation of Structure and Function in Mammals.* Granada, 1980.

Siiteri PK, MacDonald PC: Role of extraglandular es-trogen in human endocrinology. Chapter 28 in: *Hand-book of Physiology.* Section 7: Endocrinology. Vol 2, Part 1. Geiger SR, Astwood EB, Greep RO (editors). American Physiological Society, 1973.

Speroff L, Glass RH, Kase NG: *Clinical Gynecologic Endocrinology and Infertility,* 4th ed. Williams & Wilkins, 1989.

Ying, SY: Inhibins, activins, and follistatins: Gonadal proteins modulating the secretion of follicle-stimulat-ing hormone. *Endocr Rev* 1988;**9**:267.

Disorders of Ovarian Function

Goldzieher JW: Polycystic ovarian disease. Chapter 15 in: *Progress in Infertility.* Behrman SJ, Kistner RW (edi-tors). Little, Brown, 1968.

Griffin JE, Wilson JD: The syndromes of androgen re-sistance. *N Engl J Med* 1980;**302**:198.

Judd HL: Endocrinology of polycystic ovary disease. *Clin Obstet Gynecol* 1978;**21**:99.

Kirschner MA, Samojlik E, Szmal E: Clinical usefulness of plasma androstanediol glucuronide measurements in women with idiopathic hirsutism. *J Clin Endocrinol Metab* 1987;**65**:597.

Malkasian GD Jr et al: Functioning tumors of the ovary in women under 40. *Obstet Gynecol* 1965;**26**:669.

Ross GT: Disorders of the ovary and female reproductive tract. Pages 206–258 in: *Williams Textbook of Endo-crinology,* 7th ed. Wilson JD, Foster DW (editors). Saunders, 1985.

Schlechte J et al: The natural history of untreated hyper-prolactinemia: A prospective analysis. *J Clin Endo-crinol Metab* 1989;**68**:412.

Hirsutism

Andreyko JL, Monroe SE, Jaffe RB: Treatment of hir-sutism with a gonadotropin-releasing hormone agonist (nafarelin). *J Clin Endocrinol Metab* 1986;**63**:854.

Cummings DC et al: Treatment of hirsutism with spirono-lactone. *JAMA* 1982;**247**:1295.

Ferriman D, Gallwey JD: Clinical assessment of body hair growth in women. *J Clin Endocrinol Metab* 1961; **21**:1440.

Givins JR: Role of oral contraceptives in the treatment of hyperandrogenism of hirsute women. Pages 351–367 in: *Hirsutism and Virilism: Pathogenesis, Diagnosis, and Management.* Mahesh VB, Greenblatt RB (edi-tors). PSG, 1983.

Horton R, Lobo R (editors): Androgen metabolism in hir-sute and normal females. *Clin Endocrinol Metab* 1986;**15**:213.

Mahesh VB, Greenblatt RB (editors): *Hirsutism and Vir-ilism: Pathogenesis, Diagnosis, and Management.* PSG, 1983.

Pittaway DE, Maxson WS, Wentz AC: Spironolactone in combination drug therapy for unresponsive hirsutism. *Fertil Steril* 1985;**43**:878.

Raj SG et al: Normalization of testosterone levels using a low estrogen-containing oral contraceptive in women with polycystic ovarian syndrome. *Obstet Gynecol* 1982;**60**:15.

Therapeutic Use of Ovarian & Hypothalamic Hormones & Inhibitors

Andreyko JL et al: Therapeutic uses of gonadotropin-releasing hormone analogs. *Obstet Gynecol Surv* 1987;**42**:1.

Chetkowski RJ et al: Biologic effects of transdermal es-tradiol. *N Engl J Med* 1986;**314**:1615.

Couzinet B et al: Termination of early pregnancy by the progesterone antagonist RU 486 (mifepristone). *N Engl J Med* 1986;**315**:1565.

Crooij MJ et al: Termination of early pregnancy by the 3β-hydroxysteroid dehydrogenase inhibitor epostane. *N Engl J Med* 1988;**319**:813.

D'Amato G et al: Serum and bile lipid levels in a postmenopausal woman after percutaneous and oral natural estrogens. *Am J Obstet Gynecol* 1989;**169**:600.

Dmowski WP: Endocrine properties and clinical applica-tion of danazol. *Fertil Steril* 1979;**31**:237.

Hammond CS et al: Effects of long-term estrogen replace-ment therapy. *Am J Obstet Gynecol* 1979;**133**:525.

McFarlane MJ, Feinstein AR, Horwitz, RI: Diethylstilbestrol and clear cell vaginal carcinoma: Reappraisal of the epidemiologic evidence. *Am J Med* 1986;**81**:855.

Mishell DR Jr: Contraception. *N Engl J Med* 1989;**320**:777.

Nieman LK et al: The progesterone antagonist RU 486: A potential new contraceptive agent. *N Engl J Med* 1987;**316**:187.

Reid RL, Fretts R, Van Vugt DA: The theory and practice of ovulation induction with gonadotropin-releasing hormone. *Am J Obstet Gynecol* 1988;**158**:176.

Speroff L, Diczfalusy E: International symposium on contraception. *Am J Obstet Gynecol* 1987;**157**:1019.

Stampfer MJ et al: A prospective study of past use of oral contraceptive agents and risk of cardiovascular diseases. *N Engl J Med* 1988;**319**:1313.

Voss HE, Oertel G: Androgens II and antiandrogens. In: *Handbook of Experimental Pharmacology.* Vol 35, Part 2. Springer, 1974.

Menopause

Cann CE et al: Spinal mineral loss by quantitative computed tomography in oophorectomized women. *JAMA* 1980;**244**:2056.

Civitelli R et al: Bone turnover in postmenopausal osteoporosis: Effect of calcitonin treatment, *J Clin Invest* 1988;**82**:1268.

Henderson BE, Paganini-Hill A, Ross RK: Estrogen replacement therapy and protection from acute myocardial infarction. *Am J Obstet Gynecol* 1988;**159**:312.

Judd HL: Hormonal dynamics associated with the menopause. *Clin Obstet Gynecol* 1976;**19**:775.

Knopp RH, Mishell DR Jr (editors): Prevention and management of cardiovascular risk in women. *Am J Obstet Gynecol* 1988;**158**:1551.

Lindsay R et al: Bone response to termination of oestrogen treatment. *Lancet* 1978;**1**:1325.

Prough SG et al: Continuous estrogen/progestin therapy in menopause. *Am J Obstet Gynecol* 1987;**157**:1449.

Sherman BM, West JH, Korenman SG: The menopausal transition: Analysis of LH, FSH, estradiol, and progesterone concentrations during menstrual cycles of older women. *J Clin Endocrinol Metab* 1976;**42**:629.

Van Keep PA, Lauritzen C (editors): Frontiers of hormone research. In: *Ageing and Estrogens.* Vol 2. Karger, 1973.

Wolfe BM, Huff MW: The effects of combined estrogen and progestin administration on plasma lipoprotein metabolism in postmenopausal women. *J Clin Invest* 1989;**83**:40.

Hormonal Contraception

Bradley BD et al: Serum high-density-lipoprotein cholesterol in women using oral contraceptives, estrogen and progestins. *N Engl J Med* 1978;**299**:17.

Royal College of General Practitioners: *Oral Contraceptives and Health.* Pitman, 1974.

Infertility

Speroff L, Glass RH, Kase NG: *Clinical Gynecologic Endocrinology and Infertility,* 4th ed. Williams & Wilkins, 1989.

Abnormalities of Sexual Differentiation*

18

Felix A. Conte, MD, & Melvin M. Grumbach, MD

Advances in cytogenetics, experimental embryology, steroid biochemistry, and methods of evaluation of the interaction between the hypothalamus, pituitary, and gonads have helped to clarify problems of sexual differentiation. Such anomalies may occur at any stage of intrauterine maturation and can lead to gross ambisexual development or to subtle abnormalities that do not become manifest until sexual maturity is achieved.

NORMAL SEX DIFFERENTIATION

Chromosomal Sex

The normal human diploid cell contains 22 autosomal pairs of chromosomes and 2 sex chromosomes (two X or one X and one Y). Arranged serially and numbered according to size and centromeric position, they are known as a karyotype. Advances in the techniques of staining chromosomes (Fig 18–1) permit positive identification of each chromosome by its unique "banding" pattern. Bands can be produced in the region of the centromere (C bands), with the fluorescent dye quinacrine (Q bands), and with Giemsa's stain (G bands). Fluorescent banding (Fig 18–2) is particularly useful because the Y chromosome stains so brightly that it can be identified easily in both interphase and metaphase cells. The standard nomenclature for describing the human karyotype is shown in Table 18–1.

---

*This chapter is modified from the authors' Chapter 33 in Smith DR: *General Urology,* 11th ed. Lange, 1984. Figs 18–1 to 18–4, Figs 18–6 to 18–10, Fig 18–14, and Tables 18–1, 18–2, 18–4, and 18–5 are reproduced, with permission, from Grumbach MM, Conte FA: Disorders of sex differentiation. Chap 9, pp 423–514, in: *Textbook of Endocrinology,* 6th ed. Williams RH (editor). Saunders, 1981.

Acronyms Used in This Chapter	
ACTH	Adrenocorticotropic hormone
CAH	Congenital adrenal hyperplasia
DHEA	Dehydroepiandrosterone
DHT	Dihydrotestosterone
DNA	Deoxyribonucleic acid
DOC	Deoxycorticosterone
DOCA	De[s]oxycorticosterone acetate
FSH	Follicle-stimulating hormone
GH	Growth hormone
GnRH	Gonadotropin-releasing hormone
hCG	Human chorionic gonadotropin
HLA	Human leukocyte antigen
LH	Luteinizing hormone
RFLP	Restriction fragment length polymorphism
RNA	Ribonucleic acid
TDF	Testis-determining factor
TSH	Thyroid-stimulating hormone (thyrotropin)
ZFX	Zinc finger X
ZFY	Zinc finger Y

Studies in animals as well as humans with abnormalities of sexual differentiation indicate that the sex chromosomes (the X and Y chromosomes) and the autosomes carry genes that influence sexual differentiation by causing the bipotential gonad to develop either as a testis or as an ovary. Two intact and normally functioning X chromosomes, in the absence of a Y chromosome (and the genes for testicular organogenesis), lead to the formation of an ovary, whereas a Y chromosome or the presence of the male-determining region of the short arm of the Y chromosome—the "testis-determining factor" (TDF)—will lead to testicular organogenesis.

In humans there is a marked discrepancy in size between the X and Y chromosomes. There is evidence that gene dosage compensation is achieved in all persons with 2 or more X chromosomes in their genetic constitution by inactivation of all X chromosomes except one. This phenomenon is thought to be a random process that occurs in each cell in the late blastocyst stage of embryonic development. The result of this

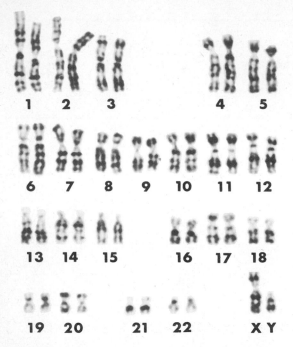

Figure 18–1. A normal 46,XY karyotype stained with Giemsa's stain to produce G bands. Note that each chromosome has a specific banding pattern.

change of DNA between the X and Y chromosomes. MIC2, a gene coding for a cell surface antigen recognized by the monoclonal antibody, 12E7, has been localized to the pseudoautosomal region of the X and Y chromosomes.

In buccal mucosal smears of 46,XX females, a sex chromatin body is evident in 20–30% of the interphase nuclei examined, whereas in normal 46,XY males, a comparable sex chromatin body is absent. In patients with more than two X chromosomes, the maximum number of sex chromatin bodies in any diploid nucleus is one less than the total number of X chromosomes. By utilizing sex chromatin and Y fluorescent staining (Figs 18–3 and 18–4), one can determine indirectly the sex chromosome complement (Table 18–2).

Sex Determination (H-Y Antigen and Testis-Determining Factor)

In 1955, Eichwald and Silmser showed that among inbred strains of mice, most male-to-female skin grafts were rejected, whereas male-to-male and female-to-female grafts survived. This phenomenon was attributed to a specific Y-linked histocompatibility locus, the H-Y antigen.

Utilizing a serologic assay for this antigen, Wachtel et al expanded the study of H-Y antigen from inbred mice to rats, guinea pigs, rabbits, and humans. They demonstrated the association of serologically determined H-Y antigen with the heterogametic sex (usually the male) in a wide range of vertebrates. In mammals, serologically determined H-Y antigen is expressed in the heterogametic male but not usually in the homogametic XX female.

Wachtel and Ohno and their associates noted the striking conservation throughout evolution of this ubiquitous minor cross-reacting plasma membrane histocompatibility antigen, its appearance early in em-

process is formation of an X chromatin body (Barr body) in the interphase cells of persons having 2 or more X chromosomes. (Fig 18–3)

The distal portion of the short arm of the X chromosome escapes inactivation and has a segment homologous to a segment on the distal portion of the Y chromosome. This segment is called the "pseudoautosomal" region; it is these 2 limited regions on the X and Y which pair during meiosis and allow for ex-

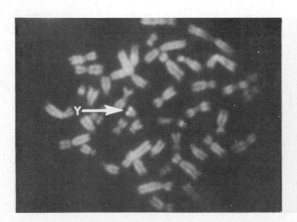
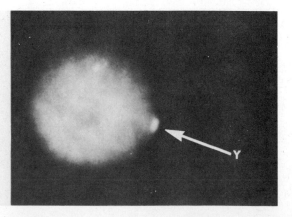

Figure 18–2. Metaphase chromosomes stained with quinacrine and examined through a fluorescence microscope. Note the bright fluorescence of the distal arms of the Y chromosome, which can also be seen in interphase cells ("Y body" at right).

Table 18–1. Nomenclature for describing the human karyotype
pertinent to designating sex chromosome abnormalities.

Paris Conference	Description	Former Nomenclature
46,XX	Normal femal karyotype	XX
46,XY	Normal male karyotype	XY
47,XXY	Karyotype with 47 chromosomes including an extra X chromosome	XXY
	Monosomy X	
45,X	Mosaic karyotype composed of 45,X and 46,XY cell lines	XO
45,X/46,XY	Short arm	XO/XY
	Long arm	
p	Deletion of the short arm of the X distal to band Xp21	p
q	Deletion of the long arm of the X distal to band Xq21	q
46,X,del (X) (qter → p21:)	Isochromosome of the long arm of X	XXp−
	Isochromosome of the short arm of X	
46,X,del (X) (pter → q21:)	Ring X chromosome	XXq−
	Translocation of the distal fluorescent portion of the Y chromosome to the	
46,X,i(Xq)	long arm of chromosome 7	XXqi
46,X,i(Xp)		XXpi
46,X,r(X)		XXr
46,X,t(Y;7) (q11;q36)		46,XYt (Yq−7q+)

bryonic development (in the 8-cell male mouse embryo), and its association with heterogametic sex. These observations led them to suggest that this phylogenetically conserved antigen was the factor responsible for inducing testicular organogenesis of the bipotential fetal gonads. They examined their hypothesis by testing patients with testicular tissue who had XX karyotypes, eg, XX males and XX true hermaphrodites. Despite the absence of a Y chromosome in these patients, serologically determined H-Y antigen was detected in all patients tested (although it is usually at lower levels than that observed in control 46,XY males). Further evidence indicated that even in the absence of a discrete Y chromosome, or karyotypic evidence of a Y-to-X chromosome, or Y-to-autosome translocation or insertion, the presence of testicular tissue was invariably associated with a positive test for serologically determined H-Y antigen.

More direct evidence for the role of serologically determined H-Y antigen in sex determination was demonstrated in vitro by Ohno and Zenzes (Fig 18–5). Using the "Moscona" technique, they exposed a suspension of single cells from newborn mouse and rat testes to anti-H-Y antibody and reported that these cells reorganized to form "follicular-like" structures rather than seminiferous tubules. Similarly, bovine and human fetal XX undifferentiated gonads formed testicularlike structures when incubated with "purified" H-Y antigen. These data, as well as the data from humans with abnormalities of sex differentiation, suggested that serologically determined H-Y antigen played a primary role in gonadal determination. In studies using an antibody to H-Y antigen, a gene locus

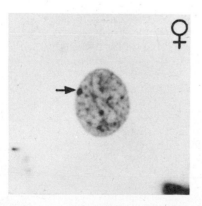

Figure 18–3. X chromatin (Barr) body in the nucleus of a buccal mucosal cell from a normal 46,XX female.

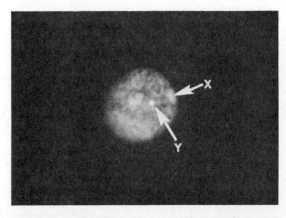

Figure 18–4. An interphase nucleus stained with quinacrine and examined by fluorescence microscopy. This cell reveals a "Y body" and an X chromatin body. The patient has a 47,XXY karyotype.

Table 18–2. Sex chromosome complement correlated with X chromatin and Y bodies in somatic interphase nuclei.[1]

Sex Chromosomes	Maximum Number in Diploid Somatic Nuclei	
	X Bodies	Y Bodies
45,XO	0	0
46,XX	1	0
46,XY	0	1
47,XXX	2	0
47,XXY	1	1
47,XYY	0	2
48,XXXX	3	0
48,XXXY	2	1
48,XXYY	1	2
49,XXXXX	4	0
49,XXXXY	3	1
49,XXXYY	2	2

[1]The maximum number of X chromatin bodies in diploid somatic nuclei is one less than the number of Xs, whereas the maximum number of Y fluorescent bodies is equivalent to the number of Ys in the chromosome constitution.

that appears to encode a protein similar to that reported by Ohno as H-Y antigen has been identified on chromosome 6 near the HLA locus.

However, the specificity, reproducibility, and quantification of the serologic assay for H-Y antigen have been questioned, and there are doubts about the putative role of serologically determined H-Y antigen in sex determination. Questions have arisen regarding the correlation between serologically determined H-Y antigen and classically defined H-Y antigen as shown by the rejection by inbred female mice of skin grafts from male mice of the same strain. Therefore, some workers now refer to serologically determined H-Y antigen as serologically determined male antigen (SDMA) or use the nomenclature H-Ys to differentiate this material from H-Y antigen assayed by skin graft rejection or by the cytotoxic T cell assay (H-Yc). The

finding of patients with Turner's syndrome who had 45,X and 46,X isochromosome X karyotypes and were H-Ys–positive was discordant with the putative role of H-Y antigen in testis determination. Recent evidence in mice and humans suggests that the genes controlling the expression of cytotoxic H-Y antigen and testicular organogenesis are linked to one another on the Y chromosome but that they are not identical. Recombinant DNA studies in 46,XX males and 46,XY females with gonadal dysgenesis have demonstrated that a small portion of the distal short arm of the Y chromosome just proximal to the pseudoautosomal (pairing) region is critical for testicular organogenesis. Researchers using the cytotoxic T cell assay have localized the H-Yc locus to the long arm of the Y chromosome, indicating that it is quite distinct from the testis-determining factor region, which is on the short arm. The H-Yc gene on the long arm of the Y chromosome has been postulated to play a role in spermatogenesis, or possibly gonadoblastoma formation, in patients with dysgenetic testes.

Page and coworkers have cloned a 230-Kb sequence from the short arm of the Y chromosome thought to contain all or some of the testis-determining factor (TDF) gene. This cloned region was found to have highly conserved DNA sequences homologous to those found on the Y chromosome of other mammals. It appears to code for a DNA-binding protein with "13 zinc finger domains" (zinc finger Y; ZFY) that may act as a transcriptional regulating factor, switching on several downstream autosomal genes, leading to testicular development in the bipotential fetal gonad. Sequences homologous to this putative TDF locus were found on the X chromosome (zinc finger X; ZFX). The zinc finger X locus does not appear to be "inactivated" during the process of X chromosome inactivation and sex chromatin formation. Further studies will be necessary to establish the characteristics and function of

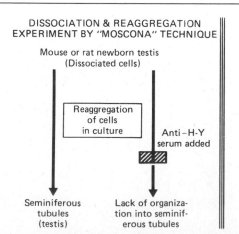

DISSOCIATION & REAGGREGATION EXPERIMENT BY "MOSCONA" TECHNIQUE

Mouse or rat newborn testis (Dissociated cells)

Reaggregation of cells in culture

Anti–H-Y serum added

Seminiferous tubules (testis)

Lack of organization into seminiferous tubules

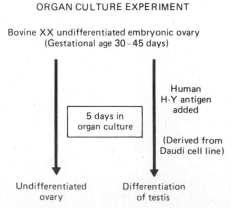

ORGAN CULTURE EXPERIMENT

Bovine XX undifferentiated embryonic ovary (Gestational age 30–45 days)

5 days in organ culture

Human H-Y antigen added

(Derived from Daudi cell line)

Undifferentiated ovary

Differentiation of testis

Figure 18–5. Diagrammatic scheme summarizing experimental evidence supporting H-Y antigen as the inducer of the testis in gonadal organogenesis.

the ZFY and ZFX genes and to test postulated models for sex determination that take into account the finding of homologous loci on the X and Y chromosomes. Nevertheless, the finding of the zinc protein gene on the Y chromosome in the region critical for testis determination is compelling albeit presumptive evidence of a role for this gene and its homologues in sex determination. The critical experiment—the transvection of the gene for ZFY into a 46,XX embryo, leading to testis determination—has not yet been reported.

TESTICULAR & OVARIAN DIFFERENTIATION

Until the 12-mm stage (approximately 42 days of gestation), the embryonic gonads of males and females are indistinguishable. By 42 days, 300–1300 primordial germ cells have seeded the undifferentiated gonad. These large cells later become oogonia and spermatogonia, and lack of these cells is incompatible with further ovarian differentiation. Under the influence of the genes that code for male sex determination (Fig 18–6), the gonad will begin testicular differentiation by 43–50 days of gestation. Leydig cells are apparent by about 60 days, and differentiation of male external genitalia occurs by 65–77 days of gestation.

In the gonad destined to be an ovary, the lack of differentiation persists. At 77–84 days, long after differentiation of the testis in the male fetus, a significant number of germ cells enter meiotic prophase to characterize the transition of oogonia into oocytes, which

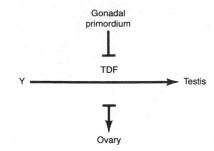

Figure 18–6. Interaction of testis-determining factor (TDF), germ cells, and somatic elements of the primordial gonad in testicular differentiation.

marks the onset of ovarian differentiation from the undifferentiated gonads (Fig 18–7).

Differentiation of Genital Ducts (Fig 18–8)

By the seventh week of intrauterine life, the fetus is equipped with the primordia of both male and female genital ducts. The müllerian ducts, if allowed to persist, form the uterine (fallopian) tubes, the uterus, the cervix, and the upper third of the vagina. The wolffian ducts, on the other hand, have the potential for differentiating into the epididymis, vas deferens, seminal vesicles, and ejaculatory ducts of the male. In the presence of a functional testis, the müllerian ducts involute under the influence of "müllerian duct inhibitory factor," a dimeric glycoprotein secreted by Sertoli cells.

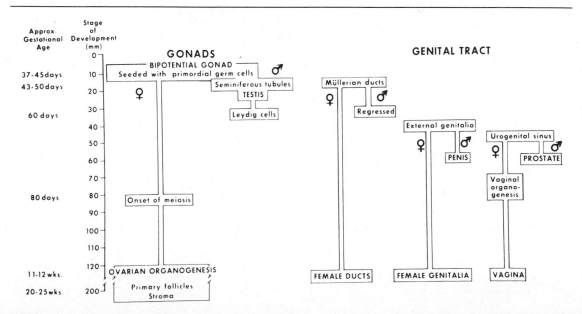

Figure 18–7. Schematic sequence of sexual differentiation in the human fetus. Note that testicular differentiation precedes all other forms of differentiation.

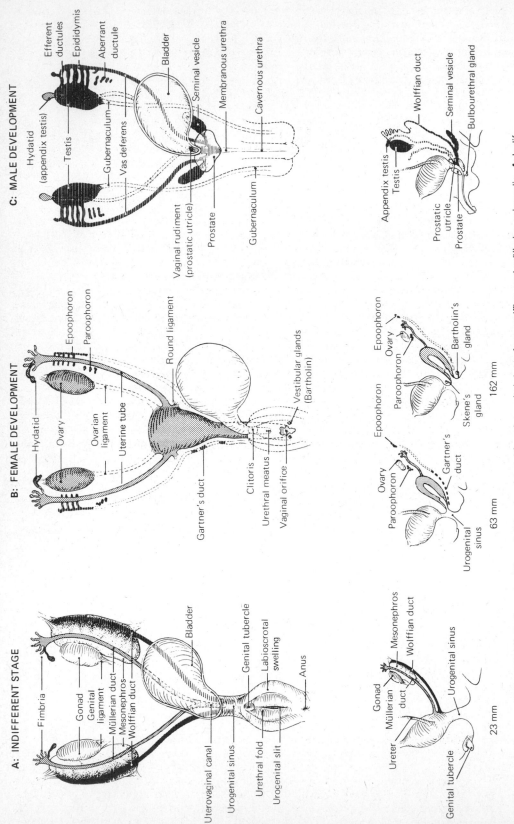

A: INDIFFERENT STAGE

Fimbria
Gonad
Genital ligament
Müllerian duct
Mesonephros
Wolffian duct
Bladder
Genital tubercle
Labioscrotal swelling
Anus
Uterovaginal canal
Urogenital sinus
Urethral fold
Urogenital slit

Gonad
Müllerian duct
Mesonephros
Wolffian duct
Ureter
Urogenital sinus
Genital tubercle

23 mm

B: FEMALE DEVELOPMENT

Hydatid
Ovary
Ovarian ligament
Uterine tube
Epoophoron
Paroophoron
Round ligament
Gartner's duct
Clitoris
Urethral meatus
Vaginal orifice
Vestibular glands (Bartholin)

Ovary
Paroophoron
Epoophoron
Paroophoron
Gartner's duct
Urogenital sinus
63 mm

Epoophoron
Ovary
Skene's gland
Bartholin's gland
162 mm

C: MALE DEVELOPMENT

Hydatid (appendix testis)
Efferent ductules
Epididymis
Aberrant ductule
Testis
Gubernaculum
Vas deferens
Bladder
Seminal vesicle
Membranous urethra
Cavernous urethra
Vaginal rudiment (prostatic utricle)
Prostate
Gubernaculum

Appendix testis
Testis
Prostatic utricle
Prostate
Wolffian duct
Seminal vesicle
Bulbourethral gland

Figure 18–8. Embryonic differentiation of male and female genital ducts from wolffian and müllerian primordia. *A*: Indifferent stage showing large mesonephric body. *B*: Female ducts. Remnants of the mesonephros and wolffian ducts are now termed the epoophoron, paroophoron, and Gartner's duct. *C*: Male ducts before descent into scrotum. The only müllerian remnant is the testicular appendix. The prostatic utricle (vagina masculina) is derived from the urogenital sinus. (Redrawn from Corning & Wilkins.)

This hormone acts "locally" to cause müllerian duct repression ipsilaterally. The differentiation of the wolffian duct is stimulated by testosterone secretion from the testis. In the presence of an ovary or in the absence of a functional fetal testis, müllerian duct differentiation occurs, and the wolffian ducts involute.

Differentiation of External Genitalia (Fig 18–9)

Up to the eighth week of fetal life, the external genitalia of both sexes are identical and have the capacity to differentiate into the genitalia of either sex. Female sex differentiation will occur in the presence of an ovary or streak gonads or if no gonad is present (Fig 18–10). Differentiation of the external genitalia along male lines depends on the action of testosterone and particularly dihydrotestosterone, the 5α-reduced metabolite of testosterone. In the male fetus, testosterone is secreted by the Leydig cells, possibly autonomously at first, thereafter under the influence of hCG, and then by stimulation from fetal pituitary LH. Masculinization of the external genitalia and urogenital sinus of the fetus results from the action of dihydrotestosterone, which is converted from testosterone in the target cells by the enzyme 5α-reductase. Dihydrotestosterone is bound to a specific protein receptor in the target cell. The transformed steroid-receptor complex binds with high affinity to specific DNA domains, initiating DNA-directed, RNA-mediated transcription and results in androgen-induced differentiation and growth of the cell. The gene that codes for the intracellular androgen-binding protein has been localized to the proximal portion of the long arm of the X chromosome. Thus, an X-linked gene controls the androgen response of all somatic cell types by specifying the androgen receptor protein.

As in the case of the genital ducts, there is an inherent tendency for the external genitalia and urogenital sinus to develop along female lines. Differentiation of the external genitalia along male lines requires androgenic stimulation early in fetal life. The testosterone metabolite dihydrotestosterone and its specific cytosol/nuclear receptor must be present to effect masculinization of the external genitalia of the fetus. Dihydrotestosterone stimulates growth of the genital tubercle, fusion of the urethral folds, and descent of the labioscrotal swellings to form the penis and scrotum. Androgens also inhibit descent and growth of the vesicovaginal septum and differentiation of the vagina. There is a critical period for action of the androgen. After about the 12th week of gestation, fusion of the labioscrotal folds will not occur even under intense androgen stimulation, although phallic growth can be induced. Impairment in the synthesis or secretion of fetal testosterone or in its conversion to dihydrotestosterone, deficient or defective androgen receptor activity, or defective production and local action of müllerian duct inhibitory factor leads to incomplete masculinization of the male fetus (Fig 18–

10). Exposure of the female fetus to abnormal amounts of androgens from either endogenous or exogenous sources, especially before the 12th week of gestation, can result in virilization of the external genitalia.

PSYCHOSEXUAL DIFFERENTIATION

Psychosexual differentiation may be classified into 4 broad categories: (1) gender identity, defined as the identification of self as either male or female; (2) gender role, ie, those aspects of behavior in which males and females differ from one another in our culture at this time; (3) gender orientation, which is the choice of erotic partner; and (4) cognitive differences.

Studies in individuals who have been reared in a sex opposite to their chromosomal or gonadal sex—as well as prenatally androgenized females with virilizing adrenal hyperplasia—provide strong evidence that gender identity is not determined primarily by sex chromosomes or prenatal sex steroid exposure. Rather, it is imprinted postnatally by words, attitudes, and comparisons of one's body with that of others. Generally, gender identity agrees with the sex of assignment in the intersex patient, provided the child is raised *unambiguously* and appropriate surgical and hormonal therapy is instituted so that the child has an unambiguous male or female phenotype. Under these circumstances, gender identity is usually established by 18–30 months of age. If at puberty discordant secondary sexual characteristics are allowed to develop and persist, some intersex individuals may develop doubts about their gender identity and request a change of sex.

Thus, it appears that gender identity may be more plastic than previously thought and that at puberty sex steroids as well as socialization play a role in the function and maintenance of gender identity. However, the weight of evidence still strongly supports environmental factors as the principal determinant of gender identity in our culture.

ABNORMAL SEX DIFFERENTIATION

Classification of Errors in Sex Differentiation (Table 18–3)

Disorders of sexual differentiation are the result of abnormalities in the complex processes of sexual differentiation, which originate in genetic information on the X and Y chromosomes as well as on the autosomes. A true hermaphrodite is defined as a person who possesses both ovarian and testicular tissue. A male pseudohermaphrodite is one whose gonads are exclusively testes but whose genital ducts or external

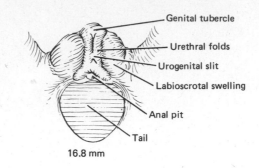

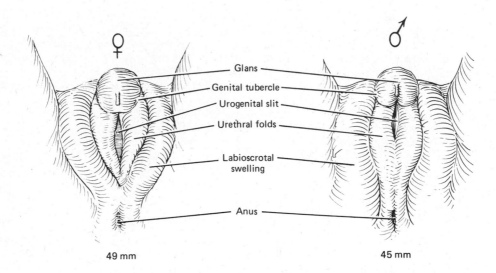

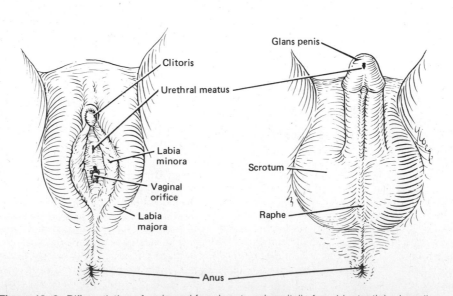

Figure 18–9. Differentiation of male and female external genitalia from bipotential primordia.

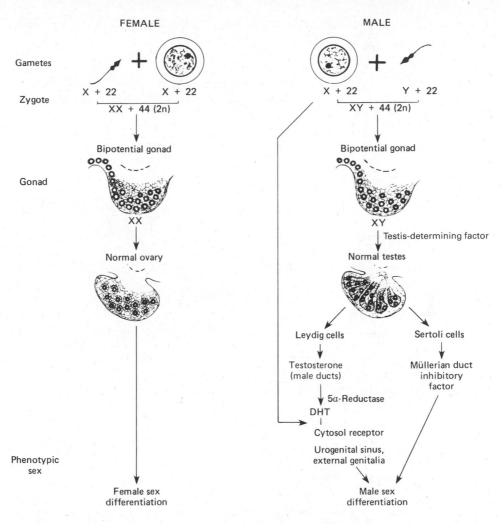

Figure 18–10. Diagrammatic summation of human sexual differentiation. DHT, dihydrotestosterone.

genitalia, or both, exhibit incomplete masculinization. A female pseudohermaphrodite is a person whose gonadal tissue is exclusively ovarian but whose genital development exhibits an ambiguous or male appearance.

SEMINIFEROUS TUBULE DYSGENESIS: CHROMATIN-POSITIVE KLINEFELTER'S SYNDROME & ITS VARIANTS

Klinefelter's syndrome is one of the most common forms of primary hypogonadism and infertility in males (see also Chapter 16). Affected patients usually have an XXY sex chromosome constitution and an X chromatin–positive buccal smear, although patients with a variety of sex chromosome constitutions, including mosaicism, have been described. Virtually all of these variants have in common the presence of at least two X chromosomes and a Y chromosome, except for the rare group in which only an XX sex chromosome complement is found.

Surveys of the prevalence of 47,XXY fetuses by karyotype analysis of unselected newborn infants indicate an incidence of about one per 1000 newborn males. The invariable clinical features of Klinefelter's syndrome in adults are a male phenotype; small, firm testes less than 3 cm in length; and azoospermia. Prepubertally, the disorder is characterized by small testes, disproportionately long legs, personality and behavioral disorders, and a lower verbal IQ score when compared to controls but no significant difference in full-scale IQ. Severe mental retardation requiring special schooling is uncommon. Gynecomastia and other signs of androgen deficiency such as diminished facial and body hair, a small phallus, poor muscular development, and a eunuchoid body habitus occur postpubertally in affected patients. Adult males with a 47,XXY karyotype tend to be taller than average, with adult

Table 18–3. Classification of anomalous sexual development.

Disorders of Gonadal Differentiation
A. Seminiferous tubule dysgenesis (Klinefelter's syndrome).
B. Syndrome of gonadal dysgenesis and its variants (Turner's syndrome).
C. Complete and incomplete forms of XX and XY gonadal dysgenesis.
D. True hermaphroditism.

Female Pseudohermaphroditism
A. Congenital virilizing adrenal hyperplasia.
B. Androgens and synthetic progestins transferred from maternal circulation.
C. Malformations of intestine and urinary tract (nonadrenal female pseudohermaphroditism).
D. Other teratologic factors.

Male Pseudohermaphroditism
A. Testicular unresponsiveness to hCG and LH (Leydig cell agenesis or hypoplasia).
B. Inborn errors of testosterone biosynthesis:
    1. Enzyme defects affecting synthesis of both corticosteroids and testosterone (variants of congenital adrenal hyperplasia).
        a. P-450scc (Cholesterol side-chain cleavage) deficiency (congenital lipoid adrenal hyperplasia).
        b. 3β-Hydroxysteroid dehydrogenase Δ^5 isomerase deficiency.
        c. P-450c17 (17α-hydroxylase) deficiency.
    2. Enzyme defects primarily affecting testosterone biosynthesis by the testes.
        a. P-450c17 (17,20lyase) deficiency.
        b. 17β-Hydroxysteroid oxidoreductase (dehydrogenase) deficiency.
C. Defects in androgen-dependent target tissues:
    1. End-organ resistance to androgenic hormones (androgen receptor and postreceptor defects).
        a. Syndrome of complete androgen resistance and its variants (testicular feminization and its variant forms).
        b. Syndrome of incomplete androgen resistance and its variants (Reifenstein's syndrome).
        c. Androgen resistance in phenotypically normal males.
    2. Defects in testosterone metabolism by peripheral tissues; 5α-reductase deficiency (pseudovaginal perineoscrotal hypospadias).
D. Dysgenetic male pseudohermaphroditism:
    1. X chromatin–negative variants of the syndrome of gonadal dysgenesis (eg, XO/XY,XYp−).
    2. Incomplete form of XY gonadal dysgenesis.
    3. Associated with degenerative renal disease (Wilms' tumor-aniridia-gonadoblastoma-mental retardation syndrome)
    4. "Vanishing testes" (embryonic testicular regression; XY agonadism →XY gonadal agenesis →rudimentary testes → anorchia).
E. Defects in synthesis, secretion, or response to müllerian duct inhibitory factor: Female genital ducts in otherwise normal men–"uteri herniae inguinale"; persisten müllerian duct syndrome.

Unclassified Forms of Abnormal Sexual Development
A. In males:
    1. Hypospadias.
    2. Ambiguous external genitalia in XY males with multiple congenital anomalies.
B. In females: Absence or anomalous development of the vagina, uterus, and uterine tubes (Rokitansky-Küster syndrome).

---

height close to the 75th percentile, mainly because of the disproportionate length of their legs. They also have an increased incidence of mild diabetes mellitus, varicose veins, chronic pulmonary disease, and carcinoma of the breast; the incidence of breast carcinoma in patients with Klinefelter's syndrome is 20 times higher than that in normal men. These patients generally have a delay in the onset of adolescence. Sexual precocity may occur owing to an hCG-secreting extragonadal polyembroma. These patients are at risk for developing malignant extragonadal germ cell tumors, including central nervous system germinoma.

The testicular lesion appears to be progressive and gonadotropin-dependent. It is characterized in the adult by extensive seminiferous tubular hyalinization and fibrosis, absent or severely deficient spermatogenesis, and pseudoadenomatous clumping of the Leydig cells. Although hyalinization of the tubules is usually extensive, it varies considerably from patient to patient

and even between testes in the same patient. Spermatogenesis is rarely found, and patients who have been reported to be fertile have been XY/XXY mosaics.

Advanced maternal age and meiotic nondisjunction have been found to play a role in the genesis of the 47,XXY karyotype. Pedigree studies indicate that both X chromosomes are of maternal origin in 67% of XXY patients.

The diagnosis of Klinefelter's syndrome is suggested by the classic phenotype and hormonal changes. It is confirmed by the finding of an X chromatin–positive buccal smear and demonstration of an XXY karyotype in blood, skin, or gonads. After puberty, levels of serum and urinary gonadotropins, especially FSH, are raised. The testosterone production rate, the total and free levels of testosterone, and the metabolic clearance rates of testosterone and estradiol tend to be low, while plasma estradiol levels are normal or high. Testicular biopsy reveals the classic findings of hyalinization of the seminiferous tubules, severe deficiency of spermatogonia, and pseudoadenomatous clumping of Leydig cells.

Treatment of patients with Klinefelter's syndrome is directed toward androgen replacement, especially in patients in whom puberty is delayed or fails to progress or in those who have subnormal testosterone levels for age and development. Testosterone therapy may help to enhance secondary sexual characteristics and sexual performance, prevent osteoporosis, and improve general well-being in most patients with Klinefelter's syndrome. Testosterone therapy should commence with 50–100 mg of testosterone enanthate in oil intramuscularly monthly and gradually increase to the adult replacement dose of 200 mg every 2 weeks. Gynecomastia is not amenable to hormone therapy but can be surgically corrected if it is severe or psychologically disturbing to the patient. Early diagnosis, support and appropriate counseling may improve the overall prognosis.

Variants of Chromatin-Positive Seminiferous Tubule Dysgenesis

A. 46,XY/47,XXY Mosaicism: This is the second most common chromosome complement associated with the Klinefelter phenotype. Mosaicism with any XY cell line may modify the clinical syndrome and result in less severe gynecomastia, as well as a lesser degree of testicular pathology. Some affected patients are fertile. Mean testosterone levels tend to be higher in XY/XXY patients than in XXY patients. In order to rule out XY/XXY mosaicism, cultures for karyotype analysis should be obtained from 2 or more tissues, and a sufficient number of cells (50 or more) should be examined from each tissue. Therapy depends on the severity of the clinical and gonadal aberrations associated with the XXY cell line.

B. 48,XXYY: Patients with this karyotype comprise 3% of chromatin-positive males. In addition to exhibiting the usual characteristics of Klinefelter's syndrome, they tend to be tall, and almost all reported patients have been mentally retarded. Therapy with testosterone is similar to that in patients with XXY Klinefelter's syndrome.

C. 48,XXXY and 49,XXXYY: All patients with these karyotypes have had significant mental retardation; developmental anomalies (short neck, epicanthal folds, radioulnar synostosis, and clinodactyly) are present in half of patients.

D. 49,XXXXY: Patients with this karyotype are more severely affected than those with a lesser number of X chromosomes. In addition to severe mental retardation, they exhibit radioulnar synostosis, epiphyseal dysplasia, hypoplastic external genitalia, and cryptorchid testes. Other anomalies such as congenital heart disease, cleft palate, strabismus, and microcephaly may be present. The facies is characteristic, with prognathism, hypertelorism, and myopia. As noted above, early diagnosis and appropriate counseling and support for the parents and child will improve the social and intellectual function of these and other patients with variations of Klinefelter's syndrome.

E. 46,XX Males: Over 200 phenotypic males with a 46,XX karyotype have been described since 1964; the incidence of 46,XX males is approximately one in 20,000 births. In general, they have a male phenotype, male psychosocial gender identity, and testes with histologic features similar to those observed in patients with a 47,XXY karyotype. At least 10% of patients have had hypospadias or ambiguous external genitalia. XX males have normal body proportions and a mean final height that is shorter than patients with an XXY karyotype or normal males but taller than normal females. As in XXY males, testosterone levels are low or low normal, gonadotropins are elevated, and spermatogenesis is impaired. Gynecomastia is present in approximately one-third of the patients.

The presence of testes and male sexual differentiation in 46,XX individuals has been a perplexing problem. However, the paradox has been clarified by the use of recombinant DNA studies utilizing Y chromosome-specific probes. Males with a 46,XX karyotype have been shown by genetic linkage studies and X chromosome restriction fragment length polymorphisms (RFLPs) to possess one X chromosome from each of their parents. Ninety percent of XX males have a Y chromosome-specific DNA segment from the distal portion of the Y short arm translocated to the distal portion of the short arm of the paternal X chromosome. This translocated segment is heterologous in length but almost always includes the 230-Kb sequence cloned by Page, which seems to code for a gene critical to male sex determination. The present data indicate that 90% of XX males are due to an abnormal X-Y terminal exchange during paternal meiosis which results in 2 products: an X chromosome with the translocated testis-determining factor from the Y chromosome and a Y chromosome deficient in this factor (the latter would result in a female with XY gonadal dysgenesis). Ten percent of XX males tested have been shown to lack Y chromosome-specific DNA sequences. These Y DNA-negative males tend to have hypospadias or have family members with true hermaphroditism. Recently, 4 XX patients have been described (3 XX males and 1 true hermaphrodite) who appear to have a Y to X translocation involving the region on the Y chromosome distal to 230 kilobase locus cloned by Page. These four patients suggests that there may be another gene(s) present on the Y chromosome distal to ZFY whose presence is critical to testis determination. However, in the same study 4 of 14 XX males had no evidence of a Y to X translocation using multiple probes for the short arm of the Y chromosome. The finding of Y-specific, DNA-negative XX males suggests that testicular determination and, thus, male differentiation can occur in the absence of a gene or genes from the Y chromosome. This could be a result of (1) mutation of a "downstream" autosomal gene involved in male sex determination; (2) mutation, deletion, or aberrant inactivation of the putative testis-determining factor homologous gene sequence on the X chromosome; or (3) circumscribed Y chromosome mosaicism (ie, that occurring only in the gonads). Further studies will be necessary to elucidate the pathogenesis of male sex determination and differentiation in those 46,XX males who lack discernible Y-to-X chromosome translocations.

SYNDROME OF GONADAL DYSGENESIS: TURNER'S SYNDROME & ITS VARIANTS

Turner's Syndrome: 45,X Gonadal Dysgenesis

One in 10,000 newborn females has a 45,X or XO sex chromosome constitution. The cardinal features of 45,X gonadal dysgenesis are a variety of somatic anomalies, sexual infantilism at puberty secondary to gonadal dysgenesis, and short stature. (See also Chapter 17.) Patients with a 45,X karyotype can be recognized in infancy usually because of lymphedema of the extremities and loose skin folds over the nape of the neck. In later life, the typical patient is often recognizable by her distinctive facies, in which micrognathia, epicanthal folds, prominent low-set ears, a fishlike mouth, and ptosis are present to varying degrees. The chest is shieldlike and the neck short, broad, and webbed (40% of patients). Additional anomalies associated with Turner's syndrome include coarctation of the aorta (10%), hypertension, renal abnormalities (50%), pigmented nevi, cubitus valgus, a tendency to keloid formation, puffiness of the dorsum of the hands

and feet, short fourth metacarpals, and recurrent otitis media. Routine intravenous urography or ultrasonography is indicated for all patients to rule out a surgically correctable renal abnormality. The internal ducts as well as the external genitalia of these patients are invariably female except in rare patients in whom Y-to-autosome translocations have been found.

Short stature is an invariable feature of the syndrome of gonadal dysgenesis. Mean final height in 45,X patients is 143 cm, with a range of 133–153 cm. Current data suggest that the short stature found in patients with the syndrome of gonadal dysgenesis is not due to a deficiency of growth hormone, somatomedin, sex steroids, or thyroid hormone. However, administration of biosynthetic human growth hormone in combination with oxandrolone therapy results in an increase in predicted final height.

Gonadal dysgenesis is another feature of patients with a 45,X sex chromosome constitution. The gonads are typically streaklike and usually contain only fibrous stroma arranged in whorls. Longitudinal studies of both basal and GnRH-evoked gonadotropin secretion in patients with gonadal dysgenesis indicate a lack of feedback inhibition of the hypothalamic-pituitary axis by the dysgenetic gonads in affected infants and children (Fig 18–11). Thus, plasma and urinary gonadotropin levels, particularly FSH levels, are high, especially during early infancy and after 10 years of age. Since ovarian function is impaired, puberty does not usually ensue spontaneously; thus, sexual infantilism is a hallmark of this syndrome. Rarely, patients with a 45,X karyotype may undergo spontaneous pubertal maturation and menarche.

A variety of disorders are associated with this syndrome, including obesity, osteoporosis, diabetes mellitus, Hashimoto's thyroiditis, rheumatoid arthri-

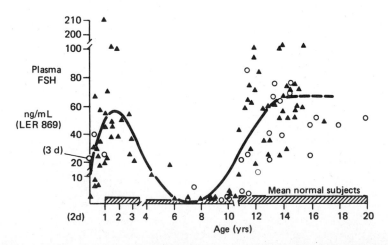

Figure 18–11. Diphasic variation in basal levels of plasma FSH (ng/mL LER 869) in patients with a 45,X karyotype (solid triangles) and patients with structural abnormalities of the X chromosome, and mosaics (open circles). Note that mean basal levels of plasma FSH in patients with gonadal dysgenesis are in the castrate range before 4 years and after 10 years of age. (Reproduced, with permission, from Grumbach MM, Conte FA, Kaplan SL: *J Clin Endocrinol Metab* 1975, **40:**670.)

tis, and inflammatory bowel disease. Because an increased incidence of bicuspid aortic valve and aortic dilatation with aneurysm formation and rupture has been reported in patients with Turner's syndrome, a routine echocardiogram is indicated in all 45,X patients.

Phenotypic females with the following features should have a buccal smear for sex chromatin or preferably a karyotype analysis: (1) short stature (>2.5 SD below the mean value per age); (2) somatic anomalies associated with the syndrome of gonadal dysgenesis; and (3) delayed adolescence and increased concentration of plasma gonadotropins. In normal XX females, 20–30% of the nuclei are sex chromatin–positive. Although a buccal smear for sex chromatin is useful, karyotype analysis should be performed for definitive diagnosis.

Therapy should be directed toward maximizing final height and inducing secondary sexual characteristics and menarche at an age commensurate with that of normal peers. The preliminary results of recent clinical trials suggest that patients treated with recombinant growth hormone (0.125 mg/kg subcutaneously 3 times a week) plus oxandrolone (0.0625 mg/kg/d by mouth) had an increase in growth rate, which was sustained over 3 years and resulted in an increase in predicted final height of 8.2 cm after 3 years of therapy. Although data on actual final heights are not yet available, it is reasonable to consider using growth hormone therapy in girls with Turner's syndrome in an attempt to augment final height.

The authors' long-term studies with low-dose estrogen therapy have not demonstrated a significant effect (positive or negative) on final height in girls with Turner's syndrome. The recommended treatment involves initiating estrogen therapy at 12–13 years of age with conjugated estrogens (0.3 mg or less) or ethinyl estradiol (5 μg) orally for the first 21 days of the calendar month. Thereafter, the dose of estrogen is gradually increased over the next 1–2 years to 0.6–1.25 mg of conjugated estrogens or 10 μg of ethinyl estradiol daily for the first 21 days of the month. The minimum dose of estrogen necessary to maintain secondary sexual characteristics and menses and prevent osteoporosis should be administered. Medroxypro-

gesterone acetate, 5 mg daily, is given on the 12th–21st days of the menstrual cycle to ensure physiologic menses and to reduce the risk of endometrial carcinoma, which is associated with unopposed estrogen stimulation. After the first year of estrogen therapy, progestin therapy is usually started.

X Chromatin–Positive Variants of the Syndrome of Gonadal Dysgenesis

Patients with structural abnormalities of the X chromosome (deletions and additions) and mosaicism with XX cell lines may manifest the somatic as well as the gonadal features of the syndrome of gonadal dysgenesis (Table 18–4). Evidence suggests that genes on both the long and short arms of the X chromosome control gonadal differentiation, whereas genes on the short arms of the X prevent the short stature and somatic anomalies that are seen in 45,X patients. In general, mosaicism with a 46,XX cell line in association with a 45,X cell line will modify the phenotype toward normal and can even result in normal gonadal function.

X Chromatin–Negative Variants of the Syndrome of Gonadal Dysgenesis

These patients usually have mosaicism with a 45,X- and a Y-bearing cell line—45,X/46,XY; 45,X/47,XXY; 45,X/46XY/47,XYY—or perhaps a structurally abnormal Y chromosome. They range from phenotypic females with the features of Turner's syndrome through patients with ambiguous genitalia to (rarely) completely virilized males with a few stigmas of Turner's syndrome. The variations in gonadal differentiation range from bilateral streaks to bilateral dysgenetic testes to apparently "normal" testes, and there may be asymmetric development, ie, a streak on one side and a dysgenetic testicle (or, rarely, a normal testis) on the other side, sometimes called "mixed gonadal dysgenesis." The development of the external genitalia as well as the internal ducts correlates well with the degree of testicular differentiation and, presumably, the capacity of the fetal testes to secrete müllerian duct inhibitory factor and testosterone.

The risk of development of gonadal tumors is great-

Table 18–4. Relationship of structural abnormalities of the X and Y to clinical manifestations of the syndrome of gonadal dysgenesis.

Type of Sex Chromosome Abnormality	Karyotype	Phenotype	Sexual Infantilism	Short Stature	Somatic Anomalies of Turner's Syndrome
Loss of an X or Y	45,XO	Female	+	+	+
Deletion of short arm of an X[1]	46,XXqi	Female	+ (occ. ±)	+	+
	46,XXp−	Female	+, ±, or −	+ (−)	+ (−)
Deletion of long arm of an X[1]	46,XXq−	Female	+	− (+)	− or (±)
Deletion of ends of both arms of an X	46,XXr	Female	− or +	+	+ or (±)
Deletion of short arm of Y	46,XYp−	Female	I	+	+

[1]In Xp− and Xq−, the extent and site of the deleted segment are variable.
Xqi = isochromosome for long arm of an X; Xp− = deletion of short arm of an X; Xpi = isochromosome for short arm of an X; Xq− = deletion of long arm of an X; Xr = ring chromosome derived from an X.

ly increased in patients with 45,X/46,XY mosaicism, and prophylactic removal of streak gonads or dysgenetic undescended testes in this syndrome is indicated. Breast development at or after the age of puberty in these patients is commonly associated with a gonadal neoplasm, usually a gonadoblastoma. Pelvic sonography, CT, or MRI scanning may be useful in screening for neoplasms in these patients. Gonadoblastomas are calcified, so that they may be visible even on a plain film of the abdomen.

The diagnosis of 45,X/46,XY mosaicism can be established by the demonstration of both 45,X and 46,XY cells in blood, skin, or gonadal tissue. The decision as to the sex of rearing of the child should be based on the age at diagnosis and the potential for normal function of the external genitalia. Patients with 45,X/46XY mosaicism ascertained by amniocentesis have been described who have normal male genitalia and normal testicular histology. Hence, the ambiguity of the genitalia invariably described in these patients is due to ascertainment bias. In patients assigned a female gender role, the gonads should be removed and the external genitalia repaired. Estrogen therapy should be initiated at the age of puberty, as in patients with a 45,X karyotype (see above). In affected infants who are assigned a male gender role, all gonadal tissue except that which appears histologically normal and is in the scrotum should be removed. Removal of the müllerian structures and repair of hypospadias are also indicated. At puberty, depending on the functional integrity of the retained gonad, androgen replacement therapy may be indicated in doses similar to those for patients with XY gonadal dysgenesis. In patients with retained scrotal testes, a repeat gonadal biopsy is indicated postpubertally to rule out the possibility of carcinoma in situ, a premalignant lesion (see below).

46,XX & 46,XY GONADAL DISGENESIS

The terms XX and XY gonadal dysgenesis have been applied to XX or XY patients who have bilateral streak gonads, a female phenotype, and no stigmas of Turner's syndrome. After puberty, they exhibit sexual infantilism, castrate levels of plasma and urinary gonadotropins, normal or tall stature, and eunuchoid proportions.

46,XX Gonadal Dysgenesis

Familial and sporadic cases of XX gonadal dysgenesis have been reported. Pedigree analysis of familial cases is consistent with autosomal recessive inheritance. However, in one family recently reported, 4 affected women had an inherited interstitial deletion of the long arm of the X chromosome involving the q21–q27 region. This region seems to contain a gene or genes "critical" to ovarian development and function. In 3 families, XX gonadal dysgenesis was associated with deafness of the sensorineural type. In several

affected groups of siblings, a spectrum of clinical findings occurred, eg, varying degrees of ovarian function, including breast development and menses followed by secondary amenorrhea. Unlike in Turner's syndrome, stature is normal. The diagnosis of 46,XX gonadal dysgenesis should be suspected in phenotypic females with sexual infantilism and normal müllerian structures who lack the somatic stigmas of the syndrome of gonadal dysgenesis (Turner's syndrome). Karyotype analysis reveals only 46,XX cells. As in Turner's syndrome, gonadotropin levels are high, estrogen levels are low, and treatment consists of cyclic estrogen replacement.

Sporadic cases of XX gonadal dysgenesis may represent a heterogeneous group of patients from a pathogenetic point of view. XX gonadal dysgenesis should be distinguished from ovarian failure due to infections such as mumps, antibodies to gonadotropin receptors, biologically inactive FSH, and gonadotropin-insensitive ovaries as well as errors in steroid (estrogen) biosynthesis.

46,XY Gonadal Dysgenesis

XY gonadal dysgenesis occurs both sporadically and in familial aggregates. Patients with the complete form of this syndrome have female external genitalia, normal or tall stature, bilateral streak gonads, müllerian duct development, sexual infantilism, eunuchoid habitus, and a 46,XY karyotype. Clitorimegaly is quite common, and in familial cases, a continuum of involvement ranging from the complete syndrome to ambiguity of the external genitalia has been described. The phenotypic difference between the complete form of XY gonadal dysgenesis and the incomplete form is due to the degree of differentiation of the testicular tissue and its functional capacity to produce testosterone and müllerian duct inhibitory factor. Postpubertally, plasma and urinary gonadotropin levels are markedly elevated.

Analysis of familial cases suggests that XY gonadal dysgenesis is transmitted as an X-linked recessive or sex-limited autosomal dominant trait. A small proportion of patients (10%) studied using Y-specific DNA probes have a deletion involving the short arm of the Y chromosome (the testis-determining factor region). The other patients in whom no deletion is evident may have (1) mutations of downstream autosomal genes involved in testicular differentiation; (2) mutations, deletions, or duplications of an X-linked gene, including the gene homologous to testis-determining factor on the X chromosome (ZFX) postulated to play a role in sex determination; or (3) mutation of the testis-determining factor gene on the Y chromosome. Sporadic cases may represent teratologic defects in gonadal morphogenesis. In addition, XY gonadal dysgenesis has been updated to be associated with camptomelic dysplasia and to be part of other dysmorphic syndromes.

Therapy for patients with 46,XY gonadal dysgenesis who have female external genitalia involves prophylactic gonadectomy at diagnosis and estrogen substitution at puberty. In the incomplete form of XY gonadal dysgenesis, assignment of a male gender role may be possible. It depends upon the degree of ambiguity of the genitalia and the potential for normal function. Prophylactic gonadectomy must be considered, since fertility is unlikely and there is an increased risk of malignant gonadal transformation in these patients. Page has suggested that there is a locus on the long arm of the Y chromosome linked closely to or identical to the locus coding for cytotoxic H-Y antigen that predisposes to the development of gonadoblastoma in patients with dysgenetic testes. Biopsy of all retained gonads should be done pre- and postpubertally in order to detect early malignant changes (carcinoma in situ). Prosthetic testes should be implanted at the time of gonadectomy, and androgen substitution therapy is instituted at the age of puberty. Testosterone enanthate in oil is utilized, beginning with 50 mg intramuscularly monthly and gradually increasing the dose over 3–4 years to a full replacement dose of 200 mg intramuscularly every 2 weeks.

TRUE HERMAPHRODITISM

True hermaphrodites have both ovarian and testicular tissue present in either the same or opposite gonads. Differentiation of the internal and external genitalia is highly variable. The external genitalia may simulate those of a male or female, but most often they are ambiguous. Cryptorchidism and hypospadias are common. A testis or ovatestis, if present, is located in the labioscrotal folds in one-third of patients, in the inguinal canal in one-third, and in the abdomen in the remaining one-third of patients. In all cases, a uterus is present, although it may be hypoplastic or unicornuate. The differentiation of the genital ducts usually follows that of the ipsilateral gonad. The ovotestis is the most common gonad found in true hermaphrodites, followed by the ovary and, least commonly, the testis. At puberty, breast development is usual in the untreated patients, and menses occur in over 50% of cases. Whereas the ovary or the ovarian portion of an ovotestis may function normally, the testis or testicular portion of an ovotestis is almost always dysgenetic.

Sixty percent of true hermaphrodites have a 46,XX karyotype, 20% have 46,XY, and about 20% have mosaicism or 46,XX/46,XY chimerism. Researchers using Y-specific DNA probes have not detected Y chromosome DNA (testis-determining factor) in the genomes of 46,XX true hermaphrodites. Thus, the pathogenesis of 46,XX true hermaphroditism cannot be explained either by Y-to-X or Y-to-autosome translocations or by low-percentage sex chromosome chimerism or mosaicism. Other possible pathogenetic mechanisms include (1) mutation of a downstream autosomal gene or genes involved in male sex determination; (2) mutation, deletion, or anomalous inactivation of the putative X-linked locus homologous to testis-

determining factor; or (3) circumscribed chimerism or mosaicism occurring only in the gonads.

The diagnosis of true hermaphroditism should be considered in all patients with ambiguous genitalia. The finding of an 46,XX/46,XY karyotype or a bilobed gonad compatible with an ovotestis in the inguinal region or labioscrotal folds suggests the diagnosis. If all other forms of male and female pseudohermaphroditism have been excluded, laparotomy and histologic confirmation of both ovarian and testicular tissue establish the diagnosis. The management of true hermaphroditism is contingent upon the age at diagnosis and a careful assessment of the functional capacity of the gonads, genital ducts, and external genitalia.

Gonadal Neoplasms in Dysgenetic Gonads

While gonadal tumors are rare in patients with Klinefelter's syndrome and 45,X gonadal dysgenesis, the prevalence of gonadal neoplasms is greatly increased in patients with certain types of dysgenetic gonads. Gonadoblastomas, dysgerminomas, seminomas, and teratomas are found most frequently. The frequency is increased (1) in 45,X/46,XY mosaicism and in patients with a structurally abnormal Y chromosome and (2) in XY gonadal dysgenesis, either with a female phenotype or with ambiguous genitalia. Prophylactic gonadectomy is advised in these 2 categories as well as in individuals with gonadal dysgenesis who manifest signs of virilization, regardless of karyotype.

The gonad should be preserved in patients who are being raised as males only if it is a histologically normal testicle that can be relocated in the scrotum. The fact that a gonad is palpable in the scrotum does not preclude malignant degeneration and dissemination, since seminomas tend to metastasize at an early stage before a local mass is obvious.

FEMALE PSEUDO-HERMAPHRODITISM

Affected individuals have normal ovaries and müllerian derivatives associated with ambiguous external genitalia. In the absence of testes, a female fetus will be masculinized if subjected to increased circulating levels of androgens derived from an extragonadal source. The degree of masculinization depends upon the stage of differentiation at the time of exposure (Fig 18–12). After 12 weeks of gestation, androgens will produce only clitoral hypertrophy. Rarely, ambiguous genitalia that superficially resemble those produced by androgens are the result of teratogenic malformations.

Congenital Adrenal Hyperplasia (Fig 18–13)

There are 6 majors types of congenital adrenal hyperplasia (CAH) all transmitted as autosomal recessive disorders. (See also Chapters 11 and 12.) The common

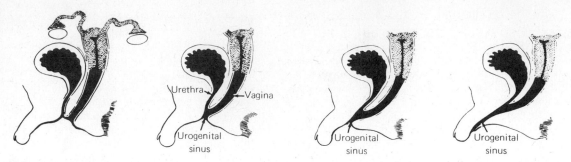

Figure 18–12. Female pseudohermaphorditism induced by prenatal exposure to androgens. Exposure after the 12th fetal week leads only to clitoral hypertrophy (diagram on left). Exposure at progressively earlier stages of differentiation (depicted from left to right in drawings) leads to retention of the urogenital sinus and labioscrotal fusion. If exposure occurs sufficiently early, the labia will fuse to form a penile urethra. (Reproduced, with permission, from Grumbach MM, Ducharme J: *Fertil Steril* 1960;**11**:757.)

denominator of all 6 types is a defect in the synthesis of cortisol that results in an increase in ACTH and then in adrenal hyperplasia. Both males and females can be affected, but males are rarely diagnosed at birth unless they have ambiguous genitalia, are salt losers and manifest adrenal crises, are identified during newborn screening, or are at risk because they have an affected sibling. Defects of types I–III are confined to the adrenal gland and produce virilization. Defects of types IV–VI have in common blocks in cortisol and sex steroid synthesis, in both the adrenals and the gonads. The latter 3 types produce primarily incomplete masculinization in the male and little or no virilization in the female (Table 18–5). Consequently, these will be

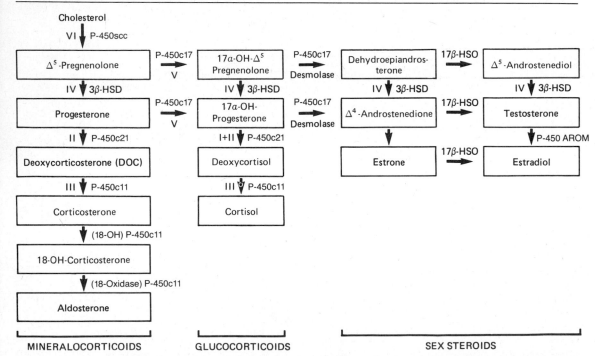

Figure 18–13. A diagrammatic representation of the steroid biosynthetic pathways in the adrenal and gonads. I to VI correspond to enzymes whose deficiency results in congenital adrenal hyperplasia. OH, hydroxy or hydroxylase; 3β-HSD, 3β-hydroxysteroid dehydrogenase/Δ⁵-isomerase; 17β-HSO, 17β-hydroxysteroid oxidoreductase (dehydrogenase); P-450scc, cholesterol side-chain cleavage, previously termed 20,22 desmolase; P-450c21, 21-hydroxylase; P-450c17, 17-hydroxylase; P-450arom, aromatase. P-450c17 also mediates 17,20 lyase activity; P-450c11, 11-hydroxylase, also mediates 18 hydroxylase and 18 oxidase reactions. (See also Figs 12–4, 12–5, and 16–2.) (Modified and reproduced, with permission, from Conte FA, Grumbach MM: Pathogenesis, classification, diagnosis, and treatment of anomalies of sex. Chapter 109 in: *Endocrinology*. DeGroot L [editor]. Grune & Stratton, 1989.)

Table 18–5. Clinical manifestations of the various types of congenital adrenal hyperplasia.

Enzymatic Defect	P-450scc Cholesterol Side-Chain Cleavage		3β-Hydroxysteroid Dehydrogenase		P-450c17 (17α-Hydroxylase)		P-450c11 (11β-Hydroxylase)		P-450c21 (21α-Hydroxylase)	
Type	VI		IV		V		III		II and I	
Chromosomal	XX	XY	XX	XY	XX	XY	XX	XY	XX	XY
External genitalia	Female	Female	Female (clitori-megaly)[1]	Ambig-uous	Female	Female or am-biguous	Ambig-uous[1]	Male	Ambig-uous[1]	Male
Postnatal virilization	− (Sexual infantilism at puberty)		±	Mild to moder-ate	− (Sexual infantilism at puberty)		+		+	
Addisonian crises	+		±		−		−		+ in 80% (type II)	
Hypertension	−		−		+		+		−	

[1]Normal female in late-onset and "cryptic" forms.

discussed primarily as forms of male pseudoherma-phroditism.

A. Type I—P450c21 Hydroxylase Deficiency With Virilization: 21-Hydroxylase activity is mediated by P-450c21, a microsomal cytochrome P-450 enzyme. A deficiency of this enzyme results in the most common type of adrenal hyperplasia, with an overall prevalence of 1:14,000 live births in Caucasians. The locus for the gene that codes for 21-hydroxylation is on the short arm of chromosome 6, close to the locus for C4 (comple-ment) between HLA-B and HLA-D. DNA hybridiza-tion analysis has detected 2 genes, designated 21-OHA and 21-OHB, in this area in tandem with the 2 genes for complement—C4A and C4B. 21-OHA is a nonfunc-tional "pseudogene," ie, it is missing criti-cal sequences and is not transcribed. Patients with P-450c21 (21α-hydroxylase) deficiency have been found to have mutations, gene conversions, or deletions in the 21-OHB gene. Seventy-five percent of patients with P-450c21 deficiency have point gene mutations or microgene conversions. The remainder of these pa-tients have gene deletions and macrogene conversions. The gene for P-450c21 (21α-hydroxylase) deficiency is not only closely linked to the HLA supergene complex, but certain specific HLA subtypes are found to be statis-tically increased in patients with 21-hydroxylase defi-ciency. These include Bw51 in the simple virilizing form and Bw47 in the salt-losing form.

The defect in P-450c21 (21α-hydroxylase) activity results in impaired cortisol synthesis, increased ACTH levels, and increased adrenal androgen and androgen precursor production. Prior to 12 weeks of gestation, high fetal androgen levels lead to a varying degree of labioscrotal fusion and clitoral enlargement in the female fetus; exposure to androgen after 12 weeks in-duces clitorimegaly alone. In the male fetus, no struc-tural abnormalities in the external genitalia are evident at birth, but the phallus may be enlarged. These pa-tients produce sufficient amounts of aldosterone to pre-vent the signs and symptoms of mineralocorticoid de-ficiency. Virilization continues after birth in untreated patients. This results in rapid growth and bone matura-tion as well as physical signs of excess androgen secre-tion (eg, acne, seborrhea, premature development of pubic or axillary hair, and phallic enlargement). True, or central, precocious puberty can occur following ini-tiation of glucocorticoid therapy in affected children with peripubertal bone ages.

Mild defects in P-450c21 (21α-hydroxylase) ac-tivity have been reported. Patients can be symptomatic (late-onset or acquired form) or asymptomatic ("cryp-tic" form). These mild forms of P-450c21 hydroxylase deficiency are HLA-linked, as is "classic" P-450c21 hydroxlyase deficiency; however, they occur much more frequently than the classic form of the disease. It has been postulated that "nonclassic" P-450c21 hy-droxylase deficiency is the most common autosomal recessive disorder, affecting 1 in 100 persons of all ethnic groups but having an incidence 2 to 3 times higher in Ashkenazi Jews and Hispanics. Females with late-onset P-450c21 hydroxylase deficiency have nor-mal female genitalia at birth and do not have an elec-trolyte abnormality. Mild virilization occurs later in childhood and adolescence, resulting in the premature development of pubic or axillary hair, slight clitoral enlargement, menstrual irregularities, acne, and hir-sutism. Affected males have normal male genitalia at birth, but later in childhood they may exhibit pre-mature pubic or axillary hair, early puberty, and short stature due to early bone maturation and epiphyseal fusion. Asymptomatic individuals who have the same biochemical abnormalities as patients with mild forms of P-450c21 hydroxylase deficiency can be detected by hormonal testing of families in which there is at least one member with symptoms.

B. Type II—P-450c21 Hydroxylase Deficiency With Virilization and Salt Loss: The salt-losing variant of P-450c21 hydroxylase deficiency accounts for about 80% of the patients with classic 21-hydroxy-lase deficiency and involves a more severe deficit of P-450c21 hydroxylase, which leads to impaired secretion of both cortisol (zona fasciculata) and aldosterone (zona glomerulosa). This results in electrolyte and fluid losses after the fifth day of life which are manifested as hyponatremia, hyperkalemia, acidosis, dehydration, and vascular collapse. Masculinization of the external genitalia of affected females tends to be more severe than that found in patients with simple P-450c21 hydroxylase deficiency. Affected males have macrogenitosomia.

The diagnosis of P-450c21 hydroxylase deficiency should always be considered (1) in patients with ambiguous genitalia who have a 46,XX karyotype and are thus female pseudohermaphrodites; (2) in apparent cryptorchid males; (3) in any infant who presents with shock, hypoglycemia, and chemical findings compatible with adrenal insufficiency; and (4) in males and females with signs of virilization prior to puberty, including premature adrenarche. In the past, the diagnosis of P-450c21 hydroxylase deficiency was based on the finding of elevated levels of 17-ketosteroids and pregnanetriol in the urine. Although still valid and useful, urinary steroid determinations have been replaced by the measurement of plasma 17-hydroxyprogesterone. The concentration of plasma 17-hydroxyprogesterone is elevated in umbilical cord blood but rapidly decreases into the range of 100–200 ng/dL (3–6 nmol/L) by 24 hours after delivery. In premature infants and in stressed full-term newborns, the levels of 17-hydroxyprogesterone are higher than those observed in nonstressed full-term infants. In patients with P-450c21 hydroxylase deficiency, the 17-hydroxyprogesterone values usually range from 3000 to 40,000 ng/dL (90–1200 nmol/L), depending on the age of the patient and the severity of P-450c21 hydroxylase deficiency. Patients with mild P-450c21 hydroxylase deficiency, ie, late-onset and "cryptic" forms, may have borderline basal 17-hydroxyprogesterone values, but they can be distinguished from heterozygotes on the basis of a more augmented 17-hydroxyprogesterone response to the parenteral administration of ACTH. Salt losers can be ascertained clinically, usually by chemical evidence of hyponatremia and hyperkalemia on a regular or low-salt diet. In these patients, aldosterone levels in both plasma and urine are low in relation to the serum sodium concentration, while plasma renin activity is elevated. HLA typing and measurement of amniotic fluid 17-hydroxyprogesterone levels have been utilized in the prenatal diagnosis of affected fetuses. There is data to indicate that prenatal therapy with dexamethasone given to the mother can ameliorate the genital ambiguity seen in affected females. Heterozygosity has been ascertained by HLA typing in informative families and by the use of ACTH-induced rises in plasma 17-hydroxyprogesterone levels. Measurement of plasma 17-hydroxyprogesterone levels using heel-stick capillary blood specimens blotted onto filter paper has been shown to be a valid screening tool for 21-hydroxylase deficiency in 3-day-old infants.

C. Type III—P-450c11 Hydroxylase Deficiency (Virilization With Hypertension): A defect in hydroxylation at C11 leads to the hypersecretion of 11-deoxycorticosterone and 11-deoxycortisol in addition to adrenal androgens. Marked heterogeneity in the clinical and hormonal manifestations of this defect have been described, including mild, late-onset, and even "cryptic" forms of this disease. Patients with this form of adrenal hyperplasia classically exhibit virilization secondary to increased androgen production and hypertension caused by increased 11-deoxycorticosterone secretion. The hypertension is not obligatory and may appear in late childhood or adolescence.

The P-450c11 hydroylase gene has been localized to the long arm of chromosome 8. This gene codes for a protein that has P-450c11 hydroxylase, 18-hydroxylase (corticosterone methyloxidase, CMO type I), and 18-oxidase (aldosterone synthetase, CMO type II) activities. Hence, mutations in this gene can produce a wide variety of clinical manifestations, from hypertension and virilization to salt wasting alone, ie, CMO type II deficiency.

Since this gene is on chromosome 8, it is not linked to HLA. ACTH stimulation tests have failed to demonstrate a consistent biochemical aberration in obligate heterozygotes thus far.

The diagnosis of P-450c11 hydroxylase deficiency can be confirmed by demonstration of elevated plasma levels of 11-deoxycortisol and 11-deoxycorticosterone and increased excretion of their metabolites in urine (mainly tetrahydro 11-deoxycortisol) either in the basal state or after the administration of ACTH.

D. Type IV—3β-Hydroxysteroid Dehydrogenase Deficiency (Male or Female Pseudohermaphroditism and Adrenal Insufficiency): See below.

E. Type V—P-450c17 Deficiency (Male Pseudohermaphroditism, Sexual Infantilism, Hypertension, and Hypokalemic Alkalosis): See below.

F. Type VI—P-450scc Side-Chain Cleavage Deficiency (Congenital Lipoid Adrenal Hyperplasia, Male Pseudohermaphroditism, Sexual Infantilism, and Adrenal Insufficiency): See below.

Treatment

Treatment of patients with adrenal hyperplasia may be divided into acute and chronic phases. In acute adrenal crises, a deficiency of both cortisol and aldosterone results in hypoglycemia, hyponatremia, hyperkalemia, hypovolemia, and shock. An infusion of 5% glucose in isotonic saline should be started immediately. In the first hour, if the patient is in shock, a saline infusion of 20 mL/kg may be given; thereafter, fluid and electrolyte replacement is calculated on the basis of deficits and standard maintenance requirements. Hydrocortisone sodium hemisuccinate, 50 mg/m^2, should be given as a bolus and another 50–100 mg/m^2 added to the infusion fluid over the first 24 hours of therapy. If hyponatremia and hyperkalemia are present, desoxycorticosterone acetate (DOCA), 1–2 mg, may be given every 12–24 hours intramuscularly (if available). The amount of DOCA and the concentration and amount of saline solution must be adjusted according to the results of frequent electrolyte determinations, assessment of the state of hydration, and blood pressure measurements. Excess DOCA and salt can result in hypokalemia, hypertension, congestive heart failure, and hypertensive encephalopathy, whereas too little salt and DOCA will fail to correct the electrolyte imbalance. If DOCA is unavailable, fludrocortisone, 0.05–0.1 mg by mouth may be given along with the intravenous saline and hydocortisone. In extreme cases of hyponatremia, hyperkalemia, and acidosis, sodium bicarbonate and a cation exchange resin, eg, sodium polystyrene sulfonate (kayexalate), may be needed.

Once the patient is stabilized and a definitive diagnosis with appropriate steroid studies has been made, the patient should receive maintenance doses of glucocorticoids to permit normal growth, development, and bone maturation (hydrocortisone, approximately 12–18 mg/m^2/d by mouth in 3 divided doses). The dose of hydrocortisone must be titered in each patient, depending on steroid hormone levels, growth, and clinical signs of steroid overdose or virilization. Salt losers need treatment with mineralocorticoid (fludrocortisone, 0.05–0.1 mg/d by mouth) and added dietary salt. The dose of mineralocorticoid should be adjusted so that the electrolytes and blood pressure, as well as the plasma renin activity, are in the normal range.

Patients with ambiguous external genitalia should have plastic repair of the external genitalia before age 1 year. Clitoral recession or clitoroplasty rather than clitoridectomy is preferred. Of major importance to the family with an affected child is the assurance that their child will grow and develop into a normal functional adult. In patients with the most common form of adrenal hyperplasia–21-hydroxylase deficiency–fertility in males and feminization, menstruation, and fertility in females can be expected with adequate treatment. Long-term psychologic guidance and support for the patient and family by the physician is essential.

Aberrant adrenal rests in the testes of males with P-450c21 hydroxylase deficiency (especially salt losers) may enlarge and may be mistaken for either adult testicular maturation or testicular neoplasms. These adrenal rests are often bilateral and are made up of cells that appear indistinguishable from Leydig cells histologically except for the fact that they lack Reinke crystalloids. The rests are usually seen in noncompliant or undertreated patients. To prevent this complication as well as the risk of adrenal crisis, pituitary hyperplasia, and adrenal carcinoma, continuous treatment with a glucocorticoid (and, if indicated, a mineralocorticoid) is recommended even in adult males.

MATERNAL ANDROGENS & PROGESTOGENS

Masculinization of the external genitalia of a female infant can occur if the mother ingested testosterone or synthetic progestational agents during the first 8 weeks of pregnancy. After the 12th week of gestation, exposure results in clitorimegaly only. Norethindrone, ethisterone, norethynodrel, and medroxyprogesterone acetate have all been implicated in masculinization. Recently, nonadrenal female pseudohermaphroditism as a consequence of the maternal ingestion of danazol, the 2,3-*d*-isoxazole derivative of 17α-ethinyl testosterone, has been described. In rare instances, masculinization of a female fetus may occur if the mother has an ovarian or adrenal tumor, congenital virilizing adrenal hyperplasia, or a luteoma of pregnancy.

The diagnosis of female pseudohermaphroditism arising from transplacental passage of androgenic steroids is based on exclusion of other forms of female pseudohermaphroditism and a history of drug exposure. Surgical correction of the genitalia, if needed, is the only therapy necessary.

Nonadrenal female pseudohermaphroditism can be associated with imperforate anus, renal anomalies, and other malformations of the lower intestine and urinary tract. Sporadic as well as familial cases have been reported.

MALE PSEUDOHERMAPHRODITISM

Male pseudohermaphrodites have gonads that are testes, but the genital ducts or external genitalia are not completely masculinized. Male pseudohermaphroditism can result from deficient testosterone secretion as a consequence of (1) a defect in testicular differentiation, (2) failure of secretion of testosterone or müllerian duct inhibitory factor, (3) failure of target tissue response to testosterone or dihydrotestosterone, and (4) failure of conversion of testosterone to dihydrotestosterone.

Testicular Unresponsiveness to hCG & LH

Male sexual differentiation is dependent upon the production of testosterone by fetal Leydig cells. Leydig cell testosterone secretion is under the influence of placental hCG during the critical period of male sexual differentiation, and, thereafter, fetal pituitary LH during gestation.

The finding of normal male sexual differentiation in XY males with anencephaly, apituitarism, or congenital hypothalamic hypopituitarism suggests that male sex differentiation can occur independently of the secretion of fetal pituitary gonadotropins.

Absence, hypoplasia, or unresponsiveness of Leydig cells to hCG-LH would result in deficient testosterone production and, consequently, male pseudohermaphroditism. The extent of the genital ambiguity is a function of the degree of testosterone deficiency. A small number of patients with absent, hypoplastic, or unresponsive Leydig cells (attributed to a lack of receptor activity for hCG-LH) have been reported, as well as an animal model—the "vet" rat. In most of the patients thus far reported, the defect resulted in female-appearing genitalia. Müllerian duct regression was complete. Basal gonadotropin levels as well as GnRH-evoked responses were elevated in postpubertal patients. Plasma 17α-hydroxyprogesterone, androstenedione, and testosterone levels were low, and hCG elicited little or no response in testosterone or its precursors. Treatment depends on the age at diagnosis and the extent of masculinization. A female sex assignment has usually been chosen in patients with female-appearing genitalia.

Inborn Errors of Testosterone Biosynthesis

Fig 18–14 demonstrates the major pathways in testosterone biosynthesis in the gonads; each step is associated with an inherited defect that results in testosterone deficiency and, consequently, male pseudohermaphroditism. (See also Chapter 16.) Steps 1, 2, and 3 are enzymatic deficiencies that occur in both the adrenals and gonads and result in defective synthesis of both corticosteroids and testosterone. Thus, they represent forms of congenital adrenal hyperplasia.

(1) P-450scc deficiency, cholesterol side-chain cleavage defect, type VI adrenal hyperplasia, congenital lipoid adrenal hyperplasia (male pseudohermaphroditism, sexual infantilism, and adrenal insufficiency): This is a very early defect in the synthesis of all steroids and results in severe adrenal and gonadal insufficiency. The P-450scc gene has been isolated, cloned, and localized to chromosome No. 15. Affected males have female (or, rarely, ambiguous) external genitalia with a blind vaginal pouch and hypoplastic male genital ducts but no müllerian derivatives; the genitalia of affected females are normal. Large lipid-laden adrenals that displace the kidneys downward may be demonstrated by intravenous urography, abdominal ultrasonography, or CT scanning. Death in early infancy from adrenal insufficiency is not uncommon. The diagnosis is confirmed by the lack of or low levels of all steroids in plasma and urine and an absent response to ACTH stimulation. Treatment involves replacement with appropriate doses of glucocorticoids and mineralocorticoids.

(2) 3β-Hydroxysteroid dehydrogenase/Δ⁵-isomerase deficiency, type IV congenital adrenal hyperplasia (male or female pseudohermaphroditism and adrenal insufficiency): 3β-Hydroxysteroid dehydrogenase deficiency is an early defect in steroid synthesis that results in inability of the adrenals and gonads to convert 3β-hydroxy-Δ⁵ steroids to 3-keto-Δ⁴ steroids. This defect in its complete form results in a deficiency of aldosterone, cortisol, testosterone, and

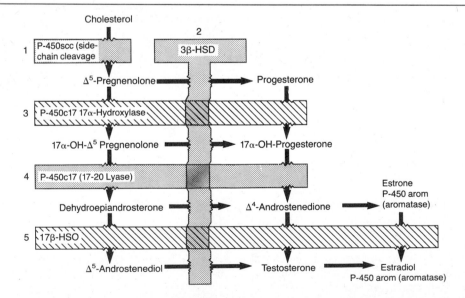

Figure 18–14. Enzymatic defects in the biosynthetic pathway for testosterone. All 5 of the enzymatic defects cause male pseudohermaphroditism in affected males. Although all of the blocks affect gonadal steroidogenesis, those at steps 1, 2, and 3 are associated with major abnormalities in the biosynthesis of glucocorticoids and mineralocorticoids in the adrenal. OH, hydroxy; 3β-HSD, 3β-hydroxysteroid dehydrogenase; 17β-HSO, 17β-hydroxysteroid oxidoreductase (dehydrogenase). Chemical names for enzymes are shown with traditional names in parentheses. (Modified and reproduced, with permission, from Conte FA, Grumbach MM: Pathogenesis, classification, diagnosis, and treatment of anomalies of sex. Chapter 109 in: *Endocrinology.* DeGroot L [editor]. Grune & Stratton, 1989.)

estradiol. Males with this defect are incompletely masculinized, and females have mild clitorimegaly. Salt loss and adrenal crises usually occur in early infancy in affected patients. Affected males may experience normal puberty except for gynecomastia. Patients with a mild—non-salt-losing—form of 3β-hydroxysteroid dehydrogenase deficiency have been described. A study of two siblings has been reported in which the XY male had perineal hypospadias and the female had normal genitalia at birth. Both presented with premature pubarche, and elevated Δ^5-17-ketosteroids were present in urine and blood; mineralocorticoid function was normal. "Nonclassic" (late-onset) forms of this defect usually present with premature pubarche, hirsutism, or both.

The diagnosis of 3β-hydroxysteroid dehydrogenase deficiency is based on finding elevated concentrations of Δ^5-pregnenolone, 17α-hydroxy-Δ^5 pregnenolone, dehydroepiandrosterone (DHEA) and its sulfate, and other 3β-hydroxy-Δ^5 steroids in the plasma and urine of patients with a consistent clinical picture. The diagnosis may be facilitated by the finding of abnormal levels of serum Δ^5-17α-hydroxypregnenolone and DHEA as well as abnormal ratios of Δ^5–Δ^4 steroids after intravenous administration of 0.25 mg of synthetic ACTH. Suppression of the increased plasma and urinary 3β-hydroxy-Δ^5 steroids by the administration of dexamethasone distinguishes 3β-hydroxysteroid dehydrogenase deficiency from a virilizing adrenal tumor. Treatment of this condition is similar to that of other forms of adrenal hyperplasia (see above).

(3) P-450c17 deficiency, 17α-hydroxylase deficiency, type V congenital adrenal hyperplasia (male pseudohermaphroditism, sexual infantilism, hypertension, and hypokalemic alkalosis): A defect in 17α-hydroxylation in the zona fasciculata of the adrenal and in the gonads results in impaired synthesis of 17α-hydroxyprogesterone and 17α-hydroxypregnenolone and, consequently, cortisol and sex steroids. The secretion of large amounts of corticosterone and deoxycorticosterone (DOC) leads to hypertension, hypokalemia, and alkalosis. Increased DOC secretion with resultant hypertension produces suppression of renin and consequently aldosterone secretion.

A single gene on chromosome No. 10 encodes both adrenal and testicular P-450c17. This enzyme catalyzes the 17-hydroxylation of pregnenolone and progesterone to 17α-hydroxypregnenolone and 17α-hydroxyprogesterone as well as their scission (with lyase) to C19 steroids, including dehydroepiandrosterone in the adrenal cortex and androstenedione in the gonads (see Figs 12–4 and 16–2).

The clinical manifestations result from the adrenal and gonadal defect. XX females have normal development of the internal ducts and external genitalia but manifest sexual infantilism with elevated gonadotropin concentrations at puberty. XY males have impaired testosterone synthesis by the fetal testes, which results in female or ambiguous genitalia. At adoles-

cence, sexual infantilism and hypertension are the hallmarks of this defect.

The diagnosis of 17α-hydroxylase deficiency should be suspected in XY males with female or ambiguous genitalia or XX females with sexual infantilism, who also manifest hypertension associated with hypokalemic alkalosis. High levels of progesterone, Δ^5-pregnenolone, DOC, and corticosterone in plasma and increased excretion of their urinary metabolites establish the diagnosis. Plasma renin activity and aldosterone secretion are markedly diminished in these patients.

The following errors affect testosterone and estrogen biosynthesis in the gonads primarily:

(4) P-450c17 deficiency (17,20-lyase deficiency): The enzyme P-450c17 mediates the 17-hydroxylation of pregnenolone and progesterone to 17α-hydroxypregnenolone and 17α-hydroxyprogesterone as well as the scission of the C17,20 bond to yield DHEA and androstenedione, respectively. Rare patients have a defect primarily in the scission of the C21 steroids to C19 steroids (DHEA and androstenedione), which results in a defect in testosterone synthesis and subsequently pseudohermaphroditism in the male and impaired sex steroid synthesis and secretion in the affected 46,XX female. Hence, affected XY individuals with 17,20-lyase deficiency have been male pseudohermaphrodites with either female or ambiguous genitalia and inguinal or intra-abdominal testes. Müllerian derivatives are absent due to secretion of müllerian duct inhibitory factor by affected fetal testes. At puberty, incomplete virilization without gynecomastia occurs. One affected 46,XX woman with sexual infantilism and elevated serum gonadotropin levels has been reported.

Patients with 17,20 lyase deficiency have low circulating levels of testosterone, androstenedione, DHEA, and estradiol. The diagnosis can be confirmed by demonstration of an increased ratio of 17α-hydroxy C21 steroids to C19 steroids (testosterone, DHEA, Δ^5-androstenediol, and androstenedione) after stimulation with ACTH or chorionic gonadotropin.

(5) 17β-Hydroxysteroid oxidoreductase (dehydrogenase) deficiency: The last step in testosterone and estradiol biosynthesis by the gonads involves the reduction of androstenedione to testosterone and estrone to estradiol. At birth, males with a deficiency of the enzyme 17β-hydroxysteroid oxidoreductase have female or mildly ambiguous external genitalia resulting from testosterone deficiency during male differentiation. They have male duct development, absent müllerian structures with a blind vaginal pouch, and inguinal or intra-abdominal testes. At puberty, progressive virilization with clitoral hypertrophy occurs, often associated with the concurrent development of gynecomastia. Plasma gonadotropin, androstenedione, and estrone levels are markedly elevated, whereas testosterone and estradiol concentrations are relatively low.

17β-Hydroxysteroid oxidoreductase deficiency should be included in the differential diagnosis of (1) male pseudohermaphrodites with absent müllerian derivatives who have no abnormality in glucocorticoid or mineralocorticoid synthesis and (2) male pseudohermaphrodites who virilize at puberty, especially if they also exhibit gynecomastia. The diagnosis of 17β-hydroxysteroid oxidoreductase deficiency can be confirmed by the demonstration of inappropriately high plasma levels of estrone and androstenedione and increased ratios of plasma androstenedione to testosterone and estrone to estradiol before and after stimulation with chorionic gonadotropin.

Management of the patients, as with other forms of male pseudohermaphroditism, depends on the age at diagnosis and the degree of ambiguity of the external genitalia. In the patient assigned a male gender identity, plastic repair of the genitalia and testosterone replacement therapy at puberty will be necessary. In patients reared as females (the usual case), the appropriate treatment is castration, followed by estrogen replacement therapy at puberty.

An interesting cohort of patients with 17-oxidoreductase deficiency has been reported from the Middle East. Undiagnosed and undetected, these male pseudohermaphrodites with apparently normal female external genitalia are raised unambiguously as females. At puberty, some degree of virilization occurs, which, in conjunction with cultural pressures in a setting that values males over females, has led to the tradition of changing to a male gender identity. Because of this, it has been suggested that early diagnosis, along with testosterone therapy to augment phallic size, hypo-spadic repair, and male gender assignment is the treatment of choice for these patients in this cohort. The relevance of this approach to other male pseudohermaphrodites with abnormalities in testosterone synthesis is uncertain; further data on the functional adequacy of the phallus after multiple hypospadial repairs, as well as on the long-term psychosexual status of these patients, is required before extrapolations can be made.

Defects in Androgen-Dependent Target Tissues

The complex mechanism of action of steroid hormones at the cellular level has recently been clarified (Fig 18–15).

Free testosterone enters the target cells and undergoes 5α reduction to dihydrotestosterone, which in turn is bound to an intracellular receptor protein; the transformed receptor protein complex is translocated into the nucleus of the target cell. In the nucleus, the receptor-dihydrotestosterone complex binds to specific DNA sites and initiates transcription. Messenger RNA is synthesized, modified, and exported to the cytoplasm of the cell, where ribosomes translate mRNA into new proteins that have an androgen effect on the cell. A lack of androgen effect at the end organ, and consequently male pseudohermaphroditism, may result from dihydrotestosterone receptor activity, abnormalities in 5α-reductase activity, transformation of the steroid-receptor complex, binding to DNA, transcription, exportation, or translation. (See also Chapter 16.)

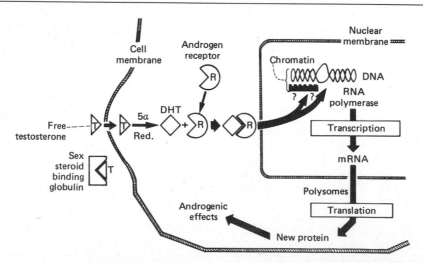

Figure 18–15. A simplified diagrammatic representation of the mechanism of action of testosterone at the target organ 5α-Red, 5α-reductase, DHT, dihydrotestosterone. (Reproduced, with permission, from Conte FA, Grumbach MM. Pathogenesis, classification, diagnosis, and treatment of anomalies of sex. Chapter 109 in: *Endocrinology*. DeGroot L [editor]. Grune & Stratton, 1989.)

End-Organ Resistance to Androgenic Hormones (Androgen Receptor & Postreceptor Defects)

A. Syndrome of Complete Androgen Resistance and Its Variants (Testicular Feminization): The syndrome of complete androgen resistance (testicular feminization) is characterized by a 46,XY karyotype, bilateral testes, female-appearing external genitalia, a blind vaginal pouch, and absent müllerian derivatives. At puberty, female secondary sexual characteristics develop, but menarche does not ensue. Pubic and axillary hair is usually sparse and in one-third of patients totally absent. Some patients have a variant form of this syndrome and exhibit slight clitoral enlargement. These patients may exhibit mild virilization in addition to the development of breasts and a female habitus.

Androgen resistance during embryogenesis prevents masculinization of the external genitalia and differentiation of the wolffian ducts. Secretion of müllerian duct inhibitory factor by the fetal Sertoli cells leads to regression of the müllerian ducts. Thus, affected patients are born with female external genitalia and a blind vaginal pouch. At puberty, androgen resistance results in augmented LH secretion with subsequent increases in testosterone and estradiol. Estradiol arises from conversion of testosterone and androstenedione as well as from direct secretion by the testes. Androgen resistance coupled with increased estradiol secretion results in the development of female secondary sexual characteristics at puberty.

Data on rodents as well as mammals indicate that androgen resistance is modulated, at least in part, by abnormalities in androgen receptor activity in androgen-sensitive tissues. Studies utilizing fibroblasts cultured from genital skin indicate that patients with complete androgen resistance are genetically heterogeneous. Patients have been described who have (1) an undetectable or low amount of androgen receptor activity, (2) a qualitatively abnormal (thermolabile, unstable, or both) androgen receptor, and (3) a normal amount of androgen receptor activity (a presumed postreceptor defect). Inheritance in all forms appears to be X-linked. X-linked genomic and cDNA clones for the androgen receptor have been isolated. The androgen receptor gene has been localized to the q11-12 region of the long arm of the X chromosome. A study of 6 patients with complete androgen resistance and absent receptor activity revealed heterogeneity. One patient was found to have a deletion of the gene involving the steroid-binding domain, while no deletion was found in the 5 other patients. These data suggest that point mutations may also result in the androgen receptor-negative form of complete androgen resistance. Further studies utilizing molecular DNA analyses will undoubtedly help to elucidate the molecular nature of the heterogeneity of androgen receptor defects and their phenotypes.

The diagnosis of complete androgen resistance can be suspected from the clinical features. Prepubertally, testislike masses in the inguinal canal or labia in a phenotypic female suggest the diagnosis. Postpubertally, the patients present with primary amenorrhea, normal breast development, and absent or sparse pubic or axillary hair. Characteristically, the concentrations of LH and testosterone are markedly elevated. This latter finding is an important hormonal feature of androgen resistance. The family history, phenotype, endocrine evaluation, androgen receptor studies, and, if necessary, the metabolic response to testosterone will help confirm the diagnosis.

Therapy of patients with complete androgen resistance involves affirmation and reinforcement of their female gender identity. Castration, either prior to or after puberty, is indicated because of the increased risk of gonadal neoplasms with age. Estrogen replacement therapy is required at the age of puberty in orchidectomized patients.

B. Syndrome of Incomplete Androgen Resistance and Its Variants (Reifenstein's Syndrome): Patients with incomplete androgen resistance manifest a wide spectrum of phenotypes as far as masculinization is concerned. The external genitalia at birth can range from ambiguous, with a blind vaginal pouch, to hypoplastic male genitalia. Müllerian duct derivatives are absent and wolffian duct derivatives present, but they are usually hypoplastic. At puberty, virilization is poor; pubic and axillary hair as well as gynecomastia are usually present. The most common phenotype postpubertally is the male with perineoscrotal hypospadias and gynecomastia. Axillary and pubic hair are normal. The testes remain small and exhibit azoospermia as a consequence of germinal cell arrest. As in the case of patients with complete androgen resistance, there are high levels of plasma LH, testosterone, and estradiol. However, the degree of feminization in these patients despite high estradiol levels is less than that found in the syndrome of complete androgen resistance.

Androgen receptor studies in these patients have primarily revealed (1) a partial deficiency of androgen receptor activity and (2) a qualitatively abnormal androgen receptor. As in the syndrome of complete androgen resistance, inheritance appears to be X-linked.

Androgen Resistance in Men With Normal Male Genitalia

Partial androgen resistance has been described in a group of infertile men who have a normal male phenotype but may exhibit gynecomastia. Unlike other patients with androgen resistance, some of these patients have normal plasma LH and testosterone levels. Infertility in otherwise normal men may be the only clinical manifestation of androgen resistance. However, infertility may not always be associated with androgen resistance. Recently, a family in which 5 males showed signs of gynecomastia and "undervirilization" was described. Receptor studies revealed a subtle qualitative abnormality, and plasma testosterone levels were elevated. Four of the 5 affected males were fertile and had fathered children. These patients may represent one extreme form of the highly variable phenotype expression of androgen resistance.

Defects in Testosterone Metabolism by Peripheral Tissues; 5α-Reductase Deficiency (Pseudovaginal Perineoscrotal Hypospadias)

The defective conversion of testosterone to dihydrotestosterone produces a unique form of male pseudohermaphroditism (Fig 18–16). At birth, ambiguous external genitalia are manifested by a small hypospadiac phallus bound down in chordee, a bifid scrotum, and a urogenital sinus that opens onto the perineum. A blind vaginal pouch is present, opening either into the urogenital sinus or onto the urethra, immediately behind the urethral orifice. The testes are either inguinal or labial. The müllerian structures are absent, and the wolffian structures are well differentiated. At puberty, affected males virilize; the voice deepens, muscle mass increases, and the phallus enlarges. The bifid scrotum becomes rugate and pigmented. The testes enlarge and descend into the labioscrotal folds, and spermatogenesis may ensue. Gynecomastia is notably absent in these patients. Of note also is the absence of acne, temporal hair recession, and hirsutism. A remarkable feature of this form of male pseudohermaphroditism has been the reported change in gender identity from female to male at puberty, primarily in affected individuals living in rural communities in the Dominican Republic.

After the onset of puberty, patients with 5α-reductase deficiency have normal to elevated testosterone levels and slightly elevated plasma concentrations of LH. As expected, plasma dihydrotesterone is low and the testosterone/dihydrotestosterone ratio is abnormally high. Apparently, lack of 5α reduction of testosterone to dihydrotestosterone in utero during the critical phases of male sex differentiation results in incomplete masculinization of the external genitalia, while testosterone-dependent wolffian structures are normally developed. The marked virilization that occurs at puberty in these patients is in sharp contrast to that which occurs in utero and is as yet not well explained. Since the androgen receptor binds both dihydrotestosterone and testosterone (but with a lower affinity), the sustained high levels of circulating testosterone attained at puberty may be a factor in the virilization achieved. In addition, the enzyme defect is incomplete, and at puberty the plasma concentration of dihydrotestosterone, while low, is detectable. Also the hormonal environment is markedly different at puberty in that large quantities of competitive steroids (estrogens and progesterone) are not present as they are in utero. In particular, high concentrations of progesterone may have an inhibiting effect on 5α-reductase activity in utero, whereas at puberty progesterone levels are low in males. 5α-Reductase deficiency is inherited as an autosomal recessive, and the enzymatic defect exhibits genetic heterogeneity.

5α-Reductase deficiency should be suspected in male pseudohermaphrodites with a blind vaginal pouch. The diagnosis can be confirmed by demonstration of an abnormally high plasma testosterone/dihydrotestosterone ratio, either under basal conditions or after hCG stimulation. Other confirmatory findings include an increased 5β/5α ratio of urinary C19 steroid metabolites of testosterone, a decreased level of 5α-reductase activity in genital skin in vitro, and decreased conversion of infused testosterone to dihydrotestosterone in vivo.

The early diagnosis of this condition is particularly critical. In view of the natural history of this disorder, a male gender assignment should be considered; consequently, dihydrotestosterone (if available) or testosterone therapy should be initiated in order to augment phallic size. Repair of hypospadias should be performed as soon as possible in infancy. In patients who are diagnosed after infancy, in whom gender identity is unequivocally female, prophylactic orchiectomy and estrogen substitution therapy may still be considered the treatment of choice until further experience with this biochemical entity and sex reversal in our culture is available.

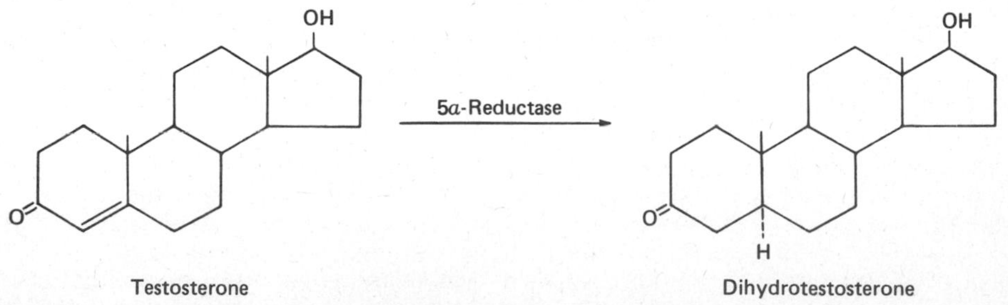

Figure 18–16. Metabolism of testosterone.

Dysgenetic Male Pseudohermaphroditism (Ambiguous Genitalia Due to Dysgenetic Gonads)

Defective gonadogenesis results in ambiguous development of the genital ducts, urogenital sinus, and external genitalia. Patients with 45,X/46,XY mosaicism, structural abnormalities of the Y chromosome, and forms of XY gonadal dysgenesis manifest defective gonadogenesis and thus defective virilization. These disorders are classified under disorders of gonadal differentiation but also are included as a subgroup of male pseudohermaphroditism.

A. Ambiguous Genitalia Associated With Degenerative Renal Disease: Several cases are recorded of male pseudohermaphroditism associated with degenerative renal disease and hypertension as well as with Wilms' tumor. In this syndrome, both the kidneys and the testes are dysgenetic, and a predisposition for renal neoplasms exists. A deletion of p13 on chromosome 11 has been found in over 30 patients with so-called Wilms' tumor-aniridia-gonadoblastoma-mental retardation syndrome. These patients also exhibit various forms of ambiguous or hypoplastic male genitalia, including bifid scrotum, hypospadias, and cryptorchidism.

B. Vanishing Testes Syndrome (Embryonic Testicular Regression Syndrome; XY Agonadism; Rudimentary Testes Syndrome; Congenital Anorchia): Cessation of testicular function during the critical phases of male sex differentiation can lead to varying clinical syndromes depending on when testicular function ceases. At one end of the clinical spectrum of these heterogeneous conditions are the XY patients in whom testicular functional deficiency occurred prior to 8 weeks of gestation, which results in female differentiation of the internal and external genitalia. At the other end of the spectrum are the patients with "anorchia" or "vanishing testes." These patients have perfectly normal male differentiation of their internal and external structures, but gonadal tissue is absent. The diagnosis of anorchia should be considered in all cryptorchid males. Administration of chorionic gonadotropin, 1000–2000 units injected intramuscularly every other day for 2 weeks (total of 7 injections), is a useful test of Leydig cell function. In the presence of normal Leydig cell function, there is a rise in plasma testosterone from concentrations of less than 20 ng/dL (0.69 nmol/L) to over 200 ng/dL (6.9 nmol/L) in prepubertal males. In infants under 4 years of age and children over 10 years of age, plasma FSH levels are a sensitive index of gonadal integrity. The gonadotropin response to a 100-μg bolus injection of GnRH can also be used to diagnose the absence of gonadal feedback on the hypothalamus and pituitary. In agonadal children, GnRH elicits a rise in LH and FSH levels that is greater than that achieved in prepubertal children with normal gonadal function. Patients with high gonadotropin levels and no testosterone response to chorionic gonadotropin are usually found to lack recognizable gonadal tissue at surgery.

Defects in the Synthesis, Secretion, or Response to Müllerian Duct Inhibitory Factor

A small number of patients have been described in whom normal male development of the external genitalia has occurred but in whom the müllerian ducts persist. The retention of müllerian structures can be ascribed to (1) failure of the Sertoli cells to synthesize müllerian duct inhibitory factor, (2) a defect in the response of the duct to that factor, or (3) possibly discordant timing of the release of that factor. This condition appears to be transmitted as an autosomal recessive trait. Therapy involves removal of the müllerian structures.

UNCLASSIFIED FORMS OF ABNORMAL SEXUAL DEVELOPMENT IN MALES

Hypospadias

Hypospadias occurs as an isolated finding in one per 1000 newborn males. It is often associated with ventral contraction and bowing of the penis, or chordee. On an embryologic basis, deficient virilization of the external genitalia implies subnormal Leydig cell function in utero, end-organ resistance, or improper chronologic correlation between hormone level and critical time for tissue response. Although in most patients there is little reason to suspect these mechanisms, recent reports in a small number of patients have suggested that simple hypospadias is associated with an abnormality in androgen receptor activity, nuclear localization, or an aberration in the maturation of the hypothalamic-pituitary-gonadal axis. Further studies are necessary to determine the role of these factors in the pathogenesis of simple hypospadias. Nonendocrine factors that affect differentiation of the primordia may be found in a variety of genetic syndromes. Aarskog prospectively studied 100 patients with hypospadias and found one patient to be a genetic female with congenital adrenal hyperplasia, 5 with sex chromosome abnormalities, and one with the incomplete form of XY gonadal dysgenesis. Nine patients were from pregnancies in which the mother had taken progestational compounds during the first trimester. Thus, a pathogenetic mechanism was found in 15% of these patients.

Microphallus

Microphallus without hypospadias can result from a heterogeneous group of disorders, but by far the most common is fetal testosterone deficiency. In the human male fetus, testosterone synthesis by the fetal Leydig cell during the critical period of male differentiation (8–12 weeks) is under the influence of placental hCG.

After midgestation, fetal pituitary LH seems to modulate fetal testosterone synthesis by the Leydig cell and, consequently, growth of the phallus. GH also appears to play a role in growth of the phallus. Thus, males with congenital hypopituitarism as well as isolated gonadotropin deficiency and "late" fetal testicular failure can present with normal male differentiation and microphallus at birth (phallus < 2 cm in length). Patients with hypothalamic hypopituitarism or pituitary aplasia may also have midline defects, hypoglycemia, and giant cell hepatitis. After appropriate evaluation of anterior pituitary function (ie, GH, ACTH, cortisol, TSH, T_4 and gonadotropins) and stabilization of the patient with hormone replacement, if necessary, an hCG stimulation test should be performed. Thereafter, a trial of testosterone therapy should be administered to all patients with microphallus before definitive gender assignment is made. Patients with fetal testosterone deficiency as a cause of their microphallus—whether due to gonadotropin deficiency or to a primary testicular disorder—respond to 25–50 mg of testosterone enanthate intramuscularly monthly for 3 months with a mean increase of 2 cm in phallic length (Fig 18–17). In the rare patient in whom a trial of testosterone therapy does not result in a reasonable increase in phallic size, castration and assignment of a female gender may then be a prudent course to follow.

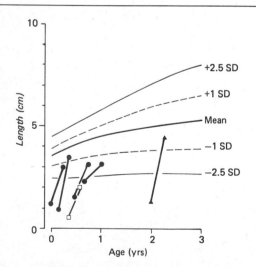

Figure 18–17. The response in phallic length to a 3-month course of testosterone in 6 patients with microphallus. Patients were under 2 years of age. Each patient was given 25 mg of testosterone enanthate in oil intramuscularly monthly for 3 months. △, □ indicate 2 patients who subsequently underwent a second course of testosterone therapy. (Reproduced, with permission, from Burstein S, Grumbach MM, Kaplan SL: Early determination of androgen-responsiveness is important in the management of microphallus. *Lancet* 1979;**2**:983.)

UNCLASSIFIED FORMS OF ABNORMAL SEXUAL DEVELOPMENT IN FEMALES

Congenital absence of the vagina occurs in one per 5000 female births. It can be associated with müllerian derivatives that vary from normal to absent. Ovarian function is usually normal. Therapy involves plastic repair of the vagina, if indicated.

MANAGEMENT OF PATIENTS WITH INTERSEX PROBLEMS

Choice of Sex
The goal of the physician in the management of patients with ambiguous genitalia is to establish a diagnosis and to assign a sex for rearing that is most compatible with a well-adjusted life and sexual adequacy. Once the sex for rearing is assigned, the gender role is reinforced by the use of appropriate surgical, hormonal, or psychologic measures. Except in female pseudohermaphrodites, ambiguities of the genitalia are caused by lesions that almost always make the patient infertile. In recommending male sex assignment, the adequacy of the size of the phallus should be the most important consideration.

Differential Diagnosis
The steps in the diagnosis of intersexuality are delineated in Figure 18–18.

Reassignment of Sex
Reassignment of sex in infancy and childhood is always a difficult psychosocial problem for the patient, the parents, and the physicians involved. While easier in infancy than after 2 years of age, it should always be undertaken with much deliberation and with provision for long-term medical and psychiatric supervision and counseling.

Reconstructive Surgery
It is desirable to initiate plastic repair of the external genitalia prior to 6–12 months of age. In children raised as females, the clitoris should be salvaged, if possible, by clitoroplasty or clitoral recession. Reconstruction of a vagina, if necessary, can be deferred until adolescence.

Removal of the gonads in children with the variant forms of gonadal dysgenesis should be performed at the time of initial repair of the external genitalia, because gonadoblastomas, seminomas, and dysgerminomas have been reported to occur during the first decade.

In a patient with testicular feminization, the gonads may be left in situ (provided they are not situated in the labia majora) to provide estrogen until late adolescence. The patient may then undergo prophylactic cas-

Diagnosis of Intersexuality

1. History: Family, pregnancy.
2. Physical examination: Palpation of inguinal region, labioscrotal folds, and rectal examination.
3. Initial studies: X chromatin pattern, karyotype analysis, serum electrolytes, 17-hydroxyprogesterone, androstenedione, dehydro-epiandrosterone, testosterone, and dihydrotestosterone. Sonogram of kidneys, ureters, and pelvic contents.
4. Provisional diagnosis: "Abnormal" external genitalia—proceed as shown below.

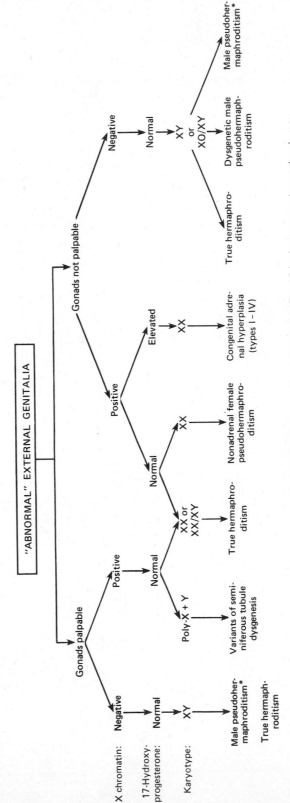

Figure 18–18. Steps in the diagnosis of intersexuality in infancy and childhood. *The 17-hydroxyprogesterone levels may be modestly elevated in patients with 3β-hydroxysteroid dehydrogenase deficiency (type IV) and are "low" in patients with 17α-hydroxylase deficiency (type V) and cholesterol side-chain cleavage deficiency (type VI). (Modified, with permission, from Grumbach MM. In: *Pediatrics*, 13th ed. Holt LE Jr, McIntosh R, Barnett HL [editors]. Appleton-Century-Crofts, 1962.)

tration, having had her female identity reinforced by normal feminization at puberty.

In patients with incomplete testicular feminization reared as females or in patients with errors of testosterone biosynthesis in whom some degree of masculinization occurs at puberty, gonadectomy should be performed prior to puberty.

Hormonal Substitution Therapy

Cyclic estrogen and progestin are used in individuals reared as females in whom a uterus is present. In males, virilization is achieved by the administration of a repository preparation of testosterone.

Psychologic Management

Sex is not a single biologic entity but the summation of many morphogenetic, functional, and psychologic potentialities. There must never be any doubt in the mind of the parent or child as to the child's true sex. Chromosomal and gonadal sex are secondary matters; the sex of rearing is paramount. With proper surgical reconstruction, hormone substitution, and continuing psychologic support, the individual whose psychosexual gender is discordant with chromosomal sex need not have any psychologic catastrophes as long as the sex of rearing is accepted with conviction by the family and others during the critical early years. These individuals should reach adulthood as well-adjusted men or women capable of normal sexual interaction, albeit usually not of procreation.

REFERENCES

Austin CR, Edwards RG (editors): *Mechanisms of Sex Differentiation in Animals and Man.* Academic Press, 1981

Bandmann HJ, Breit R, Perwin E (editors): *Klinefelter's Syndrome.* Springer-Verlag, 1984.

Conte FA, Grumbach MM: Pathogenesis, classification, diagnosis, and treatment of anomalies of sex. Chapter 109 in: *Endocrinology,* 2nd ed. DeGroot L (editor). Saunders, 1988.

Goodfellow PN, Darling SM: Genetics of sex determination in man and mouse. *Development* 1988;**102**:251.

Goodfellow PN et al (editors): The mammalian Y chromosome: Molecular search for the sex-determining factor. *Development* 1987; **101(Suppl).** [Entire issue.]

Griffen JE, Wilson JD: Disorders of sexual differentiation. In: *Campbell's Urology,* 5th ed. Walsh PG et al (editors). Saunders, 1986.

Gross DJ et al: Male pseudohermaphrodism due to 17β-hydroxysteroid dehydrogenase deficiency: Gender reassignment in early infancy. *Acta Endocrinol* 1986;**112**:238.

Grumbach MM, Conte FA: Disorders of sex differentiation. In: *Williams Textbook of Endocrinology,* 7th ed. Wilson JD, and Foster DW (editors). Saunders, 1985.

Haseltine FP, McClure ME, Goldberg EH (editors): *Genetic Markers of Sex Differentiation.* Plenum Press, 1987.

Imperato-McGinley JL et al: Androgens and the evolution of male-gender identity among male pseudohermaphrodites with 5α-reductase deficiency. *N Engl J Med* 1979; **300**:1233.

Josso N: Antimüllerian hormone: New perspectives for a sexist molecule. *Endocr Rev* 1986; **7**:421.

Lustig RH et al: Ontogeny of gonadotropin secretion in congenital anorchia: Sexual dimorphism versus syndrome of gonadal dysgenesis and diagnostic considerations. *J Urol* 1987;**138**:587.

New MI, Speiser PW: Genetics of adrenal steroid 21-hydroxylase deficiency. *Endocr Rev* 1986;**7**:331.

New MI et al: The adrenal hyperplasias. In: *The Metabolic Basis of Inherited Disease,* 6th ed. Scriver CR, Bendet AL, Sly WS (editors). McGraw-Hill, 1989.

Page DC et al: The sex-determining region of the human Y chromosome encodes a finger protein. *Cell* 1987;**51**:1091.

Serio M et al (editors): *Sexual Differentiation: Basic and Clinical Aspects.* Vol 2. Raven Press, 1984.

Simpson E et al: Separation of the genetic loci for the H-Y antigen and for testis determination on human Y chromosome. *Nature* 1987;**326**:876.

Simpson JL: *Disorders of Sexual Differentiation: Etiology and Clinical Delineation.* Academic Press, 1977.

Van Niekerk WA: *True Hermaphrodism.* Harper & Row, 1974.

Verp MS, Simpson JL: Abnormal sexual differentiation and neoplasia. *Cancer Genet Cytogenet* 1987;**25**:191.

Wachtel SS (editor): *H-Y Antigen and the Biology of Sex Determination.* Grune & Stratton, 1982.

Wilson JD et al: The androgen resistance syndromes. In: *The Metabolic Basis of Inherited Disease,* 6th ed. Scriver CR, Beaudet AL, Sly WS (editors). McGraw-Hill, 1989.

Wilson JD, Griffen JE: Disorders of Sexual Differentiation. Chap 33, page 1840, in: *Harrison's Principles of Internal Medicine,* 11th ed. Braunwald E et al (editors). McGraw-Hill, 1987.

Zenzes MT et al: Studies on the function of H-Y antigen: Dissociation and reorganization experiments on rat gonadal tissue. *Cytogenet Cell Genet* 1978;**20**:365.

Puberty

19

Dennis M. Styne, MD

Puberty is one stage in the continuing process of growth and development that begins during gestation and continues until the end of reproductive life. After an interval of childhood quiescence, hypothalamic-pituitary-gonadal activity intensifies in the peripubertal period, leading to increased secretion of gonadal sex steroids that cause secondary sexual development, the pubertal growth spurt, and fertility. Historical records show that the age at onset of certain stages of puberty in boys and girls in Western countries has steadily declined since about 1850; this is probably due to improvements in socioeconomic conditions, nutrition, and general health during that period. However, this trend has not continued during the past 4 decades in the USA.

Many factors can alter age at onset of puberty. Moderate obesity may be associated with an earlier onset of puberty, while severe, morbid obesity may delay puberty. Chronic illness and malnutrition may delay puberty. There is a significant concordance of age at menarche between mother-daughter pairs and within ethnic populations, indicating an influence of genetic factors.

Physical Changes Associated With Puberty

Descriptive standards proposed by Tanner for assessing pubertal development in males and females are in wide use. They focus attention on specific details of the examination and make it possible to objectively record subtle progression of secondary sexual development that may otherwise be overlooked.

A. Female Changes: The first sign of puberty in the female, as noted in longitudinal studies, is an increase in growth velocity that heralds the beginning of the pubertal growth spurt; girls are not usually examined frequently enough to demonstrate this change, however, so breast development is the first sign of puberty noted by most examiners. Breast development (Fig 19–1) is stimulated chiefly by ovarian estrogen secretion, although other hormones also play a part. The size and shape of the breasts may be determined by genetic and nutritional factors, but the characteristics of the stages in Figure 19–1 are the same in all females. Standards are now available for the change in nipple plateau (flat tip of

Acronyms Used in This Chapter	
AASH	Adrenal androgen-stimulating hormone
ACTH	Adrenocorticotropic hormone
DHEA	Dehydroepiandrosterone
DHEAS	Dehydroepiandrosterone sulfate
FSH	Follicle-stimulating hormone
GH	Growth hormone (somatotropin)
GnRH	Gonadotropin-releasing hormone
hCG	Human chorionic gonadotropin
hGH	Human growth hormone
LH	Luteinizing hormone
PRL	Prolactin
RIA	Radioimmunoassay
SHBG	Sex hormone-binding globulin
TSH	Thyroid-stimulating hormone (thyrotropin)

nipple) diameter during puberty. A longitudinal study demonstrated that nipple diameter changes little from stages B1 to B3 (approximately 3–4 mm) but that it enlarges substantially in subsequent stages (approximately 7.4 mm at stage B4 to 10 mm at stage B5), presumably due to increased estrogen secretion at the time of menarche. Other estrogenic features include enlargement of the labia minora and majora, dulling of the vaginal mucosa, and production of a clear or slightly whitish vaginal secretion prior to menarche. Pubic hair development (Fig 19–2) is determined primarily by adrenal and ovarian androgen secretion. Breast development and growth of pubic hair usually proceed at similar rates, but because discrepancies in rates of advancement are possible, it is best to stage breast development separately from pubic hair progression.

Uterine size and shape change with pubertal development; with prolonged estrogen stimulation, the fundus:cervix ratio increases and the uterus elongates to greater than 3 cm. Clinicians can use ultrasonography to reveal the developmental stage of the uterus by comparing the results with the available standards.

B. Male Changes: The first sign of normal puberty in boys is usually an increase in the size of the testes to greater than 2.5 cm in the longest diameter, excluding the epididymis. Most of the increase in testicular size is due to seminiferous tubular development secondary

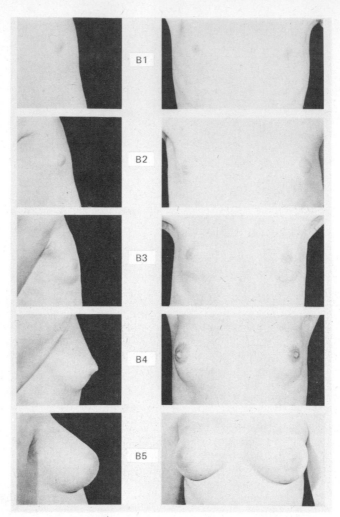

Figure 19–1. Stages of breast development, according to Marshall and Tanner. (Photographs from van Wieringen JC et al, 1971; with permission.) *Stage B1:* Preadolescent; elevation of papilla only. *Stage B2:* Breast bud stage; elevation of breast and papilla as a small mound, and enlargement of areolar diameter. *Stage B3:* Further enlargement of breast and areola, with no separation of their contours. *Stage B4:* Projection of areola and papilla to form a secondary mound above the level of the breast. *Stage B5:* Mature stage; projection of papilla only, owing to recession of the areola to the general contour of the breast. (Reproduced, with permission, from Marshall WA, Tanner JM: *Arch Dis Child* 1969;**44:**291.)

to stimulation by FSH, but a smaller component is due to Leydig cell stimulation by LH. Pubic hair development is caused by adrenal and testicular androgens and is classified separately from genital development, as noted in Figure 19–3. The appearance of spermatozoa in early morning urinary specimens, or spermarche, occurs at a mean age of 13.4 years in gonadal stage 3–4 and pubic hair stage 2–4; if puberty starts earlier or later, the age of spermarche changes accordingly.

C. Age at Onset: The limits of onset of normal secondary sexual development in 98.8% of North American children (ie, mean ± 2.5 SD) are 8–13 years for girls and 9–14 years for boys. A graphic representation of the stages of pubertal development for British children is shown in Figure 19–4; North American and British boys develop at about the same ages, but 6

months should be subtracted from these figures to correct for North American girls. Black boys develop comparably to white boys, but black girls develop earlier than white girls. (Black girls have menarche on average of 0.3 years younger than white girls.) Late onset of pubertal development may indicate hypothalamic, pituitary, or gonadal failure. The time from onset of puberty to complete adult development is also of importance; delays in reaching subsequent stages may indicate hypogonadism. Girls complete secondary sexual development in 1.5–6 years, with a mean of 4.2 years; and boys in 2–4.5 years, with a mean of 3.5 years.

D. Growth Spurt: The striking increase in growth velocity in puberty (pubertal growth spurt) is under complex endocrine control. GH and sex steroids ap-

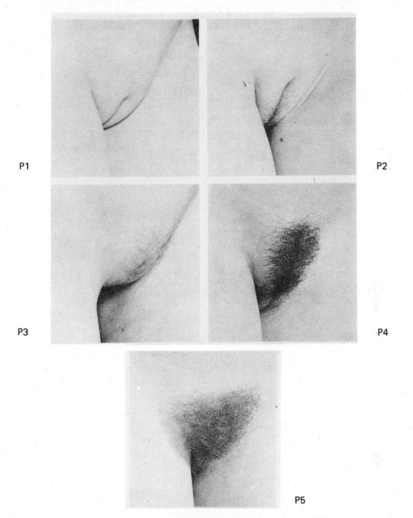

Figure 19–2. Stages of female pubic hair development, according to Marshall and Tanner. (Photographs from van Wieringen JC et al, 1971; with permission.) *Stage P1:* Preadolescent; the vellus over the pubes is no further developed than that over the anterior abdominal wall, ie, no pubic hair. *Stage P2:* Sparse growth of long, slightly pigmented, downy hair, straight or only slightly curled, appearing chiefly along the labia. This stage is difficult to see on photographs. *Stage P3:* Hair is considerably darker, coarser, and curlier. The hair spreads sparsely over the junction of the pubes. *Stage P4:* Hair is now adult in type, but the area covered by it is still considerably smaller than in most adults. There is no spread to the medial surface of the thighs. *Stage P5:* Hair is adult in quantity and type, distributed as an inverse triangle of the classic feminine pattern. Spread is to the medial surface of the thighs but not up the linea alba or elsewhere above the base of the inverse triangle. (Reproduced, with permission, from Marshall WA, Tanner JM: *Arch Dis Child* 1969;**44**:291.)

pear to be important in this process; when either or both are absent, the growth spurt is decreased or absent. Conversely, a pubertal growth spurt in a patient with precocious puberty may mask the presence of coexisting GH deficiency. In girls, the pubertal growth spurt begins in early puberty and is mostly finished by menarche. In boys, the pubertal growth spurt occurs toward the end of puberty, at an average age 2 years older than the growth spurt in girls. Total height attained during the growth spurt in girls is about 25 cm; in boys, it is about 28 cm. The mean adult height differential of 10 cm between men and women is due in part to heights already attained before the onset of the

pubertal growth spurt and in part to the height gained during the spurt.

E. Changes in Body Composition: Changes in body composition are also prominent during pubertal development. Prepubertal boys and girls start with equal lean body mass, skeletal mass, and body fat, but at maturity men have approximately 1.5 times the lean body mass, skeletal mass, and muscle mass of women, while women have 2 times as much body fat as men. Using statistical analysis of age at menarche compared to height and weight at menarche, Frisch and Revelle have postulated that menarche is related to attainment of a critical body weight or to changes in body fat percent-

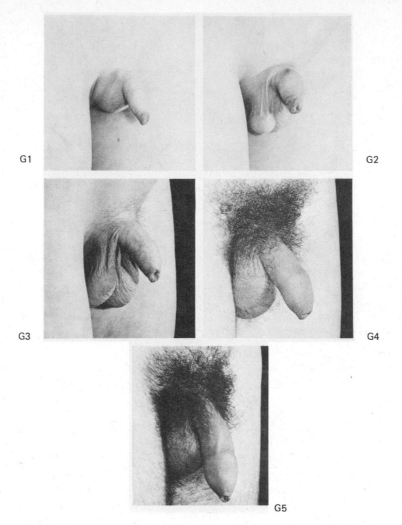

Figure 19–3. Stages of male genital development and pubic hair development, according to Marshall and Tanner. (Photographs from van Wieringen JC et al, 1971; with permission.) **Genital:** *Stage G1:* Preadolescent. Testes, scrotum, and penis are about the same size and proportion as in early childhood. *Stage G2:* The scrotum and testes have enlarged, and there is a change in the texture and some reddening of the scrotal skin. *Stage G3:* Growth of the penis has occurred, at first mainly in length but with some increase in breadth; further growth of testes and scrotum. *Stage G4:* Penis further enlarged in length and girth with development of glans. Testes and scrotum further enlarged. The scrotal skin has further darkened. *Stage G5:* Genitalia adult in size and shape. No further enlargement takes place after stage G5 is reached. **Pubic hair:** *Stage P1:* Preadolescent. The vellus over the pubes is no further developed than that over the abdominal wall, ie, no pubic hair. *Stage P2:* Sparse growth of long, slightly pigmented, downy hair, straight or only slightly curled, appearing chiefly at the base of the penis. *Stage P3:* Hair is considerably darker, coarser, and curlier and spreads sparsely over the junction of the pubes. *Stage P4:* Hair is now adult in type, but the area it covers is still considerably smaller than in most adults. There is no spread to the medial surface of the thighs. *Stage P5:* Hair is adult in quantity and type, distributed as an inverse triangle. Spread is to the medial surface of the thighs but not up the linea alba or elsewhere above the base of the inverse triangle. Most men will have further spread of pubic hair. (Modified and reproduced, with permission, from Marshall WA, Tanner JM: *Arch Dis Child* 1970;**45**:13.)

age. These theories have been criticized as being too general to be predictive in one individual.

F. Other Changes of Puberty: Other changes that are characteristic of puberty are mediated either directly or indirectly by the change in sex steroids. Bone density increases during pubertal development. Sebor-

rheic dermatitis may appear at this age. The mouth flora change and periodontal disease, rare in childhood, may appear at this stage. Growth hormone secretion increases in puberty as does secretion of IGF-1; peak IGF-1 levels are reached about 1 year after peak growth velocity and IGF-1 levels remain elevated

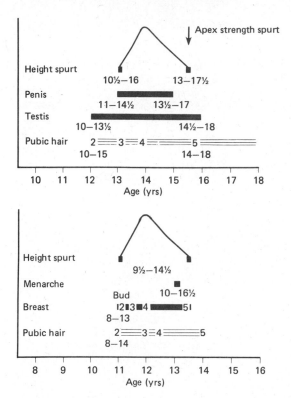

Figure 19–4. Sequence of secondary sexual development in British males (**top**) and females (**bottom**). The range of ages is indicated. (Reproduced, with permission, from Marshall WA, Tanner JM: *Arch Dis Child* 1970;**45**:13.)

above normal adult levels for up to 4 years thereafter. Insulin resistance intensifies in adolescents with insulin-dependent diabetes mellitus; this may be partly related to the increased GH levels.

Endocrine Changes From Fetal Life to Puberty

Gonadotropin secretion is caused by the hypothalamus releasing pulses of gonadotropin-releasing hormone (GnRH) into the pituitary-portal system so that it can reach the anterior pituitary gland. Control of GnRH secretion is exerted by a "hypothalamic pulse generator" in the arcuate nucleus that is sensitive to feedback control from sex steroids and inhibin, and that varies the frequency and amplitude of gonadotropin secretion during development in both sexes and during the progression of the menstrual cycle in females (see Chapter 6).

In males, luteinizing hormone (LH) stimulates the Leydig cells to secrete testosterone, while follicle-stimulating hormone (FSH) stimulates the Sertoli cells to produce a peptide called inhibin, which in turn feeds back and inhibits FSH. In females, FSH stimulates the granulosa cells to produce estrogen and the follicles to secrete inhibin, while LH appears to play little role

until menarche when it triggers ovulation and later stimulates the theca cells to secrete androgens and their precursors (see Chapter 17).

A. Fetal Life: The concept of the continuum of development between the fetus and the adult is well illustrated by the changes that occur in the hypothalamic-pituitary-gonadal axis. Gonadotropins are demonstrable in fetal pituitary glands during the first trimester, and serum FSH and LH can be measured by 12 weeks of gestation. The pituitary content of gonadotropins rises to a plateau at mid gestation. Serum concentrations of LH and FSH increase to a peak at mid gestation and then gradually decrease until term. During the first half of gestation, hypothalamic GnRH content also increases and the hypophyseal-portal circulation achieves anatomic maturity. These data are compatible with a general theory of early unrestrained GnRH secretion stimulating pituitary gonadotropin secretion, followed by the appearance of factors that inhibit GnRH release and decrease gonadotropin secretion at mid gestation. Since male fetuses have measurable serum testosterone concentrations but have lower serum gonadotropin concentrations than female fetuses, negative feedback inhibition of gonadotropin secretion by testosterone appears operative after mid gestation.

B. Changes at Birth: At term, plasma gonadotropin concentrations are suppressed, but with postnatal clearing of high circulating estrogen concentrations, negative inhibition is reduced and postnatal peaks of LH and FSH are measurable several months after birth. Testosterone concentrations may be elevated for several months after birth in males; early to mid pubertal plasma concentrations of testosterone have been documented. While episodic peaks of plasma gonadotropins may occur until 2 years of age, serum gonadotropin concentrations are low during later years in normal childhood.

C. Mid Childhood Nadir of Gonadotropin Secretion: Patients with gonadal failure—such as in the syndrome of gonadal dysgenesis (Turner's syndrome)—demonstrate an exaggeration of the normal pattern of gonadotropin secretion, with exceedingly high concentrations of LH and FSH during the first 2–4 years of life (see Chapter 18). Such patients show that negative feedback inhibition is active during childhood; without sex steroid secretion to exert inhibition, gonadotropin values are greatly elevated. Absence of inhibin probably also allows elevated FSH values in such patients. During mid childhood, healthy individuals and patients with primary hypogonadism have lower gonadotropin levels than they did in the neonatal period, but the range of gonadotropin concentrations in hypogonadal patients during mid childhood is still higher than that found in healthy children of the same age. The decrease in gonadotropin concentrations in hypogonadal children during mid childhood is incompletely understood but has been attributed to an increasing central nervous system inhibition of gonadotropin secretion during these years. (See Fig 19–11.)

D. Peripubertal Gonadotropin Increase: During the peripubertal period of endocrine change prior to secondary sexual development, gonadotropin secretion becomes less sensitive to negative feedback inhibition. Before this time a small dose of sex steroids virtually eliminates gonadotropin secretion, while afterward a far larger dose is required to suppress FSH and LH. A parallel situation occurs with opioid control of gonadotropin secretion; in prepuberty or early puberty, naltrexone, an opiate receptor antagonist, can completely suppress gonadotropin secretion due to its weak opioid effects, while after mid puberty the antiopioid effects predominate and gonadotropin secretion increases. This indicates that gonadotropin secretion is exquisitely sensitive to opiates in prepuberty or early puberty but less sensitive later. In the peripubertal period, endogenous GnRH secretion increases in amplitude and frequency during the early hours of sleep; testosterone levels rise several hours later in boys and suppress gonadotropin secretion, apparently by decreasing GnRH pulse frequency (Fig 19–5). As puberty progresses in both sexes, the peaks of LH and FSH occur more often during waking hours, and, finally, in late puberty, the peaks occur at all times. Thus, daytime samples of plasma for gonadotropin concentrations are of less value during early puberty because such sampling misses these nighttime peaks.

Most studies on gonadotropin secretion measured the gonadotropin concentrations by radioimmunoassay (RIA). However, the biologic activity of LH may change because of changes in the glycosylation and tertiary structure of gonadotropin molecules; this change may not be reflected in the RIA. Recent studies comparing immunoassayable LH (I-LH) to bioassayable LH (B-LH) suggest that the ratio of B-LH:I-LH increases with the onset of puberty and that this ratio may explain the profound endocrine changes of puberty better than the rather small changes in I-LH secretion. The full implications of this phenomenon are not yet known, and some of the B-LH:I-LH ratios obtained result from the chosen radioimmunoassay standards. Many investigators believe, however, that the measurement of biologic LH is important in the understanding of the onset of puberty.

E. Sex Steroid Secretion: Sex steroid secretion is correlated with the development of gonadotropin secretion. During the postnatal period of episodic gonadotropin secretion, plasma concentrations of gonadal steroids are occasionally elevated. This indicates the potential for secretory activity in the neonatal gonad. Later, when gonadotropin secretion decreases in mid childhood, gonadal activity decreases, but testes can still be stimulated by LH or hCG and ovaries by FSH, with resulting secretion of gonadal steroids. With the onset of puberty, plasma gonadal steroid concentrations progressively increase (Fig 19–6). While sex steroids are secreted in a diurnal rhythm in early puberty because they are bound to sex hormone-binding globulin, the half-life of sex steroids is longer than gonadotropins, so random daytime measurements of sex steroids are more helpful in determining pubertal status than similar samples for gonadotropins.

Most (97–99%) of the circulating estradiol and testosterone is associated with sex hormone-binding globulin (SHBG). The free hormone is the active fraction, but SHBG modulates the activity of the total testosterone and estradiol. Boys and girls have equal concentrations of SHBG, but because testosterone decreases SHBG and estrogen increases it, adult men have only half the concentration of SHBG that adult women have. Thus, SHBG amplifies the androgen effect in men; while adult men have 20 times the amount of plasma testosterone that adult women have, men have 40 times the amount of free testosterone (see Chapter 16).

F. GnRH Stimulation: The use of intravenous GnRH has further clarified the pattern of pubertal development (Fig 19–7). When GnRH is administered to children under 2 years of age, pituitary secretion of LH and FSH increases markedly. During the period of low basal gonadotropin secretion (age 2 to age 9 or 10 years), exogenous GnRH has less effect on LH release. By the peripubertal period, 100 μg of intravenous GnRH induces a rise in LH concentrations of greater than 15.6 mIU/ML* in boys and girls, and this response continues until adulthood. There is no signifi-

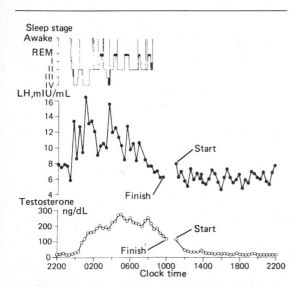

Figure 19–5. Plasma LH and testosterone measured during a 24-hour period in a 14-year-old boy in pubertal stage 2. Samples collected at night are displayed with electroencephalographic sleep stages. (Reproduced, with permission, from Boyar RM et al: *J Clin Invest* 1974;**54**:609.)

*This would be reported as 2 ng/mL (LER 960) in some laboratories. See Fig 19–6 legend.

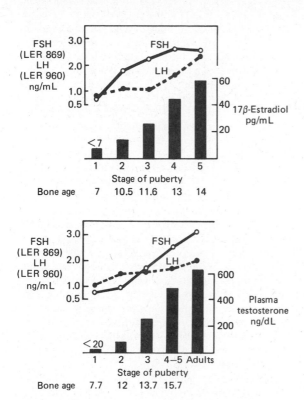

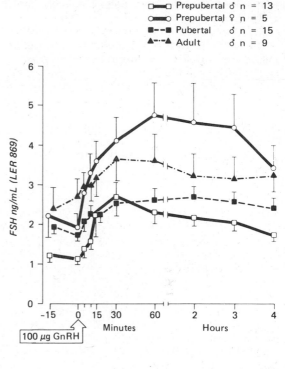

Figure 19–6. Mean plasma LH, FSH, and estradiol (girls) or testosterone (boys) correlated with stage of puberty and bone age. LER 869 and LER 960 are the reference standards for FSH and LH, respectively. The values reported here in ng/mL would be reported as mIU/mL in most laboratories. The conversion factors are as follows: for FSH (LER 869), 1 ng = 3 mIU; for LH (LER 960), 1 ng = 7.8 mIU. (Reproduced, with permission, from Grumbach MM: Onset of puberty. In: *Puberty*. Berenberg SR [editor]. H.E. Stenfert Kroese. Copyright © 1975 by Martinus Nijhoff.)

cant change in the magnitude of FSH secretion after GnRH with the onset of puberty, although females at all ages release more FSH than males.

Gonadotropins are released in secretory spurts in response to endogenous GnRH, which itself is secreted episodically about every 90–120 minutes in response to a central nervous system "pulse generator." GnRH has been administered to patients in boluses every 90 minutes, mimicking the natural secretory episodes. A prepubertal subject without significant gonadotropin peaks in the basal state will demonstrate the normal pubertal pattern of episodic secretion of gonadotropins after only a few days of GnRH boluses. Hypogonadotropic patients, who in the basal state do not have secretory episodes of gonadotropin release, have also been restored to normal episodic gonadotropin secretion and fertility by this method of pulsatile GnRH administration. Varying the timing of pulsatile GnRH administration can regulate the ratio of FSH to LH; the frequency of hypothalamic GnRH release shifts during the menstrual cycle and puberty to natu-

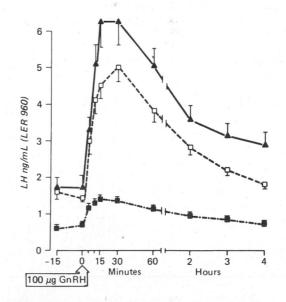

Figure 19–7. The changes in plasma FSH (**top**) and LH (**bottom**) after GnRH was administered in prepubertal, pubertal, and adult subjects. LER 869 and LER 960 are the reference standards for FSH and LH, respectively. See legend for Fig 19–6 for conversion of ng/mL to mIU/mL. (Reproduced, with permission, from Grumbach MM et al: *Control of the Onset of Puberty*. Grumbach MM, Grave GD, Mayer FE [editors]. Wiley, 1974.)

rally change the ratio. Increasing the frequency of GnRH pulses increases the LH:FSH ratio; an increased ratio is characteristic of midcycle and peripubertal dynamics. If GnRH is administered continuously rather than in pulses or if superactive analogues of GnRH are given, a brief period of increased gonadotropin secretion is followed by LH and FSH suppression.

Menarche

The last stage in hypothalamic-pituitary development is the onset of positive feedback. After mid puberty, estrogen can stimulate gonadotropin release. The frequency of pulsatile GnRH release increases during the normal menstrual cycle and raises the ratio of LH to FSH secretion. This stimulates the ovary to produce estrogen and leads to the midcycle LH surge. Even if the midcycle surge of gonadotropins is present, ovulation may not occur during the first menstrual cycles; 90% of all menstrual cycles are anovulatory in the first year after menarche, and it is not until 4–5 years after menarche that the percentage of anovulatory cycles decreases to less than 20%. In the USA, the mean age at menarche is 12.8 years (± 1.2 years SD). Menarche is closely correlated with a skeletal age of 13 years (see Chapter 8).

Adrenarche

While the hypothalamic-pituitary axis has been well characterized in recent years, our understanding of the mechanism of control of adrenal androgen secretion is still somewhat rudimentary. The adrenal cortex secretes the weak androgens dehydroepiandrosterone (DHEA), dehydroepiandrosterone sulfate (DHEAS), and androstenedione in increasing amounts at an average age of 6–7 years in girls and 7–8 years in boys (Table 19–1). A continued rise in adrenal androgen secretion persists until late puberty. Thus, adrenarche (the secretion of adrenal androgens) occurs years before gonadarche (the secretion of gonadal sex steroids). It is postulated that an adrenal androgen-stimulating hormone (AASH) secreted by the pituitary gland is responsible for adrenarche. An alternative explanation is that primary intra-adrenal changes modulate the release of androgens. The observation that patients with Addison's disease, who do not secrete adrenal androgens, and patients with premature adrenarche, who secrete increased amounts of adrenal androgens at an early age, usually enter gonadarche at a normal age suggests that age at adrenarche does not significantly influence age at gonadarche. Furthermore, patients treated with a GnRH agonist to suppress gonadotropin secretion progress through adrenarche despite their suppressed gonadarche. Measurements of urinary 17-ketosteroids reflect principally adrenal androgen secretion and not secretion of testosterone or its metabolites. Thus, urinary 17-ketosteroid levels rise considerably at adrenarche but less so at gonadarche.

Miscellaneous Metabolic Changes

The onset of puberty is associated with many changes in laboratory values that are either directly or indirectly caused by the rise in sex steroid concentrations. Thus, in boys, hematocrit rises and HDL concentration falls due to testosterone effects. In both boys and girls, alkaline phosphatase rises during the pubertal growth spurt, as does IGF-I; however, IGF-I is more closely correlated to sex steroid concentration than to growth rate. IGF-I levels peak 1 year after peak growth velocity is reached and remain elevated for 4 years thereafter even though growth rate is decreasing.

Table 19–1. Mean serum concentrations of DHEAS during childhood.[1]

	Boys		Girls	
	(µg/dL)	(µmol/L)	(µg/dL)	(µmol/L)
Chronologic age (years)				
1–6	15.4 ± 6.8	0.53 ± 0.23	24.7 ± 11.1	0.86 ± 0.38
6–8	18.8 ± 4.1	0.65 ± 0.14	30.4 ± 7.6	1.05 ± 0.26
8–10	58.6 ± 10.1	2.03 ± 0.35	117.3 ± 41.7	4.06 ± 1.44
10–12	126.4 ± 28.0	4.38 ± 0.97	112.7 ± 16.4	3.90 ± 0.57
12–14	133.4 ± 22.2	4.62 ± 0.77	168.9 ± 19.3	5.85 ± 0.67
14–16	264.3 ± 19.4	9.15 ± 0.67	253.5 ± 41.3	8.78 ± 1.43
16–20	264.1 ± 61.8	9.14 ± 2.14	232.5 ± 49.8	8.05 ± 1.72
Bone age (years)				
1–6	16.6 ± 6.1	0.57 ± 0.21	2.5 ± 2.5	0.09 ± 0.09
6–8	36.3 ± 6.7	1.25 ± 0.23	27.2 ± 9.6	0.94 ± 0.33
8–10	57.4 ± 8.5	1.98 ± 0.29	. . .	. . .
10–12	125.0 ± 22.7	4.33 ± 0.79	112.9 ± 27.6	3.91 ± 0.96
12–14	214.9 ± 30.1	7.44 ± 1.04	159.7 ± 26.3	5.53 ± 0.91
14–16	403.4 ± 99.4	14.00 ± 3.44	261.0 ± 45.0	9.04 ± 1.56
16–20	. . .	. . .	145.3 ± 32.2	5.03 ± 1.12

[1]Modified and reproduced, with permission, from Reiter EO, Fuldauer LG, Root AW: *J Pediatr* 1977;**90**:766.

DELAYED PUBERTY
OR ABSENT PUBERTY
(Sexual Infantilism)

Any girl of 13 or boy of 14 years of age with no signs of pubertal development falls more than 2.5 SD below the mean and is considered to have delayed puberty (Table 19–2). By this definition, 0.6% of the healthy population are classified as having constitutional delay in growth and adolescence. These patients need reassurance rather than treatment and will ultimately progress through the normal stages of puberty, albeit later than their peers. The examining physician must decide which patients are constitutionally delayed and which truly have organic disease. In some cases this is a difficult decision.

Constitutional Delay in Growth & Adolescence

A patient with delayed onset of secondary sexual development who has a history of always being shorter than age-matched peers but who consistently maintains a normal growth velocity for bone age and whose skeletal development is more than 2 SD less than the mean is likely to have constitutional delay in puberty (Fig 19–8). There is often a family history of a similar pattern in a parent or sibling. The subject is usually thin. These patients are at the older end of the distribution curve of age at onset of puberty. In many cases, even if they show no physical signs of puberty at the time of examination, the initial elevation of gonadal sex steroids has already begun, or their plasma LH response to intravenous GnRH is pubertal (a rise in LH of > 15.6 mIU/mL). These results suggest that sec-

Table 19–2. Classification of delayed puberty.

Constitutional delay in growth and adolescence
Hypogonadotropic hypogonadism
  Central nervous system disorders
    Tumors
    Other acquired disorders
    Congenital disorders
  Isolated gonadotropin deficiency
  Multiple pituitary hormonal deficiencies
  Miscellaneous disorders
    Prader-Willi syndrome
    Laurence-Moon-Biedl syndrome
    Chronic disease
    Weight loss
    Anorexia nervosa
    Increased physical activity in female athletes
    Hypothyroidism
Hypergonadotropic hypogonadism
  Klinefelter's syndrome
  Other forms of primary testicular failure
  Anorchia or cryptorchidism
  Turner's syndrome
  Other forms of primary ovarian failure
  Pseudo-Turner's syndrome
  XX and XY gonadal dysgenesis

---

ondary sexual development will commence within 6 months. However, in some cases, observation for endocrine or physical signs of puberty must continue for a period of months or years before the diagnosis is made. Generally, signs of puberty will appear after the patient reaches a skeletal age of 11 years (girls) or 12 years (boys). Patients with constitutional delay in adolescence will almost always manifest secondary sexual development by 18 years of chronologic age, although there is one reported case of spontaneous puberty occurring at 25 years of age (this patient may have had Kallmann's syndrome [see below and Chapter 6]). Adrenarche is characteristically delayed, along with gonadarche.

Hypogonadotropic Hypogonadism

The absent or decreased ability of the hypothalamus to secrete GnRH or of the pituitary to secrete LH and FSH leads to hypogonadotropic hypogonadism. This classification denotes an irreversible condition requiring replacement therapy. If the deficiency is limited to gonadotropins, patients are usually close to normal height for age, in contrast to the shorter patients with constitutional delay. Of course, if GH deficiency accompanies gonadotropin deficiency, severe short stature will result.

A. Central Nervous System Disorders:

1. Tumors–A tumor involving the hypothalamus or pituitary gland can interfere with hypothalamic-pituitary-gonadal function as well as the control of GH, ACTH, TSH, PRL, and vasopressin secretion. Thus, delayed puberty may be a manifestation of a central nervous system tumor accompanied by any or all of the following: GH deficiency, secondary hypothyroidism, secondary adrenal insufficiency, hyperprolactinemia, and diabetes insipidus. The combination of anterior and posterior pituitary deficiencies acquired after birth indicates the likelihood of a hypothalamic-pituitary tumor.

Craniopharyngioma is the most common type of hypothalamic-pituitary tumor leading to delay or absence of pubertal development. This neoplasm originates in Rathke's pouch but may develop into a suprasellar tumor. The peak age incidence of craniopharyngioma is between 6 and 14 years. Presenting symptoms may include headache, visual deficiency, growth failure, polyuria, and polydipsia; presenting signs may include visual defects, optic atrophy or papilledema, and clinical manifestations of gonadotropin, thyroid, and GH deficiency. Laboratory evaluation may reveal any type of anterior or posterior pituitary deficiencies. Bone age may be retarded at the time of presentation.

Calcification in the suprasellar region is the hallmark of craniopharyngiomas; 80% of cases will have calcifications on lateral skull x-ray, and a higher percentage will show this on CT or MRI scan. The tumor often presents a cystic appearance on CT or MRI scan

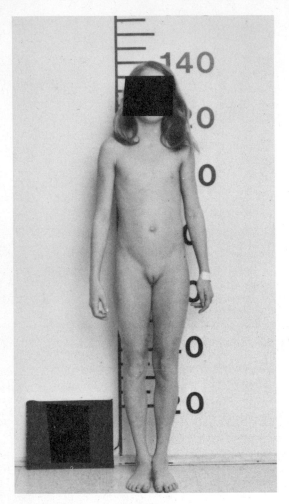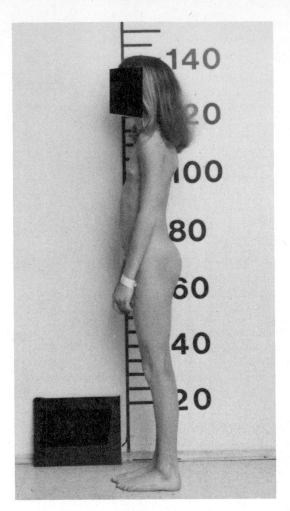

Figure 19–8. Girl 13⁴⁄₁₂ years old with constitutional delay in growth and puberty. History revealed a normal growth rate but short stature at all ages. Physical examination revealed a height of 138 cm (−4.5 SD) and a weight of 28.6 kg (−3 SD). The patient had early stage 2 breast development, with 1 cm of glandular tissue on the right breast and 2 cm on the left breast. The vaginal mucosa was dulled, and there was no pubic hair. Karyotype was 46,XX. Bone age was 10 years. After administration of GnRH, LH rose from 14.8 to 37.4 mIU/mL and FSH from 11.7 to 20.1 mIU/mL. Estradiol was 40 pg/mL. She has since spontaneously progressed through pubertal development. (Reproduced, with permission, from Styne DM, Kaplan SL: *Pediatr Clin North Am* 1979;**26**:123.)

and at the time of surgery may contain dark, cholesterol-laden fluid. The rate of growth of craniopharyngiomas is quite variable, with some indolent and some quite aggressive. Small intrasellar tumors may be resected by transsphenoidal surgery; larger ones are best treated by partial resection and radiation therapy (see Chapter 6).

Extrasellar tumors that involve the hypothalamus and produce sexual infantilism include germinomas, gliomas (sometimes with neurofibromatosis), and astrocytomas (see Chapter 6). Intrasellar tumors such as chromophobe adenomas are quite rare in children. Hyperprolactinemia, with or without a diagnosed microadenoma or galactorrhea, may delay the onset or pro-

gression of puberty; with therapy to decrease prolactin concentrations, puberty progresses.

2. Other acquired central nervous system disorders–Other acquired central nervous system disorders may lead to hypothalamic-pituitary dysfunction. Hand-Schüller-Christian disease (histiocytosis X), when involving the hypothalamus, most frequently leads to diabetes insipidus, but any other hypothalamic defect may also occur. Tuberculous or sarcoid granulomas, other postinfectious inflammatory lesions, vascular lesions, and trauma more rarely cause hypogonadotropic hypogonadism.

3. Developmental defects–Developmental defects of the central nervous system may cause hypogonadotropic hypogonadism or other types of hypothalamic dysfunction. Optic dysplasia is associated with small, hypoplastic optic disks and, in some patients, absence of the septum pellucidum on pneumoencephalography or CT or MRI scanning; associated hypothalamic deficiencies are often present. Optic hypoplasia or dysplasia must be differentiated from optic atrophy; optic atrophy implies an acquired condition and may indicate a hypothalamic-pituitary tumor. Both anterior and posterior pituitary deficiencies may occur with congenital midline defects. Early onset of such a combination suggests a congenital defect, while late onset more strongly indicates a neoplasm. Cleft palate or other midline anomalies may also be associated with hypothalamic dysfunction.

4. Radiation therapy—Central nervous system radiation therapy involving the hypothalamic-pituitary area can lead to hypogonadotropic hypogonadism with onset at 6–18 months (or sometimes longer) after treatment. Growth hormone secretion is more frequently affected than gonadotropin secretion.

B. Isolated Hormonal Deficiency: Patients who have isolated deficiency of gonadotropins but normal GH secretion tend to be of normal height for age. They will have eunuchoid proportions of increased span for height and decreased upper to lower segment ratios. Their skeletal development will be delayed for chronologic age during the teenage years.

Kallmann's syndrome is the most common form of isolated gonadotropin deficiency (Fig 19–9). Gonadotropin deficiency in these patients is associated with hypoplasia or aplasia of the olfactory lobes and hyposmia or anosmia; remarkably, they may not notice that they have no sense of smell, although olfactory testing will reveal it. This is a familial syndrome of variable manifestations in which anosmia may occur with or without hypogonadism in a given member of a kindred. Associated abnormalities in Kallmann's syndrome may affect the kidneys and bones, and patients may have undescended testes, gynecomastia, and obesity. Ultimate height is normal, although patients are delayed in reaching adult height and so are shorter

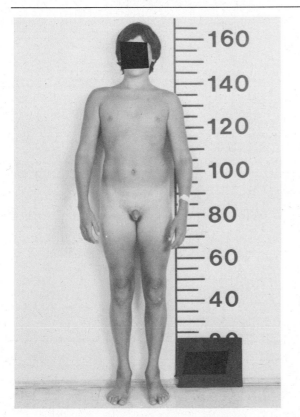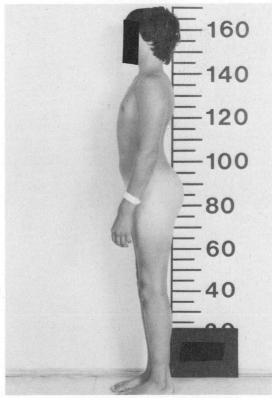

Figure 19–9. Boy 15^{10}/$_{12}$ years old with Kallmann's syndrome. His testes were originally undescended, but they descended into the scrotum after human chorionic gonadotropin treatment was given. His height was 163.9 cm (−1.5 SD), and the upper to lower segment ratio was 0.86 (eunuchoid). The penis was 6.3 × 1.8 cm. Each testis was 1 × 2 cm. Plasma LH was not detectable and rose to 5.5 mIU/mL after administration of 100 μg of GnRH; FSH rose from 3.6 mIU/mL to 7.2 mIU/mL. Testosterone did not change from 17 ng/dL. He had no ability to smell standard odors. (Reproduced, with permission, from Styne DM, Grumbach MM: *Reproductive Endocrinology.* Yen SSC, Jaffe RB [editors]. Saunders, 1978.)

than peers until the late teenage years. Kallmann's syndrome was at first believed to have an X-linked inheritance pattern, but recent reports show autosomal dominant patterns with variable penetrance.

Other cases of hypogonadotropic hypogonadism may occur sporadically or via an autosomal recessive pattern without anosmia. X-linked congenital adrenal hypoplasia is associated with hypogonadotropic hypogonadism; glycerol kinase deficiency and muscular dystrophy have also been linked to this syndrome. Some hypogonadal patients lack only LH secretion and have spermatogenesis without testosterone production (fertile eunuch syndrome); others lack only FSH.

C. Idiopathic Hypopituitary Dwarfism: Patients with congenital GH deficiency have early onset of growth failure (Fig 19–10); this feature separates them from patients with GH deficiency due to hypothalamic tumors, who usually have late onset of growth failure. Even without associated gonadotropin deficiency, untreated GH-deficient patients often have delayed onset of puberty associated with their delayed bone ages. With appropriate hGH therapy, however, onset of puberty occurs at a normal age. Patients who have combined GH and gonadotropin deficiency do not undergo puberty even when bone age reaches the pubertal stage.

Idiopathic hypopituitarism is usually sporadic but may follow an autosomal recessive or X-linked inheritance pattern. Birth injury or breech delivery is a common feature of the neonatal history of patients with idiopathic hypopituitarism.

The syndrome of microphallus (due to congenital gonadotropin deficiency) and neonatal hypoglycemic seizures (due to congenital ACTH deficiency, GH deficiency, or both) must be diagnosed and treated early to avoid mental retardation. Patients with this syndrome will not undergo spontaneous pubertal development. Testosterone in low doses (testosterone enanthate, 25 mg intramuscularly every month for 3 doses), can increase the size of the penis in infants diagnosed with congenital hypopituitarism without significantly advancing bone age. Males with isolated GH deficiency can also have microphallus; the penis will enlarge to some degree with hGH therapy in these patients. It is important to note that microphallus due to hypopituitarism is medically treatable, and sex reversal usually need not be considered (see Chapter 18).

D. Miscellaneous Disorders:

1. Prader-Willi syndrome—Prader-Willi syndrome occurs sporadically and is associated with fetal and infantile hypotonia, short stature, massive obesity, characteristic facies, small hands and feet, mental retardation, and emotional instability in patients of either sex, delayed menarche in females, and micropenis and cryptorchidism in males. In about 50% of patients, the syndrome has been associated with deletion or translocation of chromosome 15. Osteoporosis is common in these patients during the teenage years. Behavioral

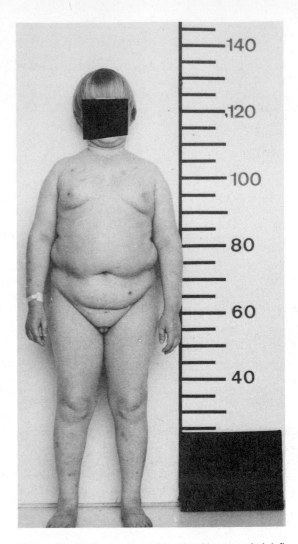

Figure 19–10. Twenty-year-old male with congenital deficiency of GH, GnRH, TSH, and ACTH. Height was 8 SD below the mean, and the phallus was 2 × 1 cm. Bone age was 10 years, and the sella turcica was small on lateral skull x-ray. LH was 1.6 mIU/mL and rose only to 4.7 mIU/mL after administration of 100 μg of GnRH. Testosterone was less than 10 ng/dL and did not rise after administration of GnRH. (Reproduced, with permission, from Styne DM, Grumbach MM: *Reproductive Endocrinology.* Yen SSC, Jaffe RB [editors]. Saunders, 1978.)

modification may improve the usual pattern of rampant weight gain.

2. Laurence-Moon-Biedl syndrome—This autosomal recessive condition is characterized by polydactyly, obesity, short stature, mental retardation, and retinitis pigmentosa. Hypogonadotropic hypogonadism or primary hypogonadism have variously been reported in affected patients.

3. Chronic disease and malnutrition—A delay in sexual maturation may be due to chronic disease or malnutrition. For example, children with severe asthma have delayed pubertal development leading to short stature during the teenage years; studies have shown that in general they ultimately reach an appropriate height. Children with other chronic disease may not fare so well in long-term follow-up. Weight loss to less than 80% of ideal weight caused by disease or voluntary dieting may result in gonadotropin deficiency; weight gain toward the ideal usually restores gonadotropin function. Delayed puberty and short stature have been reported to occur in healthy individuals who voluntarily diet because of "fear of obesity" (see Chapter 8).

4. Anorexia nervosa–Anorexia nervosa involves weight loss associated with significant psychologic disorder. Patients are usually girls who have a disturbed body image, avoid food, and often induce regurgitation after ingestion. Weight loss may be so severe as to cause a fatal complication such as immune dysfunction, fluid and electrolyte imbalance, or circulatory collapse. Primary or secondary amenorrhea is a classic finding in these patients and has been correlated with the degree of weight loss, although evidence exists that patients with anorexia nervosa may cease to menstruate before their substantial weight loss. Other endocrine abnormalities occur in anorexia nervosa such as elevated growth hormone, decreased somatomedin, decreased triiodothyronine, decreased 1,25 OH vitamin D, and elevated 24,25 OH vitamin D levels. Weight gain to the normal range for height, however, does not ensure immediate resumption of menses. There appears to be an increased incidence of anorexia nervosa in ballet dancers or students; the incidence of scoliosis and mitral valve insufficiency is also increased in these patients. Functional amenorrhea may also occur in women of normal weight, some of whom demonstrate evidence of psychologic stress. The interpretation of gonadotropin data in amenorrhea may be difficult. If the women retains the prepubertal pattern on nighttime sampling or the GnRH test, hypogonadotropic hypogonadism may be obvious. However, even if the GnRH test shows a normal pubertal pattern, cyclicity over the whole month may still be abnormal. The retention of a diurnal rhythm of gonadotropin secretion is another abnormality found in anorexia nervosa patients.

5. Increased physical activity–Girls who regularly participate in strenuous athletics, ballet dancing, etc, may have delayed thelarche, delayed menarche, and irregular or absent menstrual periods; this effect is not always related to less than ideal weight. It was reported that one patient resumed menses while she was temporarily bedridden.

6. Hypothyroidism–Hypothyroidism can delay all aspects of growth and maturation, including puberty and menarche. Conversely, severe hypothyroidism may advance the age at onset of pubertal signs in some patients (Van Wyk-Grumbach syndrome); galactor-

rhea may also occur in such patients. With thyroxine therapy, catch-up growth and resumed pubertal development and menses will occur.

Hypergonadotropic Hypogonadism

Primary gonadal failure is heralded by elevated gonadotropins due to the absence of negative feedback effects of gonadal sex steroids. The most common causes of hypergonadotropic hypogonadism are associated with karyotypic and somatic abnormalities, but isolated gonadal failure can also present with delayed puberty without other physical findings.

A. Syndrome of Seminiferous Tubule Dysgenesis (Klinefelter's Syndrome): (See Chapters 16 and 18.) The most common form of primary testicular failure is Klinefelter's syndrome (47,XXY karyotype), with an incidence of 1:1000 males. Before puberty, patients have decreased upper to lower segment ratios, increased arm span, small testes, and an increased incidence of mental retardation and personality disorders. Onset of puberty is not usually delayed, because Leydig cell function is characteristically less affected than seminiferous tubule function. Gonadotropin levels rise after the onset of puberty; the testes become firm and are rarely larger than 3.5 cm in diameter. After the onset of puberty, there are histologic changes of seminiferous tubule hyalinization and fibrosis, adenomatous changes of the Leydig cells, and impaired spermatogenesis. Gynecomastia is common, and variable degrees of male secondary sexual development are found.

Other forms of male hypergonadotropic hypogonadism are found with 46,XX/47,XXY, 48,XXYY, 48,XXXY, and 49,XXXXY karyotypes. Phenotypic males have been described with 46,XX karyotypes and some physical features of Klinefelter's syndrome.

B. Other Forms of Primary Testicular Failure: Those surviving treatment for malignant diseases form a growing category of patients with testicular failure. Chemotherapy, primarily with alkylating agents, or radiation therapy directed to the testes often leads to testicular failure; injury is more likely if the treatment is given during puberty than if it occurs in the prepubertal period. Theoretically, the use of GnRH agonists to revert the pubertal state to prepuberty may prevent testicular damage during such treatment for malignancy. The "Sertoli cell only" syndrome (germinal cell aplasia) is a congenital form of testicular failure with azoospermia and elevated FSH levels but generally normal secondary sexual characteristics, normal testosterone concentrations, and no other anomalies. Patients with Down syndrome may have elevated LH and FSH levels even in the presence of normal testosterone levels, suggesting some element of primary gonadal failure.

C. Cryptorchidism or Anorchia: Phenotypic males with a 46,XY karyotype but no palpable testes have either cryptorchidism or anorchia. Cryptorchid males should produce a rise in testosterone levels 72 hours after 2000 units of chorionic gonadotropin is given intramuscularly, and the testes may descend during 2 weeks of treatment with 2000 units given 3 times a week. Patients with increased plasma testosterone levels in response to chorionic gonadotropin but no testicular descent have cryptorchidism; their testes should be surgically brought into the scrotum to decrease the likelihood of further testicular damage due to the elevated intra-abdominal temperature or undetected tumor formation. Cryptorchid testes may have congenital abnormalities, even if brought into the scrotum early in life. Furthermore, the descended testis in a unilaterally cryptorchid boy may itself show abnormal histology; such patients have a 69% incidence of decreased sperm counts and can be infertile even with early treatment of cryptorchidism. In addition, patients undergoing orchiopexy may sustain subtle damage to the vas deferens, leading to the later production of antibodies to sperm. This may result in infertility. The diagnosis of anorchia is more difficult; in a prepubertal boy the presence of normal basal gonadotropin levels suggests the presence of testicular tissue even if the testosterone response to hCG is low, while the presence of elevated gonadotropin levels without any testosterone response to hCG suggests anorchia. Except for absent testes, patients with anorchia have normal male genital development, including wolffian duct formation and müllerian duct regression. The testes were presumably present in early fetal life during sexual differentiation but degenerated after the 13th week of gestation for unknown reasons ("vanishing testes syndrome").

D. Syndrome of Gonadal Dysgenesis (Turner's Syndrome): (See Chapters 17 and 18.) 45,X gonadal dysgenesis is associated with short stature, female phenotype with sexual infantilism, and a chromatin-negative buccal smear. Patients have "streak" gonads consisting of fibrous tissue without germ cells. Other classic but variable phenotypic features include micrognathia, "fish" mouth, ptosis, low-set or deformed ears, a broad shieldlike chest, hypoplastic areolae, a short neck with low hairline and webbing (pterygium colli), short fourth metacarpals, cubitus valgus, structural anomalies of the kidney, extensive nevi, hypoplastic nails, and cardiovascular anomalies of the left side of the heart (most commonly coarctation of the aorta). The medical history of patients with gonadal dysgenesis will often reveal small size at birth, lymphedema of the extremities, and loose posterior cervical skin folds. (The terms Bonnevie-Ullrich syndrome and infant Turner's syndrome have been applied to this neonatal appearance.) Affected patients often have a history of frequent otitis media with conductive hearing loss. Patients have no pubertal growth spurt and reach a mean final height of 142 cm. Short stature is a classic feature of Turner's syndrome but not of other forms of hypergonadotropic hypogonadism that

occur without karyotypic abnormalities. GH function is normal in Turner's syndrome, and the cause of short stature is not known. However, preliminary studies suggest that hGH treatment may improve growth rate in certain affected girls (see Chapter 18). Pubic hair may appear late and is usually sparse in distribution; thus, adrenarche progresses in Turner's syndrome even in the absence of gonadarche.

Serum gonadotropin concentrations in Turner's syndrome are high between birth and age 4 years. They decrease toward the normal range in prepubertal patients and then rise to castrate levels after age 10 years. (See Fig 18–11.)

Sex chromatin-positive variants of gonadal dysgenesis include 45,X/46,XX, 45,X/47,XXX, and 45,X/46,XX/47,XXX mosaicism with chromatin-positive buccal smears. Patients with these karyotypes may resemble patients with the classic syndrome of gonadal dysgenesis, or they may have fewer manifestations and have normal or nearly normal female phenotypes. Streak gonad formation is not invariable; some patients have had secondary sexual development, and menarche and (rarely) even pregnancy have been reported. A few patients with Turner's syndrome have benefited from the new in vitro fertilization techniques. After exogenous hormonal preparation of the patient's uterus, a fertilized ovum (possibly her sister's ovum fertilized by the patient's male partner, or an extra fertilized ovum from another couple undergoing in vitro fertilization) can be introduced into the patient's uterus. This procedure has been successful in some patients, and studies of such cases have furthered the understanding of the normal process of fertility.

Sex chromatin-negative variants of the syndrome of gonadal dysgenesis have karyotypes revealing 45,X/46,XY mosaicism. Physical features vary; some patients have the features of classic Turner's syndrome, while others may have ambiguous genitalia or even the features of phenotypic males. Gonads are dysgenetic but vary from streak gonads to functioning testes. These patients are at risk for gonadoblastoma formation. Since gonadoblastomas may secrete androgens or estrogens, patients with a gonadoblastoma may virilize or feminize as though they had functioning gonads. Gonadoblastomas may demonstrate calcification on abdominal x-ray. Malignant germ cell tumors may arise in dysgenetic testes, and orchiectomy is generally indicated. In some mosaic patients with one intact X chromosome and one chromosomal fragment, it is difficult to determine whether the fragment is derived from an X chromosome or a Y chromosome; present research into appropriate markers for the chromosome or for the presence of testis-determining factor will probably allow the future diagnosis of patients at risk for such complications.

E. Other Forms of Primary Ovarian Failure: Ovaries appear to be more resistant to the chemotherapy used in the treatment of malignant disease than are testes. Nonetheless, ovarian failure can occur with such therapy; radiation damage is common if the ovaries are not "tacked" out of the path of the beam in abdominal radiation therapy. Premature menopause has also been described in otherwise healthy girls, possibly due to the presence of antiovarian antibodies. Patients with Addison's disease may have autoimmune oophoritis as well as adrenal failure. A sex steroid biosynthetic defect due to 17α-hydroxylase deficiency will be manifested as sexual infantilism and primary amenorrhea in a phenotypic female (regardless of genotype) with hypokalemia and hypertension.

F. Pseudo-Turner's Syndrome (Noonan's Syndrome, Ullrich's Syndrome, Male Turner's Syndrome): Pseudo-Turner's syndrome is associated with manifestations of Turner's syndrome such as webbed neck, ptosis, short stature, cubitus valgus, and lymphedema, but other clinical findings such as a normal karyotype, triangular-shaped facies, pectus excavatum, right-sided heart disease, and an increased incidence of mental retardation should differentiate these patients from those with Turner's syndrome. Males may have undescended testes and variable degrees of germinal cell and Leydig cell dysfunction. Pseudo-Turner's syndrome follows an autosomal dominant pattern of inheritance with incomplete penetrance.

G. Familial and Sporadic Forms of 46,XX or 46,XY Gonadal Dysgenesis: These forms of gonadal dysgenesis are characterized by structurally normal chromosomes and streak gonads or partially functioning gonads. If there is some gonadal function, 46,XY gonadal dysgenesis may present with ambiguous genitalia or virilization at puberty. If no gonadal function is present, patients appear as phenotypic sexually infantile females. Patients with 46,XY gonadal dysgenesis and dysgenetic testes should undergo gonadectomy to eliminate the possibility of malignant germ cell tumor formation.

H. Primary Amenorrhea Associated With Normal Secondary Sexual Development: If a structural anomaly of the uterus or vagina interferes with the onset of menses but the endocrine milieu remains normal, the patient presents with primary amenorrhea in the presence of normal breast and pubic hair devel-

opment. A transverse vaginal septum will seal the uterine cavity from the vaginal orifice, leading to the retention of menstrual flow. An imperforate hymen, which develops from other embryonic abnormalities, can also cause primary amenorrhea. The Rokitansky-Küster-Hauser syndrome combines congenital absence of the vagina with abnormal development of the uterus, ranging from a rudimentary bicornuate uterus that may not open into the vaginal canal to a virtually normal uterus; surgical repair may be possible in those patients with abnormalities toward the normal end of the spectrum, and fertility has been reported. Associated abnormalities include major urinary tract anomalies and spinal or other skeletal disorders. The rarest anatomic abnormality in this group is the absence of the uterine cervix in the presence of a functional uterus.

Male pseudohermaphroditism is an alternative cause for amenorrhea in the presence of at least thelarche. The syndrome of complete androgen resistance leads to female genitalia and phenotype without axillary or pubic hair development in the presence of pubertal breast development (syndrome of testicular feminization; see Chapter 18).

Differential Diagnosis of Delayed Puberty (Table 19–3)

Young people who do not begin secondary sexual development by age 13 (girls) or age 14 (boys) and patients who do not progress through development on a timely basis (girls should menstruate within 5 years after breast budding; boys should reach stage 5 pubertal development 4½ years after onset) may have some form of hypogonadism.

If the diagnosis is not obvious on the basis of physical or historical features, the differential diagnostic process begins with determination of whether plasma gonadotropins are (1) elevated owing to primary gonadal failure or (2) decreased owing to secondary or tertiary hypogonadism or constitutional delayed puberty. If plasma gonadotropins are low, the differential diagnosis is between hypogonadotropic hypo-

Table 19–3. Differential diagnosis of delayed puberty.

	Serum Gonadotropins	Serum Gonadal Steroids	Miscellaneous
Constitutional delay in growth and adolescence	Prepubertal (low)	Low	Patient usually has short stature for chronologic age but appropriate height and growth rate for bone age. Adrenarche and gonadarche are delayed.
Hypogonadotropic hypogonadism	Prepubertal (low)	Low	Patient may have anosmia (Kallmann's syndrome) or other associated pituitary hormone deficiencies. If gonadotropin deficiency is isolated, patient usually has normal height and growth rate. Adrenarche may be normal in spite of absent gonadarche (serum DHEA sulfate may be pubertal).
Hypergonadotropic hypogonadism	Elevated	Low	Patient may have abnormal karyotype and stigmas of Turner's or Klinefelter's syndrome.

gonadism and constitutionally delayed puberty. A patient with constitutional delay may have a characteristic history of short stature for age with normal growth velocity for bone age and a family history of delayed but spontaneous puberty. The patient's mother may have had late onset of menses, or the father may have begun to shave late. Not all patients with constitutional delay are classic, and gonadotropin-deficient patients may have some features similar to those of constitutional delay in adolescence. The determination of rise in LH after administration of GnRH is helpful in differential diagnosis; secondary sexual development usually follows within 6 months of conversion to a pubertal LH response to luteinizing hormone-releasing factor. Frequent nighttime sampling (every 20 minutes through an indwelling catheter) for peaks of LH secretion during sleep is an alternative to GnRH testing. Unfortunately, the results of GnRH infusions or nighttime sampling are not always so straightforward. Patients may have pubertal responses to exogenous GnRH but not spontaneously secrete adequate gonadotropins in time to allow secondary sexual development. In females with amenorrhea, the frequency and amplitude of gonadotropin secretion may not change to allow monthly menstrual cycles. Studies have also suggested that the retention of a diurnal rhythm of gonadotropin secretion (normal in early puberty) into late puberty interferes with pubertal progression. Other methods of differential diagnosis between constitutional delay and hypogonadotropic hypogonadism have been proposed but are complex or are not definitive because the response between the 2 groups overlaps; eg, most patients with hypogonadotropic hypogonadism have lower prolactin concentrations after protirelin or chlorpromazine administration than do patients with constitutional delay. Prior infusion of GnRH or hCG with a GnRH test or the use of a potent GnRH agonist instead of native GnRH for a challenge test have also been proposed, but again results have not yet been consistent enough for clinical use.

Clinical observation for signs of pubertal development and laboratory evaluation for the onset of rising levels of sex steroids may have to continue until the patient is 18 years of age or older before the diagnosis is definite. In most cases, if spontaneous pubertal development is not noted by 18 years of age, the diagnosis is gonadotropin deficiency. Of course, the presence of neurologic impairment or other endocrine deficiency should immediately lead to investigation for central nervous system tumor or congenital defect in a patient with delayed puberty. CT or MRI scanning may be helpful in this situation.

Treatment of Delayed Puberty

A. Constitutional Delay in Growth and Adolescence:

1. Psychologic support—Patients with constitutional delay in growth and adolescence should be counseled that normal pubertal development will oc-

cur spontaneously. Peer pressure and teasing can be oppressive. Severe depression must be treated seriously, since short patients with pubertal delay have become suicidal. In some cases it helps to excuse the patient from physical education class, as the lack of development is most apparent in the locker room and the brunt of teasing occurs during such a situation.

2. Sex steroids—The teenager who is so embarrassed about his or her short stature and lack of sexual development as to have significant psychologic problems may require special help. The following treatment can be given: (1) for girls, a 3-month course of conjugated estrogen (0.3 mg) or ethinyl estradiol (5–10 μg) given orally each day for 21 days a month; or (2) for boys, a 3-month course of testosterone enanthate (100 mg) given intramuscularly once every 28 days. This treatment will elicit gratifyingly noticeable secondary sexual development and a slight increase in stature. The low dose recommended has not significantly changed final height. Such low-dose sex steroid treatment may actually promote spontaneous pubertal development after it has been discontinued. The short course of therapy may also improve patients' psychologic outlook and allow them to await spontaneous pubertal development with greater ease. Continuous gonadal steroid replacement in these patients is not indicated, as it will advance bone age and lead to epiphyseal fusion and a decrease in ultimate stature.

B. Permanent Hypogonadism: Once a patient has been diagnosed with delayed puberty due to permanent hypogonadism, either primary or secondary, replacement therapy must be considered.

Males with hypogonadism may be treated with testosterone enanthate intramuscularly every month, gradually increasing the dosage from 100 to 300 mg a month. Frequent erections may occur if the higher dose is used initially but are less likely if the dose is built up over several months. Oral halogenated testosterone or methylated testosterone is usually not recommended because of the risk of hepatocellular carcinoma or cholestatic jaundice.

Testosterone therapy may not cause adequate pubic hair development but, in patients without primary hypogonadism, hCG supplements can increase pubic hair growth due to endogenous androgen secretion.

Therapy with oxandrolone has been suggested as a method of increasing secondary sexual development and increasing growth without advancing skeletal development; such claims have not been sufficient to differentiate oxandrolone therapy from that with low-dose testosterone. Furthermore, testosterone, which can be aromatized, increases the generally low endogenous growth hormone secretion in constitutional delayed puberty to normal, while oxandrolone, which cannot be aromatized, does not increase growth hormone secretion (see Chapter 16).

Females may be treated with ethinyl estradiol (increasing from 5 to 10–20 μg/d depending upon results) or conjugated estrogens (0.3–0.625 mg/d) on days 1–21, with 5 mg of medroxyprogesterone acetate added on days 12–21 after physical signs of estrogen effect are noted or breakthrough bleeding occurs. Neither hormone is administered from day 22 to the end of the month, to allow regular withdrawal bleeding (see Chapter 17).

C. Coexisting GH Deficiency: The treatment of patients with coexisting GH deficiency requires consideration of their bone age and amount of growth left before epiphyseal fusion; if they have not yet received adequate treatment with growth hormone, sex steroid therapy may be delayed to optimize final adult height.

Constitutional delayed puberty may be associated with decreased growth hormone secretion in 24-hour profiles of spontaneous secretion or in stimulated testing. Growth hormone secretion increases when pubertal development begins, so the condition should be considered temporary. Growth hormone therapy is not proven to increase final height in those patients with normal height predictions; some studies have shown an increased growth rate in the first year of such therapy with a decreasing growth rate thereafter. Nonetheless, true growth hormone-deficient patients may have delayed puberty due to the growth hormone deficiency or to coexisting gonadotropin deficiency. Therefore, deciding whether a pubertal patient has a temporary or a permanent GH deficiency can be difficult; previous growth rate and bone age progression may indicate a long history characteristic of constitutional delay in adolescence, while a recent decrease in growth rate may suggest the onset of a brain tumor.

D. Gonadal Dysgenesis: In the past, patients with the syndrome of gonadal dysgenesis were frequently not given estrogen replacement until after age 13 years, for fear of compromising final height. It has now been demonstrated that low-dose estrogen therapy (5–10 μg of ethinyl estradiol orally) can be used to allow feminization at 12–13 years of age without decreasing final height in these patients. Low-dose estrogen will increase growth velocity, while high-dose estrogen suppresses it; even if growth velocity is increased, however, final height is reportedly not increased with estrogen. Treatment of Turner's syndrome with GH appears to be more successful (see Chapter 18).

PRECOCIOUS PUBERTY (Sexual Precocity)

The appearance of secondary sexual development before the age of 8 years in girls and 9 years in boys is greater than 2.5 SD below the mean age at onset of puberty and constitutes precocious sexual development (Table 19–4). When the cause is premature activation of the hypothalamic-pituitary axis, the diagnosis is complete (true) precocious puberty; if ectopic gonadotropin secretion occurs in boys or autonomous sex steroid secretion occurs in either sex, the diagnosis

Table 19–4. Classification of precocious puberty.

Complete (true) precocious puberty
Constitutional
Idiopathic
Central nervous system disorders
Severe hypothyroidism
Following androgen exposure
Incomplete precocious puberty
Males
Gonadotropin-secreting tumors
Excessive androgen production
Premature Leydig and germinal cell maturation
Females
Ovarian cysts
Estrogen-secreting neoplasms
Sexual precocity due to gonadotropin or sex steroid exposure
Variation in pubertal development
Premature thelarche
Premature menarche
Premature pubarche
Adolescent gynecomastia

is incomplete precocious puberty. In all forms of sexual precocity, there is an increase in growth velocity, somatic development, and skeletal maturation. When unchecked, this rapid epiphyseal development may lead to tall stature during the early phases of the disorder but to short final stature because of early epiphyseal fusion. Plasma somatomedin values may be elevated for age in the untreated state.

Complete (True) Precocious Puberty (Fig 19–11)

A. Constitutional Complete (True) Precocious Puberty: Children who demonstrate isosexual precocity at an age more than 2.5 SD below the mean may simply represent the lower reaches of the distribution curve of age at onset of puberty; often there is a familial tendency toward early puberty. True precocious puberty may rarely be due to an autosomal recessive or (in males) sex-limited autosomal dominant trait.

B. Idiopathic Complete (True) Precocious Puberty: Affected children with no familial tendency toward early development and no organic disease may be considered to have idiopathic precocious puberty. Electroencephalographic abnormalities or other evidence of neurologic dysfunction may be found in these patients. Pubertal development may follow the normal course in these patients or may wax and wane. Gonadotropin and sex steroid concentrations and response to GnRH are similar to those found in normal pubertal subjects. In idiopathic true precocious puberty, as in all forms of true isosexual precocity, testicular enlargement in boys should be the first sign; in girls, either breast development or pubic hair appearance may be first. Girls present with idiopathic precocious puberty more commonly than boys.

C. Central Nervous System Disorders:
1. Tumors–Central nervous system tumor as a cause of precocious puberty is more common in boys

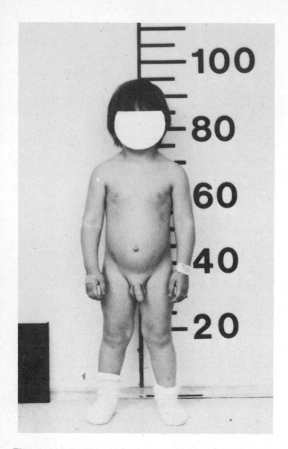

Figure 19–11. Boy 2⁵/₁₂ years of age with idiopathic true precocious puberty. By 10 months of age, he had pubic hair and phallic and testicular enlargement. At 1 year of age, his height was 4 SD above the mean; the phallus was 10 × 3.5 cm; each testis was 2.5 × 1.5 cm. Plasma LH was 14.8 mIU/mL and rose to 65.5 mIU/mL after administration of 100 μg of GnRH. Plasma testosterone was 416 ng/dL. At the time of the photograph, he had been treated with medroxyprogesterone acetate for 1½ years, with reduction of his rapid growth rate and decreased gonadotropin and testosterone secretion. His height was 95.2 cm (>2 SD above mean height for his age); plasma testosterone was 7 ng/dL, and after 100 μg of GnRH, plasma LH rose from 7 mIU/mL to 17.9 mIU/mL. (Reproduced, with permission, from Styne, DM, Grumbach MM: *Reproductive Endocrinology.* Yen SSC, Jaffe RB [editors]. Saunders, 1978.)

than in girls. Optic gliomas or hypothalamic gliomas (isolated or with neurofibromatosis), astrocytomas, ependymomas, and other central nervous system tumors may cause precocious puberty by interfering with neural pathways inhibiting GnRH secretion. Remarkably, craniopharyngiomas, which are well known to cause delayed puberty, can also trigger precocious pubertal development. Hamartomas of the tuber cinereum have been reported to contain GnRH and neurosecretory cells such as are found in the median eminence; they may cause precocious puberty by secreting GnRH. With improved methods of imaging the central

nervous system, hamartomas, with their characteristic radiographic appearance, are now being more frequently diagnosed in patients who were previously thought to have idiopathic precocious puberty. These tumors do not grow and so pose no increasing threat to the patients; surgical removal is not indicated, as hamartomas respond readily to GnRH agonist therapy. In fact, most tumors of the hypothalamic area are in critical areas of the brain, so a GnRH agonist is the treatment of choice for those nonoperable tumors that are not rapidly growing or malignant. Radiation therapy is indicated in radiosensitive tumors such as germinomas and craniopharyngiomas.

Tumors or other abnormalities of the central nervous system may cause growth hormone deficiency in association with precocious puberty. Such patients will grow much faster than isolated growth hormone–deficient patients but slower than children with classic precocious puberty. Often the growth hormone deficiency will be unmasked after successful treatment for precocious puberty. This combination must be considered during the diagnostic process so that growth hormone testing and treatment can be offered when necessary.

2. Other causes of true precocious puberty– Infectious or granulomatous conditions such as encephalitis, brain abscess, postinfectious (or postsurgical or congenital) suprasellar cysts, sarcoidosis, and tuberculous granulomas of the hypothalamus have been reported to cause true precocious puberty. Suprasellar cysts or hydrocephalus are conditions that cause precocious puberty and are particularly amenable to surgical correction. Brain trauma may be followed by either precocious or delayed puberty. Radiation therapy for acute lymphoblastic leukemia is characteristically associated with hormonal deficiency, but cases have been reported of precocious puberty occurring after such therapy. Epilepsy and mental retardation have also been associated with precocious puberty, without anatomic lesions of the central nervous system.

D. McCune-Albright Syndrome: McCune-Albright syndrome is classically manifested as a triad of irregular café au lait spots, fibrous dysplasia of long bones with cysts, and precocious puberty. However, cases have been reported that also included hyperthyroidism, adrenal nodules with Cushing's syndrome, acromegaly, hyperprolactinemia, hyperparathyroidism, hypophosphatemic hyperphosphaturic rickets, or autonomous functioning ovarian cysts in girls. Precocious puberty may be complete or incomplete; longitudinal study suggests that some patients start with incomplete precocious puberty and progress to complete precocious puberty. Long-term follow-up of McCune-Albright patients reveals a high incidence of pathologic fractures and orthopedic deformities due to the bone cysts, as well as hearing impairment due to the thickening of the temporal area of the skull.

E. Hypothyroidism: Severe untreated hypothyroidism can be associated with sexual precocity and galactorrhea (Van Wyk-Grumbach syndrome); treatment with thyroxine will correct hypothyroidism, halt precocious puberty and galactorrhea, and lower PRL levels. The cause of this syndrome is postulated to be increased gonadotropin secretion associated with the massive increase in TSH secretion.

F. Virilizing Syndromes: Patients with long-untreated virilizing adrenal hyperplasia who have advanced bone ages may manifest precocious puberty after the adrenal hyperplasia is controlled with glucocorticoids. Children with virilizing tumors or those given long-term androgen therapy may follow the same pattern when the androgen source is removed. Advanced maturation of the hypothalamic-pituitary-gonadal axis appears to occur with any excessive androgen conditions that cause advanced skeletal age.

Incomplete Precocious Puberty

A. Males: Male patients may manifest premature sexual development in the absence of hypothalamic-pituitary maturation from either (1) ectopic or autonomous secretion of hCG or LH or iatrogenic administration of chorionic gonadotropin, which can stimulate Leydig cell production of testosterone; or (2) autonomous secretion of androgens from the testes or adrenal glands or from iatrogenic administration of exogenous androgens.

1. Gonadotropin-secreting tumors–These include hepatomas or hepatoblastomas of the liver as well as teratomas or chorionepitheliomas of the mediastinum, gonads, retroperitoneum, or pineal gland and germinomas of the central nervous system. (In females, secretion of hCG will not by itself cause secondary sexual development.)

2. Autonomous androgen secretion–Secretion of androgens can occur because of inborn errors of adrenal enzymes, as in 21-hydroxylase deficiency or 11β-hydroxylase deficiency, virilizing adrenal carcinomas, interstitial cell tumors of the testes, or premature Leydig and germinal cell maturation. Newly recognized forms of late onset congenital adrenal hyperplasia, generally of the 21-hydroxylase deficiency form, may occur years after birth with no congenital or neonatal manifestations of virilization. Adrenal rest tissue may be found in the testes as a vestige of the embryonic common origin of these 2 organs; in states of ACTH excess, primarily adrenal hyperplasia, adrenal rests can enlarge and secrete adrenal androgens (see Chapter 18).

In all forms of incomplete male isosexual precocity, FSH is not elevated, and since the seminiferous tubules are not stimulated, the testes do not enlarge as much as in complete sexual precocity. If incomplete sexual precocity is due to a testicular tumor, the testes may be large, asymmetric, and irregular in contour. Symmetric bilateral moderate enlargement of the testes suggests gonadotropin-independent premature maturation of Leydig and germinal cells, which is a sex-limited dominant condition. The testes are somewhat smaller in this condition than in true precocious puberty but are still greater than 2.5 cm in diameter. In boys with premature Leydig and germinal cell maturation, plasma testosterone levels are in the pubertal range but plasma gonadotropin levels and the LH response to exogenous GnRH are in the prepubertal range because the autonomous testosterone secretion suppresses endogenous GnRH release. The differential diagnosis rests between a testosterone-secreting tumor of the adrenal, a testosterone-secreting Leydig cell neoplasm, and premature Leydig and germinal cell maturation.

B. Females: Female patients with incomplete isosexual precocity have a source of excessive estrogens. In all cases of autonomous estrogen secretion or ingestion, serum LH and FSH levels should be low.

1. Follicular cysts–If follicular cysts are large enough, they can secrete sufficient estrogen to cause breast development and even vaginal withdrawal bleeding; some girls have recurrent cysts that lead to several episodes of vaginal bleeding. Patients with cysts may have levels of serum estrogen high enough to mimic a tumor. Larger follicular cysts can twist on their pedicles and infarct, causing symptoms of acute abdomen in addition to the precocious estrogen effects.

2. Granulosa or theca cell tumors–These tumors of the ovaries secrete estrogen and are palpable in 80% of cases. Gonadoblastomas found in streak gonads, lipoid tumors, cystadenomas, and ovarian carcinomas are rare ovarian sources of estrogens or androgens.

3. Adrenal rest tissue–Adrenal rest tissue has long been known to cause testicular enlargement and androgen secretion in boys, particularly with associated increased ACTH secretion. Recently, however, a girl with an ovarian adrenal rest was reported to have hypertension, precocious puberty, Cushing's syndrome, and ovarian enlargement.

4. Exogenous estrogen administration–Ingestion of estrogen-containing substances or even cutaneous absorption of estrogen from cosmetics can cause feminization in children. Recent epidemics of gynecomastia and precocious thelarche in Puerto Rico and Italy have variously been attributed to ingestion of estrogen-contaminated food, estrogens in the environment, or undetermined causes. One outbreak of gynecomastia in boys and precocious thelarche in girls in Bahrain was traced to a cow that received continuous estrogen treatment to assure continued milk production.

5. Virilization in girls–Excess androgen effect can be caused by premature adrenarche or more significant pathologic conditions such as congenital or late onset adrenal hyperplasia or adrenal or ovarian tumors. Adrenal hyperplasia can be diagnosed by elevated 17 OH progesterone concentrations. Both adrenal and ovarian tumors generally secrete testosterone, while adrenal tumors secrete DHEA as well. The source of the tumor may be difficult to differentiate if it only produces testosterone; MRI or CT scanning may be inadequate to diagnose the tumor's organ of origin and selective venous sampling may be needed.

Variations in Pubertal Development

A. Premature Thelarche: The term "premature thelarche" denotes unilateral or bilateral breast enlargement without other signs of androgen or estrogen secretion of puberty. Patients are usually under 3 years of age; the breast enlargement may regress within months or remain until actual pubertal development occurs at a normal age. Nipple development and vaginal mucosal signs of estrogen effect are usually absent. Premature thelarche may be caused by brief episodes of estrogen secretion from ovarian cysts. Plasma estrogen levels are usually low in this disorder, possibly because blood samples are drawn after the initiating secretory event.

B. Premature Menarche: A recent report described a group of girls who began to menstruate at an early age without showing any other signs of estrogen effect. An unproved theory suggests that they may have been manifesting increased uterine sensitivity to estrogen. In this group menses stopped with 1–6 years and normal pubertal progression occurred thereafter.

C. Premature Adrenarche: The term "premature adrenarche" denotes the early appearance of pubic or axillary hair without other signs of virilization or puberty. This nonprogressive disorder is compatible with a normal age at onset of other signs of puberty. It is more common in girls than in boys and usually is found in children over 6 years of age. Plasma DHEAS and urinary 17-ketosteroids are elevated to stage 2 pubertal levels, which are higher than normally found in this age group. Bone and height ages may be slightly advanced for chronologic age. Patients may have abnormal electroencephalographic tracings without other signs of neurologic dysfunction. The presenting symptoms of late onset adrenal hyperplasia may be similar to those of premature adrenarche.

D. Adolescent Gynecomastia: This may be unilateral or bilateral and usually begins in boys in stage 2–3 of puberty, regressing about 2 years later. Plasma estrogen and testosterone concentrations are normal, but the estradiol:testosterone ratio may be elevated and SHBG concentrations may be high. Reassurance is usually all that is required, but some severely affected patients with extremely prominent breast development will require reduction mammoplasty if psychologic distress is extreme. Some pathologic conditions such as Klinefelter's and Reifenstein's syndromes and the syndrome of incomplete androgen resistance are also associated with gynecomastia; these disorders should be clearly differentiated from the gynecomastia of normal puberty in males.

Differential Diagnosis of Precocious Puberty

The history and physical examination should be directed toward eliciting pertinent findings that may confirm one of the diagnostic possibilities discussed above. A recent and disturbing finding is that children undergoing frequent genital examination were noted to perceive the process as equivalent to sexual abuse; clearly, the utmost consideration must be extended to the child during the examination. Gonadotropin and sex steroid concentrations should be determined to distinguish between gonadotropin-mediated secondary sexual development (gonadotropin and sex steroid levels elevated) or autonomous secretion or exogenous administration of gonadal steroids (gonadotropin levels suppressed and sex steroid levels elevated).

If plasma LH (or hCG) levels are quite high in a boy or a pregnancy screening test is positive, the likely diagnosis is an extrapituitary hCG-secreting tumor. If no abdominal source of hCG is found, a CT or MRI scan of the head is indicated to evaluate the possibility of a germinoma of the pineal.

If plasma sex steroid levels are very high and gonadotropin levels low, an autonomous source of gonadal steroid secretion must be assumed. If plasma gonadotropin and sex steroid levels are in the pubertal range, the most likely diagnosis is complete precocious puberty. In such patients, the GnRH test will usually result in a rise in LH levels compatible with normal puberty and will thus confirm the diagnosis (Table 19–5).

The presence of true or complete precocious puberty may indicate the presence of a hypothalamic tumor. Boys more often than girls have central nervous system tumors associated with complete precocious puberty. Skull x-rays are not usually helpful, but CT or MRI scanning is indicated in children with true precocious puberty. The present generation of CT and MRI scanners can make thin cuts through the hypothalamic-pituitary area with good resolution; small hypothalamic hamartomas are now being diagnosed more frequently.

Treatment of Precocious Puberty

A. Complete Precocious Puberty:

1. Medroxyprogesterone–In the USA, medical treatment of true precocious puberty was most commonly accomplished with medroxyprogesterone acetate, a progestational agent that reduces gonadotropin secretion by negative feedback. In girls, medroxyprogesterone will stop menses and breast development; in boys, it will decrease testicular size, decrease erection frequency, and modify aggressive behavior. Growth velocity and skeletal maturation may also be reduced with adequate dosage. In animal studies, medroxyprogesterone has caused breast nodules in beagles; in humans, no conclusive case of breast cancer associated with medroxyprogesterone administration has been noted. Since medroxyprogesterone has

Table 19–5. Differential diagnosis of precocious puberty.

	Serum Gonadotropin Concentrations	LH Response to GnRH	Serum Sex Steroid Concentrations	Gonadal Size	Miscellaneous
Complete (true) pre-cocious puberty	Pubertal.	Pubertal pattern.	Pubertal values.	Normal pubertal enlargement of testes in males.	CT or MRI scan of head to rule out a central nervous system tumor.
Incomplete pre-cocious puberty **Males** Gonadotropin-secreting tumor	High hCG or LH (positive pregnancy test).	High basal LH that does not rise with GnRH.	High or pubertal values.	Slight to moderate enlargement of testes.	Hepatic tumor must be considered. CT or MRI scan of head if gonadotropin-secreting central nervous system tumor suspected.
Leydig cell tumor	Prepubertal (low).	Prepubertal or suppressed pattern.	Extremely high testosterone.	Irregular asymmetric enlargement of testes.	
Gonadotropin-independent sexual precocity with premature Leydig and germinal cell maturation	Prepubertal (low).	Prepubertal or suppressed pattern.	Pubertal or higher values.	Testes larger than 2.5 cm but smaller than expected for stage of pubertal development.	Often found in sex-limited dominant patterns.
Females Granulosa cell tumor (follicular cysts may be similar to presentation)	Prepubertal (low).	Prepubertal or suppressed pattern.	Extremely high estradiol.	Ovarian enlargement on physical, CT, or sonographic examination.	Granulosa cell tumor is usually palpable on rectal examination.
Follicular cyst	Prepubertal (low).	Prepubertal pattern of LH. FSH secretion may rise above normal range.	Estradiol may be normally low or quite high, depending upon the stage of cyst formation or regression.	Cysts may be visible on sonogram.	Withdrawal bleeding may occur when estrogen levels decrease. Cysts may recur.

glucocorticoidlike effects, it suppresses ACTH and corticosteroid secretion and, with larger doses, a cushingoid appearance may develop. Medroxyprogesterone has not yet been approved for use in precocious puberty, so the preparation must be considered experimental treatment for this disorder. The dosage is 10–20 mg orally twice daily or 100 mg/m^2 intramuscularly weekly or fortnightly. In Europe, cyproterone acetate was used for the same indications as medroxyprogesterone acetate in the USA. Recent reports have shown that cyproterone acetate has little effect on the final height of treated patients.

2. Gonadotropin-Releasing hormone agonists—A new primary treatment for precocious puberty due to a central nervous system lesion has now been established, although it is not yet approved in the USA. Chronic use of highly potent and long-acting analogues of GnRH has been shown to down-regulate GnRH receptors and reduce pituitary gland response to GnRH, thereby causing decreased secretion of gonadotropin and sex steroids. This suppressive effect is reversed after therapy is discontinued. This treatment has rapidly stopped the progression of signs of sexual precocity in numerous children studied at many centers. Treatment of idiopathic precocious puberty and precocious puberty caused by hamartomas of the tuber cinereum, neoplasms of the central nervous system, or long-term androgen exposure has been successful. Results were mixed when patients with Mc-Cune-Albright syndrome were treated with GnRH agonists because some patients had central precocious puberty while others had incomplete precocious puberty that did not respond to GnRH agonists. The GnRH agonists are given daily subcutaneously or by intranasal insufflation; the successful use of these agents in microcapsules that are injected every 3 weeks suggests that an improved method of delivery is feasible. Numerous agents with varying potencies are used at different centers. Because of these differing potencies, it is possible that patients may only be partially treated, and therefore their response to GnRH may be only partially suppressed. Such a patient may appear to have arrested pubertal development while they are actually secreting low but significant levels of sex steroids, so that their bone age is advancing while their growth rate is suppressed. Side effects have generally been limited to allergic skin reaction and elevation of immunoglobulins directed to the agent. However, at least one child manifested a significant anaphylactic reaction to an injection. GnRH agonists promise to become the preferred treatment for true precocious puberty.

3. Psychologic support–Psychologic support is important for patients with sexual precocity. The somatic changes or menses will frighten some children and may make them the object of ridicule. These patients do not experience social maturation to match their physical development, although their peers, teachers, and relatives will tend to treat them as if they were older because of their large size. Thus, supportive counseling must be offered to both patient and family. Preliminary evidence indicates that children with precocious puberty have an increased incidence of sexual abuse, so appropriate precautions are necessary.

B. Incomplete Precocious Puberty: Treatment of the disorders discussed above under incomplete precocious puberty is directed toward the underlying tumor or abnormality rather than toward the signs of precocious puberty. If the primary cause is controlled, signs of sexual development will be halted in progression or may even regress.

Males with familial Leydig cell maturation will not respond to GnRH agonist therapy, but some have improved with medroxyprogesterone acetate. Recently, 4 boys were successfully treated with ketoconazole, which can block 17–20 lyase and therefore decrease testosterone production. After initial control with ketoconazole, the boys developed true precocious puberty, because prolonged exposure to androgens matured the hypothalamic-pituitary axis; treatment with GnRH agonist then effectively halted this pubertal progression. Males with McCune-Albright syndrome have had their incomplete precocious puberty controlled with testolactone. Girls with recurrent estrogen-secreting ovarian cyst formation may have a decreased incidence of cysts with medroxyprogesterone acetate therapy. GnRH agonist may be effective in such cases. Surgical removal of such ovarian cysts is unnecessary with such medical therapy available.

Precocious thelarche or adrenarche requires no treatment, as both are self-limited benign conditions. No therapy has been reported for premature menarche, although GnRH agonists or medroxyprogesterone acetate would seem to be possibilities. Severe cases of adolescent gynecomastia have been treated by testolactone and dihydrotestosterone heptanoate with success, suggesting that less surgery will be necessary for chronic cases in the future.

REFERENCES

General

Styne DM: Puberty. In: *Pediatric Endocrinology for the House Officer.* Styne DM (editor). Williams & Wilkins, 1988.

Styne DM, Grumbach MM: Puberty in the male and female: Its physiology and disorders. Pages 313–384 in: *Reproductive Endocrinology,* 2nd ed. Yen SSC, Jaffe RB (editors). Saunders, 1986.

Wilkins L: *The Diagnosis and Treatment of Endocrine Disorders in Childhood and Adolescence,* 2nd ed. Thomas, 1965.

Physical Changes Associated With Puberty

Bayley N, Pinneau SF: Tables for predicting adult height from skeletal age: Revised for use with the Greulich-Pyle standards. *J Pediatr* 1952;**40:**423.

Greulich WW, Pyle SI: *Radiographic Atlas of Skeletal Development of the Hand and Wrist,* 2nd ed. Stanford Univ Press, 1959.

Harlan WR, Harlan EA, Grillo GP: Secondary sex characteristics of girls 12 to 17 years of age: The U.S. Health Examination Survey. *J Pediatr* 1980;**96:**1074.

Harlan WR et al: Secondary sex characteristics of boys 12 to 17 years of age: The U.S. Health Examination Survey. *J Pediatr* 1979;**95:**293.

Marshall JC, Kelch RP: Low dose pulsatile gonadotropin-releasing hormone in anorexia nervosa: A model of human pubertal development. *J Clin Endocrinol Metab* 1979;**49:**712.

Marshall WA, Tanner JM: Variations in the pattern of pubertal changes in boys. *Arch Dis Child* 1970;**45:**13.

Marshall WA, Tanner JM: Variations in the pattern of pubertal changes in girls. *Arch Dis Child* 1969;**44:**291.

Nielsen CT et al: Onset of the release of spermatozoa (spermarche) in boys in relation to age, testicular growth, pubic hair, and height. *J Clin Endocrinol Metab* 1986;**62:**532.

Rohn RD: Nipple (papilla) development in puberty: Longitudinal observations in girls. *Pediatrics* 1987;**79:**745.

Tanner JM et al: The adolescent growth spurt of boys and girls of the Harpenden Growth Study. *Ann Hum Biol* 1976;**3:**109.

Van Wieringen JC et al: *Growth Diagrams 1965 Netherlands: Second National Survey on 0–24 Year Olds.* Groningen, Netherlands Institute for Preventive Medicine TNO Leiden, Wolters-Noordhoff Publishing, 1971.

Endocrine Changes From Fetal Life to Puberty

Boyar RM et al: Simultaneous augmented secretion of luteinizing hormone and testosterone during sleep. *J Clin Invest* 1974;**54**:609.

Cara JF, Rosenfield RL, Furlanetto RW: A longitudinal study of the relationship of plasma somatomedin-C concentration to the pubertal growth spurt. *Am J Dis Child* 1987;**141**:562.

Corley KP et al: Estimation of GnRH pulse amplitude during pubertal development. *Pediatr Res* 1981;**15**:157.

Faiman C, Winter JSD: Gonadotropins and sex hormone patterns in puberty: Clinical data. Pages 32–61 in: *Control of the Onset of Puberty*. Grumbach MM, Grave GD, Mayer FE (editors). Wiley, 1974.

Forest MG, de Peretti E, Bertrand J: Hypothalamic-pituitary-gonadal relationships in man from birth to puberty. *Clin Endocrinol* 1976;**5**:551.

Grumbach MM et al: Hypothalamic-pituitary regulation of puberty in man: Evidence and concepts derived from clinical research. Pages 115–166 in: *Control of the Onset of Puberty*. Grumbach MM, Grave GD, Mayer FE (editors). Wiley, 1974.

Hale PM et al: Increased luteinizing hormone pulse frequency during sleep in early to midpubertal boys: Effects of testosterone infusion. *J Clin Endocrinol Metab* 1988;**66**:785.

Harris DA et al: Somatomedin-C in normal puberty and in true precocious puberty before and after treatment with a potent LRF agonist: Evidence for an effect of estrogen and testosterone on somatomedin-C concentrations. *J Clin Endocrinol Metab* 1985;**61**:152.

Kaplan SL, Grumbach MM, Aubert ML: The ontogenesis of pituitary hormones and hypothalamic factors in the human fetus: Maturation of central nervous system regulation of anterior pituitary function. *Recent Prog Horm Res* 1976;**32**:161.

Kirkland RT et al: Decrease in plasma high-density lipoprotein cholesterol levels at puberty in boys with delayed adolescence: Correlation with plasma testosterone levels. *JAMA* 1987;**257**:502.

Link K et al: The effect of androgens on the pulsatile release and the twenty-four-hour mean concentration of growth hormone in peripubertal males. *J Clin Endocrinol Metab* 1986;**62**:159.

Luna AM et al: Somatomedins in adolescence: A cross-sectional study of the effect of puberty on plasma insulin-like growth factor I and II levels. *J Clin Endocrinol Metab* 1983;**57**:268.

Mauras N, Veldhuis JD, Rogol AD: Role of endogenous opiates in pubertal maturation: Opposing actions of naltrexone in prepubertal and late pubertal boys. *J Clin Endocrinol Metab* 1986;**62**:1256.

Reame N et al: Pulsatile gonadotropin secretion during the human menstrual cycle: Evidence for altered frequency of gonadotropin-releasing hormone secretion. *J Clin Endocrinol Metab* 1984;**59**:328.

Reiter EO et al: Responsivity of pituitary gonadotropes to luteinizing hormone–releasing factors in idiopathic precocious puberty, precocious thelarche, and precocious adrenarche. *Pediatr Res* 1975;**9**:111.

Rosenthal SM, Grumbach MM, Kaplan SL: Gonado tropin-independent familial sexual precocity with premature Leydig and germinal cell maturation (familial testotoxicosis): Effects of a potent luteinizing hormone–releasing factor agonist and medroxyprogesterone acetate therapy in four cases. *J Clin Endocrinol Metab* 1983;**57**:571.

Roth, JC, Grumbach MM, Kaplan SL: Effect of synthetic luteinizing hormone–releasing factor on serum testosterone and gonadotropins in prepubertal, pubertal and adult males. *J Clin Endocrinol Metab* 1973;**37**:680.

Sizonenko PC et al: Hormonal changes in puberty. 2. Correlation of serum luteinizing hormone and follicle-stimulating hormone with stages of puberty and bone age in normal girls. *Pediatr Res* 1970;**4**:36.

Sklar CA et al: Human chorionic gonadotropin–secreting pineal tumor: Relation to pathogenesis and sex limitation of sexual precocity. *J Clin Endocrinol Metab* 1981;**53**:656.

Wildt L, Marshall G, Knobil E: Experimental induction of puberty in the infantile female rhesus monkey. *Science* 1980;**207**:1373.

Adrenarche

Attanasio A et al: Plasma adrenocorticotropin, cortisol, and dehydroepiandrosterone response to corticotropin-releasing factor in normal children during pubertal development. *Pediatr Res* 1987;**22**:41.

Grumbach MM et al: Clinical disorders of adrenal function and puberty: An assessment of the role of the adrenal cortex in normal and abnormal puberty in man and evidence for an ACTH-like pituitary adrenal androgen stimulating hormone. In: *The Endocrine Function of the Human Adrenal Cortex*. Serio M (editor). Academic Press, 1977.

Jarow JP et al: Elevation of serum gonadotropins establishes the diagnosis of anorchism in prepubertal boys with bilateral cryptorchidism. *J Urol* 1986;**136**:227.

Reiter EO, Fuldauer VG, Root AW: Secretion of the adrenal androgen, dehydroepiandrosterone sulfate, during normal infancy, childhood, and adolescence, in sick infants and in children with endocrinologic abnormalities. *J Pediatr* 1977;**90**:766.

Sklar CA, Kaplan SL, Grumbach MM: Evidence for dissociation between adrenarche and gonadarche: Studies in patients with idiopathic precocious puberty, gonadal dysgenesis, isolated gonadotropin deficiency, and constitutionally delayed growth and adolescence. *J Clin Endocrinol Metab* 1980;**51**:548.

Delayed Puberty & Sexual Infantilism

Connors MH, Styne DM: Familial functional anorchism: A review of etiology and management. *J Urol* 1985;**133**:1049.

Frisch RE, Wyshak G, Vincent L: Delayed menarche and amenorrhea in ballet dancers. *N Engl J Med* 1980;**303**:17.

Griffin JE et al: Congenital absence of the vagina: The Mayer-Rokitansky-Kuster-Hauser syndrome. *Ann Intern Med* 1976;**85**:224.

Grumbach MM, Conte FA: Disorders of sexual differentiation. Pages 312–401 in: *Williams Textbook of Endocrinology*, 7th ed. Wilson JD, Foster DW (editors). Saunders, 1985.

Kaplan SL, Grumbach MM, Hoyt WF: A syndrome of hypopituitary dwarfism, hypoplasia of optic nerves, and malformation of prosencephalon: Report of 6 patients. *Pediatr Res* 1970;**4**:480.

Patton ML, Woolf PD: Hyperprolactinemia and delayed puberty: A report of three cases and their response to therapy. *Pediatrics* 1983;**71**:572.

Pugliese MT et al: Fears of obesity: A cause of short stature and delayed puberty. *N Engl J Med* 1983;**309**:513.

Rivkees SA, Crawford JD: The relationship of gonadal activity and chemotherapy-induced gonadal damage. *JAMA* 1988;**259**:2123.

Santoro N, Filicori M, Crowley WF Jr: Hypogonadotropic disorders in men and women: Diagnosis and therapy with pulsatile gonadotropin-releasing hormone. *Endocr Rev* 1986;**7**:11.

Schwabe AD et al: Anorexia nervosa. *Ann Intern Med* 1981;**94**:371.

Shulman DI et al: Hypothalamic-pituitary dysfunction in primary empty sella syndrome in childhood. *J Pediatr* 1986;**108**:540.

Sklar CA et al: Hormonal and metabolic abnormalities associated with central nervous system germinoma in children and adolescents and the effect of therapy: Report of 10 patients. *J Clin Endocrinol Metab* 1981;**52**:9.

Thomsett MJ et al: Endocrine and neurologic outcome in childhood craniopharyngioma: Review of effect of treatment in 42 patients. *J Pediatr* 1980;**97**:728.

Van Dop C et al: Isolated gonadotropin deficiency in boys: Clinical characteristics and growth. *J Pediatr* 1987;**111**:684.

Wilson DM et al: Effects of testosterone therapy for pubertal delay. *Am J Dis Child* 1988;**142**:96.

Sexual Precocity

Boepple PA et al: Use of a potent, long-acting agonist of gonadotropin-releasing hormone in the treatment of precocious puberty. *Endocr Rev* 1986;**7**:24.

Bongiovanni AM: An epidemic of premature thelarche in Puerto Rico. *J Pediatr* 1983;**103**:245.

Cacciari E et al: How many cases of true precocious puberty in girls are idiopathic? *J Pediatr* 1983;**102**:357.

Eberle AJ, Sparrow JT, Keenan BS: Treatment of persistent pubertal gynecomastia with dihydrotestosterone heptanoate. *J Pediatr* 1986;**109**:144.

Egli CA et al: Pituitary gonadotropin-independent male-limited autosomal dominant sexual precocity in nine generations: Familial testotoxicosis. *J Pediatr* 1985;**106**:33.

Feuillan PP et al: Treatment of precocious puberty in the McCune-Albright syndrome with the aromatase inhibitor testolactone. *N Engl J Med* 1986;**315**:1115.

Herman-Giddens ME, Sandler AD, Friedman NE: Sexual precocity in girls: An association with sexual abuse? *Am J Dis Child* 1988;**142**:431.

Hochman HI, Judge DM, Reichlin S: Precocious puberty and hypothalamic hamartoma. *Pediatrics* 1981;**67**:236.

Holland FJ et al: Ketoconazole in the management of precocious puberty not responsive to LHRH-analogue therapy. *N Engl J Med* 1985;**312**:1023.

Holland FJ, Kirsch SE, Selby R: Gonadotropin-independent precocious puberty ("testotoxicosis"): Influence of maturational status on response to ketoconazole. *J Clin Endocrinol Metab* 1987;**64**:328.

Judge DM et al: Hypothalamic hamartoma: A source of luteinizing hormone–releasing factor in precocious puberty. *N Engl J Med* 1977;**296**:7.

Lee PA, Van Dop C, Migeon CJ: McCune-Albright syndrome: Long-term follow-up. *JAMA* 1986;**256**:2980.

Mills JL et al: Premature thelarche: Natural history and etiologic investigation. *Am J Dis Child* 1981;**135**:743.

Pescovitz OH et al: The NIH experience with precocious puberty: Diagnostic subgroups and response to short-term luteinizing hormone–releasing hormone analogue therapy. *J Pediatr* 1986;**108**:47.

Pescovitz OH et al: True precocious puberty complicating congenital adrenal hyperplasia: Treatment with a luteinizing hormone–releasing hormone analog. *J Clin Endocrinol Metab* 1984;**58**:847.

Reiter EU et al: Male-limited familial precocious puberty in three generations. *N Engl J Med* 1984;**311**:515.

Styne DW et al: Treatment of true precocious puberty with a potent luteinizing hormone–releasing factor agonist: Effect on growth, sexual maturation, pelvic sonography, and the hypothalamic-pituitary-gonadal axis. *J Clin Endocrinol Metab* 1985;**61**:142.

Van Wyk JJ, Grumbach MM: Syndrome of precocious menstruation and galactorrhea in juvenile hypothyroidism: An example of hormonal overlap in pituitary feedback. *J Pediatr* 1960;**57**:416.

The Endocrinology of Pregnancy

20

Mary C. Martin, MD, Robert N. Taylor, MD, PhD, & Philip G. Hoffman, Jr., MD, PhD*

Throughout pregnancy, the fetal-placental unit secretes protein and steroid hormones into the mother's bloodstream, and these apparently or actually alter the function of every endocrine gland in her body. Both clinically and in the laboratory, pregnancy can mimic hyperthyroidism, Cushing's disease, pituitary adenoma, diabetes mellitus, and polycystic ovary syndrome.

The endocrine changes associated with pregnancy are adaptive, allowing the mother to nurture the developing fetus. Although maternal reserves are usually adequate, occasionally, as in the case of gestational diabetes or hypertensive disease of pregnancy, a woman may develop overt signs of disease as a direct result of pregnancy.

Aside from creating a satisfactory maternal environment for fetal development, the placenta serves as an endocrine gland as well as a respiratory, alimentary, and excretory organ. Measurements of fetal-placental products in the maternal serum provide one means of assessing the health of the developing fetus. This chapter will consider the changes in maternal endocrine function in pregnancy and during parturition as well as fetal endocrine development. The chapter concludes with a discussion of some endocrine disorders complicating pregnancy.

CONCEPTION & IMPLANTATION

Fertilization

In fertile women, ovulation occurs approximately 12–16 days after the onset of the previous menses. The ovum must be fertilized within 24–48 hours if conception is to result. For about 48 hours around ovulation, cervical mucus is copious, nonviscous, and slightly alkaline and forms a gel matrix that acts as a filter and conduit for sperm. Following intercourse, sperm that are to survive penetrate the cervical mucus within minutes and can remain viable there until the mucus character changes, approximately 24 hours following ovulation. Sperm begin appearing in the outer third of the uterine tube (the ampulla) 5–10 minutes after

---

Acronyms Used in This Chapter

ACTH	Adrenocorticotropic hormone
cAMP	Cyclic adenosine monophosphate
CBG	Corticosteroid-binding globulin
CST	Contraction stress test
DHEA	Dehydroepiandrosterone
DOC	Deoxycorticosterone
EGF	Epidermal growth factor
FGF	Fibroblast growth factor
FSH	Follicle-stimulating hormone
GnRH	Gonadotropin-releasing hormone
hCG	Human chorionic gonadotropin
hCGnRH	Human chorionic gonadotropin–releasing hormone
hCS	Human chorionic somatomammotropin
hGH	Human growth hormone
hPL	Human placental lactogen
hPRL	Human prolactin
IGFs	Insulin-like growth factors
LATS	Long-acting thyroid stimulator
LH	Luteinizing hormone
L/S	Lecithin/sphingomyelin (ratio)
NST	Nonstress test
PDGF	Platelet-derived growth factor
SHBG	Sex hormone–binding globulin
TBG	Thyroid hormone–binding globulin
TRH	Thyrotropin-releasing hormone
TSH	Thyroid-stimulating hormone (thyrotropin)
TSI	Thyroid-stimulating immunoglobulin

---

coitus and continue to migrate to this location from the cervix for about 24–48 hours. Of the 200×10^6 sperm that are deposited in the vaginal fornices, only approximately 200 reach the distal uterine tube. Fertilization normally occurs in the ampulla.

Implantation

Implantation in the uterus does not occur until 6 or 7 days later, when the conceptus is a blastocyst of 1000–10,000 cells. In most pregnancies, the dates of ovulation and implantation are not known. Weeks of gestation ("gestational age") are by convention calculated from the first day of the last menstrual period. Within 24 hours after implantation, or at about 3 weeks of gestation, human chorionic gonadotropin (hCG) is de-

---

*deceased

SYSTEM	HORMONE	PATTERN	AVERAGE PEAK CONCENTRATION (TIME)
Placenta and corpus luteum	Progesterone	Rises to term.	190 ng/mL (552 nmol/L) (term)
	17-Hydroxy-progester-one	Peaks at 5 weeks, then declines.	6 ng/mL (19 nmol/L) (5 weeks)
Adrenal	Cortisol	Increases to 3 times prepregnancy values at term.	300 ng/mL (0.83 μmol/L) (term)
	Aldosterone	Plateaus at 34 weeks with small rise near term.	100 ng/mL (277 nmol/L)
	DOC	Increases to 10 times prepregnancy value at term.	1200 pg/mL (3.48 nmol/L) (term)
Thyroid	Total T_4	Increases during first trimester, then plateaus.	150 ng/mL (193 pmol/L)
	Free T_4	Unchanged.	30 pg/mL (38.6 pmol/L)
	Total T_3	Increases during first trimester, then plateaus.	2 ng/mL (3.1 nmol/L)
	Free T_3	Unchanged.	4 pg/mL (5.1 pmol/L)

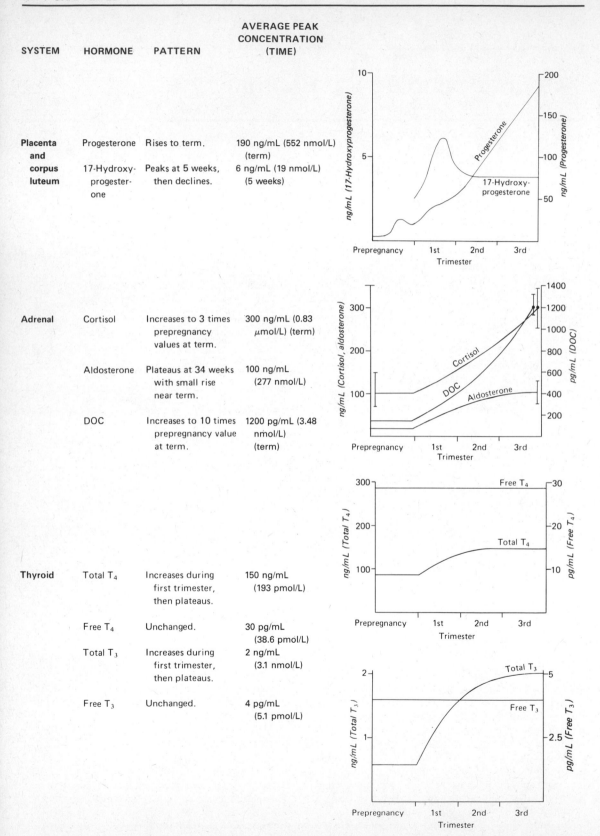

Figure 20–1. Maternal serum hormone changes during pregnancy.

SYSTEM	HORMONE	PATTERN	AVERAGE PEAK CONCENTRATION (TIME)
Anterior pituitary	GH	Unchanged.	
	LH, FSH	Low, basal levels.	
	ACTH	Unchanged.	
	TSH	Unchanged.	
	PRL	Rise to term.	≈200 ng/mL (200 μg/L) (term)
Placental proteins	hCG	Peaks at 10 weeks, then decreases to a lower plateau.	5 μg/mL (5 μg/L) (end of first trimester)
	hCS	Rises with placental weight.	5–25 μg/mL (5–25μg/L) (term)
Fetoplacental estrogens	Estradiol	Increases to term.	15–17 ng/mL (55–62 nmol/L) (term)
	Estriol	Increases to term.	12–15 ng/mL (42–52 nmol/L) (term)
	Estrone	Increases to term.	5–7 ng/mL (18.5–26 nmol/L) (term)
	Estetrol	Increases to term.	4–5 ng/mL (13.1–16.4 nmol/L) (term)
Fetoplacental androgens	Testosterone	Rises to 10 times prepregnancy values.	≈2000 pg/mL (6.9 nmol/L) (term)
	DHEA	Falls during pregnancy.	5 ng/mL (17.3 nmol/L) (prepregnancy)
	Androstenedione	Small increase.	2.6 ng/mL (9.0 nmol/L) (term)

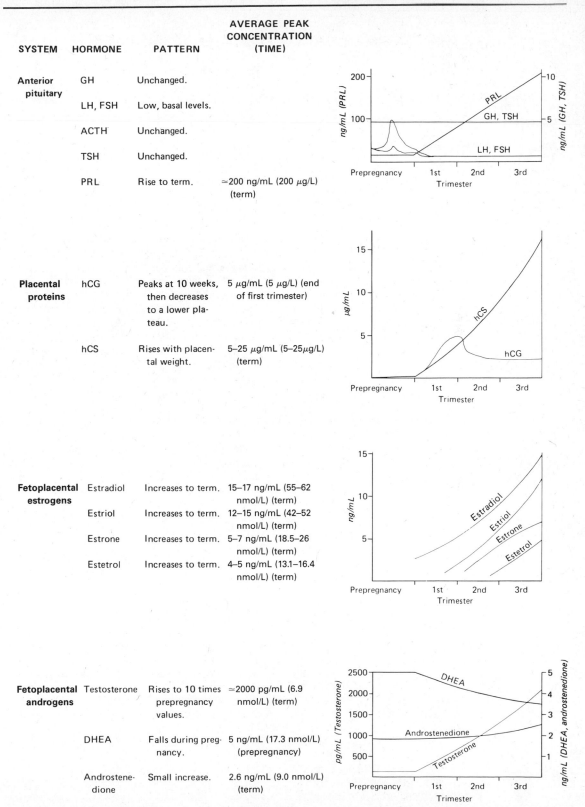

Figure 20–1 (cont'd). Maternal serum hormone changes during pregnancy.

tectable in maternal serum. Under the influence of hCG, the corpus luteum continues to secrete steroid hormones in increasing quantities. Without effective implantation and subsequent hCG production, the corpus luteum survives for only about 14 days following ovulation.

Symptoms of Pregnancy

Breast tenderness, fatigue, nausea, absence of menstruation, softening of the uterus, and a sustained elevation of basal body temperature are all attributable to hormone production by the corpus luteum and developing placenta.

Ovarian Hormones of Pregnancy

The hormones produced by the corpus luteum include progesterone, 17-hydroxyprogesterone, and estradiol. The indispensability of the corpus luteum in early pregnancy has been demonstrated by ablation studies, in which luteectomy or oophorectomy before 42 days of gestation results in precipitous decreases in levels of serum progesterone and estradiol, followed by abortion. Exogenous progesterone will prevent abortion, proving that progesterone alone is required for maintenance of early pregnancy. After about the seventh gestational week, the corpus luteum can be removed without subsequent abortion, owing to increasing progesterone production by the placenta.

Because the placenta does not produce appreciable amounts of 17-hydroxyprogesterone, this steroid provides a marker of corpus luteum function. As shown in Fig 20–1, the serum concentrations of estrogens and total progesterone exhibit a steady increase, but the concentration of 17-hydroxyprogesterone rises and then declines to low levels that persist for the duration of the pregnancy. The decline of corpus luteum function occurs despite the continued production of hCG; in fact, corpus luteum production of 17-hydroxyprogesterone declines while hCG is still rising to maximal levels.

Another marker of corpus luteum function is the polypeptide hormone relaxin, a dipeptide with a molecular mass of about 6000. It is similar in its tertiary structure to insulin. Relaxin becomes detectable at about the same time as hCG begins to rise, and it maintains a maximum maternal serum concentration of about 1 ng/mL during the first trimester. The serum concentration then falls approximately 20% and is constant for the remainder of the pregnancy.

Pharmacologically, relaxin ripens the cervix, softens the pubic symphysis, and acts synergistically with progesterone to inhibit uterine contractions. A major physiologic role for relaxin in human gestation, however, is doubtful, since luteectomy after 7 weeks of gestation does not interfere with gestation in spite of undetectable relaxin levels. Extraluteal production of relaxin by the decidua and placenta has been demonstrated.

FETAL-PLACENTAL-DECIDUAL UNIT

The function of the placenta is to establish effective communication between the mother and the developing fetus while maintaining the immune and genetic integrity of both individuals. Initially, the placenta functions autonomously. By the end of the first trimester, however, the fetal endocrine system is sufficiently developed to influence placental function and to provide some hormone precursors to the placenta. From this time, it is useful to consider the conceptus as the fetal-placental unit.

The placenta and the fetal-placental unit will be considered in 3 separate but related categories: as sources of secretion of protein and steroid hormones into the maternal circulation; as participants in the control of fetal endocrine function, growth, and development; and as selective barriers governing the interaction between fetal and maternal systems.

Seven days after fertilization, implantation begins. The trophoblast invades the endometrium, and 2 layers of developing placenta can be demonstrated. The mature syncytiotrophoblast adjacent to the endometrium is derived from the precursor cytotrophoblast. The syncytiotrophoblast is the major source of hormone production, containing the cellular machinery needed for synthesis, packaging, and secretion of both steroid and polypeptide hormones. It is in direct contact with the maternal circulation and the decidua.

The decidua is the endometrium of pregnancy. Recent investigation has shown that the decidual cells are capable of synthesizing a variety of polypeptide hormones, including prolactin (hPRL) and relaxin. The importance of the role of the decidua as an endocrine organ has not been established, but its role as a source of prostaglandins during labor is certain (see Endocrine Control of Parturition, below).

POLYPEPTIDE HORMONES

Human Chorionic Gonadotropin

The first measurable product of the placenta is chorionic gonadotropin (hCG). hCG is a glycoprotein consisting of about 237 amino acids. It is quite similar in structure to the pituitary glycoproteins in that it consists of 2 chains: an alpha chain, which is species-specific; and a beta chain, which determines receptor interaction and ultimate biologic effect. The alpha chain is almost identical in sequence to the alpha chains of the hormonal glycoproteins TSH, FSH, and LH. The beta chain has significant sequence homology with LH but is not identical; of the 145 amino acids in β-hCG, 97 (67%) are identical to those of β-LH. In addition, the placental hormone has a carboxy-terminal segment of 30 amino acids not found in the pituitary LH molecule. Carbohydrate constitutes approximately 30% by weight of each subunit. Sialic acid alone accounts for 10% of the weight of the molecule and confers a high degree of resistance to degradation.

In the early weeks of pregnancy, the concentration of hCG doubles every 1.7–2 days, and serial measurements provide a sensitive index of early trophoblast function. Maternal plasma hCG peaks at about 100,000 mIU/mL (100,000 IU/L) during the 10th gestational week and then declines gradually to about 10,000 mIU/mL (10,000 IU/L) in the third trimester.

These characteristics of hCG all contribute to the possibility of diagnosing pregnancy several days before any symptoms occur or a menstrual period has been missed. Without the long plasma half-life of hCG (approximately 24 hours), the tiny mass of cells comprising the blastocyst could not produce sufficient hormone to be detected in the peripheral circulation within 24 hours of implantation. The unique β-carboxy-terminal segment of hCG has been isolated, and an antibody has been raised against it in rabbits. The beta subunit assay for hCG that uses this antibody does not cross-react significantly with any of the pituitary glycoproteins. As little as 5 mIU/mL (1 ng/mL) of hCG in plasma can be detected without interference from the higher levels of LH, FSH, and TSH. The reliable sensitivities of commonly available pregnancy tests are summarized in Table 20–1.

Like its pituitary counterpart LH, hCG is luteotropic, and the corpus luteum has high-affinity receptors for hCG. The stimulation of increased amounts of progesterone production by corpus luteum cells can be demonstrated in vitro and is mediated by the cAMP system. hCG has been shown to enhance placental conversion of maternal low-density lipid cholesterol to pregnenolone and progesterone. The hCG molecule also demonstrates TSH-like activity, but the biologic significance of this activity in normal pregnancy is modest, because hCG has only 1/4000 the potency of TSH.

The concentration of hCG in the fetal circulation is less than 1% of that found in the maternal compartment. However, there is evidence that fetal hCG is an important regulator of the development of the fetal adrenal and gonad during the first trimester.

hCG is also produced by trophoblastic neoplasms such as hydatidiform mole and choriocarcinoma, and the concentration of hCG or its beta subunit is used as a tumor marker, for diagnosis, and for monitoring the success or failure of chemotherapy in these disorders. Women with very high hCG levels due to trophoblastic disease may become clinically hyperthyroid and revert to euthyroidism as hCG is reduced during chemotherapy.

Somatomammotropin

A second placental polypeptide hormone, also with homology to a pituitary protein, is termed placental lactogen (hPL) or chorionic somatomammotropin (hCS). hCS is detectable in the early trophoblast, but detectable serum concentrations are not reached until 4–5 gestational weeks. hCS is a protein of about 190 amino acids whose primary, secondary, and tertiary structures are similar to those of human growth hormone (hGH). The 2 molecules cross-react in immunoassays and in some receptor and bioassay systems. However, hCS has only some of the biologic activities of hGH. Like hGH, hCS is diabetogenic, but it has minimal growth-promoting activity as measured by standard hGH bioassays. hCS also shares many structural features with human prolactin (hPRL) and is a potent stimulator of pigeon crop sac growth. hCS appears to have greater intrinsic lactogenic activity than hGH.

The physiologic role of hCS during pregnancy remains controversial, and normal pregnancy without detectable hCS production has been reported. Although not clearly shown to be a mammotropic agent, hCS contributes to altered glucose metabolism and mobilization of free fatty acids; causes of hyperinsulinemic response to glucose loads; and contributes to the peripheral insulin resistance characteristic of pregnancy. Factors that regulate the synthesis or release of hCS from the syncytiotrophoblast have not been fully determined, but prolonged fasting and insulin-induced hypoglycemia raise hCS concentrations. hCS production is roughly proportionate to placental mass. Actual production rates may reach as much as 1–1.5 g/d. The disappearance curve shows multiple components but yields a serum half-life of 15–30 minutes. Serum hCS concentration has been proposed as an indicator of the continued health of the placenta and has been used to monitor intrauterine growth retardation and fetal jeopardy. It was hoped that chronically low hCS or acute drops in its concentrations would be clinically useful in predicting placental compromise in pregnancies complicated by chronic hypertension, preeclampsia, intrauterine growth retardation, or postmaturity. Concentrations of hCS are indeed low in verified placental insufficiency, but the range of normal values is wide, and serial determinations are necessary. hCS determinations have largely been replaced by biophysical profiles, which are more sensitive indicators of fetal jeopardy. In conditions such as diabetes, in which fetal jeopardy occurs with normal placental

Table 20–1. Relative sensitivity of various pregnancy tests.

Test	Sensitivity (mIU/mL or IU/L)	Time Required (hours)	Reliable Detection After Ovulation (days)
Agglutination inhibition			
Slide test	1500–3000	0.5	28–30
Tube test	200–1000	2	14–30
Radioimmunoassay	5–50	1–36	8–14
Radioreceptor assay	200	1–3	14–17

function, serum concentrations of hCS are of no predictive value.

Other Chorionic Peptide Hormones and Growth Factors

Other chorionic peptides have been identified, but their functions have not yet been defined. One of these proteins is a glycoprotein with partial sequence and functional homology to TSH. Its existence as a separate entity from hCG has been debated in the literature, with some reports suggesting that chorionic TSH is a protein with a molecular weight of about 28,000, structurally different from hCG, with weak thyrotropic activity. Similarly, ACTH-like, lipotropinlike, and endorphinlike peptides have been isolated from placenta, but they have low biologic potency and undetermined physiologic roles. A chorionic FSH–like protein has also been isolated from placenta but has not yet been detected in plasma. Good evidence now exists that the cytotrophoblast produces a human chorionic gonadotropin–releasing hormone (hCGnRH) that is biologically and immunologically indistinguishable from the hypothalamic GnRH. The release of hCG from the syncytiotrophoblast may be under the direct control of this factor, in a fashion analogous to the hypothalamic control of anterior pituitary secretion of gonadotropins. Preliminary evidence is also available for similar paracrine control of syncytiotrophoblastic release of TSH, somatostatin, and corticotropin by analogous cytotrophoblastic releasing hormones. Multiple peptide growth factors, including fibroblast growth factor (FGF), epidermal growth factor (EGF), platelet-derived growth factor (PDGF), and the insulinlike growth factors (IGFs), have all been isolated from placental tissue.

STEROID HORMONES

In contrast to the impressive synthetic capability exhibited in the production of placental proteins, the placenta does not appear to have the capability to synthesize steroids de novo. All steroids produced by the placenta are derived from maternal or fetal precursor steroids.

No tissue, however, even remotely approaches the syncytiotrophoblast in its capacity to efficiently interconvert steroids. This activity is demonstrable even in the preimplantation blastocyst, and by the seventh gestational week, when the corpus luteum has undergone relative senescence, the placenta becomes the dominant source of steroid hormones.

Progesterone

The placenta relies on maternal cholesterol as its substrate for progesterone production. Fetal death has no immediate influence on progesterone production, suggesting that the fetus is a negligible source of substrate. The placenta cleaves the cholesterol side chain, yielding pregnenolone, which in turn is partially isomerized to progesterone; 250–350 mg of progesterone is produced daily by the third trimester, and most enters the maternal circulation. The maternal plasma concentration of progesterone rises progressively throughout pregnancy and appears to be independent of factors that normally regulate steroid synthesis and secretion. Whereas exogenous hCG increases progesterone production in pregnancy, hypophysectomy has no effect. Administration of ACTH or cortisol does not influence progesterone concentrations, nor does adrenalectomy or oophorectomy do so after 7 weeks.

Progesterone is necessary for establishment and maintenance of pregnancy. Insufficient corpus luteum production of progesterone may contribute to failure of implantation, and luteal phase deficiency is implicated in some cases of infertility and recurrent pregnancy loss. Furthermore, progesterone contributes to maintaining a relatively quiescent state of the myometrium. In some animals, such as the rabbit or sheep, labor is heralded by a decrease in progesterone concentration, and the administration of progesterone in these species can delay labor indefinitely. Progesterone is also active as an immunosuppressive agent in some systems and inhibits T cell–mediated tissue rejection. Thus, high local concentrations of progesterone may contribute to immunologic tolerance by the uterus of invading embryonic trophoblast tissue.

Estrogens

Estrogen production by the placenta also depends on circulating precursors, but in this case both fetal and maternal steroids are important sources. Most of the estrogens are derived from fetal androgens, primarily dehydroepiandrosterone sulfate (DHEA sulfate). Fetal DHEA sulfate, produced mainly by the fetal adrenal, is converted by placental sulfatase to the free dehydroepiandrosterone (DHEA) and then, through enzymatic pathways common to steroid-producing tissues, to androsterone and testosterone. These androgens are finally aromatized by the placenta to estrone and estradiol, respectively.

The greater part of fetal DHEA sulfate is metabolized to produce a third estrogen: estriol. While serum estrone and estradiol concentrations are increased during pregnancy about 50-fold over their maximal pre-pregnancy values, estriol increases approximately 1000-fold. The key step in estriol synthesis is 16α-hydroxylation of the steroid molecule (see Fig 17–4). The substrate for the reaction is primarily fetal DHEA sulfate, and the vast majority of the production of the 16α-hydroxy-DHEA sulfate occurs in the fetal adrenal and liver, not in maternal or placental tissues. The final steps of desulfation and aromatization to estriol occur in the placenta. Maternal serum or urinary estriol measurements, unlike measurements of progesterone or hCS, reflect fetal as well as placental function. Normal estriol production, therefore, reflects the integrity of fetal circulation and metabolism as well as adequacy of the placenta. Rising serum or urinary estriol concentrations are the best available biochemical indicator of fetal well-being. When estriol is assayed daily, a significant drop (>50%) may be a sensitive early indicator of fetal jeopardy.

There are many circumstances in which altered estriol production does not signal fetal compromise but is instead the result of congenital derangements or iatrogenic intervention. Maternal estriol remains low in pregnancies with placental sulfatase deficiency and in cases of fetal anencephaly. In the first case, DHEA sulfate cannot be hydrolyzed; in the second, little fetal DHEA is produced because fetal adrenal stimulation by ACTH is lacking. Maternal administration of glucocorticoids inhibits fetal ACTH and lowers maternal estriol. Administration of DHEA to the mother during a healthy pregnancy increases estriol production. Antibiotic therapy can reduce estriol by interfering with maternal reabsorption of estriol from the gut.

Estetrol, an estrogen with a fourth hydroxyl at the 15 position, is unique to pregnancy, but at present it is not clear that determinations of estetrol offer any clinical advantage over estriol measurements.

MATERNAL ADAPTATION TO PREGNANCY

As a successful "parasite," the fetal-placental unit manipulates the maternal "host" for its own gain but normally avoids imposing excessive stress that would jeopardize the "host" and thus the "parasite" itself. The prodigious production of polypeptide and steroid hormones by the fetal-placental unit directly or indirectly results in physiologic adaptations of virtually every maternal organ system. These alterations are summarized in Fig 20–2. Most of the commonly measured maternal endocrine function tests are radically changed. In some cases, true physiologic alteration has occurred; in others, the changes are due to increased production of specific serum binding proteins by the liver or to decreased serum levels of albumin. Additionally, some hormonal changes are mediated by altered clearance rates owing to increased glomerular filtration, decreased hepatic excretion of anions, or metabolic clearance of steroid and protein hormones by the placenta. The changes in endocrine function tests are summarized in Table 20–2. Failure to recognize normal pregnancy-induced alterations in endocrine function tests can lead to unnecessary diagnostic tests and therapy that may be seriously detrimental to mother and fetus.

Maternal Pituitary Gland

The mother's anterior pituitary gland hormones have little influence on pregnancy after implantation has occurred. The gland itself enlarges by about one-third, with the major component of this increase being hyperplasia of the lactotrophs in response to the high plasma estrogens. PRL, the product of the lactotrophs, is the only anterior pituitary hormone that rises progressively during pregnancy, with contributions from both the anterior pituitary and the decidua. In spite of the high serum concentrations, pulsatile release of PRL and nocturnal and food-induced increases persist. Hence, the normal neuroendocrine regulatory mechanisms appear to be intact. Pituitary ACTH and TSH secretion remain unchanged. Serum FSH and LH fall to the lower limits of detectability and are unresponsive to GnRH stimulation. hGH concentrations are not significantly different from nonpregnant levels, but pituitary response to provocative testing is markedly altered. hGH response to hypoglycemia and arginine infusion is enhanced but thereafter becomes depressed. Established pregnancy can continue in the face of hypophysectomy, and in women hypophysectomized prior to pregnancy, induction of ovulation and normal pregnancy can be achieved with appropriate replacement therapy. In cases of primary pituitary hyperfunction, the fetus is not affected.

Maternal Thyroid Gland

The thyroid becomes palpably enlarged during the first trimester, and a bruit may be present. [131]I uptake and thyroid iodide clearance are increased. These changes are due in large part to the increased renal clearance of iodide, which causes a relative iodine deficiency. While total serum thyroxine is elevated as a result of increased thyroid hormone–binding globulin (TBG), free thyroxine and triiodothyronine are normal (Fig 20–1).

Maternal Parathyroid Gland

The net calcium requirement imposed by fetal skeletal development is estimated to be about 30 g by term. This is met by hyperplasia of the parathyroid glands and elevated serum levels of parathyroid hormone. The maternal serum calcium concentration declines to a nadir at 28–32 weeks, largely owing to the hypoalbuminemia of pregnancy. Ionized calcium is maintained at normal concentrations.

Maternal Pancreas

The nutritional demands of the fetus require alteration of maternal metabolic homeostatic control, which results in both structural and functional changes in the maternal pancreas. The size of pancreatic islets increases, and insulin-secreting β cells undergo hyperplasia. Basal levels of insulin are lower or unchanged in early pregnancy but increase during the second trimester. Thereafter, pregnancy is a hyperinsulinemic state, with resistance to the peripheral metabolic effects of insulin. The increased concentration of insulin has been shown to be a result of increased secretion rather than decreased metabolic clearance. The measured half-life for insulin is unchanged in pregnant women. The effects of pregnancy on the pancreas can

SYSTEM	PARAMETER	PATTERN
Cardiovascular	Rate	Gradually increases 20%.
	Blood pressure	Gradually decreases 10% by 34 weeks, then increases to prepregnancy values.
	Stroke volume	Increases to maximum at 19 weeks, then plateaus.
	Cardiac output	Rises rapidly by 20%, then gradually increases an additional 10% by 28 weeks.
	Peripheral venous distention	Progressive increase to term.
	Peripheral vascular resistance	Progressive decrease to term.
Pulmonary	Respiratory rate	Unchanged.
	Tidal volume	Increases by 30–40%.
	Expiratory reserve	Gradual decrease.
	Vital capacity	Unchanged.
	Respiratory minute volume	Increases by 40%.
Blood	Volume	Increases by 50% in second trimester.
	Hematocrit	Decreases slightly.
	Fibrinogen	Increases.
	Electrolytes	Unchanged.
Gastrointestinal	Sphincter tone	Decreases.
	Gastric emptying time	Increases.

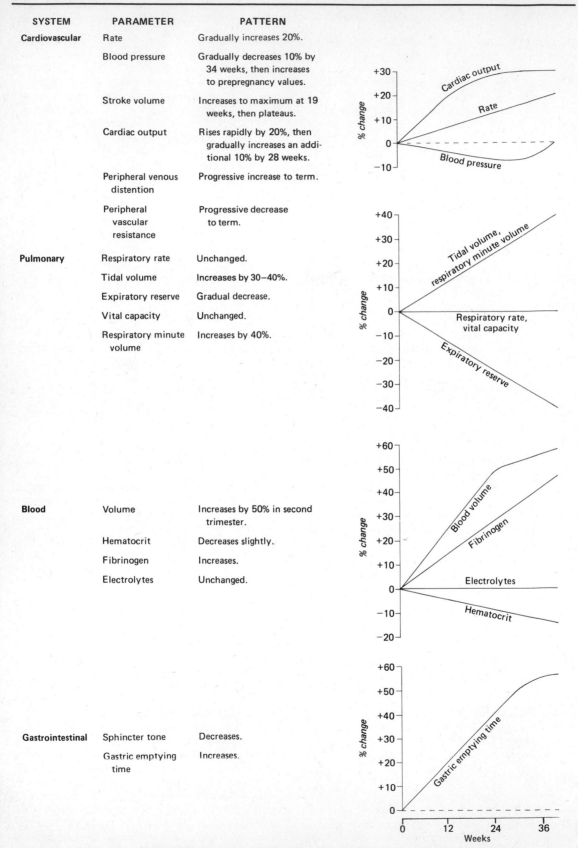

Figure 20–2. Maternal physiologic changes during pregnancy.

SYSTEM	PARAMETER	PATTERN
Renal	Renal flow	Increases 25–50%.
	Glomerular filtration rate	Increases early, then plateaus.
Weight	Uterine weight	Increases from about 60–70 g to about 900–1200 g.
	Body weight	Average 11-kg (25-lb) increase.

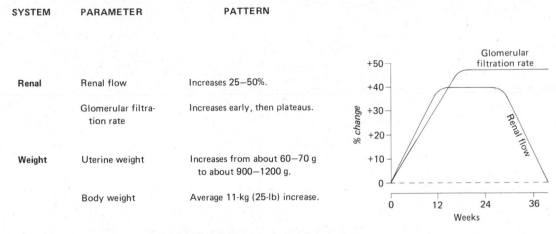

Figure 20–2 (cont'd). Maternal physiologic change during pregnancy.

be mimicked by appropriate treatment with estrogen, progesterone, hCS, and corticosteroids.

Pancreatic production of glucagon remains responsive to usual stimuli and is suppressed by glucose loading, although the degree of responsiveness has not been well evaluated.

Table 20–2. Effect of pregnancy on endocrine function tests.

	Test	Result
Pituitary FSH, LH	GnRH stimulation	Unresponsive from third gestational week until puerperium.
GH	Insulin tolerance test	Response increases during the first half of pregnancy and then is blunted until the puerperium.
	Arginine stimulation	Hyperstimulation during the first and second trimesters, then suppression
TSH	TRH stimulation	Response unchanged.
Pancreas Insulin	Glucose tolerance	Peak glucose increases, and glucose concentration remains elevated longer.
	Glucose challenge	Insulin concentration increases to higher peak levels.
	Arginine infusion	Insulin response is blunted in mid to late pregnancy.
Adrenal Cortisol	ACTH infusion	Exaggerated cortisol and 17-hydroxycorticosterone responses.
	Metyrapone	Diminished response.
Mineralo- corti- coids	ACTH infusion	No DOC response.
	Dexamethasone suppression	No DOC response.

The major role of insulin and glucagon is the control of concentrations of nutrients, specifically glucose, amino acids, and fatty acids. These concentrations are regulated during pregnancy primarily for fetal needs, and the pre- and postfeeding levels cause pancreatic responses that act to support the fetal economy. Insulin is not transported across the placenta but rather exerts its effects on transportable metabolites. Peak insulin secretion in response to meals is accelerated, and glucose tolerance curves are characteristically altered. Fasting glucose levels are maintained at low normal levels. Excess carbohydrate is converted to fat, and fat is readily mobilized during decreased caloric intake.

Amino acid metabolism is also altered during pregnancy, at the expense of maternal needs. Hypoglycemia, hypoinsulinemia, and hyperketonuria do not cause an augmented hepatic gluconeogenesis. The key amino acid substrate, alanine, is diminished by mechanisms as yet unknown.

The normal result of pregnancy, then is to reduce glucose levels modestly but to reserve glucose for fetal needs while maternal energy requirements are met increasingly by the peripheral metabolism of fatty acids. These changes in energy metabolism are beneficial to the fetus and innocuous to the mother with an adequate diet. Even modest fasting, however, causes ketosis, which is potentially injurious to the fetus.

Maternal Adrenal Cortex

A. Glucocorticoids: Plasma cortisol concentrations increase to 3 times nonpregnant levels by the third trimester. Most of the increase can be accounted for by a doubling of corticosteroid-binding globulin (CBG). The increased estrogen levels of pregnancy account for the increase in CBG, which, in turn, is sufficient to account for decreased catabolism of cortisol by the liver. The result is a doubling of the half-life of plasma cortisol. The actual production of cortisol by the zona fasciculata is reduced by about 20%.

The net effect of these changes, however, is an increase in plasma free cortisol, which is approximately doubled by late pregnancy. Whether this increase is mediated through ACTH or by other mechanisms is not known. In spite of cortisol concentrations approaching those found in Cushing's syndrome, diurnal variation in plasma cortisol is maintained. The elevated free cortisol probably contributes to the insulin resistance of pregnancy and possibly to the appearance of striae, but most signs of hypercortisolism do not occur in pregnancy. It is possible that high progesterone levels act as a glucocorticoid antagonist and prevent some cortisol effects.

B. Mineralocorticoids and the Renin-Angiotensin System: Serum aldosterone is markedly elevated in pregnancy. The increase is due to an 8- to 10-fold increased production of aldosterone by the zona glomerulosa and not to increased binding or decreased clearance. The peak in aldosterone production is reached by mid pregnancy and is maintained until delivery. Renin substrate is increased owing to the influence of estrogen on hepatic synthesis, and renin also is increased.

The increases in both renin and renin substrate inevitably lead to increases in renin activity and angiotensin. In spite of these dramatic changes, normal pregnant women show few signs of hyperaldosteronism. There is no tendency to hypokalemia or hypernatremia, and blood pressure at mid pregnancy—when changes in the aldosterone-renin-angiotensin system are maximal—tends to be lower than in the nonpregnant state. It has been suggested that edema of late pregnancy may be due to these changes, but hyperaldosteronism in nonpregnant women leads to hypertension, not edema.

Although the quantitative aspects of this apparent paradox are not fully understood, a qualitative explanation is possible. Progesterone is an effective competitive inhibitor of mineralocorticoids in the distal renal tubules. Exogenous progesterone (but not synthetic progestins) is natriuretic and potassium-sparing in intact humans, whereas it has no effect in adrenalectomized subjects not receiving mineralocorticoids. Progesterone also blunts the response of the kidney to exogenous aldosterone—thus, the increases in renin and aldosterone may simply be an appropriate response to the high gestational levels of progesterone. The concomitant increase in angiotensin II as a result of increased plasma renin activity apparently does not normally result in hypertension, because of diminished sensitivity of the maternal vascular system to angiotensin. Even during the first trimester, exogenous angiotensin provokes less of a rise in blood pressure than in the nonpregnant state.

It is clear that the high levels of renin, angiotensin, and aldosterone in pregnant women are subject to the usual feedback controls, because they respond appropriately to changes in posture, dietary sodium, and water loading and restriction in qualitatively the same way as they do in nonpregnant women. Finally, in patients with pregnancy-induced hypertension in the second half of pregnancy, serum renin, aldosterone, and angiotensin levels are lower than in normal pregnancy, thus ruling out any primary role for the renin-angiotensin system in this disorder.

Production of the mineralocorticoid 11-deoxycorticosterone (DOC) rises throughout pregnancy, and plasma levels 6–10 times normal are achieved by term. In contrast to the nonpregnant state, DOC production in pregnancy is unaffected by ACTH or glucocorticoid administration. The source of DOC appears to be conversion of progesterone to DOC in peripheral tissue. DOC is not elevated in hypertensive disorders of pregnancy.

C. Androgens: In normal pregnancy, the maternal production of androgens is slightly increased. The most important determinant of plasma levels of specific androgens, however, appears to be whether or not the androgen binds to sex hormone–binding globulin (SHBG). Testosterone, which binds avidly to SHBG, increases to the normal male range by the end of the first trimester, but free testosterone levels are actually lower than in the nonpregnant state. Dehydroepiandrosterone sulfate (DHEA sulfate) does not bind significantly to SHBG, and plasma concentrations of DHEA sulfate actually decrease during pregnancy. The desulfation of DHEA sulfate by the placenta and the conversion of DHEA sulfate to estrogens by the fetal-placental unit are also important factors in its increased metabolic clearance.

FETAL ENDOCRINOLOGY

Because of the inaccessibility of the fetus, much of our information about fetal endocrinology is derived indirectly. Most early studies of fetal endocrinology relied upon observations of infants with congenital disorders or inferences from ablation studies or acute experiments in mammals. The development of effective cell culture methods and sensitive radiolabeled assay systems and the ability to achieve stable preparations of chronically catheterized monkey fetuses have increased our understanding of the dynamics of intrauterine endocrine events.

Study of the fetal endocrine system is further complicated by the multiplicity of sources of the various hormones. The fetus is exposed to maternal and placental hormones as well as to those it produces itself. Amniotic fluid contains a variety of hormones of mixed fetal and maternal origin, and these hormones are of uncertain importance. Study of the isolated fetus, even if possible, would thus be of little physiologic relevance.

A final pitfall in the study of fetal endocrine systems relates to the process of development itself. Inferences from the behavior of adult endocrine systems are not transferable to the fetus, because target organs, receptors, modulators, and regulators develop at different times. Thus, the role of a particular hormone in the fetal economy at any one point in gestation may bear little or no relationship to its role in postnatal life.

Dating of events in fetal development is usually given in "fetal weeks," which begin at the time of ovulation. Thus, fetal age is always 2 weeks less than gestational age.

Fetal Anterior Pituitary Hormones

The characteristic anterior pituitary cell types are discernible as early as 8–10 fetal weeks, and all of the hormones of the adult anterior pituitary are extractable from the fetal adenohypophysis by 12 weeks. Similarly, the hypothalamic hormones thyrotropin-releasing hormone (TRH), gonadotropin-releasing hormone (GnRH), and somatostatin are present by 8–10 weeks. The direct circulatory connection between hypothalamus and pituitary develops later, with capillary invasion initially visible at about 16 weeks.

The role of the fetal pituitary in organogenesis of various target organs during the first trimester appears to be negligible. None of the pituitary hormones are released into the fetal circulation in large quantities until after 20 fetal weeks. Even growth hormone (GH) appears not to be influential, and in fact total absence of GH is consistent with normal development at birth. Development of the gonads and adrenals during the first trimester appears to be directed by hCG rather than by fetal trophic hormones, and the development of the thyroid glands during the first trimester occurs independently of TSH production by the fetus.

During the second trimester, there is a marked increase in secretion of all of the anterior pituitary hormones, which coincides with maturation of the hypophyseal portal system. Observations include a marked rise in production of GH and an increase in fetal serum TSH, with a concomitant increase in fetal thyroidal iodine uptake. Gonadotropin production also increases, with the female achieving higher FSH levels in both pituitary and serum than does the male. The fetal gonadotropins do not direct the events of early gonadal development but are essential for normal development of the differentiated gonads and external genitalia. ACTH rises significantly during the second trimester and assumes an increasing role in directing the maturation of the differentiated adrenal, as shown by the anencephalic fetus, in which the fetal zone of the adrenal undergoes atrophy after 20 weeks. Fetal PRL secretion also increases after the 20th fetal week, but the functional significance of this hormone, if any, is unknown.

During the third trimester, maturation of feedback systems modulating hypothalamic release signals causes serum concentrations of all of the pituitary hormones except PRL to decline.

Fetal Posterior Pituitary Hormones

Vasopressin and oxytocin are demonstrable by 12–18 weeks in the fetal posterior pituitary gland and correlate with the development of their sites of production, the supraoptic and paraventricular nuclei. The hormone content of the gland increases toward term, with no evidence of feedback control.

During labor, umbilical artery oxytocin is higher than umbilical vein oxytocin. It has been suggested that the fetal posterior pituitary may contribute to the onset or maintenance of labor.

Fetal Thyroid Gland

The thyroid gland develops at about the same stage in development as the pituitary. Initial first-trimester development occurs in the absence of detectable TSH. By 12 weeks the thyroid is capable of iodine-concentrating activity and thyroid hormone synthesis.

During the second trimester, TRH, TSH, and free T_4 all begin to rise. The maturation of feedback mechanisms is suggested by the subsequent plateau of TSH at about 20 fetal weeks. Fetal T_3 and reverse T_3 do not become detectable until the third trimester. The hormone produced in largest amount throughout fetal life is T_4, with the metabolically active T_3 and its inactive derivative, reverse T_3, rising in parallel to T_4 during the third trimester. At birth, conversion of T_4 to T_3 becomes demonstrable.

The development of thyroid hormones occurs independently of maternal systems, and very little placental transfer of thyroid hormone occurs in physiologic concentrations. This prevents maternal thyroid disorders from affecting the fetal compartment but also prevents effective therapy for fetal hypothyroidism through maternal supplementation. Goitrogenic agents such as propylthiouracil are transferred across the placenta and may induce fetal hypothyroidism and goiter.

The function of the fetal thyroid hormones appears crucial to somatic growth and for successful neonatal adaptation.

Fetal Parathyroid Gland

The fetal parathyroid is capable of synthesizing parathyroid hormone by the end of the first trimester. However, the placenta actively transports calcium into the fetal compartment, and the fetus remains relatively hypercalcemic throughout gestation. This contributes to a suppression of parathyroid hormone, and fetal serum levels in umbilical cord have been reported to be low or undetectable. Fetal serum calcitonin levels are elevated, enhancing bone accretion. Fetal vitamin D levels reflect maternal levels but do not appear to be significant in fetal calcium metabolism.

Fetal Adrenal Cortex

The fetal adrenal differs anatomically and functionally from the adult gland. The cortex is identifiable as early as 4 weeks of fetal age, and by the seventh week, steroidogenic activity can be detected in the inner zone layers.

By 20 weeks, the adrenal cortex has increased to a mass that is considerably larger than its relative postnatal size. During gestation, it occupies as much as 0.5% of total body volume, and most of this tissue is composed of a unique fetal zone that subsequently regresses or is transformed into the definitive (adult) zone during the early neonatal period. The inner fetal zone is responsible for the majority of steroids produced during fetal life and comprises 80% of the mass of the adrenal. During the second trimester, the inner fetal zone continues to grow, while the outer zone remains relatively undifferentiated. At about 25 weeks, the definitive (adult) zone develops more rapidly and begins to produce steroids, ultimately assuming the principal role in steroid synthesis during the early postnatal weeks. This transfer of function is accompanied by involution of the fetal zone, which is completed during the first months of neonatal life.

Fetal Gonads

The testis is a detectable structure by about 6 fetal weeks. The interstitial or Leydig cells, which synthesize fetal testosterone, are functional at this same stage. The maximal production of testosterone coincides with the maximal production of hCG by the placenta; binding of hCG to fetal testes with stimulation of testosterone release has been demonstrated. Other fetal testicular products of importance are the reduced testosterone metabolite dihydrotestosterone and müllerian duct inhibitory factor. Dihydrotestosterone is responsible for development of the external genital structures, whereas müllerian duct inhibitory factor prevents development of female internal structures.

Little is known about fetal ovarian function. By 7–8 weeks of intrauterine life, the ovaries become recognizable, but their importance in fetal physiology has not been established, and the significance of the steroids produced by the ovaries remains unclear.

ENDOCRINE CONTROL OF PARTURITION

During the last few weeks of normal pregnancy, 2 processes herald approaching labor. Uterine contractions, usually painless, become increasingly frequent, and the lower uterine segment and cervix become softer and thinner, a process known as effacement, or "ripening." Although false alarms are not uncommon, the onset of true labor is usually fairly abrupt, with the establishment of regular contractions every 2–5 minutes, leading to delivery in less than 24 hours. There is a huge literature describing the physiologic and biochemical events that occur during human labor, but the key inciting event has eluded detection. For sheep, it is

the fetus that controls the onset of labor. The initial measurable event is an increase in fetal plasma cortisol, which, in turn, alters placental steroid production, resulting in a drop in progesterone. Cortisol reliably induces labor in sheep, but in humans, glucocorticoids do not induce labor and there is no detectable drop in plasma progesterone prior to labor. Furthermore, exogenous progesterone does not prevent labor in humans.

The difficulty in identifying a *single* initiating event in human labor suggests that there is more than one. Approaching the matter in a different way, one could ask: What are the factors responsible for maintenance of pregnancy, and how can they fail?

Sex Steroids

Progesterone is essential for maintenance of early pregnancy, and withdrawal of progesterone leads to termination of pregnancy. Progesterone causes hyperpolarization of the myometrium, decreasing the amplitude of action potentials and preventing effective contractions. In various experimental systems, progesterone decreases alpha-adrenergic receptors, stimulates cAMP production, and inhibits oxytocin receptor synthesis. Progesterone also inhibits estrogen receptor synthesis, promotes the storage of prostaglandin precursors in the decidua and fetal membranes, and stabilizes the lysosomes containing prostaglandin-synthesizing enzymes. Estrogen opposes progesterone in these actions and may have an independent role in ripening the uterine cervix and promoting uterine contractility. Thus, the estrogen:progesterone ratio may be an important parameter. In a small series of patients, an increase in the estrogen:progesterone ratio has been shown to precede labor. Thus, for some individuals, a drop in progesterone or an increase in estrogen may initiate labor. The cause of the change in steroids may be placental maturation or a signal from the fetus, but there are not data to support either thesis. It has been shown that an increase in the estrogen:progesterone ratio increases the number of myometrial gap junctions; this finding may explain the coordinate, effective contractions that characterize true labor as opposed to the nonpainful, ineffective contractions of false labor.

Oxytocin

Oxytocin infusion is commonly used to induce or augment labor. Both maternal and fetal oxytocin levels increase spontaneously during labor, but neither has been convincingly shown to increase prior to labor. Data in animals suggest that oxytocin's role in initiation of labor is due to increased sensitivity of the uterus to oxytocin rather than increased plasma concentrations of the hormone. Even women with diabetes insipidus are able to deliver without oxytocin augmentation; thus a maternal source of the hormone is not indispensable.

Prostaglandins

Prostaglandin $F_{2\alpha}$ administered intra-amniotically or intravenously is an effective abortifacient as early as 14 weeks of gestation. Prostaglandin E_2 administered by vagina will induce labor in most women in the third trimester. The amnion and chorion contain high concentrations of arachidonic acid, and the decidua contains active prostaglandin synthetase. Prostaglandins are almost certainly involved in maintenance of labor once it is established. They also probably are important in initiating labor in some circumstances, such as in amnionitis or when the membranes are "stripped" by the physician. They probably are part of the "final common pathway" of labor.

Prostaglandin synthetase inhibitors abolish premature labor, but their clinical usefulness has been restricted by their simultaneous effect of closing the ductus arteriosus, which can lead to fetal pulmonary hypertension.

Catecholamines

Catecholamines with α_2-adrenergic activity cause uterine contractions, whereas β_2-adrenergics inhibit labor. Progesterone increases the ratio of beta receptors to alpha receptors in myometrium, thus favoring continued gestation. There is no evidence that changes in catecholamines or their receptors initiate labor, but it is likely that such changes help sustain labor once initiated. The beta-adrenergic drug ritodrine has proved to be a valuable agent in the management of premature labor. Alpha-adrenergic agents have not been useful in inducing labor, because of their cardiovascular side effects.

ENDOCRINOLOGY OF THE PUERPERIUM

Extirpation of any active endocrine organ leads to compensatory changes in other organs and systems. Delivery of the infant and placenta causes both immediate and long-term adjustment to loss of the pregnancy hormones. The sudden withdrawal of fetal-placental hormones at delivery permits determination of their serum half-lives and some evaluation of their function during pregnancy.

Physiologic & Anatomic Changes

Some of the physiologic and anatomic adjustments that take place after delivery are hormone-dependent, whereas others are themselves responsible for hormonal changes. For example, major readjustments of the cardiovascular system occur in response to the normal blood losses associated with delivery and to loss of the low-resistance placental shunt. By the third postpartum day, blood volume is estimated to decline to about 84% of predelivery values. These cardiovascular changes influence renal and liver clearance of hormones.

Reproductive Tract Changes

The uterus decreases progressively in size at the rate of about 500 g/wk and continues to be palpable abdominally until about 2 weeks postpartum, when it reoccupies its position entirely within the pelvis. Nonpregnant size and weight (60–70 g) are reached by 6 weeks. The reversal of myometrial hypertrophy occurs with a decrease in size of individual myometrial cells rather than by reduction in number. Uterine discharge also changes progressively during this period, with the mixture of fresh blood and decidua becoming a serous transudate and then ceasing in 3–6 weeks.

The endometrium, which is sloughed at the time of delivery, regenerates rapidly; by the seventh day, there is restoration of surface epithelium, except at the placental site. By the second week after delivery, the endometrium resembles normal proliferative-phase endometrium, except for the characteristic hyalinized decidual areas. The earliest documented appearance of a secretory endometrium occurred on day 44 in one series of daily biopsies. These rapid regenerative changes do not apply to the area of placental implantation, which requires much longer for restoration and retains pathognomonic histologic evidence of placentation indefinitely.

The cervix and vagina also recover rapidly from the effects of pregnancy, labor, and delivery. The cervix regains tone over the first week; by 6 weeks postpartum, it usually exhibits complete healing of lesions sustained at the time of delivery. Histologically, involution may continue beyond 6 weeks, with stromal edema, leukocytic infiltration, and glandular hyperplasia still apparent. Similarly, the vagina regains muscular tone following delivery, and rugae appear as early as 3 weeks. However, in women who nurse, the vaginal mucosa may remain atrophic for months, sometimes resulting in dyspareunia and a watery discharge.

Endocrine Changes

A. Steroids: With expulsion of the placenta, the steroid levels decline precipitously, their half-lives being measured in minutes or hours. As a consequence of continued low-level production by the corpus luteum, progesterone does not reach basal prenatal levels as rapidly as does estradiol. Plasma progesterone falls to luteal-phase levels within 24 hours after delivery but to follicular-phase levels only after several days. Removal of the corpus luteum results in a fall to follicular levels within 24 hours. Estradiol reaches follicular-phase levels within 1–3 days after delivery.

B. Pituitary Hormones: The pituitary gland, which enlarges during pregnancy owing primarily to an increase in lactotrophs, does not diminish in size until after lactation ceases. Secretion of FSH and LH continues to be suppressed during the early weeks of the puerperium, and stimulus with bolus doses of GnRH results in subnormal release of LH and FSH.

Over the ensuing weeks, responsiveness to GnRH gradually returns to normal, and most women exhibit follicular-phase serum levels of LH and FSH by the third or fourth postpartum week.

C. Prolactin: Serum prolactin (PRL), which rises throughout pregnancy, falls with the onset of labor and then exhibits variable patterns of secretion depending upon whether breast feeding occurs. Delivery is associated with a surge in PRL, which is followed by a rapid fall in serum concentrations over 7–14 days in the nonlactating mother.

In nonlactating women, the return of normal cyclic function and ovulation may be expected as soon as the second postpartum month, with the initial ovulation occurring at an average of 9–10 weeks postpartum. In lactating women, PRL usually causes a persistence of anovulation. Surges of PRL are believed to act on the hypothalamus to inhibit GnRH secretion. Administration of exogenous GnRH during this time induces normal pituitary responsiveness, and occasional ovulation may occur spontaneously even during lactation. The average time for ovulation in women who have lactated for at least 3 months is about 17 weeks. The percentage of nonlactating women who have resumed menstruation increases linearly up to 12 weeks, by which time 70% will have restored menses. In contrast, the linear increase for lactating women exhibits a much shallower slope, and 70% of lactating women will have menstruated by about 36 weeks.

Lactation

Development of the breast alveolar lobules occurs throughout pregnancy. This period of mammogenesis requires the concerted participation of estrogen, progesterone, PRL, GH, and glucocorticoids. hCS may also play a role but is not indispensable. Milk secretion in the puerperium is associated with further enlargement of the lobules, followed by synthesis of milk constituents such as lactose and casein.

Lactation requires PRL, insulin, and adrenal steroids. It does not occur until unconjugated estrogens fall to nonpregnant levels at about 36–48 hours postpartum.

PRL is essential to milk production. Its action involves induced synthesis of large numbers of PRL receptors; these appear to be autoregulated by PRL, since PRL increases receptor levels in cell culture and since bromocriptine, a PRL inhibitor, causes a decrease in both PRL and its receptors. In the absence of PRL, milk secretion does not take place; but even in the presence of high levels of PRL during the third trimester, milk secretion does not take place until after delivery, owing to the blocking effect of high levels of estrogen.

Galactopoiesis, or the process of continued milk secretion, is also dependent upon the function and integration of several hormones. Evidence from GH-deficient dwarfs and hypothyroid patients suggests that GH and thyroid hormone are not required.

Milk secretion requires the additional stimulus of emptying of the breast. A neural arc must be activated for continued milk secretion. Milk ejection occurs in response to a surge of oxytocin, which induces a contractile response in the smooth muscle surrounding the gland ductules. Oxytocin release is occasioned by stimuli of a visual, psychologic, or physical nature that prepare the mother for suckling.

INHIBITION OF LACTATION

There are relatively few contraindications to breast-feeding. Among these are purulent mastitis; breast cancer; and ingestion of medications such as chemotherapeutic agents or radioactive iodide, which are secreted in breast milk. The major indication for suppression of lactation is personal preference on the part of mothers unwilling or unable to breast-feed. Methods of suppression of lactation include avoidance of breast stimulation; use of estrogens, androgens, or both; and use of dopamine agonists to inhibit PRL secretion. If avoidance of breast stimulation is used alone, about 50% of women will have significant engorgement and pain. This discomfort led to the practice of seeking pharmacologic means of preventing engorgement. Estrogen, combinations of estrogen and androgen, and synthetic antiestrogens such as clomiphene have all been promoted for this use. Their mechanism of action is not established but is believed to be at the level of the breast as opposed to the pituitary or hypothalamus. Estrogens alone are only slightly more effective than placebo. Problems associated with the administration of large doses of estrogenic compounds include occasional rebound lactation following therapy and the increased risk of thromboembolic complications in patients already at risk due to parturition itself. Estrogen-androgen combinations may act at the pituitary level as well, and results of controlled studies suggest they may provide greater relief than placebo or estrogen alone. These steroids must be given at the time of delivery, because effectiveness diminishes after even 1 or 2 hours have elapsed. Rebound lactation may occur. Virilization has not been reported despite the use of large doses of androgens. Clomiphene and tamoxifen have been reported to provide relief in more than 90% of cases, with minimal side effects; these drugs are believed to act primarily by reducing serum PRL. Bromocriptine mesylate, a dopamine agonist that effectively inhibits PRL secretion, is 97% effective in inhibiting both engorgement and secretion. A 14-day course of 2.5 mg orally twice daily is recommended. A third week of 2.5 mg daily is suggested by some. Only 3% of patients have sufficient side effects (nausea or dizziness) to require early cessation of therapy. Mild rebound lactation requiring only supportive therapy or an additional 7-day course of the drug occurs in one out of 4 patients.

In summary, where suppression of lactation is required, avoidance of stimulation will be effective in 60–70% of women. A single injection of a combination of testosterone and estradiol valerate given immediately at delivery has a high success rate, but there is risk of rebound lactation. Inhibition of PRL with dopamine agonists is most effective when initiated immediately postpartum and usually requires at least 2 weeks of therapy.

ENDOCRINE DISORDERS & PREGNANCY

PREGNANCY & PITUITARY ADENOMAS

In women of reproductive age, small tumors of the anterior pituitary are not uncommon (see also Chapter 6). While most are nonfunctional and asymptomatic, the most common symptom of pituitary microadenomas is amenorrhea, frequently accompanied by galactorrhea. In the past, few affected women became pregnant, but now most can be made to ovulate and to conceive with the aid of clomiphene citrate, menotropins and hCG, or bromocriptine. Before ovulation is induced in any patient, serum PRL should be determined. If it is elevated, the sella turcica should be evaluated by magnetic resonance imaging (MRI) or by high-resolution CT scanning with contrast. About 10% of women with secondary amenorrhea will be found to have adenomas, while 20–50% of women with amenorrhea and galactorrhea will have detectable tumors.

The effect of pregnancy on pituitary adenomas depends on the size of the adenoma. Among 215 women with microadenomas (< 10 mm in diameter), fewer than 1% developed progressive visual field defects, 5% developed headaches, and none experienced more serious neurologic sequelae. Of 60 patients who had macroadenomas and became pregnant, 20% developed abnormal changes in their visual fields or other neurologic signs, usually in the first half of their pregnancies. Many of these required therapy. Monitoring of patients with known PRL-secreting adenomas during pregnancy is primarily based on clinical examination. The normal gestational increase in PRL may obscure the increase attributable to the adenoma, and radiographic procedures are undesirable in pregnancy.

Visual disturbances are usually experienced as "clumsiness" and are objectively found to be due to visual field changes. The most frequent findings is bitemporal hemianopia, but in advanced cases the defect can progress to concentric contraction of fields and enlargement of the blind spot.

Since the pituitary normally increases in size during pregnancy, headaches are common and bitemporal hemianopia not uncommon in patients with adenomas. These changes almost always revert to normal after delivery, so that aggressive therapy for known pituitary adenomas is not indicated except in cases of rapidly progressive visual loss.

Management

Management of the pregnant woman with a small adenoma includes early ophthalmologic consultation for formal visual field mapping and repeat examinations once a month or every other month throughout pregnancy.

If visual field disturbances are minimal, pregnancy may be allowed to proceed to term. If symptoms become progressively more severe and the fetus is mature, labor should be induced. If symptoms are severe and the fetus is immature, management may consist of transsphenoidal resection of the adenoma or medical treatment with bromocriptine. While bromocriptine inhibits both fetal and maternal pituitary PRL secretion, it does not affect decidual PRL secretion. At present, bromocriptine appears not to be teratogenic, and no adverse fetal effects have been reported. It should, of course, be used with caution in pregnancy, but in most cases it is probably preferable to surgery. Radiation therapy should not be used in pregnancy.

Management of PRL-secreting tumors in women who want to become pregnant is controversial. Surgical resection by surgeons with experience in transsphenoidal procedures results in reduction of PRL levels and resumption of normal ovulation in 60–80% of women with microadenomas and 30–50% of women with macroadenomas. The incidence of recurrence is at least 10–15% and will probably increase with further follow-up. Bromocriptine is usually well tolerated and is successful in achieving normal menstrual cycles and lowering PRL levels in 40–80% of patients. Bromocriptine also causes a marked decrease in tumor size, but the original size of the tumor is usually regained within days or weeks after discontinuing therapy. In the case of large tumors, combined medical and surgical management may often be appropriate. Radiation therapy has an important role in arresting growth of tumors that are resistant to other management, particularly large tumors that involve the cavernous sinuses and tumors that secrete both GH and PRL (see Chapter 6).

Prognosis & Follow-Up

There appears to be no increase in obstetric complications associated with pituitary adenomas, and no fetal jeopardy. The rate of prematurity increases in women with tumors requiring therapy, but this is probably due to aggressive intervention rather than to spontaneous premature labor.

The postpartum period is characterized by rapid relief of even severe symptoms, with less than 4% of untreated tumors developing permanent sequelae. In some cases, tumors improve following pregnancy, with normalization or lowering of PRL relative to pre-pregnancy values. Management should include radiography and assessment of PRL levels 4–6 weeks after delivery. There are no contraindications to breastfeeding.

PREGNANCY & BREAST CANCER

Breast cancer complicates one in 1500–5000 pregnancies. Only one-sixth of breast cancers occur in women of reproductive age, but of these, one in 7 is diagnosed during pregnancy or the puerperium. Pregnancy and breast cancer have long been considered such an ominous combination that only one in 20 young women who have had breast cancer have later become pregnant. It now appears, however, that pregnancy has little effect on growth of breast cancer, though it presents problems of detection and management of the cancer (see Chapter 26).

Influence of Pregnancy on Breast Cancer

Pregnancy is not an etiologic factor in breast cancer. Indeed, there is good evidence that pregnancy at an early age actually reduces the risk of developing mammary cancer, and multiple pregnancies may also make the disease less likely. Moreover, contemporary concepts of the rate of tumor growth suggest that a tumor becomes clinically evident only 8–10 years after its inception. Thus, a tumor cannot arise and be discovered during the same pregnancy. In view of the increased glandular proliferation and blood flow and marked increase in lymph flow that occur during pregnancy, it could be argued that pregnancy accelerates the appearance of previously subclinical diseases, but this has not been demonstrated.

Probably the most important influence of pregnancy on breast cancer is the delay it may cause in making the diagnosis and starting therapy. In some series, the interval between initial symptoms and treatment was 6–7 months longer than in the absence of pregnancy. The increased density of the breasts in pregnancy makes small masses less apparent; and even when masses are found, both the patient and the physician are apt to attribute them to expected physiologic changes in pregnancy. Larger tumors may be misdiagnosed as galactoceles, and inflammatory carcinoma in the puerperium is liable to be misdiagnosed as mastitis.

At the time of diagnosis, 60% of pregnancy-associated breast cancers have metastasized to regional lymph nodes, and an additional 20% have distant metastases. Stage for stage, however, salvage rates following appropriate therapy are comparable to those achieved in nonpregnant patients. Termination of pregnancy, either by abortion or by early delivery, does not influence maternal survival.

Pregnancy After Treatment for Cancer

Pregnancy following definitive treatment of breast cancer has no adverse effect on survival. Indeed, women who become pregnant following stage I or II breast cancer have a somewhat better 5-year survival rate than matched controls who did not become pregnant but who survived at least as long as their match before becoming pregnant.

Women who have had breast cancer are frequently advised to avoid pregnancy for 5 years. Because most fertile women with breast cancer are in their mid 30s, such a plan virtually precludes pregnancy. Because pregnancy is not known to influence the rate of cancer recurrence, the only reasons for proscribing pregnancy are to avoid the possibility that management of a recurrence will be complicated by the pregnancy or to avoid the problem of producing motherless children. For a couple strongly desiring pregnancy, these risks may become acceptable in a much shorter time than 5 years, especially if the original lesion was small and the spread of disease minimal.

Estrogen in Cancer

Determinations of soluble estrogen and progesterone receptors are frequently used in breast cancer to predict whether the tumor is likely to respond to endocrine therapy. There is also evidence that the presence of estrogen receptor-positive tumors is correlated with a lower risk of early recurrence. In the pregnant patient, however, high progesterone levels inhibit estrogen and progesterone receptor synthesis, and high levels of both hormones cause their receptors to become tightly associated with the nuclear fraction. Thus, when soluble receptors are quantified, all breast cancers arising in pregnancy appear to be receptor-negative, making such measurements in pregnancy at best worthless and at worst dangerously misleading. The introduction of immunohistochemical assays, which allow identification of occupied nuclear receptors, may lead to a more reliable assessment.

Early Diagnosis

It is clear that early diagnosis of breast cancer in pregnancy gives the best chance of improved survival. Self-examination should be encouraged in spite of the anxiety it will cause, and thorough breast examinations should be performed periodically throughout pregnancy, not just at the initial examination. Even mildly suspicious lesions should be investigated if they persist for 1–2 weeks; waiting for a lesion to grow before further investigation is not acceptable practice. If a woman has discovered a small mass, her assessment should be accepted even if the physician cannot feel the mass by the usual techniques. Small lesions that would otherwise be missed can often be felt if soap and water are used for lubrication. Cytologic examination of fine-needle aspirates is probably the best technique for investigating discrete lesions. If any question persists, ultrasonography or low-dose mammography should be employed. Unless one is very experienced with evaluating early breast carcinomas, consultation with a surgical oncologist is always in order.

Treatment of Breast Cancer in Pregnancy

Once the diagnosis of cancer is made, the patient must be treated surgically without delay. In view of the large percentage of patients with positive nodes, the procedure should be one that provides adequate sampling of the axillary nodes, such as modified radical mastectomy. Simple mastectomy with axillary irradiation should be avoided. Therapeutic abortion is not routinely indicated. If, on the basis of surgical staging, adjuvant therapy is considered advisable, the decision must be made either to terminate the pregnancy by abortion or early delivery or to postpone therapy. Since delay in treatment is the principal known reason for the poorer prognosis of breast cancer in pregnancy, delivery should be accomplished as soon as there is a substantial probability of good fetal outcome—usually at 32–34 weeks. Most forms of cytotoxic therapy are absolutely contraindicated in pregnancy. Radiation can be given with appropriate shielding, but the dose to the fetus will not be negligible.

HYPERTENSIVE DISORDERS OF PREGNANCY

Hypertension associated with pregnancy is generally categorized as chronic, in which elevated blood pressures are clinically recognized prior to the 20th week of pregnancy, or gestational, when the onset is beyond 20 weeks of gestation. If the latter is complicated by proteinuria and generalized edema, the triad is referred to as preeclampsia. When seizures accompany this syndrome, the condition is termed eclampsia. The incidence of preeclampsia is about 7%. Women at highest risk include primigravidas under 18 years old, multiparous women over 35 years old, black women, and women with twin gestations, diabetes, hydramnios, or prepregnancy hypertension. About half of women with prepregnancy hypertension develop exacerbations of hypertension in the third trimester.

Course of Hypertension in Pregnancy

In normal pregnancies, as well as those complicated by mild essential hypertension, diastolic blood pressure decreases 10–15 mm Hg in the second trimester. Hypertensive patients first seen at that time may be mistakenly identified as having preeclampsia when the blood pressure again increases in the third trimester.

Clinically, preeclampsia usually appears after the 32nd week of gestation and, most frequently, during labor. In severe cases, especially those complicated by essential hypertension, acute rises in blood pressure may occur as early as 26 weeks. If hypertension appears in the first or early second trimester, it is associated either with gestational trophoblastic disease or an underlying disorder such as an acute flare-up of lupus nephritis. Occasionally, the onset of hypertension is recognized during the 24 hours following delivery.

In normal pregnancies, all of the components of the renin-angiotensin-aldosterone system are markedly elevated. In pregnancies complicated by chronic hypertension or preeclampsia, these components are reduced toward normal nonpregnant levels, suggesting an appropriate feedback response. The most consistent finding in women with hypertension in pregnancy is the increased sensitivity to angiotensin, in contrast to reduced sensitivity to angiotensin that is characteristic of normal pregnancy. Arteriolar constriction in response to angiotensin and other pressors is diminished during normal pregnancy from the first trimester until delivery. In pregnancies destined to be complicated by hypertension, there is a gradual *increase* in arteriolar response to angiotensin that becomes statistically significant by 18–22 weeks of gestation—long before changes in blood pressure are detectable. The cause of this increase in vascular sensitivity to angiotensin is not known. It has been suggested that endothelial cell dysfunction may explain many of the pathophysiologic features of preeclampsia.

Symptoms & Signs

Signs of preeclampsia include a rise in diastolic pressure by 15 mm Hg or more over first trimester values, and proteinuria exceeding 500 mg daily. Symptoms include headaches, visual disturbances, and epigastric pain. Eclampsia may occur even with mild elevation of blood pressure and is associated with a maternal mortality rate as high as 10%. Deaths occur most frequently from cerebral hemorrhage, renal failure, disseminated intravascular coagulopathy, acute pulmonary edema, or hepatic failure. The fetal perinatal mortality rate is in excess of 30%, and the risk of perinatal morbidity due to hypoxia is even higher.

Treatment of Preeclampsia

The only definitive therapy for preeclampsia is delivery. If a modest increase in blood pressure first occurs in association with proteinuria at 32–36 weeks of gestation, bed rest, preferably in the left lateral decubitus position, is frequently effective in temporarily inducing diuresis and controlling progression of the disease, thus gaining time for the developing fetus. If labor occurs or induction of labor is attempted, parenteral magnesium sulfate should be used to prevent seizures and should be continued for 24 hours following delivery. Moderate hypertension need not be treated with antihypertensive agents; however, diastolic blood pressure above 120 mm Hg must be controlled to reduce the risk of intracranial hemorrhage. The agent of choice is hydralazine, 5 mg intravenously at 15- to 20-minute intervals, until the diastolic pressure is approximately 100 mm Hg. If hydralazine is unsuccessful, diazoxide or nitroprusside may be used, but these agents are rarely required.

Treatment of Chronic Hypertension

Women with chronic hypertension who become pregnant require special management. Chesley's recommendations are probably the best:

(1) Diastolic pressures under 100 mm Hg should not be treated. However, if a woman is receiving antihypertensive therapy when first seen in pregnancy, therapy should be continued. If she is taking propranolol, consideration may be given to switching to a more specific β_1-antagonist such as metoprolol or atenolol. The rare patient who has been taking ganglionic blockers should receive another form of therapy instead. Owing to a transient decrease in blood volume and placental perfusion associated with thiazide diuretics, use of these agents should usually not be initiated during pregnancy; however, if a woman is already receiving such therapy, it may be continued.

(2) Diastolic pressures above 100 mm Hg discovered during pregnancy call for antihypertensive management. Initial therapy should be with methyldopa, 250 mg orally at bedtime. This may be increased 1 g twice daily as required. If unacceptable drowsiness lasting more than 2–3 days occurs, the dosage may be reduced, and hydralazine, beginning at 10 mg orally twice daily and increasing up to 100 mg twice daily, may be added. If hydralazine is not tolerated, prazosin may be gradually added to the methyldopa therapy.

(3) Accelerated hypertension at any stage of gestation should be managed with bed rest and, if necessary, intravenous hydralazine. Unless diastolic pressure can be reduced to 110 mm Hg promptly, delivery should be performed regardless of gestational age.

Prognosis

The prognosis for hypertensive cardiovascular disease in later life in women with preeclampsia depends on the patient's age and parity. Preeclampsia in the young primigravida is not associated with an increased risk of hypertension in later pregnancies or in later life. Hypertension in later pregnancies is associated with an increased risk of chronic hypertension in later life. However, if the hypertensive pregnancy was related to multiple gestation or trophoblastic disease, there is no increased risk of later hypertension.

HYPERTHYROIDISM IN PREGNANCY

Pregnancy mimics hyperthyroidism. There is thyroid enlargement, increased cardiac output, and peripheral vasodilatation. Owing to the increase in thyroid hormone–binding globulin (TBG), total serum thyroxine is in the range expected for hyperthyroidism. Free thyroxine, the free thyroxine index, and TSH levels, however, remain in the normal range (see Chapter 10).

True hyperthyroidism complicates one or 2 per 1000 pregnancies. The most common form of hyperthyroidism during pregnancy is Graves' disease. Hyperthyroidism is associated with an increased risk of premature delivery (11–25%) and may modestly increase the risk of early abortion. In Graves' disease, thyroid-stimulating immunoglobulin (TSI), also known as long-acting thyroid stimulator (LATS), a 7S globulin, crosses the placenta and may cause fetal goiter and transient neonatal hyperthyroidism, but these effects do not seriously jeopardize the fetus.

Treatment

The treatment of maternal hyperthyroidism is complicated by pregnancy. Radioiodides are strictly contraindicated. Iodide therapy can lead to huge fetal goiter and is contraindicated except as acute therapy to prevent thyroid storm before thyroid surgery. All antithyroid drugs cross the placenta and may cause fetal hypothyroidism and goiter or cretinism in the newborn. However, propylthiouracil in doses of 300 mg/d or less has been shown to be reasonably safe, although even at low doses about 10% of newborns will have a detectable goiter. Propranolol has been used to control maternal cardiovascular symptoms but may result in fetal bradycardia, growth retardation, premature labor, and neonatal respiratory depression. Partial or total thyroidectomy, especially in the second trimester, is a reasonably safe procedure except for the risk of premature labor.

A. Propylthiouracil: A reasonable plan of management is to begin therapy with propylthiouracil in doses high enough to bring the free T_4 index into the mildly hyperthyroid range and then to taper the dose gradually. Giving thyroxine along with propylthiouracil in the hope that it will cross the placenta in sufficient quantities to prevent fetal hypothyroidism is not effective and serves only to increase the amount of propylthiouracil required. If the maintenance dose of propylthiouracil is above 300 mg/d, serious consideration should be given to partial thyroidectomy.

B. Propranolol: Propranolol may be used transiently to ameliorate cardiovascular symptoms while control is being achieved.

Management of Newborn

Newborns should be observed carefully. In infants of mothers given propylthiouracil, even equivocal evidence of hypothyroidism is an indication for thyroxine replacement therapy. Neonatal Graves' disease, which may present as late as 2 weeks after delivery, requires intensive therapy (see Chapter 10).

HYPOTHYROIDISM IN PREGNANCY

Hypothyroidism is uncommon in pregnancy, since most women with the untreated disorder are oligo-ovulatory. As a practical matter, women taking thyroid medication at the time of conception should be maintained on the same dose throughout pregnancy, whether or not the obstetrician believes thyroid replacement was originally indicated. Physiologic doses of thyroid are innocuous, but maternal hypothyroidism may be hazardous to the developing fetus. The correlation between maternal and fetal thyroid status is poor, and hypothyroid mothers frequently deliver euthyroid infants. The strongest correlation between maternal and newborn hypothyroidism occurs in areas where endemic goiter due to iodide deficiency is common. In these regions, dietary iodide supplementation in addition to thyroid hormone treatment of the mother may be of the greatest importance in preventing cretinism.

DIABETES MELLITUS & PREGNANCY
John L. Kitzmiller, MD

Hormone & Fuel Balance During Normal Pregnancy

Pregnancy produces major changes in the homeostasis of all metabolic fuels and in this way affects the management of diabetes. Plasma concentrations of glucose in the **postabsorptive state** decline as pregnancy advances, because of increasing placental uptake of glucose and a probable limitation on hepatic glucose output. Therefore, fasting hypoglycemia is more common during pregnancy. Gluconeogenesis could be limited by a relative lack of the major substrate alanine. The plasma concentration of alanine has been shown in some studies to be lower during pregnancy, probably as a result of placental uptake and a restraint on proteolysis. Although fat deposition is accentuated in early pregnancy, lipolysis is enhanced by human placental lactogen (hPL) later in gestation, and more glycerol and free fatty acids are released in the postabsorptive state. Ketogenesis is thus accentuated in the postabsorptive state during pregnancy, probably secondary to increased provision of substrate free fatty acids and hormonal effects on the maternal liver cells.

The balance of metabolic fuels is also different in the **fed state** during pregnancy. Despite hyperinsulinism in normal pregnancy, the disposal of glucose is impaired, producing somewhat higher maternal blood levels. The contra-insulin effects of gestation have been related to hPL, progesterone, and cortisol. The

disappearance in plasma of administered insulin is not greater during pregnancy, despite the presence of placental insulin receptors and degrading enzymes. Glucagon is well suppressed by glucose during pregnancy, and secretory responses of glucagon to amino acids are not increased above nonpregnant levels. After meals, more glucose is converted to triglyceride in pregnant compared with nonpregnant animals, which would tend to conserve calories and enhance fat deposition. Insulin resistance during pregnancy apparently does not extend to the lipogenic and antilipolytic effects of the hormone.

Overview of Diabetes During Pregnancy

Diabetic pregnant women have been classified on the basis of duration and severity of diabetes (Table 20–3). A classification system (White) was originally used for prognosis of perinatal outcome and to determine obstetric management. Because the perinatal mortality rate has declined dramatically for many reasons in women in all classes, the system is now used mainly to describe and compare populations of diabetic pregnant women. However, certain characteristics of patients are still pertinent. The risk of complications is minimal if gestational diabetes is well controlled by diet alone, and these patients may be otherwise managed as normal pregnant women. Class B patients, whose insulin dependence is of recent onset, will probably have residual islet B cell function, and control of hyperglycemia may be easier than in class C or D patients. Finally, the most complicated and difficult pregnancies occur in women with renal, retinal, or cardiovascular disease.

The hormonal and metabolic effects of pregnancy are associated with increased risks of both hypoglycemic reactions and ketoacidosis. Increasing amounts of insulin are usually required to control hyperglycemia throughout gestation.

If diabetes is poorly controlled in the first weeks of pregnancy, the risks of spontaneous abortion and congenital malformation of the infant are increased. Later in pregnancy, polyhydramnios is also common in women with poorly controlled diabetes and may lead to preterm delivery. Fetal distress may develop in the third trimester if diabetic control has been inadequate. Careful fetal monitoring must be used to prevent stillbirth. The high incidence of fetal macrosomia (birth weight > 90th percentile for gestational age) increases the potential for traumatic vaginal delivery; primary cesarean deliveries are more common in these cases. Fetal intrauterine growth retardation may occur in diabetic women with vascular disease.

Other neonatal risks include respiratory distress syndrome, hypoglycemia, hyperbilirubinemia, hypocalcemia, and poor feeding; however, these problems are limited to the first days of life, and childhood development is usually normal. Despite these possible

Table 20–3. Classification of diabetes during pregnancy (Priscilla White).

Class	Characteristics	Implications
Gestational diabetes	Abnormal glucose tolerance during pregnancy; postprandial hyperglycemia during pregnancy.	Diagnosis before 30 weeks' gestation important to prevent macrosomia. Treat with diet adequate in calories to prevent maternal weight loss. Goal is postprandial blood glucose <130 mg/dL (7.2 mmol/L) at 1 hour or <105 mg/dL (5.8 mmol/L) at 2 hours. If insulin is necessary, manage as in classes B, C, and D.
A	Chemical diabetes diagnosed before pregnancy; managed by diet alone; any age at onset.	Management as for gestational diabetes.
B	Insulin treatment or oral hypoglycemic agent used before pregnancy; onset at age 20 or older; duration <10 years.	Some endogenous insulin secretion may persist. Fetal and neonatal risks same as in classes C and D, as is management; can be type I or II.
C	Onset at age 10–20, or duration 10–20 years.	Insulin-deficient diabetes of juvenile onset; type I.
D	Onset before age 10, or duration >20 years, or chronic hypertension (not preeclampsia), or background retinopathy (tiny hemorrhages).	Fetal macrosomia or intrauterine growth retardation possible. Retinal microaneurysms, dot hemorrhages, and exudates may progress during pregnancy, then regress after delivery.
F	Diabetic nephropathy with proteinuria.	Anemia and hypertension common; proteinuria increases in third trimester, declines after delivery. Fetal intrauterine growth retardation common; perinatal survival about 90% under optimal conditions; bed rest necessary.
H	Coronary artery disease.	Serious maternal risk.
R	Proliferative retinopathy.	Neovascularization, with risk of vitreous hemorrhage or retinal detachment; laser photocoagulation useful; abortion usually not necessary. With active process of neovascularization, prevent bearing-down efforts.

complications, diabetic women now have a 97–98% chance of delivering a healthy child if they adhere to a program of careful management and surveillance.

In the following sections, the convention used for designating the number of weeks of gestation is the number of weeks from the last menstrual period.

Gestational Diabetes

The hormonal and metabolic changes of pregnancy result in the diagnosis of glucose intolerance during the second half of gestation in 2–3% of pregnant women. Criteria for diagnosis are given in Table 20–4. Gestational diabetes may result from inadequate insulin response to carbohydrate load, from excessive resistance to the action of insulin, or from both. Once the diagnosis has been made, the patient should be placed on a diabetic diet modified for pregnancy: 25–35 kcal/kg ideal weight, 40–55% carbohydrate, 20% protein, and 25–40% fat. Calories are distributed over 3 meals and 3 snacks (Table 20–5). The goal of therapy is not weight reduction but prevention of both fasting and postprandial hyperglycemia. If 1-hour or 2-hour postprandial glucose values are consistently greater than 130 or 105 mg/dL (7.2 or 5.8 mmol/L), therapy is begun with human insulin, and the patient is managed as if insulin-dependent.

The risk of developing overt diabetes later in life is influenced by body weight. Follow-up studies indicate that 5–15% of nonobese gestational diabetics will need treatment in 5–20 years, compared to 35–50% of gestational diabetic women with a body weight greater than 120% of ideal. This suggests the possibility of preventive benefits of achieving weight loss after pregnancy and lactation.

Table 20–4. Diagnosis of gestational diabetes.

Screening with glucose loading test:
  Indications: (1) Screen all gravidas or (2) screen all gravidas who are overweight[1] or over 25 years of age (misses 10% of cases) plus all gravidas with glycosuria, a family history of diabetes (in parents, siblings, aunts, or uncles), or a history of stillbirth or macrosomic infant (misses 40% of cases).
  Procedure: Give 50 g of glucose by mouth at 24–26 weeks' gestation. Measure plasma glucose 1 hour later. If value exceeds 130 mg/dL (7.2 mmol/L) give the oral glucose tolerance test.
Oral glucose tolerance test:
  Procedure: Give 100 g of glucose by mouth. Normal values for plasma or serum glucose[2] are as follows:
    fasting, 105 mg/dL (5.8 mmol/L)
    1 hour, 190 mg/dL (10.5 mmol/L)
    2 hours, 165 mg/dL (9.2 mmol/L)
    3 hours, 145 mg/dL (8.0 mmol/L)
  Results are abnormal if 2 values are elevated above limits listed.
  Caution: Glucose should not be given if fasting blood glucose is >130 mg/dL.

[1]Overweight = height under 165 cm with weight over 68 kg (<5 ft 5 in, >150 lb) in first trimester; height over 165 cm with weight over 81 kg (>5 ft 5 in, >180 lb) in first trimester.
[2]Criteria of National Diabetes Data Group (NIH). (See *Diabetes* 1979;**28**:1039.)

Table 20–5. Management of diet for patients with gestational diabetes.

---

(1) Assess present pattern of food consumption.
(2) Balance calories with optimal weight gain.
    (a) Caloric intake: 25–35 kcal/kg ideal weight.
    (b) Weight gain: 0.45 kg (1 lb) per month during the first trimester; 0.2–0.35 kg (0.5–0.75 lb) per week during the second and third trimesters.
(3) Distribute calories and carbohydrates over 3 meals and 3 snacks; evening snack to include complex carbohydrate and at least one meat exchange.
(4) Use food exchanges to assess the amount of carbohydrate, protein, and fat:
    (a) Carbohydrate: 40–55% of calories or ≥150 g/d.
    (b) Protein: 20% of calories or ≥74 g/d.
    (c) Fat: 25–40% of calories.
(5) Emphasize high-fiber, complex carbohydrate foods.
(6) Identify individual glycemic responses to certain foods.
(7) Tailor eating plans to personal needs.

Insulin Management

The goal of insulin therapy during pregnancy is to prevent both fasting and postprandial hyperglycemia and to avoid debilitating hypoglycemic reactions. Maternal hyperglycemia is associated with fetal macrosomia and delayed lung maturation. Most experts believe that one should aim for fasting plasma glucose levels below 105 mg/dL (5.8 mmol/L) and postprandial levels below 140 mg/dL (7.8 mmol/L). Self-monitoring of capillary blood glucose at home with glucose oxidase strips and portable reflectance colorimeters has proved a reliable means of helping patients monitor the course of therapy. Since glycosylated hemoglobin correlates with mean daily capillary blood glucose over a few weeks during pregnancy, sequential measurement will provide another indicator of long-term control. Yet because insulin dosage must be frequently adjusted up or down during the metabolically dynamic state of pregnancy, capillary blood glucose must be measured several times each day to assist in the "fine-tuning" of insulin management.

Most pregnant insulin-dependent patients will require at least 2 injections of about a 1:2 mixture of regular and intermediate insulin each day in order to prevent fasting and postprandial hyperglycemia. The usual practice is to give two-thirds of the insulin before breakfast and one-third before supper (Table 20–6). More stringent regimens of administering regular subcutaneous insulin 4–6 times each day, or continuously with a portable insulin pump, may be necessary to achieve normoglycemia in some patients.

Hypoglycemia reactions are more frequent and sometimes more severe in early pregnancy. Therefore, patients must keep glucagon on hand, and a member of the household must be instructed in the technique of injection. Hypoglycemic reactions have not been associated with fetal death or congenital anomalies.

Fetal Development & Growth

Major congenital anomalies are those which may severely affect the life of the individual or require major surgery for correction. The incidence of major congenital anomalies in infants of diabetic mothers is 6–12%, compared with 2% in infants of a nondiabetic population. While perinatal deaths due to stillbirth and respiratory distress syndrome have declined in pregnancies complicated by diabetes, the proportion of fetal and neonatal deaths ascribed to congenital anomalies has risen to 50–80%. The types of anomalies most common in infants of diabetic mothers and their presumed time of occurrence during embryonic development are listed in Table 20–7. It is apparent that any intervention to reduce the incidence of major congenital anomalies must be applied very early in pregnancy. The additional finding that the excess risk of anomalies is associated with the group of diabetic women with elevated glycosylated hemoglobin early in pregnancy suggests that poor diabetic control is related to the risk of major congenital anomalies in infants of diabetic mothers. Protocols of intensive diabetic management instituted prior to conception and continued through early pregnancy have resulted in significant reduction in the frequency of anomalies. This means that primary care physicians treating diabetic women of reproductive age must evaluate them for the possibility of becoming pregnant and inform them of the risks related to the level of hyperglycemia.

Table 20–6. Illustration of use of home blood glucose monitoring to determine insulin dosage during pregnancy.

Self-Monitored Capillary Blood Glucose		Insulin Doses
Fasting blood glucose	148 mg/dL (8.2 mmol/L)	14 units regular, 28 units intermediate
1 h after breakfast	206 mg/dL (11.4 mmol/L)	
1 h after lunch	152 mg/dL (8.4 mmol/L)	
1 h after supper	198 mg/dL (11.0 mmol/L)	9 units regular, 10 units intermediate
2–4 AM	142 mg/dL (7.9 mmol/L)	

Suggested changes based on pattern of blood glucose values over 2–3 days: slight increases in presupper intermediate insulin to control fasting blood glucose next day, in morning regular insulin to control postbreakfast glucose, and in presupper regular insulin to control postsupper hyperglycemia. Dose of morning intermediate insulin is adequate to control early afternoon blood glucose. When dose of presupper intermediate insulin is increased, patient should test to detect and prevent nocturnal hypoglycemia. One-hour postprandial testing is advised to detect the probable peaks of glycemic excursions. Patient should also test when symptoms of hypoglycemia appear.

Table 20–7. Congenital malformations in infants of diabetic mothers.[1]

	Ratio of Incidences Diabetic vs Control Group	Latest Gestational Age for Occurrence (Weeks After Menstruation)
Caudal regression	252	5
Anencephaly	3	6
Spina bifida, hydro-cephalus, or other central nervous system defects	2	6
Cardiac anomalies	4	
Transposition of great vessels		7
Ventricular septal defect		8
Atrial septal defect		8
Anal/rectal atresia	3	8
Renal anomalies	5	
Agenesis	6	7
Cystic kidney	4	7
Ureter duplex	23	7
Situs inversus	84	6

[1]Modified and reproduced, with permission, from Kucera J: Rate and type of congenital anomalies among offspring of diabetic women. *J Reprod Med* 1971;**7**:61; and Mills JL, Baker L, Goldman AS: Malformations in infants of diabetic mothers occur before the seventh gestational week: Implications for treatment. *Diabetes* 1979;**28**:292.

Ultrasonography in the first half of pregnancy may detect neural tube defects (anencephaly, meningomyelocele) that occur with a higher than normal incidence in infants of diabetic mothers. The physician should also screen all insulin-dependent pregnant women for elevated serum alpha-fetoprotein levels at 14–16 weeks of gestation to detect other cases of neural tube defects. Later in pregnancy, sophisticated ultrasonographic examinations may detect congenital heart defects or other anomalies.

The initial ultrasonographic examination at 18–20 weeks confirms the dating of gestation, and subsequent examinations at 26 and 36 weeks measure fetal growth. Many of these infants are large for dates, ie, macrosomic infants with increased fat stores, increased length, and increased abdomen-to-head or thorax-to-head ratios. The hypothesis that fetal macrosomia results from the causal chain of maternal hyperglycemia → fetal hyperglycemia → fetal hyperinsulinemia → fetal macrosomia has long been debated. Excess insulin increases fetal fat deposition. Macrosomic infants of diabetic mothers have significantly higher concentrations of C peptide in their cord sera or

amniotic fluid (representing endogenous insulin secretion) than do infants of diabetic mothers with birth weights appropriate for gestational age. The determinants of fetal hyperinsulinemia throughout pregnancy may not be simply maternal hyperglycemia, however. Other metabolic substrates that cross the placenta and are insulinogenic (eg, branched-chain amino acids) may play a role in fetal macrosomia, and transplacental lipids could contribute to fat deposition.

The degree of maternal glycemia is related to birth weights of infants of diabetic mothers, as adjusted for gestational age. This suggests that prevention of maternal hyperglycemia throughout pregnancy may reduce the incidence of macrosomia. Pilot studies of highly selected patients have shown this to be the case in many but not all instances. The metabolic and nutritional determinants of birth weights of infants of diabetic mothers other than maternal glucose are under study.

Polyhydramnios is an excess volume of amniotic fluid (> 1000 mL, often > 3000 mL). It may cause severe discomfort or premature labor and is most often associated with fetal macrosomia. The excess volume of amniotic fluid was not related to the concentration of glucose or other solutes in amniotic fluid or to excess fetal urine output as measured by change in bladder size by means of ultrasonography in one study. Additional possible factors in causation of polyhydramnios in diabetic pregnancies include fetal swallowing, decidual and amniotic fluid PRL, and as yet unknown determinants of the complicated multicompartmental intrauterine transfer of water. However, diuretics do little to mobilize excessive amniotic fluid. Polyhydramnios is rare in women with well-controlled diabetes.

In contrast to fetal macrosomia, the fetus of a woman with diabetes of long duration and vascular disease may suffer intrauterine growth retardation. This problem is apparently related to inadequate uteroplacental perfusion. All body diameters may be below normal or ultrasonographic measurements; oligohydramnios is common; and after 30 weeks of gestation, maternal plasma or urinary estriol levels are usually below the 95% confidence limits for stage of gestation.

Obstetric Management

Not long ago the incidence of apparently sudden intrauterine fetal demise in the third trimester of diabetic pregnancies was at least 5%. Since the risk increased as pregnancies approached term, preterm delivery was instituted but risk and neonatal death from respiratory distress syndrome increased. Curiously, the cause of stillbirth was usually not obvious. The risk was greater with poor diabetic control, and the incidence of fetal death exceeded 50% with ketoacidosis. Some instances of fetal demise were associated with preeclampsia, which is a common complication of diabetic pregnancy. Fetal death was also associated with pyelonephritis, which is now largely prevented by screening for and treating asymptomatic bacteriuria. Other than these known risk factors, one can speculate that fetal distress was related to (1) a combination of relative fetal hypoxia and hyperglycemia or (2) fetal myocardial dysfunction.

Advances during the past decade have led to techniques for detecting fetal distress and preventing stillbirth. The infrequency of fetal movement as noted in fetal activity determinations (<4/h) may indicate fetal jeopardy. More quantitative studies of fetal activity patterns using ultrasonography are now available.

Maternal estriol assays were also used for fetal evaluation, based on the knowledge that placental production of estriol is dependent on precursors from the fetal adrenals. It has been demonstrated that the maternal 24-hour urine estriol level correlates with the mass of the fetal-placental unit and that a 40% or greater drop in maternal plasma or urinary estriol level usually precedes fetal demise in pregnancies complicated by diabetes. However, estriol monitoring has been replaced by biophysical assessment at most centers.

The primary mode of fetal assessment is antepartum fetal heart rate monitoring. The presence of fetal heart rate accelerations and good long-range variability on the nonstress test (NST) and the absence of late decelerations (lower rate persists after the contraction subsides) on the contraction stress test (CST) almost always suggest that the fetus is well oxygenated and has a low risk of dying within several days. However, the predictive value of normal test results is only valid for a short duration in diabetic women with unstable metabolic control or hypertension. Generally, the NST and CST are sensitive screening tests, and abnormal results in these tests of fetal heart monitoring will overestimate the diagnosis of fetal distress. Therefore, some authorities require that additional evidence of fetal distress (by biophysical ultrasonographic assessment) be obtained before intervention in preterm pregnancies can be recommended.

Insulin-dependent diabetic patients were usually admitted to the hospital at 36 weeks' gestation or earlier for fetal monitoring and careful control of diabetes. However, normotensive women achieving very good control (fasting blood glucose about 100 mg/dL, 1-hour postprandial blood glucose <140 mg/dL) with self-monitoring of blood glucose levels have no excess risk of fetal distress and do not require antepartum admission to the hospital.

Unless maternal or fetal complications arise, the goal for the termination of pregnancy should be 38 weeks or even later, in order to reduce neonatal morbidity from preterm deliveries. On the other hand, the obstetrician may wish to induce labor before 38 weeks if he or she is concerned about increasing fetal weight. Before the delivery decision is made, fetal pulmonary maturity should be determined. The standard test for pulmonary maturity is the lecithin/sphingomyelin (L/S) ratio, in which a value greater than 2 indicates a low risk for respiratory distress syndrome. However,

in pregnancies complicated by diabetes, many authors have reported a false-positive rate of 6–12% with L/S values between 2 and 3. The reason for the discrepancy is unknown, but the lowest risk for respiratory distress syndrome is attained by delaying delivery (if possible) until the L/S ratio becomes abnormally high (>3.5). The false-negative rate for L/S ratios of 1.5–2.0 is at least 50% in nondiabetic pregnancies (ie, delivery occurs within 72 hours, but respiratory distress syndrome does not develop). Other amniotic fluid assays (eg, measurement of phosphatidylglycerol) can be used to evaluate the risk for respiratory distress syndrome. If phosphatidylglycerol is present in the amniotic fluid, the risk is low even if the L/S ratio is below 3.5.

Once fetal lung maturity is likely, the route of delivery must be selected based on the usual obstetric indications. If the fetus seems large (> 4200 g) on clinical and ultrasonographic or CT pelvimetric examination, cesarean section probably should be performed because of the possibility of shoulder dystocia. Otherwise, induction of labor is reasonable, because maternal and peripartum risks are fewer following vaginal delivery. Once labor is under way, continuous fetal heart rate monitoring (with scalp pH backup measurements) must be performed.

Traditional insulin management for labor and delivery has been to give only one-third to one-half the prepregnancy dose in the morning. The diabetic parturient may be unusually sensitive to insulin during active labor and delivery, and insulin shock is possible if delivery occurs sooner than anticipated. Protocols for continuous low-dose intravenous insulin administration during labor or prior to cesarean delivery are now used to achieve stringent control of blood glucose in order to reduce the incidence of intrapartum fetal distress and neonatal metabolic problems. A cord blood glucose level at delivery correlates positively with the higher maternal levels, and there does not seem to be an upper limit on placental transfer of glucose. During labor, maternal plasma glucose can usually be kept below 100 mg/dL (5.6 mmol/L) with 1–2 units of regular insulin and 7.5 g of dextrose given intravenously every hour. If cesarean section is necessary, insulin management is similar, and infants do equally well with general, spinal, or epidural anesthesia. Nonetheless, the anesthesiologist should be cautioned against the administration of copious glucose-containing intravenous solutions.

Neonatal Morbidity

Planning for the care of infants of diabetic mothers should begin prior to delivery, with participation by the neonatologist in decisions about timing and management of delivery. The pediatrician must be in attendance to know of antenatal problems, to assess the need for resuscitation, and to determine major congenital anomalies.

Infants of diabetic mothers have an increased risk of respiratory distress syndrome compared with infants of matched nondiabetic mothers. Possible reasons include abnormal production of pulmonary surfactant or connective tissue changes leading to decreased pulmonary compliance. However, in recent years, the incidence of respiratory distress syndrome has declined from 24% to 5%, probably related to use of the L/S ratio and delivery of most infants at term (see above). The diagnosis of respiratory distress syndrome is based on clinical signs (grunting, retraction, respiratory rate > 60/min), typical findings on chest x-ray (diffuse reticulogranular pattern and air bronchogram), and an increased oxygen requirement (to maintain the P_{aO2} at 50–70 mm Hg) for more than 48 hours with no other identified cause of respiratory difficulty (heart disease, infection). Survival of infants with respiratory distress syndrome has dramatically improved as a result of advances in ventilation therapy.

Hypoglycemia is common in the first 48 hours after delivery and is defined as blood glucose below 30 mg/dL (1.7 mmol/L) regardless of gestational age. The symptomatic infant may be lethargic rather than jittery, and hypoglycemia may be associated with apnea, tachypnea, cyanosis, or seizures. Hypoglycemia has been related to elevated fetal insulin levels during and after delivery. Nevertheless, infants of diabetic mothers may also have deficient catecholamine and glucagon secretion, and the hypoglycemia may be related to diminished hepatic glucose production and oxidation of free fatty acids. The neonatologist attempts to prevent hypoglycemia in "well" infants with early feedings of 10% dextrose in water by bottle or gavage by 1 hour of age. If this is not successful, treatment with intravenous dextrose solutions is indicated. Rigid control of diabetes to prevent fetal hyperglycemia may reduce the incidence of neonatal hypoglycemia. There are usually no long-term sequelae of episodes of neonatal hypoglycemia.

Other frequent problems in infants of diabetic mothers include hypocalcemia (< 7 mg/dL [1.75 mmol/L]), hyperbilirubinemia (> 15 mg/dL [256 μmol/L]), polycythemia (central hematocrit > 70%), and poor feeding. Further investigation is necessary to determine the cause of these problems. Better control of the maternal diabetic state in the future should reduce their incidence.

REFERENCES

General

Burrow GN, Ferris TF (editors): *Medical Complications During Pregnancy*, 2nd ed. Saunders, 1982.

Chez RA (editor): Fetal and placental endocrinology. *Clin Obstet Gynecol* 1980;**23**:719.

Goebelsmann U: Protein and steroid hormones in pregnancy. *J Reprod Med* 1979;**23**:166.

Jaffe RB: Endocrine-metabolic alterations induced by pregnancy. Chap 24–26, pp 735–788, in: *Reproductive Endocrinology: Physiology, Pathophysiology, and Clinical Management*, 2nd ed. Yen SSC, Jaffe RB (editors). Saunders, 1986.

Milne JA (editor): The physiologic response to pregnancy in health and disease. Proceedings of a symposium arranged by the Department of Obstetrics and Gynaecology, University of Cambridge, Sept 15–16, 1978. *Postgrad Med J* 1979;**55**:293. [Entire issue.]

Tulchinsky D, Ryan KJ (editors): *Maternal-Fetal Endocrinology*. Saunders, 1980.

Chorionic Proteins & Pregnancy Tests

Derman R, Edelman DA, Berger GS: Current status of immunologic pregnancy tests. *Int J Gynaecol Obstet* 1979;**17**:190.

Fisher DA: Maternal-fetal thyroid function in pregnancy. *Clin Perinatol* 1983;**10**:615.

Harada A et al: Comparison of thyroid stimulators and thyroid hormone concentrations in the sera of pregnant women. *J Clin Endocrinol Metab* 1979;**48**:793.

Healy DL, Hodgen GD: The endocrinology of human endometrium. *Obstet Gynecol Surv* 1983;**38**:509.

Horne CHW, Nisbet AD: Pregnancy proteins: A review. *Invest Cell Pathol* 1979;**2**:217.

Hsueh AJW, Jones PBC: Gonadotropin-releasing hormone: Extrapituitary actions and paracrine control mechanisms. *Annu Rev Physiol* 1983;**45**:83.

Siler-Khodr TM: Hypothalamic-like releasing hormones of the placenta. *Clin Perinatol* 1983;**10**:533.

Weiss G: Relaxin. *Annu Rev Physiol* 1984;**46**:43.

Steroid Hormones

Bammann BL, Coulam CB, Jiang NS: Total and free testosterone during pregnancy. *Am J Obstet Gynecol* 1980;**137**:293.

Buster JE: Gestational changes in steroid hormone biosynthesis, secretion, metabolism, and action. *Clin Perinatol* 1983;**10**:527.

Laatikainen T et al: Fetal and maternal serum levels of steroid sulfates, unconjugated steroids and prolactin at term pregnancy and in early spontaneous labor. *J Clin Endocrinol Metab* 1980;**50**:489.

Lind T: Clinical chemistry of pregnancy. *Adv Clin Chem* 1980;**21**:1.

Nolten WE, Holt LH, Rueckert PA: Desoxycorticosterone in normal pregnancy. 3. Evidence of a fetal source of desoxycorticosterone. *Am J Obstet Gynecol* 1981;**139**:477.

Parker CR et al: Hormone production during pregnancy in the primigravid patient. 2. Plasma levels of desoxycorticosterone throughout pregnancy of normal women and women who developed pregnancy-induced hypertension. *Am J Obstet* 1980;**138**:626.

Schrader WT: New model for steroid hormone receptors? *Nature* 1984;**308**:17.

Siiteri PK et al: Progesterone and maintenance of pregnancy: Is progesterone nature's immunosuppressant? *Ann NY Acad Sci* 1977;**286**:384.

Fetal Endocrinology

Jaffe RB: Fetoplacental endocrine and metabolic physiology. *Clin Perinatol* 1983;**10**:669.

Serón-Ferré M, Jaffe RB: The fetal adrenal gland. *Annu Rev Physiol* 1981;**43**:141.

Parturition

Challis JRG: Endocrinology of late pregnancy and parturition. In: *Reproductive Physiology, III, International Review of Physiology.* Vol 22. Greep RO (editor). University Park Press, 1980.

Fuchs AR: Hormonal control of myometrial function during pregnancy and parturition. *Acta Endocrinol [Suppl]* 1978;**89**:1.

Garfield RE et al: Hormonal control of GAP junction formation in sheep myometrium during parturition. *Biol Reprod* 1979;**21**:999.

Liggins GC: Initiation of parturition. *Br Med Bull* 1979; **35**:145.

Liggins GC et al: Control of parturition in man. *Biol Reprod* 1977;**16**:39.

Ryan KJ: New concepts in hormonal control of parturition. *Biol Reprod* 1977;**16**:88.

Thorburn G, Challis JRG: Endocrine control of parturition. *Physiol Rev* 1979;**59**:863.

Puerperium & Lactation

Duchesne C, Leke R: Bromocriptine mesylate for prevention of postpartum lactation. *Obstet Gynecol* 1981;**57**:464.

Harrison RG: Suppression of lactation. *Semin Perinatol* 1979;**3**:287.

Monheit AG, Cousins L, Resnick R: The puerperium, anatomic and physiologic readjustments. *Clin Obstet Gynecol* 1980;**23**:973.

Tucker HA: Endocrinology of lactation. *Semin Perinatol* 1979;**3**:199.

Vance ML, Evans WS, Thorner MO: Bromocriptine. *Ann Intern Med* 1984;**100**:78.

Vorherr H: Hormonal and biochemical changes of pituitary and breast during pregnancy. *Semin Perinatol* 1979;**3**:193.

Pituitary Adenomas

Barbieri RL, Ryan KJ: Bromocriptine: Endocrine pharmacology and therapeutic applications. *Fertil Steril* 1983;**39**:727.

Johnston DG et al: Hyperprolactinemia: Long-term effects of bromocriptine. *Am J Med* 1983;**75**:868.

Marshall JR: Pregnancy in patients with prolactin-producing pituitary tumors. *Clin Obstet Gynecol* 1980; **23**:453.

Breast Cancer & Pregnancy

Bottles K, Taylor RN: Diagnosis of breast masses in pregnancy and lactating women by aspiration cytology. *Obstet Gynecol* 1985;**66(3 Suppl)**:76S.

Cooper DR, Butterfield J: Pregnancy subsequent to mastectomy for cancer of the breast. *Ann Surg* 1970; **171**:429.

Donegan WL: Breast cancer and pregnancy. *Obstet Gynecol* 1977;**50**:244.

Hochman A, Schreiber H: Pregnancy and cancer of the breast. *Obstet Gynecol* 1953;**2**:268.

Holleb AJ, Farrow JH: The relation of carcinoma of the breast and pregnancy in 283 patients. *Surg Gynecol Obstet* 1962;**115**:65.

Wynder EL, Bross IJ, Hirayama T: A study of the epidemiology of cancer of the breast. *Cancer* 1960;**13**:559.

Zinns JS: The association of pregnancy and breast cancer. *J Reprod Med* 1979;**22**:297.

Hypertensive Disorders

Carr BR, Gant NF: The endocrinology of pregnancy-induced hypertension. *Clin Perinatol* 1983;**10**:737.

Chesley LC: The control of hypertension in pregnancy. *Obstet Gynecol Annu* 1981;**10**:67.

Roberts JM: Pregnancy-related hypertension. Pages 703–752 in: *Maternal-Fetal Medicine: Principles and Practice.* Creasy RK, Resnick R (editors). Saunders, 1984.

Rodgers GM, Taylor RN, Roberts JM: Preeclampsia is associated with a serum factor cytotoxic to human endothelial cells. *Am J Obstet Gynecol* 1988;**159**:908.

Sullivan JM: The hypertensive diseases of pregnancy and their management. *Adv Intern Med* 1982;**27**:407.

Symonds EM: The renin-angiotensin system in pregnancy. *Obstet Gynecol Annu* 1981;**10**:45.

Wilson M et al: Blood pressure, the renin-aldosterone system and sex steroids throughout normal pregnancy. *Am J Med* 1980;**68**:97.

Worley AJ et al: Vascular responsiveness to pressor agents during human pregnancy. *J Reprod Med* 1979;**23**:115.

Hyperthyroidism in Pregnancy

Burrow GN: Hyperthyroidism during pregnancy. *N Engl J Med* 1978;**298**:150.

Cheron RG et al: Neonatal thyroid function after propylthiouracil therapy for maternal Graves' disease. *N Engl J Med* 1981;**304**:525.

Diabetes Mellitus & Pregnancy

Algert S, Shragg P, Hollingsworth DR: Moderate caloric restriction in obese women with gestational diabetes. *Obstet Gynecol* 1985;**65**:487.

Bochner CJ et al: Early third-trimester ultrasound screening in gestational diabetes to determine the risk of macrosomia and labor dystocia at term. *Am J Obstet Gynecol* 1987;**157**:703.

Cheney C, Shragg P, Hollingsworth D: Demonstration of heterogeneity in gestational diabetes by a 400-kcal breakfast meal tolerance test. *Obstet Gynecol* 1985; **65**:17.

Cousins L: Pregnancy complications among diabetic women. *Obstet Gyneol Surv* 1987;**42**:140.

Dibble CM et al: Effect of pregnancy on diabetic retinopathy. *Obstet Gynecol* 1982;**59**:699.

Ericksson UJ: Congenital malformations in diabetic animal models: A review. *Diabetes Res* 1984;**1**:57.

Fuhrmann K et al: Prevention of congenital malformations in infants of insulin-dependent diabetic mothers. *Diabetes Care* 1983;**6**:219.

Gabbe SG et al: Management and outcome of class A diabetes mellitus. *Am J Obstet Gynecol* 1977;**127**:465.

Gabbe SG et al: Management and outcome of pregnancy in diabetes mellitus, classes B to R. *Am J Obstet Gynecol* 1977;**129**:723.

Jovanovic L. Peterson CM: Optimal insulin delivery for the pregnant diabetic patient. *Diabetes Care* 1982;**5 (Suppl)**:24.

Kitzmiller JL: The endocrine pancreas and maternal metabolism. Pages 56–83 in: *Maternal-Fetal Endocrinology*. Tulchinsky DT, Ryan KJ (editors). Saunders, 1980.

Kitzmiller JL et al: Diabetic nephropathy and perinatal outcome. *Am J Obstet Gynecol* 1981;**141:**741.

Kitzmiller JL et al: Diabetic pregnancy and perinatal morbidity. *Am J Obstet Gynecol* 1978;**131:**560.

Kitzmiller JL et al: Measurement of fetal shoulder width with computed tomography in diabetic women. *Obstet Gynecol* 1987;**70:**941.

Landon MB et al: Neonatal morbidity in pregnancy complicated by diabetes mellitus: predictive value of maternal glycemic profiles. *Am J Obstet Gynecol* 1987; **156:**1089.

Langer O et al: Gestational diabetes: insulin requirements in pregnancy. *Am J Obstet Gynecol* 1987;**157:**669.

Miller E et al: Elevated maternal hemoglobin A_{1C} in early pregnancy and major congenital anomalies in infants of diabetic mothers. *N Engl J Med* 1981;**304:**1331.

Mills JL, Baker L, Goldman AS: Malformations in infants of diabetic mothers occur before the seventh gestational week: Implications for treatment. *Diabetes* 1979;**28:**292.

Miodovnik M et al: Elevated maternal glycohemoglobin in early pregnancy and spontaneous abortion among insulin-dependent diabetic women. *Am J Obstet Gynecol* 1985;**153:**439.

Moloney JBM, Drury MI: The effect of pregnancy on the natural course of diabetic retinopathy. *Am J Ophthalmol* 1982;**93:**745.

Mueller-Heubach E et al: Lecithin/sphingomyelin ratio in amniotic fluid and its value for the prediction of neonatal respiratory distress syndrome in pregnant diabetic women. *Am J Obstet Gynecol* 1978;**130:**28.

O'Sullivan JB: Body weight and subsequent diabetes mellitus. *JAMA* 1982;**248:**949.

O'Sullivan JB et al: Medical treatment of the gestational diabetic. *Obstet Gynecol* 1974;**43:**817.

Reece EA, Coustan DR, (editors): *Diabetes Mellitus in Pregnancy*. Churchill Livingston, 1988.

Roversi GD et al: The intensive care of perinatal risk in pregnant diabetics: A new therapeutic scheme for the best control of maternal disease. *J Perinatal Med* 1973;**1:**114.

White P: Diabetes mellitus in pregnancy. *Clin Perinatol* 1974;**1:**331.

Ylinen K et al: Risk of minor and major fetal malformations in diabetics with high haemoglobin A_{1C} values in early pregnancy. *Br J Med* 1984;**289:**345.

Regulatory Peptides of the Gut

21

Sean J. Mulvihill, MD, Clifford W. Deveney, MD, Lawrence W. Way, MD, & Haile T. Debas, MD

The origins of gastrointestinal endocrinology can be traced to experiments performed by William Bayliss and Ernest Starling at University College in London in 1902. They showed that acidification of the duodenum or the denervated jejunum stimulated exocrine pancreatic secretion in anesthetized dogs. Furthermore, intravenous injection of an extract of jejunal, but not ileal, mucosa similarly stimulated pancreatic secretion. They postulated the presence of a chemical messenger, which they termed secretin, within the duodenal and jejunal mucosa. Starling later went on to define chemical messengers as substances "carried from the organ where they are produced to the organ where they affect by means of the bloodstream." He called these messengers hormones, a word suggested by William Hardy. Thus began the physiologic era of gastrointestinal endocrinology, in which hormones such as gastrin, secretin, and cholecystokinin were discovered through their physiologic actions. Only later were these substances isolated and characterized.

Since the early 1970s, in what could be termed the "biochemical era" of gastrointestinal endocrinology, about 30 new peptides have been described through biochemical purification of extracts of gastrointestinal mucosa. The discovery that many of these peptides are located in the central nervous system and in enteric neurons, in addition to being found in specialized endocrine cells of the gastrointestinal tract, has led to the concept of a brain-gut axis (see below). Recently, recombinant DNA technology has been used to identify gastrointestinal peptides in the absence of physiologic or biochemical information. The presence of calcitonin gene-related peptide (CGRP) in many neural tissues, including those of the gut, was identified in this manner after an examination of the calcitonin gene suggested the presence of a second peptide sequence.

The physiologic importance of many of the newly discovered peptides is unclear. Unlike in other endocrine systems, in which specific kinds of endocrine cells are concentrated into distinct organs, those of the gut are widely dispersed. Furthermore, disease states attributable to disorders of gut endocrine cells are rare and, in fact, there are as yet no known deficiency states. In other endocrine organs, such as the thyroid

Acronyms Used in This Chapter	
ACTH	Adrenocorticotropic hormone
APUD	Amine precursor uptake and decarboxylation
BLI	Bombesin-like immunoreactivity
CCK	Cholecystokinin
CGRP	Calcitonin gene-related peptide
CRH	Corticotropin-releasing hormone
DNA	Deoxyribonucleic acid
GH	Growth hormone
GIP	Glucose-dependent insulin-releasing peptide (gastric inhibitory peptide)
GRH	Growth hormone-releasing hormone
GRP	Gastrin-releasing peptide
5-HIAA	5-Hydroxyindoleacetic acid
MEN	Multiple endocrine neoplasia
MSH	Melanocyte-stimulating hormone
NPY	Neuropeptide Y
NSE	Neuronal-specific enolase
PHI	Peptide histidine isoleucine
PHM	Peptide histidine methionine
PP	Pancreatic polypeptide
PRL	Prolactin
PTH	Parathyroid hormone
PYY	Peptide YY
TRH	Thyrotropin-releasing hormone
VIP	Vasoactive intestinal polypeptide
WDHA	Watery diarrhea, hypokalemia, and achlorhydria

and adrenal, disorders of function have provided natural models for physiologic study, but this is uncommon in the gastrointestinal tract.

Modes of Gut Peptide Delivery (Table 21–1)

Gastrointestinal hormones regulate digestion by influencing gastrointestinal secretion, absorption, motility, and blood flow. These hormones are delivered to their sites of action in 3 ways: Some circulate in the bloodstream in order to affect the target cell (**endocrine communication**). Some are released into the interstitial fluid and affect nearby cells (**paracrine**

Table 21–1. Gastrointestinal hormones.

	Mode of Delivery[1]			
	E	N	P	Major Action
Gastrin	+	(+)	−	Gastric acid and pepsin secretion.
Cholecystokinin (CCK)	(+)	(+)	−	Pancreatic amylase secretion.
Secretin	+	−	−	Pancreatic bicarbonate secretion.
Gastric inhibitory polypeptide (GIP)	+	−	−	Enhances glucose-mediated insulin release. Inhibits gastric acid secretion.
Vasoactive intestinal polypeptide (VIP)	−	+	(−)	Smooth muscle relaxation. Stimulates pancreatic bicarbonate secretion.
Motilin	(+)	−	−	Initiates interdigestive intestinal motility.
Somatostatin	+	+	(+)	Numerous inhibitory effects.
Pancreatic polypeptide (PP)	(+)	−	(+)	Inhibits pancreatic bicarbonate and protein secretion.
Enkephalins	−	+	(+)	Opiatelike actions.
Substance P	−	+	(+)	Physiologic actions uncertain.
Gastrin-releasing peptide (GRP)[2]	−	+	(+)	Stimulates release of gastrin and CCK.
Neurotensin	−	+	(+)	Physiologic actions unknown.
Enteroglucagon	(+)	(+)	(+)	Physiologic actions unknown.
Peptide YY (PYY)	(+)	(−)	(+)	Inhibits pancreatic bicarbonate and protein secretion.
Neuropeptide Y	−	+	−	
Calcitonin gene-related peptide (CGRP)	−	+	(−)	Stimulates acid secretion and somatostatin release

[1]E = endocrine; N = neurocrine; P = paracrine; ( ) = suggested but not proved; + = yes; − = no.
[2]Gastrin-releasing peptide (GRP) is probably the mammalian form of bombesin and is responsible for bombesinlike immunoreactivity (BLI).

communication). Still others, within neurons, act as neurotransmitters or neuromodulators (**neurocrine communication**) (Fig 21–1; see also Chapter 5). A peptide may have more than one mode of delivery. For example, somatostatin has an endocrine function, it is present in neurons, and it also exercises paracrine actions in the gastric body and antrum. Because of their various modes of delivery, it may be preferable to refer to these substances as regulatory peptides rather than as hormones.

To prove that a substance has a possible endocrine function in the gastrointestinal tract, 2 criteria must be met: (1) blood levels of the substance must rise after a meal, and (2) infusion of the substance at a rate that reproduces postprandial blood levels must elicit a physiologic response from the target organ. Only a handful of peptides meet these criteria in the gastrointestinal tract: gastrin, for stimulation of gastric acid and pepsin secretion; secretin, for stimulation of pancreatic bicarbonate secretion; cholecystokinin (CCK), for stimulation of gallbladder contraction and pancreatic enzyme secretion; somatostatin, for inhibition of gastric acid secretion; and gastric inhibitory polypeptide (GIP), for stimulation of insulin release. It is possible that other peptides such as motilin (for stimulation of the interdigestive migratory motor complex) and pancreatic polypeptide (PP), (for inhibition of pancreatic bicarbonate and protein secretion) also act as hormones, but most gut peptides serve as neurocrine or paracrine agents. It has been difficult to prove that these agents have important regulatory activities on digestive processes, because there is no way to measure the concentrations of these locally acting agents at their presumed sites of action.

Cellular Mechanisms of Action

The actions of most gastrointestinal peptide hormones are mediated by membrane-bound receptors. These receptors are proteins whose synthesis is subject to regulation, often by the hormone itself. In the best-studied examples, such as gastrin, CCK, and somatostatin, there is down-regulation of receptor concentrations by high plasma levels of the hormone. This may be due to alterations in synthesis, function, or degradation of the receptor. Hormone-receptor affinity can be quantified by measurement of binding in the presence of varying concentrations of the hormone. There is some evidence, particularly in the case of CCK, that there may be 2 classes of receptor—one with low affinity and high capacity and one with high affinity and low capacity.

Binding to the cell membrane receptors activates one of 2 major intracellular pathways and stimulates cell function. These pathways have been termed second messengers (see Chapter 1). The effects of some hormones (eg, gastrin, CCK, and the neurotransmitter acetylcholine) are due to the release of intracellular calcium from stores in rough endoplasmic reticulum. The peptide-receptor complex activates membrane-bound phospholipase C, which converts inositol diphosphate to inositol triphosphate and diacylglycerol. Inositol triphosphate mobilizes calcium from stores in the rough endoplasmic reticulum and increases cytosolic calcium levels by increasing membrane permeability. This free intracellular calcium binds to the calcium receptor protein, calmodulin, activating phosphoprotein kinase to phosphorylate protein. Other peptides, such as secretin, vasoactive intestinal polypeptide (VIP), glucagon, and the paracrine substance histamine, activate adenylate cyclase, the enzyme responsible for catalyzing the conversion of ATP to

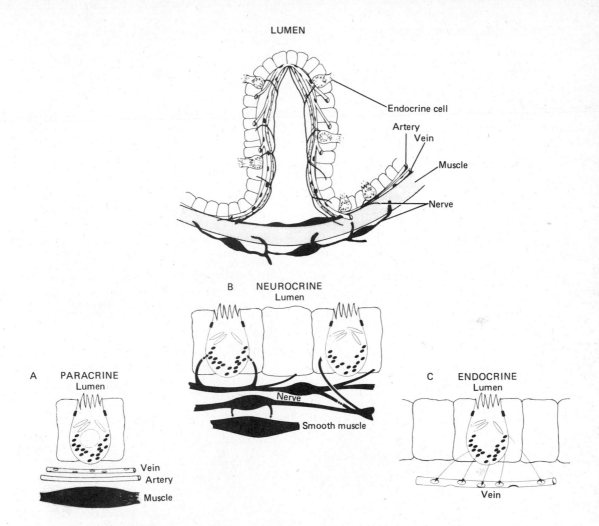

Figure 21–1. Schematic representation of the wall of the small intestine. Note the close proximity of endocrine cells and nerves to mucosal cells, blood vessels, and smooth muscle. Anatomically, local release of hormone by endocrine cells or nerves could affect secretion and absorption (mucosal cells), motility (muscle), and blood flow (blood vessels). *A:* Paracrine communication—release of a messenger locally to affect adjacent cells. *B:* Neurocrine communication—release of messenger by nerves to affect mucosal cells, other endocrine cells, or smooth muscle of both small intestine and blood vessels. *C:* Endocrine communication—release of messenger into the blood to act as a circulating hormone.

cyclic AMP (cAMP). cAMP is a second messenger that activates protein kinases, which stimulate cellular function. These 2 second messenger systems, intracellular calcium and cAMP, are distinct in their early steps but may cause similar changes in intracellular processes. For example, in the parietal cell, histamine, acting through the generation of intracellular cAMP, and acetylcholine, acting through the release of intracellular calcium, both stimulate the H^+, K^+-ATPase in canalicular membranes, resulting in the secretion of H^+ to the extracellular space. The mechanism of action of some gut peptides, including somatostatin, epidermal growth factor, and insulin, are unknown. In the case of somatostatin, there is evidence for multiple sites of intracellular action.

Structure of Gastrointestinal Peptide Hormones

All gut regulatory substances, with 2 possible exceptions (serotonin and melatonin) are polypeptides. Many exhibit homology, which allows them to be grouped into families (Table 21–2). Most of these peptides are probably synthesized as precursor molecules, with posttranslational processing to their active forms. Tatemoto and Mutt have taken advantage of the common phenylalanine-amine carboxyl terminus to isolate and characterize an entire family of gut peptides, including peptide YY (PYY), neuropeptide Y (NPY), and others. The amino acid sequence for most gut peptides is now known and, in many instances, the gene sequence has also been determined.

Table 21–2. Gastrointestinal peptide families.

Family	Peptides
Gastrin	Gastrin
	CCK
Secretin	Secretin
	VIP
	PHI
	PHM
	Glucagon
	GIP
PP	PP
	PYY
	NPY
Others	Motilin
	Neurotensin
	Somatostatin
	GRP
	Substance P
	Galanin

Distribution of Gut Peptides

Gut peptides are located in specialized endocrine cells widely dispersed throughout the gastrointestinal tract. The cells are distinguished by a clear cytoplasm and prominent basal acidophilic granules. Most gut endocrine cells are triangular, with a broad base and narrow apex, usually with a brush border facing the intestinal lumen (Fig 21–2). Immunocytochemical studies suggest that each cell manufactures and secretes just one peptide. Most gut peptides are found in enteric neurons, where they probably act as neurotransmitters or neurocrine agents. The bodies of enteric neurons are located within the gut wall, usually in the submucosal or myenteric plexus, from which their pathways extend to cells of the mucosa, smooth muscle, blood vessels, and other endocrine cells. It is likely that these peptidergic neurons exert local control over digestive processes, such as absorption, secretion, motility, and blood flow. Table 21–3 summarizes the distribution of gut peptides in their respective cells.

Brain-Gut Axis

Many of the peptides originally isolated from the gut are also found in the brain, and vice versa. Table 21–4 lists the peptides of this brain-gut axis. The reason for the dual localization of these peptides is not known. In the central nervous system, gut peptides are thought to be important in the regulation of bodily functions, eg,

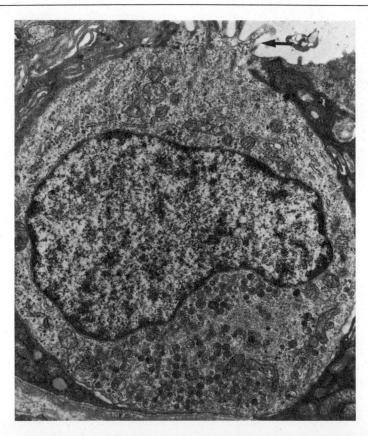

Figure 21–2. Typical endocrine cell of the gut. The arrow points to the brush border, which is at the cell apex and is open to the lumen of the gut. Granules at the cell base contain a peptide messenger, which in this cell is gastrin (G cell). (Reproduced, with permission, from Lechago J: Endocrine cells of the gastrointestinal tract and their pathology. *Pathol Annu* 1978;**13**:329.)

Table 21–3. Distribution of gastrointestinal hormones.[1]

	Endocrine Cell[2]	Localization	Localized in Gut Nerves
Gastrin	G	Gastric antrum, duodenum	No
CCK	I	Duodenum, jejunum	Yes
Secretin	S	Duodenum, jejunum	No
GIP	K	Small bowel	No
VIP	D_1	Pancreas	Yes
Motilin	EC_2	Small bowel	No
Substance P	EC_1	Entire gastrointestinal tract	Yes
Neurotensin	N	Ileum	No
Somatostatin	D	Stomach, duodenum, pancreas	Yes
Enkephalins	. . .	Stomach, duodenum, gallbladder	Yes
GRP	. . .	Stomach, duodenum	Yes
PP	D_2F	Pancreas	No
Enteroglucagon	A	Pancreas	No
	L	Small intestine	
PYY	. . .	Small intestine, colon	No
CGRP	. . .	Entire gastrointestinal tract	Yes
NPY	. . .	Small intestine	Yes

[1]Note that several peptides are found both in nerves and in endocrine cells. VIP has been found only in nerves and is probably not present in endocrine cells.
[2]Endocrine cells identified with a specific hormone are identified by a letter. EC = enterochromaffin cell. The cells containing enkephalins and PYY have yet to be named.

satiety (CCK), thermoregulation (bombesin), and inhibition of acid secretion (thyrotropin-releasing hormone [TRH], bombesin, and opiates).

APUD Concept

The cytochemical and ultrastructural characteristics of gastrointestinal endocrine cells were described by Pearse in 1966. These cells were similar in their ability to produce peptide hormones and biogenic amines (epinephrine, norepinephrine, dopamine, and serotonin) and to actively absorb amine precursors and convert them to amines. It was speculated that the uptake of 5-hydroxytryptophan and conversion of 5-hydroxytryptamine (serotonin) was linked to the production of peptide hormones. Most of the cells possessing these characteristics are found in the gut or central nervous system (hypothalamus, pituitary axis, and pineal gland), but they are also present in the thyroid (calcitonin cell), parathyroid, and placenta. Pearse referred to them as APUD cells from their char-

Table 21–4. Peptides found in the brain and gut (brain-gut axis).

Originally Found in Brain	Originally Found in Gut
Substance P	CCK
Thyrotropin-releasing hormone (TRH)	Gastrin
Somatostatin	Secretin
Enkephalins	VIP
CGRP	Glucagon
Corticotropin-releasing hormone (CRH)	PHI
	PP
	PYY
	NPY
	Bombesin
	GRP
	Neurotensin
	Insulin

acteristic amine handling (**amine precursor uptake and decarboxylation**). It was postulated that APUD cells originated from the primitive neural crest.

Whether all APUD cells actually come from the neural crest is not known. Studies using quail and chick embryos have disputed the claim that the APUD cells of the gastrointestinal tract originate from neural ectoderm. However, the endocrine cells of the gastrointestinal tract and pancreas contain an enzyme specific to neural cells (neuronal-specific enolase, NSE), which supports the postulate of a common neural origin. Regardless of their origin, it is clear that the endocrine cells of the gut are remarkably similar to other cells of the hypothalamic-pituitary axis and to neurons within the gut wall, and the gut endocrine cells are considered to be neuroendocrinologically programmed.

The APUD concept assumes that all cells that produce and release peptide hormones have a common embryologic origin. Even though its validity has been challenged, the concept is appealing because it posits a common origin for gut and central nervous system cells with almost identical cytochemical characteristics (storage of peptides) and cellular functions (release of peptide messengers). It helps clarify why identical peptides are synthesized, stored, and released by gut epithelial cells, neurons of the gastrointestinal tract, and nerve cells in the central nervous system. Peptide-releasing neurons and peptide-releasing epithelial cells actually have the same function—release of a chemical messenger (see Chapter 27).

GASTRIN

In 1905, Edkins discovered a potent gastric acid secretagogue in extracts of antral mucosa and named it gastrin. However, he could not exclude the possibility that the extract contained histamine, and for many years it was not known whether Edkins' gastrin was truly different from histamine. The existence of gastrin was firmly established in the early 1960s when Gregory et al isolated the peptide, identified its amino acid sequence, and synthesized the hormone. Because of the availability of pure synthetic gastrin and the relative ease with which physiologic concentrations can be measured by radioimmunoassay, gastrin is the best-studied gastrointestinal hormone.

Biochemistry & Distribution

There are presently 3 known biologically active forms of the gastrin molecule: a 14-amino-acid (G14), a 17-amino-acid (G17), and a 34-amino-acid (G34) peptide. They are also known as "mini gastrin," "little gastrin," and "big gastrin." Their 14 carboxy-terminal residues are identical, and G34 also contains the entire G17 sequence. In each form of gastrin, the tyrosine moiety in the sixth position from the carboxyl terminus may be sulfated or unsulfated, an alteration with no effect on range of action or potency. Digestion of big gastrin (G34) with trypsin cleaves 2 lysyl residues and releases little gastrin (G17). A molecule larger than G34, called component I or "big big gastrin," has also been discovered. Although the structure of component I has not been completely deciphered, tryptic digestion of this compound also releases G17, suggesting that component I consists of G17 joined at the N terminus with basic amino acids to a larger peptide.

G17 accounts for most of the gastrin in antral G cells; G34 predominates in serum, however, because it has a longer half-life. G17 is presumed to be the physiologically most important form of gastrin. The significance of the larger forms is not known, but it appears that many peptide hormones may be synthesized as a larger molecule containing the active fragment and that the precursor molecule is cleaved at positions where basic amino acids occur. A similar process occurs with proinsulin and insulin.

Both the human and porcine genes that encode for gastrin have been characterized. In the pig, a precursor cDNA to gastrin corresponds to an mRNA sequence of 312 nucleotides, which codes for a preprogastrin of 104 amino acids. The corresponding human mRNA codes for a preprogastrin of 101 amino acids. The entire human gene, which includes 2 introns, is 4100 base pairs long. Gastrin is secreted in an inactive form with a glycine extension at the carboxyl terminus. Conversion into the active form requires the presence of a deaminizing enzyme.

The carboxyl terminus of gastrin is responsible for its biologic activity. In fact, the carboxy-terminal tetrapeptide alone (gastrin tetrapeptide) displays the full range of actions, although it is only about one-sixth as potent on a molar basis as G17 for stimulation of acid secretion. G17 is about 3 times more potent than G34.

Gastrin and CCK have 5 identical carboxy-terminal amino acids (Fig 21–3). For CCK, 7 carboxy-terminal peptides are necessary for full biologic activity, whereas for gastrin, only the 4-carboxy-terminal amino acids

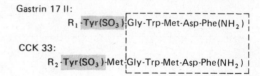

The gastrin-cholecystokinin family

Figure 21–3. Gastrin and cholecystokinin possess identical carboxy-terminal pentapeptides. However, the tyrosine is 7 amino acids from the carboxyl end of CCK and must be sulfated for maximal potency. The tyrosine is 6 positions from the carboxyl end in gastrin and need not be sulfated for maximal potency. R_1 and R_2 represent the amino terminal sequences for gastrin and CCK.

are necessary. The effects of gastrin and CCK are similar to the extent that both hormones stimulate gastric acid and pancreatic enzyme secretion and contraction of the gallbladder. However, their potency for eliciting these responses differs considerably. Gastrin is a strong stimulant of acid secretion and a weak stimulant of enzyme secretion and gallbladder contraction, while the relative potency of CCK for these actions is reversed. These differences are determined by the position of the tyrosine molecule located near the carboxyl end of the molecule. In gastrin, tyrosine is the sixth amino acid from the carboxyl end, while in CCK it is the seventh. For CCK-like activity, the tyrosine must be sulfated, but whether or not the tyrosine is sulfated does not affect the activity of gastrin.

Gastrin is synthesized and stored in the G cell. Ninety percent of gastrointestinal gastrin is found in the gastric antrum, and most of the remainder is in the duodenum. Under normal conditions, there is virtually no gastrin in the pancreas, although pancreatic endocrine tumors often produce gastrin.

Measurement & Release

Serum concentrations of gastrin range from 10 to 50 pmol/L. The concentration is often expressed as picograms of G17 per milliliter, since G17 is used as the standard. Because gastrin is present in other forms in serum, however, this is not entirely precise. Owing to the molecular heterogeneity of gastrin, antibodies used for immunoassay must measure G17 and G34 both in the sulfated and in the nonsulfated forms. Clinical laboratories use an antibody that recognizes all forms of gastrin, and the results are expressed as total gastrin in serum.

Serum gastrin concentrations increase by 20–40 pmol/L 30–60 minutes postprandially. Partially digested proteins, peptides, and amino acids in the antrum release gastrin, while carbohydrates and fats do not. Other stimulants of gastrin release include calcium and bombesin, or the mammalian counterpart of bombesin, gastrin-releasing peptide (GRP). The half-life in the circulation for G17 is 3–6 minutes and for G34 about 15 minutes.

Gastrin release is inhibited by antral acidification. Substantial inhibition occurs at pH 2.5, and release is abolished at pH 1. Secretion, glucagon, VIP, GIP, calcitonin, and somatostatin inhibit the release of meal-stimulated gastrin, but whether these are physiologic actions is unknown.

There is evidence for the presence of cholinergic mechanisms that both stimulate and inhibit gastrin release. Vagal stimulation by electrical current, insulin hypoglycemia, or injection of 2-deoxyglucose releases gastrin. However, cholinergic blockade with atropine enhances meal-stimulated gastrin release independently of gastric pH, which suggests the presence of a cholinergic (ie, vagal) mechanism that suppresses gastrin release. One hypothesis to explain vagal inhibition of gastrin release views the G cell as under the simultaneous influence of nearby somatostatin-producing cells and bombesin-containing postganglionic neurons. The former blocks gastrin release (a paracrine effect), and the latter stimulates gastrin release. Atropine (or vagotomy) blocks meal-stimulated somatostatin release but does not affect bombesin release, which results in an exaggerated postprandial gastrin response.

Gastrin is not preferentially metabolized by the liver but appears to be removed across capillary beds in tissues throughout the body. It is metabolized by the kidneys and does not appear as an immunologically reactive peptide in the urine.

Actions

The only certain actions of gastrin that occur at physiologic levels are stimulation of gastric acid and pepsin secretion. Gastrin evokes acid secretion by several mechanisms, one of which is release of histamine from cells near the parietal cells. The histamine then acts directly on parietal cells to cause acid secretion. Gastrin-stimulated histamine release in gastric mucosa has been documented in vivo and in vitro. H_2 receptor antagonists completely inhibit gastrin-stimulated acid secretion in vivo, which implies that a major portion of gastrin-stimulated acid secretion is mediated through histamine. There is also evidence, however, that gastrin acts directly on parietal cells to stimulate acid secretion. For example, there are gastrin receptors on parietal cells, and gastrin induces intracellular changes that do not occur in response to histamine. Furthermore, gastrin potentiates the action of histamine on acid secretion.

Increased gastric mucosal blood flow may be caused directly by gastrin or may be secondary to increased acid secretion. Gastrin also has a trophic effect on gastric mucosa and pancreas. Several other actions have been ascribed to gastrin, such as contraction of the lower esophageal sphincter and secretion of water and electrolytes by the jejunum, but they are not seen at physiologic concentrations. Excess amounts of gastrin secreted by pancreatic tumors (gastrinoma) cause acid hypersecretion and severe peptic ulcer disease.

CHOLECYSTOKININ

In 1928, Ivy and Oldberg observed that instillation of fat into the small intestine caused the gallbladder to contract. They postulated a hormonal mechanism and named the mediator cholecystokinin (CCK). In the early 1940s, Harper and Raper discovered a substance in extracts of duodenal mucosa that stimulated the secretion of enzyme-rich juice by the pancreas and called the substance pancreozymin. In 1964, Jorpes et al found that increasing purification of a single extract from porcine small intestine proportionally increased its potency for gallbladder contraction and pancreatic enzyme secretion, indicating that the 2 actions were properties of a single hormone. Previously, the term cholecystokinin had been used for the gallbladder effects and pancreozymin for the pancreatic effects; but because the former were discovered first, the hormone is now referred to simply as cholecystokinin, or CCK. In 1971, Mutt and Jorpes reported the amino acid sequence of CCK.

Biochemistry & Distribution

CCK exists in several molecular forms. Peptides containing 58, 39, 33, and 8 amino acids have been isolated and studied and are called CCK58, CCK39, CCK33, and CCK8, respectively. The carboxy-terminal octapeptide sequences are identical for all molecular forms of CCK. The CCK33 molecule is susceptible to tryptic digestion at positions 1, 6, 11, 21, and 25. Tryptic digestion at position 25 produces CCK8.

Like gastrin, CCK is probably synthesized as a precursor, with CCK39 and CCK33 representing progressive steps in the creation of CCK8. All of the biologic actions are contained in the terminal octapeptide, which is 4–6 times more potent than CCK33 on a molar basis. Sulfation of the tyrosine moiety in position 7 from the carboxyl terminus is necessary for full biologic potency. The human gene for CCK consists of a sequence of 345 base pairs that codes for a preprocholecystokinin of 115 amino acids.

CCK is located in the duodenum and proximal jejunum within the mucosal I cell. It is also found in the central nervous system, in the myenteric plexus of the intestine, and in nerves supplying the urinary bladder and uterus.

Measurement & Release

Development of a radioimmunoassay for CCK has been difficult, principally because iodination alters the CCK molecule. Several investigators have reported the ability to measure serum levels of CCK by radioimmunoassay. Others have developed an in vitro bioassay using dispersed pancreatic acini. Serum levels of CCK increase within 10 minutes postprandially and remain elevated for at least 2 hours. Fasting CCK levels vary from 0 to 20 pmol/L and postprandial levels from 20 to 100 pmol/L, depending on the immunoassay used. It is presently unclear whether CCK8 or CCK33 is the major circulating form. Levels measured by bioassay are lower than those measured by radioimmunoassay.

Like gastrin, CCK circulates in several forms. Since CCK8 is 5–6 times more potent than CCK33, it will be necessary to measure these 2 forms separately in order to interpret the significance of the concentration of CCK in blood.

The half-life of CCK in blood is 2.5–7 minutes. CCK is taken up and degraded in the capillary beds of most organs (eg, lung, spleen, liver, intestine, stomach, and kidney). It is released by intraduodenal food, amino acids, fatty acids, calcium, and acid. Cholinergic neural mechanisms enhance CCK release in response to luminal stimulants. Phenylalanine and tryptophan are the most potent amino acids for release of CCK. For fatty acids to be effective, they must be more than 9 carbons long, and potency increases up to a chain length of 18 carbons. The magnitude of the CCK response to amino acids and fatty acids is also proportionate to the length of intestine perfused. The presence of increasing concentrations of bile acids in the intestine progressively inhibits the CCK-like effects of luminal stimuli but has no effect on the response to intravenous CCK. This suggests that bile acids block the release of endogenous CCK and that this constitutes a mechanism which allows the gallbladder to relax again in the late stages after a meal.

Actions

Gallbladder contraction and pancreatic enzyme secretion are the only actions of CCK presently accepted as physiologic. CCK also affects motor function of the gastrointestinal tract; has a trophic effect on the pancreas; and induces satiety in several species, including humans. Intact vagal innervation is necessary for the latter effect. The presence of CCK in gut neurons as well as endocrine cells suggests that CCK acts in a neurocrine or paracrine manner in addition to its endocrine function.

The actions of CCK on smooth muscle include contraction of the gallbladder and stimulation of antral and intestinal motility to produce delayed gastric emptying. CCK has been shown to both relax and contract the lower esophageal sphincter and the sphincter of Oddi. A possible explanation for this apparent conflict is that CCK acts as a neurotransmitter to stimulate postganglionic inhibitory neurons to cause sphincter relaxation and also acts directly on the smooth muscle to produce contraction. The observed effect (relaxation or contraction) would depend upon which system predominates. CCK acts directly on the smooth muscle of gallbladder and sphincter of Oddi and indirectly through cholinergic nerves on the smooth muscle of the small intestine.

The secretory actions of CCK include stimulation of pancreatic enzyme secretion, hepatic bile secretion, and Brunner's gland secretion. CCK also stimulates release of insulin and pancreatic polypeptide from the pancreas and calcitonin from the thyroid. Intraperito-neal injections of CCK33 or CCK8 cause early satiety in rats.

Hypertrophy of the pancreas is produced by intraperitoneal injections of CCK8. The number of acinar, ductal, and B cells (of the islets of Langerhans) is increased. The effect entails both cellular hypertrophy and hyperplasia. While there is good evidence that the effect of CCK on gallbladder contraction, sphincter of Oddi relaxation, pancreatic enzyme secretion, and gastric smooth muscle contraction occurs under physiologic conditions, it remains to be seen whether other effects occur at physiologic levels of CCK.

SECRETIN

Secretin was the first hormone discovered when Bayliss and Starling demonstrated that intravenous injection of acid extracts of jejunum stimulated secretion of water and bicarbonate from the pancreas. Secretin was purified by Jorpes and Mutt in 1961, and its amino acid sequence was identified in 1966.

Biochemistry & Distribution

Unlike most other hormones, secretin has been identified in only one form. It is a basic 27-amino-acid polypeptide containing 4 arginine residues and one histidine residue. Fourteen of the 27 amino acids in secretin occupy the same position as in glucagon. Secretin also shows structural similarities to GIP, VIP, peptide histidine isoleucine (PHI), and peptide histidine methionine (PHM), and these peptides are known as the secretin-glucagon family (Table 21–2). The entire molecule of secretin is necessary for biologic activity. Secretin is found in S cells in the duodenum and proximal jejunum and in the central nervous system.

Measurement & Release

Secretin is difficult to label with radioactive iodine, because the molecule lacks a tyrosine residue. This problem has been solved by iodination under conditions that label histidine or by using a synthetic secretin analogue in which tyrosine has been substituted for one of the other amino acids. Most immunoassays for secretin are too insensitive to measure changes in serum levels. Furthermore, secretin is highly unstable in solution, so that special measures must be taken to protect against degradation. The most sensitive immunoassays for secretin have reported fasting serum values of 1–5 pmol/L, but it has not been possible to measure changes after a meal.

The only known stimulus for secretin release is duodenal acidification, which causes an increase in serum levels within minutes. Small increments follow rapid drops in duodenal pH. The threshold for secretin release is a duodenal pH of less than 4.5. Infusion of bile salt into the duodenum also causes a small increase in serum levels of secretin. Other substances such as fats, alcohols, glucose, and amino acids do not release secretin if the pH of the duodenum is kept constant. Neither vagotomy nor atropinization alters the secretin response to intraduodenal acid. Vagotomy may indirectly affect secretin release by elevating duodenal pH. The half-life of secretin in blood is 3–7.5 minutes.

Actions

Secretin stimulates pancreatic bicarbonate and water secretion at physiologic levels. Because serum levels are so low, there is some question about whether circulating secretin can account for the postprandial increase in pancreatic bicarbonate and water secretion. Nevertheless, small increases in serum secretin do correlate positively with increases in the output of pancreatic bicarbonate and water. Furthermore, small amounts of secretin infused intravenously to mimic the physiologic changes in serum levels produce a corresponding increase in pancreatic water and bicarbonate secretion. Therefore, it is probably correct to conclude that secretin has a physiologic effect on pancreatic water and bicarbonate secretion. CCK markedly potentiates the effect of secretin on pancreatic secretion. In physiologic circumstances (ie, after a meal), CCK is released in amounts sufficient to enhance the effect of secretin. Although infusion of secretin can inhibit meal-stimulated gastrin release and gastric acid secretion, these effects are not seen with physiologic amounts of secretin.

Clinical Uses

Secretin is used clinically to evaluate pancreatic function, to obtain specimens of pancreatic juice for cytologic study, and as a provocative agent for the release of gastrin from gastrinomas. When used for clinical tests, secretin is measured in clinical units (4000 clinical units = 1 mg).

To evaluate **pancreatic function,** a Dreiling tube is placed in the duodenum to aspirate pancreatic secretions, and secretin (1 clinical unit/kg body weight) is injected intravenously. Duodenal juice is collected over eight 10-minute periods, and volume and bicarbonate concentration are measured. A maximal bicarbonate concentration of less than 90 meq/L and a flow of less than 2 mL/kg body weight over 80 minutes are diagnostic of impaired pancreatic function. Secretin may also be used to stimulate secretion of pancreatic juice for examination for malignant cells. The juice may be collected through a duodenal tube or by direct endoscopic cannulation of the pancreatic duct. A description of the use of secretin in the diagnosis of gastrinoma appears in the section of gastrinoma (see below).

GASTRIC INHIBITORY POLYPEPTIDE

Biochemistry & Distribution

Gastric inhibitory polypeptide (GIP) was first isolated in 1971, and it has subsequently been synthesized. GIP is a 42-amino-acid polypeptide with a structure similar to those of secretin, glucagon, and VIP. GIP has been found in serum in larger molecular forms that may represent precursors of the 42-amino-acid hormone. GIP is found in mucosal cells in the duodenum, jejunum, and ileum; the highest concentrations are in the jejunum. These cells, termed K cells, are most abundant in the microvilli and upper crypts of the small intestine. GIP may also be found in pancreatic islet A cells containing glucagon.

Measurement & Release

Basal levels of GIP are in the range of 250 pg/mL (50 pmol/L). GIP release is stimulated by ingestion of food, with a peak of approximately 1000 pg/mL (200 pmol/L) occurring 60 minutes postprandially. GIP remains elevated for about 3 hours. The most potent stimuli for release of GIP are intraluminal glucose and triglyceride, and the magnitude of the response is dose-dependent. Ingestion of glucose produces an increase within 60 minutes, while ingestion of fat produces an increase within 120–150 minutes. The response to glucose is dependent on glucose absorption. The half-life of GIP in plasma is about 20 minutes. Release of GIP may also be modulated by adrenergic stimulation, calcium, and glucagon.

Actions

Physiologic doses of GIP given intravenously increase the insulin response to glucose, but the effect is dependent on the presence of elevated blood glucose levels. This has prompted some to suggest that GIP be renamed **glucose-dependent insulin-releasing polypeptide.** Thus, GIP may function as an internal secretion, or "incretion," enhancing insulin release and glucose disposal during periods of hyperglycemia. GIP also inhibits gastrin release and gastric acid secretion, but it is unlikely that these effects occur at physiologic levels of the hormone. The amino-terminal portion of the molecule is essential for the effect on insulin, and the carboxy-terminal portion is essential for the gastric effect. GIP in physiologic doses causes secretion of fluid and electrolytes by the ileal mucosa, but the importance of this is not known.

VASOACTIVE INTESTINAL POLYPEPTIDE

Biochemistry & Distribution

Vasoactive intestinal polypeptide (VIP) was first isolated in 1970 by Said and Mutt from porcine small intestine. Its structure has been determined, and it has been synthesized. VIP is colocalized on a gene with peptide histidine isoleucine (PHI). VIP is a basic 28-amino-acid peptide with strong homology to PHI, PHM, secretin, glucagon, GIP, and GRP. In addition, it has a close structural relationship to helospectin and helodermin, which occur in the venom of Gila monsters. This suggests that, as a highly conserved molecule, it has important biologic activity.

VIP is distributed in a wide range of neurons in the gut, the central nervous system, and the urogenital tract. It is not present in gut endocrine cells, except in lower vertebrates. It probably functions as a neurocrine agent, and its presence in neurons with processes extending to mucosal cells, smooth muscle, and blood vessels VIP affects local secretion, motility, and blood flow.

Measurement & Release

Fasting serum levels of VIP are low (> 7 pmol/L) and do not increase much postprandially. VIP concentrations in venous effluent from the gut increase with electrical stimulation, esophageal distension, and mechanical stimulation of intestinal mucosa. The half-life of VIP in blood is about one minute in humans.

Actions

The most important physiologic actions of VIP are probably relaxation of the lower esophageal sphincter, receptive relaxation of the gastric fundus, and relaxation of the anal sphincter. Additionally, VIP increases gut blood flow and is responsible for penile erection. When infused intravenously, VIP inhibits pentagastrin and histamine-stimulated gastric acid and pepsin secretion. It stimulates lipolysis, glycogenolysis, and secretion by the small intestine and pancreas.

Abnormally large amounts of VIP produced by islet cell tumors of the pancreas are at least partly responsible for the manifestations of the pancreatic cholera (WDHA) syndrome (discussed in a subsequent section). The diarrhea in this condition is due to secretion of voluminous amounts of fluid by the small intestine.

SUBSTANCE P

Substance P was discovered by Von Euler and Gaddum in 1931 and was the first peptide found in both brain and gut. Little further research was done on substance P until 1970, when Chang and Leeman isolated and purified it from the brain. The amino acid sequence is known, and it has been synthesized.

Biochemistry & Distribution

Substance P is an 11-amino-acid polypeptide, of which the 5 carboxy-terminal amino acids are required for biologic action. There appear to be larger precursor forms in serum. The gene encoding substance P has been cloned and sequenced. Two distinct mRNA sequences have been identified, one coding for substance P and the other coding for a tachykinin known as **substance K** (also called neurokinin-α or neuromedin-L).

Substance P is distributed throughout the body, with the highest concentrations occurring in the gut and nervous system. High concentrations are also found in structures along the brainstem (eg, hypothalamus, substantia nigra). In the spinal cord, it is concentrated mainly in sensory areas. In the gut, substance P has

been found in nerve plexuses and enterochromaffin cells.

Measurement & Release

Substance P is released from enteric neurons in response to electrical stimulation, serotonin, and CCK. The normal serum concentration of substance P is about 70 pmol/L, most of which is of enteric origin. Substance P is not released into the blood except in disease states (eg, carcinoid syndrome and dumping syndrome). It probably acts through neurocrine or paracrine mechanisms.

Actions

The major action of substance P is stimulation of smooth muscle contraction of the gut. Part of the contraction is tetrodotoxin-sensitive, which suggests that substance P acts through a neural reflex. Since contraction is not completely blocked by tetrodotoxin, substance P is also thought to act directly on the muscle. Intravenous infusion of substance P increases intestinal motility and stimulates pancreatic exocrine and salivary gland secretion and gallbladder contraction. Cell bodies of substance P–containing nerves are located in the myenteric plexus, and the axons are scattered throughout the smooth muscle, suggesting that it may have an effect on intestinal motility. Because it is present in plexuses, substance P may also serve as an excitatory transmitter in afferent neurons of the gut. It also causes vasodilatation and the release of histamine from mast cells.

Substance P is thought to act as a neurotransmitter or modulator of sensory input in the spinal cord and specifically to have a role in the central transmission of pain impulses. In the brain, substance P stimulates secretion of prolactin (PRL) and growth hormone (GH).

ENKEPHALINS

The enkephalins are neuropeptides closely related to other central nervous system opiate peptides, the α and β-endorphins. The endorphins and enkephalins bind to opiate receptors found in the brain and gut.

Biochemistry & Distribution

Each of the 2 enkephalins in the gastrointestinal tract, met-enkephalin and leu-enkaphalin, contains 5 amino acids and differs only at the terminal –COOH residue, which is either methionine or leucine. Three distinct genes have been identified that code for opiate peptides. The pro-opiomelanocortin gene gives rise to ACTH, MSH, and β-endorphin. Its expression in the enteric nervous system is poorly understood. A second gene codes for precursor molecules of met-enkephalin and leu-enkephalin. There is direct evidence of synthesis of these peptides within myenteric neurons in the gut. A third gene codes for precursor molecules of dynorphin, β-neoendorphin, and leu-enkephalin.

Enkephalins are located in cells in the stomach, duodenum, and gallbladder as well as in nerves. Enkephalin-containing cells are numerous in the gastrointestinal tract, and their distribution in nerves is similar to that of substance P.

Measurement & Release

Enkephalins have not been detected in plasma or serum. They are rapidly destroyed in blood, which makes it unlikely that they act as circulating hormones. The normal stimulus for the release of enkephalins is unclear. It is likely that they function as neurocrine or paracrine agents within the gut wall. Specific and nonspecific degrading enzymes have been found in the interstitial fluid and lymphatic channels of the gut.

Actions

When infused intravenously, enkephalins have the same actions as morphine. In the central nervous system, they cause analgesia, sedation, respiratory depression, muscular rigidity, and emesis. In the gastrointestinal tract, the most prominent manifestation of intravenous enkephalin infusion is constipation. However, motor activity in all parts of the gut is affected. In stomach, duodenum, and jejunum, enkephalins initially cause increased contractions, followed by distention and atony. In the colon, they produce segmental areas of contraction without peristalsis and sustained contraction of the anal sphincter.

Infusion of enkephalins increases histamine-stimulated gastric acid and pepsin secretion and inhibits secretin-stimulated bicarbonate secretion from the pancreas. Enkephalins also decrease mesenteric vascular resistance and increase intestinal blood flow.

NEUROTENSIN

Neurotensin was discovered accidentally during isolation of substance P from the hypothalamus when a fraction of the extract was found to produce vasodilatation and hypotension. The term neurotensin originated from its neurologic origin and its hypotensive properties.

Biochemistry & Distribution

Neurotensin is a 13-amino-acid polypeptide that has been synthesized. It is found extensively in nerve cells in the central nervous system. In the gut, it is located in the N cells of the ileum and is almost absent from nerve fibers. The carboxy-terminal segment of the molecule is responsible for the biologic activity of neurotensin.

Measurement & Release

Release after a meal has been documented, but the half-life in serum is very short. Immunoassay for neurotensin is available in only a few laboratories.

Actions

The physiologic actions of neurotensin are not known. Neurotensin is a kinin and causes hypotension and vasodilatation and contraction of various smooth muscle groups. It decreases gastric acid secretion and peristaltic activity in the gastrointestinal tract. Because gastric acid secretion can be blocked by vagal denervation, it is probably mediated through the vagi. Neurotensin binds to mast cells, and since many of its effects are histaminelike (ie, hypotension, hypoglycemia, increased vascular permeability, smooth muscle contraction), neurotensin may act by releasing histamine. An exaggerated postprandial release of neurotensin has been reported to occur in patients with dumping syndrome. Experimentally, intravenous infusion of neurotensin inhibits gastrin-stimulated but not histamine-stimulated acid secretion. It also delays gastric emptying.

MOTILIN

The existence of motilin was postulated by Brown et al in 1966, when they observed that alkalinization of the duodenum in dogs produced contractions in denervated pouches of the body of the stomach. Similar contractions followed injection of an impure preparation of CCK but not of pure CCK. Subsequently, motilin was isolated from the crude CCK extract, purified, and identified.

Biochemistry & Distribution

Motilin is a 22-amino-acid polypeptide. It has been synthesized, and ample quantities are available for immunoassays and physiologic studies. There is at least one larger form of motilin.

Motilin is located in endocrine cells in the mucosa of the duodenum, proximal jejunum, antrum, and fundus. It is often seen with serotonin in enterochromaffin cells. It is also present in nerves throughout the gut.

Measurement & Release

The concentration of motilin in blood ranges from 4 to 350 pmol/L, with a median of about 60 pmol/L. Motilin is released into the blood in cyclic fashion in fasting dogs; if the same is true in humans, it would explain the variations reported in basal levels.

Serum motilin concentrations do not rise postprandially. In fact, a protein meal depresses serum levels.

Actions

Intravenous infusion of motilin stimulates pepsin secretion from the stomach and increases the rate of intestinal transit. In vitro, motilin causes contraction of duodenal, ileal, colonic, and gallbladder smooth muscle. Its actions are most pronounced on duodenal smooth muscle, where it is 100 times as potent as acetylcholine. The actions of motilin on smooth muscle are not blocked by atropine, phentolamine, propranolol, cimetidine, or chlorpheniramine; this suggests that the hormone acts directly on motilin receptors in the muscle. Smooth muscle other than from the gut does not respond to motilin.

In the fasting state, the smooth muscle of the stomach and small bowel displays electrical activity termed the **interdigestive migrating myoelectric complex.** There are 4 phases (I-IV), and muscular contraction occurs in phases III and IV. In fasting dogs, phase III and IV myoelectric activity occurs at 90- to 120-minute intervals, beginning in the duodenum and propagating over 60–80 minutes to the distal ileum. Phase III and IV myoelectric activity coincides with a peristaltic wave, which propels enteric contents distally during fasting. The cyclic occurrence of phase III and IV myoelectric activity coincides with increases in serum motilin levels. Conversely, intravenous infusion of motilin produces phase III myoelectric activity in the duodenum. These observations implicate motilin in the cyclic peristalsis that occurs between meals.

Motilin has been shown to be about as potent as CCK in stimulation of gallbladder contraction, and because an effect is seen with serum levels within the physiologic range, motilin may participate in the control of gallbladder emptying, particularly in the fasting state.

SOMATOSTATIN

Somatostatin was first isolated from the hypothalamus, where it was found to inhibit the release of GH. Somatostatin was subsequently found in large amounts in endocrine cells of the stomach and pancreas and in nerve fibers in the gut mucosa. It is the preeminent inhibitory peptide of the gut.

Biochemistry & Distribution

Somatostatin is a cyclic 14-amino-acid polypeptide. It has been synthesized, and antisomatostatin antibodies have been generated. Somatostatin also occurs in at least one larger form containing 28 amino acids, which is probably a precursor of the 14-amino-acid molecule.

Somatostatin is found in the central nervous system as well as in the gastrointestinal tract, where it is present in both endocrine and nerve cells. In the gastrointestinal tract, somatostatin is most prominent in endocrine cells within the mucosa of the gastric antrum and in the D cells of the pancreatic islets.

The gene sequence for somatostatin is known, and the structure of the human somatostatin precursor has been deduced from the cDNA sequence. The gene is located on chromosome No. 3. Preprosomatostatin contains 116 amino acids, with posttranslational processing occuring at both the amino- and carboxy-terminal regions. The sequence of the tetradecapeptide somatostatin is strongly conserved.

Measurement & Release

Antibodies have proved useful in localizing somatostatin in the gastrointestinal tract and in the measurement of serum levels. By selective cannulation of the venous drainage of the gastric fundus, antrum, and pancreas, somatostatin release has been demonstrated in anesthetized dogs following intragastric instillation of fat, glucose, and amino acids.

Actions

The principal actions of somatostatin are inhibitory. It inhibits the release of gastrin, secretin, motilin, CCK, GIP, insulin, and glucagon as well as of GH. It also inhibits gastric acid and pancreatic exocrine secretion; gallbladder contraction; gastric emptying; small bowel absorption of amino acids, glucose, and triglycerides; and the release of acetylcholine from cholinergic nerves.

Because its inhibitory effects are so diffuse, somatostatin is unlikely to act as a circulating hormone. However, in physiologic levels, circulating somatostatin delays gallbladder and gastric emptying, decreases glucose uptake from the gut, and decreases gastric acid secretion. The evidence for a paracrine function for somatostatin is indirect and is based on the location of somatostatin-containing cells and the actions of somatostatin. For example, somatostatin is found near parietal cells and antral G cells and is a potent inhibitor of gastrin release and gastric acid secretion. Somatostatin is contained in the D cells of the pancreatic islets and inhibits the release of insulin and glucagon from the islets. (See also Chapter 5).

PEPTIDE YY

Peptide YY (PYY) was so named because it has tyrosine residues at the amino and carboxyl ends of the molecule, and the symbol for tyrosine is Y.

Biochemistry & Distribution

PYY is a 36-amino-acid peptide that contains 5 tyrosine molecules and has several sequence similarities to pancreatic polypeptide (PP). PYY is present in mucosal endocrine cells in the small bowel and colon, with highest concentrations in the ileum and colon.

Measurement & Release

Information on the release of PYY is meager. Serum levels of PYY increase to 200–300 pg/mL postprandially in dogs.

Actions

Intravenous infusion of PYY (10–20 pmol/kg) inhibits pancreatic secretion of bicarbonate and enzymes. The inhibition occurs at low doses, but it is not yet known whether the action is physiologic.

BOMBESIN & GASTRIN-RELEASING PEPTIDE

Bombesin belongs to a group of peptides found in the skin of frogs. Bombesinlike immunoreactivity (BLI) has been detected in mammalian brain and gut, but the actual molecule in mammals is probably gastrin-releasing peptide (GRP). The 10 carboxy-terminal peptides are nearly identical in GRP and bombesin, and these 10 peptides are responsible for their biologic activity.

Biochemistry & Distribution

Bombesin obtained from frog skin is a 14-amino-acid polypeptide. It belongs to a group of homologous peptides (litorin, ranatensin, and alytensin) obtained from the same source. It bears no similarity to other mammalian hormones. GRP is a 27-amino-acid polypeptide isolated from mammalian gut. It has a carboxy-terminal decapeptide almost identical to that of bombesin. The human GRP gene has been cloned from a patient with carcinoid metastasized to the lungs. It encodes a precursor molecule of 148 amino acids, termed preproGRP, which undergoes posttranslational processing to the active 27-amino-acid form.

BLI is seen throughout the gut in nerves and endocrine cells. It is most concentrated in the antral and duodenal mucosa and is present also in fine nerve fibers in the gut wall. The distribution of GRP in mammals is similar to that of bombesin.

Measurement & Release

Little or no change in plasma GRP concentrations occurs postprandially. In anesthetized pigs, marked release of GRP occurs in the venous outflow of the stomach in response to electrical vagal stimulation. The neuronal origin and mechanism of release of GRP support its function as a neurotransmitter.

Actions

The physiologic actions of bombesin are not definitely known. When infused intravenously, bombesin stimulates release of gastrin and CCK and inhibits release of VIP. It also causes pancreatic secretion of amylase, which occurs independently of CCK release. Finally, it contracts smooth muscle of the gallbladder, duodenum, and stomach.

Because BLI is present in the antrum and duodenum and because bombesin given experimentally releases gastrin and CCK, bombesin has been postulated to act as a neurotransmitter that releases these hormones. In the brain, it may play a role in thermoregulation and pain perception.

PANCREATIC POLYPEPTIDE

Biochemistry & Distribution

Pancreatic polypeptide (PP) was first discovered during attempts to isolate insulin from chicken pancreas in 1968. It is a 36-amino-acid peptide with a carboxy-terminal tyrosine amide. Small differences in the amino acid sequence are present among the species that have been studied, including chicken, pig, cow, rat, and human. The PP gene has been characterized. It codes for a 95-amino-acid prepropancreatic polypeptide that undergoes posttranslational processing to the active form. In the pancreas, PP is found in the islets as well as in cells in close association with the acini. The concentrations of PP in the head of the pancreas are greater than in the tail; this distribution is the opposite of that of glucagon. PP is probably present in the brain.

Measurement & Release

Basal plasma PP concentrations in humans average 12 pmol/L and increase somewhat with age. The most potent stimulant of PP release is a protein meal. This appears to be vagally mediated, although additional hormonal mechanisms are probably involved. These mechanisms are, as yet, poorly defined.

Actions

The major physiologic action of PP is inhibition of bicarbonate and protein secretion. It also causes relaxation of the gallbladder and a decrease in hepatic bile secretion. Intravenous infusion of PP does not affect acid secretion, carbohydrate or lipid metabolism, or the release of other hormones. PP levels may be elevated in patients with several kinds of hormone-secreting tumors (eg, gastrinoma, VIPoma). This is not a consistent finding, however, and thus the value of PP as a tumor marker is limited.

ENTEROGLUCAGON

Biochemistry & Distribution

The best known form of glucagon is a 29-amino-acid peptide found mainly in the pancreatic A cells. A number of other larger forms exist in the gut, including glicentin and enteroglucagon. They all are present within the same gene sequence and share amino-terminal homology. Forms of glucagon have been found in the intestinal mucosa, stomach, salivary gland, and brain.

Measurement & Release

Measurement of serum levels of enteroglucagon is imprecise, owing to the presence of multiple molecular forms of cross-reactivity of antibody assays with pancreatic glucagon. Ileal fat perfusion appears to be the most important stimulant of enteroglucagon release.

Actions

The intestinal forms of glucagon are much less potent than pancreatic glucagon in the regulation of hepatic glucose production. It has been postulated that enteroglucagon is an important trophic factor for small intestinal mucosa.

HORMONAL ABNORMALITIES IN DISEASES OF THE GASTROINTESTINAL TRACT

Although gastrointestinal peptide hormones are clearly important in the regulation of digestion, their role in disease states of the gut is less clear. Unlike in other endocrine systems, no proven deficiency states of gut peptides exist. A number of excess states have been identified and are reviewed in this section.

DUODENAL ULCER

On the average, patients with duodenal ulcer deliver excess acid and pepsin into the duodenum and secrete more acid in response to gastrin or histamine than do subjects without duodenal ulcer. Consequently, the search for hormonal abnormalities in duodenal ulcer has centered around mechanisms that control gastric acid secretion, neutralization of gastric acid in the duodenum, and the rate of gastric emptying (ie, the rate of delivery of gastric acid into the duodenum). Hormones that may affect acid secretion or duodenal pH are listed in Table 21–5.

The role of gastrin in duodenal ulcer disease has been the most extensively investigated. Neither basal serum levels of gastrin nor the individual components (G17 and G34) are elevated in patients with duodenal ulcer, and the number of G (gastrin-secreting) cells in the antrum is normal. However, the gastrin response to a meal and to hypoglycemia is greater than normal and more prolonged in these patients. Furthermore, inhibition of gastrin release following antral acidification is less effective in these patients. In fact, the exaggerated gastrin response in duodenal ulcer disease may be explained by a blunted negative feedback response to antral acidification.

Acid secretion is greater than normal at any given dose of gastrin in ulcer patients; ie, the parietal cells have a heightened sensitivity to stimulation. In summary, most patients with duodenal ulcer have 2 abnormalities in gastrin metabolism: (1) increased gastrin response to a meal and (2) increased sensitivity of the parietal cells to stimulation by gastrin.

Basal Hypergastrinemia

There are 7 uncommon causes of basal hypergastrinemia associated with duodenal ulcer: gastrinoma, hypercalcemia, massive small bowel resection, renal failure, gastric outlet obstruction, antral G cell hyperplasia, and antral exclusion. In the evaluation of a patient with duodenal ulcer, one should measure gastrin levels, and if hypergastrinemia is present, these conditions should be considered.

A. Gastrinoma: Patients with gastrinoma have autogenous production of large amounts of gastrin by a tumor. The result is excessive acid secretion and severe ulcer disease. Treatment, as discussed in detail later in this chapter, consists of administering H_2 receptor antagonists or performing tumor resection or total gastrectomy.

B. Hypercalcemia: Patients with hypercalcemia may secrete increased amounts of gastrin and gastric acid. In patients with hyperparathyroidism, removal of a parathyroid adenoma with return of the serum calcium level to normal usually also allows the serum gastrin and gastric acid secretion to become normal. However, the relationship between hypercalcemia and duodenal ulcer disease is not close, and in general, if severe duodenal ulcer disease is present in a patient with hyperparathyroidism, the cause is more likely to be gastrinoma (as part of multiple endocrine neoplasia [MEN] syndrome type I) than a direct effect of hypercalcemia.

C. Extensive Small Bowel Resection: People who have had extensive small bowel resections often secrete increased amounts of gastric acid and have elevated gastrin levels. Although this could be a result of decreased degradation of gastrin, it more likely reflects loss of an enterogastrone (a hormone from the intestine that inhibits gastrin release and gastric acid secretion). The increased acid secretion that follows enterectomy usually subsides within a few months, so that treatment with H_2 blocking agents is usually sufficient.

D. Renal Failure: Renal failure may be accompanied by hypergastrinemia and gastric hyperacidity, probably because of decreased catabolism of the large molecular forms of gastrin by the diseased kidneys. Treatment consists of antacids and H_2 blocking agents.

E. Gastric Outlet Obstruction: Hypergastrinemia in association with gastric outlet obstruction is probably caused by antral distention. Tube decompres-

Table 21–5. Hormones that may affect acid secretion or duodenal pH.

Action	Stimulation	Inhibition
Acid secretion	Gastrin CCK	VIP GIP Somatostatin Secretin
Gastrin release	Bombesin GRP	Secretin Somatostatin VIP GIP Glucagon
Pancreatic bicarbonate secretion	CCK Secretin VIP	PP Somatostatin
Delay of gastric emptying of acid into duodenum	CCK	

sion of the stomach usually results in a return of the gastrin levels to normal.

F. Antral G Cell Hyperplasia: Rare patients have hypergastrinemia from hyperactivity of the G cells, a condition referred to as antral G cell hyperplasia. Treatment consists of H_2 blocking agents or antrectomy.

G. Excluded Antrum Syndrome: In the past, surgeons would occasionally divide the antrum proximal to the pylorus in an attempt to simplify surgical treatment of duodenal ulcer disease. The proximal stomach was reconstructed as a Billroth II gastrojejunostomy, and the divided end of the antrum was oversewn, leaving it excluded from the influence of acid secreted by the parietal cell mucosa in the remaining body and fundus. The isolated antrum would occasionally produce large amounts of gastrin, resulting in a syndrome similar to gastrinoma. Since surgeons long ago abandoned this operation and since the phenomenon does not occur if only a small amount of antral mucosa is accidentally left attached to the duodenum, the excluded antrum syndrome is exceedingly rare nowadays.

Effects of Other Hormones

Bombesin or **GRP** releases gastrin and is not inhibited by antral acidification. GRP is present in the antral mucosa and may serve as a physiologic stimulus for gastrin release. Theoretically, excess GRP could produce the effects that characterize duodenal ulcer disease, ie, the exaggerated gastrin response to a meal and the diminished inhibition of gastrin release by acid.

CCK is a weak agonist of acid secretion, but it has a strong potentiating influence on pancreatic bicarbonate secretion and delays gastric emptying. Pancreatic bicarbonate neutralizes acid in the duodenum, and the rate of gastric emptying governs delivery of acid to the duodenum. It is unlikely that CCK could contribute to ulcer formation by directly stimulating acid secretion. However, low CCK levels could be involved by allowing more rapid emptying of acid into the duodenum and decreasing bicarbonate secretion.

Secretin inhibits meal-stimulated gastrin released and gastric acid secretion in pharmacologic doses, but secretin is liberated in such small quantities that it could have little effect on the stomach. Secretin does, however, stimulate pancreatic bicarbonate secretion, and duodenal acidification stimulates secretin release. Although abnormalities in secretin could contribute to ulcer formation, studies comparing secretin release in patients with ulcer and in normal subjects have given conflicting results. In fact, excessive duodenal acidification is usually associated with increased secretin levels.

GIP inhibits acid secretion in response to many stimuli, and GIP levels increase after a meal. However, postprandial GIP levels are higher in patients with ulcer than in controls.

VIP inhibits gastric acid secretion and stimulates pancreatic secretion, but the serum levels are low and do not change after a meal.

Somatostatin inhibits gastrin release and gastric acid secretion in response to virtually all stimuli. The location of somatostatin in antral cells near the G cells suggests that it may serve as a paracrine inhibitor of gastric acid secretion. It is possible that decreased somatostatin activity contributes to duodenal ulcer formation, but experiments testing this possibility are inconclusive.

CELIAC SPRUE DISEASE

In sprue, the villi of the proximal small intestine are fewer, shortened, and blunted—changes that substantially decrease the absorptive area. Malabsorption of protein, carbohydrate, and fat is the result. Fat malabsorption may be aggravated by hormonal abnormalities. Postprandial gallbladder contraction is delayed and incomplete in sprue, and pancreatic exocrine function in response to intraluminal stimuli is decreased. Exogenous administration of CCK or secretin in patients with sprue evokes normal responses in the gallbladder and pancreas, suggesting that the defect is in the release of these hormones. One report has documented decreased postprandial CCK levels in patients with sprue.

The abnormal gallbladder contraction results in decreased bile flow and bile salt concentrations in the intestine, and decreased stimulation of the pancreas lowers pancreatic enzyme concentrations. The end result is impaired micelle formation and fat absorption. While decreased intestinal surface area is probably the principal cause of malabsorption in sprue, these hormonal abnormalities enhance the malabsorption defect.

MOTILITY DISORDERS OF THE GASTROINTESTINAL TRACT

Stimulation of sympathetic nerves normally relaxes the gut, and stimulation of parasympathetic nerves causes it to contract. If both adrenergic and cholinergic receptors are blocked, nerve stimulation causes muscle relaxation.

Hirschsprung's disease is characterized by absence of neurons in a segment of distal colon. The affected colon is contracted, the muscular coat is hypertrophied, and the lumen is narrow. The colon proximally is dilated as a consequence of chronic partial obstruction. The concentrations of VIP and substance P as well as the numbers of nerves containing VIP and substance P are greatly decreased in the contracted segment. The present view is that the neurologic abnormality responsible for Hirschsprung's disease consists of loss of the relaxing influences of peptidergic VIP and substance P neurons.

Conceivably, other abnormalities of peptidergic neurons could contribute to other motility disorders such as pyloric stenosis, achalasia, and chronic idiopathic intestinal pseudoobstruction.

APUDOMAS

Apudoma is the general term for tumors of gut endocrine cells that secrete peptide hormones. The tumors may be very small and difficult to detect even at laparotomy.

Most apudomas are found in the pancreas, but a few occur in the wall of the duodenum or the retroperitoneum. Apudomas probably arise from pleuripotential stem cells (nesidioblasts) present in pancreatic ducts. Origin in such a cell could explain why many apudomas contain more than one type of endocrine cell and secrete more than one hormone. For example, VIPomas often secrete PP in addition to VIP. Insulin, gastrin, serotonin, substance P, PP, VIP, glucagon, enteroglucagon, and somatostatin have been found to be synthesized and secreted by different apudomas.

Although apudomas often secrete more than one peptide, they are usually named after the one most responsible for the clinical manifestations. Thus, a gastrin-secreting tumor is a gastrinoma and a VIP-secreting tumor a VIPoma. The incidence of other endocrine tumors in patients with gastrinoma is about 10–20%; in patients with insulinoma, 4%.

Wermer's syndrome is an autosomal dominant inherited condition in which 2 or more endocrine glands become hyperplastic or undergo tumor formation. Wermer's syndrome is also called multiple endocrine neoplasia (MEN) type I. In MEN type I, the pancreas, pituitary, and parathyroid glands are most often involved, and the most common pancreatic tumors are gastrinoma, insulinoma, and VIPoma. MEN type IIa, also known as **Sipple's syndrome,** consists of medullary carcinoma of the thyroid, pneochromocytoma, and hyperparathyroidism (see Chapter 28). The tumors are always multiple and diffuse in both MEN type I and MEN type IIa.

The diagnosis of apudoma is most often made by finding an elevated level of a hormone in the blood, and the usual conclusion is that the patient has a hormone-secreting tumor, most probably in the pancreas. Because the tumor is often difficult to find at laparotomy, preoperative localization is helpful. Pancreatic arteriography is occasionally useful in locating insulinomas but rarely so with gastrinomas. Ultrasonography and CT scanning have been disappointing. Selective sampling of hormone levels in venous outflow from the pancreas is now being studied to determine its value. The technique entails percutaneous puncture of the liver and threading a catheter into the splanchnic tributaries of the portal vein. Hormone levels in blood draining the tail, body, and head of the pancreas can be measured, and the point where a sharp increase in concentration is detected indicates where the tumor is located.

Tumor resection is the preferred treatment for apudomas, but many of them are malignant or multifocal and cannot be cured in this way. When resection is not possible, gastrinoma may be treated by gastrectomy (removing the target organ) or with H_2 blocking agents. However, for other hormone-producing tumors (eg, insulinoma or VIPoma), it is not possible to direct therapy at the target organ, and antitumor drugs are the only alternative to resection.

Fifty percent of apudomas found at operation are malignant, and most of these are unresectable. The chemotherapeutic agent most often used to treat malignant islet cell tumors is streptozocin, a nitrosourea derivative that inhibits DNA synthesis. The drug is usually given intravenously, but for treating hepatic metastases it may be infused directly in the hepatic artery. Streptozocin has been used to treat malignant gastrinomas, VIPomas, and glucagonomas. It produces a favorable response in about 50% of patients.

ZOLLINGER-ELLISON SYNDROME (Gastrinoma)

Zollinger-Ellison syndrome consists of gastric acid hypersecretion caused by a gastrin-producing tumor (gastrinoma). Although the normal pancreas does not contain appreciable amounts of gastrin, most gastrinomas occur in the pancreas; others are found submucosally in the duodenum and rarely in the antrum. The gastrin-producing lesions in the pancreas are non–B islet cell carcinomas (60%), solitary adenomas (25%), and hyperplasia or microadenomas (10%); the remaining cases (5%) are due to solitary submucosal gastrinomas in the first or second portion of the duodenum. The tumors, which may be as small as 2–3 mm, are often difficult to find. In about one-third of cases, the tumor cannot be located at laparotomy.

The diagnosis of cancer can be made only by finding metastases or blood vessel invasion, because the histologic pattern is similar for benign and malignant tumors. In most patients with malignant gastrinomas, the manifestations of hypergastrinemia (ie, severe peptic ulcer disease) are a far greater threat to health than are those of malignant growth and spread.

About a third of patients have other endocrine tumors—most commonly of the parathyroid and pituitary glands. When associated with tumors in other endocrine organs, the condition is known as MEN type I.

Clinical Findings

The symptoms in patients with gastrinoma are principally due to acid hypersecretion, and most of them are manifestations of peptic ulcer disease. Some patients with gastrinoma have severe diarrhea from the large amounts of acid entering the duodenum that may (1) destroy pancreatic lipase and produce steatorrhea, (2) damage the small bowel mucosa, and (3) overload the intestine with gastric and pancreatic secretions. About 5% of patients present with diarrhea only.

Ulcer symptoms are often refractory to large doses of antacids. Hemorrhage, perforation, and obstruction are common complications. Marginal ulcers often appear after surgical procedures that would cure the ordinary ulcer diathesis.

Diagnosis

Hypergastrinemia in the presence of acid hypersecretion is almost pathognomonic of gastrinoma. Because gastrin levels are normally inversely proportionate to gastric acid levels, many conditions that result in an increased gastric pH will allow the serum gastrin concentration to rise. Examples are pernicious anemia, atrophic gastritis, gastric ulcer, and postvagotomy state. In addition, use of H_2 blocking agents or antacids may increase the serum gastrin concentration, and these agents should be avoided for 24 hours before making gastrin measurements. It is often helpful to measure gastric acid secretion to rule out H^+ hyposecretion as a cause of hypergastrinemia.

A. Measurement of Serum Gastrin: Serum gastrin levels should be measured in any patient suspected of harboring a gastrinoma and in any patient whose ulcer disease is severe enough to warrant consideration of surgical treatment. In most laboratories, the normal gastrin value is less than 200 pg/mL. Patients with gastrinoma have levels that usually exceed 500 pg/mL, and they may reach 10,000 pg/mL or more. Patients with borderline gastrin values (200–500 pg/mL) whose acid secretion is in the range associated with ordinary duodenal ulcer disease should have a secretin provocative test. After administration of secretin, 2 units/kg as a bolus, a rise in the gastrin level of 150 pg/mL within 15 minutes is diagnostic (Table 21–6). Calcium given intravenously has also been used for this purpose, but secretin is both safer and more reliable. Postprandially, the serum gastrin levels do not change appreciably in patients with gastrinoma, whereas in normal subjects they double within 30 minutes.

Marked basal acid hypersecretion (> 15 meq H^+ per hour) occurs in most patients with Zollinger-Ellison syndrome who have an intact stomach. In a patient with a previous gastrectomy, a basal acid output of 5 meq/h or more would be highly suggestive. Since the parietal cells are already under near-maximal stimulation from hypergastrinemia, there is little increase in acid secretion following an injection of betazole (Histalog) or pentagastrin, and the ratio of basal to maximal acid output (BAO/MAO) characteristically exceeds 0.6.

Hypergastrinemia and gastric acid hypersecretion may be seen in gastric outlet obstruction, retained antrum after Billroth II gastrojejunostomy, and antral

Table 21–6. Provocative tests for gastrin release.[1]

Syndrome or Illness	Secretin Test	Calcium Test	Standard Meal
Duodenal ulcer without gastrinoma	Negative	Negative	Positive
Gastric outlet obstruction	Negative	Negative	
Retained antrum	Negative	±	±
Antral gastrin cell hyperactivity	Negative	Positive	Positive
Gastrinoma	Positive	Positive	Negative

[1]For secretin test, positive = increase in gastrin > 150 pg/mL; for calcium test, positive = increase in gastrin > 300 pg/mL; for standard meal, positive = change in gastrin > 80% of basal.

gastrin cell hyperactivity (hyperplasia). These conditions may be differentiated from gastrinoma by use of the calcium, secretin, and standard meal provocative tests. Large increases in serum gastrin levels after calcium or secretin and little change after a meal are characteristic of gastrinoma (Table 21–6). Because associated hyperparathyroidism is so common, all patients with gastrinoma should have their serum calcium concentration measured.

B. X-Ray Findings: An upper gastrointestinal series usually shows ulceration in the duodenal bulb, although ulcers sometimes appear in the distal duodenum or proximal jejunum. The presence of ulcers in these distal ("ectopic") locations is nearly diagnostic of gastrinoma. The stomach contains prominent rugal folds, and secretions are present in the lumen despite the overnight fast. The duodenum may be dilated and exhibit hyperactive peristalsis. Edema may be detected in the small bowel mucosa. The barium flocculates in the intestine, and transit time is accelerated. Selective angiography, transhepatic portal vein blood sampling, or CT scanning can sometimes demonstrate the pancreatic tumor, but misleading results are common with each.

Treatment

A. Operative Treatment: The optimal treatment for gastrinoma is surgical resection, but this measure is curative in only about 20% of patients. Nonetheless, tumor resection should be attempted in all fit patients without preoperative evidence of unresectable metastases and without MEN-1 syndrome. Although proximal gastric vagotomy reduces the dose of antisecretory agents required to inhibit acid secretion, it has little place in therapy at present. Total gastrectomy, the mainstay of surgical therapy of gastrinoma in the past, has largely been supplanted by the use of antisecretory agents. Total gastrectomy is advisable only in patients whose disease cannot be controlled either with symptomatic measures (see below) or by tumor resection.

B. Symptomatic Measures: The goal of medical therapy for gastrinoma is to inhibit gastric acid secretion. Histamine H_2 receptor antagonists such as cimetidine, ranitidine, and famotidine are effective in the short term, but progressively higher doses are usually required. Inhibition of basal acid secretion to less than 10 mmol/h is required for successful control of symptoms. The long-term failure rate with histamine H_2 receptor blockade is high. Omeprazole, a long-acting inhibitor of the parietal cell H^+, K^+-ATPase, is more potent than histamine H_2 receptor antagonists in inhibiting acid secretion. It is effective in the treatment of gastrinoma. A long-acting somatostatin analogue (octreotide) inhibits gastrin release, gastric acid secretion, and diarrhea in patients with gastrinoma. It may have occasional application in patients refractory to histamine H_2 receptor antagonists or omeprazole.

PANCREATIC CHOLERA
(WDHA Syndrome: Watery Diarrhea, Hypokalemia, & Achlorhydria; VIPoma, or Verner-Morrison Syndrome)

Pancreatic cholera is characterized by profuse watery diarrhea, massive fecal loss of potassium, low serum potassium concentration, and extreme weakness. Gastric acid secretion is usually low or absent even after stimulation with betazole or pentagastrin. Stool volume averages about 5 L/d during acute episodes and contains over 300 meq/L of potassium (20 times normal). Severe metabolic acidosis frequently results from loss of bicarbonate in the stool. Many patients are hypercalcemic, possibly from secretion by the tumor of a PTH-like substance. Abnormal glucose tolerance may result from hypokalemia and altered sensitivity to insulin. Patients who complain of severe diarrhea must be carefully studied for other causes before the diagnosis of WDHA syndrome is seriously entertained. Chronic laxative abuse is a frequent explanation.

Pathogenesis
WDHA syndrome is characterized by enormous jejunal secretion (instead of absorption) of water and electrolytes. The colon and ileum appear to function normally, but they are overwhelmed by the fluid load.

The hormone most often associated with WDHA syndrome is vasoactive intestinal polypeptide (VIP). In addition to VIP, 5-hydroxytryptamine (serotonin), substance P, calcitonin, PP, and some of the prostaglandins may cause diarrhea when present in high concentrations in the blood. High prostaglandin E_2 levels have been reported in some patients with WDHA syndrome, and in rare patients symptoms are abolished by indomethacin, a prostaglandin synthetase inhibitor.

Because about 80% of patients have high serum VIP levels, VIP is considered to be the principal mediator of this syndrome. In these patients, successful treatment is accompanied by a fall in serum VIP levels to normal. An intravenous infusion of VIP produces diarrhea in pigs and in humans when the blood concentration reaches levels similar to those in patients with this syndrome.

Diagnosis
The presence of severe watery secretory diarrhea and hypokalemia with normal or low gastric acid secretion should lead one to suspect this disease. Other causes of diarrhea such as malabsorption, infection, and surreptitious laxative use should be ruled out.

The presence of hypercalcemia and abnormal results in the oral glucose test tend to reinforce the diagnosis. A high VIP level is essentially diagnostic, but a normal level does not exclude WDHA syndrome.

The diagnosis may be confirmed at operation by finding a pancreatic islet cell tumor or a retroperitoneal neural tumor. In a substantial number of patients, no tumor is found.

Treatment
The optimal treatment for VIPoma is surgical resection, which is possible in about 50% of patients. In the absence of a visible tumor, some patients have been cured by distal or subtotal pancreatectomy. The pathologic finding in these patients has been pancreatic islet cell hyperplasia. Palliative therapy includes cytotoxic chemotherapy (usually streptozotocin plus fluorouracil), indomethacin, and a somatostatin analogue.

GLUCAGONOMA

Glucagonoma syndrome is characterized by a migratory necrolytic dermatitis (usually involving the legs and perineum), weight loss, stomatitis, hypoaminoacidemia, anemia, and mild diabetes mellitus. Visual scotomas and changes in visual acuity have been reported in some cases. The age range is 20–70 years, and the condition is more common in women. The diagnosis is usually suspected from the distinctive skin lesion; in fact, the presence of a prominent rash in a patient with diabetes mellitus should be enough to raise suspicions. Confirmation of the diagnosis depends on demonstration of elevated serum glucagon levels. It may be possible to demonstrate the tumor by arteriography or CT scanning.

Glucagonomas arise from A_2 cells in the pancreatic islets. About 25% are benign and confined to the pancreas. The remainder have metastasized by the time of diagnosis, most often to the liver, lymph nodes, adrenal glands, or vertebrae. A few cases have been the result of islet cell hyperplasia.

Surgical removal of the primary lesion and metastases is indicated if technically feasible. Even if it is not possible to remove all of the tumor deposits, considerable palliation may result from subtotal removal. Streptozocin, decarbazine, and somatostatin analogues are effective palliative agents for unresectable lesions. The clinical course generally parallels changes in serum levels of glucagon in response to therapy.

SOMATOSTATINOMA

Somatostatinomas are rare tumors characterized by diabetes mellitus (usually mild), diarrhea and malabsorption, and dilatation of the gallbladder (usually with cholelithiasis). High levels of calcitonin and IgM have been present in the serum in some patients. The syndrome results from secretion of somatostatin by an islet cell tumor of the pancreas, which in most cases is malignant and accompanied by hepatic metastases. The diagnosis may be made by recognizing the clinical syndrome and measuring increased concentrations of somatostatin in the serum. In most cases, however, the somatostatin syndrome has been unsuspected until histologic evidence of metastatic islet cell carcinoma has been obtained. Surgery is indicated if the disease is localized. More often, chemotherapy with streptozocin, dacarbazine, doxorubicin, etc, is the only treatment possible.

PANCREATIC POLYPEPTIDE-PRODUCING TUMORS (PPomas)

A few tumors of the pancreas have been found to produce pancreatic polypeptide (PP). Since PP produces few (if any) symptoms, the clinical manifestations in patients with PPomas have been chiefly due to direct effects of the tumor (eg, abdominal pain, weight loss). The tumor is malignant in 50% of cases. Treatment consists of tumor resection.

CARCINOID TUMORS & CARCINOID SYNDROME

Carcinoid tumors arise from enterochromaffin cells. They are often multiple and may appear anywhere in the gut from the gastroesophageal junction to the anus. In general, carcinoid tumors less than 1 cm in diameter are benign, and those greater than 1 cm in diameter are malignant. In the gastrointestinal tract, their propensity for malignant change depends upon their location. For example, fewer than 10% of the appendiceal or rectal carcinoids are malignant, whereas 30% of ileal and 60% of colonic (excluding rectal) carcinoids are malignant. Carcinoid tumors may also occur in the bronchi or ovaries. Local resection is adequate treatment for benign lesions, and wide excision including the lymphatic drainage is recommended for malignant ones.

Because carcinoids in different locations behave dif-

ferently and probably have different secretory products, it is appropriate to categorize them as foregut (bronchus and stomach), midgut (small intestine and colon), or hindgut (rectum) tumors. Hindgut carcinoids synthesize no specific by-products, and they do not stain with silver salts (ie, they are argentaffin- and argyrophil-negative). Foregut carcinoids secrete 5-hydroxytryptophan and are argentaffin-negative and argyrophil-positive. Midgut tumors secrete 5-hydroxytryptamine and are both argentaffin- and argyrophil-positive.

Carcinoid syndrome is caused by release of 5-hydroxytryptamine (serotonin) and other substances from enterochromaffin tumors. The syndrome is also occasionally caused by other tumors, such as oat cell carcinoma and medullary carcinoma of the thyroid. Because the humoral substances liberated by carcinoids are deactivated during one passage through the liver, the presence of the syndrome implies either a primary lesion draining into the systemic circulation or hepatic metastasis from a gastrointestinal lesion.

The tumors responsible for the syndrome arise in the ileum (45%), bronchus (30%), ovary (10%), stomach (5%), and other sites rarely. Fortunately, only 1% of patients with a gastrointestinal carcinoid manifest the carcinoid syndrome.

Etiology

The symptoms of carcinoid syndrome are probably caused by more than one substance, though serotonin is the most firmly established one. Carcinoid tumors contain large amounts of serotonin, and serum levels are markedly elevated in patients with this syndrome. When given intravenously, serotonin produces diarrhea and hypotension but not flushing, which is more likely caused by substance P–related peptides (the tachykinins) or perhaps prostaglandins or dopamine. The evidence is as yet inconclusive.

Clinical Findings

The most common symptoms are flushing of the head and neck and diarrhea. The flushing attacks last a few minutes and may be accompanied by hypotension. The attacks may be provoked by emotional stress, ingestion of particular foods, straining at stool, etc. Diarrhea is often severe and may be debilitating. Both flushing and diarrhea occur in the majority of patients. About 35% of patients develop endocardial fibrosis of the tricuspid and pulmonary valves. Retroperitoneal fibrosis, arthritis, and bronchial asthma also occur but less frequently.

Diagnosis

The most useful diagnostic test for carcinoid tumors is measurement of urinary 5-hydroxyindoleacetic acid (5-HIAA), a breakdown product of serotonin. Measurement of serotonin, histamine, prostaglandin, and bradykinin levels in blood may also be of use, but these tests are difficult to perform and are not available in most laboratories.

Once the diagnosis is established, it is important to localize the tumor. If it is outside the gastrointestinal tract, it may be benign. If the syndrome is secondary to a gastrointestinal carcinoid, 60% of patients have a tumor of the ileum or jejunum with metastases to the liver. Small bowel contrast studies and arteriography help to localize these tumors.

Treatment

A. Operative Treatment: Even though systemic symptoms usually imply the presence of hepatic metastases and an incurable lesion, patients with carcinoid syndrome should be surgically explored to confirm that a gastrointestinal carcinoid is the cause of the syndrome. To prevent future bleeding and bowel obstruction, all primary tumor that can be resected safely should be removed. In selected cases, hepatic metastases may be treated by a limited hepatic resection (ie, lobectomy), which may reduce symptoms and occasionally may cure the disease.

B. Symptomatic Measures: Pharmacologic treatment should be aimed at minimizing diarrhea and flushing. Diarrhea can often be controlled by diphenoxylate with atropine (Lomotil), paregoric, or codeine. Specific antiserotonin agents such as methysergide and cyproheptadine are also used, but flushing is usually not meliorated by these drugs. Phenoxybenzamine (Dibenzyline) (an alpha-adrenergic blocker), glucocorticoids, methyldopa (a decarboxylase inhibitor), and phenothiazines have all been used with some success to control flushing. Treatment with a long-acting analogue of somatostatin (octreotide) results in successful long-term palliation of symptoms in about 80% of patients. Additionally, somatostatin reverses the life-threatening hypotension seen in carcinoid crisis.

C. Antitumor Chemotherapy: Because these tumors are slow-growing and may produce minimal symptoms, cytotoxic drugs are not given for early disease that is minimally symptomatic. Remissions can be achieved in about 20–70% of patients by use of cancer chemotherapeutic agents. The most successful regimen consists of streptozocin plus fluorouracil. Other agents with potential antitumor activity include doxorubicin, dacarbazine, and interferon. Hepatic artery chemoembolization has produced long-lasting palliation in a few patients.

Prognosis

The 5-year survival rate for patients with metastases is 20%. However, the cure rate for surgical resection of localized disease is good. If only regional nodes are involved, the 5-year survival rate is 65%; if the tumor is locally invasive without lymph node involvement, the 5-year survival rate is 95%. The 5-year survival rates associated with different tumor sites are 99% for appendix, 87% for lung, 50% for small intestine and colon, and 83% for rectum and rectosigmoid.

MISCELLANEOUS GASTROINTESTINAL TUMORS

Other islet cell tumors have been reported that produce neurotensin, CCK, vasopressin, a GH-releasing factor, ACTH, and MSH.

REFERENCES

General

Bishop AE et al: Peptidergic nerves. *Scand J Gastroenterol* 1982;**17(Suppl 71):**43.

Buchanan KD: Gastrointestinal hormones: General concepts. *Clin Endocrinol Metab* 1979;**8:**249.

Furness JB et al: Detection and characterisation of neurotransmitters, particularly peptides, in the gastrointestinal tract. *Scand J Gastroenterol* 1982;**17(Suppl 71):**61.

Gershon MD, Erde SM: The nervous system of the gut. *Gastroenterology* 1981;**80:**1571.

Krieger D: Brain peptides: What, where and why? *Science* 1983;**222:**975.

Larsson LI: Pathology of gastrointestinal endocrine cells. *Scand J Gastroenterol* 1979;**14(Suppl 53):**1.

Polak JM, Bloom SR: Regulatory peptides: Key factors in the control of bodily function. *Br Med J* 1983;**286:**1461.

Solcia E et al: The diffuse endocrine-paracrine system of the gut in health and disease: Ultrastructural features. *Scand J Gatroenterol* 1981;**16(Suppl 70):**11.

Strauss E: Radioimmunoassay of gastrointestinal hormones. *Gastroenterology* 1978;**74:**141.

Sundler F et al: Peptidergic nervous systems in the gut. *Clin Gastroenterol* 1980;**9:**517.

Thompson J, Marx M: Gastrointestinal hormones. *Curr Probl Surg* 1984;**12:**1.

Walsh JH: Gastrointestinal hormones. In: *Physiology of the Gastrointestinal Tract,* 2nd ed. Johnson LR et al (editors). Raven Press, 1987.

Weinbeck M, Erckenbrecht J: The control of gastrointestinal motility in GI hormones. *Clin Gastroenterol* 1982;**11:**523.

Welbourn RB et al: Tumors of the neuroendocrine system (APUD cell tumors—apudomas). *Curr Probl Surg* 1984;**11:**1.

Gastrin

Chew CS, Hersey S: Gastrin stimulation of isolated gastric glands. *Am J Physiol* 1982;**242:**G504.

Mulholland MW, Debas HT: Physiology and pathophysiology of gastrin: A review. *Surgery* 1988;**103:**135.

Soll A et al: Gastrin receptors on isolated canine parietal cells. *J Clin Invest* 1984;**73:**1434.

Sygano K, Aponte GW, Yamada T: Identification and

characterization of glycine-extended posttranslational processing intermediates of progastrin in porcine stomach. *J Biol Chem* 1985;**260**:11724.

Wiborg O et al: Structure of a human gastrin gene. *Proc Natl Acad Sci USA* 1984;**81**:1067.

Cholecystokinin

Anika SM et al: Cholecystokinin and satiety in pigs. *Am J Physiol* 1981;**240**:310.

Calam J, Ellis A, Dockray GJ: Identification and measurement of molecular variants of cholecystokinin in duodenal mucosa and plasma. *J Clin Invest* 1982;**169**:218.

Deschenes RJ et al: Cloning and sequence analysis of a cDNA encoding rat preprocholecystokinin. *Proc Natl Acad Sci USA* 1984;**81**:726.

Dockray GJ: The physiology of cholecystokinin. *Brain Gut* 1982;**38**:253.

Gosnell B, Hsiao S: Cholecystokinin satiety and orosensory feedback. *Physiol Behav* 1981;**27**:153.

Wiener I et al: Release of cholecystokinin in man: Correlation of blood levels with gallbladder function. *Ann Surg* 1981;**194**:321.

Secretin

Gyr K et al: Plasma secretin and pancreatic response to various stimulants including a meal. *Am J Physiol* 1984;**246**:G535.

Hacki WH: Secretin. *Clin Gastroenterol* 1980;**9**:609.

Kleibeuker J et al: Role of endogenous secretin on acid-induced inhibition of human gastrin function. *J Clin Invest* 1984;**73**:526.

Mutt V, Jorpes J, Magnusson S: Structure of porcine secretin: The amino acid sequence. *Eur J Biochem* 1970;**15**:513.

Gastric Inhibitory Polypeptide

Brown JC: Gastric inhibitory polypeptide. *Monogr Endocrinol* 1982;**24**:1.

Cataland S: Physiology of GIP in man. In: *Gut Hormones,* 2nd ed. Bloom SR (editor). Churchill Livingstone, 1981.

Sarson D, Hayter R, Blood S: The pharmacokinetics of porcine glucose-dependent insulinotropic polypeptide (GIP) in man. *Eur J Clin Invest* 1982;**12**:457.

Vasoactive Intestinal Polypeptide

Biancani P, Walsh J, Behar J: Vasoactive intestinal polypeptide: A neurotransmitter for esophageal sphincter relaxation. *J Clin Invest* 1984;**73**:963.

Fahrenkrug J: Vasoactive intestinal polypeptide: Functional aspects. *Br Med Bull* 1982;**38**:265.

Itoh N et al: Human preprovasoactive intestinal polypeptide contains a novel PHI-27-like peptide, PHM-27. *Nature* 1983;**304**:547.

Krejs G et al: Effect of VIP infusion in water and ion transport in the human jejunum. *Gastroenterology* 1980;**78**:722.

Said SI: Vasoactive intestinal polypeptide (VIP): Current status. *Peptides* 1984;**5**:145.

Substance P

Couture R, Regori D: Mini review: Smooth muscle pharmacology of substance P. *Pharmacology* 1982; **24**:1.

Nawa H et al: Nucleotide sequences of cloned cDNAs for two types of bovine brain substance P precursor. *Nature* 1983;**306**:32.

Pearse AGE, Polak JM: Immunocytochemical localization of substance P in mammalian intestine. *Histochemistry* 1975;**41**:373.

Reynolds J, Ouyang A, Cohen S: A lower esophageal sphincter reflex involving substance P. *Am J Physiol* 1984;**246**:G346.

Enkephalins

Ambinder RF, Schuster MM: Endorphins: New gut peptides with a familiar face. *Gastroenterology* 1979; **77**:1132.

Nakanishi S et al: Nucleotide sequence of cloned cDNA for bovine corticotropin-β-lipotropin precursor. *Nature* 1979;**278**:423.

Polak J et al: Enkephalin-like immunoreactivity in the human gastrointestinal tract. *Lancet* 1972;**1**:972.

Neurotensin

Brown DR, Miller RJ: Neurotensin. *Br Med Bull* 1982;**38**:239.

Miller RJ: Neurotensin as a gastrointestinal hormone. *Med Biol* 1981;**59**:65.

Motilin

Adachi H et al: Mechanism of the excitatory action of motilin on isolated rabbit intestine. *Gastroenterology* 1981;**80**:783.

Fox JE: Motilin: An update. *Life Sci* 1984;**35**:695.

Poitros P et al: Motilin-independent ectopic fronts of the interdigestive myoelectric complex in dogs. *Am J Physiol* 1980;**239**:215.

Somatostatin

Armiuro A et al: Somatostatin: Abundance of immunoreactive hormone in rat stomach and pancreas. *Science* 1975;**189**:1007.

Reichlin S: Somatostatin. (2 parts.) *N Engl J Med* 1983;**309**:1495, 1556.

Shen LP, Rutter WJ: Sequence of the human somatostatin I gene. *Science* 1984;**224**:168.

Toro MJ et al: Mechanism of action of somatostatin. *Horm Res* 1988;**29**:59.

Peptide YY

Adrian TE et al: Human distribution and release of a putative new gut hormone, peptide YY. *Gastroenterology* 1985;**89**:1070.

Tatemoto K: Isolation and characterization of peptide YY (PYY), a candidate gut hormone that inhibits pancreatic exocrine secretion. *Proc Natl Acad Sci USA* 1982;**79**:2514.

Bombesin & Gastrin-Releasing Peptide

Erspamer V et al: Occurrence and polymorphism of bombesin-like peptides in the gastrointestinal tract of birds and mammals. *Gut* 1979;**20**:1047.

Inoue K et al: Effect of gastrin-releasing peptide on the release of gastrointestinal hormones in dogs. *Physiologist* 1982;**25**:218.

McDonald T et al: Characterization of a gastrin-releasing peptide from porcine non-antral gastric tissue. *Biochem Biophys Res Commun* 1979;**90**:227.

McDonald T et al: A qualitative comparison of canine

plasma gastroenterohepatic hormone response to bombesin and the porcine gastrin-releasing peptide (GRP). *Regul Pept* 1981;**2:**293.

Spindel ER et al: Cloning and characterization of cDNAs encoding human gastrin-releasing peptide. *Proc Natl Acad Sci USA* 1984;**81:**5699.

Walsh JH et al: Bombesin-like peptides in mammals. *Fed Proc* 1979;**38:**2315.

Pancreatic Polypeptide

Adrian TE et al: Inhibition of secretin-stimulated pancreatic secretion by pancreatic polypeptide. *Gut* 1979;**20:**37.

Lonovics J et al: Pancreatic polypeptide: A review. *Arch Surg* 1981;**116:**1256.

Takeuchi T, Yamada T: Isolation of a cDNA clone encoding pancreatic polypeptide. *Proc Natl Acad Sci USA* 1985;**82:**1536.

Taylor IL et al: Pancreatic polypeptide metabolism and effect on pancreatic secretion in dogs. *Gastroenterology* 1979;**76:**524.

Enteroglucagon

Holst JJ: Gut glucagon, enteroglucagon, gut glucagonlike immunoreactivity, glicentin: Current status. *Gastroenterology* 1983;**84:**1602.

Lund PK et al: Pancreatic preproglucagon cDNA contains two glucagon-related coding sequences arranged in tandem. *Proc Natl Acad Sci USA* 1982;**79:**345.

Hormonal Abnormalities in Diseases of the Gastrointestinal Tract

Besterman HS et al: Gut hormone profile in coeliac disease. *Lancet* 1978;**1:**785.

Chajvialle JAP et al: Somatostatin in mucosa of stomach and duodenum in gastroduodenal disease. *Gastroenterology* 1978;**75:**13.

Debas HT: Clinical significance of gastrointestinal hormones. *Adv Surg* 1987;**21:**157.

Mulvihill S et al: The use of somatostatin and its analogs in the treatment of surgical disorders. *Surgery* 1986; **100:**467.

Taylor IL: Gastrointestinal hormones in the pathogenesis of peptic ulcer disease. *Clin Gastroenterol* 1984;**13:**355.

Zollinger-Ellison Syndrome

Ellison EC et al: Observations on the effect of a somatostatin analog in the Zollinger-Ellison syndrome: Implications for the treatment of apudomas. *Surgery* 1986;**100:**437.

Lamers CB et al: Omeprazole in Zollinger-Ellison syndrome: Effects of a single dose and of long-term treatment in patients resistant to histamine H_2-receptor antagonists. *N Engl J Med* 1984;**310:**758.

Maton PN et al: Medical management of patients with Zollinger-Ellison syndrome who have had previous gastric surgery: A prospective study. *Gastroenterology* 1988;**94:**294.

Norton JA et al: Aggressive resection of metastatic disease in selected patients with malignant gastrinoma. *Ann Surg* 1986;**203:**352.

Wolfe MM, Jensen RT: Zollinger-Ellison syndrome: Current concepts in diagnosis and management. *N Engl J Med* 1987;**317:**1200.

Zollinger RM: Gastrinoma: Factors influencing prognosis. *Surgery* 1985;**97:**49.

Pancreatic Cholera

Field M, Chang E: Pancreatic cholera: Is the diarrhea due to VIP? *N Engl J Med* 1983;**309:**1513.

Kahn CR et al: Pancreatic cholera: Beneficial effects of treatment with streptozotocin. *N Engl J Med* 1975; **292:**941.

Kane M, O'Dorisio T, Krejs G: Production of secretory diarrhea by intravenous infusion of vasoactive intestinal polypeptide. *N Engl J Med* 1983;**309:**1482.

Krejs GJ: VIPoma syndrome. *Am J Med* 1987;**82(Suppl 5B):**37.

Krejs GJ et al: Effect of VIP infusion on water and ion transport in the human jejunum. *Gastroenterology* 1980;**78:**722.

Mekhjian HS, O'Dorisio TM: VIPoma syndrome. *Semin Oncol* 1987;**14:**282.

Rood RP et al: Pancreatic cholera syndrome due to a vasoactive intestinal polypeptide-producing tumor: Further insights into the pathophysiology. *Gastroenterology* 1988;**94:**813.

Yamaguchi K et al: The WDHA syndrome: Clinical and laboratory data on 28 Japanese cases. *Peptides* 1984;**5:**415.

Glucagonoma

Bloom SR, Polak JM: Glucagonoma syndrome. *Am J Med* 1987;**82(Suppl 5B):**25.

Cavallo-Perin P et al: A combined glucagonoma and VIPoma syndrome: First pathologic and clinical report. *Cancer* 1988;**62:**2576.

Leichter SB: Clinical and metabolic aspects of glucagonoma. *Medicine* 1980;**59:**100.

Prinz RA et al: Operative and chemotherapeutic management of malignant glucagon-producing tumors. *Surgery* 1981;**90:**713.

Stacpoole PW: The glucagonoma syndrome: Clinical features, diagnosis, and treatment. *Endocr Rev* 1981; **76:**125.

Pancreatic Polypeptide-Producing Tumors (PPomas)

Strodel WE et al: Pancreatic polypeptide-producing tumors: Silent lesions of the pancreas? *Arch Surg* 1984;**119:**508.

Somatostatinoma

Axelrod L et al: Malignant somatostatinoma: Clinical features and metabolic studies. *J Clin Endocrinol Metab* 1981;**52:**886.

Harris GJ, Tio F, Cruz AB Jr: Somatostatinoma: A case report and review of the literature. *J Surg Oncol* 1987;**36:**8.

Krejs GJ et al: Somatostatinoma syndrome: Biochemical, morphologic and clinical features. *N Engl J Med* 1979;**301:**285.

Vinik AI et al: Somatostatinomas, PPomas, neurotensinomas. *Semin Oncol* 1987;**14:**263.

Carcinoid Tumors & Carcinoid Syndrome

Codd JE, Drozda J, Merjavy J: Palliation of carcinoid heart disease. *Arch Surg* 1987;**122:**1076.

Hodgson HJ: Controlling the carcinoid syndrome. *Br Med J* 1988;**297**:1213.

Kvols LK et al: Treatment of the malignant carcinoid syndrome: Evaluation of a long-acting somatostatin analogue. *N Engl J Med* 1986;**315**:663.

Maton, PN: The carcinoid syndrome. *JAMA* 1988; **260**:1602.

Norheim I et al: Malignant carcinoid tumors: An analysis of 103 patients with regard to tumor localization, hormone production, and survival. *Ann Surg* 1986;**206**:115.

Oberg K, Funa K, Alm G: Effects of leukocyte interferon on clinical symptoms and hormone levels in patients with mid-gut carcinoid tumors and carcinoid syndrome. *N Engl J Med* 1983;**309**:129.

Thompson GB et al: Carcinoid tumors of the gastrointestinal tract: Presentation, management, and prognosis. *Surgery* 1985;**98**:1054.

22

Pancreatic Hormones & Diabetes Mellitus

John H. Karam, MD, Patricia R. Salber, MD, & Peter H. Forsham, MD

I. THE ENDOCRINE PANCREAS

The pancreas is made up of 2 functionally different organs: the **exocrine pancreas,** the major digestive gland of the body; and the **endocrine pancreas,** the source of insulin, glucagon, somatostatin, and pancreatic polypeptide. Whereas the major role of the products of the exocrine pancreas (the digestive enzymes) is the processing of ingested foodstuffs so that they become available for absorption, the hormones of the endocrine pancreas modulate every other aspect of cellular nutrition from rate of adsorption of foodstuffs to cellular storage or metabolism of nutrients. Dysfunction of the endocrine pancreas or abnormal responses to its hormones by target tissues result in serious disturbances in nutrient homeostasis, including the important clinical syndromes grouped under the name of **diabetes mellitus.**

ANATOMY & HISTOLOGY

The endocrine pancreas consists of hundreds of thousands of small endocrine glands—the islets of Langerhans—scattered within the glandular substance of the exocrine pancreas. The islet volume comprises about 2–3% of the total mass of the pancreas and weighs about 1–2 g in adult humans.

At least 4 cell types—A, B, D, and F—have been identified in the islets (Table 22–1). These cell types are not distributed uniformly throughout the pancreas. The F cell, which secretes pancreatic polypeptide (PP), has been found primarily in islets in the posterior portion (posterior lobe) of the head, a discrete lobe of the pancreas separated from the anterior portion by a fascial partition. This lobe originates in the primordial ventral bud as opposed to the dorsal bud. The posterior lobe receives its blood supply from the superior mes-

Acronyms Used in This Chapter	
ADA	American Diabetes Association
ADH	Antidiuretic hormone (vasopressin)
ADP	Adenosine diphosphate
ATP	Adenosine triphosphate
cAMP	Cyclic adenosine monophosphate
CCK	Cholecystokinin
cGMP	Cyclic guanosine monophosphate
DNA	Deoxyribonucleic acid
FDA	Food and Drug Administration
GH	Growth hormone
GI	Glycemic index
GIP	Gastric inhibitory polypeptide
GLP-1	Glucagonlike peptide 1
GLP-2	Glucagonlike peptide 2
HDL	High-density lipoprotein(s)
5-HIAA	5-Hydroxyindoleacetic acid
HLA	Human leukocyte antigen
IDDM	Insulin-dependent diabetes mellitus
MODY	Maturity-onset diabetes of the young
NIDDM	Non–insulin-dependent diabetes mellitus
NPH	Neutral protamine Hagedorn
PP	Pancreatic polypeptide
PZI	Protamine zinc insulin
RNA	Ribonucleic acid
UGDP	University Group Diabetes Program
VLDL	Very low density lipoprotein(s)

enteric artery; the remainder of the pancreas derives most of its blood flow from the celiac artery.

Islets in the posterior lobe area consist of 80–85% F cells, 15–20% B cells, and less than 0.5% glucagon-producing A cells. The pancreatic polypeptide cell volume varies with age and sex—the volume tends to be larger in men and in older persons. In contrast to the posterior lobe, the PP-poor islets located in the tail, body, and *anterior* portion of the head of the pancreas, arising from the embryonic dorsal bud, contain predominantly insulin-secreting B cells (70–80% of the islet cells), with approximately 20% of the cells being

Table 22–1. Cell types in pancreatic islets of Langerhans.

Cell Types	Approximate % of Islet Volume		Secretory Products
	Dorsally Derived (anterior head, body, tail)	**Ventrally Derived (posterior portion of head)**	
A cell (α)	20%	<0.5%	Glucagon, proglucagon, glucagon-like peptides (GLP-1 and GLP-2)
B cell (β)	70–80%	15–20%	Insulin, C peptide, proinsulin
D cell (δ)	3–5%	<1%	Somatostatin
F cell (PP cell)	<2%	80–85%	Pancreatic polypeptide

glucagon-secreting A cells and about 3–5% D cells that produce somatostatin. A typical islet from this part of the pancreas is depicted in Figure 22–1.

Islet Vascularization

The islets are richly vascularized, receiving 5–10 times the blood flow of a comparable portion of exocrine pancreatic tissues. The direction of the blood flow within the islet has been postulated to play a role in carrying insulin secreted from the central region of an islet to its peripheral zone, where the insulin modulates and decreases glucagon release from A cells, which are mainly located in the periphery of islets.

HORMONES OF THE ENDOCRINE PANCREAS

1. INSULIN

Biosynthesis

The human insulin gene is located on the short arm of chromosome 11. A precursor molecule, **preproinsulin,** a long-chain peptide of MW 11,500, is produced by DNA/RNA-directed synthesis in the rough endoplasmic reticulum of pancreatic B cells (Fig 22–2). It is cleaved by microsomal enzymes to **proinsulin** (MW about 9000) almost immediately after synthesis. Proin-

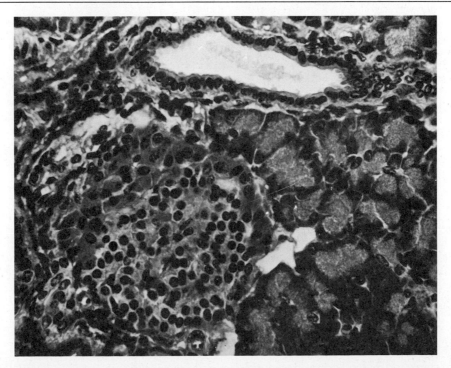

Figure 22–1. Photomicrograph of a section of the pancreas. In the islet of Langerhans, A cells appear mainly in the periphery as large cells with dark cytoplasm. Some D cells are also present in the periphery, while the central core is composed chiefly of B cells. (Reproduced, with permission, from Junqueira LC, Carneiro J, Long JA: *Basic Histology,* 5th ed. Lange, 1986.)

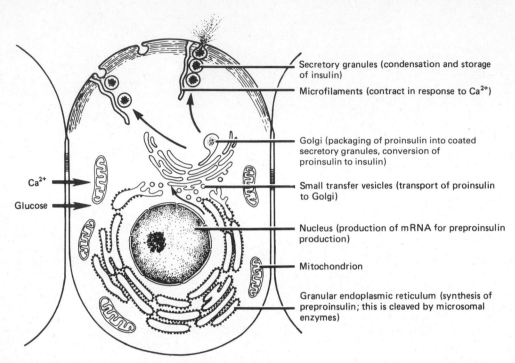

Figure 22–2. Structural components of the pancreatic B cell involved in glucose-induced biosynthesis and release. Schematic representation of secretory granular alignment on microfilament "tracks" that contract in response to calcium. (Based on data presented by Orci L: A portrait of the pancreatic B cell. *Diabetologia* 1974;**10**:163.) (Modified and reproduced, with permission, from Junqueira LC, Carneiro J, Long JA: *Basic Histology*, 5th ed. Lange, 1986.)

sulin (Fig 22–3) is transported to the Golgi apparatus, where packaging into clathrin-coated secretory granules takes place. Maturation of the secretory granule is associated with loss of the clathrin coating and conversion of proinsulin into **insulin** and a smaller connecting peptide, or **C peptide,** by proteolytic cleavage at 2 sites along the peptide chain. Normal mature (uncoated) secretory granules contain insulin and C peptide in equimolar amounts and only small quantities of proinsulin, a small portion of which consists of partially cleaved intermediates.

Biochemistry

Proinsulin (Fig 22–3) consists of a single chain of 86 amino acids, which includes the A and B chains of the insulin molecule plus a connecting segment of 35 amino acids. Converting enzymes (probably trypsin-like and carboxypeptidase-B–like proteases) cleave off 2 pairs of dibasic amino acids (3 arginines and one lysine) from the proinsulin molecule as shown in Figure 22–3. The result is a 51-amino-acid insulin molecule and a 31-amino-acid residue, the C peptide.

A small amount of proinsulin produced by the pancreas escapes cleavage and is secreted intact into the bloodstream, along with insulin and C peptide. Most anti-insulin sera used in the standard immunoassay for

insulin cross-react with proinsulin; about 3–5% of immunoreactive insulin extracted from human pancreas is actually proinsulin. Because proinsulin is not removed by the liver, it has a half-life 3–4 times that of insulin. This allows proinsulin to accumulate in the blood, where it accounts for 12–20% of the circulating immunoreactive "insulin" in the basal state in humans. Human proinsulin has about 7–8% of the biologic activity of insulin. The kidney is the principal site of proinsulin degradation.

Partially cleaved proinsulin molecules probably do not gain access to the bloodstream in significant quantity. However, families with such abnormal circulating insulins have been described.

C peptide, the 31-amino-acid residue (MW 3000) formed during cleavage of insulin from proinsulin, has no known biologic activity. It is released from the B cells in equimolar amounts with insulin. It is not removed by the liver but is degraded or excreted chiefly by the kidney. It has a half-life 3–4 times that of insulin. In the basal state after an overnight fast, the average concentration of C peptide may be as high as 1000 pmol/L.

Insulin is a protein consisting of 51 amino acids contained within 2 peptide chains: an A chain, with 21 amino acids; and a B chain, with 30 amino acids. The chains are connected by 2 disulfide bridges as shown in

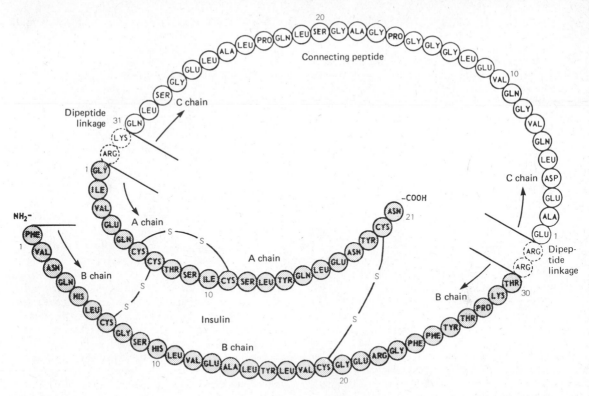

Figure 22–3. Structure of human proinsulin C peptides and insulin molecules connected at 2 sites by dipeptide links.

Figure 22–3. In addition, there is an intrachain disulfide bridge that links positions 6 and 11 in the A chain. The molecular weight of human insulin is 5808.

Human insulin differs only slightly in amino acid composition from the 2 mammalian insulins presently used for therapeutic insulin replacement. Pork insulin differs from human by only one amino acid—alanine instead of threonine at the carboxyl terminus of the B chain (position B 30). Beef insulin differs by 3 amino acids—alanine instead of threonine at A 8 as well as the B 30 position and valine instead of isoleucine at A 10.

Endogenous insulin has a circulatory half-life of 3–5 minutes. It is catabolized chiefly by insulinases in liver, kidney, and placenta. Approximately 50% of insulin is removed in a single pass through the liver.

Secretion

The human pancreas secretes about 40–50 units of insulin per day in normal adults. The basal concentration of insulin in the blood of fasting humans averages 10 μU/mL (0.4 ng/mL, or 69 pmol/L). In normal control subjects, insulin seldom rises above 100 μU/mL (690 pmol/L) after standard meals. There is an increase in peripheral insulin concentration beginning 8–10 minutes after ingestion of food and reaching peak concentration in peripheral blood by 30–45 minutes. This is followed by a rapid decline in postprandial plasma glucose concentration, which returns to baseline values by 90–120 minutes (Fig 22–4).

Basal insulin secretion, which occurs in the absence of exogenous stimuli, is the quantity of insulin secreted in the fasting state. Although it is known that plasma glucose levels below 80–100 mg/dL (4.4–5.6 mmol/L) do not stimulate insulin release, it has also

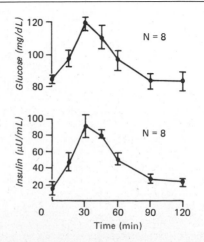

Figure 22–4. Plasma glucose and insulin response to a standard 530-kcal breakfast in normal subjects.

been demonstrated that the presence of glucose is necessary (in in vitro systems) for most other known regulators of insulin secretion to be effective.

Stimulated insulin secretion is that which occurs in response to exogenous stimuli. In vivo, this is the response of the B cell to ingested meals. Glucose is the most potent stimulant of insulin release. The exact mechanism of action of glucose on the B cell remains to be clarified. The perfused rat pancreas has demonstrated a biphasic release of insulin in response to glucose (Fig 22–5). When the glucose concentration in the system is increased suddenly, an initial short-lived burst of insulin release occurs (the **early phase**); if the glucose concentration is held at this level, the insulin release gradually falls off and then begins to rise again to a steady level (the **late phase**). However, sustained levels of high glucose stimulation (4 hr or more in vitro or > 24 hr in vivo) results in a reversible desensitization of the B cell response to glucose but not to other stimuli.

Currently, the mechanism of action of glucose-stimulated insulin release is not well understood. There is evidence that glucose may act through a membrane-bound glucose receptor; however, despite extensive research in this area, no such glucose receptor has been identified on the B cell. There is a greater body of data suggesting that *metabolism* of glucose is essential in stimulating insulin release. Indeed, agents such as 2-deoxyglucose that inhibit the metabolism of glucose interfere with release of insulin.

Insulin release has been shown to require calcium. It has been proposed that mature insulin-containing granules in the B cell attach linearly to microtubules that contract after exposure to high intracellular calcium, thereby ejecting the granules (Fig 22–2). The following effects of glucose on calcium ion movement have been demonstrated: (1) Calcium uptake is increased by glucose stimulation of the B cell. (2) Calcium efflux from the cell is retarded by some action of glucose. (3) Mobilization of calcium from mitochondrial compartments occurs secondary to cAMP induction by glucose.

cAMP is another important modulator of insulin release. As mentioned above, glucose has been shown to directly induce cAMP formation. Furthermore, many nonglucose stimuli to insulin release are known to increase intracellular cAMP. Elevations of cAMP, however, will not stimulate insulin release in the absence of glucose.

Other factors involved in the regulation of insulin secretion are summarized in Table 22–2. These factors can be divided into 3 categories: **direct stimulants,** which are known to stimulate insulin release directly; **amplifiers,** which appear to potentiate the response of the B cell to glucose; and **inhibitors.** The action of the amplifier substances, many of which are gastrointestinal hormones stimulated by ingestion of meals, explains the observation that insulin response to an ingested meal is greater than the response of intravenously administered substrates.

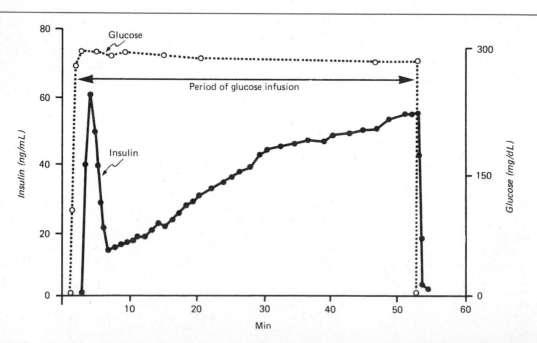

Figure 22–5. Multiphasic response of the in vitro perfused pancreas during constant stimulation with glucose. (Modified from Grodsky GM et al: Further studies on the dynamic aspects of insulin release in vitro with evidence for a 2-compartmental storage system. *Acta Diabetol Lat* 1969;**6[Suppl 1]:**554.)

Table 22–2. Regulation of insulin release in humans.

Stimulants of insulin release
 Glucose, mannose
 Leucine
 Vagal stimulation
 Sulfonylureas
Amplifiers of glucose-induced insulin release
 1. Enteric hormones:
  Gastrin inhibitory polypeptide
  Cholecystokinin
  Secretin, gastrin
 2. Neural amplifiers: Beta-adrenergic stimulation
 3. Amino acids: Arginine
Inhibitors of insulin release
 Neural: Alpha-adrenergic effect of catecholamines
 Humoral: Somatostatin
 Drugs: Diazoxide, phenytoin, vinblastine, colchicine

Insulin Receptors & Insulin Action

Insulin action begins with binding of insulin to a receptor on the surface of the target cell membrane. Many cells of the body appear to have specific cell surface insulin receptors. In fat, liver, and muscle cells, binding of insulin to these receptors is associated with the biologic response of these tissues to the hormone. These receptors bind insulin rapidly, with high specificity and with an affinity high enough to bind picomolar amounts.

It has recently been demonstrated that insulin receptors are membrane glycoproteins composed of 2 subunits, a larger alpha subunit (molecular weight 130,000), which extends extracellularly and is involved in binding the insulin molecule, and a smaller beta subunit (molecular weight 90,000), which is predominantly cytoplasmic and contains a kinase that becomes activated during insulin binding and results in autophosphorylation of the beta subunit itself. After insulin is bound to its receptor, a number of insulin-receptor complexes are internalized.

Two models for insulin action have been proposed. One involves a cascade of phosphorylations emanating from the activated kinase region that induces an intracellular compartment of proteins, including the glucose transporter, transferrin, the low-density lipoprotein receptor, and the insulinlike growth factor II (IGF-II) receptor, to move to the cell surface. When these proteins, which are sequestered intracellularly during the postabsorptive period, move to the cell surface during feeding they facilitate transport of nutrients into insulin target tissues and can promote growth by giving circulating IGF-II access to a cell surface receptor. Within this model, genetic defects distal to the insulin receptor could result in "postreceptor" insulin resistance. Possible defects include abnormalities in the enzymes responsible for phosphorylation of the glucose transporter protein, mutation of the glucose transporter itself, or abnormalities in its processing. Moreover, abnormalities in phosphatase enzymes might account for a delay in the normal restoration of the insulin receptor to its surface membrane locus, resulting in resistance to the further action of insulin. A second model invokes the hydrolysis of a membrane glycolipid by insulin-stimulated phospholipase C activity. Potential "second messengers" such as inositol monophosphate, glucosamine, or diacylglycerol may mediate the intracellular response to insulin, with diacylglycerol promoting intracellular phosphorylations by activating protein kinase C (see Fig 1–17).

Abnormalities of insulin receptors—in concentration, affinity, or both—will affect insulin action. **"Down-regulation"** is a phenomenon in which the number of insulin receptors is decreased in response to chronically elevated circulating insulin levels, probably by increased intracellular degradation. When insulin levels are low, on the other hand, receptor binding is up-regulated. Conditions associated with high insulin levels and lowered insulin binding to the receptor include obesity, high intake of carbohydrates, and (perhaps) chronic exogenous overinsulinization. Conditions associated with low insulin levels and increased insulin binding include exercise and fasting. The presence of excess amounts of cortisol decreases insulin binding to the receptor, although it is not clear if this is a direct effect of the hormone itself or one that is mediated through accompanying increases in the insulin level.

Metabolic Effects of Insulin

The major function of insulin is to promote **storage of ingested nutrients.** Although insulin directly or indirectly affects the function of almost every tissue in the body, the discussion here will be limited to a brief overview of the effects of insulin on the 3 major tissues specialized for energy storage: liver, muscle, and adipose tissue. In addition, the **paracrine effects** of insulin will be discussed briefly. The section on hormonal control of nutrient metabolism (see below) presents a detailed discussion of the effects of insulin and glucagon on the regulation of intermediary metabolism.

A. Paracrine Effects: The effects of the products of endocrine cells on surrounding cells are termed "paracrine" effects, in contrast to actions that take place at sites distant from the secreting cells, which are termed "endocrine" effects (see Fig 5–1). Paracrine effects of the B and D cells on the close-lying A cells (Fig 22–1) are of considerable importance in the endocrine pancreas. The first target cells reached by insulin are the pancreatic A cells at the periphery of the pancreatic islets. In the presence of insulin, A cell secretion of glucagon is reduced. In addition, somatostatin, which is released from D cells in response to most of the same stimuli that provoke insulin release, also acts to inhibit glucagon secretion.

Because glucose stimulates only B and D cells (whose products then inhibit A cells) whereas amino acids stimulate glucagon as well as insulin, the type and amounts of islet hormones released during a meal depend on the ratio of ingested carbohydrate to protein. The higher the carbohydrate content of a meal, the less glucagon will be released by any amino acids absorbed. In contrast, a predominantly protein meal will result in relatively greater glucagon secretion, because amino acids are less effective at stimulating insulin release in the absence of concurrent hyperglycemia but are potent stimulators of A cells.

B. Endocrine Effects: (Table 22–3.)

1. Liver–The first major organ reached by insulin via the bloodstream is the liver. Insulin exerts its action on the liver in 2 major ways:

a. Insulin promotes anabolism–Insulin promotes glycogen synthesis and storage at the same time it inhibits glycogen breakdown. These effects are mediated by changes in the activity of enzymes in the glycogen synthesis pathway (see below). The liver has a maximum storage capacity of 100–110 g of glycogen, or approximately 440 kcal of energy.

Insulin increases both protein and triglyceride synthesis and VLDL formation by the liver. It also inhibits gluconeogenesis and promotes glycolysis through its effects on enzymes of the glycolytic pathway.

b. Insulin inhibits catabolism–Insulin acts to reverse the catabolic events of the postabsorptive state by inhibiting hepatic glycogenolysis, ketogenesis, and gluconeogenesis.

2. Muscle–Insulin promotes protein synthesis in muscle by increasing amino acid transport as well as by stimulating ribosomal protein synthesis. In addition, insulin promotes glycogen synthesis to replace glycogen stores expended by muscle activity. This is accomplished by increasing glucose transport into the muscle cell, enhancing the activity of glycogen synthetase, and inhibiting the activity of glycogen phos-

phorylase. Approximately 500–600 g of glycogen is stored in the muscle tissue of a 70-kg man, but because of the lack of glucose 6-phosphatase in this tissue, it cannot be used as a source of blood glucose.

3. Adipose tissue–Fat, in the form of triglyceride, is the most efficient means of storing energy. It provides 9 kcal per gram of stored substrate, as opposed to the 4 kcal/g generally provided by protein or carbohydrate. In the typical 70-kg man, the energy content of adipose tissue is about 100,000 kcal.

Insulin acts to promote triglyceride storage in adipocytes by a number of mechanisms: (1) It induces the production of lipoprotein lipase (this is the lipoprotein lipase that is bound to endothelial cells in adipose tissue and other vascular beds), which leads to hydrolysis of triglycerides from circulating lipoproteins. (2) By increasing glucose transport into fat cells, insulin increases the availability of α-glycerol phosphate, a substance used in the esterification of free fatty acids into triglycerides. (3) Insulin inhibits intracellular lipolysis of stored triglyceride by inhibiting intracellular lipase (also called "hormone-sensitive lipoprotein lipase").

2. GLUCAGON

Biochemistry

Pancreatic glucagon, whose gene is located on human chromosome 2, is a single-chain polypeptide consisting of 29 amino acids with a molecular weight of 3485 (Fig 22–6). It is synthesized in the A cells on the islets of Langerhans and derived from a large 160-amino-acid precursor molecule that is 5–6 times larger than glucagon. Within this proglucagon molecule are several other peptides connected in tandem: glicentin-related peptide, glucagon, glucagonlike peptide 1 (GLP-1), and glucagonlike peptide 2 (GLP-2). The combination of glicentin-related peptide with glucagon consists of 69 amino acids and comprises the hormone glicentin, which is predominantly secreted from the intestine and not the pancreas. Both GLP-1 and GLP-2 increase after meals. An endogenous natural

Table 22–3. Endocrine effects of insulin.

Effects on liver
  Anabolic effects:
    Promotes glycogenesis
    Increases synthesis of triglycerides, cholesterol, and VLDL.
    Increases protein synthesis
    Promotes glycolysis.
  Anticatabolic effects:
    Inhibits glycogenolysis.
    Inhibits ketogenesis.
    Inhibits gluconeogenesis.
Effects on muscle
  Promotes protein synthesis:
    Increases amino acid transport.
    Stimulates ribosomal protein synthesis.
  Promotes glycogen synthesis:
    Increases glucose transport.
    Enhances activity of glycogen synthetase.
    Inhibits activity of glycogen phosphorylase.
Effects on fat
  Promotes triglyceride storage:
    Induces lipoprotein lipase, making fatty acids available for absorption into fat cells.
    Increases glucose transport into fat cells, thus increasing availability of α-glycerol phosphate for triglyceride synthesis.
    Inhibits intracellular lipolysis.

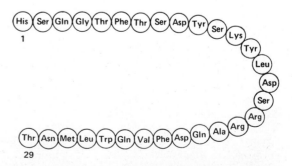

Figure 22–6. Amino acid sequence of glucagon polypeptide. (Reproduced, with permission, from Katzung BG [editor]: *Basic & Clinical Pharmacology,* 4th ed. Appleton & Lange, 1989.)

derivative of GLP-1, with the first 6 of its 37 amino acids absent (GLP-1 [7-37]), is an extremely potent stimulator of pancreatic B cells. It is several times more potent than glucagon itself as an insulinotropic secretagogue, whereas intact GLP-1 (1-37) and GLP-2 do not stimulate insulin secretion. In healthy humans, the average fasting plasma immunoreactive glucagon level is 75 pg/mL (25 pmol/L). Only 30–40% of this is actually pancreatic glucagon, the remainder being a heterogeneous composite of larger molecular-weight molecules with glucagon immunoreactivity such as proglucagon, glicentin, GLP-1, and GLP-2. The circulation half-life of pancreatic glucagon is 3–6 minutes. Glucagon is mainly removed by the liver and kidney.

Secretion

Glucagon secretion is inhibited by glucose—in contrast to the effect of glucose on insulin secretion. There are conflicting data about whether the effect of glucose is a direct one on the A cell or whether it is mediated via release of insulin or somatostatin, both of which are known to inhibit the A cell directly (see above).

Many amino acids stimulate glucagon release, although there are differences in their ability to do so. Some, such as arginine, release both glucagon and insulin; others (eg, alanine) stimulate primarily glucagon release. Leucine, a good stimulant for insulin release, does not stimulate glucagon. Other substances that promote glucagon release are catecholamines, the gastrointestinal hormones (cholecystokinin [CCK], gastrin, and gastric inhibitory polypeptide [GIP]), and glucocorticoids. Both sympathetic and parasympathetic (vagal) stimulation promote glucagon release; this is especially important in augmenting the response of the A cell to hypoglycemia. High levels of circulating fatty acid are associated with suppression of glucagon secretion.

Action of Glucagon

In contrast to insulin, which promotes energy storage in a variety of tissues, glucagon is a humoral mechanism for making energy available to the tissues between meals, when ingested food is not available for absorption. Glucagon stimulates the breakdown of stored glycogen, maintains hepatic output of glucose from amino acid precursors (gluconeogenesis), and promotes hepatic output of ketone bodies from fatty acid precursors (ketogenesis). The liver, because of its geographic proximity to the pancreas, represents the major target organ for glucagon, with portal vein glucagon concentrations reaching as high as 300–500 pg/mL (100–166 pmol/L). Binding of glucagon to its receptor on hepatocytes results in activation of adenylate cyclase and generation of cAMP, which both promotes glycogenolysis and stimulates gluconeogenesis. Uptake of alanine by liver cells is facilitated by glucagon, and fatty acids are directed away from re-esterification to triglycerides and toward ketogenic pathways (see below). It is unclear whether physiologic levels of glucagon affect tissues other than the liver.

3. SOMATOSTATIN

The gene for somatostatin is on the long arm of chromosome 3. It codes for a 116-amino-acid peptide, preprosomatostatin, from whose carboxyl terminus is cleaved the hormone somatostatin, a 14-amino-acid cyclic polypeptide with a molecular weight of 1640 (Fig 22–7). It is present in D cells at the periphery of the human islet (Fig 22–1). It was first identified in the hypothalamus and owes its name to its ability to inhibit release of growth hormone (pituitary somatotropin). Since that time, somatostatin has been identified in a number of tissues, including many areas of the brain,

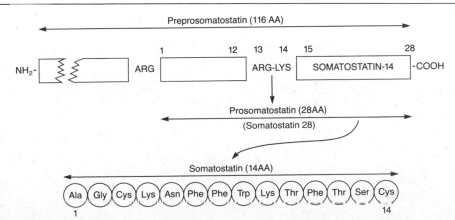

Figure 22–7. Amino acid sequence of somatostatin and its cleavage from dibasic amino acid residue in prosomatostatin and preprosomatostatin.

the gastrointestinal tract, and the pancreas. In the central nervous system and the pancreas, somatostatin-14 predominates, but approximately 5–10% of the somatostatinlike immunoreactivity is due to a 28-amino-acid peptide, somatostatin-28 (prosomatostatin). This consists of an N-terminal region of 14 amino acids and a carboxy-terminal segment containing somatostatin-14. In small intestine, the larger molecule is more prevalent, with 70–75% of the hormone having 28 amino acids and only 25–30% being somatostatin-14. Unlike most prohormones, the larger peptide somatostatin-28 is 10 times more potent than somatostatin-14 in inhibiting growth hormone and insulin.

Almost every known stimulator of release of insulin from pancreatic B cells also promotes somatostatin release from D cells. This includes glucose, arginine, gastrointestinal hormones, and tolbutamide. The importance of circulating somatostatin is unclear, since a major role of this peptide may be as a paracrine regulator of the pancreatic islet and the tissues of the gastrointestinal tract (see Chapter 21). Physiologic levels of somatostatin in humans seldom exceed 80 pg/mL (49 pmol/L). The metabolic clearance of exogenously infused somatostatin in humans is extremely rapid; the half-life of the hormone is less than 3 minutes.

Somatostatin acts in several ways to restrain the movement of nutrients from the intestinal tract into the circulation. It prolongs gastric emptying time, decreases gastric acid and gastrin production, diminishes pancreatic exocrine secretion, decreases splanchnic blood flow, and retards xylose absorption. Neutralization of circulating somatostatin with antisomatostatin serum is associated with enhanced nutrient absorption in dogs. This implies that at least some of the effects of somatostatin are truly endocrine, as opposed to the paracrine effects discussed earlier.

4. PANCREATIC POLYPEPTIDE

Pancreatic polypeptide (PP) is found in F cells located chiefly in islets in the posterior portion of the head of the pancreas. PP is a 36-amino-acid peptide with a molecular weight of 4200. Little is known about its biosynthesis. Circulating levels of the peptide increase in response to a mixed meal; however, intravenous infusion of glucose or triglyceride does not produce such a rise, and intravenous amino acids cause only a small increase. Vagotomy abolishes the response to an ingested meal.

In healthy subjects, basal levels of PP average 24 ± 4 pmol/L and may become elevated owing to a variety of factors including old age, alcohol abuse, diarrhea, chronic renal failure, hypoglycemia, or inflammatory disorders. Values above 300 pmol/L are found in most patients with pancreatic endocrine tumors such as glucagonoma or VIPoma and in all patients with tumors of the pancreatic F cell. As many as 20% of patients with insulinoma and one-third of those with gastrinomas also have pancreatic polypeptide plasma concentrations of greater than 300 pmol/L.

The physiologic action of PP is unknown. It is discussed further in Chapter 21.

HORMONAL CONTROL OF NUTRIENT METABOLISM

Hormones are important in every aspect of nutrient flux, from ingestion of foodstuffs to the ultimate assimilation of nutrients through biochemical processes at the intracellular level.

Hormones are important in regulating appetite and thus food-seeking behavior. Somatostatin, insulin, glucagon, CCK, cortisol, thyroid hormones, and estrogens have all been shown to play roles in regulating appetite in animal studies. Somatostatin and the gastrointestinal hormones are important modulators of rates of digestion and absorption, both by direct effects on the gut itself and by their effects on the exocrine pancreas and gallbladder (see Chapter 21). Once absorption of nutrients has taken place, insulin plays a crucial role in promoting movement of these circulating nutrients into target cells. Insulin enhances entry of glucose into skeletal muscle, cardiac muscle, and adipose tissue but does not appear to be necessary for glucose transport into liver or brain cells. Transport of certain amino acids, fatty acids, potassium, and magnesium is also stimulated in the presence of insulin. Gut hormones, particularly GIP, as well as vagally mediated neural signals act to potentiate the release of insulin in response to absorbed nutrients. The effects of a meal on the release of glucagon depend on the summation of a number of factors: (1) stimulation of glucagon release by absorbed amino acids, gastrointestinal hormones, and vagal stimulation, versus (2) inhibition of glucagon by postprandial hyperglycemia and concomitant insulin and somatostatin release. Circulating plasma glucagon usually shows little change after a mixed meal because of these opposing factors.

The ultimate fate of the 3 major classes of absorbed nutrients—carbohydrates (especially glucose), amino acids, and triglycerides—depends on the hormonal milieu of the individual. This hormonal milieu, in turn, is dependent on the nutrient status of the person (fed versus short-term fast). In simplified terms, the fed state is characterized by a relatively high insulin:glucagon ratio, whereas the preprandial or fasted state is characterized by a relatively lower insulin:glucagon ratio. The starving state has a number of unique features that are beyond the scope of this discussion.

EFFECT OF INSULIN & GLUCAGON ON FUEL METABOLISM

A summary of the key steps in fuel metabolism of nutrients is presented in Fig 22–8. After glucose enters the hepatic cell, it may be converted to glycogen for storage or it may enter the glycolytic pathway and be broken down to pyruvate, with production of a readily available form of energy, ATP. In the presence of adequate intracellular oxygenation, pyruvate enters the mitochondria and participates in the tricarboxylic acid cycle, with the ultimate production of even larger quantities of ATP. Fats enter cells as free fatty acids and may then be stored as triglycerides or broken down by beta oxidation into acetyl-CoA, which can then enter the tricarboxylic acid cycle and be used to produce ATP. Amino acids can be used to synthesize necessary structural and secreted proteins after entry into cells—or, conversely, proteins in cells can be broken down, some of the amino acids can be used for the production of energy, or can serve as precursors for gluconeogenesis.

Insulin and glucagon affect many different steps of fuel metabolism. Their diverse roles can best be understood by clarifying a few general principles. First, insulin is primarily an **anabolic** hormone. It enhances storage of nutrients such as glycogen, triglycerides, and protein by promoting glycogenesis, fatty acid synthesis, protein synthesis, and glycolysis (which makes available building blocks for fat and protein synthesis). Glucagon, on the other hand, functions primarily to **protect the organism from hypoglycemia** by stimulating gluconeogenesis and glycogenolysis.

The second general principle is that there are **2 types of control** of metabolism by these hormones. One type is rapid (minutes to hours) and is mediated by hormone-induced changes in the catalytic properties of key enzymes by phosphorylation-dephosphorylation. The other type of control is slower (hours to days) and involves induction of the synthesis of key enzymes by the hormone. The first type of control involves a change in enzyme kinetics; the second involves a change in the amount of enzyme without a change in the kinetics.

1. HORMONE-INDUCED CHANGES IN ENZYME KINETICS

The enzymes affected by hormone-induced changes in phosphorylation-dephosphorylation belong to a class of enzymes called **interconvertible enzymes.** The interconvertible enzymes that are important in intermediary metabolism are listed in Table 22–4. Insulin stimulates the **dephosphorylation** of these enzymes, whereas glucagon stimulates the **phosphorylation** of the same enzymes. Most of these enzymes are activated by dephosphorylation. Exceptions include glycogen phosphorylase, fructose 2,6-bisphos-

phatase, and hormone-sensitive lipoprotein lipase of adipose cells, all of which are active in the phosphorylated form.

The mechanism of phosphorylation-dephosphorylation of glycogen phosphorylase (Fig 22–9) has been well studied and will be described in detail. It is important to remember in this example that glycogen phosphorylase is one of the enzymes that is active (rather than inactive) in the phosphorylated form. Glucagon binds to a specific receptor on the outer side of the liver cell membrane. The hormone-receptor interaction leads to activation of adenylate cyclase, an enzyme bound to the cytoplasmic side of the plasma membrane. Adenylate cyclase then utilizes intracellular ATP to produce the "second messenger" cAMP. This cyclic nucleotide activates a cAMP-dependent protein kinase, an enzyme whose function is to phosphorylate other proteins. (This enzyme is also called phosphorylase kinase kinase, since it phosphorylates the enzyme phosphorylase kinase.) Phosphorylase kinase is activated when it is phosphorylated and inactivated when it is dephosphorylated. In its active (phosphorylated) form, it phosphorylates the enzyme glycogen phosphorylase (phosphorylase b in Fig 22–9). As stated above, this enzyme is also active in its phosphorylated form, catalyzing the breakdown of glycogen into glucose 1-phosphate.

Insulin, probably via an intracellular messenger, promotes the dephosphorylation of the interconvertible enzymes; in the above example, insulin acts by opposing the action of cAMP. In addition, insulin probably increases the activity of specific phosphatases that directly catalyze dephosphorylation of the phosphorylated interconvertible enzymes. Glycogen synthetase, glycogen phosphorylase (via phosphorylase kinase), and pyruvate kinase are all known to be regulated via a cAMP-dependent protein kinase. The mechanism of regulation of the other interconvertible enzymes is still unknown.

Hormonally mediated phosphorylation and dephosphorylation are important regulators of several key steps in fuel metabolism, eg, the conversion of fructose 6-phosphate into fructose 1,6-bisphosphate. As can be seen in Figure 22–8, this step is catalyzed by 6-phosphofructo 1-kinase. The reverse step is catalyzed by fructose 1,6-bisphosphatase (Fig 22–8). The activity of these 2 enzymes is controlled by the level of another metabolite of the glycolytic pathway, fructose 2,6-bisphosphate, which is formed by the phosphorylation of fructose 6-phosphate. High levels of fructose 2,6-bisphosphate stimulate the activity of 6-phosphofructo 1-kinase and inhibit the activity of fructose 1,6 bisphosphatase, thus promoting glycolysis and inhibiting gluconeogenesis. The formation of fructose 2,6-bisphosphate is controlled, in turn, by a remarkable protein (a so-called tandem enzyme) that has 2 different enzyme activities. The enzyme activity that promotes phosphorylation of fructose 6-phosphate

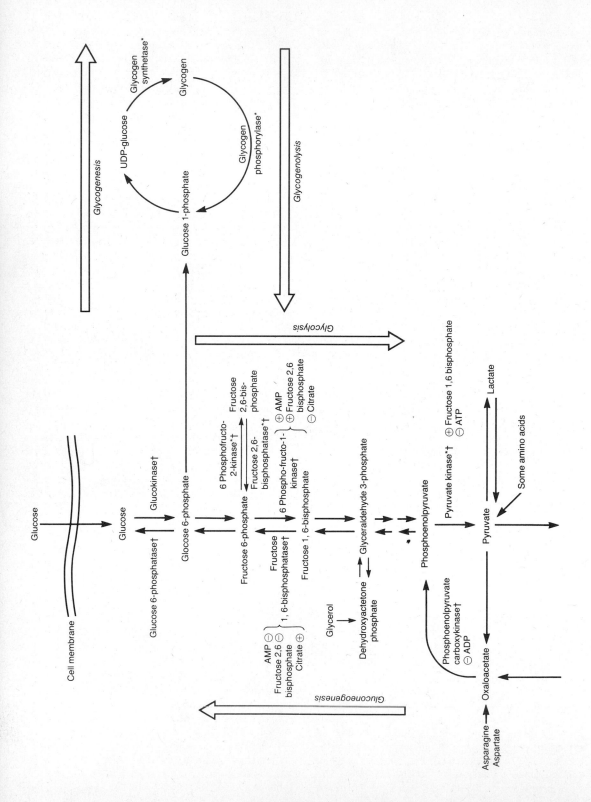

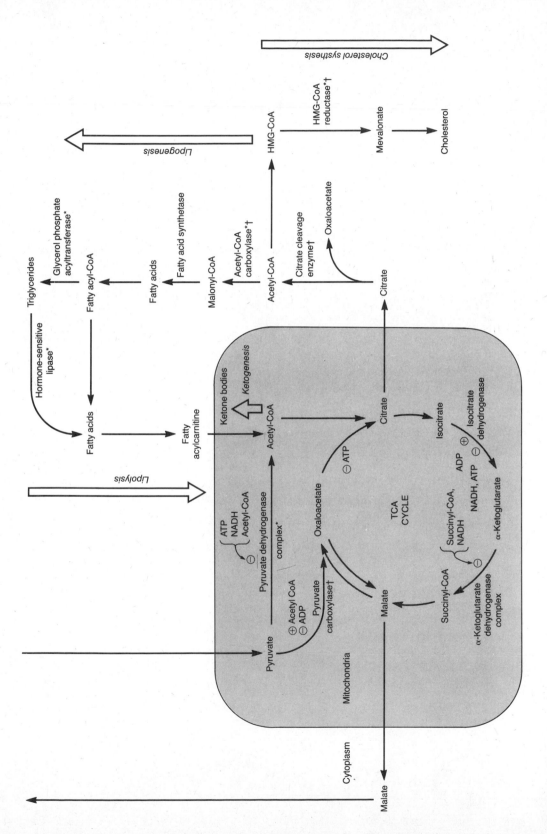

Figure 22–8. Interrelationship of fat and carbohydrate metabolism in normal energy homeostasis in the liver. Major functional pathways depicted by hollow arrows. Enzymes with asterisks are the interconvertible enzymes that are phosphorylated or dephosphorylated depending on the ratio of insulin to glucagon. Enzymes with daggers are induced or repressed depending on the ratio of insulin to glucagon. UDP, uridine diphosphate; HMG-CoA, hydroxymethylglutaryl-CoA; ATP, adenosine triphosphate; NADH, nicotinamide adenine dinucleotide (reduced form); TCA, tricarboxylic acid; ADP, adenosine diphosphate.

Table 22–4. Interconvertible enzymes important in intermediary metabolism.[1]

6-Phosphofructo 2-kinase/fructose 2,6-bisphosphatase[2]
Pyruvate kinase (L isoenzyme)[3]
Pyruvate dehydrogenase complex
Acetyl-CoA carboxylase
Glycerol phosphate acyltransferase
HMG-CoA reductase
Glycogen synthetase
Glycogen phosphorylase
Hormone-sensitive lipoprotein lipase of adipose cells

[1] All of these enzymes except glycogen phosphorylase and hormone-sensitive lipoprotein lipase of adipose cells are **active** in the dephosphorylated form and **inactive** in the phosphorylated form. Glucagon promotes phosphorylation of these enzymes; insulin promotes their dephosphorylation.

[2] In the liver, dephosphorylation activates 6-phosphofructo 2-kinase but inactivates fructose 2,6-bisphosphatase activity of this tandem enzyme (see text). In muscle, epinephrine-induced phosphorylation activates the kinase.

[3] The liver contains the L isoenzyme of pyruvate kinase. The M isoenzyme of pyruvate kinase found in muscle and brain is *not* reversibly phosphorylated.

into fructose 2,6-bisphosphate is 6-phosphofructo 2-kinase; the activity that promotes dephosphorylation of fructose 2,6-bisphosphate is called fructose 6-bisphosphatase. Dephosphorylation of this enzyme, which occurs in the presence of a high insulin:glucagon ratio, enhances the kinase activity and inhibits the phosphatase activity, thus promoting glycolysis. A low insulin:glucagon ratio, on the other hand, activates the fructose 2,6-bisphosphatase and inhibits the 6-phosphofructo 2-kinase activity, thus promoting gluconeogenesis.

2. HORMONE-INDUCED CHANGES IN ENZYME QUANTITY

Table 22–5 lists the enzymes shown to be affected by alterations in the ratio of insulin to glucagon.

Glucokinase, 6-phosphofructo 1-kinase, 6-phosphofructo 2-kinase, and pyruvate kinase (all enzymes that promote breakdown of glucose) are induced in the

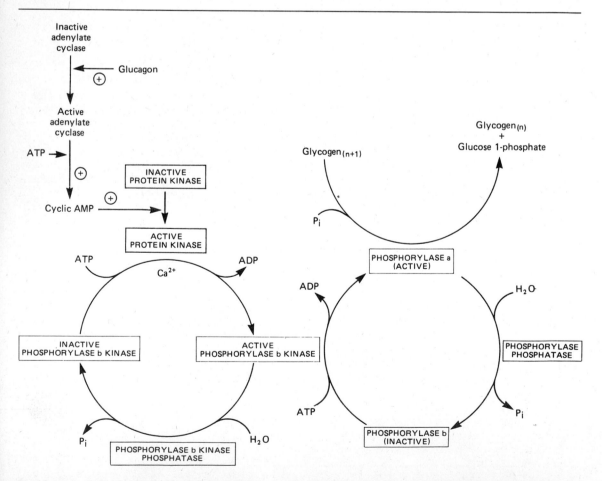

Figure 22–9. Control of phosphorylase by glucagon. n = number of glucose residues. (Modified and reproduced, with permission, from Martin DW Jr, Mayes PA, Rodwell VW: *Harper's Review of Biochemistry,* 20th ed. Lange, 1985.)

Table 22–5. Enzymes induced or repressed by insulin or glucagon.

Enzymes induced by a high insulin:glucagon ratio and repressed by a low insulin:glucagon ratio:
 Glucokinase
 6-Phosphofructo 1-kinase
 6-Phosphofructo 2-kinase (fructose 2,6-bisphosphatase)
 Citrate cleavage enzyme
 Acetyl-CoA carboxylase
 HMG-CoA reductase
 Pyruvate kinase
Enzymes induced by a low insulin:glucagon ratio and repressed by a high insulin:glucagon ratio:
 Glucose 6-phosphatase
 Fructose 1,6-bisphosphatase
 Phosphoenolpyruvate carboxykinase

presence of high insulin:glucagon ratios and repressed when the ratio is low. Glucose 6-phosphatase, fructose 1,6-bisphosphatase, and phosphoenolpyruvate carboxykinase (the enzymes that promote gluconeogenesis), on the other hand, are repressed in the presence of high circulating insulin and low circulating glucagon and induced when the levels of glucagon are relatively increased in comparison with insulin levels. The significance of these effects is discussed in the following section.

3. INSULIN & GLUCAGON CONTROL OF FUEL METABOLISM

The details of hormonal control of nutrient metabolism vary depending on the tissue involved. The differences between tissues arise because of differences in the hormone sensitivity of enzymes involved or because of the presence or absence of the enzyme system or of insulin receptors in a particular tissue. A complete discussion of fuel metabolism is beyond the scope of this text, and only a review of events in key tissues will be offered. Enzymes discussed below are indicated by asterisks and daggers in Figure 22–8.

Fed State
A. Liver: In the fed state, the insulin:glucagon ratio is relatively high, and the liver is both glycogenic and lipogenic.

Glycogenesis (glycogen formation) is enhanced by the activation of glycogen synthetase through its hormone-induced dephosphorylation. On the other hand, the simultaneous dephosphorylation of glycogen phosphorylase inactivates the enzyme, thus inhibiting glycogen breakdown. Concurrent inhibition of breakdown and stimulation of glycogen formation avoids a glycogenesis-glycogenolysis "futile cycle" and leads to glycogen storage.

Insulin promotes **lipogenesis** indirectly, by stimulation of glycolysis (which makes available precursors of fatty acid synthesis); and directly, by stimulation of

enzymes in the pathway of fatty acid and cholesterol synthesis. Glycolysis is stimulated by the **dephosphorylation** of phosphofructokinase, pyruvate kinase, and pyruvate dehydrogenase as well as induction of glucokinase, phosphofructokinase, and pyruvate kinase. All of the above tend to increase the utilization of glucose in the glycolytic pathway, which leads to an accumulation of acetyl-CoA. In the fed state, there is a high ratio of ATP to ADP + AMP and of NADH to ADP, both of which slow down the tricarboxylic acid cycle (Fig 22–8). Acetyl-CoA leaves the mitochondria via citrate and participates in the synthesis of fats and cholesterol rather than entering the tricarboxylic acid cycle for the production of more ATP. The fat and cholesterol synthetic activities are directly accelerated by the dephosphorylation (activation) of acetyl-CoA carboxylase and glycerol phosphate acyltransferase and by HMG-CoA reductase, respectively.

The high insulin:glucagon ratio is also associated with a reduction in activity of the gluconeogenic enzymes (pyruvate carboxylase, phosphoenolpyruvate carboxykinase, fructose 1,6-bisphosphatase, and glucose 6-phosphatase), which inhibits glucose production via reversal of the glycolytic pathway and thus prevents a gluconeogenic-glycolytic "futile cycle." (This is analogous to the situation described above for glycogen synthesis.)

The net effect, then, of the elevated insulin:glucagon ratio in the well-fed state is storage of nutrient energy as glycogen and fats.

B. Adipose Tissue: In the fed state, lipogenesis is favored in adipose tissue because pyruvate kinase, pyruvate dehydrogenase, acetyl-CoA carboxylase, and glycerol phosphate acyltransferase are in their dephosphorylated state and thus active. In addition, an enzyme that is specific to adipose tissue, **hormone-sensitive lipoprotein lipase,** is (like glycogen phosphorylase; see above) inactive in the dephosphorylated state, thereby reinforcing the lipogenic state and inhibiting the lipolytic pathway.

Fasted State
A. Liver: In the postabsorptive or fasting state and in starvation, the ratio of insulin to glucagon is low, which results in production of the phosphorylated form of the interconvertible enzymes. As noted above, all of these liver enzymes except glycogen phosphorylase are inactive in the phosphorylated state. Hence, glycolysis, glycogenesis, lipogenesis, and cholesterol synthesis are inhibited. On the other hand, **glycogenolysis** is enhanced.

The increase in glucagon and decrease in insulin levels also result in an increase in activity of the gluconeogenic enzymes pyruvate carboxylase, phosphoenolpyruvate carboxykinase, fructose 1,6-bisphosphatase, and glucose 6-phosphatase. The activity of glycolytic enzymes—glucokinase, phosphofructokinase, and pyruvate kinase—are reduced. This serves the dual purpose of inhibiting the glycolytic pathway and increasing gluconeogenesis, thereby ensuring a continuous supply of glucose by the liver to the blood and peripheral tissues.

B. Adipose Tissue: Phosphorylation of the interconvertible enzymes of fat and cholesterol synthesis (acetyl-CoA carboxylase, glycerol phosphate acyltransferase, and HMG-CoA reductase) also leads to their inactivation, thereby favoring fatty acid oxidation (beta oxidation) to acetyl-CoA and the availability of this intermediate for ketogenesis. Furthermore, beta oxidation of fatty acids leads to the production of NADH, which suppresses the tricarboxylic acid cycle (Fig 22–8) and thus promotes the production of ketone bodies as the end product of fatty acid breakdown.

Again, in the starved state, the reduced insulin:glucagon ratio results in the phosphorylation (inactivation) of the interconvertible enzymes of glycolysis and fat and cholesterol synthesis and the activation of hormone-sensitive lipoprotein lipase, shutting down lipogenesis and cholesterol synthesis and promoting lipolysis and fatty acid oxidation. Adipose tissue lacks the enzymes that mediate glycogenesis, glycogenolysis, and gluconeogenesis.

C. Muscle: The same events occur as in liver in the fasted state, except that muscle lacks gluconeogenic enzymes and has no glucose 6-phosphatase and therefore cannot produce free glucose. The liver is the main source of free glucose in the postabsorptive state, with the kidney playing a minor role.

II. DIABETES MELLITUS

Clinical diabetes mellitus is a syndrome of disordered metabolism with inappropriate hyperglycemia due either to an absolute deficiency of insulin secretion or a reduction in the biologic effectiveness of insulin (or both).

CLASSIFICATION

Traditionally, diabetes has been classified according to the patient's age at onset of symptoms (juvenile-onset versus adult-onset). In 1979, the NIH Diabetes Data Group recommended that diabetes mellitus be classified into one of 2 major types according to dependence on exogenous insulin. Most patients with diabetes fall into one of 2 major categories: **insulin-dependent** (type I) or **non–insulin-dependent** (type II) diabetes mellitus (Table 22–6).

TYPE I: INSULIN-DEPENDENT DIABETES MELLITUS (IDDM)

Type I is a severe form of diabetes mellitus and is associated with ketosis in the untreated state. About 10–20% of diabetics in North America and Europe are of the insulin-dependent type. It is most common in young individuals but occurs occasionally in nonobese adults. It is a catabolic disorder in which circulating insulin is virtually absent, plasma glucagon is elevated, and the pancreatic B cells fail to respond to all known insulinogenic stimuli. In the absence of insulin, the 3 main target tissues of insulin (liver, muscle, and fat) not only fail to appropriately take up absorbed nutrients but continue to deliver glucose, amino acids, and fatty acids into the bloodstream from their respective storage depots. Furthermore, alterations in fat metabolism lead to the production and accumulation of ketones. This inappropriate persistence of the fasted state postprandially can be reversed by the administration of insulin.

Genetics of Type I Diabetes

Studies in monozygotic twins suggest that genetic influences are less marked in type I diabetes than in type II diabetes. Only 50% of identical twins of type I diabetic patients will develop the disease. This also suggests that an environmental factor is required for induction of diabetes in these cases. In contrast, the identical twin of a type II diabetic will usually develop diabetes within a year of onset of the disease in the sibling.

Type I diabetes is believed to result from an infectious or toxic environmental insult to the pancreatic B cells in genetically predisposed persons. Environmental factors that have been associated with altered pancreatic islet cell function include viruses (mumps, rubella, coxsackievirus B4), toxic chemical agents such as Vacor (a nitrophenylurea rat poison), and other destructive cytotoxins such as hydrogen cyanide from spoiled tapioca or cassava root.

Type I diabetes is strongly associated with an increased frequency of certain HLA antigens. These antigens are glycoproteins found on cell surfaces of all cells except red blood cells and sperm. They allow the immune system to distinguish other body cells from foreign invaders such as viruses, bacteria, or fungi. The predominant HLA antigens associated with type I diabetes vary in different racial groups. Thus, HLA-B8, -B15, -B18, -Cw3, -DR3, and -DR4 occur with increased frequency on leukocytes of Caucasian diabetics, whereas only HLA-DR3 and -DR4 appear to be correlated with type I diabetes in Asians, Africans, and Latin-Americans. Either HLA-DR3 or -DR4 occur in about 95% of Caucasian type I diabetics, compared to 45–50% of Caucasian controls. It has been shown that HLA-DQ genes are even more specific markers of susceptibility to type I diabetes, since a particular variety (HLA-DQw3.2) is invariably found in the HLA-DR4

Table 22–6. Clinical classification of diabetes mellitus.

	Ketosis	Islet Cell Antibodies	HLA Associ-ation	Estimated Prevalence (% of All Diabetics)	Treatment
Insulin-dependent diabetes (IDDM, type I)	Marked	Usually present at onset.	Yes	10–20%	1. Insulin. 2. Diet.
Non–insulin-dependent diabetes (NIDDM, type II)	Absent	Absent	No	80–90%	
Nonobese NIDDM				15% of NIDDM patients	Eucaloric diet alone or diet plus sulfonylurea or insulin.
Obese NIDDM				85% of NIDDM patients	1. Weight reduction. 2. Hypocaloric diet plus sulfonylureas or insulin *for symptomatic control only.*
Gestational diabetes					See Chapter 20.
Secondary diabetes: diabetes mellitus and impaired glucose tolerance secondary to or associated with other conditions, eg, pancreatic disease, drug toxicity, endocrine disorders, genetic disease, insulin receptor abnormalities with acanthosis nigricans.					Treatment varies according to the specific condition. In general, removal or correction of offending agent if possible, diet, and insulin are the foundation of treatment. See text for details.

patients with type I diabetes while a "protective" gene (HLA-DQw3.1), which has an aspartic acid encoded in region 57 of the HLA-DQ beta chain, is prevalent in the HLA-DR4 controls. Moreover, HLA-DR2, which is generally protective against type I diabetes, seems to be so by virtue of its linkage to HLA-DQ genes containing aspartic acid at position 57 of their beta chains.

A plausible theory that explains the association of HLA types with type I diabetes is as follows: The HLA antigens are located close to the immune response genes on chromosome 6; there may be a functional link. An initial viral infection of the pancreatic B cells is aggravated by an immune deficiency that leads to a greater infiltration and destruction of the B cells by the virus. This could enhance the release of sensitizing proteins from the B cells with the consequent production of cytotoxic lymphocytes and autoantibodies, resulting in excessive B cell destruction ("autoaggression"). Thus, it is possible that the HLA marker denotes either a hypoimmune or hyperimmune response (or a mixture of both) whose ultimate outcome is excessive loss of pancreatic B cells. Alternatively, rather than a functional link, a "diabetes gene" may be in linkage disequilibrium with certain subtypes of the HLA-DR3 and -DR4 regions of chromosome 6.

Circulating islet cell autoantibodies, virtually absent in nondiabetics, have been detected in as many as 85% of type I diabetics tested in the first few weeks of onset of diabetes. Moreover, when sensitive immunoassays are used, the majority of these patients also have detectable antibodies to insulin prior to receiving insulin therapy. The high prevalence of these islet cell and insulin autoantibodies in type I diabetes, as well as in certain of their siblings who later develop overt diabetes, supports the concept that autoimmune mecha-

nisms may contribute significantly to progressive B cell destruction.

A genetic link to chromosome 11 has been identified in type I diabetes. Comparison of the size of a polymorphic DNA locus flanking the 5′ region of the insulin gene on chromosome 11 revealed that 88% of the alleles in a Caucasian population of type I diabetics were in a "small" class of about 570 base pairs, while 12% of the alleles were in a larger class (averaging 2470 base pairs). In contrast, only 67% of the alleles in nondiabetic Caucasian controls were in the "small" class, and 33% were in the larger class of alleles. This polymorphic locus does not seem either to encode a protein or to affect insulin gene expression, but it may represent a marker for a linked gene relating to B cell replication or function that influences susceptibility to type I diabetes.

Immunosuppression in the Treatment of Recent-Onset Type I Diabetes

Since the destruction of B cells in type I diabetes is a progressive, immune-mediated process, clinical trials with immunosuppressive therapy at the onset of type I diabetes have been initiated. In one study of 310 type I diabetics in Canada and Europe who are receiving cyclosporine, an inhibitor of T cell function, a partial remission, wherein insulin requirements have been reduced or eliminated, has been maintained in 50–60%, but none have a completely normalized carbohydrate tolerance. The hazards of cyclosporine, including its nephrotoxicity, remain a concern, particularly since immunotherapy apparently cannot be discontinued without reexacerbation of B cell destruction. A consensus meeting in 1987 concluded that while residual

B cell function can be preserved to some extent, the results from controlled trials were not significant enough to justify the clinical use of cyclosporine.

More specific strategies for immunosuppression, such as the use of monoclonal antibodies against particular T cell products, may reduce the hazards of long-term immunotherapy. A new highly selective immunosuppressant, ciamexon, has the advantage of not suppressing resistance against infection and not promoting tumor growth while proving effective in delaying the onset diabetes in animal models. It is being studied in Europe, in a double-blind controlled trial involving 120 type I diabetics at 20 centers.

Other nonimmunosuppressive therapeutic modalities under investigation include probucol, which tends to quench free radicals that have been implicated as a means of T-lymphocyte cytotoxicity, and nicotinamide, an inhibitor of poly(ADP-ribose) synthetase, an enzyme whose repair of DNA injury tends to deplete the cell of its vital supply of NAD.

Subgroups of Type I Diabetes

In Britain, a subclassification of type I diabetes has been suggested. One subgroup, termed Ia, accounts for 80% of type I diabetics. These patients have islet cell autoantibodies only transiently, at the onset of their disease; they seldom have any other associated autoimmune phenomena. The most common HLA types in this subgroup are B15 and DR4. A viral infection appears to be mainly responsible for the B cell destruction in these patients.

Subgroup Ib accounts for the remainder of insulin-dependent diabetic patients. These patients have islet cell autoantibodies that tend to persist in high titers. Associated autoimmune disorders of the thyroid and adrenal cortex occur frequently; hypogonadism and pernicious anemia are also found. Immune destruction of pancreatic B cells appears to be responsible for the development of the disease (see Chapter 28). Most of these patients are female, and the most frequent HLA types are HLA-B8 and HLA-DR3.

TYPE II: NON–INSULIN-DEPENDENT DIABETES MELLITUS (NIDDM)

Type II diabetes, which comprises a heterogeneous group of the milder forms of diabetes, occurs predominantly in adults but may occasionally have its onset in childhood.

Type II diabetes is defined mainly in *negative* terms. It is a *non*ketotic form of diabetes which is *not* linked to HLA markers on the sixth chromosome and is *not* associated with islet cell autoantibodies. The patients are *not* dependent on exogenous insulin therapy to sustain life—thus the name, *non*–insulin-dependent diabetes mellitus. An element of tissue insensitivity to insulin has been noted in most NIDDM patients. Possible mechanisms for this are shown in Table 22–7.

Table 22–7. Factors reducing response to insulin.[1]

Prereceptor inhibitors: Insulin antibodies
Receptor inhibitors:
  Insulin receptor autoantibodies
  "Down-regulation" of receptors by hyperinsulinism:
    Primary hyperinsulinism (B cell adenoma)
    Hyperinsulinism secondary to a postreceptor defect
    (obesity, Cushing's syndrome, acromegaly, pregnancy)
    or prolonged hyperglycemia (diabetes mellitus, post–
    glucose tolerance test)
Postreceptor influences:
  Poor responsiveness of principal target organs; obesity;
    hepatic disease; muscle inactivity
  Hormonal excess: glucocorticoids, growth hormone, oral
    contraceptive agents, progesterone, human chorionic
    somatomammotropin, catecholamines, thyroxine

[1] Reproduced, with permission, from Krupp MA, Chatton MJ, Tierney LM Jr (editors): *Current Medical Diagnosis & Treatment 1986*. Lange, 1986.

Subgroups of Type II Diabetes

Type II diabetics can be distributed on the basis of body weight into obese or nonobese subtypes. Currently, it is impossible to identify diagnostic characteristics that allow further clear-cut separation into more specific subtypes. Circulating insulin levels are presently considered too variable to be of use in classification.

Among this "non–type I" group are a wide assortment of heterogeneous disorders. These include rare instances in which a defective insulin gene produces a biologically inadequate abnormal insulin or a proinsulin that is not transformed to insulin in the B cell. Receptor blocks to insulin action have been demonstrated in some cases. In most patients with type II diabetes, the cause of the disorder is presently undefined although both a defect in insulin secretion and a defect in insulin action at the postreceptor level are generally present.

Obese NIDDM

Up to 85% of type II diabetics are obese. These patients have an insensitivity to endogenous insulin that is positively correlated with the presence of an abdominal distribution of fat, producing an abnormally high waist to hip ratio. In addition, distended adipocytes and overnourished liver and muscle cells may also resist the deposition of additional glycogen and triglycerides in their storage depots. Hyperplasia of pancreatic B cells is often present and probably accounts for the normal or exaggerated insulin responses to glucose and other stimuli seen in the milder forms of this disease. In more severe cases, secondary (but potentially reversible) failure of pancreatic B cell secretion may result after exposure to prolonged fasting hyperglycemia. This phenomenon has been called "desensitization." It is selective for glucose, and the B cell recovers sensitivity to glucose stimulation once the sustained hyperglycemia is corrected by any form of therapy, including diet therapy, sulfonylureas, and insulin.

A major cause of the observed resistance to insulin in target tissues of obese patients is believed to be a postreceptor defect in insulin action. This is associated with overdistended storage depots and a reduced ability to clear nutrients from the circulation after meals. Consequent hyperinsulinism can further enhance insulin resistance by down-regulation of insulin receptors. Furthermore, when hyperglycemia becomes sustained, a specific glucose transporter protein in insulin target tissue also becomes down-regulated after continuous activation. This contributes to further defects in postreceptor insulin action, thereby aggravating the hyperglycemia.

When overfeeding is corrected so that storage depots become less saturated, the cycle is interrupted. Insulin sensitivity improves and is further normalized by a reduction in both the hyperinsulinism and the hyperglycemia.

Nonobese NIDDM

Approximately 15% of patients with NIDDM are nonobese diabetics. In most of these patients, impaired insulin action at the postreceptor level and an absent or delayed early phase of insulin release in response to glucose can be demonstrated. However, other insulinogenic stimuli, such as acute infusion of amino acids, intravenous tolbutamide, or intramuscular glucagon, often remain effective in eliciting acute insulin release.

The hyperglycemia in patients with nonobese NIDDM often responds to dietary therapy or to oral hypoglycemic agents. Occasionally, insulin therapy is required to achieve satisfactory glycemic control even though it is not needed to prevent ketoacidosis.

While most nonobese NIDDM patients cannot be subclassified, several discrete subtypes are suggested in a small proportion of patients on the basis of genetic characteristics:

A. NIDDM Occurring in Late Childhood or Young Adulthood:

1. Autosomal dominant nonobese NIDDM—A specific subclass of nonobese NIDDM includes patients with "maturity-onset diabetes of the young" (MODY, or Mason type). These patients have mild hyperglycemia with onset in late childhood or young adulthood. Their strong family history of a mild form of diabetes occurring in one parent and in one-half of the parent's offspring suggests an autosomal dominant transmission.

2. Type II diabetes of early onset—A high familial prevalence of type II diabetes has been noted in patients whose age at onset of mild diabetes is 25–40 years. Epidemiologic studies suggest that this familial prevalence is due to inheritance of diabetogenic genes from both parents (homozygous state). When only one parent passes on the diabetogenic gene (heterozygous state), its later expression as clinical diabetes may require additional genetic or environmental factors (eg, aging, obesity). Thus, 2 heterozygous parents may or may not each develop diabetes after age 40 years, but as many as 75% of their offspring are at high risk of developing diabetes, with as many as 25% of them becoming diabetic before age 40 years.

B. Mutant Insulins: Recently, 8 families have been identified as having abnormal circulating forms of insulin. In 3 of these families, there is impaired cleavage of the proinsulin molecule; in the other 5 families, abnormalities of the insulin molecule itself have been reported (Table 22–8).

Analysis of the insulin gene, circulating insulin, and clinical features of family members in these cases indicates that individuals with mutant insulin are heterozygous for this defect, with both a normal and an abnormal insulin molecule being equally expressed. However, because the abnormal insulin binds to receptors poorly, it has very low biologic activity and accumulates in the blood to exceed the concentration of the normal insulin. This decreased removal rate of mutant insulin results in hyperinsulinemia after overnight fasting and a subnormal molar ratio of C peptide to immunoreactive insulin. Diabetes mellitus may or may not be present in association with mutant insulin, depending on the concentration and bioactivity of circulating normal and abnormal insulins and on the insulin responsiveness of peripheral tissues. Since there is no obvious resistance to insulin in any of these cases, it appears that abnormal insulin does not interfere with binding of normal insulin to receptors; therefore, a feature of this syndrome is the normal response to exogenously administered insulin.

1. Abnormalities of the proinsulin molecule—A partially cleaved intermediate of proinsulin comprising up to 90% of circulating insulin immunoreactivity has been described in 2 families, one from Japan and one from Boston. Both families seem to have similar defects, with the arginine in position 65 being replaced by another amino acid and thereby interfering with cleavage of the C peptide from the A chain of insulin. However, mild diabetes mellitus was present only in the 3 affected members of the family from Japan; it was not present in 17 affected members of the large kindred in Boston, despite a similar mutation of the insulin gene.

In a third family, hyperproinsulinemia was reported in 5 members. Although one of the 5 members (a 12-

Table 22–8. Mutant insulins and proinsulins.

Name	Amino Acid Substitution
Insulin Chicago (USA)	B 25 (Phe → Leu)
Insulin Los Angeles (USA)	B 24 (Phe → Ser)
Insulin Wakayama (Japan) I, II, III (3 families)	A 3 (Val → Leu)
Proinsulin Tokyo (Japan)	Arg 65 (Arg → His)
Proinsulin Boston (USA)	Arg 65 (Arg → ?)
Proinsulin Providence (USA)	B 10 (His → Asp)

year-old girl) had borderline glucose intolerance, the other 4 had normal blood glucose levels. In this family, a mutation in the insulin gene coding for histidine at B 10 results in substitution of an aspartic acid, inducing a conformational change that prevents conversion of proinsulin to insulin.

2. Abnormalities of the insulin molecule–Genetic defects in insulin synthesis have resulted in substitutions of leucine for phenylalanine at position B 25 ("insulin Chicago") and serine for phenylalanine at position B 24 ("insulin Los Angeles"). (See Fig 22–3). The observation that there was loss of a normal restriction endonuclease cleavage site in the area of the insulin gene coding for B 24 and B 25 phenylalanine was used in conjunction with results of high-performance liquid chromatographic analysis of circulating insulin to establish the nature of the mutant insulin in affected family members. Glucose tolerance ranged from normal to overtly diabetic in affected individuals, who were generally nonobese and had subnormal molar ratios of C peptide to immunoreactive insulin.

In Japan, a mutant insulin with a substitution of leucine for the normal valine at A 3 was initially described in Wakayama but was subsequently identified in the adjacent Osaka region in 2 other families who had no documented relationship.

"NIDDM" Diabetics Who May Be Type I Diabetics in Remission

The current classification of diabetes mellitus has been widely accepted throughout the world, but its deficiencies are apparent in many cases. A subgroup that has been difficult to place in the current "therapeutic" classification is made up of those type I diabetics who remain in temporary remission for up to 2 years. A history of ketoacidosis with the finding of islet cell autoantibodies at the onset of the diabetes—and an HLA pattern that includes HLA-B8, -B15, -DR3, or -DR4—would indicate that these patients have type I diabetes from an etiologic standpoint even though they may be temporarily not "insulin-dependent."

SECONDARY DIABETES

As noted in Table 22–6, there is a diverse group of disorders characterized by the association of diabetes with another condition. Only a few of the many types of secondary diabetes will be discussed here.

Pancreatic Disease

Surgical removal of the pancreas, pancreatic disease due to chronic alcoholism, and other forms of pancreatitis are associated with many of the clinical characteristics of insulin-dependent diabetes mellitus, because the primary abnormality is insulin deficiency. There is, however, a greater tendency to develop insulin-induced hypoglycemia, probably because of the

concomitant lack of the counterregulatory hormone glucagon. At least two-thirds of the pancreas must be destroyed to develop the clinical syndrome. It is usually associated with exocrine pancreatic insufficiency as well.

Drug Toxicity

Many drugs are associated with carbohydrate intolerance or frank diabetes mellitus. Some act by interfering with insulin release from the B cells (thiazides, phenytoin, beta-adrenergic blockers such as propranolol, and calcium channel blockers), some by inducing insulin resistance (glucocorticoids and oral contraceptive pills), and some by causing B cell destruction (pentamidine).

Endocrine Disorders

Excess production of certain hormones (GH [acromegaly], glucocorticoids [Cushing's syndrome or disease], catecholamines [pheochromocytoma], glucagon [glucagonoma], or pancreatic somatostatin [somatostatinoma]) can produce the syndrome of NIDDM by a number of mechanisms. In all but the last instance (somatostatinoma), peripheral responsiveness to insulin is impaired. In addition, excess of catecholamines or somatostatin decreases insulin release from B cells.

Insulin-Resistant Diabetes With Acanthosis Nigricans

Patients with the rare syndrome of extreme insulin resistance associated with acanthosis nigricans can be divided into 2 groups on the basis of clinical and laboratory manifestations. **Group A** consists of younger women with androgenic features (hirsutism, amenorrhea, polycystic ovaries) in whom insulin receptors are deficient in number. Point mutations in the insulin receptor gene have been shown to produce this syndrome. **Group B** consists of older people, mostly women, in whom immunologic disease is suspected. They have a high erythrocyte sedimentation rate, DNA autoantibodies, and a circulating immunoglobulin that binds to insulin receptors, thereby reducing their affinity for insulin.

In both of the above groups, carbohydrate tolerance may at times be normal, and in most cases ketoacidosis does not develop despite severe insulin resistance and diabetes. Occasionally, spontaneous remission of insulin resistance and diabetes occurs, particularly in the group A patients. In neither of the above groups is insulin therapy very effective.

Other Forms of Secondary Diabetes

Other rare diseases associated with insulin receptor or postreceptor abnormalities include leprechaunism, ataxia-telangiectasia, Prader-Willi syndrome, and certain forms of myotonic dystrophy.

CLINICAL FEATURES OF DIABETES MELLITUS

The principal clinical features of the 2 major types of diabetes mellitus are listed for comparison in Table 22–9.

TYPE I DIABETES (IDDM)

IDDM patients present with a characteristic symptom complex, as outlined below. An absolute deficiency of insulin results in excessive accumulation of circulating glucose and fatty acids, with consequent hyperosmolality and hyperketonemia. The severity of the insulin deficiency and the acuteness with which the catabolic state develops determine the intensity of the osmotic and ketotic excess.

Clinical Features

A. Symptoms: Increased urination is a consequence of osmotic diuresis secondary to sustained hyperglycemia. This results in a loss of glucose as well as free water and electrolytes in the urine. Nocturnal enuresis due to polyuria may signal the onset of diabetes in very young children. Thirst is a consequence of the hyperosmolar state, as is blurred vision, which often develops as the lenses and retinas are exposed to hyperosmolar fluids.

Weight loss despite normal or increased appetite is a common feature of IDDM when it develops subacutely over a period of weeks. The weight loss is initially due to depletion of water, glycogen, and triglyceride stores. Chronic weight loss due to reduced muscle mass occurs as amino acids are diverted to form glucose and ketone bodies.

Lowered plasma volume produces dizziness and weakness due to postural hypotension when sitting or standing. Total body potassium loss and the general catabolism of muscle protein contribute to the weakness.

Paresthesias may be present at the time of diagnosis of type I diabetes, particularly when the onset is subacute. They reflect a temporary dysfunction of peripheral sensory nerves and usually clear as insulin replacement restores glycemic levels closer to normal; thus, their presence suggests neurotoxicity from sustained hyperglycemia.

When insulin deficiency is severe and of acute onset, the above symptoms progress in an accelerated manner. Ketoacidosis exacerbates the dehydration and hyperosmolality by producing anorexia, nausea, and vomiting, thus interfering with oral fluid replacement. As plasma osmolality exceeds 330 mosm/L (normal, 285–295 mosm/L), impaired consciousness ensues. With progression of acidosis to a pH of 7.1 or less, deep breathing with a rapid ventilatory rate (Kussmaul respiration) occurs as the body attempts to eliminate carbonic acid. With worsening acidosis (to pH 7 or less), the cardiovascular system may be unable to maintain compensatory vasoconstriction; severe circulatory collapse may result.

B. Signs: The patient's level of consciousness can vary depending on the degree of hyperosmolality. When insulin deficiency develops relatively slowly and sufficient water intake is maintained to permit renal excretion of glucose and appropriate dilution of extracellular sodium chloride concentration, patients remain relatively alert and physical findings may be minimal. When vomiting occurs in response to worsening ketoacidosis, dehydration progresses and compensatory mechanisms become inadequate to keep plasma osmolality below 330 mosm/L. Under these circumstances, stupor or even coma may occur. Evidence of dehydration in a stuporous patient, with rapid deep breathing and the fruity breath odor of acetone, suggests the diagnosis of diabetic ketoacidosis.

Postural hypotension indicates a depleted plasma volume; hypotension in the recumbent position is a serious prognostic sign. Loss of subcutaneous fat and muscle wasting are features of more slowly developing insulin deficiency. In occasional patients with slow, insidious onset of insulin deficiency, subcutaneous fat may be considerably depleted. An enlarged liver, eruptive xanthomas on the flexor surface of the limbs and on the buttocks, and lipemia retinalis indicate that chronic insulin deficiency has resulted in chylomicronemia, with circulating triglycerides elevated usually to over 2000 mg/dL (see Chapter 24).

TYPE II DIABETES (NIDDM)

NIDDM patients also present with characteristic signs and symptoms. The presence of obesity or a strongly positive family history of mild diabetes also suggests a high risk for the development of type II diabetes.

Table 22–9. Clinical features of diabetes.[1]

	Diabetes Type I (IDDM)	Diabetes Type II (NIDDM)
Polyuria and thirst	++	+
Weakness or fatigue	++	+
Polyphagia with weight loss	++	−
Recurrent blurred vision	+	++
Vulvovaginitis or pruritus	+	++
Peripheral neuropathy	+	++
Nocturnal enuresis	++	−
Often asymptomatic	−	++

[1]Reproduced, with permission, from Krupp MA, Chatton MJ, Tierney LM Jr (editors): *Current Medical Diagnosis & Treatment 1986.* Lange, 1986.

Clinical Features

A. Symptoms: The classic symptoms of polyuria, thirst, recurrent blurred vision, paresthesias, and fatigue are manifestations of hyperglycemia and osmotic diuresis and are therefore common to both forms of diabetes. However, many patients with type II diabetes have an insidious onset of hyperglycemia and may be relatively asymptomatic initially. This is particularly true in obese patients, whose diabetes may be detected only after glycosuria or hyperglycemia is noted during routine laboratory studies. Chronic skin infections are common. Generalized pruritus and symptoms of vaginitis are frequently the initial complaints of women with NIDDM. Diabetes should be suspected in women with chronic candidal vulvovaginitis as well as in those who have delivered large infants (> 9 lb, or 4.1 kg) or have had polyhydramnios, preeclampsia, or unexplained fetal losses. Occasionally, a man with previously undiagnosed diabetes may present with impotence.

B. Signs: Nonobese patients with this mild form of diabetes often have no characteristic physical findings at the time of diagnosis. Obese diabetics may have any variety of fat distribution; however, diabetes seems to be more often associated in both men and women with localization of fat deposits on the upper part of the body (particularly the abdomen, chest, neck, and face) and relatively less fat on the appendages, which may be quite muscular. This centripetal fat distribution has been termed "android" and is characterized by a high waist to hip ratio. It differs from the more centrifugal "gynecoid" form of obesity, in which fat is localized more in the hips and thighs and less in the upper parts of the trunk. Refined radiographic techniques of assessing abdominal fat distribution with CT scans has documented that a "visceral" obesity, due to accumulation of fat in the omental and mesenteric regions, correlates with insulin resistance, whereas fat predominantly in subcutaneous tissues of the abdomen has little, if any, association with insulin insensitivity. Mild hypertension may be present in obese diabetics, particularly when the "android" form of obesity is predominant. In women, candidal vaginitis with a reddened, inflamed vulvar area and a profuse whitish discharge may herald the presence of diabetes.

LABORATORY FINDINGS IN DIABETES MELLITUS

Tests of urine glucose and ketone bodies as well as whole blood or plasma glucose measured in samples obtained under basal conditions and after glucose administration are very important in evaluation of the diabetic patient. Tests for glycosylated hemoglobin have proved useful in both initial evaluation and in assessment of the effectiveness of therapeutic management. In certain circumstances, measurements of insulin or C peptide levels and levels of other hormones involved in carbohydrate homeostasis (eg, glucagon, GH) may be useful. In view of the increased risk of atherosclerosis in diabetics, estimates of serum cholesterol, including its beneficial HDL fraction (HDL$_2$), and triglycerides may be helpful.

URINALYSIS

Glycosuria

Several problems are associated with using urine glucose as an index of blood glucose, regardless of the method employed. First of all, the glucose concentration in bladder urine reflects the blood glucose at the time the urine was formed. Therefore, the first voided specimen in the morning contains glucose that was excreted throughout the night and does not reflect the morning blood glucose at all. Some improvement in the correlation of urine glucose to blood glucose can be obtained if the patient "double voids"—that is, empties the bladder completely, discards that sample, and then urinates again about one-half hour later, testing only the second specimen for glucose content. However, difficulty in completely emptying the bladder (large residual volumes), problems in understanding the instructions, and the inconvenience impair the usefulness of this test. Self-monitoring of blood glucose has replaced urine glucose testing in most patients with IDDM and in many patients with NIDDM (particularly those receiving insulin therapy).

Several commercial products are available for determining the presence and amount of glucose in urine. The older and more cumbersome bedside assessment of glycosuria with Clinitest tablets has generally been replaced by the dipstick method, which is rapid, convenient, and glucose-specific. This method consists of paper strips (Clinistix, Diastix, Tes-Tape) impregnated with enzymes (glucose oxidase and hydrogen peroxidase) and a chromogenic dye that is colorless in the reduced state. Enzymatic generation of hydrogen peroxide oxidizes the dye to produce colors whose intensity depends on the glucose concentration. These dipsticks are sensitive to as little as 0.1% glucose (100 mg/dL) but do not react with the smaller amounts of glucose normally present in urine. The strips are subject to deterioration if exposed to air, moisture, and extreme heat and must be kept in tightly closed containers except when in use. False-negative results may be obtained in the presence of alkaptonuria and when certain substances such as salicylic acid or ascorbic acid are ingested in excess. All of these false-negative results occur because of the interference of strong reducing agents with oxidation of the chromogen.

Differential Diagnosis of Glycosuria (Sugar in the Urine)

Although glycosuria reflects hyperglycemia in over 90% of patients, 2 major classes of nondiabetic glycosuria must be considered:

A. Nondiabetic Glycosuria Due to Glucose: This occurs when glucose appears in the urine despite a normal amount of glucose in the blood. Disorders associated with abnormalities in renal glucose handling include Fanconi's syndrome (an autosomal dominant genetic disorder), dysfunction of the proximal renal tubule, chronic renal failure, and a benign familial disorder of the renal tubule manifest only by a defect in renal glucose reabsorption (occurs predominantly in males).

In addition, glycosuria is relatively common in pregnancy as a consequence of the increased load of glucose presented to the tubules by the elevated glomerular filtration rate during pregnancy. As many as 50% of pregnant women normally have demonstrable sugar in the urine, especially after the first trimester. This sugar is almost always glucose except during the late weeks of pregnancy, when lactose may be present (see below).

B. Nondiabetic Glycosuria Due to Sugars Other Than Glucose: Occasionally, a sugar other than glucose is excreted in the urine. Lactosuria during the late stages of pregnancy and the period of lactation is the most common example. Much rarer are other conditions in which inborn errors of metabolism allow fructose, galactose, or a pentose (1-xylose) to be excreted in the urine. Testing the urine with glucose-specific strips will help differentiate true glycosuria from other glycosurias.

Ketonuria

In the absence of adequate insulin, 3 major "ketone bodies" are formed and excreted into the urine: β-hydroxybutyric acid, acetoacetic acid, and acetone (see also Serum Ketone Determinations, below). Commercial products are available to test for the presence of ketones in the urine. Acetest tablets, Ketostix, and Keto-Diastix utilize a nitroprusside reaction that measures only acetone and acetoacetate. Therefore, these tests can be misleading if β-hydroxybutyric acid is the predominant ketone present. Ketostix and Keto-Diastix have short shelf-lives once the containers are opened and thus may give false-negative results.

Other conditions besides diabetic ketoacidosis may cause ketone bodies to appear in the urine; these include starvation, high-fat diets, alcoholic ketoacidosis, fever, and other conditions in which metabolic requirements are increased.

Proteinuria

Proteinuria as noted on a routine dipstick examination of the urine is often the first sign of renal complications of diabetes. If proteinuria is detected, a 24-hour urine collection should be analyzed to quantify the degree of proteinuria (normal individuals excrete < 150 mg of protein per day) and the rate of urinary creatinine excretion; at the same time, serum creatinine levels should be determined so that the creatinine clearance (an estimate of the glomerular filtration rate) can be calculated. In some cases, heavy proteinuria (3.5 g/d) develops later, along with other features of nephrotic syndrome such as edema, hypoalbuminemia, and hypercholesterolemia.

Microalbuminuria

Urinary albumin can now be detected in microgram concentrations using a radioimmunoassay method that is more sensitive than the dipstick method, whose minimal detection limit is 0.3–0.5%. Conventional 24-hour urine collections, in addition to being inconvenient for patients, also show wide variability of albumin excretion, since several factors such as sustained upright posture, dietary protein, and exercise tend to increase albumin excretion rates. For these reasons, many clinics prefer to screen patients with a timed *overnight* urine collection beginning at bedtime, when the urine is discarded and the time recorded. The collection is ended at the time the bladder is emptied the next morning, and this urine, as well as any other urine voided overnight, is assayed for albumin. Normal subjects excrete less than 15 μg/min during overnight urine collections; values of 20 μg/min or higher represent abnormal microalbuminuria, which may be an early predictor of the development of diabetic nephropathy.

BLOOD GLUCOSE TESTING

Normal Values

The normal fasting *whole blood* glucose varies from 60 to 110 mg/dL (3.3–6.1 mmol/L). Plasma or serum levels are 10–15% higher because structural components of blood cells are absent, so that more glucose is present per unit volume. Thus, the normal range of fasting plasma or serum glucose is 70–120 mg/dL (3.9–6.7 mmol/L). Plasma or serum glucose measurements are more frequently used clinically because they are independent of the hematocrit, more closely approach the glucose level in the interstitial tissue spaces, and lend themselves to automated analytic procedures. Whole blood glucose determinations are used in spot testing of glucose in emergency situations and also in the procedures for self-monitoring of capillary blood glucose, a technique that has become widely accepted in the management of diabetes mellitus (see below).

The accepted normal range of blood or plasma glucose requires a correction for age of 1 mg/dL (0.056 mmol/L) per year of age past 60. Thus, fasting plasma glucose in elderly nondiabetics will range from 80 to 150 mg/dL (4.4–8.3 mmol/L).

Venous Blood Samples

Samples should be collected in tubes containing sodium fluoride, which prevents glycolysis in the blood sample that would artifactually lower the measured glucose level. If such tubes are not available, samples must be centrifuged within 30 minutes of collection and the plasma or serum stored at 4 °C.

The laboratory methods regularly used for determining plasma glucose utilize enzymatic methods (such as glucose oxidase or hexokinase), colorimetric methods (such as o-toluidine), or automated methods. The automated methods utilize reduction of copper or iron compounds by reducing sugars in dialyzed serum. They are convenient but are not specific for glucose, since they react with other reducing substances (which are elevated in azotemia or with high ascorbic acid intake).

Capillary Blood Samples

There are several paper strip (glucose oxidase) methods for measuring capillary whole blood glucose. All have been adapted for use with portable, battery-operated reflectance meters that give a digital readout. One test strip kit, Chemstrip bG, provides a color chart for visual comparison and estimation of the blood glucose range. More conventional reflectance meters (eg, Glucometer, Glucoscan, Glucochek, Diascan, or Accuchek) require exact timing by the operator as well as careful removal of all traces of blood from the strip prior to reading the color. Newer devices (eg, One Touch, ExacTech) have eliminated these 2 potential sources of technical error by providing automatic timing and allowing colorimeter quantitation without removal of the blood. To monitor their own blood glucose levels, patients must prick their fingers with a small lancet (eg, Monolet), which can be facilitated by a small plastic trigger device (eg, Autolet, Penlet). With proper instruction in technique, patients can obtain accurate and reliable measurements of their own blood glucose levels, which are indispensable to the proper long-term management of their diabetes. These methods are also of great value to health care professionals in the management of seriously ill diabetic patients.

SERUM KETONE DETERMINATIONS

As noted above in the section on ketonuria, there are 3 major ketone bodies: β-hydroxybutyrate (often the most prevalent ketone in diabetic ketoacidosis), acetoacetate, and acetone. The same testing materials used for determining urine ketones may be used to measure serum (or plasma) ketones. When a few drops of serum are placed on a crushed Acetest tablet, the appearance of a purple color indicates the presence of ketones. A strongly positive reaction in undiluted serum correlates with a serum ketone concentration of at least 4 mmol/L. It must be kept in mind that Acetest tablets (as well as Ketostix and Keto-Diastix) utilize the nitroprusside reaction, which measures only acetoacetate and acetone. Specific enzymatic techniques are available to quantitate each of the ketone acids, but these techniques are cumbersome and not necessary in most clinical situations.

GLYCOSYLATED HEMOGLOBIN ASSAYS

Glycohemoglobin is produced by a ketoamine reaction between glucose and the N-terminal amino acid of both beta chains of the hemoglobin molecule. The major form of glycohemoglobin is hemoglobin A_{1c}, which normally comprises only 4–6% of total hemoglobin. The remaining glycohemoglobins (2–4% of total hemoglobin) contain phosphorylated glucose or fructose and are termed hemoglobin A_{1a} and A_{1b}, respectively. The hemoglobin A_{1c} fraction is abnormally elevated in diabetics with chronic hyperglycemia and appears to correlate positively with metabolic control. Specific assays for hemoglobin A_{1c} are technically less convenient than assays for total glycohemoglobin and offer little advantage for clinical purposes. Therefore, most laboratories measure the sum of these 3 glycohemoglobins and report it simply as hemoglobin A_1 or "glycohemoglobin."

The glycosylation of hemoglobin is dependent on the concentration of blood glucose. The reaction is not reversible, so that the half-life of glycosylated hemoglobin relates to the life span of red cells (which normally circulate for up to 120 days). Thus, glycohemoglobin generally reflects the state of glycemia over the preceding 8–12 weeks, thus providing a method of assessing chronic diabetic control. A glycosylated hemoglobin close to the normal range (5–8%) would reflect good control during the preceding 2–3 months, whereas a glycosylated hemoglobin in the range of 12–15% would reflect poor control during the same period.

Conditions Interfering With Glycohemoglobin Measurements (Table 22–10)

The most common laboratory error in measuring glycohemoglobins occurs when chromatographic methods measure an acutely generated intermediary aldimine in blood (prehemoglobin A_{1c}), which fluctuates directly with the prevailing blood glucose level. This artifact can falsely elevate glycohemoglobin by as much as 1–2% during an episode of acute hyperglycemia. It can be eliminated either by washing the red blood cells with saline prior to assay or by dialyzing the hemolysate prior to chromatography. Other substances that falsely elevate "glycohemoglobin" are carbamylated hemoglobin and hemoglobin F; the former is seen in association with uremia, and the latter circulates in some adults with genetic or hematologic

Table 22–10. Factors interfering with chromatographic measurement of glycohemoglobins.

Substances causing falsely high values
  Prehemoglobin A_{1c} (reversible aldimine intermediate)
  Carbamylated hemogloin (uremia)
  Hemoglobin F
Conditions causing falsely low values
  Hemoglobinopathies (hemoglobin C, D, and S)
  Reduced life span of erythrocytes
    Hemorrhage or therapeutic phlebotomies
    Hemolytic disorders

---

disorders. In these cases, more intricate methodology such as thiobarbituric acid colorimetry or isoelectric focusing is required to distinguish hemoglobin A_{1c} from the interfering substance.

Hemoglobinopathies such as those associated with hemoglobin C, D, and S will cause falsely low values, since their glycosylated products elute only partially from chromatographic columns. In addition, these hemoglobinopathies are often associated with hemolytic anemias that shorten the life span of red blood cells, thereby further lowering glycohemoglobin measurements. Falsely low values are also seen in patients with chronic or acute blood loss from hemorrhage or phlebotomies and in diabetic patients with hemochromatosis; under these conditions, measurements of glycohemoglobin are not valid for assessment of diabetic therapy.

Glycohemoglobin assays suffer from the lack of universally available reference standards. However, in a reliable laboratory where reversible aldimines (prehemoglobin A_{1c}) are routinely removed prior to chromatography, they are useful in assessing the effectiveness of diabetic therapy and particularly helpful in evaluating the reliability of a patient's self-monitoring records of urine or blood glucose values. A glycosylated hemoglobin test is presently being evaluated for diagnostic screening purposes, and while the test is generally too insensitive to rule out impaired glucose tolerance, a value above the normal range is generally a specific indicator of diabetes mellitus.

When abnormal hemoglobins or hemolytic states affect the interpretation of glycohemoglobin results or when a narrower time frame is required, eg, when ascertaining glycemic control at the time of conception in a diabetic woman who has recently become pregnant, serum fructosamine assays offer some advantage. Serum fructosamine is formed by nonenzymatic glycosylation of serum proteins (predominantly albumin). Since serum albumin has a much shorter half-life than hemoglobin, serum fructosamine generally reflects the state of glycemic control for only the preceding 2 weeks. In most circumstances, however, glycohemoglobin assays remain the preferred method for assessing long-term glycemic control in diabetic patients.

CAPILLARY MORPHOMETRY

The basement membrane of capillaries from skeletal muscle tissue of the quadriceps area is abnormally thickened in adults with overt spontaneous diabetes (fasting hyperglycemia of 140 mg/dL [7.8 mmol/L] or more). Capillary morphometry appears to be less discriminatory in diabetic children, being normal in as many as 60% of those below age 18. Evidence of the reversibility of capillary basement membrane thickening after near-normalization of glycemia with intensive therapy suggests that this thickening in diabetes is a consequence of long-term hyperglycemia, although the rapidity and severity of its progression may vary according to an individual's genetic predisposition.

DIAGNOSIS OF DIABETES MELLITUS

SIMPLE DIAGNOSTIC TEST BY FASTING PLASMA GLUCOSE

A fasting plasma glucose value above 140 mg/dL (7.8 mmol/L) on more than one occasion establishes the diagnosis of diabetes mellitus. The sample for fasting plasma glucose is best drawn in the morning after an overnight fast.

ORAL GLUCOSE TOLERANCE TEST

An oral glucose tolerance test is only rarely indicated, since the criteria for a positive test are still poor, being based on a nonhospitalized group of active young people who are not really comparable to any bedridden, ill, or aging population. In the past, oral glucose tolerance testing led to the overdiagnosis of diabetes. The much more rigid criteria currently recommended (see interpretation, below) should alleviate this tendency for overdiagnosis and improve the utility of the test.

If the fasting plasma glucose is between 120 and 140 mg/dL, an oral glucose tolerance test may be considered, especially in men with impotence or women who have delivered infants above 9 lb (4.1 kg) birth weight or have had recurrent vaginal yeast infections.

Preparation for Test

In order to optimize insulin secretion and effectiveness, especially when patients have been on a low-carbohydrate diet, a minimum of 150–200 g of carbohydrate per day should be included in the diet for 3 days preceding the test. The patient should eat nothing after midnight prior to the test day.

Testing Procedure

Adults are given 75 g of glucose in 300 mL of water; children are given 1.75 g of glucose per kilogram of ideal body weight. The glucose load is consumed within 5 minutes. Blood samples for plasma glucose are obtained at 0, 30, 60, 90, and 120 minutes after ingestion of glucose.

Interpretation

An oral glucose tolerance test is normal if the fasting venous plasma glucose value is less than 115 mg/dL (6.4 mmol/L), the 2-hour value falls below 140 mg/dL (7.8 mmol/L), and the value in none of the samples exceeds 200 mg/dL (11.1 mmol/L). A 2-hour value of greater than 200 mg/dL (11.1 mmol/L) in addition to one other value greater than 200 mg/dL (11.1 mmol/L) is diagnostic of diabetes mellitus. The diagnosis of "impaired glucose tolerance" is reserved for values between the upper limits of normal and those values diagnostic for diabetes. False-positive results may occur in patients who are malnourished at test time, bedridden, or afflicted with an infection or severe emotional stress. Diuretics, oral contraceptives, glucocorticoids, excess thyroxine, phenytoin, nicotinic acid, and some of the psychotropic drugs may also cause false-positive results.

INSULIN LEVELS

To measure insulin levels during the glucose tolerance test, serum or plasma must be separated within 30 minutes after collection of the specimen and frozen prior to assay. Normal immunoreactive insulin levels range from 5–20 μU/mL in the fasting state, reach 50–130 μU/mL at 1 hour, and usually return to levels below 30 μU/mL by 2 hours. Insulin levels are rarely of clinical usefulness during glucose tolerance testing for the following reasons: When fasting glucose levels exceed 120 mg/dL (6.7 mmol/L), B cells generally have reduced responsiveness to further degrees of hyperglycemia regardless of the type of diabetes. When fasting glucose levels are below 120 mg/dL (6.7 mmol/L), late hyperinsulinism may occur as a result of insulin resistance in type II diabetes; however, it also may occur even in mild forms or in the early phases of type I diabetes when sluggish early insulin release results in late hyperglycemia that may stimulate excessive insulin secretion at 2 hours.

INTRAVENOUS GLUCOSE TOLERANCE TEST

The intravenous glucose tolerance test is performed by giving a rapid infusion of glucose followed by serial plasma glucose measurements to determine the disappearance rate of glucose per minute. The disappearance rate reflects the patient's ability to dispose of a glucose load. This test is generally used to evaluate glucose tolerance in patients with gastrointestinal abnormalities (such as malabsorption). Caution should be used in interpreting the results, because the test bypasses normal glucose absorption and associated changes in gastrointestinal hormones that are important in carbohydrate metabolism. Furthermore, the test is relatively insensitive, and adequate criteria for diagnosis of diabetes have not been established for the various age groups.

Preparation for Test

Preparation is the same as for the oral glucose tolerance test (see above).

Testing Procedure

Intravenous access is established, and the patient is given a bolus of 50 g of glucose per 1.7 m^2 body surface area (or 0.5 g/kg of ideal body weight) as a 25% or 50% solution over 2–3 minutes. Timing begins with injection. Samples for plasma glucose determination are obtained from an indwelling needle in the opposite arm at 0, 10, 15, 20, and 30 minutes. The plasma glucose values are plotted on semilogarithmic paper against time. K, a rate constant that reflects the rate of fall of blood glucose in percent per minute, is calculated by determining the time necessary for the glucose concentration to fall by one-half ($t_{1/2}$) and using the following equation:

$$K \text{ (glucose)} = \frac{0.693}{t_{1/2}} \times 100$$

The average K value for a nondiabetic patient is approximately 1.72% per minute; this value declines with age but remains above 1.3% per minute. Diabetic patients almost always have a K value of less than 1% per minute.

TREATMENT OF DIABETES

Rational therapy of diabetes requires the application of principles derived from current knowledge concerning both the nature of the particular type of diabetes and the mechanism of action, efficacy, and safety of the available treatment regimens: diet, oral hypoglycemic drugs, and insulin. Controversy continues about what constitutes the best therapeutic regimen. Fundamental to this controversy is the still conflicting evidence about whether microangiopathy is related exclusively to the existence and duration of hyperglycemia or whether it reflects a separate coexisting genetic disorder. The weight of current evidence tends to favor the former view, though a genetic predisposition may potentiate glucotoxic manifestations.

The recommendations of the Executive Committee of the American Diabetes Association are to try to restore known metabolic derangements to normal in an attempt to retard (if not prevent) the progression of microvascular disease. One should aim at simulating a normal physiologic status by administering insulin in such a manner as to provide a continuous low basal level of circulating insulin and produce an 8- to 10-fold rise in plasma insulin concentration with the average meal. Care should be taken to avoid administration of excessive insulin that might down-regulate the insulin receptors in target tissues or induce hypoglycemia that will then call forth insulin antagonists which would reduce subsequent insulin activity. To achieve these goals, the patient, in cooperation with the physician, must make adjustments in diet, exercise, and, if indicated, hypoglycemic agents.

AVAILABLE TREATMENT REGIMENS

1. DIET

A proper diet remains a fundamental element of therapy in all patients with diabetes. However, in over half of cases, diabetics fail to follow their diet. The reasons include unnecessary complexity of dietary instructions and poor understanding of the goals of dietary control by the patient and physician.

Exchange lists for meal planning can be obtained from the American Diabetes Association (ADA; 1660 Duke Street, Alexandria, Virginia 22314) and its affiliate associations or from the American Dietetic Association (430 North Michigan Avenue, Chicago 60611). The ADA diet stresses caloric restriction as the major method of achieving or maintaining ideal weight, with a fat intake of 35% or less of total calories. Furthermore, it is recommended that saturated fat be reduced to only one-third of this amount by substitution of unsaturated fats for saturated fats and by substitution of poultry, veal, and fish for red meats as the major protein source. At the same time, cholesterol is restricted to less than 300 mg daily. Complex carbohydrates may be consumed liberally (as much as 50% of total calories) as long as refined and simple sugars are limited.

Prescribing the Diet

A. Type I Diabetes (IDDM): In type I diabetes, total calories are calculated to maintain ideal body weight. In the typical patient, insulin is administered at least twice a day, often as a mixture of a short-acting and an intermediate-acting insulin. Meals should be adjusted accordingly in an effort to match food intake with insulin action. Breakfast should be eaten within $\frac{1}{2}$–1 hour of the morning insulin dose (especially if short-acting insulin is administered at this time). A

carbohydrate snack should be eaten 3 hours later and lunch no later than 5 hours after the morning insulin dose. A midafternoon carbohydrate snack is given 7–8 hours after the morning insulin. Dinner should follow the second injection by $\frac{1}{2}$–$1\frac{1}{2}$ hours, depending on whether a short-acting insulin is administered at this time. A bedtime snack high in protein and low in carbohydrate should be given 3 hours after the evening insulin in order to provide a slow influx of carbohydrate from metabolized protein during most of the night. When multiple insulin injections are prescribed, greater flexibility with regard to timing of meals is possible.

B. Type II Diabetes (NIDDM): In type II diabetes, patients are often at least mildly obese. Treatment requires a vigorous program to achieve weight reduction. A fall in fasting blood sugar may follow caloric restriction prior to any significant weight loss. Weight reduction is an elusive goal that can be achieved and maintained only by close supervision of the obese patient and a supervised exercise program. The total amount of calories prescribed must take into account the patient's ideal body weight, life-style, and activity level. A diet consisting of no more than 600 kcal daily may be appropriate for a sedentary patient who is overweight, but a mildly active person can lose weight on a diet of up to 1400 kcal.

Special Considerations in Dietary Control

A. Dietary Fiber: Plant components such as cellulose, gum, and pectin are indigestible by humans and are termed dietary "fiber." **Insoluble fibers** such as cellulose or hemicellulose, as found in bran, tend to increase intestinal transit time and may have beneficial effects on colonic function. In contrast, **soluble fibers** such as gums and pectins, as found in beans, oatmeal, or apple skin, tend to decrease gastric and intestinal transit so that glucose absorption is slower and hyperglycemia is diminished. Although the ADA diet does not require insoluble fiber supplements such as added bran, it recommends foods such as oatmeal, cereals, and beans with relatively high soluble fiber content as stable components of the diet in diabetics. High soluble fiber content in the diet may also have a favorable effect on blood cholesterol levels.

B. Glycemic Index: Jenkins et al have attempted to quantitate the relative glycemic contribution of different carbohydrate foods and have suggested the use of a "glycemic index" (GI) in which the area of blood glucose (plotted on a graph) generated over a 3-hour period following ingestion of a test food containing 50 g of carbohydrate is compared with the area plotted after giving a similar quantity of reference food such as glucose or white bread:

$$GI = \frac{\text{Blood glucose area of test food}}{\text{Blood glucose area of reference food}} \times 100$$

White bread is preferred to glucose as a reference standard because it is more palatable and has less tendency to slow gastric emptying by high tonicity, as happens when glucose solution is used.

Differences in GI were noted in normal subjects and diabetics when various foods were compared. In comparison to white bread, which was assigned an index of 100, the mean GI for other foods was as follows: baked potato, 135; table sugar (sucrose), 86; spaghetti, 66; kidney beans, 54; ice cream, 52; and lentils, 43. Some investigators have questioned whether the GI for a food ingested alone is meaningful, since the GI may become altered considerably by the presence of fats and protein when the food is consumed in a mixed meal.

Further studies of the reproducibility of the GI in the same person and the relation of a particular food's GI to its insulinotropic action on pancreatic B cells are needed before the utility of the GI in prescribing diabetic diets can be appropriately assessed. At present, however, it appears that small amounts of sucrose—particularly when taken with high-fiber substances such as cereals or whole-grain breads—may have no greater glycemic effects than comparable portions of starch from potatoes, rice, or bread.

C. Sweeteners: The nonnutritive sweetener **saccharin** continues to be available in certain foods and beverages despite recent warnings by the FDA about its potential long-term bladder carcinogenicity. A committee of the National Academy of Sciences recommended restrictions in the use of saccharin in children and pregnant women. The panel felt that physicians might be best suited to determine on an individual basis its comparative benefit versus risk for patients with diabetes or obesity.

Aspartame may prove to be the safest sweetener for use in diabetics; it consists of 2 major amino acids, aspartic acid and phenylalanine, which combine to produce a nutritive sweetener 180 times as sweet as sucrose. A major limitation is its heat lability, which precludes its use in baking or cooking.

Other sweeteners such as sorbitol and fructose have recently gained popularity. Except for acute diarrhea induced by ingestion of large amounts of sorbitol-containing foods, their relative risk has yet to be established. **Fructose** represents a "natural" sugar substance that is a highly effective sweetener which induces only slight increases in plasma glucose levels and does not require insulin for its utilization.

D. Starch Blockers: The FDA has decided that enzymatic antagonists of amylase and sucrase (alpha-glucosidase inhibitors) can no longer be classified as "foods" but must be classified as drugs. At present, clinical trials are in progress to ascertain the efficacy and safety of these substances in reducing postprandial hyperglycemia in diabetes. They have not proved effective as an adjunct to weight reduction in the management of obesity.

2. ORAL HYPOGLYCEMIC DRUGS (Sulfonylureas & Biguanides)

There are 2 major types of oral hypoglycemic drugs: the sulfonylureas and the biguanides. The modes of action of the 2 types are quite different. In 1977, the United States Department of Health, Education, and Welfare recommended discontinuing general use of phenformin, the only biguanide available in the USA. It was considered to be a health hazard because of its reported association with the development of lactic acidosis. Recently, clinical trials with another biguanide, metformin, have been initiated. This agent is said to be less likely to produce lactic acidosis.

Sulfonylureas

Currently, the sulfonylureas are the only oral hypoglycemic drugs approved for use in the USA. This group of drugs contains a sulfonic acid–urea nucleus that can be modified by chemical substitutions to produce agents that have similar qualitative actions but differ widely in potency. The proposed mechanisms of action of the sulfonylureas include (1) augmentation of insulin release from pancreatic B cells and (2) increased insulin binding to insulin receptors.

A. Mechanism of Action: Specific receptors on the surface of pancreatic B cells bind sulfonylureas in the rank order of their insulinotropic potency (glyburide with the greatest affinity and tolbutamide with the least). It has been proposed that activation of these receptors closes potassium channels, resulting in depolarization of the B cell. This depolarized state permits calcium to enter the cell and actively promote insulin release. Controversy persists, however, whether this well-documented insulinotropic action during acute administration is sufficient to explain adequately the hypoglycemic effect of sulfonylureas during chronic therapy. Additional extrapancreatic effects of sulfonylureas, such as their potentiation of the peripheral effects of insulin at the receptor or postreceptor level, have been invoked to account for their continued effectiveness during long-term treatment despite a lack of demonstrable increase in insulin secretion. However, several clinical trials have failed to demonstrate any therapeutic benefit on long-term glycemic control when sulfonylureas are added to insulin therapy in the patient with IDDM. These observations suggest that in vitro evidence for a potentiation by sulfonylureas of the peripheral effects of insulin may have little clinical relevance.

B. Indications: Sulfonylureas are not indicated in ketosis-prone type I diabetic patients, since these drugs require functioning pancreatic B cells to produce their effect on blood glucose. Moreover, clinical trials show no benefit from the use of sulfonylureas as an adjunct to insulin replacement in type I diabetic patients. The sulfonylureas seem most appropriate for use in the nonobese patient with mild maturity-onset diabetes whose hyperglycemia has not responded to diet therapy. In obese patients with mild diabetes and slight to moderate peripheral insensitivity to levels of circulating insulin, the primary emphasis should be on weight reduction. When hyperglycemia in obese diabetics has been more severe, with consequent impairment of pancreatic B cell function, sulfonylureas may improve glycemic control until concurrent measures such as diet, exercise, and weight reduction can sustain the improvement without the need for oral drugs.

C. Sulfonylureas Currently Available in the USA: (See Table 22–11.)

1. Tolbutamide (Orinase)–Tolbutamide is supplied in tablets of 250 and 500 mg. It is rapidly oxidized in the liver to an inactive form. Because its duration of effect is short (6–10 hours), it is usually administered in divided doses (eg, 500 mg before each meal and at bedtime). The usually daily dose is 1.5–3 g; some patients, however, require only 250–500 mg daily. Acute toxic reactions are rare, with skin rashes occurring most commonly. Because of its short duration of action, which is independent of renal function, tolbutamide is probably the safest agent to use in elderly patients in whom hypoglycemia would be a particularly serious risk. Prolonged hypoglycemia has been reported rarely, mainly in patients receiving certain drugs (eg, dicumarol, phenylbutazone, or sulfonamides) that compete with sulfonylureas for hepatic oxidation, resulting in maintenance of high levels of unmetabolized active sulfonylureas in the circulation.

2. Chlorpropamide (Diabinese)–This drug is supplied in tablets of 100 and 250 mg. It has a half-life of 32 hours and a duration of action of up to 60 hours. It is slowly metabolized by the liver, with approximately 20–30% excreted unchanged in the urine. Since the metabolites retain hypoglycemic activity, elimination of the biologic effect is almost completely dependent on renal excretion, so that its use is contraindicated in patients with renal insufficiency. The average maintenance dose is 250 mg daily (range, 100–500 mg), given as a single dose in the morning. Chlorpropamide is a potent agent that is occasionally effective in controlling hyperglycemia in NIDDM despite the failure of maximum therapeutic doses of other less potent sulfonylureas such as tolbutamide, tolazamide, and acetohexamide. A potential hazard in the use of this drug is development of prolonged hypoglycemia, which occurs more commonly with the use of chlorpropamide than with the shorter-acting oral hypoglycemic agents. Elderly patients, especially those with reduced renal function, are at greatest risk for development of hypoglycemia with chlorpropamide, and the drug should probably not be used in patients over 65 years of age. Doses in excess of 500 mg/d increase the risk of jaundice, which does not occur with the usual dose of 250 mg or less. About 15% of patients taking chlorpropamide develop a facial flush when they drink alcohol, and occasionally they may develop a full-blown disulfiramlike reaction, with nausea, vomiting, weakness, and even syncope. There appears to be a genetic predisposition to the development of this reaction.

Other side effects of chlorpropamide include water retention and the development of hyponatremia, effects that are mediated through an ADH mechanism. The hyponatremia is generally a benign condition with

Table 22–11. Sulfonylureas.[1]

	Chemical Structure	Daily Dose	Duration of Action (hours)
Tolbutamide (Orinase)	H_3C—〈 〉—SO_2—NH—C(=O)—NH—$(CH_2)_3$—CH_3	1500–3000 mg in divided doses	6–12
Tolazamide (Tolinase)	H_3C—〈 〉—SO_2—NH—C(=O)—NH—N〈 〉	200–1000 mg as single dose or in divided doses	12–24
Acetohexamide (Dymelor)	H_3C—C(=O)—〈 〉—SO_2—NH—C(=O)—NH—〈 〉	250–1500 mg as single dose or in divided doses	12–24
Chlorpropamide (Diabinese)	Cl—〈 〉—SO_2—NH—C(=O)—NH—$(CH_2)_2$—CH_3	100–500 as single dose	Up to 60
Glyburide (glibenclamide; DiaBeta, Micronase)	Cl, C(=O)—NH—$(CH_2)_2$—〈 〉—SO_2—NH—C(=O)—NH—〈 〉, OCH_3	2.5–20 mg	10–24
Glipizide (glydiazinamide; Glucotrol)	N, H_3C, C(=O)—NH—$(CH_2)_2$—〈 〉—SO_2—NH—C(=O)—NH—〈 〉	2.5–40 mg	3–8

[1] Modified slightly and reproduced, with permission, from Katzung BG (editor): *Basic & Clinical Pharmacology*, 2nd ed. Lange, 1984.

sodium values between 125 and 130 meq/L, but occasional cases of symptomatic hyponatremia with sodium concentrations below 125 meq/L have been reported, particularly when concomitant diuretic therapy is being used. Chlorpropamide stimulates ADH secretion and also potentiates its action at the renal tubule. Its antidiuretic effect is somewhat unusual, since 3 other sulfonylureas (acetohexamide, tolazamide, and glyburide) appear to facilitate water excretion in humans. Hematologic toxicity (transient leukopenia, thrombocytopenia) occurs in less than 1% of patients.

3. Tolazamide (Tolinase)–Tolazamide is supplied in tablets of 100, 250, and 500 mg. The average daily dose is 200–1000 mg, given in one or 2 doses. It is comparable to chlorpropamide in potency but is devoid of disulfiramlike or water-retaining effects. Tolazamide is more slowly absorbed than the other sulfonylureas, with effects on blood glucose not appearing for several hours. Its duration of action may last up to 20 hours, with maximal hypoglycemic effect occurring between the fourth and 14th hours. Tolazamide is metabolized to several compounds that retain hypoglycemic effects. If more than 500 mg/d is required, the dose should be divided and given twice daily. Doses larger than 1000 mg/d do not improve the degree of glycemic control.

4. Acetohexamide (Dymelor)–This agent is supplied in tablets of 250 and 500 mg. Its duration of action is about 10–16 hours (intermediate in duration of action between tolbutamide and chlorpropamide). The usual daily dose is 250–1500 mg given in one or 2 doses. Liver metabolism is rapid, but an active metabolite is produced and excreted by the kidney.

5. Second-generation sulfonylureas–In April, 1984, the FDA approved 2 potent sulfonylurea compounds, glyburide and glipizide. These agents have similar chemical structures, with cyclic carbon rings at each end of the sulfonylurea nucleus; this causes them to be highly potent (100-fold more potent than tolbutamide). The drugs should be used with caution in patients with cardiovascular disease as well as in elderly patients, in whom hypoglycemia would be especially dangerous. Neither glyburide nor glipizide should be prescribed to patients with hepatic or renal impairment, since a reduced clearance of these drugs from the blood would greatly increase the risk of hypoglycemia.

Diabetic patients who have not responded to tolbutamide or even tolazamide often—but not always—respond to the more potent first-generation sulfonylurea, chlorpropamide, or to either of the second-generation sulfonylureas. Unfortunately, substantial glycemic benefit has not always resulted when a maximum therapeutic dose of chlorpropamide or tolazamide has been replaced with that of a second-generation drug.

a. Glyburide (glibenclamide; DiaBeta, Micronase)–Glyburide is supplied in tablets containing 1.25, 2.5, and 5 mg. The usual starting dose is 2.5 mg/d, and the average maintenance dose is 5–10 mg/d

given as a single morning dose. If patients are going to respond to glyburide, they generally do so at doses of 10 mg/d or less, given once daily. If they fail to respond to 10 mg/d, it is uncommon for an increase in dosage to result in improved glycemic control. Maintenance doses higher than 20 mg/d are not recommended. Glyburide is metabolized in the liver into products with such low hypoglycemic activity that they are considered clinically unimportant. Although assays specific for the unmetabolized compound suggest a plasma half-life of only 1–2 hours, the biologic effects of glyburide clearly persist for 24 hours after a single morning dose in diabetic patients.

Glyburide does not cause water retention, as chlorpropamide does, and even slightly enhances free water clearance. Glyburide has few adverse effects other than its potential for causing hypoglycemia. It is particularly hazardous in patients over 65 years of age, in whom serious, protracted, and even fatal hypoglycemia can occur even with relatively small daily doses. Drugs with a shorter half-life, eg, tolbutamide or possibly glipizide, are preferable in the treatment of type II diabetes in the elderly patient.

b. Glipizide (glydiazinamide; Glucotrol)– Glipizide is supplied in tablets containing 5 and 10 mg. For maximum effect in reducing postprandial hyperglycemia, this agent should be ingested 30 minutes before breakfast, since rapid absorption is delayed when the drug is taken with food. The recommended starting dose is 5 mg/d, with up to 15 mg/d given as a single daily dose. When higher daily doses are required, they should be divided and given before meals. The maximum recommended dose is 40 mg/d.

At least 90% of glipizide is metabolized in the liver to inactive products, and 10% is excreted unchanged in the urine. Glipizide therapy is thus contraindicated in patients who have hepatic or renal impairment and who would therefore be at high risk for hypoglycemia, but because of its lower potency and shorter half-life, it is preferable to glyburide in elderly patients.

Biguanides

Unlike sulfonylureas, the biguanides (Table 22–12) do not require functioning pancreatic B cells for reduction of hyperglycemia. They are believed to act by retarding absorption of nutrients from the intestine, decreasing hepatic gluconeogenesis, and facilitating insulin binding to receptors on insulin target tissues. Use of **phenformin** was discontinued in the USA because of its association with the development of lactic acidosis in patients with coexisting liver or kidney disease. Also of note was lack of documentation of any long-term efficacy of this drug in treating diabetes. Biguanides continue to be used in many countries throughout the world. **Metformin,** a biguanide reported to be less likely to produce lactic acidosis, has generally replaced phenformin in the treatment of diabetiels.

Table 22–12. Biguanides in clinical use outside the USA.[1]

	$R-\underset{\underset{NH}{\|}}{C}-\underset{\|}{\overset{\overset{H}{\underset{\|}{N}}}{}}-\underset{\underset{NH}{\|}}{C}-NH_2$	Daily Dose	Duration of Action (hours)
Phenformin	⬡—$(CH_2)_2$—NH—	0.05–0.1 g as single dose or in divided doses as timed disintegration capsules	8–14
Buformin	$CH_3-(CH_2)_3$—NH—	0.05–0.3 g in divided doses	...
Metformin	$(CH_3)_2$—N—	1–3 g in divided doses	...

*Reproduced, with permission, from Katzung BG (editor): *Basic & Clinical Pharmacology,* 2nd ed. Lange, 1984.

Efficacy & Safety of Oral Hypoglycemic Agents

The University Group Diabetes Program (UGDP) reported that the number of deaths due to cardiovascular disease in diabetic patients treated with tolbutamide or phenformin was excessive when compared to either insulin-treated patients or to patients receiving placebos. Controversy persists about the validity of the conclusions reached by the UGDP because of the heterogeneity of the population studied, its preponderance of obese subjects, and certain features of the experimental design, such as the use of a fixed dose of oral drug and lack of control for cigarette smoking. At present, a warning label outlining their cardiovascular risk is inserted in each packet of sulfonylureas dispensed. However, the ADA places no restrictions on their use.

3. INSULIN

Insulin is indicated for type I diabetics as well as for those type II diabetics whose hyperglycemia does not respond to diet therapy and oral hypoglycemic drugs.

Insulin replacement in patients with type I diabetes has been less than optimal because it is not possible to completely reproduce the normal physiologic pattern of insulin secretion into the portal vein. The problem of achieving optimal insulin delivery remains unsolved with the present state of technology. Subcutaneous injections do not reproduce the physiologic patterns of insulin secretion; however, with the help of appropriate modifications of diet and exercise and careful monitoring of capillary blood glucose levels at home, it is possible to achieve acceptable control of blood glucose by using multiple injections of mixtures of short- and intermediate-acting insulins. In some patients, a portable insulin infusion pump or a single injection of a long-acting insulin may be required for optimal control.

With the development of highly purified human insulin preparations, immunogenicity has been markedly reduced, thereby decreasing the incidence of therapeutic complications such as insulin allergy, immune insulin resistance, and localized lipoatrophy at the injection site.

Characteristics of Currently Available Insulin Preparations

Commercial insulin preparations differ with regard to the animal species from which they are obtained; their purity, concentration, and solubility; and their time of onset and duration of biologic action (Tables 22–13 and 22–14; Fig 22–10). In 1988 more than 40 different formations of insulin were available in the USA.

A. Species of Insulin: Because the supply of human or pork insulin is too limited to satisfy the demand for insulin in the USA, most commercial insulins are composed of beef insulin or mixtures of beef and pork insulin. Beef insulin, which differs by 3 amino acids from human insulin, is more antigenic than pork insulin, which differs from human insulin by just one amino acid. The standard preparation of Iletin I (Lilly) is a mixture of 70% beef and 30% pork insulin, whereas the highly purified Iletin II insulins are available as either beef or pork insulin. Human insulin can now be

Table 22–13. Summary of bioavailability characteristics of the insulins.

	Insulin Type	Onset	Peak Action	Duration
Short-acting	Regular, Actrapid, Velosulin	15–30 minutes	1–3 hours	5–7 hours
	Semilente, Semitard	30–60 minutes	4–6 hours	12–16 hours
Intermediate-acting	Lente, Lentard, Monotard	2–4 hours	8–10 hours	18–24 hours
	NPH, Insulatard, Protaphane			
Long-acting	Ultralente, Ultratard, PZI	4–5 hours	8–14 hours	25–36 hours

Table 22–14. Insulin preparations available in the USA.[1]

	Species Source	Concentration
Short-acting		
Standard[2]		
Regular Iletin I (Lilly)	Beef and pork	U40, U100
Regular (Novo Nordisk)	Pork	U40, U100
Semilente Iletin I (Lilly)	Beef and pork	U40, U100
Semilente (Novo Nordisk)	Beef	U40, U100
"Purified"[3]		
Regular Humulin (Lilly)	Human	U100
Regular Iletin II (Lilly)	Pork or beef	U100, U500[4]
Novolin-R (Novo Nordisk)	Human	U100
Velosulin (Nordisk)	Pork or human	U100
Semitard (Novo Nordisk)	Pork	U100
Intermediate-acting		
Standard[2]		
NPH Iletin I (Lilly)	Beef and pork	U40, U100
Lente Iletin I (Lilly)	Beef and pork	U40, U100
Isophane NPH (Novo Nordisk)	Beef and pork	U40, U100
Lente (Novo Nordisk)	Beef	U40, U100
"Purified"[3]		
NPH Humulin (Lilly)	Human	U100
NPH Iletin II (Lilly)	Pork or beef	U100
Lente Humulin (Lilly)	Human	U100
Lente Iletin II (Lilly)	Pork or beef	U100
Novolin-N (NPH) (Novo Nordisk)	Human	U100
Lentard (Novo Nordisk)	Beef and pork	U100
Novolin-L (Lente) (Novo Nordisk)	Human	U100
Insulatard NPH (Nordisk)	Pork or human	U100
Pre-mixed Insulins		
Mixtard (Nordisk)	Pork or human	U100
Novolin 70:30 (Novo Nordisk)	Human	U100
Humulin-70:30 (Lilly)	Human	U100
Long-acting		
Standard[2]		
Ultralente Iletin I (Lilly)	Beef and pork	U40, U100
PZI Iletin I (Lilly)	Beef and pork	U40, U100
Ultralente (Novo Nordisk)	Beef	U100
PZI (Novo Nordisk)	Beef and pork	U40, U100
"Purified"[3]		
PZI Iletin II (Lilly)	Pork or beef	U100
Ultratard (Novo Nordisk)	Beef	U100
Humulin-U (Lilly)	Human	U100

[1]Modified and reproduced, with permission, from Krupp MA, Chatton MJ, Tierney LM Jr (editors): *Current Medical Diagnosis & Treatment 1986.* Lange, 1986.
[2]Greater than 10 but less than 25 ppm proinsulin.
[3]Less than 10 ppm proinsulin.
[4]U500 available only as pork insulin.

produced by recombinant DNA techniques (biosynthetic human insulin) or by enzymatic conversion of pork insulin to human insulin (semisynthetic human insulin), in which alanine, the terminal amino acid on the beta chain of pork insulin, is replaced by threonine. Human insulin prepared by the recombinant DNA method is available for clinical use as Humulin (Lilly) and dispensed as either Regular(R), NPH(N), or Lente(L). Human insulin prepared by enzymatic conversion of pork insulin is marketed as Novolin by Novo Nordisk and as Velosulin-Human by Nordisk. Novolin-R is a rapid-acting soluble form of human insulin. Novolin-L is a zinc suspension with an intermediate duration of action similar to that of Novolin-N, which is an isophane suspension of human insulin with protamine. Since human insulin tends to be slightly more hydrophilic than beef insulin, an ultralente formulation of human insulin with the required degree of insolubility characteristic of beef insulin has only recently been produced.

B. Purity of Insulin: (Table 22–14.) Improvements in purification techniques with Sephadex gel columns have reduced or eliminated contamination with proteins having molecular weights greater than that of insulin (eg, proinsulin). Although these contaminants were biologically inactive, they were capable of inducing anti-insulin antibodies. The degree of purification in which proinsulin contamination is greater than 10 ppm but less than 25 ppm justifies their present labeling as "new improved single peak insulin." When the proinsulin content is reduced to less than 10 ppm, manufacturers are entitled by FDA regulations to label the insulin **"purified."** These "purified" insulins are generally available as a monospecies of pork or beef or human insulin (Table 22–14); however, a monocomponent beef and pork mixture is also available (Lentard, Novo Nordisk).

The more highly purified insulins currently in use preserve their potency quite well; therefore, refrigeration while in use is not necessary. During travel, reserve supplies of insulin can be readily transported for weeks without significant loss of potency provided they are protected from extremes of heat or cold.

Concentrations of Insulin

At present, most insulins in the USA are available in a concentration of 100 units/mL (U100); all are dispensed in 10-mL vials. To accommodate children and the occasional adult who may require small quantities of insulin, a U40 (40 units/mL) insulin continues to be available. However, with the popularity of the "low-dose" (0.5-mL and 0.3-mL) disposable insulin syringes, there is less need for U40 insulin, since U100 can now be measured accurately in doses as low as 1 or 2 units. For use in rare cases of severe insulin resistance in which large quantities of insulin are required, a limited supply of U500 (500 units/mL) regular insulin is available from Lilly (pork, Iletin II).

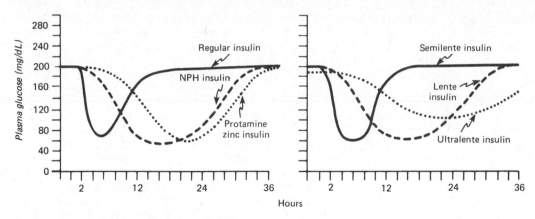

Figure 22–10. Extent and duration of action of various types of insulin (in a fasting diabetic). (Reproduced, with permission, from Katzung BG [editor]: *Basic & Clinical Pharmacology,* 2nd ed. Lange, 1984.)

Bioavailability Characteristics

Three principal types of insulin are available: (1) short-acting insulin, with rapid onset of action; (2) intermediate-acting; and (3) long-acting, with slow onset of action (Table 22–13; Fig 11–10). Short-acting (unmodified) insulin is a crystalline zinc insulin with a neutral pH in soluble form; it is dispensed as a *clear* solution. All other commercial insulins have been specifically modified to obtain more prolonged action. They are dispensed as opaque suspensions at neutral pH with either protamine (derived from fish sperm) in phosphate buffer (protamine zinc insulin and NPH) or varying concentrations of zinc in acetate buffer (ultralente, semilente, and lente insulins), rendering the insulin insoluble.

As noted above, conventional insulin therapy relies on combinations of short-acting and either intermediate-acting or long-acting insulin. The characteristics of these various insulins are discussed below and summarized in Table 22–13. It is important to recognize that values given for time of onset of action, peak effect, and duration of action are only approximate ones and that there is great variability in these parameters from patient to patient and even in a given patient depending on the size of the dose, the site of injection, the degree of exercise, the avidity of circulating anti-insulin antibodies, and other less well defined variables.

A. Short-Acting Insulins:

1. Regular insulin–Regular insulins (Regular Iletin I or II, or Humulin [Lilly], Insulin Injection Actrapid or Novolin-R [Novo Nordisk], Velosulin [Nordisk]) are short-acting, soluble crystalline zinc insulins whose hypoglycemic effect appears within 15 minutes after subcutaneous injection, peaks at 1–3 hours, and lasts for about 5–7 hours when usual quantities, eg, 5–15 units, are administered. Regular insulin is the only type that can be administered intravenously or used in continuous subcutaneous infusion pumps. It is particularly useful in the treatment of dia-

betic ketoacidosis and when the insulin requirement is changing rapidly, such as after surgery or during acute infections.

Regular insulin produced by Squibb-Novo and Lilly is dispensed without a buffer, but when it is used in reservoirs or infusion pumps, stability is improved when regular insulin is buffered with disodium phosphate, as in Velosulin (Nordisk). A special formation of Humulin Buffered Regular (Lilly) is designated for use only in infusion pumps.

2. Semilente Insulin–(Semilente [Lilly], Semitard [Novo Nordisk]) These insulins are an amorphous (or microcrystalline) form of insulin and zinc in acetate buffer. The onset of action is 30–60 minutes, peak action is reached at 6 hours, and the duration of action is 12–16 hours. Most physicians prefer to prescribe regular insulin rather than the semilente series, because of the more prompt onset of action of regular insulin when injected before meals.

B. Intermediate-Acting Insulins:

1. Lente insulin–This is a mixture of 30% semilente with 70% ultralente insulin (Lente Iletin I and II and Humulin-L [Lilly], Lente Insulin [beef], Monotard [pork], Lentard [beef-pork], and Novolin-L [Novo Nordisk]). Its onset of action is delayed to 2–4 hours, and its peak response is generally reached in about 8–10 hours. Because its duration of action is often less than 24 hours (with a range of 18–24 hours), most patients require at least 2 injections daily to maintain a sustained insulin effect. The supernatant of the lente suspension contains an excess of zinc ions, which may precipitate regular insulin if it is added to lente.

2. NPH (neutral protamine Hagedorn, or isophane) insulin–(NPH Iletin I and II or Humulin-N [Lilly], NPH Insulin Protaphane and Novolin-N [Novo Nordisk], Insulatard NPH [pork or human] [Nordisk]) NPH is an intermediate-acting insulin in which the onset of action is delayed by combining 2 parts of soluble crystalline zinc insulin with one part protamine zinc insulin. The mixture is reported to have equivalent concentrations of protamine and insulin, so that neither is in excess ("isophane"). The peak action and duration of action of NPH insulin are similar to those of lente insulin, however, in contrast to lente insulin, regular insulin retains its solubility and independent rapid action when mixed with NPH.

Flocculation of suspended particles may occasionally "frost" the sides of a bottle of NPH insulin or "clump" within bottles from which multiple small doses are withdrawn over a prolonged period. These bottles generally have been kept at room temperature and subjected to recurrent agitation. Patients should be vigilant for early signs of frosting or clumping of the NPH insulin, because it indicates a pronounced loss of potency. Several cases of diabetic ketoacidosis have been reported in IDDM patients who had been inadvertently injecting this denatured insulin.

C. Long-Acting Insulins:

1. Ultralente–(Iletin I Ultralente [Lilly], Ultratard [Novo Nordisk]) Ultralente is a long-acting crystalline suspension of insulin whose onset of action is quite delayed, with peak effects at 8–14 hours and a duration of action of up to 36 hours. Beef insulin is less soluble than pork insulin, producing larger crystals and thus assuring a prolonged action. Beef insulin has thus been preferred in producing the ultralente insulins. Ultratard (Novo Nordisk) is a pure beef insulin, whereas Ultralente Iletin I is 70% beef and 30% pork. Recently, a human insulin formulation (Humulin-U, [Lilly]) whose pharmacokinetics are similar to those of beef insulin (except for a slightly shorter duration of action (24–28 hours rather than 28–36 hours) has been developed. Ultralente is increasingly used in association with multiple preprandial injections of regular insulin in an attempt to establish optimal control in IDDM patients. Its very slow onset of action and prolonged duration (Fig 22–10) have led to its use in providing a basal level of insulin comparable to that achieved by basal endogenous secretion or by the overnight infusion rate programmed into insulin pumps.

2. Protamine zinc insulin (PZI)–This modified insulin was the first long-acting insulin available. The addition of protamine to insulin produced an insulin with poor solubility and therefore slow absorption. The very long duration of action of PZI limits its usefulness. In addition, it contains an excess of protamine, which binds to any crystalline insulin added to the same syringe and thus converts the short-acting insulin to long-acting protamine insulin. Because of these problems, PZI is seldom used in the USA.

D. Premixed Insulins: As a convenience to patients, particularly those with impaired visual acuity or hand coordination, premixed insulin preparations with fixed ratios of 70% NPH insulin and 30% regular insulin are available. These include Mixtard pork or human insulin (Nordisk), Novolin 70:30 (Novo Nordisk) and Humulin 70:30.

Methods of Insulin Administration

A. Insulin Syringes and Needles: Disposable plastic syringes with needles attached are available in 1-mL, 0.5-mL, and 0.3-mL sizes. Their finely honed 27- or 28-gauge attached needles have greatly reduced the pain of injections. They are light, not susceptible to damage, and convenient when traveling. Moreover, their clear markings and tight plungers allow accurate measurement of insulin dosage. In cases where very low insulin doses are prescribed, specially calibrated 0.3-mL and 0.5-mL disposable syringes facilitate accurate measurement of U100 insulin in doses up to 50 units. These "low-dose" syringes have become increasingly popular because it is now recommended that diabetics not take more than 50 units of insulin in a single injection except in the rare instance of extreme insulin resistance. Several recent reports indicate that "disposable" syringes may be reused until blunting of the needle occurs (usually after 3–5 injections). Wiping the needle with a clean alcohol swab, reapplying the needle guard, and refrigeration after use appear to maintain adequate sterility to avoid infection. A concern, however, arises from a recent report that flecks of silicone may become suspended in insulin bottles into which disposable syringes have been repeatedly inserted; the silicone flecks seem to reduce the activity of the insulin.

B. Mixing Insulin: Since intermediate insulin requires several hours to reach adequate therapeutic levels, supplements of regular insulin are generally added preprandially in IDDM patients. Recent reports caution that insulin mixtures containing increased proportions of lente to regular insulins retards the rapid action of admixed regular insulin. The excess zinc in lente insulin binds the soluble insulin and partially blunts its action, particularly when a relatively small proportion of regular insulin is mixed with lente (eg, one part regular to 1.5 or more parts lente). NPH preparations do not delay absorption of admixed regular insulin. They are therefore preferable to lente when mixtures of intermediate and regular insulins are prescribed. For convenience, regular and NPH insulin may be mixed together in the same syringe and injected subcutaneously in split dosage before breakfast and supper.

When mixing insulin, it is necessary to inject into both bottles a quantity of air equivalent to the volume of insulin being withdrawn. Traditionally, regular insulin is withdrawn first, and the longer-action insulin is then added to the syringe. Care must be taken to avoid contaminating either insulin bottle with insulin of the different type. The injection is preferably given immediately after loading the syringe, and no attempt should be made to mix the insulins in the syringe.

C. Sites for Injection: Any part of the body covered by loose skin can be used as an injection site, including the abdomen, thighs, upper arms, flanks, and upper outer quadrants of the buttocks. In general, regular insulin is absorbed more rapidly from upper regions of the body such as the deltoid area or the abdomen rather than from the thighs or buttocks. Exercise appears to facilitate insulin absorption when the injection site is adjacent to the exercising muscle. Rotation of sites continues to be recommended to avoid delayed absorption when fibrosis or lipohypertrophy occurs owing to repeated use of a single site. However, considerable variability of absorption rates from different sites, particularly with exercise, may contribute to the instability of glycemic control in certain IDDM patients if injection sites are rotated indiscriminately over different areas of the body. Consequently, health professionals recommend limiting injection sites to a single region of the body and rotating sites within that region. It is possible that some of the stability of glycemic control achieved by infusion pumps may be related to the constancy of the site of infusion from day to day. For most patients the abdomen is the recommended site for injection, since it provides a considerable area in which to rotate sites and there may be less variability of absorption with exercise than when the thigh or deltoid areas are used.

D. Insulin Delivery Systems: Efforts to administer insulin by **"closed loop" systems** (glucose-controlled insulin infusion systems [Biostator]) have been successful in acute situations such as diabetic ketoacidosis or during surgery. However, chronic use is precluded by the bulkiness of the computerized pump and by the need for continuous aspiration of blood for the external glucose sensor that activates the appropriate insulin or glucose infusion.

Many small portable **"open loop" devices** for the delivery of insulin are on the market. These devices contain an insulin reservoir and a pump programmed to deliver regular insulin (by either a subcutaneous, intravenous, or intraperitoneal route) at a previously determined rate; they do not contain a glucose sensor. With improved methods for self-monitoring of *blood* glucose at home (see below), these pump systems have become very useful for managing some diabetic patients. However, there have been reports of numerous acute complications, such as infection at the catheter site and ketoacidosis due to kinking of the tube attached to the insulin reservoir. At present, conventional methods of insulin administration, with multiple subcutaneous injections of mixtures of a rapid and either an intermediate-acting or long-acting insulin, can provide glycemic control almost as effectively as the open loop systems in most patients with IDDM who self-monitor their blood glucose levels accurately and regularly.

To facilitate treatment of patients who are adhering to a regimen of multiple preprandial injections of regular insulin that supplement a single injection of long-acting insulin delivered by a conventional syringe, portable **pen injectors** have been introduced. These pen-sized devices (Novo-Pen, Insuject) contain cartridges of U100 regular human insulin and retractable needles and eliminate the need to carry an insulin bottle and syringes during the day.

Intranasally administered soluble insulin is rapidly absorbed when given along with a detergent substance to facilitate adsorption. Preliminary clinical trials have demonstrated its efficacy in reducing postprandial hyperglycemia in insulin-dependent diabetics. Further studies are in progress to assess its usefulness as an insulin delivery system in treating diabetic patients.

Pancreatic islet cells have been successfully transplanted in genetically similar strains of rodents with experimental diabetes; however, this approach has not yet been successful in humans because of immunologic rejection of the tissue. Similarly, **whole pancreas transplants** have generally proved unsatisfactory in treating the insulin-dependent (type I) patient because of the hazards of prolonged antirejection therapy.

STEPS IN THE MANAGEMENT OF THE DIABETIC PATIENT

Diagnostic Examination

A. History and Physical Examination: A complete history is taken and physical examination is performed for diagnostic purposes and to rule out the presence of coexisting or complicating disease. Nutritional status should be noted, particularly if catabolic features such as progressive weight loss are present despite a normal or increased food intake. The family history should include not only the incidence but also the age at onset of diabetes in other members of the family, and it should be noted whether affected family members were obese and whether they required insulin. Other factors that increase cardiovascular risk, such as a smoking history, presence of hypertension or hyperlipidemia, or oral contraceptive pill use should be documented.

A careful physical examination should include baseline height and weight, pulse rate, and blood pressure. If obesity is present, it should be characterized as to its distribution and a waist to hip ratio should be recorded. All peripheral arterial pulses should be examined, noting whether bruits or other signs of atherosclerotic disease are present. Neurologic and ophthalmologic examinations should be performed, with emphasis on investigation of abnormalities that may be related to diabetes, such as neovascularization of the retina or stocking/glove sensory loss in the extremities.

B. Laboratory Diagnosis: (See also Laboratory Findings in Diabetes Mellitus, above.) Laboratory diagnosis should include documentation of the presence of fasting hyperglycemia (plasma glucose > 140 mg/dL [7.7 mmol/L]) or postprandial (post–glucose tolerance test) values consistently above 200 mg/dL (11.1 mmol/L). An attempt should be made to characterize the diabetes as IDDM or NIDDM, based on the

Instructions in the Care of the Feet for Persons With Diabetes Mellitus or Vascular Disturbances*

Hygiene of the Feet

(1) Wash feet daily with mild soap and lukewarm water. Dry thoroughly between the toes by pressure. Do not rub vigorously, as this is apt to break the delicate skin.

(2) When feet are thoroughly dry, rub well with vegetable oil to keep them soft, prevent excess friction, remove scales, and prevent dryness. Care must be taken to prevent foot tenderness.

(3) If the feet become too soft and tender, rub them with alcohol about once a week.

(4) When rubbing the feet, always rub upward from the tips of the toes. If varicose veins are present, massage the feet very gently; never massage the legs.

(5) If the toenails are brittle and dry, soften them by soaking for one-half hour each night in lukewarm water containing 1 tbsp of powdered sodium borate (borax) per quart. Follow this by rubbing around the nails with vegetable oil. Clean around the nails with an orangewood stick. If the nails become too long, file them with an emery board. File them straight across and no shorter than the underlying soft tissues of the toe. Never cut the corners of the nails. (The podiatrist should be informed if a patient has diabetes.)

(6) Wear low-heeled shoes of soft leather that fit the shape of the feet correctly. The shoes should have wide toes that will cause no pressure, fit close in the arch, and grip the heels snugly. Wear new shoes one-half hour only on the first day and increase by 1 hour each day following. Wear thick, warm, loose stockings.

Treatment of Corns & Calluses

(1) Corns and calluses are due to friction and pressure, most often from improperly fitted shoes and stockings. Wear shoes that fit properly and cause no friction or pressure.

(2) To remove excess calluses or corns, soak the feet in lukewarm (not hot) water, using a mild soap, for about 10 minutes and then rub off the excess tissue with a towel or file. Do not tear it off. Under no circumstances must the skin become irritated.

(3) Do not cut corns or calluses. If they need attention, it is safer to see a podiatrist.

(4) Prevent callus formation under the ball of the foot (a) by exercises, such as curling and stretching the toes several times a day; (b) by finishing each step on the toes and not on the ball of the foot; and (c) by wearing shoes that are not too short and that do not have high heels.

Aids in Treatment of Impaired Circulation (Cold Feet)

(1) Never use tobacco in any form. Tobacco contracts blood vessels and so reduces circulation.

(2) Keep warm. Wear warm stockings and other clothing. Cold contracts blood vessels and reduces circulation.

(3) Do not wear circular garters, which compress blood vessels and reduce blood flow.

(4) Do not sit with the legs crossed. This may compress the leg arteries and shut off the blood supply to the feet.

(5) If the weight of the bedclothes is uncomfortable, place a pillow under the covers at the foot of the bed.

(6) Do not apply any medication to the feet without directions from a physician. Some medicines are too strong for feet with poor circulation.

(7) Do not apply heat in the form of hot water, hot water bottles, or heating pads without a physician's consent. Even moderate heat can injure the skin if circulation is poor.

(8) If the feet are moist or the patient has a tendency to develop athlete's foot, a prophylactic dusting powder should be used on the feet and in shoes and stockings daily. Change shoes and stockings at least daily or oftener.

Treatment of Abrasions of the Skin

(1) Proper first-aid treatment is of the utmost importance even in apparently minor injuries. Consult a physician immediately for any redness, blistering, pain, or swelling. Any break in the skin may become ulcerous or gangrenous unless properly treated by a physician.

(2) Dermatophytosis (athlete's foot), which begins with peeling and itching between the toes or discoloration or thickening of the toenails, should be treated immediately by a physician or podiatrist.

(3) Avoid strong irritating antiseptics such as tincture of iodine.

(4) As soon as possible after any injury, cover the area with sterile gauze, which may be purchased at drugstores. Only fine paper tape or cellulose tape (Scotch Tape) should be used on the skin if adhesive retention of the gauze is required.

(5) Elevate and, as much as possible until recovery, avoid using the foot.

---

*Reproduced, with permission, from Krupp MA, Chatton MJ, Tierney LM Jr (editors): *Current Medical Diagnosis & Treatment 1986.* Lange, 1986.

clinical features present and on whether or not ketonuria accompanies the glycosuria. With current emphasis on home blood glucose monitoring, laborious attempts to document the renal threshold for glucose are no longer necessary in the initial evaluation of diabetic patients, particularly since "double-voided" urine specimens are difficult to obtain and since acceptable control of glycemia now allows only rare episodes of glycosuria.

Other baseline laboratory measurements that should be made part of the record include either glycohemoglobin or hemoglobin A_{1c}, total and HDL cholesterol, plasma triglycerides, electrocardiogram, chest x-ray, complete blood count, complete urinalysis, and renal function studies (serum creatinine, blood urea nitrogen, and, if possible, creatinine clearance).

Patient Education

Education is the most important task of the physician who provides care to diabetic patients. It must be remembered that education is necessary not only for newly diagnosed diabetic patients and their families but also for patients with diabetes of any duration who may never have been properly educated about their disorder or who may not be aware of advances in diabetes management. The "teaching curriculum" should include explanations of the nature of diabetes, its potential acute and chronic complications, and information on how these complications can be prevented or at least recognized and treated early. The importance of self-monitoring of blood glucose should be emphasized, particularly in all insulin-requiring diabetic patients, and instructions on proper testing and on recording of data should be provided. Patients should be taught to use algorithms to adjust the timing and quantity of their insulin dose, food, and exercise in response to their recorded blood glucose values, so that optimal blood glucose control is achieved. Patients must be helped to accept the fact that they have diabetes; until this difficult adjustment has been made, efforts to cope with the disorder are likely to be futile. Counseling should be directed at avoidance of extremes such as compulsive rigidity or self-destructive neglect. All patients should be made aware of community agencies (Diabetes Association chapters, etc.) that serve as resources for continuing education.

A. Diet Instruction: All diabetic patients should receive individual instruction on diet, as described earlier in this chapter. Unrestricted diets are not advised for insulin-requiring diabetics. Until new methods of insulin replacement are available to provide more normal patterns of insulin delivery in response to metabolic demands, multiple small feedings restricted in simple sugars will continue to be recommended.

B. Insulin: Give the patient an understanding of the actions of the various insulins and the methods of administration of insulin. Since infections, particularly pyogenic ones with fever and toxemia, provoke a marked increase in insulin requirements, patients must be taught how to appropriately administer supplemental regular insulin as needed to correct hyperglycemia during infections. Patients and their families or friends should also be taught to recognize signs and symptoms of hypoglycemia and how to institute appropriate therapy for hypoglycemic reactions (see Acute Complications of Diabetes Mellitus, below).

C. Hypoglycemic Agents: Information must be provided on the principles of hypoglycemic therapy (including information about time of onset, peak action, and duration of action of any pharmacologic agent being used). Patients should be made aware of the maximum recommended dose of the sulfonylureas that they are taking and should learn to inquire about possible drug interactions whenever any new medications are added to their regimens.

D. Effect of Exercise: Exercise increases the effectiveness of insulin, and regular daily moderate exercise is an excellent means of improving utilization of fats and carbohydrates in diabetic patients. A judicious balance of the size and frequency of meals with moderate regular exercise can often stabilize the insulin dosage in diabetics who tend to slip out of control easily. Strenuous exercise, however, can precipitate hypoglycemia in an unprepared patient, and diabetics must therefore be taught to reduce their insulin dosage or take supplemental carbohydrate in anticipation of strenuous activity. Injection of insulin into a site farthest away from the muscles most involved in exercise may help meliorate exercise-induced hypoglycemia, since insulin injected to exercising muscle is much more rapidly mobilized. With more knowledge regarding the relationship between caloric intake and expenditure and insulin requirements, the patient can become liberated from much of the regimentation imposed by the disorder.

E. Good Hygiene: All diabetic patients must receive adequate instruction on personal hygiene, especially with regard to care of the feet (see p 625), skin, and teeth.

F. Infections: Infections with fever and severe illness provoke the release of high levels of insulin antagonists that will bring about a marked increase in insulin requirements. It is essential to limit the period of infection, since infection raises the blood glucose level and this, in turn, immobilizes the general defense mechanisms that the body uses against bacterial and even viral organisms. Thus, the early and sufficient use of bactericidal antibiotics is imperative. Type I diabetics must be taught how to supplement the regimen with regular insulin if persistent glycosuria and ketonuria occur—especially if associated with infection. Patients must understand that insulin therapy should never be withheld in the presence of gastric upset and vomiting if glycosuria with ketonuria is present. When food intake is limited by nausea or vomiting, the patient should take ginger ale, apple juice, or grape juice in small sips and should notify the physician in case supplemental intravenous fluids might be required.

G. Self-Monitoring: Patients in whom labile diabetes is difficult to control should receive instructions on techniques for self-monitoring of blood glucose (see below). They should be encouraged to keep careful records of their glucose measurements and instructed on appropriate measures to correct for emerging patterns of hyperglycemia as well as to prevent recurrent episodes of hypoglycemia. Self-monitoring instructs patients on the glycemic effects of specific foods and exercise and alleviates the likelihood of unexpected episodes of severe hypoglycemia. Moreover, when combined with an appropriate algorithm for therapy so that patients can respond appropriately to the various effects of glycemia, self-monitoring allows for greater flexibility in life-style and enables patients to be more fully in control of their diabetes.

H. Identification Bracelet: All patients receiving hypoglycemic therapy should wear a Medic-Alert bracelet or necklace that clearly states that insulin or an oral sulfonylurea drug is being taken. A card in the wallet or purse is less useful, since legal problems may arise if a victim's person and belongings are searched without permission. (Information on how to obtain a Medic-Alert identification device can be obtained from the Medic-Alert Foundation, PO Box 1009, Turlock, CA 95380.)

I. Restrictions on Occupation: Certain occupations potentially hazardous to the diabetic patient or others will continue to be prohibited (eg, piloting airplanes, operating cranes).

Avoidance of Stress & Emotional Turmoil

Prevention of psychologic turmoil is of great importance in the control of diabetes, particularly when the disease is difficult to stabilize. One reason blood glucose control in diabetics may be particularly sensitive to emotional upset is that their pancreatic A cells are hyperresponsive to physiologic levels of epinephrine, producing excessive levels of glucagon with consequent hyperglycemia.

Specific Therapy

Treatment must be individualized depending on the specific needs of each patient. Certain general principles of management pertaining to each type of diabetes are outlined below.

A. Type I Diabetes (IDDM): IDDM patients require replacement therapy with exogenous insulin. This should be instituted under conditions of an individualized diabetic diet with multiple feedings and normal daily activities so that an appropriate dosage regimen can be developed.

At the onset of diabetes, many type I patients recover some pancreatic B cell function and may temporarily need only low doses of exogenous insulin to supplement their own endogenous insulin secretion. This is known as the "honeymoon period." Within 8 weeks to 2 years, however, most of these patients show either absent or negligible pancreatic B cell function.

At this point, these patients may be instructed to take a "conventional" regimen of 2 injections of insulin mixtures (a short-acting combined with intermediate-acting NPH insulin). Alternatively, if more flexibility with meal intervals and exercise is desired, multiple preprandial small injections of regular insulin may be prescribed along with a bedtime injection of long-acting or intermediate-acting insulin. Self-monitoring of blood glucose levels is the recommended means of determining the adjustment of insulin dosage and the modulation of food intake and exercise in type I diabetes.

1. Conventional insulin therapy (split doses of insulin mixtures)– A conventional insulin regimen in a 70-kg patient taking 2200 kcal divided into 6 feedings might be 10 units of regular and 10 units of NPH insulin in the morning and 8 units of regular and 8 units of NPH insulin in the evening. The morning blood glucose level gives a measure of the effectiveness of NPH insulin administered the previous evening; the noon level reflects the effects of the morning regular insulin; and the 5 PM and 9 PM levels represent the effects of the morning NPH and the evening regular insulins, respectively. A properly educated patient should be taught to adjust insulin dosage by observing the pattern of recorded self-monitored blood glucose levels and correlating it with the approximate duration of action and the time of peak effect after injection of the various insulin preparations (Table 22–13). Adjustments should be made gradually, preferably not more often than every 2 or 3 days if possible.

Certain caveats should be kept in mind regarding insulin treatment. Considerable variations in absorption and bioavailability exist, even when the same dose is injected in the same region on different days in the same individual. Such variation often can be minimized by injecting smaller quantities of insulin at each dose and consequently using multiple doses. Also, a given insulin dose may undergo considerable differences in pharmacokinetics in different individuals, either because of insulin antibodies that bind insulin with different avidity, or for other as yet unknown reasons.

2. Intensive multiple-dose insulin therapy– While split doses of insulin mixtures daily have improved the quality of glycemic control as compared to single injections of intermediate insulin in type I diabetics, blood glucose values throughout the day are often not optimal, and nocturnal hypoglycemia may result from attempts to achieve euglycemia. In cases in which conventional split doses of insulin mixtures cannot maintain near-normalization of blood glucose without hypoglycemia (particularly at night), multiple injections of insulin may be required. An increasingly popular regimen consists of reducing or omitting the evening dose of intermediate insulin and adding a portion of it at bedtime. For example, 10 units of regular insulin mixed with 10 units of NPH insulin might be prescribed in the morning, 8–10 units of regular insulin before the evening meal, and 6 units of NPH at bedtime.

To further reduce variation in absorption kinetics, which is aggravated when ratios of insulin in mixtures are altered on different days, a multiple injection regimen that avoids mixing insulin has been devised. The patient administers small doses of regular insulin more frequently (eg, 4 times a day) and one injection of a long-acting insulin at bedtime (eg, ultralente insulin). Both of these multiple-dose regimens give greater flexibility regarding meal patterns and content than conventional therapy with split doses of insulin mixtures and are helpful in reducing the frequency and severity of hypoglycemia in patients attempting near-normalization of blood glucose.

3. Intensive insulin therapy using insulin pumps–Several types of portable battery-operated "open loop" devices have been marketed to deliver insulin continuously (see Methods of Insulin Administration, above). These generally infuse insulin through a needle or catheter implanted subcutaneously in the abdomen. A basal infusion rate of regular insulin is provided over a 24-hour period, and this is augmented by a bolus of regular insulin prior to meals. In addition, since insulin requirements appear to increase slightly in the early dawn period in the majority of patients with type I diabetes, most pumps also have adjustable basal rates that can be programmed to rise automatically at 6 AM. Unbuffered regular insulins such as Humulin-R, Iletin I and II, or Novolin-R have been associated with frequent blockage of pump tubing due to precipitation of the insulin. Accordingly, only insulin buffered with phosphate such as Velosulin or the specially issued Humulin Buffered Regular (for pump use only) have been recommended for use in insulin infusion pumps.

The use of pumps requires knowledgeable and compliant patients who can be depended on to monitor their blood glucose levels as often as 4 times daily. The indwelling needle or catheter should be changed every 48 hours to reduce the risk of infection, and patients should be alert for symptoms of sudden deterioration of glycemic control, due to pump blockage, pump failure, or leakage of insulin from the tubing. The selection of dosage is usually based on providing 40–50% of the estimated daily dose of insulin as the basal infusion rate and the remaining amount divided as intermittent boluses given prior to meals to control postprandial metabolism. For example, in a 70-kg patient requiring 40–45 units of insulin a day, 20 units of regular insulin would be administered as a basal infusion of 0.8 unit/h, with the remaining units administered as follows: 7–8 units before breakfast, 5–6 units before lunch, 6–8 units before supper, and 0–2 units prior to a bedtime snack. The results of blood glucose monitoring as well as the extent of physical activity and dietary intake will all contribute to fine-tuning the proper dosage of insulin administered at various meals and basally.

4. Selection of patients for intensive insulin therapy–Patient selection is difficult, and exact criteria are controversial. Patients should be highly mo-

tivated and willing to monitor their blood glucose levels several times daily and record the results. They should not have impaired adrenergic responses to hypoglycemia, as is often seen with autonomic neuropathy, since this reduces their awareness of being hypoglycemic and increases the risk of severe hypoglycemic episodes. Finally, if nonproliferative ("background") or proliferative retinopathy is present, intensive insulin therapy should be initiated slowly and with careful attention to possible progression of retinal disease (see Ophthalmologic Complications, below).

5. Self-monitoring of blood glucose levels–Monitoring of capillary glucose levels has greatly improved glycemic control by enabling patients to alter their dietary intake or insulin dose to maintain glycemic ranges below the renal threshold for glycosuria. This has been particularly helpful at bedtime to determine whether supplementary feedings are required to avoid nocturnal hypoglycemia.

Self-monitoring of blood glucose levels is particularly helpful in managing diabetes in the following groups: patients with brittle diabetes; patients who are attempting ideal glycemic control, such as during pregnancy; and patients with impaired or absent early warning of hypoglycemic episodes. Self-monitoring is useful in educating patients about the glycemic effects of specific foods in their diet and reduces the likelihood of unexpected episodes of severe hypoglycemia in insulin-treated diabetics.

There are 3 essential elements to self-monitoring of blood glucose: (1) obtaining the blood specimen, (2) applying the specimen to enzyme-impregnated strips capable of discriminating the glucose level, and (3) reading the glucose level from the test strip. Each of these will be discussed briefly.

The patient may obtain a capillary blood sample from the fingertip by means of a lancet designed for this purpose. The patient should be taught how to clean the site and how to rapidly pierce the skin to obtain a drop of blood. Automatic spring-loaded devices such as the Autolet or Penlet are useful in simplifying the finger-pricking technique and ensuring an adequate blood sample.

The drop of blood is then applied to the appropriate area of an enzyme-impregnated strip such as the Dextrostix, Chemstrip bG, or Glucostix. It is important to follow the instructions for each type of strip. The strips vary with respect to the area necessary to cover with the blood drop, washing technique, and timing of the procedure.

Chemstrip bG results can be visually interpreted by comparing the colors obtained on the strip with the color chart supplied by the manufacturer. For patients who have difficulty with color discrimination or who prefer more exact results, devices with automated digital readouts are available to quantitate the color changes (Glucometer, Glucoscan, Accu-Chek bG, Diascan, One Touch, or ExacTech). These devices vary in cost, ease of use, portability, and strip compatibility.

Newer meters such as One Touch, and particularly ExacTech, are more compact and have the distinct advantage of automatically timing the entire reaction as well as obviating the need to wipe off the strip, thereby reducing the potential for technical error. The physician should learn the advantages and disadvantages of these devices and help the patient make an appropriate choice.

Initially, blood glucose levels should be checked at least 4 times a day in patients with type I diabetes. Generally, these measurements are taken before each meal and at bedtime. Once these levels are brought into an acceptable range, the patient should continue to check blood glucose levels at least twice daily. In addition, patients should be taught to check their blood glucose level whenever they develop symptoms that could represent a hypoglycemic episode. All blood glucose levels and their timing and corresponding insulin doses should be recorded in an organized fashion and brought with the patient for physician review during regularly scheduled check-ups; such personal blood glucose logs are commercially available.

6. Management of early morning hyperglycemia in IDDM patients–

a. Etiology and diagnosis–One of the more difficult therapeutic problems in managing patients with IDDM is determining the proper adjustment of insulin dose when the early morning blood glucose level is high before breakfast. Prebreakfast hyperglycemia is sometimes due to the **Somogyi effect,** in which nocturnal hypoglycemia evokes a surge of counterregulatory hormones to produce high blood glucose levels by 7 AM. If this is the case, lowering the evening dose of intermediate insulin is indicated. However, a more common cause of prebreakfast hyperglycemia is the **waning of circulating insulin levels,** which requires use of more (rather than less) intermediate insulin in the evening. These 2 phenomena are not mutually exclusive and can occur together to produce a greater magnitude of hyperglycemia in affected patients with IDDM. A third phenomenon—the recently described **"dawn phenomenon"**—has been reported to occur in as many as 75% of IDDM patients and in the majority of NIDDM patients and normal subjects as well. It is characterized by a reduced tissue sensitivity to insulin between 5 AM and 8 AM (dawn), and apparently is evoked by spikes of growth hormone released hours before, at onset of sleep. When the "dawn phenomenon" occurs alone, it may produce only mild hyperglycemia in the early morning; however, when it is associated with either or both of the other phenomena, it can further aggravate the hyperglycemia (Table 22–15). Diagnosis of the cause of prebreakfast hyperglycemia can be facilitated by asking the patient to self-monitor blood glucose levels at 3 AM in addition to monitoring at the usual times, bedtime and 7 AM. When this was done (see Havlin and Cryer reference), the Somogyi effect was found to be much less prevalent and of lower magnitude as a cause of prebreakfast hyperglycemia than had been previously suspected. In insulin-treated patients, serum levels of free immunoreactive insulin (particularly in the basal or low ranges) are difficult to quantitate accurately because of technical interference. In specialized research laboratories, however, these levels have been measured in hospitalized patients with prebreakfast hyperglycemia (Table 22–15).

b. Treatment–When a particular pattern emerges from monitoring blood glucose levels at 10 PM, 3 AM, and 7 AM, appropriate therapeutic measures can be taken. Prebreakfast hyperglycemia due to the Somogyi effect can be treated by either reducing the dose of intermediate insulin, giving a portion of it at bedtime, or supplying more food at bedtime. When the "dawn phenomenon" alone is present, shifting a portion of the intermediate insulin from dinnertime to bedtime often suffices; or when insulin pumps are used, the basal infusion rate can be stepped up appropriately (eg, from 0.8 unit/h to 1 unit/h) from 6 AM until breakfast. Finally, in cases in which the circulating insulin level is waning, either increasing the evening insulin dose or shifting it from dinnertime to bedtime (or both) may be efficacious.

B. Type II Diabetes (NIDDM): The principles of therapy are less well defined in this heterogeneous group of diabetic patients than is the case with type I

Table 22–15. Typical patterns of overnight blood glucose levels and serum free immunoreactive insulin levels in prebreakfast hyperglycemia due to various causes in patients with IDDM.

	Blood Glucose Levels (mg/dL)			Serum Free Immunoreactive Insulin Levels (μU/mL)		
	10 PM	**3 AM**	**7 AM**	**10 PM**	**3 AM**	**7 AM**
Somogyi effect	90	40	200	High	Slightly high	Normal
"Dawn phenomenon"	110	110	150	Normal	Normal	Normal
Waning of circulating insulin levels plus "dawn phenomenon"	110	190	220	Normal	Low	Low
Waning of circulating insulin levels plus "dawn phenomenon" plus Somogyi effect	110	40	380	High	Normal	Low

diabetes. Therapeutic recommendations are based upon the relative contributions of B cell insufficiency and insulin insensitivity in individual patients.

1. The obese patient—The most common type of diabetic patient is the obese diabetic with insulin insensitivity. Characteristically, these patients have normal or increased basal levels of circulating insulin, and in the presence of mild hyperglycemia they are capable of responding to a glucose load with insulin secretion. However, as hyperglycemia progresses, the insulin response to a glucose load decreases. This refractoriness of the B cell is primarily related to the hyperglycemic stimulation, since other B cell–stimulating agents such as sulfonylureas, arginine, and glucagon still provoke rapid insulin release.

a. Weight reduction—One of the primary modes of therapy in the obese type II diabetic patient is weight reduction. Normalization of glycemia can be achieved by reducing adipose stores, with consequent restoration of tissue sensitivity to insulin. A combination of caloric restriction, increased exercise, modification of behavior, and consistent reinforcement of good eating habits is required if a weight reduction program is to be successful. Knowledge of the symptoms of diabetes and an understanding of the risks and complications of diabetes often increase the patient's motivation for weight reduction. Even so, significant weight loss is seldom achieved in the morbidly obese patient; there is a variable effectiveness in moderately obese patients depending on the enthusiasm of the therapist and the motivation of the patient.

b. Hypoglycemic agents—Hypoglycemic agents, including insulin as well as the oral hypoglycemic drugs are generally *not* indicated for long-term use in the obese patient with mild diabetes. A weight reduction program can be disrupted by real or imagined hypoglycemic reactions when insulin therapy is used, and weight gain is quite common in the insulin-treated obese diabetic patient. It is also possible that administration of insulin to an obese patient who already has excessive circulating levels may maintain insulin insensitivity through down-regulation of receptor sites and by interference with catabolic mechanisms during caloric deprivation. The obese diabetic who has been previously treated with conventional beef-pork insulin, often in high doses and in an interrupted fashion, may occasionally develop immune insulin resistance (see below). This not only increases the requirements for exogenous insulin but may further impair the effectiveness of endogenous insulin because of cross-reacting antibodies; on occasion, this can even precipitate ketoacidosis. Fortunately, this complication is presently much less common due to greater use of less immunogenic human insulins.

Oral sulfonylureas, therefore, are more appropriate than insulin for *symptomatic* moderately severe diabetes in an obese patient. If sulfonylurea therapy (combined with a weight reduction regimen) is inadequate to control symptoms of hyperglycemia (eg, noc-

turia, blurred vision, or candidal vulvovaginitis) insulin therapy may be necessary, directed at elimination of symptoms rather than restoration of euglycemia. Use of a sulfonylurea agent or insulin to supplement a weight reduction program should be for a limited period (weeks or months) to meliorate hyperglycemic symptoms until sufficient weight reduction has occurred to keep the patient symptom-free.

2. The nonobese patient—In the nonobese NIDDM diabetic with moderately severe hyperglycemia, pancreatic B cells are refractory to glucose stimulation. Peripheral insulin resistance is also detectable but is considerably less intense than in obese diabetics who have a comparable degree of hyperglycemia; it is also of less therapeutic import, since insulin-treated nonobese patients do not generally need an excessive dosage of insulin.

a. Diet—If hyperglycemia is mild (fasting blood glucose levels of < 200 mg/dL [11.1 mmol/L]), normal metabolic control can occasionally be restored by a diet devoid of simple sugars and with calories calculated to maintain ideal body weight. Restriction of saturated fats and cholesterol is also strongly advised. The standard ADA diet with its recommended exchange list should be prescribed for these nonobese NIDDM patients.

b. Oral hypoglycemic agents—When diet therapy alone is not sufficient to correct hyperglycemia, a trial of sulfonylurea drugs is indicated to supplement the dietary regimen. The controversies raised by the UGDP (see Efficacy and Safety of Oral Hypoglycemic Agents, above) apply mainly to obese patients with relatively mild diabetes (who represented the great majority of patients in that study), and there are few data on which to base an assessment of the risk-benefit ratio of sulfonylureas in nonobese patients with fasting hyperglycemia above 140 mg/dL (7.8 mmol/L). Therefore, once their efficacy is demonstrated in these patients and since there is no evidence suggesting harm to them, it seems reasonable to continue the use of sulfonylureas as long as they remain effective in controlling hyperglycemia. The degree of control to aim for remains arbitrary at present; however, data from the United Kingdom and from studies of Pima Indians suggest that maintaining postprandial plasma glucose levels below 200 mg/dL (11.1 mmol/L) seems to spare NIDDM patients from increased risk of severe retinopathy or vascular complications. Once the dosage of sulfonylurea reaches the upper recommended limit in a compliant patient without maintaining plasma glucose below 200 mg/dL (11.1 mmol/L) throughout the day, insulin therapy is indicated.

c. Insulin—A single dose of intermediate-acting insulin may suffice to supplement endogenous insulin secretion in nonobese NIDDM patients who require insulin therapy. This is in contrast to type I diabetics, who can seldom be rendered euglycemic unless multiple injections or a continuous infusion of insulin is employed. Many nonobese patients with mild insulinopenia can have their glycohemoglobin levels brought into the normal range with relatively small doses of insulin and with no suggestion of nocturnal hypoglycemia. Occasional patients with more severe insulinopenia may require split doses of insulin.

d. Therapeutic combinations of sulfonylureas with insulin—Both nonobese and obese NIDDM patients usually show a modest glycemic improvement with a regimen combining sulfonylurea drugs and insulin, but this improvement can generally be achieved with insulin therapy alone. At present, there is no overall consensus regarding how these agents should be combined. One proposed regimen adds a bedtime intermediate-acting insulin to reduce excessive nocturnal hepatic glucose output in NIDDM patients who are responding poorly on maximal doses of sulfonylureas, but most diabetologists recommend stopping the sulfonylureas in these circumstances and changing over to insulin therapy alone. Only in the case of NIDDM patients requiring excessive amounts of insulin (>100 units/d) is it considered a reasonable option to add sulfonylureas to improve glycemic control rather than prescribing inordinately high insulin doses.

In IDDM patients, the absence of glycemic improvement or reduction in insulin dose when sulfonylureas are added to the insulin regimen suggests that the predominant effect of sulfonylureas is their insulinotropic action, and that any effect on potentiation of insulin action is limited to in vitro systems and of little clinical importance. In NIDDM patients, observations of an improvement in insulin action during sulfonylurea therapy need not be a direct "extrapancreatic" effect but could be explained by improved endogenous insulin release, since other means of reducing hyperglycemia (eg, diet therapy or insulin administration) have been equally effective in decreasing insulin resistance.

Immunopathology of Insulin Therapy

At least 5 molecular classes of insulin antibodies are produced during the course of insulin therapy: IgA, IgD, IgE, IgG, and IgM. Even though the use of highly purified pork and human insulins has considerably reduced the immunogenicity of insulin, many diabetics continue to be treated with mixed beef-pork insulins (Table 22–14). These beef-containing insulins usually induce antibodies to insulin after about 2–3 weeks of therapy.

A. Insulin Allergy: Insulin allergy, a hypersensitivity reaction of the immediate type, is a rare condition in which local or systemic urticaria occurs immediately after insulin injection. This reaction is due to histamine release from tissue mast cells sensitized by adherence of IgE antibodies to insulin. In severe cases, anaphylaxis can occur. The appearance of a subcutaneous nodule at the site of insulin injection, occurring several hours after the injection and lasting for up to 24 hours, has been attributed to an IgG-mediated

complement-binding Arthus reaction. Because sensitivity was often due to noninsulin protein contaminants, the highly purified insulins have markedly reduced the incidence of insulin allergy, especially of the local variety. When allergy to beef insulin is present, a species change (eg, to pure pork insulin or to human insulin) may correct the problem. Antihistamines, corticosteroids, and even desensitization may be required, especially for systemic hypersensitivity in an insulin-dependent patient. A commercial kit containing various dilutions of pure beef or pure pork insulin for allergy testing and insulin desensitization is available from the Eli Lilly Company, although requests for its use have greatly diminished, as more human insulins are being prescribed from the outset of insulin therapy.

B. Immune Insulin Resistance: Except for some patients initially treated with highly purified pork or human insulin, all patients who receive insulin develop a low titer of circulating IgG antibodies to insulin, and this neutralizes to a small extent the rapid action of insulin. In some diabetic patients with a history of intermittent exposure to insulin therapy—and especially those with some degree of tissue insensitivity to insulin (such as obese NIDDM patients)—a high titer of circulating IgG antibodies to insulin develops. This results in extremely high insulin requirements, often to more than 200 units/d. This frequently is a self-limited condition and may clear spontaneously after several months. However, in cases where the circulating antibody is specifically more reactive to beef insulin, switching to a less antigenic highly purified pork insulin or human insulin may make possible a dramatic reduction in insulin dosage or at least may shorten the duration of immune resistance. In immune resistance that responds poorly to a change of insulin species, a trial of oral prednisone (40–60 mg/d for 3–7 days) may improve the response to human insulin. In NIDDM patients, whose excessive circulating insulin antibodies do not completely neutralize endogenous (human) insulin, the foreign insulin can be discontinued and the patient maintained on oral sulfonylureas combined with diet therapy.

C. Lipodystrophy at Injection Sites: Rarely, a disfiguring atrophy of subcutaneous fatty tissue occurs at the site of insulin injection. Although the cause of this complication is obscure, it seems to represent a form of immune reaction, particularly since it occurs predominantly in females and is associated with lymphocyte infiltration in the lipoatrophic area. This complication has become even less common since the development of highly purified insulin preparations of neutral pH. Injection of highly purified preparations of insulin directly into the atrophic area often results in restoration of normal contours.

Lipohypertrophy, on the other hand, is not a consequence of immune responses; rather, it seems to be due to the pharmacologic effects of depositing insulin in the same location repeatedly. It can occur with purified insulins and is best treated with localized liposuction of the hypertrophic areas by an experienced plastic surgeon. It is prevented by rotation of injection sites.

ACUTE COMPLICATIONS OF DIABETES MELLITUS

HYPOGLYCEMIA

Hypoglycemic reactions (see below and Chapter 23) are the most common complications that occur in insulin-treated diabetic patients. They may also occur in patients taking oral sulfonylureas, especially older patients or those with impaired liver or kidney function treated with long-acting and highly potent agents such as chlorpropamide or glyburide. Hypoglycemia may result from delay in taking a meal or from unusual physical exertion without supplemental calories or a decrease in insulin dose.

Clinical Features

Signs and symptoms of hypoglycemia may be divided into those resulting from neuroglycopenia (insufficient glucose for normal central nervous system function leading to confusion and coma) and those resulting from stimulation of the autonomic nervous system. There is great variation in the pattern of hypoglycemic signs and symptoms from patient to patient; however, individual patients tend to experience the same pattern from episode to episode. In older diabetics, autonomic responses are less frequent, so that hypoglycemia may be manifested only by signs and symptoms of neuroglycopenia. The gradual onset of hypoglycemia with intermediate-acting or long-acting insulin also makes recognition more difficult in older patients.

A. Neuroglycopenia: Signs and symptoms of neuroglycopenia include mental confusion with impaired abstract and, later, concrete thought processes; this may be followed by bizarre antagonistic behavior. Stupor, coma, and even death may occur with profound hypoglycemia. Full recovery of central nervous system function does not always occur if treatment is delayed.

B. Autonomic Hyperactivity: Signs and symptoms of autonomic hyperactivity can be both adrenergic (tachycardia, palpitations, sweating, tremulousness) and parasympathetic (nausea, hunger). Except for sweating, most of the sympathetic symptoms of hypoglycemia are blunted in patients receiving beta-blocking agents for angina or hypertension. Though not absolutely contraindicated, these drugs must be used with great caution in insulin-requiring diabetics.

Treatment

All of the manifestations of hypoglycemia are rapidly relieved by glucose administration. Because of the danger of insulin reactions, diabetic patients should carry packets of table sugar or a candy roll at all times for use at the onset of hypoglycemic symptoms. Tablets containing 3 g of glucose are available (dextrosol). The educated patient soon learns to take the amount of glucose needed to correct symptoms without ingesting excessive quantities of orange juice or candy, which can provoke very high glycemic levels. Family members or friends of the patient should be provided with a glucagon emergency kit (Lilly), which contains a syringe, diluent, and a 1-mg ampule of glucagon that can be injected intramuscularly if the patient is found unconscious; these kits are available by prescription. Detailed instructions in the use of glucagon are an essential part of the diabetic education program.

A. The Conscious Patient: Patients with symptoms of hypoglycemia who are conscious and able to swallow should eat or drink orange juice, glucose tablets, or any sugar-containing beverage or food except pure fructose (which does not cross the blood-brain barrier).

B. The Unconscious Patient: In general, oral feeding is contraindicated in stuporous or unconscious patients. If trained personnel are not available to administer intravenous glucose, the treatment of choice is for a family member or friend to administer 1 mg of glucagon intramuscularly (see above), which will usually restore the patient to consciousness within 10–15 minutes; the patient should then be given an oral form of sugar to ingest. If glucagon is not available, small amounts of honey, syrup, or glucose gel (Glutose) can be rubbed into the buccal mucosa. Rectal administration of syrup or honey (30 mL per 500 mL of warm water) has also been used effectively.

COMA

Coma is a *medical emergency* calling for immediate evaluation to determine its cause so that proper therapy can be started. There are several causes of coma that result directly from diabetes mellitus or its treatment. When evaluating a comatose diabetic patient, these must be considered *in addition* to the myriad causes included in the differential diagnosis of coma (cerebrovascular accidents, head trauma, intoxication with alcohol or other drugs, etc.)

Etiologic Classification of Diabetic Coma

The causes of coma resulting directly from diabetes mellitus or its treatment include the following:

A. Hyperglycemic Coma: Hyperglycemic coma may be associated with either severe insulin deficiency (diabetic ketoacidosis) or with mild to moderate insulin deficiency (hyperglycemic, hyperosmolar, non-ketotic coma).

B. Hypoglycemic Coma: This results from excessive doses of insulin or oral hypoglycemic agents (see above).

C. Lactic Acidosis: Lactic acidosis in diabetics is particularly apt to occur in association with severe tissue anoxia, sepsis, or cardiovascular collapse.

Emergency Management of Coma

The standard approach to *any comatose patient* is outlined below. Prompt action is required.

(1) Establish an airway.

(2) Establish intravenous access. About 30 mL of blood should be drawn and sent for complete blood count, serum electrolyte determinations, renal function and liver function tests, and blood glucose measurements.

(3) Administer 50 mL of 50% dextrose in water to all comatose patients, unless bedside monitoring of blood glucose shows marked hyperglycemia. This will rapidly reverse hypoglycemic coma and will not significantly alter the ultimate course of the mildly hyperglycemic patient. Since hypoglycemic blood left on an enzyme-impregnated glucose oxidase strip for longer than 1 minute (which can occur in the hectic atmosphere of an emergency situation) will give falsely elevated values, it is probably best not to withhold administration of intravenous dextrose to undiagnosed comatose patients in the absence of marked hyperglycemia (240 mg/dL or more).

(4) Administer 1 ampule (0.4 mg) of naloxone intravenously and 100 mg of thiamine intravenously.

Diagnosis of Coma

After emergency measures have been instituted, a careful history (from family, friends, paramedics, etc), physical examination, and laboratory evaluation are required to resolve the differential diagnosis. Patients in deep coma from a hyperosmolar nonketotic state or from hypoglycemia are generally flaccid and have quiet breathing—in contrast to patients with acidosis, whose respirations are rapid and deep if the pH of arterial blood has dropped to 7.1 or below. When hypoglycemia is a cause of the coma, hypothermia is usually present and the state of hydration is usually normal. Although the clinical laboratory remains the final arbiter in confirming the diagnosis, a rapid *estimation* of blood glucose and ketones can be obtained by the use of enzyme-impregnated glucose oxidase strips and crushed Acetest tablets (see Laboratory Findings in Diabetes Mellitus, above). Table 22–16 is a summary of some laboratory abnormalities found in diabetic patients with coma attributable to diabetes or its treatment. The individual clinical syndromes are discussed in detail on the following pages.

1. DIABETIC KETOACIDOSIS

This acute complication of diabetes mellitus may be the first manifestation of previously undiagnosed diabetes, or it may be the result of failure of a known diabetic to take adequate exogenous insulin. In either case, precipitating factors, such as infection, should be searched for and treated appropriately. Poor compliance, either for psychological reasons or because of inadequate patient education, is probably the most common cause of diabetic ketoacidosis, particularly when episodes are recurrent. In adolescents with type I diabetes, recurrent episodes of severe ketoacidosis often indicate the need for counseling to alter this behavior.

Diabetic ketoacidosis has been found to be one of the more common serious complications of insulin pump therapy, occurring in approximately one per 80 patient months of treatment. Many patients who monitor capillary blood glucose regularly ignore urine ketone measurements, which would signal the possibility of insulin leakage or pump failure before serious illness develops.

Table 22–16. Summary of some laboratory abnormalities in patients with coma directly attributable to diabetes or its treatment.

	Urine		Plasma			
	Glucose	**Acetone**	**Glucose**	**Bicarbonate**	**Acetone**	**Osmolality**
Hyperglycemic, hyperosmolar coma Diabetic ketoacidosis	++ to ++++	++++	High	Low	++++	+++
Hyperglycemic nonketotic coma	++ to ++++	0 or +[1]	High	Normal or slightly low[2]	0	++++
Hypoglycemia	0[3]	0 or +	Low	Normal	0	Normal
Lactic acidosis	0 or +	0 or +	Normal, low, or high	Low	0 or +	Normal

[1]A small degree of ketonuria may be present if the patient is severely stressed or has not been eating because of illness.
[2]Patient may be acidotic if there is severe volume depletion with cardiovascular collapse or if sepsis is present.
[3]Leftover urine in bladder might still contain sugar from earlier hyperglycemia.

Pathogenesis

Acute insulin deficiency results in rapid mobilization of energy from stores in muscle and fat depots, leading to an increased flux of amino acids to the liver for conversion to glucose and of fatty acids for conversion to ketones (acetoacetate, β-hydroxybutyrate, and acetone). In addition to this increased availability of precursor, there is a direct effect of the low insulin:glucagon ratio on the liver that promotes increased production of ketones. In response to both the acute insulin deficiency and the metabolic stress of ketosis, the levels of insulin-antagonistic hormones (corticosteroids, catecholamines, glucagon, and GH) are consistently elevated. Furthermore, in the absence of insulin, peripheral utilization of glucose and ketones is reduced. The combination of increased production and decreased utilization leads to an accumulation of these substances in blood, with plasma glucose levels reaching 500 mg/dL (27.8 mmol/L) or more and plasma ketones reaching levels of 8–15 mmol/L or more.

The hyperglycemia causes osmotic diuresis leading to depletion of intravascular volume. As this progresses, impaired renal blood flow reduces the kidney's ability to excrete glucose, and hyperosmolality is worsened. Severe hyperosmolality (> 330 mosm) correlates closely with central nervous system depression and coma.

In a similar manner, impaired renal excretion of hydrogen ions aggravates the metabolic acidosis that occurs as a result of the accumulation of the ketone acids, β-hydroxybutyrate and acetoacetate. The accumulation of ketones may cause vomiting, which exacerbates the intravascular volume depletion. In addition, prolonged acidosis can compromise cardiac output and reduce vascular tone. The result may be severe cardiovascular collapse with generation of lactic acid, which then adds to the already existent metabolic acidosis (Fig 22–11).

Clinical Findings

A. Symptoms and Signs: As opposed to the acute onset of hypoglycemic coma, the appearance of diabetic ketoacidosis is usually preceded by a day or more of polyuria and polydipsia associated with marked fatigue, nausea, and vomiting. Eventually, mental stupor ensues and can progress to frank coma. On physical examination, evidence of dehydration in a stuporous patient with rapid and deep respirations and the "fruity" breath odor of acetone would strongly suggest the diagnosis. Postural hypotension with tachycardia indicates profound dehydration and salt depletion.

B. Laboratory Findings: Four-plus glycosuria, strong ketonuria, hyperglycemia, ketonemia, low arterial blood pH, and low plasma bicarbonate are typical laboratory findings in diabetic ketoacidosis. Serum potassium is usually normal or slightly elevated (5–8 meq/L) despite total body potassium depletion, because of the shift of potassium from the intra- to extracellular spaces that occurs in systemic acidosis. The average total body potassium deficit resulting from osmotic diuresis, acidosis, and gastrointestinal losses is about 5–10 meq/kg body weight. Similarly, serum phosphate is elevated (6–7 mg/dL), but total body phosphate is generally depleted. Serum sodium may be slightly reduced (to about 125–130 meq/L) because of expansion of plasma volume by glucose. (For every 100 mg/dL of plasma glucose above normal, serum sodium decreases by 1.6 meq/L.) Serum osmolality can be directly measured by standard tests of freezing-point depression or can be estimated by calculating the molarity of sodium, chloride, and glucose in the serum. A convenient formula for estimating serum osmolality is as follows (physiologic values in humans are generally between 280–300 mosm/L):

$$\text{mosm/L} = 2\,[\text{Na}^+] + \frac{\text{glucose (mg/dL)}}{18} + \frac{\text{BUN (mg/dL)}}{2.8}$$

These calculated estimates are usually 10–20 mosm/L lower than values recorded by standard cryoscopic techniques. Blood urea nitrogen and serum creatinine are invariably elevated because of dehydration. In the presence of keto acids, values from multichannel chemical analysis of serum creatinine are falsely elevated and therefore quite unreliable. However, most laboratories can correct for these interfering chromogens by using a more specific method if asked to do so.

In about 90% of cases, serum amylase is elevated. However, this often represents salivary as well as pancreatic amylase and correlates poorly with symptoms of pancreatitis, such as pain and vomiting. Therefore, in patients with diabetic ketoacidosis, an elevated serum amylase does not justify a diagnosis of acute pancreatitis; serum lipase may be useful if the diagnosis of pancreatitis is being seriously considered.

C. Data Recording on a Flow Sheet: The need for frequent evaluation of the patient's status cannot be overemphasized. Patients with moderately severe diabetic ketoacidosis (pH < 7.2) are best managed in an intensive care unit. Essential baseline blood chemistries include glucose, ketones, electrolytes, arterial blood gases, blood urea nitrogen, and serum creatinine. Typically, the patient with moderately severe diabetic ketoacidosis will have a plasma glucose of 350–900 mg/dL (19.4–50 mmol/L), the presence of serum ketones at a dilution of 1:8 or greater, slight hyponatremia of 130 meq/L, hyperkalemia of 5–8 meq/L, hyperphosphatemia of 6–7 mg/dL, and an elevated blood urea nitrogen and creatinine. Acidosis may be severe (pH ranging from 6.9 to 7.2 and bicarbonate ranging from 5 to 10 meq/L); P_{CO2} is low (15–20 mm Hg) from hyperventilation.

A comprehensive flow sheet that includes vital signs, serial laboratory data, and therapeutic interventions should be meticulously maintained by the physi-

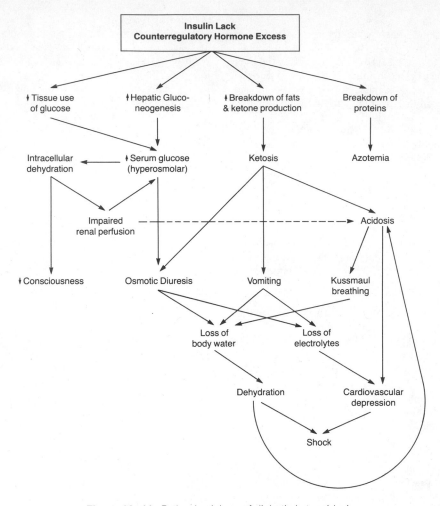

Figure 22–11. Pathophysiology of diabetic ketoacidosis.

cian responsible for the patient's care. Plasma glucose should be recorded hourly and electrolytes and pH at least every 2–3 hours during the initial treatment period. Insulin therapy is greatly facilitated when plasma glucose results are available within a few minutes of sampling. This can be achieved by the use of such instruments as the Beckman or Yellow Springs glucose analyzers. Recently developed reflectance meters designed for bedside glucose measurements of capillary blood glucose are also sufficiently accurate for use in this situation (see Blood Glucose Testing, above). Fluid intake and output as well as details of insulin therapy and the administration of other medications should also be carefully recorded on the flow sheet.

Treatment

A. Immediate Resuscitation and Emergency Measures: If the patient is stuporous or comatose, immediately institute the emergency measures outlined in the section on coma (see above). Once the diagnosis of diabetic ketoacidosis is established, a

rapid intravenous bolus of 0.3 unit of regular insulin per kilogram of body weight should be given. This will inhibit both gluconeogenesis and ketogenesis while promoting utilization of glucose and ketoacids. Administration of at least 1 L of normal saline (in an adult patient) in the first 1–2 hours is recommended initially to help restore plasma volume and stabilize blood pressure while acutely reducing the hyperosmolar state. In addition, by improving renal plasma flow, fluid replacement also restores the renal capacity to excrete hydrogen ions, thereby meliorating the acidosis as well. If arterial blood pH is less than 7.1, intravenous bicarbonate should be administered (details of administration are outlined below). Gastric intubation is recommended in the comatose patient to prevent vomiting and aspiration that may occur as a result of gastric atony, a common complication of diabetic ketoacidosis. An indwelling bladder catheter is required in all comatose patients but should be avoided, if possible, in a fully cooperative diabetic patient because of the risk of bladder infection. In patients with preexisting cardiac or renal failure or those in severe cardiovascular collapse, a central venous pressure catheter or a Swan-Ganz catheter should be inserted to evaluate the degree of hypovolemia and to monitor subsequent fluid administration.

B. Specific Measures: Each case must be managed individually depending on the specific abnormalities present and subsequent response to initial therapy.

1. Insulin—Only regular insulin, and preferably human insulin, should be used in the management of diabetic ketoacidosis. As noted above, a "loading" dose of 0.3 unit/kg body weight of regular insulin is given initially as an intravenous bolus followed by 0.1 unit/kg/h, either continuously infused or injected intramuscularly. Doses of insulin as low as 0.1 unit/kg, given hourly either by slow intravenous drip or intramuscularly, are as effective in most cases as the much higher doses previously recommended, and they appear to be safer. When a continuous infusion of insulin is used, 25 units of regular human insulin should be placed in 250 mL of physiologic saline and the first 50 mL of solution flushed through to saturate the tubing before connecting it to the intravenous line. An I-Vac or Harvard pump provides a reliable infusion rate. The insulin dose should be "piggy-backed" into the fluid line so the rate of fluid replacement can be changed without altering the insulin delivery rate. For optimal effects, continuous low-dose insulin infusions should always be preceded by a rapid intravenous loading dose of regular insulin, 0.3 unit/kg, to prime the tissue insulin receptors. If the plasma glucose level fails to fall at least 10% in the first hour, a repeat loading dose is recommended. Insulin therapy is greatly facilitated when plasma glucose can be measured within a few minutes of sampling. Rarely, a patient with insulin resistance is encountered; this requires doubling the insulin dose every 2–4 hours if hyperglycemia does not improve after the first 2 doses of insulin.

Insulin therapy, either as a continuous infusion or as injections given every 1–2 hours, should be continued until arterial pH has normalized.

2. Fluid replacement—In most adult patients, the fluid deficit is 4–5 L. Initially, normal saline is preferred for restoration of plasma volume and, as noted above, should be infused rapidly to provide 1 L/h over the first 1–2 hours. After the first 2 L of fluid have been given, the fluid should be changed to 0.45% saline solution given at a rate of 300–400 mL/h; this is because water loss exceeds sodium loss in uncontrolled diabetes with osmotic diuresis. When blood glucose falls to approximately 250 mg/dL, the fluids should be changed to a 5% glucose solution to maintain plasma glucose in the range of 250–300 mg/dL. This will prevent the development of hypoglycemia and reduce the likelihood of cerebral edema, which could result from too rapid decline of blood glucose. Intensive insulin therapy should be continued until metabolic acidosis is corrected.

3. Sodium bicarbonate—The use of sodium bicarbonate in management of diabetic ketoacidosis has been questioned by some because of the following potential consequences: (1) development of hypokalemia from rapid shift of potassium into cells; (2) tissue anoxia from reduced dissociation of oxygen from hemoglobin when acidosis is rapidly reversed (leftward shift of the oxygen dissociation curve); and (3) cerebral acidosis resulting from lowering of cerebrospinal fluid pH. It must be emphasized, however, that these considerations are less important when severe acidosis exists. It is therefore recommended that bicarbonate be administered to diabetic patients in ketoacidosis if the arterial blood pH is less than 7.1 or if hypotension, arrhythmia, or coma is present along with an arterial blood pH of less than 7.1.

One to 2 ampules of sodium bicarbonate (one ampule contains 44 meq/50 mL) should be added to 1 L of 0.45% saline. (*Note:* Addition of sodium bicarbonate to 0.9% saline would produce a markedly hypertonic solution that could aggravate the hyperosmolar state already present.) This should be administered rapidly (over the first hour). It can be repeated until the arterial pH reaches 7.1 **but should not be given if pH is 7.1 or greater.** As noted earlier, serious consideration should be given to placement of a central venous or Swan-Ganz catheter when administering fluids to severely ill patients with cardiovascular compromise.

4. Potassium—Total body potassium loss from polyuria and vomiting may be as high as 200 meq. However, because of shifts of potassium from cells into the extracellular space as a consequence of acidosis, serum potassium is usually normal to slightly elevated prior to institution of treatment. As the acidosis is corrected, potassium flows back into the cells, and hypokalemia can develop if potassium replacement is not instituted. If the patient is not uremic and has an adequate urine output, potassium chloride in doses of 10–30 meq/h should be infused during the second and third hours after beginning therapy as soon as the acidosis starts to resolve. Replacement should be started sooner if the initial serum potassium is inappropriately normal or low. Cooperative patients with only mild ketoacidosis may receive part or all of their potassium replacement orally.

An ECG can be of help in monitoring the patient's potassium status: high peaked T waves are a sign of hyperkalemia, and flattened T waves with U waves are a sign of hypokalemia.

5. Phosphate—Because severe hypophosphatemia also develops during insulin therapy of diabetic ketoacidosis, some of the potassium can be replaced as the phosphate salt. Correction of hypophosphatemia helps to restore the buffering capacity of the plasma, thereby facilitating renal excretion of hydrogen. It also corrects the impaired oxygen dissociation from hemoglobin by regenerating 2,3-diphosphoglycerate. However, a randomized study in which phosphate was replaced in only half of a group of 18 patients with diabetic ketoacidosis did not show any apparent clinical benefit from phosphate administration. Moreover, attempts to use the phosphate salt of potassium as the sole means of replacing potassium have led to a number of reported cases of severe hypocalcemia with tetany. To minimize the risk of inducing tetany from too rapid replacement of phosphate, the average deficit of 40–50 mmol of phosphate should be replaced intravenously at a rate *no greater than 3–4 mmol/h* in a 60- to 70-kg person. A stock solution (Abbott) provides a mixture of 1.12 g KH_2PO_4 and 1.18 g K_2HPO_4 in a 5-mL single-dose vial (this equals 22 mmol of potassium and 15 mmol of phosphate). One-half of this vial (2.5 mL) should be added to 1 L of either 0.45% saline or 5% dextrose in water. Two liters of this solution, infused at a rate of 400 mL/h, will correct the phosphate deficit at the optimal rate of 3 mmol/h while providing 4.4 meq of potassium per hour. (Additional potassium should be administered as potassium chloride to provide a total of 10–30 meq of potassium per hour, as noted above.) If the serum phosphate remains below 2.5 mg/dL after this infusion, a repeat 5-hour infusion can be given.

It remains controversial whether phosphate replacement is beneficial. Several clinics prohibit its use in the routine treatment of diabetic ketoacidosis, since the risk of inducing hypocalcemia is thought to outweigh its potential benefits. However, potential hazards of phosphate replacement can be greatly reduced by administering phosphate at a rate no greater than 3–4 mmol/h. To prevent errors of overreplacement, phosphate should be administered separately rather than included as a component of potassium replacement.

Prognosis

Insulin and fluid and electrolyte replacement combined with careful monitoring of patients' clinical and laboratory responses to therapy have dramatically reduced the morbidity and mortality rates of diabetic ketoacidosis. However, this complication still represents a potential threat to survival, especially in older people with cardiovascular disease. Even in specialized centers, the mortality rate may approach 5–10%. Therefore, physicians treating diabetic ketoacidosis must not be lured into adopting "cookbook" approaches that lessen their attentiveness to changes in the patient's condition. Signs to be watched for include failure of improvement in mental status after a period of treatment, continued hypotension with minimal urine flow, or prolonged ileus (which may suggest bowel infarction). Laboratory abnormalities to be watched include failure of blood glucose to fall by 80–100 mg/dL during the initial therapeutic period, failure to increase serum bicarbonate or arterial pH appropriately, serum potassium above 6 or below 2.8 meq/L, and electrocardiographic evidence of cardiac arrhythmias. Any of these signs call for a careful search for the cause of the abnormality and prompt specific therapy.

Disposition

After recovery and stabilization, patients should receive intensive detailed instruction about how to avoid this potentially disastrous complication of diabetes mellitus. They should be taught to recognize the early symptoms and signs of ketoacidosis.

Urine ketones should be measured in patients with signs of infection or in those using an insulin pump when capillary blood glucose is unexpectedly and persistently high. When heavy ketonuria and glycosuria persist on several successive examinations, supplemental regular insulin should be administered and liquid foods such as lightly salted tomato juice and broth should be ingested to replenish fluids and electrolytes. Patients should be instructed to contact the physician if ketonuria persists, and especially if vomiting develops or if appropriate adjustment of the infusion rate on an insulin pump does not correct the hyperglycemia and ketonuria.

2. HYPERGLYCEMIC, HYPEROSMOLAR, NONKETOTIC STATE

This form of hyperglycemic coma is characterized by severe hyperglycemia, hyperosmolality, and dehydration in the absence of significant ketosis. It occurs in patients with mild or occult diabetes, who are usually middle-aged to elderly. Underlying renal insufficiency or congestive heart failure is common, and the presence of either worsens the prognosis. A precipitating event such as pneumonia, cerebrovascular accident, myocardial infarction, burns, or recent operation can often be identified. Certain drugs, such as phenytoin, diazoxide, glucocorticoids, and thiazide diuretics, have been implicated in its development, as have procedures associated with glucose loading, eg, peritoneal dialysis.

Pathogenesis

A partial or relative insulin deficiency may initiate the syndrome by reducing glucose utilization by muscle, fat, and the liver while at the same time inducing hyperglucagonemia and increasing hepatic glucose output. The result is hyperglycemia that leads to glycosuria and osmotic diuresis with obligatory water loss. The presence of even small amounts of insulin is believed to prevent the development of ketosis by inhibiting lipolysis in the adipose stores. Therefore even though a low insulin:glucagon ratio promotes ketogenesis in the liver, the limited availability of precursor free fatty acids from the periphery restricts the rate at which ketones are formed. If a patient is unable to maintain adequate fluid intake because of an associated acute or chronic illness or has suffered excessive fluid loss (eg, from burns or therapy with diuretics), marked dehydration results. As plasma volume contracts, renal insufficiency develops; this, then, limits renal glucose excretion and contributes markedly to the rise in serum glucose and osmolality. Hyperosmolality causes mental confusion, and when the serum osmolality reaches approximately 330 mosm/L, coma may ensue.

Clinical Findings

A. Symptoms and Signs: The onset of the hyperglycemic, hyperosmolar, nonketotic state may be insidious, preceded for days or weeks by symptoms of weakness, polyuria, and polydipsia. A history of reduced fluid intake is common, whether due to inappropriate absence of thirst, gastrointestinal upset, or, in the case of elderly or bedridden patients, lack of access to water. A history of ingestion of large quantities of glucose-containing fluids, such as soft drinks or orange juice, can occasionally be obtained; these patients are usually less hyperosmolar than those in whom fluid intake was restricted. The absence of toxic features of ketoacidosis may retard recognition of the syndrome and thus delay institution of therapy until dehydration is profound. Because of this delay in diagnosis, the hyperglycemia, hyperosmolality, and dehydration in hyperglycemic, hyperosmolar, nonketotic coma is often more severe than in diabetic ketoacidosis.

Physical examination will reveal the presence of profound dehydration (orthostatic fall in blood pressure and rise in pulse, supine tachycardia or even frank shock, dry mucous membranes, decreased skin turgor). The patient may be lethargic, confused, or comatose. Kussmaul respirations are absent unless the precipitating event for the hyperosmolar state has also led to the development of metabolic acidosis (eg, sepsis or myocardial infarction with shock).

B. Laboratory Findings: Severe hyperglycemia is present, with blood glucose values ranging from 800 to as high as 2400 mg/dL (44.4–133.2 mmol/L). In mild cases, where dehydration is less severe, dilutional hyponatremia as well as urinary sodium losses may reduce serum sodium to about 120–125 meq/L*—this protects, to some extent, against extreme hyperosmolality. Once dehydration progresses further, however, serum sodium can exceed 140 meq/L, producing serum osmolalities of 330–440 mosm/L† (normal, 280–295 mosm/L). Ketosis is usually absent or mild; however, a small degree of ketonuria may be present if the patient has not been eating because of illness. Acidosis is not a part of the hyperglycemic, hyperosmolar state, but it may be present (usually lactic acidosis) because of other acute underlying conditions (sepsis, acute renal failure, myocardial infarction, etc). (See Lactic Acidosis, below.)

---

*See p 634 for formula used in correcting hyponatremia due to hyperglycemia.
†A convenient method for estimating serum osmolality is provided on p 634.

Treatment

There are some differences in fluid, insulin, and electrolyte replacement in this disorder, as compared to diabetic ketoacidosis. However, in common with the treatment of ketoacidotic patients, careful monitoring of the patient's clinical and laboratory response to therapy is essential.

A. Fluid Replacement: Fluid replacement is of paramount importance in treating nonketotic hyperglycemic coma. If circulatory collapse is present, fluid therapy should be initiated with isotonic saline. In all other cases, initial replacement with hypotonic (usually 0.45%) saline is preferable, because these patients are hyperosmolar with excess solute in the vascular compartment. As much as 4–6 L of fluid may be required in the first 8–10 hours. Careful monitoring of fluid quantity and type, urine output, blood pressure, and pulse is essential. Placement of a central venous pressure or Swan-Ganz catheter should be strongly considered to guide replacement of fluid, especially if the patient is elderly or has underlying renal or cardiac disease. Because insulin therapy will decrease plasma glucose and therefore serum osmolality, a change to isotonic saline may be necessary at some time during treatment in order to maintain an adequate blood pressure and a urine output of at least 50 mL/h. Once blood glucose reaches 250 mg/dL, 5% dextrose in 0.45% or 0.9% saline solution should be substituted for the sugar-free fluids. When consciousness returns, oral fluids should be encouraged.

B. Electrolyte Replacement: Hyperkalemia is less marked and much less potassium is lost in the urine during the osmotic diuresis of hyperglycemic, hyperosmolar, nonketotic coma than in diabetic ketoacidosis. There is, therefore, less severe total potassium depletion, and less potassium replacement is needed to restore potassium stores to normal. However, because the initial serum potassium usually is not elevated and because it declines rapidly as insulin therapy allows glucose and potassium to enter cells, it is recommended that potassium replacement be initiated earlier than in ketotic patients: 10 meq of potassium chloride can be added to the *initial* liter of fluid administered if the initial serum potassium is not elevated and if the patient is making urine. When hypophosphatemia develops during insulin therapy, phosphate replacement can be given intravenously with the same precautions as those outlined for ketoacidotic patients (see above). If the patient is awake and cooperative, part or all of the potassium and phosphate replacement can be given orally.

C. Insulin Therapy: In general, less insulin is required to reduce the hyperglycemia of nonketotic patients than is the case for patients in diabetic ketoacidosis. In fact, fluid replacement alone can decrease glucose levels considerably. An initial dose of 15 units of regular insulin given intravenously and 15 units given intramuscularly is usually quite effective in lowering blood glucose. In most cases, subsequent doses need not be greater than 10–25 units every 4 hours. (Insulin should be given intramuscularly or intravenously until the patient has stabilized; it may then be given subcutaneously.) Some patients—especially those who are severely ill because of other underlying diseases—may require continuous intravenous administration of insulin (in a manner similar to that described for ketoacidosis) with careful monitoring, preferably in an intensive care setting.

D. Search for the Precipitating Event: The physician must initiate a careful search for the event that precipitated the episode of hyperglycemic, hyperosmolar, nonketotic coma if it is not obvious after the initial history and physical examination. Chest x-rays and cultures of blood, urine, and other body fluids should be obtained to look for occult sources of sepsis; empiric antibiotic coverage should be considered in the seriously ill patient. Cardiac enzymes and serial ECGs can be ordered to look for evidence of "silent" myocardial infarction.

Prognosis

The overall mortality rate of hyperglycemic, hyperosmolar, nonketotic coma is over 10 times that of diabetic ketoacidosis, chiefly because of its higher incidence in older patients, who may have compromised cardiovascular systems or associated major illnesses. (When patients are matched for age, the prognoses of these 2 forms of hyperosmolar coma are reasonably comparable.)

Disposition

After the patient is stabilized, the appropriate form of long-term management of the diabetes must be determined. This must include patient education on how to recognize situations (gastrointestinal upset, infection) that will predispose to recurrence of hyperglycemic, hyperosmolar, nonketotic coma as well as detailed information on how to prevent the escalating dehydration (small sips of sugar-free liquids, increase in usual hypoglycemic therapy, or early contact with the physician) that culminates in hyperosmolar coma. For a detailed discussion of therapeutic alternatives for type II diabetic patients, see Steps in the Management of the Diabetic Patient (above).

3. HYPOGLYCEMIC COMA

Hypoglycemia is a common complication of insulin replacement therapy in diabetic patients. In most cases, it is detected and treated by patients or their families before coma results. However, it remains the most frequent cause of coma in the insulin-treated diabetic patient. In addition, it can occur in any patient taking oral sulfonylurea drugs, particularly if the patient is elderly, has renal or liver disease, or is taking

certain other medications that alter metabolism of the sulfonylureas (eg, phenylbutazone, sulfonamides, or coumarin derivatives). It occurs more frequently with the use of long-acting sulfonylureas than when shorter-acting agents are used.

Clinical Findings & Treatment

The clinical findings and emergency treatment of hypoglycemia are discussed above.

Prognosis

Many patients who arrive at emergency rooms in hypoglycemic coma appear to recover fully; however, profound hypoglycemia or delays in therapy can result in permanent neurologic deficit or even death. Furthermore, repeated episodes of hypoglycemia may have a cumulative adverse effect on intellectual functioning.

Disposition

The physician should carefully review with the patient the events leading up to the hypoglycemic episode. Associated use of other medications, as well as alcohol or narcotics, should be noted. Careful attention should be paid to diet, exercise pattern, insulin or sulfonylurea dosage, and general compliance with the prescribed diabetes treatment regimen. Any factors thought to have contributed to the development of the episode should be identified and recommendations made in order to prevent recurrences of this potentially disastrous complication of diabetes therapy.

If the patient is hypoglycemic from use of a long-acting oral hypoglycemic agent (eg, chlorpropamide or glyburide) or a long-acting insulin, admission to hospital for treatment with continuous intravenous glucose and careful monitoring of blood glucose is indicated.

4. LACTIC ACIDOSIS

When severely ill diabetic patients present with profound acidosis but relatively low or undetectable levels of ketoacids in plasma, the presence of excessive plasma lactate (> 6 mmol/L) should be considered, especially if other causes of acidosis such as uremia are not present.

Pathogenesis

Lactic acid is the end product of anaerobic metabolism of glucose. Normally, the principal sources of this acid are the erythrocytes (which lack the enzymes for aerobic oxidation), skeletal muscle, skin, and brain. The chief pathway for removal of lactic acid is by hepatic (and to some degree renal) uptake for conversion first to pyruvate and eventually back to glucose, a process that requires oxygen. Lactic acidosis occurs when excess lactic acid accumulates in the blood. This can be the result of overproduction (tissue hypoxia), deficient removal (hepatic failure), or both (circulatory collapse). Patients with lactic acidosis are usually severely ill, with problems such as myocardial infarction with shock, sepsis, hemorrhage, severe anemia, carbon monoxide poisoning, severe pulmonary disease, severe liver disease, or cyanide poisoning. Phenformin, an oral hypoglycemic agent no longer available in the USA, has been reported to cause lactic acidosis, especially in patients with altered lactate or phenformin metabolism. In addition, lactic acidosis has been reported after the use of salicylates, sodium nitroprusside, intravenous fructose, sorbitol, ethanol, and other substances.

Clinical Findings

A. Symptoms and Signs: The main clinical features of lactic acidosis are marked hyperventilation and mental confusion, which may progress to stupor or coma. When lactic acidosis is secondary to tissue hypoxia or vascular collapse, the clinical presentation is variable, being that of the prevailing catastrophic illness. In the rare instance of idiopathic or spontaneous lactic acidosis, the onset is rapid (usually over a few hours), the cardiopulmonary status is stable, and mentation may be relatively normal.

B. Laboratory Findings: Plasma glucose can be low, normal, or high in diabetic patients with lactic acidosis, but usually it is moderately elevated. Plasma bicarbonate and arterial pH are quite low. An anion gap will be present (calculated by subtracting the sum of the plasma bicarbonate and chloride from the plasma sodium; normal is 12–16). Ketones are usually absent from plasma, but small amounts may be present in urine if the patient has not been eating recently. Other causes of "anion gap" metabolic acidosis should be excluded—eg, uremia, diabetic or alcoholic ketoacidosis, and salicylate, methanol, ethylene glycol, or paraldehyde intoxication. In the absence of azotemia, hyperphosphatemia may be a clue to the presence of lactic acidosis.

The diagnosis is confirmed by demonstrating, in a sample of blood that is promptly chilled and separated, a plasma lactate concentration of 6 mmol/L or higher (normal is about 1 mmol/L). Failure to rapidly chill the sample and separate the plasma can lead to falsely high plasma lactate values as a result of continued glycolysis by the red blood cells. Frozen plasma remains stable for subsequent assay.

Treatment

The cornerstone of therapy is aggressive treatment of the precipitating cause. An adequate airway and good oxygenation should be ensured. If hypotension is present, fluids and, if appropriate, pressor agents must be given to restore tissue perfusion. Appropriate cultures and empiric antibiotic coverage should be instituted in any seriously ill patient with lactic acidosis in whom the cause is not immediately apparent. Alkalinization with intravenous sodium bicarbonate to keep the pH above 7.2 has been recommended in the emergency treatment of severe lactic acidosis. However, there is no evidence that the mortality rate is favorably affected by administering bicarbonate and the matter is at present controversial, particularly because of the hazards associated with bicarbonate therapy. Dichloroacetate, an anion that facilitates pyruvate removal by activating pyruvate dehydrogenase, reverses certain types of lactic acidosis in animals and may prove useful in treating lactic acidosis in humans.

CHRONIC COMPLICATIONS OF DIABETES MELLITUS (Table 22–17)

In most patients with diabetes, a number of pathologic changes occur at variable intervals during the course of the disease. Although they are termed complications, this is really a misnomer, because these changes are really parts of the diabetic state, ie, its late clinical manifestations. These changes involve the vascular system for the most part; however, they also occur in the nerves, the skin, and the lens. Abnormalities in lipoprotein metabolism are also common.

Classifications of Diabetic Vascular Disease

Diabetic vascular disease is conveniently divided into 2 main categories: microvascular disease and macrovascular disease.

A. Microvascular Disease: Disease of the smallest blood vessels, the capillary and the precapillary arterioles, is manifested mainly by thickening of the capillary basement membrane. Microvascular disease involving the retina leads to diabetic retinopathy, and disease involving the kidney causes diabetic nephropathy. Small vessel disease may also involve the heart; recently, cardiomegaly with heart failure has been described in diabetic patients with patent coronary arteries.

B. Macrovascular Disease: Large vessel disease in diabetes is essentially an accelerated form of atherosclerosis. It accounts for the increased incidence of myocardial infarction, stroke, and peripheral gangrene in diabetic patients. Just as in the case of atherosclerosis in the general population, the exact cause of accelerated atherosclerosis in the diabetic population remains unclear. Abnormalities in vessel walls, platelets and other components of the clotting system, red blood cells, and lipid metabolism have all been postulated to play a role. In addition, there is evidence that coexistent risk factors such as cigarette smoking and hyper-

Table 22–17. Chronic complications of diabetes mellitus.

Eyes
Diabetic retinopathy
  Nonproliferative (background)
  Proliferative
Cataracts
  Subcapsular (snowflake)
  Nuclear (senile)

Kidneys
Intracapillary glomerulosclerosis
  Diffuse
  Nodular
Infection
  Pyelonephritis
  Perinephric abscess
  Renal papillary necrosis
Renal tubular necrosis
  Following dye studies (urograms, arteriograms)

Nervous system
Peripheral neuropathy
  Distal, symmetric sensory loss
  Motor neuropathy
    Foot drop, wrist drop
    Mononeuropathy multiplex (diabetic amyotrophy)
Cranial neuropathy
  Cranial nerves III, IV, VI, VII
Autonomic neuropathy
  Postural hypotension
  Resting tachycardia
  Loss of sweating
  Gastrointestinal neuropathy
    Gastroparesis
    Diabetic diarrhea
  Urinary bladder atony
  Impotence (may also be secondary to pelvic vascular disease)

Skin
Diabetic dermopathy (shin spots)
Necrobiosis lipoidica diabeticorum
Candidiasis
Foot and leg ulcers
  Neurotropic
  Ischemic

Cardiovascular system
Heart disease
  Myocardial infarction
  Cardiomyopathy
Gangrene of the feet
  Ischemic ulcers
  Osteomyelitis

Bones and joints
Diabetic cheirarthropathy
Dupuytren's contracture
Charcot joint

Unusual infections
Necrotizing fasciitis
Necrotizing myositis
Mucor meningitis
Emphysematous cholecystitis
Malignant otitis externa

tension may be important in determining the course of the disease.

In addition to the above complications, diabetic patients have an increased incidence of certain types of infections and may handle their infections less well than the general population.

Prevalence of Chronic Complications by Type of Diabetes

Although all of the known complications of diabetes can be found in both types of the disease, some are more common in one type than in the other. Renal failure due to severe microvascular nephropathy is the major cause of death in patients with type I diabetes, whereas macrovascular disease is the leading cause in type II. Although blindness occurs in both types, it occurs more commonly as a result of severe proliferative retinopathy, vitreous hemorrhages, and retinal detachment in type I disease, whereas macular edema and ischemia or cataracts are the usual cause in type II. Similarly, although diabetic neuropathy is common in both type I and type II diabetes, severe autonomic neuropathy with gastroparesis, diabetic diarrhea, resting tachycardia, and postural hypotension is much more common in type I.

Relationship of Glycemic Control to Development of Chronic Complications

The cause of chronic microvascular complications in diabetic patients remains unresolved. However, it has been recently documented (see Finegold reference) that impaired metabolic control can initiate microvascular disease in patients with acquired diabetes. In this case, Korean patients developed chronic hyperglycemia after attempting suicide with Vacor, a rodenticide with potent toxicity for pancreatic B cells. These patients were examined 6–7 years after developing permanent diabetes, and more than one-half showed thickened capillary basement membranes, 44% showed retinopathy, and 28% showed proteinuria.

In patients with idiopathic diabetes mellitus however, there is still uncertainty about whether strict blood glucose control significantly alters the incidence of diabetic complications. There are 2 main reasons for this uncertainty: (1) past inability to safely achieve glycemic control that approaches normality and (2) present inability to accurately assess the degree of glycemic control being achieved. The use of improved delivery systems with highly purified insulins and especially the development of accurate methods for self-monitoring of blood glucose have now made "tight" glycemic control a possibility. Combined with newer methods for evaluating control, such as glycohemoglobin measurements, these developments may soon allow resolution of this important issue.

A prospective randomized trial involving 21 clinical centers (the Diabetes Control and Complications Trial) has been initiated by the National Institutes of Health to determine if tight glycemic control over a period of 7–10 years can prevent or delay the development of diabetic retinopathy or nephropathy in patients with IDDM.

In addition to this "prevention" trial, 2 short-term

"intervention" trials (the Steno Study Group and the Kroc Collaborative Study Group) agreed that intensified metabolic control does not retard the progression of mild nonproliferative retinopathy in IDDM patients. Of concern was the observation in both studies that tight glycemic control appeared to even accelerate the progression of retinopathy. Although retinal deterioration was only transient in some patients and in no case was visual acuity reduced by the accelerated progression of retinopathy, these results suggest that caution should be exercised in restoring euglycemia rapidly in patients with established retinopathy. These observations are supported by a recent study reporting no difference in the progression of diabetic retinopathy during a 2-year follow-up in IDDM patients who achieved normal glycohemoglobins after successful pancreatic transplantation, compared to a matched group with elevated glycohemoglobins in whom an attempted pancreas transplant was unsuccessful.

The Kroc Collaborative Study Group reported that in patients with established diabetic nephropathy, tight glycemic control did not retard the progression of renal disease, even though in earlier stages of renal involvement microalbuminuria was reduced considerably by near-normalization of blood glucose levels. The Steno Study Group observed that in IDDM patients with incipient diabetic nephropathy characterized by microalbuminuria, strict metabolic control with an insulin pump resulted in a smaller increase in albumin excretion than that which occurred in a conventionally treated group with higher glycohemoglobins.

An additional encouraging finding in regard to therapeutic intervention, as reported by Raskin et al, is that the thickness of the quadriceps capillary basement membrane was significantly reduced in IDDM patients whose glycemia was tightly controlled by intensive insulin therapy, whereas no significant change in thickness was seen in conventionally treated IDDM patients with only fair control of glycemia.

SPECIFIC CHRONIC COMPLICATIONS OF DIABETES MELLITUS (Table 22–17)

1. OPHTHALMOLOGIC COMPLICATIONS

Diabetic Retinopathy

For early detection of diabetic retinopathy, patients who have had type I diabetes for more than 5 years and *all* non–insulin dependent diabetic patients should be referred to an ophthalmologist for examination and follow-up. When hypertension is present in a patient with diabetes, it should be treated vigorously, since hypertension is associated with an increased incidence and accelerated progression of diabetic retinopathy.

A. Pathogenesis and Clinical Findings: Two main categories of diabetic retinopathy exist: nonproliferative and proliferative.

Nonproliferative ("background") retinopathy represents the earliest stage of retinal involvement by diabetes and is characterized by such changes as microaneurysms, dot hemorrhages, exudates, and retinal edema. During this stage, the retinal capillaries leak proteins, lipids, or red cells into the retina. When this process occurs in the macula, the area of greatest concentration of visual cells, there will be interference with visual acuity; this is the most common cause of visual impairment in type II diabetes.

Proliferative retinopathy involves the growth of new capillaries and fibrous tissue within the retina and into the vitreous chamber. It is a consequence of small vessel occlusion, which causes retinal hypoxia; this in turn stimulates new vessel growth. Proliferative retinopathy can occur in both types of diabetes but is more common in type I, developing about 7–10 years after onset of symptoms. Vision is usually normal until vitreous hemorrhage or retinal detachment occurs.

B. Treatment: Once maculopathy or proliferative changes are detected, panretinal xenon or argon laser photocoagulation therapy is indicated. Destroying retinal tissue with photocoagulation means that surviving tissue receives a greater share of the available oxygen supply, thereby abolishing hypoxic stimulation of new vessel growth. Results of a large-scale clinical trial (the Diabetic Retinopathy Study) have verified the effectiveness of photocoagulation, particularly when recent vitreous hemorrhages have occurred or when extensive new vessels are located near the optic disk.

The best results with photocoagulation are achieved if proliferative retinopathy is detected early. This is best done by obtaining a baseline fluorescein angiogram within 5–10 years after onset of type I diabetes and then repeating this study at intervals of 1–5 years, depending on the severity of the retinal involvement found.

Pituitary ablation, which has been associated with delay in progression of severe retinopathy in the past, is rarely used today because photocoagulation therapy is just as effective and avoids the risks associated with destruction of the pituitary. Occasional cases of rapidly progressive ("florid") proliferative retinopathy in type I adolescent diabetics have been reported in which photocoagulation was less effective than pituitary ablation in preventing blindness. While further studies are needed to confirm this observation, transsphenoidal hypophysectomy remains a possible therapy for the adolescent with severe progressive retinopathy.

Cataracts

Two types of cataracts occur in diabetic patients: subcapsular and senile. **Subcapsular cataract** occurs predominantly in type I diabetics, may come on fairly rapidly, and has a significant correlation with the hyperglycemia of uncontrolled diabetes. This type of cataract has a flocculent or "snowflake" appearance and develops just below the lens capsule.

Senile cataract represents a sclerotic change of the lens nucleus. It is by far the most common type of cataract found in either diabetic or nondiabetic adults and tends to occur at a younger age in diabetic patients.

Two separate abnormalities found in diabetic patients, both of which are related to elevated blood glucose levels, may contribute to the formation of cataracts: (1) glycosylation of the lens protein and (2) an excess of sorbitol, which is formed from the increased quantities of glucose found in the insulin-independent lens. Accumulation of sorbitol leads to osmotic changes in the lens that ultimately result in fibrosis and cataract formation.

2. RENAL COMPLICATIONS

Diabetic Nephropathy

A. Pathogenesis and Clinical Findings: About 4000 cases of end-stage renal disease due to diabetic nephropathy occur annually among diabetic patients in the USA. Capillary basement membrane thickening of renal glomeruli produces varying degrees of glomerulosclerosis and renal insufficiency. Diffuse glomerulosclerosis is more common than nodular intercapillary glomerulosclerosis (Kimmelstiel-Wilson lesions); both produce heavy proteinuria.

Microalbuminuria (albumin overnight excretion rate > 30 μg/min) is associated with a markedly increased risk of subsequent renal failure. Careful glycemic control, as well as a low-protein diet (0.6 g/kg/d), have been reported to reduce both the hyperfiltration and the elevated microalbuminuria in patients in the early stages of diabetes and in those with incipient diabetic nephropathy. Antihypertensive therapy also decreases microalbuminuria, and clinical trials with inhibitors of angiotensin I converting enzyme (eg, enalapril, 20 mg/d) show a reduction of microalbuminuria in diabetic patients even in the absence of hypertension. Clinically, diabetic renal disease is heralded by the onset of proteinuria, which can sometimes progress to a full-blown nephrotic syndrome, with hypoalbuminemia, hypertension, edema, and an increase in circulating low density and very low density lipoproteins. This is followed by the development of progressive renal failure, usually within 5 years after onset of proteinuria. Unlike all other renal disorders, the proteinuria of diabetic nephropathy does not diminish as renal failure progresses—patients continue to excrete 10–11 g daily as creatinine clearance diminishes. Also, there is an elevation in the tubular maximum of glucose reabsorption (and, therefore, of the threshold at which glycosuria appears) with advancing renal failure.

B. Treatment: Hemodialysis has been of limited success in the treatment of renal failure due to diabetic nephropathy, primarily because of progression of large-vessel disease with resultant death and disability from stroke and myocardial infarction. Growing experience with chronic ambulatory peritoneal dialysis suggests that it may be a more convenient method of providing adequate dialysis with a lower incidence of complications.

Renal transplantation, especially from related donors, is often successful. For patients with compatible donors and no contraindications (such as severe cardiovascular disease), it is the treatment of choice.

Necrotizing Papillitis

This unusual complication of pyelonephritis occurs primarily in diabetic patients. It is characterized by fever, flank pain, pyuria, and sloughing of renal papillae in the urine. It is treated by intravenous administration of appropriate antibiotics.

Renal Decompensation After Radiographic Dyes

The use of radiographic contrast agents in diabetic patients with reduced creatinine clearance has been associated with the development of acute renal failure. Diabetic patients with normal renal function do not appear to be at increased risk for contrast nephropathy. If a contrast study is considered essential, patients with a serum creatinine of 1.5–2.5 mg/dL should be adequately hydrated before the procedure, other nephrotoxic agents should be avoided, and only the newer, less osmolar contrast agents should be used. Among these are iohexol and iopamidol, which are nonionic, and therefore osmolality is reduced to one-half that of conventional ionized compounds with the same iodine content. Although they are 15–25 times more costly, these newer contrast substances are safer than the ionic substances, whose hyperosmolarity accounts for much of the nephrotoxicity in patients with compromised renal function. After the procedure, serum creatinine should be followed closely. Radiographic contrast material should not be given to a patient with a serum creatinine greater than 3 mg/dL.

3. NEUROLOGIC COMPLICATIONS (Diabetic Neuropathy)

Peripheral and autonomic neuropathy are the 2 most common complications of both types of diabetes. Their pathogenesis is poorly understood. Some lesions, such as the acute cranial nerve palsies and diabetic amyotrophy, have been attributed to ischemic infarction of the involved peripheral nerve. The much more common symmetric sensory and motor peripheral neuropathies and autonomic neuropathy are felt to be due to metabolic or osmotic toxicity somehow related to hyperglycemia.

Unfortunately, there is no consistently effective treatment for any of the neuropathies. It remains to be demonstrated definitively whether normalization of blood glucose levels can prevent development and progression of this devastating complication.

Peripheral Sensory Neuropathy

A. Pathogenesis and Clinical Findings: Sensory loss is commonly preceded by months or years of paresthesias such as tingling, itching, and increasing pain. The pains can vary from mild paresthesias to severe shooting pains and may be more severe at night. Discomfort of the lower extremities can be incapacitating at times. Radicular pains in the chest and the abdominal area may be extremely difficult to distinguish from pain due to an intrathoracic or intra-abdominal source. Eventually, patients develop numbness, and tactile sensations decrease. The sensory loss is generally bilateral, symmetric, and associated with dulled perception of vibration, pain, and temperature, particularly in the lower extremities, but also evident in the hands. Sensory nerve conduction is delayed in peripheral nerves, and ankle jerks may be absent. Newly developed neurothesiometer devices are being utilized to characterize the threshold levels for pain and touch, so that signs of sensory defects can be detected earlier and patients with higher risk for neuropathic foot ulcers can be identified. Because all of these sensory disturbances are made worse by pressure applied to the involved nerves, symptoms may appear first in nerves that are entrapped, such as the median nerve in carpal tunnel syndrome or the nerves around the ankle.

Characteristic syndromes that develop in diabetic patients with sensory neuropathy and are related to their failure to perceive trauma include osteopathy of the distal hand and foot, deformity of the knee or ankle (so-called Charcot joint), and neuropathic ulceration of the foot.

B. Treatment: Amitriptyline (50–75 mg at bedtime) has produced remarkable improvement in the lower extremity pain in some patients with sensory neuropathy. Dramatic relief has often occurred within 48–72 hours, and the side effect of mild to moderate drowsiness generally improves with time. This drug should be discontinued if there is no improvement after 4–5 days of therapy.

It is essential that diabetic patients with peripheral neuropathy receive detailed instructions in foot care (see p 625). Special custom-made shoes are usually required to redistribute weight evenly over an insensitive foot, particularly when it has been deformed by surgery, by asymptomatic fractures, or by Charcot joint.

Motor Neuropathy

Symmetric motor neuropathy occurs much less frequently than sensory neuropathy and is associated with delayed motor nerve conduction and muscle weakness and atrophy. Its pathogenesis is presumed to be similar to that of sensory loss. Mononeuropathy develops when there is vascular occlusion of a specific nerve trunk; if more than one nerve trunk is involved, the syndrome of **mononeuritis multiplex** occurs. Motor neuropathy is manifested by an abrupt onset of weakness in a distribution that reflects the nerve involved (eg, peroneal nerve involvement produces foot drop). A surprising number of these neuropathies improve after 6–8 weeks. Reversible **cranial nerve palsies** can occur and may present as lid ptosis (cranial nerve III), lateral deviation of the eye (IV), inability to move the eye laterally (VI), or facial paralysis (Bell's palsy) (VII). Acute pain and weakness of thigh muscles bilaterally can occur with progressive wasting and weight loss. This has been termed **diabetic amyotrophy** and is more common in elderly men. Again, the prognosis is good, with recovery of motor function over weeks to months.

Autonomic Neuropathy

Neuropathy of the autonomic nervous system is common in patients with diabetes of long duration and can be a very disconcerting clinical problem. It can affect many diverse visceral functions. With autonomic neuropathy, there is evidence of postural hypotension, resting fixed tachycardia, decreased cardiovascular responses to the Valsalva maneuver, gastroparesis, alternating bouts of diarrhea (often nocturnal) and constipation, difficulty in emptying the bladder, and impotence.

Impotence due to neuropathy differs from the psychogenic variety in that the latter may be intermittent (erections occur under special circumstances), whereas diabetic impotence is usually persistent. To distinguish neuropathic or psychogenic impotence from the impotence caused by aortoiliac occlusive disease or vasulopathy, papaverine is injected into the corpus cavernosum. If the blood supply is competent, a penile erection will occur. Urinary incontinence, with large volumes of residual urine, and retrograde ejaculation can also result from pelvic neuropathy.

Gastroparesis should be a diagnostic consideration in insulin-dependent diabetic patients who develop unexpected fluctuations and variability in their blood glucose levels after meals. Involvement of the gastrointestinal system may be manifested by nausea, vomiting, and postprandial fullness (from gastric atony); symptoms of reflux or dysphagia (from esophageal involvement); constipation and recurrent diarrhea, especially at night (from involvement of the small bowel and colon); and fecal incontinence (from anal sphincter dysfunction). Gallbladder function is altered, and this enhances stone formation.

Therapy is difficult and must be directed specifically at each abnormality. Use of Jobst fitted stockings, tilting the head of the bed, and arising slowly from the supine position are useful in minimizing symptoms of

orthostatic hypotension. Some patients may require the addition of a mineralocorticoid such as fludrocortisone acetate (0.05–0.2 mg twice daily). Metoclopramide has been of some help in treating diabetic gastroparesis over the short term, but its effectiveness seems to diminish over time. It is a dopamine antagonist with central antiemetic effects as well as cholinergic action to facilitate gastric emptying. It can be given intravenously (10–20 mg) or orally (20 mg of liquid metoclopramide) before breakfast and supper. Drowsiness is its major adverse effect. Bethanechol (Urecholine) has also been used for gastroparesis (as well as for an atonic urinary bladder) because of its anticholinergic effects.

Diabetic diarrhea is occasionally aggravated by bacterial overgrowth from stasis in the small intestine, and a trial of broad-spectrum antibiotics may give relief. If this does not help, symptomatic relief can sometimes be achieved with antidiarrheal agents such as diphenoxylate with atropine (Lomotil) or loperamide (Imodium). Metamucil and other bulk-providing agents may relieve either the diarrhea or the constipation phases, which often alternate. Beta-lactulose is useful in managing severe constipation. Bethanechol has occasionally improved emptying of the **atonic urinary bladder.** When **impotence** is due to neuropathy, penile implants can be considered (see Chapter 16).

Aldose reductase inhibitors have been generally disappointing, with only marginal therapeutic results in either autonomic or peripheral diabetic neuropathy and a relatively high incidence of toxic side effects such as skin rash and neutropenia.

4. CARDIOVASCULAR COMPLICATIONS

Heart Disease

Microangiopathy has recently been recognized to occur in the heart and may explain the existence of congestive cardiomyopathies found in diabetic patients without demonstrable coronary artery disease. Much more commonly, however, heart failure in the diabetic is a consequence of coronary atherosclerosis. Myocardial infarction is 3–5 times more common in diabetic patients than in age-matched controls and is the leading cause of death in patients with type II diabetes. A loss of the protection against myocardial infarction usually present in women during the age of childbearing is particularly evident in diabetic women. The exact reason for the increased incidence of atherosclerosis in diabetics is not clear. It may be a consequence of hyperlipidemia; abnormalities of platelet adhesiveness or coagulation factors (or both); or hypertension.

Peripheral Vascular Disease

Atherosclerosis is markedly accelerated in the larger arteries. It is often diffuse, with localized enhancement in certain areas of turbulent blood flow, such as at the bifurcation of the aorta or other large vessels. Clinical manifestations of peripheral vascular disease include ischemia of the lower extremities, impotence, and intestinal angina.

The incidence of **gangrene of the feet** in diabetics is 30 times that in age-matched controls. The factors responsible for its development, in addition to peripheral vascular disease, are small vessel disease, peripheral neuropathy with loss of both pain sensation and neurogenic inflammatory response, and secondary infection. In two-thirds of patients with ischemic gangrene, pedal pulses are not palpable. In the remaining one-third who have palpable pulses, reduced blood flow through these vessels can be demonstrated by plethysmographic or Doppler ultrasound examination. Prevention of foot injury is imperative, and certain principles that should be emphasized are outlined on p 625. Agents that reduce peripheral blood flow such as tobacco and propranolol should be avoided. Control of other risk factors such as hypertension is essential. Patients should be advised to seek immediate medical care if a diabetic foot ulcer develops. Improvement in peripheral blood flow with endarterectomy and bypass operations is possible in certain patients.

5. SKIN CHANGES

Diabetic dermopathy is characterized by atrophic brown spots on the skin, usually in the pretibial area ("shin spots"). These changes may be a consequence of increased glycosylation of tissue proteins or vasculopathy. Eruptive xanthomas may develop in some poorly controlled diabetics who have marked hypertriglyceridemia. A rare skin complication, necrobiosis lipoidica diabeticorum, occurs predominantly on the shins and is characterized by marked thinning of the skin which allows the subcutaneous vessels to be seen as though through tissue paper. An element of vascular occlusion is generally present.

6. BONE & JOINT COMPLICATIONS

Bone and joint complications are generally attributed to metabolic or vascular sequelae of diabetes of long standing.

Juvenile Diabetic "Cheirarthropathy"

This is a syndrome of chronic progressive stiffness of the hand secondary to contracture and tightening of the skin over the joints. It is characterized by inability to flatten the palms against a flat surface. It usually occurs within 5–6 years after onset of type I diabetes. It is believed to be due to glycosylation of collagen and perhaps other proteins in connective tissue.

Dupuytren's Contracture

This consists of nodular thickening of the palmar fascia of the hand, producing a clawlike deformity. Although not specific to diabetes, when it occurs in a diabetic patient it may be the result of ischemic necrosis and secondary scarring of connective tissue as a consequence of diabetic microangiopathy.

Bone Demineralization

Bone demineralization has been reported to occur with increased frequency in diabetic patients. Bone density, as measured by photon absorption in the forearms, is 10–20% below normal in diabetics as compared to appropriately matched controls. Diabetes mellitus, however, does not seem to be associated with clinically important osteopenia, since there is no increase in the occurrence of skeletal fractures.

Joint Abnormalities

Bursitis, particularly of the shoulders and hips, occurs more frequently than expected in patients with diabetes. Gout also has a higher than expected incidence, especially in obese diabetics.

7. INFECTION

Certain types of infection, such as bacteriuria, candidal esophagitis, and candidal vaginitis, occur more frequently in diabetic patients than in nondiabetic matched controls. There are also several unusual infections that occur almost exclusively in diabetics (eg, emphysematous cholecystitis, mucormycosis, malignant otitis externa). As noted above, atherosclerosis with peripheral vascular disease is very common in the diabetic population, and the resultant ischemia undoubtedly plays a role in the frequent lower extremity infections seen in these patients.

SURGERY IN THE DIABETIC PATIENT

Surgery represents a stress situation during which most of the insulin antagonists (catecholamines, GH, corticosteroids) are mobilized. In the diabetic patient, this can lead to a worsening of hyperglycemia and perhaps even ketoacidosis. The aim of medical management of diabetics during the perioperative period is to minimize these stress-induced changes. Recommendations for management depend both on the patient's usual diabetic regimen and on the type of surgery (major or minor) to be done.

DIABETICS REGULATED BY DIET ALONE

No special precautions must be taken unless diabetic control is markedly disturbed by the procedure. If this occurs, small amounts of regular insulin twice a day will establish euglycemia in a patient whose food intake is adequate. Human insulin is recommended, since it sensitizes the patient least—ie, anaphylactic complications are very rare, and patients are less likely to be sensitized to the future use of insulin.

DIABETICS TAKING ORAL HYPOGLYCEMIC AGENTS

When oral medications are allowed, these agents should be administered in the usual doses in the perioperative period. Carbohydrates should be supplied orally or by intravenous infusion of dextrose in water, with careful monitoring of blood glucose levels to avoid hypoglycemia or extremes of hyperglycemia. As in the case of diet-controlled diabetes, human insulin can be substituted if symptomatic hyperglycemia or ketosis develops.

DIABETICS TAKING INSULIN

Patients taking insulin represent the only serious challenge to management of diabetes when surgery is necessary. However, with careful attention to changes in the clinical or laboratory picture, most diabetic patients can be managed successfully.

Minor Surgery

For minor surgery requiring only local or spinal anesthesia or intravenous administration of a very transient anesthetic, half of the usual dose of insulin should be given in the morning. The patient should be placed early on the operating room schedule. A constant drip of 5% dextrose in water (at a rate of approximately 5 g of glucose per hour) should be infused if delays are necessary. Blood glucose levels should be checked at regular intervals.

Major Surgery

The night before major surgery, a 9 PM bedtime snack is given. Thereafter, the patient should receive nothing by mouth. On the morning of surgery, the usual morning subcutaneous insulin dose is omitted; instead, 10 units of regular insulin is added to 1 L of 5% dextrose in water, and this is infused intravenously at a rate of 100–180 mL/h. This will give the patient 1–1.8 units of insulin per hour, which, except in the most severe cases, will generally keep the blood glucose within the range of 100–250 mg/dL (5.5–

13.9 mmol/L). The infusion may be continued for several days if necessary. Plasma glucose or blood glucose should be determined every 2 to 4 hours to be sure metabolic control is adequate. If it is not, adjustments in the ratio of insulin to dextrose in the intravenous solution can be made.

After surgery, when the patient has resumed an adequate oral intake, intravenous administration of insulin and dextrose can be stopped. Two hours after discontinuing the intravenous insulin, subcutaneous administration of insulin can be resumed. Insulin needs may vary in the first several days after surgery because of continuing postoperative stresses and because of variable caloric intake. In this situation, multiple doses of regular insulin guided by blood glucose determinations can keep the patient in acceptable metabolic control. Routine "sliding scale" insulin orders based on urine glucose should be avoided in this setting.

PROGNOSIS FOR PATIENTS WITH DIABETES MELLITUS

The period between 10 and 20 years after the onset of diabetes seems to be a critical one. If the patient survives this period without fulminating microvascular complications, there is a strong likelihood that reasonably good health will continue. Currently, the prospect for retarding the progression of diabetic complications is good because of benefits derived from laser photocoagulation, improved results from dialysis and renal transplantation, and better treatment of the foot problems associated with diabetes. Newer methods for delivering purified insulins and for monitoring blood glucose at home have improved the overall outlook for patients with diabetes mellitus; however, it is clear that the diabetic patient's intelligence, motivation, and awareness of potential complications of the disease are major factors contributing to a successful outcome.

REFERENCES

The Endocrine Pancreas

Adrian TE et al: Secretion of pancreatic polypeptide in patients with pancreatic endocrine tumors. *N Engl J Med* 1986;**315:**287.

Bloom SR, Polak JM: Somatostatin. *Br Med J* 1987; **295:**288.

Ebert R, Creutzfeldt W: Gastrointestinal peptides and insulin secretion. *Diabetes Metab Rev* 1987;**3:**1.

Gepts W, In't-Veld PA: Islet morphologic changes. *Diabetes Metab Rev* 1987;**3:**859.

Hellerström C: The life story of the pancreatic B cell. *Diabetologia* 1984;**26:**393.

Howell SL: The mechanism of insulin secretion. *Diabetologia* 1984;**26:**319.

McCullough AJ et al: Effect of graded intraduodenal glucose infusions on the release and physiological actions of gastric inhibitory polypeptide. *J Clin Endocrinol Metab* 1983;**56:**234.

Orskov C et al: Pancreatic and intestinal processing of proglucagon in man. *Diabetologia* 1987;**30:**874.

Pipeleers G: The biosociology of pancreatic B cells. *Diabetologia* 1987;**30:**277.

Pipeleers DG et al: Interplay of nutrients and hormones in the regulation of glucagon release. *Endocrinology* 1985;**117:**817.

Reichlin S: Somatostatin. (2 parts.) *N Engl J Med* 1983;**309:**1495, 1556.

Williams JA, Goldfine ID: The insulin-pancreatic acinar axis: A review. *Diabetes* 1985;**34:**980.

Diagnosis, Classification, & Pathophysiology of Diabetes Mellitus

Bell GI, Horita S, Karam JH: A polymorphic locus near the human insulin gene is associated with insulin-dependent diabetes mellitus. *Diabetes* 1984;**33:**176.

Bennett PH: The diagnosis of diabetes: New international classification and diagnostic criteria. *Annu Rev Med* 1983;**34:**295.

DeFronzo RA: The triumvirate: Beta-cell, muscle, liver. A collusion responsible for NIDDM. *Diabetes* 1988;**37:**667.

Eisenbarth GS: Genes, generator of diversity, glycoconjugates, and autoimmune beta-cell insufficiency in type I diabetes. *Diabetes* 1987;**36:**355.

Flier JS: Insulin receptors and insulin resistance. *Annu Rev Med* 1983;**34:**145.

Fujioka S et al: Contribution of intra-abdominal fat accumulation to the impairment of glucose and lipid metabolism in human obesity. *Metabolism* 1987;**36:**54.

Garvey WT et al: Role of glucose transporters in the cellular insulin resistance of type II non-insulin-dependent diabetes mellitus. *J Clin Invest* 1988;**81:**1528.

Goldfine ID: The insulin receptor: Molecular biology and transmembrane signaling. *Endocr Rev* 1987;**8:**235.

Lernmark A: Molecular biology of type I (insulin-dependent) diabetes mellitus. *Diabetologia* 1985;**28:**195.

Nanjo K et al: Insulin Wakayama: Familial mutant insulin syndrome in Japan. *Diabetologia* 1987;**30:**87.

Permutt MA et al: Insulin gene structure and function: A review of studies using recombinant DNA methodology. *Diabetes Care* 1984;**7:**386.

Rotter JI, Rimoin DL: The genetics of the glucose intolerance disorders. *Am J Med* 1981;**70:**116.

Schade DS et al: The etiology of incapacitating, brittle diabetes. *Diabetes Care* 1985;**8:**12.

Srikanta S et al: First-degree relatives of patients with type I diabetes mellitus: Islet cell antibodies and abnormal insulin secretion. *N Engl J Med* 1985;**313:**461.

Tager HS: Abnormal products of the human insulin gene. *Diabetes* 1984;**33:**693.

Todd JA, Bell JI, McDevitt HO: HLA-DQ β gene contributes to susceptibility and resistance to insulin-dependent diabetes mellitus. *Nature* 1987;**329:**599.

Treatment of Diabetes Mellitus

Abraira C, Derler J: Large variations of sucrose in constant carbohydrate diets in type II diabetes. *Am J Med* 1988;**84:**193.

Alberti KG, Gries FA: Management of non-insulin-dependent diabetes mellitus in Europe: A concensus view. *Diabetic Med* 1988;**5:**275.

Bettmann MA: Radiographic contrast agents: A perspective. (Editorial.) *N Engl J Med* 1987;**317:**891.

Binder C et al: Insulin pharmacokinetics. *Diabetes Care* 1984;**7:**188.

Bolli GB et al: Glucose counterregulation and waning of insulin in the Somogyi phenomenon (posthypoglycemic hyperglycemia). *N Engl J Med* 1984;**311:**1214.

Bougnères PF et al: Factors associated with early remission of type I diabetes in children treated with cyclosporine. *N Engl J Med* 1988;**318:**663.

Boyd AE III: Sulfonylurea receptors, ion channels, and fruit flies. *Diabetes* 1988;**37:**847.

Brink SJ, Stewart C: Insulin pump treatment in insulin-dependent diabetes mellitus: Children, adolescents, and young adults. *JAMA* 1986;**255:**617.

Coustan DR et al: A randomized clinical trial of the insulin pump vs intensive conventional therapy in diabetic pregnancies. *JAMA* 1986;**255:**631.

Cryer PE, White NH, Santiago JV: The relevance of glucose counterregulatory systems to patients with insulin-dependent diabetes mellitus. *Endocr Rev* 1986;**7:**131.

Diabetes Control and Complications Trial (DCCT): Results of feasibility study. *Diabetes Care* 1987;**10:**1.

Fineberg SE et al: Effects of species of origin, purification levels, and formulation on insulin immunogenicity. *Diabetes* 1983;**32:**592.

Garvey WT et al: The effect of insulin treatment on insulin secretion and insulin action in type II diabetes mellitus. *Diabetes* 1985;**34:**222.

Genuth S: Treating diabetes with both insulin and sulfonylurea drugs: What is the value? *Clin Diabetes* 1987;**5:**73.

Havlin CE, Cryer PE: Nocturnal hypoglycemia does not commonly result in major morning hyperglycemia in patients with diabetes mellitus. *Diabetes Care* 1987;**10:**141.

Heine RJ et al: Absorption kinetics and action profiles of mixtures of short- and intermediate-acting insulins. *Diabetologia* 1984;**27:**558.

Herold KC, Rubenstein AH: Immunosuppression for insulin-dependent diabetes. (Editorial.) *N Engl J Med* 1988;**318:**701.

Kadowaki T et al: Chlorpropamide-induced hyponatremia: Incidence and risk factors. *Diabetes Care* 1983;**6:**468.

Karam JH, Etzwiler DD (editors): International Symposium on Human Insulin. *Diabetes Care* 1983;**6(Suppl 1):**1.

Karam JH, Root RK: Therapeutic dilemmas in type II diabetes mellitus: Improving and maintaining beta cell and insulin sensitivity. *West J Med* 1988;**148:**685.

Kolterman OG et al: The acute and chronic effects of

sulfonylurea therapy in type II diabetic subjects. *Diabetes* 1984;**33:**346.

The Kroc Collaborative Study Group: Blood glucose control and the evolution of diabetic retinopathy and albuminuria: A multicenter trial. *N Engl J Med* 1984;**311:**365.

Lebovitz HE (editor): *Physician's Guide to Non-Insulin-Dependent* (Type II) *Diabetes: Diagnosis and Treatment,* 2nd ed. American Diabetes Association, 1988.

Little RR et al: Relationship of glycosylated hemoglobin to oral glucose tolerance: Implications for diabetes screening. *Diabetes* 1988;**37:**60.

Lockwood DH, Gerich JE, Goldfine I: Symposium on effects of oral hypoglycemic agents on receptor and postreceptor actions of insulin. *Diabetes Care* 1984;**7(Suppl 1):**1.

Mazze RS et al: Reliability of blood glucose monitoring by patients with diabetes mellitus. *Am J Med* 1984;**77:**211.

Mecklenburg RS et al: Long-term metabolic control with insulin pump therapy: Report of experience with 127 patients. *N Engl J Med* 1985;**313:**465.

Melander A: Clinical pharmacology of sulfonylureas. *Metabolism* 1987;**36(2 Suppl 1):**12.

Mills JL et al: Lack of relation of increased malformation rates in infants of diabetic mothers to glycemic control during organogenesis. *N Engl J Med* 1988;**318:**671.

Mirouze J: Insulin treatment: A non-stop revolution. *Diabeto-logia* 1983;**25:**209.

Nathan DM, Roussell A, Godine JE: Glyburide or insulin for metabolic control in non-insulin-dependent diabetes mellitus: A randomized, double-blind study. *Ann Intern Med* 1988;**108:**334.

Nathan DM et al: The clinical information value of the glycosylated hemoglobin assay. *N Engl J Med* 1984;**310:**341.

Nolte MS et al: Reduced solubility of short-acting soluble insulins when mixed with longer-acting insulins. *Diabetes* 1983;**32:**1177.

Nuttal FQ: The high-carbohydrate diet in diabetes management. *Adv Intern Med* 1988;**33:**165.

O'Rahilly S et al: Type II diabetes of early onset: A distinct clinical and genetic syndrome? *Br Med J* 1987;**294:**923.

Owens DR: Effects of oral sulfonylureas on the spectrum of defects in non-insulin-dependent diabetes mellitus. *Am J Med* 1985;**79(Suppl 2B):**27.

Perriello G, De Feo P, Bolli GB: The dawn phenomenon: Nocturnal blood glucose homeostasis in insulin-dependent diabetes mellitus. *Diabetic Med* 1988;**5:**13.

Raskin P et al: The effect of diabetic control on the width of skeletal-muscle capillary basement membrane in patients with type I diabetes mellitus. *N Engl J Med* 1983;**309:**1546.

Richter EA, Ruderman NB, Schneider SH: Diabetes and exercise. *Am J Med* 1981;**70:**201.

Rizza RA: New modes of insulin administration: Do they have a role in clinical diabetes? *Ann Intern Med* 1986;**105:**126.

Sutherland D, Kendall D: Pancreas transplantation. *West J Med* 1985;**143:**845.

Teutsch SM et al: Mortality among diabetic patients using continuous subcutaneous insulin-infusion pumps. *N Engl J Med* 1984;**310:**361.

Tordjman KM et al: Failure of nocturnal hypoglycemia to cause fasting hyperglycemia in patients with insulin-dependent diabetes mellitus. *N Engl J Med* 1987;**317:**1552.

Yki-Järvinen H et al: Clinical benefits and mechanisms of a sustained response to intermittent insulin therapy in type 2 diabetic patients with secondary drug failure. *Am J Med* 1988;**84:**185.

Young CW: Rationale for glycemic control. *Am J Med* 1985;**79(Suppl 3B):**8.

Acute Complications of Diabetes Mellitus

Adrogué HJ et al: Plasma acid-base patterns in diabetic ketoacidosis. *N Engl J Med* 1982;**307:**1603.

Bending JJ, Pickup JC, Keen H: Frequency of diabetic ketoacidosis and hypoglycemic coma during treatment with continuous subcutaneous insulin infusion. *Am J Med* 1985;**79:**685.

Brown, RH et al: Caveat on fluid replacement in hyperglycemic hyperosmolar nonketotic coma. *Diabetes Care* 1978;**1:**305.

Casparie AF, Elving LD: Severe hypoglycemia in diabetic patients: Frequency, causes, prevention. *Diabetes Care* 1985;**8:**141.

Clements RS, Vourganti B: Fatal diabetic ketoacidosis: Major causes and approaches to their prevention. *Diabetes Care* 1978;**1:**314.

Cohen RD, Woods HF: Lactic acidosis revisited. *Diabetes* 1983;**32:**181.

Fisher JN, Kitabchi AE: A randomized study of phosphate therapy in the treatment of diabetic ketoacidosis. *J Clin Endocrinol Metab* 1983;**57:**177.

Flexner CW et al: Repeated hospitalization for diabetic ketoacidosis: The game of "Sartoris." *Am J Med* 1984;**76:**691.

Foster, DW, McGarry JD: The metabolic derangements and treatment of diabetic ketoacidosis. *N Engl J Med* 1983;**309:**159.

Fulop M: The treatment of severely uncontrolled diabetes mellitus. *Adv Intern Med* 1984;**29:**327.

Keller U, Berger W: Prevention of hypophosphatemia by phosphate infusion during treatment of diabetic ketoacidosis and hyperosmolar coma. *Diabetes* 1980;**29:**87.

Krane EJ et al: Subclinical brain swelling in children during treatment of diabetic ketoacidosis. *N Engl J Med* 1985;**312:**1147.

Kreisberg RA: Pathogenesis and management of lactic acidosis. *Annu Rev Med* 1984;**35:**181.

Morris LR, Murphy MB, Kitabchi AE: Bicarbonate therapy in severe diabetic ketoacidosis. *Ann Intern Med* 1986;**105:**836.

Narins RG, Cohen JJ: Bicarbonate therapy for organic acidosis: The case for its continued use. *Ann Intern Med* 1987;**106:**615.

Peterson CM, Javanovic L: *The Diabetes Self-Care Method.* Simon & Schuster, 1984.

Salzman R et al: Intranasal aerosolized insulin: Mixed-meal studies and long-term use in type I diabetes. *N Engl J Med* 1985;**312:**1078.

Schade DS, Eaton RP: Diabetic ketoacidosis: Pathogenesis, prevention and therapy. *Clin Endocrinol Metab* 1983;**13:**332.

Stacpoole PW: Lactic acidosis: The case against bicarbonate therapy. *Ann Intern Med* 1986;**105:**276.

Sutherland DE, Goetz FC, Najarian JS: Pancreas transplants from related donors. *Transplantation* 1984;**38:**625.

Wachtel TJ, Silliman RA, Lamberton P: Predisposing factors for the diabetic hyperosmolar state. (Letter.) *Arch Intern Med* 1988;**148:**747.

Chronic Complications of Diabetes Mellitus

Ai E, Coonan P: The treatment of diabetic retinopathy. *Annu Rev Med* 1987;**38:**279.

Bradley WE (editor): Aspects of diabetic autonomic neuropathy. (Symposium.) *Ann Intern Med* 1980;**92:**289.

Brownlee M, Cerami A, Vlassara H: Advanced glycosylation end products in tissue and the biochemical basis of diabetic complications. *N Engl J Med* 1988;**318:**1315.

Christlieb AR: The hypertensions of diabetes. *Diabetes Care* 1982;**5:**50.

Cogan DG et al: Aldose reductase and complications of diabetes. *Ann Intern Med* 1984;**101:**82.

Dunn FL: Hyperlipidemia and diabetes. *Med Clin North Am* 1982;**66:**1347.

Feingold KR et al: Muscle capillary basement membrane width in patients with vacor-induced diabetes mellitus. *J Clin Invest* 1986;**78:**102.

Feingold KR, Siperstein MD: Diabetic vascular disease. *Adv Intern Med* 1986;**31:**309.

Ganda OP: Pathogenesis of macrovascular disease in the human diabetic. *Diabetes* 1980;**29:**931.

Goetz FC et al: Renal transplantation in diabetes. *Clin Endocrinol Metab* 1986;**15:**807.

Greene DA, Lattimer SA, Sima AA: Are disturbances of sorbitol, phosphoinositide, and Na^+-K^+-ATPose regulation involved in pathogenesis of diabetic neuropathy? *Diabetes* 1988;**37:**688.

LoGerfo FW, Coffman D: Vascular and microvascular disease of the foot in diabetes: Implications for foot care. *N Engl J Med* 1984;**311:**1615.

Mauer SM et al: Structural functional relationships in diabetic nephropathy. *J Clin Invest* 1984;**74:**1143.

McCulloch DK et al: The prevalence of diabetic impotence. *Diabetologia* 1980;**18:**279.

Mogensen CE: Management of diabetic renal involvement and disease. *Lancet* 1988;**1:**867.

Parkhouse N, Le Quesne PM: Impaired neurogenic vascular response in patients with diabetes and neuropathic foot lesions. *N Engl J Med* 1988;**318:**1306.

Ramsay RC et al: Progression of diabetic retinopathy after pancreas transplanation for insulin-dependent diabetes mellitus. *N Engl J Med* 1988;**318:**208.

Raskin P, Rosenstock J: Blood glucose control and diabetic complications. *Ann Intern Med* 1986;**105:**254.

Rosenbloom AL et al: Limited joint mobility in childhood diabetes: Family studies. *Diabetes Care* 1983;**6:**370.

Sidenius P: The axonopathy of diabetic neuropathy. *Diabetes* 1982;**31:**356.

Viberti G, Keen H: The patterns of proteinuria in diabetes mellitus: Relevance to pathogenesis and prevention of diabetic nephropathy. *Diabetes* 1984;**33:**686.

Ward JD: The diabetic leg. *Diabetologia* 1982;**22:**141.

Wheat LJ: Infection and diabetes mellitus. *Diabetes Care* 1980;**3:**187.

Wiseman MJ et al: Effect of blood glucose on increased glomerular filtration rate and kidney size in insulin-dependent diabetes. *N Engl J Med* 1985;**312:**617.

Zatz R et al: Predominance of hemodynamic rather than metabolic factors in the pathogenesis of diabetic glomerulopathy. *Proc Natl Acad Sci USA* 1985;**82:**5963.

Hypoglycemic Disorders

23

Clinton W. Young, MD, & John H. Karam, MD

Circulating plasma glucose concentrations are kept within a relatively narrow range by a complex system of interrelated neural, humoral, and cellular controls. Under the usual metabolic conditions, the central nervous system is wholly dependent on plasma glucose and counteracts declining blood glucose concentrations with a carefully programmed response. This is often associated with a sensation of hunger; and, as the brain receives insufficient glucose to meet its metabolic needs (neuroglycopenia), an autonomic response is triggered to mobilize storage depots of glycogen and fat. Hepatic glycogen reserves directly supply the central nervous system with glucose, which is carried across the blood-brain barrier by a specific glucose transport system, while the mobilization of fatty acids from triglyceride depots provides energy for the large mass of skeletal and cardiac muscle, renal cortex, liver, and other tissues that utilize fatty acids as their basic fuel, thus sparing glucose for use by the tissues of the central nervous system.

PATHOPHYSIOLOGY OF THE COUNTERREGULATORY RESPONSE TO NEUROGLYCOPENIA

The plasma concentration of glucose that will signal the need by the central nervous system to mobilize energy reserves depends on a number of factors, such as the status of blood flow to the brain, the integrity of cerebral tissue, the prevailing arterial level of plasma glucose, the rapidity with which plasma glucose concentration falls, and the availability of alternative metabolic fuels. In most healthy people, hypoglycemic symptoms occur at plasma glucose levels below 45 mg/dL (2.5 mmol/L) (blood glucose < 40 mg/dL [2.2 mmol/L]). However, in elderly people with compromised cerebral blood supply, neuroglycopenic manifestations may be provoked at slightly higher plasma glucose levels. Patients with chronic hyperglycemia, eg, those with poorly controlled insulin-dependent diabetes mellitus, may experience symptoms of neuroglucopenia at considerably higher plasma glucose concentrations than persons without diabetes. This has been attributed to a "down-regulated" glucose transport system across the blood-brain barrier. Conversely, in patients exposed to chronic hypoglycemia, eg, those with an insulin-secreting tumor or those with diabetes who are receiving excessively "tight" glycemic control with an insulin pump, "up-regulation" of the glucose transporters may explain the greater tolerance of hypoglycemia without manifesting symptoms of neuroglucopenia.

Restoring and maintaining an adequate supply of glucose for cerebral function proceeds by a series of neurogenic events that act directly to raise the plasma glucose concentration and to stimulate hormonal responses that augment the adrenergic mobilization of energy stores (Table 23–1).

Hormonal Response to Hypoglycemia

A. Insulin: Endogenous insulin secretion is lowered both by reduced glucose stimulation to the pancreatic B cell and by sympathetic nervous system inhibition from a combination of alpha-adrenergic neural effects and increased circulating catecholamine levels. This reactive insulinopenia facilitates the mobilization of energy from existing energy stores (glycogenolysis and lipolysis), increases hepatic enzymes involved in gluconeogenesis and ketogenesis, and at the same time prevents muscle tissue from consuming the blood glucose being released from the liver (see Chapter 22).

B. Catecholamines: Circulating catecholamines and norepinephrine produced at sympathetic nerve endings provide muscle tissue with alternative sources of fuel by activating beta-adrenergic receptors—resulting in mobilization of muscle glycogen—and by providing increased plasma free fatty acids from lipolysis of adipocyte triglyceride.

C. Glucagon: Plasma glucagon is released by the beta-adrenergic effects of both sympathetic innervation and circulating catecholamines on pancreatic A cells as well as by the direct stimulation of A cells by the low plasma glucose concentration itself. This glucagon release increases hepatic output of glucose by direct glycogenolysis as well as by facilitating the activity of gluconeogenic enzymes. As shown in Figure 23–1, plasma glucagon appears to be the key counterregulato-

651

Table 23–1. Sympathetic nervous system response
to hypoglycemia.

Alpha-Adrenergic Effects
  Inhibition of endogenous insulin release.
  Increase in cerebral blood flow (peripheral vasoconstriction).
Beta-Adrenergic Effects
  Hepatic and muscle glycogenolysis.
  Stimulation of plasma glucagon release.
  Lipolysis to raise plasma free fatty acids.
  Impairment of glucose uptake by muscle tissue.
  Increase in cerebral blood flow (increase in cardiac output).
Adrenomedullary Discharge of Catecholamines
  Augmentation of all of the above alpha- and beta-adrenergic effects.

ry hormone affecting recovery from acute hypoglycemia in humans, with the adrenergic-catecholamine response representing a major backup system.

D. Corticotropin and Hydrocortisone: Pituitary ACTH is released in association with the sympathetic nervous system stimulation by neuroglycopenia. This results in elevation of plasma cortisol levels, which permissively facilitates lipolysis and actively promotes protein catabolism and conversion of amino acids to glucose by the liver.

E. Growth Hormone: Pituitary growth hormone is also released in response to falling plasma glucose levels. Its role in counteracting hypoglycemia is less

well defined, but it is known to antagonize the action of insulin on glucose utilization in muscle cells and to directly activate lipolysis by adipocytes.

Maintenance of Euglycemia in the Postabsorptive State

Glucose absorption from the gastrointestinal tract ceases by 5–8 hours after a meal. During the "postabsorptive state" immediately following, glucose must be produced endogenously from previously stored nutrients to meet the requirements of the central nervous system. The liver is the central organ involved in this process, producing the 125 mg of glucose per minute required by the brain as well as an additional 25 mg/min for other glucose-dependent tissues—predominantly blood cell elements. This is initially provided by the breakdown of stored hepatic glycogen. However, because these reserves are limited to 80–100 g, they begin to be depleted several hours into the postabsorptive state. Thereafter, hepatic glucose production is augmented by gluconeogenesis—the formation of glucose from amino acids, lactate, and glycerol. These substrates are delivered to the liver from peripheral stores: Muscle and other structural tissues supply amino acids, mainly alanine; blood cell elements supply lactate, the end product of glycolytic metabolism; and adipose tissue supplies glycerol from lipolysis of triglyceride. In addition, oxidation of the free fatty acids released from adipose cells during

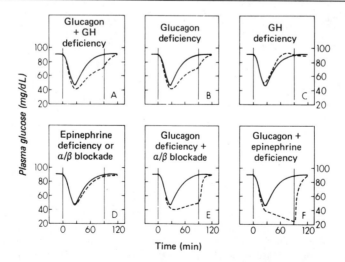

Figure 23–1. Solid lines show changes in plasma glucose that occur in normal subjects in response to insulin administration. Note the rapid recovery of glucose levels mediated by intact counterregulatory mechanisms. The dashed lines show the response to insulin-induced hypoglycemia in patients with deficiencies of the counterregulatory mechanisms induced as follows: **A:** Somatostatin infusion (inhibits both glucagon and growth hormone [GH] release). **B:** Somatostatin infusion plus GH infusion (now with functional isolated glucagon deficiency). **C:** Somatostatin infusion plus glucagon infusion (isolated GH deficiency). Note return of glucose response to normal, implying that glucagon is the main counterregulatory hormone. **D:** Bilateral adrenalectomy, leading to epinephrine deficiency, or infusion of phentolamine plus propranolol (alpha and beta blockers, respectively). Note that such deficiencies cause no major abnormality in response to induced hypoglycemia when glucagon is present. **E and F:** Sympathetic modulation (by phentolamine plus propranolol in E and by bilateral adrenalectomy in F), which seriously impairs the ability to respond to hypoglycemia in the patient made glucagon-deficient by somatostatin infusion. (Reproduced, with permission, from Cryer PE: Glucose counterregulation in man. *Diabetes* 1981:**30**:261.)

Table 23–2. Hormonal changes to maintain euglycemia in the postabsorptive state.

Decreased Insulin Secretion
Increases hepatic glycogenolysis.
Increases lipolysis.
Increases hepatic gluconeogenesis.
Decreases muscle uptake of glucose.
Increased Glucagon Secretion
Increases hepatic glycogenolysis.
Facilitates hepatic gluconeogenesis.
Increased Cortisol Secretion
Facilitates lipolysis.
Increases protein catabolism.
Augments hepatic gluconeogenesis.

Table 23–3. Common causes of symptomatic hypoglycemia.

Fasting
A. With Hyperinsulinism:
Insulin reaction.
Sulfonylurea overdose.
Surreptitious insulin or sulfonylurea administration.
Autoimmune hypoglycemia (idiopathic insulin antibodies, insulin receptor autoantibodies).
Pentamidine-induced hypoglycemia.
Pancreatic B cell tumors.
B. Without Hyperinsulinism:
Severe hepatic dysfunction.
Chronic renal insufficiency.
Inanition, ketotic hypoglycemia of childhood.
Hypocortisolism.
Alcohol use.
Nonpancreatic tumors.
Inborn errors of carbohydrate metabolism (glycogen storage disease, gluconeogenic enzyme deficiencies).
Nonfasting
Alimentary.
Functional.
Occult diabetes.
Ethanol.
Leucine sensitivity.
Hereditary fructose intolerance.
Galactosemia.
Newborn infant of diabetic mother.

lipolysis supplies the energy required for gluconeogenesis and provides ketone bodies, acetoacetate, and β-hydroxybutyrate, which can serve as alternative metabolic fuels for the central nervous system during periods of prolonged fasting.

Hormonal changes that begin early in the postabsorptive state regulate the enzymatic steps necessary for hepatic glycogenolysis and gluconeogenesis and ensure the delivery of the necessary substrate (Table 23–2). An appropriate fall in circulating insulin levels is most important; elevations in the counterregulatory hormones glucagon, cortisol, and growth hormone are less critical.

In summary, numerous endocrine and metabolic events interact to provide a continuous source of fuel for proper functioning of the central nervous system. Malfunction of any of these mechanisms can lead to symptomatic hypoglycemia.

CLASSIFICATION OF HYPOGLYCEMIC DISORDERS

Symptomatic Hypoglycemia

A clinical classification of the more common causes of symptomatic hypoglycemia in adults is presented in Table 23–3. (The inborn errors of metabolism that produce hypoglycemia in infants and children are mentioned but will not be discussed in detail in this chapter.) This classification is useful in directing diagnostic considerations.

Symptomatic **fasting hypoglycemia** is a serious and potentially life-threatening problem warranting thorough evaluation. Conditions that produce inappropriate fasting hyperinsulinism are the most common cause of fasting hypoglycemia in otherwise healthy adults. These include insulin-secreting pancreatic B cell tumors and iatrogenic or surreptitious administration of insulin or sulfonylureas. In patients with illnesses that produce symptomatic fasting hypoglycemia despite appropriately suppressed insulin levels, the clinical picture is dominated by the signs and symptoms of the primary disease, with hypoglycemia often only a late or associated manifestation.

This is in contrast to patients with inappropriate hyperinsulinism, who usually appear healthy between hypoglycemic episodes.

Symptoms of **nonfasting hypoglycemia** in adults, although distressing to the patient, do not imply serious illness or warrant extensive evaluation. Overstimulation of the B cells postprandially as a result of accelerated glucose absorption after rapid gastric emptying may result in too rapid disposal of glucose, with resulting symptoms of sympathetic nervous system hyperactivity. Other than in patients who have had gastric surgery, this diagnosis may be difficult to establish.

Asymptomatic Hypoglycemia

Hypoglycemia may be seen during prolonged fasting, strenuous exercise, or pregnancy or may occur as a laboratory artifact. In normal men, plasma glucose does not fall below 55 mg/dL (3 mmol/L) during a 72-hour fast. However, for reasons that are not clear, normal women may experience a fall to levels as low as 30 mg/dL (1.7 mmol/L) despite a marked suppression of circulating insulin to less than 6 μU/mL. They remain asymptomatic in spite of this degree of hypoglycemia, presumably because ketogenesis is able to satisfy the energy needs of the central nervous system. Basal plasma glucose declines progressively during normal pregnancy, and hypoglycemic levels may be reached during prolonged fasting. This may be a consequence of a continuous fetal consumption of glucose and diminished availability of the gluconeogenic substrate alanine. The cause of these diminished alanine levels in pregnancy is unclear. The greatly increased glucose consumption by skeletal muscle that occurs during prolonged strenuous exercise may lead to hypoglycemia despite increases in hepatic glucose production. Whether the hypoglycemia in this circumstance contributes to fatigue or other symptoms in distance runners is unknown.

In vitro consumption of glucose by blood cell elements may give rise to laboratory values in the hypoglycemic range. This is most commonly seen when an insufficient amount of the metabolic inhibitor sodium fluoride is added to specimens containing increased numbers of leukocytes (as in leukemia and leukemoid reactions).

CLINICAL PRESENTATION OF HYPOGLYCEMIA

Regardless of the cause, hypoglycemia presents certain common features characterized by **Whipple's triad:** (1) symptoms and signs of hypoglycemia, (2) an associated plasma glucose level of 45 mg/dL (2.5 mmol/L) or less, and (3) reversibility of symptoms upon administration of glucose.

The symptoms and signs of hypoglycemia are the consequences of neuroglycopenia. They vary depending on the degree of hypoglycemia, the age of the patient, and the rapidity of the decline. In diabetic patients treated with insulin, a precipitous fall in plasma glucose from hyperglycemia toward euglycemia may produce neuroglucopenic symptoms.

A. Acute Hypoglycemia: A rapid fall in plasma glucose (> 1 mg/dL/min [> 0.06 mmol/L/min]) to low levels often accompanies conditions associated with arterial hyperinsulinism—a condition that leads to increased peripheral glucose uptake and decreased hepatic glucose output. In diabetics, excessive absorption of exogenous insulin either from overtreatment or from rapid mobilization from an injection site during exercise may be responsible. In nondiabetics, reactive hypersecretion of insulin may be the cause, as in postgastrectomy patients with rapid gastric emptying time. The symptoms include anxiety, tremulousness, and feelings of unnaturalness or detachment. These are usually accompanied by palpitations, tachycardia, sweating, and hunger and can progress to neurologic sequelae of ataxia, coma, or convulsions.

B. Subacute and Chronic Hypoglycemia: A relatively slow fall in plasma glucose accompanies conditions caused primarily by a reduction in hepatic glucose output in response to hyperinsulinism (predominantly within the portal vein [insulinoma]), to the inappropriately sustained effects of long-acting insulin preparations on the liver in the postabsorptive state, or to metabolic derangements of liver functions (eg, alcohol hypoglycemia). Symptoms due to hypoglycemia in patients with these conditions may be less apparent, particularly because symptoms of sympathetic overactivity are usually absent. These patients develop progressive confusion, inappropriate behavior, lethargy, and drowsiness. If the patient does not eat, seizures or coma may develop, although this is not inevitable, and spontaneous recovery can occur. Because these patients are seldom aware of their degree of functional impairment, a history should be obtained from relatives or friends who have observed the episode. Except for hypothermia (often seen during hypoglycemic coma), there are no identifying characteristics on physical examination. Hypoglycemia will often be misdiagnosed as a seizure disorder, transient ischemic attack, or personality disorder.

Documentation of Low Plasma Glucose Values

With the specific laboratory methods now available, it has been arbitrarily decided that fasting hypoglycemia is present when plasma glucose is 45 mg/dL (2.5 mmol/L) or less after an overnight fast (corresponding to a blood glucose level of 40 mg/dL [2.2 mmol/L] or less). In the fasting state, there is no substantial difference between arterial, venous, or capillary blood samples (in contrast to nonfasting hyperglycemia, in which arteriovenous glucose differences may be considerable because of arterial hyperinsulinism and consequent increases in glucose uptake across capillary beds).

The development of glucose oxidase–hydrogen peroxidase paper strips has been of great value for a rapid estimate of blood glucose levels, particularly for insulin-treated diabetics undergoing home monitoring. In emergency room or hospital settings, the paper strips are helpful in the differential diagnosis of coma, particularly when used with a reflectance meter, but a sample should also be sent to the laboratory for definitive diagnosis. Although therapeutic decisions to administer glucose can be based on the paper strip results alone in an emergency situation, variability due to exposure to air or aging makes them less dependable as the sole laboratory indicator for a definitive diagnosis of hypoglycemia.

Reversibility of Clinical Manifestations of Hypoglycemia With Treatment

Because prolonged hypoglycemia may cause permanent brain damage and death, prompt recognition and treatment are mandatory. (It is prudent to consider the possibility of hypoglycemic coma in most unconscious patients.)

The goal of therapy is to restore normal levels of plasma glucose as rapidly as possible. If the patient is conscious and able to swallow, glucose-containing foods such as candy, orange juice with added sugar, and cookies should be quickly ingested. Fructose, found in many nutrient low-calorie sweeteners for diabetics, should not be used, because although it can be metabolized by neurons, it lacks a transport system and therefore does not cross the blood-brain barrier.

If the patient is unconscious, rapid restoration of plasma glucose must be accomplished by giving 20–

50 mL of 50% dextrose intravenously over 1–3 minutes (the treatment of choice) or, when intravenous glucose is not available, 1 mg of glucagon intramuscularly or intravenously. Families or friends of insulin-treated diabetics should be instructed in the administration of glucagon intramuscularly for emergency treatment at home. Attempts to feed the patient or to apply glucose-containing jelly to the oral mucosa should be avoided because of the danger of aspiration.

When consciousness is restored, oral feedings should begin immediately. Periodic blood glucose surveillance after a hypoglycemic episode may be needed for 12–24 hours to ensure maintenance of euglycemia. Prevention of recurrent hypoglycemic attacks depends upon proper diagnosis and management of the specific underlying disorder.

SPECIFIC HYPOGLYCEMIC DISORDERS

SYMPTOMATIC FASTING HYPOGLYCEMIA WITH HYPERINSULINISM

1. INSULIN REACTION

It is not surprising that insulin-treated diabetics make up the bulk of the patient population with symptomatic hypoglycemia. Present methods of insulin delivery rely upon subcutaneous depots of mixtures of soluble and insoluble insulin whose absorption varies with the site of injection and the degree of exercise in surrounding muscles. Variations in physical and emotional stresses can alter the response of patients to insulin, as can the cyclic hormonal changes relating to menstruation. A deficient glucagon response to hypoglycemia in diabetes compounds the problem, as does the lack of awareness of hypoglycemic symptoms in older patients and in those with neuropathy, which reduces or obliterates the autonomic responses to hypoglycemia.

Once the patient's acute hypoglycemic episode is managed, the physician should carefully examine possible correctable factors that may have contributed to the insulin reaction:

Inadequate Food Intake

An insufficient quantity of food or a missed meal is one of the commonest causes of hypoglycemia in insulin-treated diabetics. Until improved insulin delivery systems are available, patients attempting to achieve satisfactory glycemic control should self-monitor their blood glucose levels and eat 3 regular meals as well as small midmorning, midafternoon, and bedtime snacks, particularly when they are receiving 2 or more injections of insulin mixtures daily.

Exercise

The insulin-treated diabetic is especially prone to exercise-induced hypoglycemia. In nondiabetics, the enhancement of skeletal muscle glucose uptake (a 20- to 30-fold increase over basal uptake) is compensated for by enhanced hepatic glucose production. This is mediated primarily by a fall in circulating insulin levels consequent to an exercise-induced catecholamine discharge, which inhibits B cell secretion. Such regulation is impossible in the insulin-treated diabetic, whose subcutaneous depot not only continues to release insulin during exercise but also shows an accelerated absorption rate when the injection site is in close proximity to the muscles being exercised. When this occurs, increased levels of circulating insulin compromise the hepatic output of glucose. To prevent hypoglycemia, insulin-treated diabetics must be advised to avoid injections into areas adjacent to muscles most involved in the particular exercise and either to eat supplementary carbohydrate before exercising or to reduce their insulin dose appropriately.

Impaired Glucose Counterregulation in Diabetics

Most patients with insulin-dependent diabetes have a deficient glucagon response to hypoglycemia. They are thus solely dependent on epinephrine to recover from hypoglycemia. Some patients, especially those with long-standing diabetes or autonomic neuropathy, lack both a glucagon and an epinephrine response and are virtually defenseless against insulin-induced hypoglycemia. Insulin infusion tests can be used to identify these alterations in glucose counterregulation; however, at present these tests are cumbersome, and their ability to accurately predict which patients will suffer frequent severe and prolonged hypoglycemic episodes is yet to be established. Easier and more reliable methods of identifying such patients are needed. The ability of a patient to spontaneously recover from hypoglycemia may determine whether or not aggressive attempts to maintain euglycemia are associated with undue risk.

Some patients who originally had a normal counterregulatory response to hypoglycemia (except for glucagon) lose this protective response when insulin therapy is intensified to achieve tight control. The mechanisms for this reduction of hormonal response are unknown but may be related to "up-regulated" mechanisms of glucose transport across the blood-brain barrier induced by relatively low circulating blood glucose levels.

Inadvertent or Deliberate Insulin Overdosage in Diabetics

Excessive insulin may be administered inadvertently by patients with poor vision or inadequate instruction or understanding of dosage and injection technique. The widespread use of highly concentrated U100 insulin enhances the likelihood of overdosage with relatively small excesses of administered insulin.

Deliberate overdosage may occur in certain maladjusted patients, particularly adolescents, who wish to gain special attention from their families or escape tensions at school or work.

Miscellaneous Causes of Hypoglycemia in Insulin-Treated Diabetics

A. Stress: Physical stresses, such as intercurrent illnesses, infection, and surgery, or psychic stresses often require an increased insulin dosage to control hyperglycemia. Reduction to prestress doses is necessary to avoid subsequent hypoglycemia when the stresses have abated.

B. Hypocortisolism: In patients with insulin-dependent diabetes who have otherwise unexplained hypoglycemic attacks, reduced insulin requirements may indicate unusual causes (eg, Addison's disease).

C. Diabetic Gastroparesis: Unexplained episodes of postprandial hypoglycemia in insulin-dependent diabetics may be due to delayed gastric emptying consequent to autonomic neuropathy. This diagnosis can be established by appropriate radiologic studies of gastric motility using liquid or solid test meals.

D. Pregnancy: Pregnancy, with high fetal glucose consumption, decreases insulin requirements in the first trimester.

E. Renal Insufficiency: Renal insufficiency, through impairment of insulin degradation while hepatic gluconeogenesis and food intake are often reduced, also requires a reduction in insulin dosage.

F. Drugs: Numerous pharmacologic agents may potentiate the effects of insulin and predispose to hypoglycemia. Common offenders include ethanol, salicylates, and beta-adrenergic blocking drugs.

Beta blockade inhibits fatty acid and gluconeogenic substrate release and reduces plasma glucagon levels; furthermore, the symptomatic response is altered, because tachycardia is blocked while hazardous elevations of blood pressure may result during hypoglycemia in response to the unopposed alpha-adrenergic stimulation from circulating catecholamines and neurogenic sympathetic discharge. However, symptoms of sweating, hunger, and uneasiness are not masked by beta-blocking drugs and remain indicators of hypoglycemia in the aware patient.

2. SULFONYLUREA OVERDOSE

Any of the sulfonylureas may produce hypoglycemia. Chlorpropamide (Diabinese), with its prolonged half-life (35 hours), is a common offender. Older patients, especially those with impaired hepatic or renal function, are particularly susceptible to sulfonylurea-induced hypoglycemia: Liver dysfunction prolongs the hypoglycemic activity of tolbutamide (Orinase), acetohexamide (Dymelor), and tolazamide (Tolinase), as well as that of the second-generation compounds, glyburide (DiaBeta, Micronase) and glipizide (Glucotrol); renal insufficiency perpetuates the blood glucose–lowering effects of many sulfonylureas, especially chlorpropamide and glyburide. Elderly patients with gradually decreasing creatinine clearance seem to be more at risk for prolonged and severe hypoglycemia when treated with chlorpropamide or glyburide and less so when treated with shorter-acting agents such as tolbutamide or glipizide. In the presence of other pharmacologic agents such as dicumarol, phenylbutazone, or certain sulfonamides, the hypoglycemic effects of sulfonylureas may be markedly prolonged.

3. SURREPTITIOUS INSULIN OR SULFONYLUREA ADMINISTRATION (Factitious Hypoglycemia)

Factitious hypoglycemia should be suspected in any patient with access to insulin or sulfonylurea drugs. It is most commonly seen in health professionals and diabetic patients or their relatives. The reasons for self-induced hypoglycemia vary, with many patients having severe psychiatric disturbances or a need for attention.

When insulin is used to induce hypoglycemia, an elevated serum insulin level often raises suspicion of an insulin-producing pancreatic B cell tumor. It may be difficult to prove that the insulin is of exogenous origin. The triad of hypoglycemia, high immunoreactive insulin levels, and suppressed plasma C-peptide immunoreactivity* is pathognomonic of exogenous insulin administration. Technical difficulties in measuring immunoreactive insulin, caused by the inappropriate presence of circulating antibodies (usually seen only in insulin-treated individuals) will generally support the diagnosis of factitious hypoglycemia. However, the absence of detectable insulin antibodies does not rule out the possibility of exogenous insulin administration, especially with the advent of human insulins with low immunogenicity in humans.

When sulfonylurea abuse is suspected, plasma or urine should be screened for its presence. Hyperinsulinism may not persist despite sustained hypoglycemia from a sulfonylurea overdose.

Treatment of factitious hypoglycemia involves psychiatric therapy and social counseling.

4. AUTOIMMUNE HYPOGLYCEMIA

In recent years, a rare autoimmune disorder has been reported in which patients have circulating in-

---

*C peptide, a major portion of the connecting chain in amino acids in proinsulin, remains intact during the conversion of proinsulin to insulin (see Chapter 22).

sulin antibodies and the paradoxic feature of hypoglycemia. While many of these patients may be surreptitiously administering insulin, an increasing number of case reports have not been able to document exogenous insulin as the inducer of the insulin antibodies. Hypoglycemia is attributed to a sudden dissociation of insulin-antibody immune complexes, releasing free insulin.

Hypoglycemia due to insulin receptor autoantibodies is also an extremely rare syndrome, reported in only 6 patients. All of these patients have also had episodes of insulin-resistant diabetes and acanthosis nigricans. Their hypoglycemia is attributed to an agonistic action of the antibody on the insulin receptor. Balance between the antagonistic and agonistic effects of the antibody determines whether insulin-resistant diabetes or hypoglycemia occurs. Hypoglycemia was found to respond to glucorticoid therapy but not to plasmapheresis or immunosuppression.

5. PENTAMIDINE-INDUCED HYPOGLYCEMIA

With the increasing use of pentamidine for treatment of *Pneumocystis carinii* infection in patients with acquired immunodeficiency syndrome (AIDS), more reports of pentamidine-induced hypoglycemia are appearing. The cause of acute hyperglycemia appears to be the drug's lytic effect on B cells, which produces acute hyperinsulinemia followed by insulinopenia and diabetes. Physicians treating patients with pentamidine should be aware of the potential complication of acute hypoglycemia.

6. PANCREATIC B CELL TUMORS

Spontaneous fasting hypoglycemia in an otherwise healthy adult is most commonly due to **insulinoma,** an insulin-secreting tumor of the islets of Langerhans. Eighty percent of these tumors are single and benign; 10% are malignant (if metastases are identified); and the remaining 10% are multiple, with scattered micro- or macroadenomas interspersed within normal islet tissue. (As with some other endocrine tumors, histologic differentiation between benign and malignant cells is difficult, and close follow-up is necessary to ensure the absence of metastases.) Diffuse B cell hyperplasia has rarely been documented as a cause of hypoglycemia in adults.

These adenomas may be familial and have been found in conjunction with tumors of the parathyroid glands and the pituitary (multiple endocrine neoplasia type I). (See Chapter 28.) Ninety-nine percent of them are located within the pancreas and less than 1% in ectopic pancreatic tissue.

These tumors may appear at any age, although they are most common in the fourth to sixth decades. There is no sex predilection.

Clinical Findings

The signs and symptoms are predominantly those of subacute neuroglycopenia rather than adrenergic discharge. The typical picture is that of recurrent central nervous system dysfunction at times of exercise or fasting. The preponderance of neurologic symptoms rather than those commonly associated with hypoglycemia (adrenergic symptoms) often leads to delayed diagnosis following prolonged psychiatric care or treatment for seizure disorders or transient ischemic attacks. Some patients learn to relieve or prevent their symptoms by taking frequent feedings. Obesity may be the result; however, obesity is seen in less than 30% of patients with insulin-secreting tumors.

Diagnosis of Insulinoma

B cell tumors do not reduce secretion in the presence of hypoglycemia, and a serum insulin level of 10 μ/mL or more with concomitant plasma glucose values below 45 mg/dL (2.5 mmol/L) suggests an insulinoma. Other causes of hyperinsulinemic hypoglycemia must be considered, however, such as surreptitious administration of insulin or sulfonylureas.

A. Insulin Assay: Because the insulin radioimmunoassay is crucial in diagnosing insulin-secreting tumors, it is important to be aware of certain limitations in its use. It detects not only human but also beef and pork insulins, and a high level may therefore indicate either endogenous or exogenous insulin. (C-peptide measurements are necessary to make this distinction.) In addition, the assay is of no value in patients who have ever taken insulin, as virtually all will have developed low-titer insulin antibodies that will interfere. Falsely low or elevated values will result, depending on the method used. Collection of samples is also important: If they are not frozen immediately, falsely low values will result, because the insulin molecule will undergo proteolytic digestion.

B. Suppression Tests: Failure of endogenous insulin secretion to be suppressed in the presence of hypoglycemia is the hallmark of an insulin-secreting tumor. The most reliable suppression test is the prolonged supervised fast in hospitalized subjects, and this remains the preferred diagnostic maneuver in the workup of suspected insulinomas.

In normal men, the blood glucose value will not fall below 55 mg/dL (3.1 mmol/L) during a 72-hour fast, while insulin levels fall below 10 μ/mL; in some normal women, however, plasma glucose may fall below 30 mg/dL (1.7 mmol/L) (lower limits have not been established), while serum insulin levels also fall appropriately. (These women remain asymptomatic despite this degree of hypoglycemia, presumably because ketogenesis is able to provide sufficient fuel for the central nervous system.) Calculation of ratios of insulin (in μU/mL) to plasma glucose (in mg/dL) is useful diagnostically. Nonobese normal subjects maintain a ratio of less than 0.25; obese subjects may have an elevated ratio, but hypoglycemia does not occur with fasting. Virtually all patients with insulin-secreting islet cell tumors will have an abnormal insulin:glucose ratio at some time during a 72-hour fast. The majority of these will experience progressive and symptomatic fasting hypoglycemia with associated elevated insulin levels within 24–36 hours and no evidence of ketonuria. However, an occasional patient will not demonstrate hypoglycemia until 72 hours have elapsed. Brisk exercise during the fast may help precipitate hypoglycemia. Once symptoms of hypoglycemia occur, plasma glucose should be obtained and the fast immediately terminated if plasma glucose is below 45 mg/dL (2.5 mmol/L).

C. Stimulation Tests: A variety of stimulation tests with intravenous tolbutamide, glucagon, or calcium have been devised to demonstrate exaggerated and prolonged insulin secretion. However, because insulin-secreting tumors have a wide range of granular content and degrees of differentiation, they are variably responsive to these secretagogues. Thus, absence of an excessive insulin secretory response during any of these stimulation tests does not rule out the presence of an insulinoma. In addition, the tests may be extremely hazardous to patients with responsive tumors by inducing prolonged and refractory hypoglycemia. (None of these secretagogues should be given to a patient when hypoglycemia is present.) The following stimulation tests should be reserved for the difficult case in which results of a prolonged fast are equivocal. They can also be useful for screening when the index of suspicion for an insulin-secreting tumor is low.

1. Tolbutamide stimulation test–One gram of sodium tolbutamide dissolved in 20 mL of distilled water is infused intravenously over 2 minutes. Serum insulin is measured every 5 minutes for 15 minutes; a level exceeding 195 μU/mL during this time suggests an insulin-secreting tumor. However, this response is seen in only 60% or less of patients with insulinomas, and false-positive results may occur (eg, with obesity or hepatic disease). Continuation of the test beyond 15 minutes will uncover additional patients with insulinomas by demonstrating prolonged elevations of insulin; however, hazardous hypoglycemia may result.

2. Glucagon stimulation test–One milligram of glucagon is given intravenously, and serum insulin levels are measured every 5 minutes for 15 minutes. A level exceeding 135 μU/mL suggests an insulin-secreting tumor. However, only approximately 50% of patients with insulinomas will demonstrate this hyperinsulinism, and false-positive results may occur. When an exaggerated increase in serum insulin occurs, the hyperglycemic effect of glucagon may be subnormal, and profound hypoglycemia may subsequently develop by 60 minutes.

D. Oral Glucose Tolerance Test: The oral glucose tolerance test is of no value in the diagnosis of insulin-secreting tumors.

A common misconception is that patients with insulinomas will have flat glucose tolerance curves, because the tumor will discharge insulin in response to oral glucose. In fact, most insulinomas respond poorly, and curves typical of diabetes are more common. In those rare tumors that do release insulin in response to glucose, a flat curve may result; however, this is also seen in normal subjects.

E. Euglycemic Clamp: Continuous blood glucose monitoring with feedback-controlled dextrose infusion by an artificial pancreas has been used to demonstrate excessive dextrose requirements to maintain fasting euglycemia in insulinoma patients. This test remains experimental; however, it has the advantage of avoiding hypoglycemia during a supervised fast.

F. Proinsulin Measurements: In contrast to normal subjects, whose proinsulin concentration is less than 20% of the total immunoreactive insulin, patients with insulinoma have elevated levels of proinsulin that represent 30–90% of total immunoreactive insulin. Sensitive new assays for human proinsulin that incorporate specific monoclonal antibodies offer considerable potential in the evaluation of patients with suspected insulinoma.

G. Glycohemoglobin Measurements: Low glycohemoglobin values have been reported in occasional cases of insulinoma, reflecting the presence of chronic hypoglycemia. However, the diagnostic usefulness of glycohemoglobin measurements is limited by the relatively low sensitivity of this test as well as poor accuracy at the lower range of normal in many of the assays. In addition, it is nonspecific for hypoglycemia, with low levels being found in certain hemoglobinopathies and hemolytic states.

H. Tumor Localization Studies:

1. Imaging studies–The diagnosis of an insulin-secreting tumor is dependent on biochemical testing. Since most tumors are too small (80% are < 2 cm) to localize by either ultrasonography, CT scanning, or magnetic resonance imaging a negative result will not be conclusive.

Arteriography is presently the most effective method for preoperative localization of small tumors, particularly if catheterization of small arterial branches and subbranches of the celiac artery (selective and subselective arteriography) is combined with subtraction and magnification methods. However, even with these advances, arteriography is seldom helpful enough to outweigh its disadvantages, and it remains a painful and relatively imprecise procedure that exposes insulinoma patients to the risk of hypoglycemia and the discomfort of several hours of invasive and expensive radiography. In most cases, a tumor mass large enough to "blush" on arteriography is large enough for an experienced surgeon to identify by direct visualization or palpation. In addition, false-positive and false-negative results are so common that reliance on operative localization by an experienced surgeon has preempted the use of arteriography in a growing number of medical centers.

Small tumors within the pancreas that are not palpable at laparotomy have been localized using intra-operative ultrasound in which a transducer is wrapped in a sterile rubber glove and passed over the exposed pancreatic surface.

2. Transhepatic portal vein sampling–Demonstration of insulin gradients or "step-ups" in insulin concentration in the pancreatic venous effluent can be effective in localizing small insulin-secreting tumors. The procedure entails percutaneous transhepatic portal vein catheterization under local anesthesia with subsequent cannulation of the splenic vein. Samples for insulin are obtained along the splenic and portal venous systems in an attempt to show a gradient of 300 μU/mL or more of insulin concentration that would evidence a tumor. Results may be equivocal, however, because of the high rate of blood flow in these venous systems and the consequent dilution of insulin values. In addition, this uncomfortable procedure is not without complications; bile leakage, intraperitoneal hemorrhage, and infection have been reported. Since diazoxide would interfere with this test, it should be discontinued for at least 48–72 hours before sampling. An infusion of dextrose may be required, therefore, and patients should be closely monitored during the procedure to avoid hypoglycemia (as well as hyperglycemia, which could affect insulin gradients). Venous sampling is indicated for cases in which hypoglycemia does not respond to diazoxide (see below), so that surgical removal of the insulinoma is therefore mandated. In this instance, only

an angiographer with extensive experience in the technique should perform the procedure.

Treatment of Insulinoma

The treatment of choice for insulin-secreting tumors is surgical resection. A flow diagram for the approach to these patients is shown in Figure 23–2.

A. Surgical Treatment: Tumor resection should be performed only by surgeons with extensive experience with islet cell tumors, since these tumors may be small and difficult to recognize. An 85% success rate has been reported without localization procedures if surgeons have prior experience with insulinomas.

1. Preoperative management–

a. Trial of diazoxide–Oral diazoxide (Proglycem), a potent inhibitor of insulin secretion, will maintain euglycemia in most patients with insulin-secreting tumors. Doses of 300–400 mg/d (divided) will usually suffice, but an occasional patient will require up to 800 mg/d. Side effects include edema due to sodium retention (which generally necessitates concomitant thiazide administration), gastric irritation, and mild hirsutism.

b. Selection of patients–Patients who remain euglycemic on diazoxide may be operated on by an experienced surgeon, without attempts at preoperative tumor localization. However, intraoperative ultrasound should be available on call in case an insulinoma is not palpated after exposure and mobilization of the pan-

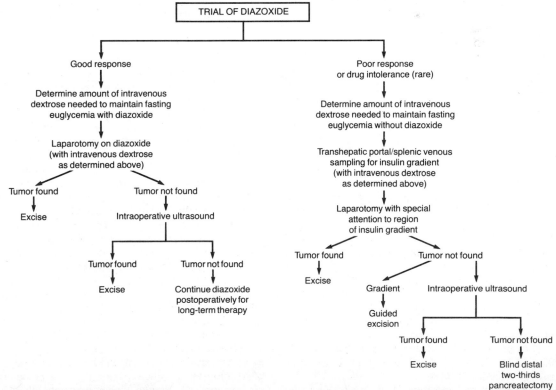

Figure 23–2. Management of patients with confirmed diagnosis of insulinoma.

creas. Patients who do not respond to diazoxide or cannot tolerate its side effects are candidates for venous sampling studies in an attempt to localize the tumor preoperatively, since failure to successfully remove the tumor has a poorer prognosis in patients in whom diazoxide therapy is not effective.

2. Treatment during surgery–

a. Glucose need during surgery–To estimate glucose needs during surgery, 5 or 10% dextrose should be infused a day or so before surgery to determine the approximate rate of glucose administration needed to maintain euglycemia. This amount can then be prescribed on the day of surgery; counterregulatory stress responses during surgery should ensure that additional glucose will probably not be required. However, plasma glucose should be monitored frequently to regulate glucose replacement during surgery, especially during manipulation of the pancreas.

b. Diazoxide–Diazoxide should be administered preoperatively as well as on the day of surgery in patients who are responsive to it, since the drug greatly reduces the need for glucose supplements and the risk of hypoglycemia during surgery while not masking the glycemic rise indicative of surgical cure.

3. Postoperative hyperglycemia–Postoperatively, several days of hyperglycemia may ensue. This is due to a combination of factors, including edema and inflammation of the pancreas after surgery, high levels of counterregulatory hormones induced by the procedure, chronic down-regulation of insulin receptors by the previously high circulating insulin levels in the tumor, and perhaps suppression of normal pancreatic B cells by long-standing hypoglycemia. Small subcutaneous doses of regular insulin may be prescribed every 4–6 hours if plasma glucose exceeds 300 mg/dL (16.7 mmol/L), but in most cases pancreatic insulin secretion recovers after 48–72 hours and very little insulin replacement is required.

4. Failure to find the tumor at operation–In approximately 10% of patients with biochemically demonstrated autonomous insulin secretion, no tumor can be found at exploratory laparotomy. The tumor will most likely be in the head of the pancreas, as this is the most difficult area for the surgeon to mobilize and explore; therefore, blind distal two-thirds pancreatectomy is seldom successful. If intraoperative ultrasound does not identify a tumor, it is best to let the prior response to diazoxide therapy dictate the proper procedure (Fig 23–2). If the patient has responded to diazoxide, this can be continued indefinitely. If the patient has not responded or is intolerant of diazoxide therapy, and if preoperative venous sampling has not been helpful in localizing a tumor, then—and only then—a blind distal two-thirds pancreatectomy should be performed. This procedure has a success rate of only 25%.

B. Medical Treatment: Diazoxide therapy is the treatment of choice in patients with inoperable functioning islet cell carcinomas and in those who are poor candidates for operation. Many patients have been maintained on long-term (> 10 years) diazoxide therapy without apparent ill effects. Frequent carbohydrate feedings (every 2–3 hours) can also be helpful in maintaining euglycemia, although obesity may become a problem.

When patients are unable to tolerate diazoxide because of side effects such as gastrointestinal upset, hirsutism, or edema, a calcium channel blocker such as verapamil (80 mg given orally every 8 hours) may be beneficial in view of its inhibitory effect on insulin release from insulinoma cells.

A potent long-acting synthetic octapeptide analogue of somatostatin (octreotide, [Sandoz]) has been used to inhibit release of hormones from a number of endocrine tumors, including inoperable insulinomas. When hypoglycemia persists after attempted surgical removal of the insulinoma and if diazoxide or verapamil is poorly tolerated or ineffective, a trial of 50 μg of octreotide injected subcutaneously twice daily may control the hypoglycemic episodes in conjunction with multiple small carbohydrate feedings.

Streptozocin has proved beneficial in patients with islet cell carcinomas, and effective doses have been achieved without the undue renal toxicity that characterized early experience. Benign tumors appear to respond poorly, if at all.

SYMPTOMATIC FASTING HYPOGLYCEMIA WITHOUT HYPERINSULINISM

1. DISORDERS ASSOCIATED WITH LOW HEPATIC GLUCOSE OUTPUT

Reduced hepatic gluconeogenesis can result from a direct loss of hepatic tissue (acute yellow atrophy from fulminating viral or toxic damage); from disorders reducing amino acid supply to hepatic parenchyma (severe muscle wasting and inanition from anorexia nervosa, chronic starvation, uremia, and glucocorticoid deficit from adrenocortical deficiency); or from inborn errors of carbohydrate metabolism affecting glycogenolytic or gluconeogenic enzymes.

2. ETHANOL HYPOGLYCEMIA

Ethanol impairs hepatic gluconeogenesis but has no effect on hepatic glycogenolysis. In the patient who is imbibing ethanol but not eating, fasting hypoglycemia may occur after hepatic glycogen stores have been depleted (within 8–12 hours of a fast). No correlation exists between the blood ethanol levels and the degree of hypoglycemia, which may occur while blood ethanol levels are declining. It should be noted that ethanol-induced fasting hypoglycemia may occur at ethanol levels as low as 45 mg/dL (10 mmol/L)—considerably below most states' legal standards (100 mg/dL [21.7 mmol/L]) for being "under the influence." Most patients present with neuroglycopenic symptoms, which may be difficult to differentiate from the neurotoxic effects of the alcohol. These symptoms in a patient whose breath smells of alcohol may be mistaken for alcoholic stupor. Intravenous dextrose should be administered promptly to all such stuporous or comatose patients. Because hepatic glycogen stores have been depleted by the time hypoglycemia occurs, parenteral glucagon will not be effective. Adequate food intake during alcohol ingestion will prevent this type of hypoglycemia.

3. NONPANCREATIC TUMORS

A variety of nonpancreatic tumors have been found to cause fasting hypoglycemia. Most are large and mesenchymal in origin, retroperitoneal fibrosarcoma being the classic prototype. However, hepatocellular carcinomas, adrenal cortical carcinomas, hypernephromas, gastrointestinal tumors, lymphomas and leukemias, and a variety of other tumors have also been reported. The mechanisms by which these tumors produce hypoglycemia are not entirely clear. None has been unequivocally shown to secrete insulin; thus, true ectopic hyperinsulinemia probably does not exist. Up to 50% of these tumors have been reported to secrete low-molecular-weight peptides with insulinlike activity. These NSILA peptides (so-called because of their nonsuppressible insulinlike activity) include human insulinlike growth factors and some of the somatomedins. Whether further refinement in the assays for these peptides will allow the demonstration of NSILA in all cases of nonpancreatic tumors that are associated with hypoglycemia remains to be seen. Treatment is aimed toward the primary tumor, with supportive therapy using frequent feedings. Diazoxide is ineffective in reversing the hypoglycemia caused by these tumors.

NONFASTING HYPOGLYCEMIA (Reactive Hypoglycemia)

Reactive hypoglycemia may be classified as early (within 2–3 hours of a meal) or late (at 3–5 hours). Early (alimentary) hypoglycemia occurs when there is a rapid discharge of ingested carbohydrate into the small bowel followed by rapid glucose absorption and hyperinsulinism. It may be seen after gastrointestinal surgery and is notably associated with the "dumping syndrome" after gastrectomy; occasionally, it is functional and may result from overactivity of the parasympathetic nervous system mediated via the vagus nerve. Late hypoglycemia (occult diabetes) is caused by a delay in early insulin release, which then results in exaggeration of initial hyperglycemia during a glucose tolerance test. As a consequence, an exaggerated insulin response produces late hypoglycemia. Early or late hypoglycemia may also occur as a consequence of ethanol's potentiation of the insulin-secretory response to glucose, as when sugar-containing soft drinks are used as mixers to dilute alcohol in beverages (gin and tonic, rum and cola).

1. POSTGASTRECTOMY ALIMENTARY HYPOGLYCEMIA

Reactive hypoglycemia after gastrectomy is a consequence of hyperinsulinism. This results from rapid gastric emptying of ingested food, which produces overstimulation of vagal reflexes and overproduction of beta-cytotrophic gastrointestinal hormones, causing arterial hyperinsulinism and consequent acute hypoglycemia. The symptoms are caused by adrenergic hyperactivity in response to the rapidly falling plasma glucose. Treatment is properly directed at avoiding this sequence of events by more frequent feedings with smaller portions of less rapidly assimilated carbohydrate and more slowly absorbed fat or protein. Occasionally, anticholinergic drugs such as propantheline (15 mg orally 4 times daily) may be useful in reducing vagal overactivity.

2. FUNCTIONAL ALIMENTARY HYPOGLYCEMIA

Early alimentary-type reactive hypoglycemia in a patient who has not undergone surgery is classified as functional. It is most often associated with chronic fatigue, anxiety, irritability, weakness, poor concentration, decreased libido, headaches, hunger after meals, and tremulousness. Whether or not hypoglycemia actually accounts for these symptoms or actually occurs at all is difficult to prove.

The usual sequence of events is that the patient presents with a number of nonspecific complaints. Normal laboratory findings and a normal physical examination confirm the initial impression that organic disease is not present, and the symptoms are then attributed to the stresses of modern living. The only form of therapy usually given is reassurance or a mild tranquilizer. When this fails to be of benefit, the patient seeks help elsewhere. Inevitably, the question of hypoglycemia is raised—frequently by the patient, who has heard of the diagnosis from friends or relatives with similar symptoms or has read of it in the lay press. The diagnosis is often supported by the demonstration of hypoglycemia with symptoms during a 5-hour oral glucose tolerance test.

Unfortunately, the precipitation of hypoglycemia with or without symptoms during oral glucose tolerance testing does not distinguish between normal and "hypoglycemic" patients. As many as one-third or more of normal subjects who have never had any symptoms will develop hypoglycemia with or without symptoms during a 5-hour glucose tolerance test. In addition, many patients will develop symptoms in the absence of hypoglycemia. Thus, the test's non-specificity makes it a highly unreliable tool that is no longer recommended for evaluating patients with suspected episodes of postprandial hypoglycemia. In 1983, Hogan et al reported that ingestion of a mixed meal did not produce hypoglycemia in 33 patients who had been diagnosed as having reactive hypoglycemia on the basis of oral glucose tolerance testing; this attempt to increase specificity for the diagnosis of reactive hypoglycemia may have resulted in loss of sensitivity.

For increased diagnostic reliability, hypoglycemia should be documented during a spontaneous symptomatic episode in routine daily activity. However, attempts to demonstrate this are almost never successful. Patients should be instructed in the proper use of Chemstrip bG, whose color development is stable enough to allow test strips to be saved and brought to the physician's office for documentation up to 72 hours after the measurement was made. Personality evaluation suggestive of hyperkinetic compulsive behavior in thin, anxious patients is often found.

The foregoing discussion should not be taken to imply that functional reactive hypoglycemia does not occur—merely that at present we have no reliable means of diagnosing it. There is no harm (and there is occasional benefit) in reducing or eliminating the content of refined sugars in the patient's diet while increasing the frequency and reducing the size of meals. However, it should not be expected that these maneuvers will cure the asthenia, since the reflex response to hypoglycemia is only a possibly aggravating feature of a generalized primary hyperactivity. Counseling and support and mild sedation should be the mainstays in therapy, with dietary manipulation only an adjunct.

3. LATE HYPOGLYCEMIA (Occult Diabetes)

This condition is characterized by delay in early insulin release from pancreatic B cells, resulting in initial exaggeration of hyperglycemia during a glucose tolerance test. In response to this hyperglycemia, an exaggerated insulin release produces late hypoglycemia 4–5 hours after ingestion of glucose. These patients are usually quite different from those with early hypoglycemia, being more phlegmatic and often obese and frequently having a family history of diabetes mellitus. In the obese, treatment is directed at reduction to ideal weight. These patients often respond to reduced intake of refined sugars with multiple, spaced small feedings high in dietary fiber. They should be considered early diabetics and advised to have periodic medical evaluations.

REFERENCES

Amiel SA et al: Defective glucose counterregulation after strict glycemic control of insulin-dependent diabetes mellitus. *N Engl J Med* 1987;**316**:1376.

Berger M et al: Functional and morphological characterization of human insulinomas. *Diabetes* 1983;**32**:921.

Boyle PJ et al: Plasma glucose concentrations at the onset of hypoglycemic symptoms in patients with poorly controlled diabetes and in nondiabetics. *N Engl J Med* 1988;**318**:1487.

Cohen RM, Camus F: Update on insulinomas or the case of the missing (pro)insulinoma. *Diabetes Care* 1988; **11**:506.

Cryer PE, White NH, Santiago JV: The relevance of glucose counterregulatory systems to patients with insulin-dependent diabetes mellitus. *Endocr Rev* 1986;**7**:131.

Dons RF et al: Anomalous glucose and insulin responses in patients with insulinoma: Caveats for diagnosis. *Arch Intern Med* 1985;**145**:1861.

Feingold KR: Hypoglycemia: A pitfall of insulin therapy. *West J Med* 1983;**139**:688.

Fischer KF, Lees JA, Newman JH: Hypoglycemia in hospitalized patients: Causes and outcomes. *N Engl J Med* 1986;**315**:1245.

Grunberger G et al: Factitious hypoglycemia due to surreptitious administration of insulin: Diagnosis, treatment, and long-term follow-up. *Ann Intern Med* 1988;**108**:252.

Hogan MJ et al: Oral glucose tolerance test compared with a mixed meal in the diagnosis of reactive hypoglycemia. *Mayo Clin Proc* 1983;**58**:491.

Kvols LK et al: Treatment of metastatic islet cell carcinoma with a somatostatin analogue (SMS 201–995). *Ann Intern Med* 1987;**17**:162.

Merimee TJ: Insulin-like growth factors in patients with non-islet cell tumors and hypoglycemia. *Metabolism* 1986; **35**:360.

Rifkin MD, Weiss SM: Intraoperative sonographic identification of nonpalpable pancreatic masses. *J Ultrasound Med* 1984;**3**:409.

Service FJ (editor): *Hypoglycemia Disorders: Pathogenesis, Diagnosis and Treatment.* GK Hall, 1983.

Simonson DC et al: Intensive insulin therapy reduces counterregulatory hormone responses to hypoglycemia in patients with type I diabetes. *Ann Intern Med* 1985;**103**:184.

Taylor SI et al: Hypoglycemia associated with antibodies to the insulin receptor. *N Engl J Med* 1982;**307**:1422.

Ulbrecht JS et al: Insulinoma in a 94-year-old woman: Long-term therapy with verapamil. *Diabetes Care* 1986;**9**:186.

Waskin H et al: Risk factors for hypoglycemia associated with pentamidine therapy for *Pneumocystis* pneumonia. *JAMA* 1988;**260**:345.

Williams HE: Alcoholic hypoglycemia and ketoacidosis. *Med Clin North Am* 1984;**68**:33.

Disorders of Lipoprotein Metabolism

24

John P. Kane, MD, PhD, & Mary J. Malloy, MD

The clinical importance of hyperlipoproteinemia derives chiefly from the role of lipoproteins in atherogenesis. However, the greatly increased risk of acute pancreatitis associated with severe hypertriglyceridemia is an additional indication for intervention. Detection and characterization of hyperlipoproteinemia is important for selection of appropriate treatment and may provide clues to underlying primary clinical disorders.

Arteriosclerosis

Arteriosclerosis is the leading cause of death in the USA. Abundant epidemiologic evidence establishes the multifactorial character of this disease and indicates that the effects of the multiple risk factors are at least additive. Risk factors that have been convincingly identified for atherosclerosis of the coronary arteries are hyperlipidemia, arterial hypertension, cigarette smoking, diabetes mellitus, physical inactivity, and decreased levels of high-density lipoproteins (HDL) in plasma. Coronary atheromas are complex lesions containing cellular elements, collagen, and lipids. It is clear, however, that the progression of the lesion is chiefly attributable to its content of unesterified cholesterol and cholesteryl esters. It is now firmly established that the cholesterol in the atheroma is delivered to the site by circulating lipoproteins. Epidemiologic evidence indicates that the atherogenic lipoproteins are the low-density (LDL), intermediate-density (IDL), very low density (VLDL), and Lp(a) species, all of which contain the B-100 apolipoprotein. In animal models, hypertension is associated with increased access of lipoprotein to the subintimal region. Smoking may accelerate the process of atherogenesis chiefly through its influence on blood platelets, though it is also associated with decreased levels of HDL in plasma. Increased platelet interaction at sites of damaged endothelium leads to release of platelet-derived growth factor (PDGF), which stimulates migration of cells of smooth muscle origin into the lesion, where they proliferate. Macrophages endocytose atherogenic lipoproteins. Although these cells can secrete cholesterol in a discoidal micelle for retrieval from peripheral sites, the macrophages may break down and liberate cholesteryl esters into the extracellular matrix. The inverse rela-

Acronyms Used in This Chapter	
ACAT	Acyl-CoA:cholesterol acyltransferase
Apo-	Apolipoprotein
CETP	Cholesteryl ester transfer protein
CoA	Coenzyme A
FFA	Free fatty acids
HDL	High-density lipoprotein(s)
HMG-CoA	Hydroxymethylglutaryl-CoA
IDDM	Insulin-dependent diabetes mellitus
IDL	Intermediate-density lipoprotein(s)
LCAT	Lecithin:cholesterol acyltransferase
LDL	Low-density lipoprotein(s)
Lp(a)	A specific high-molecular-weight glycoprotein. Also applies to lipoprotein species containing this protein.
LPL	Lipoprotein lipase
NIDDM	Non–insulin-dependent diabetes mellitus
PDGF	Platelet-derived growth factor
VLDL	Very low density lipoprotein(s)

tionship between plasma HDL levels and the rate of atherogenesis probably reflects the involvement of at least certain species of HDL in the movement of cholesterol away from the atheroma.

Reversal of Atherosclerosis

A number of studies in animals, including higher primates, indicate that atherosclerotic coronary disease resulting from diet-induced hyperlipidemia is reversible when levels of lipoproteins in plasma are restored to normal. These findings support the concept that the atheroma is a dynamic lesion. The striking similarity of the lesions induced in primates to early lesions occurring in human coronary arteries suggests that the progression of human lesions could also be retarded or perhaps that regression could occur if hyperlipidemia were controlled. The results of several recent intervention studies in humans indicate that the progression of atheromas in coronary and femoral arteries can indeed be retarded by moderate reductions of levels of atherogenic lipoproteins in serum. More effective treatments that are emerging may be capable of at least partial reversal of atheromas.

It should be noted that average levels of LDL in plasma in the United States population are considerably higher than in many other nations, where the levels appear to approach the biologic norm for humans. This probably accounts in large part for the markedly higher incidence of coronary vascular disease in industrialized Western nations and suggests that dietary changes that reduce lipoprotein levels toward normal would be beneficial.

OVERVIEW OF LIPID TRANSPORT

The Plasma Lipoproteins

Because all the lipids of plasma are relatively insoluble in water, they are transported in association with proteins. The simplest complexes are those formed between unesterified, or free, fatty acids (FFA) and albumin, which serve to carry the FFA from peripheral adipocytes to other tissues. Similarly, lysolecithins (phospholipids formed when 1 mol of fatty acid is removed from lecithin) are bound to albumin.

The remainder of the plasma lipids are transported in lipoprotein complexes (Table 24–1). All of the major lipoproteins of plasma are spherical, and each has a core region containing hydrophobic lipids. The principal core lipids are cholesteryl esters and triglycerides (Fig 24–1). Triglycerides predominate in the cores of the chylomicrons, which transport newly absorbed lipids from the intestine, and in the cores of the very low density lipoproteins, which originate in the liver. The relative content of cholesteryl ester is increased in remnants derived from these 2 classes of lipoproteins, and cholesteryl esters predominate in the cores of low-density and high-density lipoproteins. Surrounding the core in each type of lipoprotein is a stabilizing monolayer containing amphiphilic (detergentlike) lipids, chiefly phospholipids and unesterified cholesterol (frequently termed free cholesterol). Proteins called apolipoproteins, which are noncovalently bound to the lipids, are mostly located in or on this surface monolayer.

B Apolipoproteins

Several of the lipoproteins contain proteins of very high molecular weight known as the B apolipoproteins, which behave like intrinsic proteins of cell membranes. Unlike the smaller apolipoproteins, the B apolipoproteins do not migrate from one lipoprotein particle to another. The B apolipoproteins of intestinal and hepatic origin are different. They are now described by numbers in a centile system based on the relative apparent molecular weights of the different species. Thus, VLDL contain the B-100 protein, which is retained in the formation of LDL from VLDL remnants by the liver. The intestinal B protein, B-48, is found in chylomicrons and their remnant particles but is completely absent from LDL.

Other Apolipoproteins

In addition to the B apolipoproteins, the following apolipoproteins are present in lipoproteins. (The distribution of these proteins in the different lipoproteins is shown in Table 24–1.)

(1) C apolipoproteins: These are low-molecular-weight (700–10,000) proteins that equilibrate rapidly among the lipoproteins. There are 3 distinct species with unique amino acid sequences, designated C-I, C-II, and C-III. Apolipoprotein C-II has been identified as a requisite cofactor for lipoprotein lipase.

(2) E apolipoproteins: At least 2 normal isoforms (E-3 and E-4) of this MW-35,000 protein appear to be the products of allelic genes. Normal individuals thus may have either or both isoforms, which share with B-100 protein the property of interacting with certain high-affinity receptors (B-100:E receptors) on cell membranes. Another isoform (E-2) lacks this property. About 15% of individuals of European extraction are heterozygous for this isoform.

(3) Apolipoprotein A-1: This protein of MW 28,300 is the major apolipoprotein of HDL; it is also present in chylomicrons and is the most abundant of the apolipoproteins of human serum (about 125 mg/dL). It is a cofactor for lecithin:cholesterol acyltransferase (LCAT).

Table 24–1. Lipoproteins of human serum.

Lipoprotein	Electrophoretic Mobility in Agarose Gel	Density Interval g/cm³	Predominant Core Lipids	Diameter	Apolipoproteins in Order of Quantitative Importance
High-density (HDL)	Alpha	1.21–1.063	Cholesteryl ester	7.5–10.5 nm	A-I, A-II, C, E, D
Low-density (LDL)	Beta	1.063–1.019	Cholesteryl ester	~21.5 nm	B-100, B-74, B-26
Intermediate-density (IDL)	Beta	1.019–1.006	Cholesteryl ester, triglyceride	25–30 nm	B-100, some C and E
Very low density (VLDL)	Prebeta; some "slow prebeta"	<1.006	Triglyceride	30–100 nm	B-100, C, E
Chylomicrons	Remain at origin	<1.006	Triglyceride	80–500 nm	B-48, C, E, A-I, A-II, A-IV, proline-rich apoprotein
Lp(a)	Prebeta	1.04–1.08	Cholesteryl ester	21–30 nm	B-100, Lp(a)

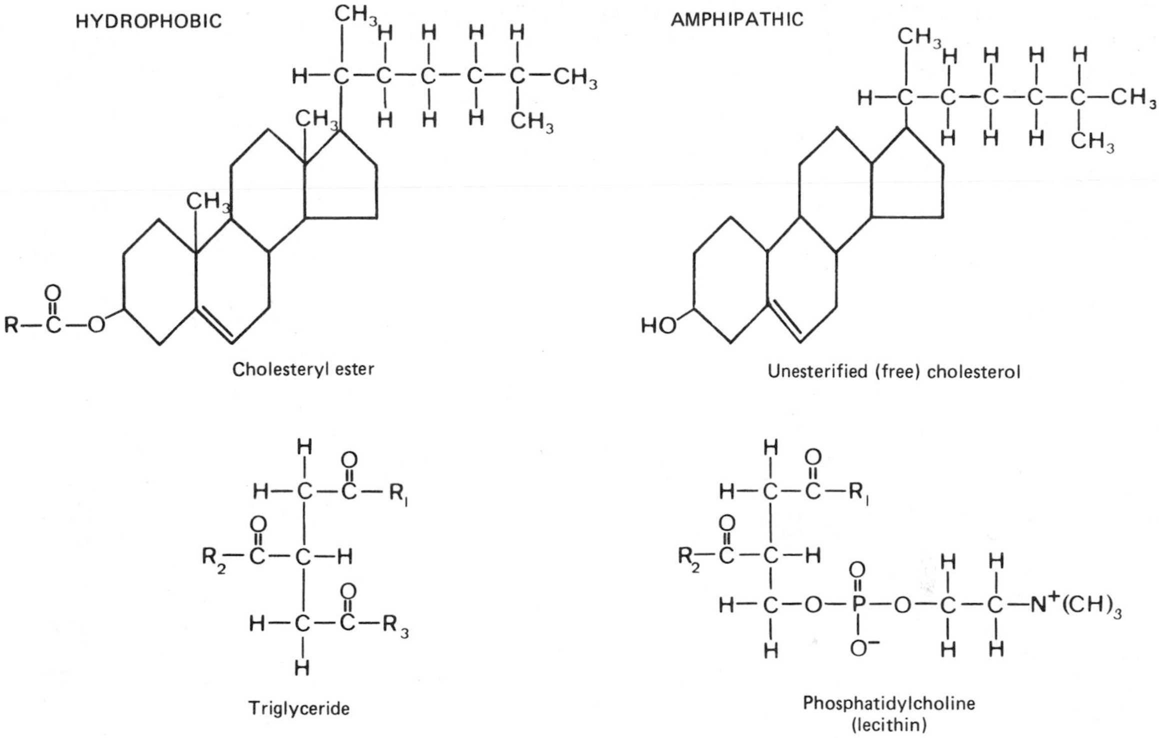

Figure 24–1. Major lipids of plasma lipoproteins. R = hydrocarbon chain of a fatty acid.

(4) Apolipoprotein A-II: This protein of MW 17,400 is an important constituent of HDL. It contains cysteine, which permits the formation of disulfide-bridged dimers with apo-E.

(5) D apolipoprotein: This heavily glycosylated protein of MW 19,000 is involved with LCAT in the centripetal transport of cholesterol.

(6) Apolipoprotein A-IV: This protein of MW 46,000 is chiefly associated with chylomicrons.

(7) Proline-rich protein: This protein of MW 74,000 is associated with chylomicrons and occurs also as a multimer in plasma that is not associated with lipoproteins.

(8) Lp(a) protein: This high-molecular-weight (200,000–750,000) glycoprotein, which has a high degree of sequence homology with plasminogen, is found as a disulfide-bridged dimer with apo-B-100 in LDL-like species of lipoproteins (Lp(a) lipoproteins).

Absorption of Dietary Fat; Secretion of Chylomicrons

Dietary triglycerides are largely hydrolyzed in the intestine to β-monoglyceride and fatty acids by pancreatic lipase. This enzyme requires activation by bile acids and a protein cofactor. The partial glycerides and fatty acids form micelles that are absorbed by intestinal epithelial cells. Within these cells, the fatty acids are reesterified with the monoglyceride to form triglycer-ides. Some dietary cholesterol absorbed with the micelles is esterified by the acyl-CoA:cholesterol acyltransferase (ACAT) system, and some appears as free cholesterol in the surface monolayers of the chylomicrons. Droplets of triglyceride containing small amounts of cholesteryl esters form in the vesicles of the Golgi apparatus. Phospholipids and free cholesterol form a surface monolayer. Some of the phospholipid originates in bile, some is from dietary sources, and some is synthesized by the intestine. Newly synthesized apo-B-48, apo-A-I, and apo-A-II are added, and the nascent chylomicron emerges into the extracellular lymph space (Fig 24–2). Chylomicrons have diameters ranging from about 60 nm to 500 nm. Once in the lymph spaces, the new chylomicron begins to exchange surface components with HDL, acquiring apo-C and apo-E and losing phospholipids. This process continues as the chylomicron is carried via the intestinal lymphatics to the thoracic duct and thence into the bloodstream. Increased triglyceride transport from the intestine results chiefly in an increase of particle diameter of chylomicrons rather than increased numbers of particles.

Formation of Very Low Density Lipoproteins

The liver exports triglycerides to peripheral tissues in the cores of VLDL (Fig 24–3). These triglycerides

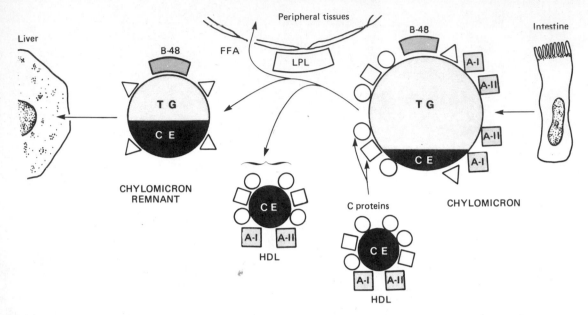

Figure 24–2. Metabolism of chylomicrons. TG = triglyceride; CE = cholesteryl esters; A-I, A-II, B-48, and C proteins = apolipoproteins. See text for details.

are synthesized in liver from free fatty acids abstracted from plasma and from fatty acids synthesized de novo. Acetyl-CoA for de novo synthesis is derived from the catabolism of carbohydrate, certain amino acids, and acetate formed by oxidation of ethanol. Several major features distinguish VLDL from chylomicrons. The only B apolipoprotein of VLDL is B-100, and VLDL contain none of the major apolipoproteins of HDL. Whereas the intestine produces only very limited amounts of apo-C, the liver secretes the bulk of these proteins with newly formed VLDL. Upon reaching the plasma, the VLDL acquire still more apo-C from HDL and yield phospholipid in exchange. Release of VLDL by liver is increased by any condition that results in increased flux of FFA to liver in the absence of increased ketogenesis. Increased caloric intake, ingestion of ethanol, and the administration of estrogens all greatly stimulate release of VLDL from liver and are important causative factors in clinical disorders resulting in elevated levels of triglycerides in plasma.

Metabolism of Triglyceride-Rich Lipoproteins in Plasma

A. Hydrolysis by Lipoprotein Lipase: Fatty acids derived from the triglycerides of chylomicrons and VLDL are delivered to tissues predominantly through a common pathway involving hydrolysis by the lipoprotein lipase (LPL) system. Alternative pathways of low efficiency also degrade triglyceride-rich lipoproteins in peripheral tissues. These pathways can account for a larger than normal fraction of the degradation of VLDL and chylomicrons in patients with hypertriglyceridemia. Over three-fourths of the FFA

derived during hydrolysis of triglycerides by LPL enters tissue directly. The remainder enters the pool of plasma FFA. Lipoprotein lipase is bound to capillary endothelium in heart, skeletal muscle, adipose tissue, mammary gland, and other tissues. The hydrolysis of triglycerides thus takes place within the vascular compartment. Removal of the first 2 fatty acids from the triglyceride appears to be mediated by LPL (triglyceridase and diglyceridase activities), whereas a separate monoglyceridase enzyme system is required for the last step.

B. Biologic Regulators of Lipoprotein Lipase: When glucose levels in plasma are elevated and the release of insulin is stimulated, LPL activity in adipose tissue increases, and fatty acids derived from triglycerides of circulating lipoproteins are stored. During prolonged fasting, however, LPL activity of adipose tissue falls to undetectable levels, completely preventing storage of fatty acids from VLDL and chylomicrons. Heparin, a mucopolysaccharide, is a cofactor for LPL. When heparin is given intravenously in doses of 0.1–0.2 mg/kg, LPL activity is displaced into plasma. This permits its in vitro measurement. An additional obligatory cofactor is apo-C-II. Normally, the content of this apolipoprotein in plasma is far in excess of that required for activation of the LPL system.

C. Formation of Lipoprotein Remnants: Hydrolysis by LPL results in progressive depletion of the content of triglycerides in the hydrophobic core regions of chylomicrons and VLDL, producing a progressive decrease in particle diameter. Amphiphilic lipids from the surface monolayer are transported to HDL directly and also indirectly via membranes of cells, principally

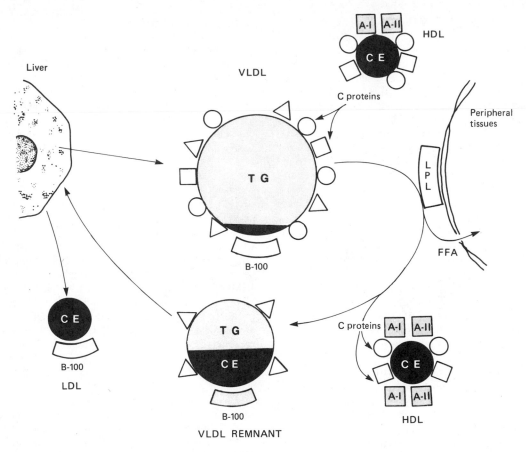

Figure 24–3. Metabolism of VLDL. TG = triglyceride; CE = cholesteryl esters; A-I, A-II, B-48, and C proteins = apolipoproteins. See text for details.

erythrocytes. This maintains an appropriate core: monolayer relationship for spheres of smaller diameters. During this process, apo-C—and, to a lesser extent, apo-E—are transferred to HDL. The products of this series of events are "remnant" lipoproteins containing their original complement of apo-B, a portion of the original amount of apo-E, and little apo-C. In the case of chylomicrons, apo-A-I and apo-A-II also leave the particles and become part of the circulating mass of HDL. The remnant particles of VLDL are 25–30 nm in diameter, and those of chylomicrons are up to 80 nm in diameter. Remnant particles are found both in the d < 1.006 g/cm³ fraction of plasma and in the IDL fraction (1.006 < d < 1.019 g/cm³). They have lost about 70% of their original complement of triglyceride but are enriched in cholesteryl esters.

D. Fate of Lipoprotein Remnants: Chylomicron remnants are removed from blood quantitatively by high-affinity, receptor-mediated endocytosis in the liver. The receptors appear to interact with apo-E on the lipoproteins. The lipid constituents enter hepatic pools, and the B-48 protein appears to be degraded completely. The cholesterol derived from chylomicron

remnants is the major mediator of feedback control of cholesterol biosynthesis in liver. Some VLDL remnants are removed from blood via the B-100:E receptors (see below) and are degraded. Those which escape uptake are transformed into LDL. Thus, the rate of removal of VLDL remnants by liver is a determinant of LDL production. The process of formation of LDL involves the removal of essentially all of the residual triglycerides and a portion of the cholesteryl esters and amphipathic lipids. The LDL particles contain chiefly cholesteryl esters in their core regions. They retain the B-100 protein but only traces of other apolipoproteins. In normal individuals, a major fraction of VLDL is converted to LDL, and all of the LDL apo-B comes from VLDL. In certain hypertriglyceridemic states, conversion of VLDL to LDL is decreased.

The fact that LDL originate from the metabolism of VLDL remnants suggests that increases of LDL in plasma can arise from an increased rate of secretion of precursor VLDL as well as from decreased catabolism of LDL. The formation of LDL from VLDL may also contribute to the clinical phenomenon referred to as the "beta shift." This is an increase of LDL (beta-lipoprotein) as hypertriglyceridemia resolves. A classic example of the beta shift occurs following institution of adequate insulin treatment in ketoacidotic diabetes with lipemia. Insulin induces increased lipoprotein lipase activity, resulting in rapid conversion of VLDL to LDL. Because of its longer half-life, the LDL accumulates in plasma. Elevated levels of LDL may persist beyond the time when levels of triglyceride-rich lipoproteins have returned to normal.

E. Half-Lives of Lipoproteins: Normally, the half-life of chylomicron apo-B in plasma is 5–20 minutes; that of the apo-B in VLDL is 1–3 hours; and that of LDL is about 2½ days. At triglyceride levels of 800–1000 mg/dL, the lipoprotein lipase mechanism is at kinetic saturation; therefore, increases in the input of triglyceride-rich lipoproteins into plasma at those levels rapidly result in much higher levels.

F. Effect of Dietary Fat Restriction: Individuals consuming a typical North American diet (with about 45% of calories as fat) transport 75–100 g or more of triglyceride per day into plasma in chylomicrons, whereas the liver exports 10–30 g of triglyceride in VLDL. Thus, the flux of triglyceride into plasma can be influenced most acutely by restriction of dietary fat. When the removal mechanisms involving lipoprotein lipase are saturated and plasma triglyceride levels are measured in thousands of milligrams per deciliter, acute restriction of dietary triglyceride intake will usually produce a significant reduction in triglyceride levels. This intervention is important in the lipemic patient with impending pancreatitis. If symptoms suggest that an attack of pancreatitis is imminent, all oral intake should be eliminated and the patient should be maintained on parenteral glucose until the symptoms subside and triglyceride levels decrease to less than 1000 mg/dL.

Catabolism of Low-Density Lipoproteins

A. Endocytosis via Specific High-Affinity Receptors: The catabolism of LDL appears to proceed by several mechanisms. The best-understood of these is a regulated adsorptive endocytosis mediated by high-affinity receptors in "coated pits" on the cell membranes of virtually all types of cells but most importantly hepatocytes (Fig 24–4). The receptors bind the apo-B protein of LDL. Because they also bind apo-E, they are called B-100:E receptors. The coated pit regions invaginate into the cell, forming endocytotic vesicles that fuse with lysosomes. The apo-B of the LDL is degraded to amino acids, and the receptor returns to the cell membrane. The cholesteryl esters of the LDL core are hydrolyzed to yield free cholesterol, which passes to the cytosol, where it is utilized in the production of cell membrane bilayers. Free cholesterol suppresses the activity of hydroxymethylglutaryl-CoA (HMG-CoA) reductase, a rate-limiting enzyme in the biosynthetic pathway for cholesterol. Thus, the intake of cholesterol by this pathway decreases the formation of new cholesterol in the cell. Cholesterol in excess of need for membrane synthesis is esterified by the acyl-CoA:cholesterol acyltransferase (ACAT) system for storage. In addition to suppression of cholesterol biosynthesis, the entry of cholesterol via the LDL pathway leads to down-regulation of LDL receptors, resulting in decreased uptake and catabolism of LDL.

B. Other Pathways: In addition to the high-affinity receptor-mediated pathway of degradation, LDL appear to be catabolized by at least 2 additional pathways. Macrophages take up chemically or physically altered LDL by a high-capacity mechanism that is apparently not subject to feedback control. This mechanism resembles the uptake of other altered serum pro-

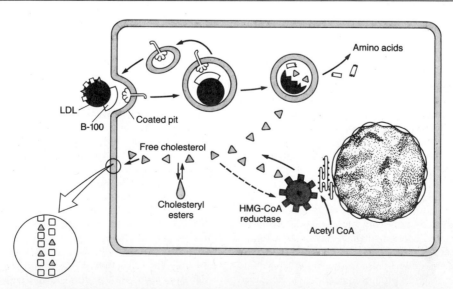

Figure 24–4. Cholesterol homeostasis in the cell. See text for details.

teins. The biologic significance of this pathway remains unclear, because the chemical alterations of LDL that may occur in vivo have not yet been determined. LDL are also taken up by many types of cells by a low-affinity process.

Metabolism of High-Density Lipoproteins

High-density lipoproteins, like the other major lipoproteins, have cholesteryl ester-filled core regions. On the basis of their flotation properties, there appear to be 2 major subclasses of HDL: HDL_3, of density 1.21–1.125, are about 7.5–10.5 nm in diameter; and HDL_2, of density 1.125–1.063, are about 9.5–10.5 nm in diameter. Males and females have nearly equal amounts of HDL_3 in their serum (about 300 mg/dL of total lipid and protein mass). Women, however, have greater amounts of HDL_2 than do men (about 80 mg/dL versus about 36 mg/dL). There is epidemiologic evidence that the inverse relationship between coronary risk and HDL levels is chiefly dependent upon the content of HDL_2 in plasma. Other evidence indicates that a number of subspecies of HDL exist which may have individual roles in lipid metabolism. Among these is a newly recognized particle with prebeta-electrophoretic mobility that appears to be involved in the retrieval of cholesterol from peripheral tissues.

A. Sources of HDL: Both the liver and intestine produce HDL apolipoproteins, which appear to organize with lipids into the native species of HDL in lymph and plasma. HDL acquire cholesteryl esters by the action of LCAT. This enzyme transfers 1 mol of fatty acid from a lecithin molecule to the hydroxyl group of unesterified cholesterol, forming cholesteryl ester, which then enters the hydrophobic region between the lamellae of the bilayer. Lysolecithin, formed by transfer of the fatty acid from lecithin, leaves the lipoprotein complex, binds to albumin, and is transported to various tissues, where it is reacylated to form lecithin. The process of transesterification by LCAT rapidly forms sufficient cholesteryl ester to fill the hydrophobic core region to a spherical shape.

LCAT enzyme is secreted by liver. In severe hepatic parenchymal disease, levels of this enzyme in plasma are low and esterification of cholesterol is impeded, leading to the accumulation of free cholesterol in lipoproteins and in membranes of erythrocytes and other cells. Excess free cholesterol in the membranes of erythrocytes transforms them into the target cells classically associated with hepatic disease.

As hydrolysis of triglycerides in chylomicrons and VLDL proceeds, phospholipids and cholesterol are transferred to HDL particles.

B. Metabolic Roles for HDL: Several metabolic roles for HDL are now recognized. These lipoproteins serve as carriers for the C apolipoproteins, transferring them to nascent VLDL and chylomicrons. HDL as well as LDL deliver cholesterol to the adrenal cortex

and gonads in support of steroidogenesis. HDL play a major role in the centripetal transport of cholesterol— ie, the transport of surplus cholesterol away from peripheral tissues. Although this process is not fully understood, it appears that several subspecies of HDL are involved. Unesterified cholesterol is acquired from the membranes of peripheral tissues and is esterified by LCAT. The resulting cholesteryl esters, predominantly cholesteryl linoleate, are then transferred to LDL and to triglyceride-rich lipoproteins. Remnants of chylomicrons and a significant fraction of VLDL remnants and LDL are taken up by liver, providing for transport of the newly formed cholesteryl esters to hepatocytes. Recently, it has been discovered that the processes of esterification and transfer are mediated by a species of lipoprotein that comprises only a small fraction of total HDL. In addition to lipids, this particle contains apo-A-I and LCAT. The apo-A-I is a cofactor for LCAT. Two other proteins, apo-II and cholesteryl ester transfer protein (CETP) appear to be involved in the transfer of the cholesteryl esters to recipient lipoproteins. At least one subspecies of HDL is involved in transferring free cholesterol from tissues to the esterification transfer particle.

C. Catabolism of HDL: The pathways of catabolism of HDL are not yet known. Radiochemical studies indicate that apo-A-I and apo-A-II are removed from plasma synchronously and that a portion of the degradation occurs in liver. Because degradation by perfused rat livers is slower than for the intact animal, it must be presumed that peripheral tissues contribute substantially to the catabolism of HDL.

The Cholesterol Economy

Cholesterol is an essential constituent of the plasma membranes of mammalian cells and of the myelin sheath. It is also required for adrenal and gonadal steroidogenesis and for the production of bile acids by the liver. Virtually all nucleated mammalian cells can synthesize cholesterol, commencing with acetyl-CoA. Formation of HMG-CoA is the initial step. The first committed step, mediated by HMG-CoA reductase, is the formation of mevalonic acid from HMG-CoA. Mevalonic acid is then metabolized via a series of isoprenoid intermediaries to squalene, which cyclizes to form a series of sterols leading to cholesterol. A small amount of the mevalonate is converted eventually to the important isoprenoid substances ubiquinone, dolichol, and isopentenyl pyrophosphate. The portion of the pathway leading to cholesterol synthesis is tightly regulated by cholesterol, or some metabolite of cholesterol, which suppresses the activity of HMG-CoA reductase. Thus, the cells have the ability to produce cholesterol to the extent that their requirements are not met by that derived from circulating lipoproteins. Cholesteryl esters stored in cells serve as an immediate reserve of cholesterol. Large requirements for cholesterol result from rapid proliferation of cells with attendant need for elaboration of cell membranes. Hepatocytes and intestinal epithelial cells require large amounts of cholesterol for secretion of lipoproteins. In addition to these requirements, cells appear to be constantly transferring cholesterol to circulating lipoproteins, chiefly HDL. A relatively small amount of cholesterol is lost from the body in desquamated skin and through the loss of intestinal epithelial cells in the stool. The net daily loss of cholesterol from the gut, derived both from biliary cholesterol and from desquamated epithelial cells, is about 50 mg. In addition, about 2% of the mass of bile acids secreted into the intestine are lost in the stool, equivalent to about 250 mg of cholesterol.

Cholesterol is acquired from the diet as well as from endogenous synthesis. Humans, unlike many other species, do not absorb dietary cholesterol quantitatively; however, at normal levels of intake, about one-third of the amount ingested reaches the bloodstream. Most of this cholesterol is transported to liver in chylomicron remnants, leading to suppression of hepatic cholesterogenesis. Recent evidence suggests that individuals may differ substantially in the effect of dietary cholesterol on serum lipoproteins, reflecting in part differences in the efficiency of absorption of cholesterol. The range of cholesterol content in the usual North American diet is 0.4–2 g/d or more. In many parts of the world, the average daily intake of cholesterol is below 0.2 g.

DIFFERENTIATION OF DISORDERS OF LIPOPROTEIN METABOLISM

Laboratory Analyses of Lipids & Lipoproteins

Because chylomicrons normally may be present in plasma up to 12 hours after a meal, they contribute triglyceride to the total measured during that period, raising the triglyceride concentration to as much as 600 mg/dL (6.9 mmol/L). However, this alimentary lipemia can be substantially prolonged if alcohol is consumed with the meal. Thus, serum lipids and lipoproteins should be measured after a fast of 14 hours or more. If blood glucose is not to be measured, patients may have fruit juice and black coffee with sugar (which provide no triglyceride) for breakfast.

A. Inspection: Much useful information is gained from inspection of the serum, especially before and after overnight refrigeration. As a screening technique, this will identify sera in which triglycerides need to be measured. Opalescence is due to light scattering by large triglyceride-rich lipoproteins. Serum begins to appear hazy when the level of triglycerides reaches 200 mg/dL (2.3 mmol/L), about the point at which clinical significance begins. The presence of chylomicrons is readily detected, because they form a white supernatant layer. A further observation made on serum, which is critical to the detection of the uncommon cases in which binding of immunoglobulins to lipoproteins takes place, is the formation of a curdlike lipoprotein aggregate or a snowy precipitate as serum cools. If one of these disorders is suspected, blood should be kept at 37 °C during the formation of the clot and separation of the serum, because the critical temperatures for precipitation of the cryoglobulin complex may be higher than room temperature.

B. Laboratory Techniques: The cholesterol and triglyceride contents of serum can be measured by several chemical techniques that provide reliable results. These measurements are an essential minimum for differentiation of disorders of lipoprotein metabolism. The usual methods determine unesterified and esterified cholesterol together, so that the reported value is the total content of cholesterol in serum. In most cases, electrophoresis of lipoproteins contributes little additional information; thus, this technique is not a necessary part of the routine laboratory examination. The exception is the identification of lipoproteins found in familial dysbetalipoproteinemia. The best electrophoretic separation of lipoproteins is made in agarose gel. The most complete characterization of a patient's lipoproteins is achieved by measurement of the cholesterol and triglyceride contents and electrophoretic behavior of individual lipoprotein fractions, separated by sequential preparative ultracentrifugation, a technique usually available only in research laboratories. However, the content of high-density lipoproteins can be measured in many laboratories using a technique in which HDL are the only lipoproteins that remain in solution after treatment of the serum with heparin and manganese. The cholesterol content of the solution is taken as HDL cholesterol. Albeit rapid, the results of this technique tend to be unacceptably variable unless rigid quality control is exercised. The prognostic implications of small changes in HDL cholesterol make such controls necessary.

An important determinant of the content of cholesteryl esters in HDL is the amount of triglyceride-rich lipoproteins to which the HDL are exposed in plasma. Triglycerides from these lipoproteins exchange into the core regions of HDL, displacing cholesteryl esters and leading to an inverse logarithmic dependence of HDL cholesterol level upon the plasma triglycerides. Thus, the HDL cholesterol value cannot be interpreted without knowledge of the level of serum triglycerides. For example, a level of HDL that would normally contain 45 mg/dL (1.17 mmol/L) of cholesterol would contain 37 mg/dL (0.96 mmol/L) when the triglycerides were 200 mg/dL (2.3 mmol/L) and 30 mg/dL (0.78 mmol/L) when they reach 500 mg/dL (5.7 mmol/L). In certain forms of hypertriglyceridemia, there may also be a moderate decrease in the protein-phospholipid vehicle of HDL, but the principal effect on the measurement of HDL cholesterol levels remains the exchange of triglycerides for cholesteryl esters.

More sophisticated tests of composition of isolated lipoprotein fractions are of use in certain instances.

The most important of these is analysis of the ratio of cholesterol to triglycerides by chemical techniques and of the apolipoproteins of VLDL by isoelectric focusing. The latter allows the identification of deficiency of the normal isoforms of apo-E, the underlying molecular defect in familial dysbetalipoproteinemia. In this disorder, there is an unusually high content of cholesterol in the VLDL. Quantitative measurement of the apolipoproteins of VLDL can be made by electrophoresis in agarose gel (following delipidation by tetramethylurea) or by immunochemical analysis. A number of immunoassays for various apolipoproteins are available.

Clinical Differentiation of Abnormal Patterns of Plasma Lipoproteins

A. Preliminary Screening: The first step in the diagnosis of hyperlipidemia is the determination that levels of lipids in serum are abnormal. Serum cholesterol and triglyceride levels are both continuously distributed in the population; therefore, some arbitrary levels must be established to define significant hyperlipidemia. The greater the departure from these norms, the greater will be the clinical importance of the hyperlipidemia. Selection of these arbitrary values should not imply that the levels of circulating lipids prevalent in most of the population in Western countries are without risk. As indicated in the introductory paragraphs, average levels of LDL in these populations appear to be well above the biologic ideal and may be a major etiologic factor underlying the increased incidence of atherosclerotic vascular disease in Western societies. Epidemiologic studies in Europe and the USA have shown that there is a progressive increase in risk of coronary artery disease as levels of serum cholesterol increase above 180 mg/dL (4.68 mmol/L). Present evidence would indicate that physicians should at least encourage patients at risk to eat diets low in saturated fats and cholesterol in order to minimize the burden of LDL in plasma.

The National Cholesterol Education Program has developed guidelines for treatment of hypercholesterolemia in adults (Table 24–2). Although criteria for triglycerides have not been established, levels above 198 mg/dL (2.18 mmol/L) merit investigation. One abnormality associated with increased risk of coronary artery disease that will not be detected if only cases with hyperlipidemia are studied is hypoalphalipoproteinemia, or deficiency of HDL. Many of the affected individuals have normal levels of both cholesterol and triglycerides in serum and no clinical stigmas to draw the attention of the physician. The argument has been offered that detection of these individuals is unavailing, because there is little that can currently be done to modify levels of HDL in serum. Appreciation that hypoalphalipoproteinemia is present, however, is important if for no other reason than to underscore the importance of controlling other risk factors and perhaps the

Table 24–2. National Cholesterol Education Program: Adult Treatment Guidelines (1987).[1]

	Total Cholesterol		LDL Cholesterol	
	mg/dL	mmol/L	mg/dL	mmol/L
Desirable	<200	<5.2	<130	<3.38
Borderline-High[2]	200–239	5.2–6.2	130–159	3.38–4.13
High	≥240	≥6.24	≥160	≥4.16

[1]Modified and reproduced, with permission, from Katzung BG (editor): *Basic & Clinical Pharmacology,* 4th ed. Appleton & Lange, 1989.
[2]Consider as high if coronary heart disease or more than 2 risk factors are present.

avoidance of factors that reduce HDL levels, such as cigarette smoking and the use of some drugs.

B. Identification of Abnormal Patterns: The second step in investigation of hyperlipidemia is determination of the species of lipoproteins that account for the increased content of lipids in serum. In some cases, multiple species may be involved; in others, qualitative properties of the lipoproteins are of diagnostic importance. After identifying the pattern of the lipoprotein abnormality, the physician must search for underlying disorders that cause secondary hyperlipidemias of similar pattern. Such disorders may be the sole cause of the lipoprotein abnormality or may aggravate primary disorders of lipoprotein metabolism. The differentiation of specific primary disorders usually requires additional clinical and genetic information.

The following diagnostic protocol, based upon initial measurement of cholesterol and triglycerides in serum after a 14-hour fast, supplemented by observation of serum and by additional laboratory measurements where essential, will serve as a practical guide in identifying abnormal patterns of lipoprotein distribution. The term "hyperlipidemia" denotes high levels of any class of lipoprotein; "hyperlipemia" denotes high levels of any of the triglyceride-rich lipoproteins.

Case 1. Serum Cholesterol Levels Increased; Triglycerides Normal:

(a) If the serum cholesterol level is modestly elevated (up to 260 mg/dL [6.76 mmol/L]), the HDL cholesterol level should be measured. Hyperalphalipoproteinemia (elevated levels of HDL in serum) may account for the observed increase in serum cholesterol level. Hyperalphalipoproteinemia is not associated with disease processes. The LDL cholesterol level in serum (in mg/dL) may be estimated by subtracting the HDL cholesterol level and the estimated cholesterol contribution of VLDL from the total serum cholesterol level. The VLDL cholesterol is approximated as one-fifth of the serum triglyceride level.

LDL cholesterol =

$$\text{Total cholesterol} - \left(\frac{\text{TG}}{5} + \text{HDL cholesterol}\right)$$

Calculated values of LDL cholesterol over 130 mg/dL (3.38 mmol/L) are clinically significant.

(b) Because HDL almost never contribute more than 120 mg/dL (3.12 mmol/L) of cholesterol, serum cholesterol levels in excess of 260 mg/dL (6.76 mmol/L) always represent significant hyperlipidemia. Unless the patient has obstructive hepatic disease, the abnormality may be assumed to be due to an increase in low-density lipoproteins. The abnormal lipoprotein of cholestasis, like LDL, is selectively rich in cholesterol. It can be differentiated because it has gamma mobility on electrophoresis in agarose gel and because it stains metachromatically with Sudan black.

Case 2. Predominant Increase of Triglycerides in Serum; Moderate Increase in Cholesterol Level May Be Present: Here it is apparent that the primary abnormality is an increase in the triglyceride-rich VLDL (hyperprebetalipoproteinemia) or chylomicrons (chylomicronemia), or both (mixed lipemia). Because both VLDL and chylomicrons contain free cholesterol in their surface monolayers and a small amount of cholesteryl ester in their cores, the total cholesterol level in serum may be increased, though to a much smaller extent than is the serum triglyceride level. The contribution of cholesterol in these lipoproteins to the total in serum is about 8–25% of the triglyceride content. Low levels of LDL cholesterol often seen in hypertriglyceridemia may largely offset the increase in cholesterol due to the triglyceride-rich lipoproteins, especially in primary chylomicronemia. A white supernatant layer in serum refrigerated overnight reveals the presence of chylomicrons. Because VLDL and chylomicrons compete as substrates in a common removal pathway, chylomicrons will nearly always be present when triglyceride levels exceed 1000 mg/dL (11.5 mmol/L).

Case 3. Cholesterol and Triglyceride Levels in Serum Both Elevated: This pattern can be the result of either of 2 abnormal lipoprotein distributions. One of these is a combined increase of VLDL (prebeta-lipoproteins), which provide most of the increase in triglycerides, and LDL (beta-lipoproteins), which account for the bulk of the increase in cholesterol in serum. This pattern is termed combined hyperlipidemia and is one of the 3 phenotypic patterns encountered in kindreds with the disorder termed familial combined or familial multiple type hyperlipidemia. The second distribution is an increase of remnant lipoproteins derived from VLDL and chylomicrons. These lipoprotein particles have been partially depleted of triglyceride by lipoprotein lipase and have been enriched with cholesteryl esters by the LCAT system, such that the total content of cholesterol in serum is similar to that of triglycerides. This pattern is almost always an expression of familial dysbetalipoproteinemia. Differentiation of these 2 patterns requires application of additional diagnostic tests. Presumptive differentiation can be made with high-quality agarose gel electrophoresis. In combined hyperlipidemia, the prebeta- and beta-lipoprotein bands are both increased in staining intensity, but each has its typical electrophoretic mobility, and they are well resolved from one another. Preparative ultracentrifugation of serum in this disorder shows elevated levels of both VLDL and LDL. In contrast, the remnant particles in dysbetalipoproteinemia are distributed in a "broad beta" pattern that obscures the resolution of beta- and prebeta-lipoprotein bands. A substantial portion of the triglyceride-rich lipoproteins shows beta-electrophoretic mobility after separation from serum in the ultracentrifuge (at a density of 1.006 g/cm³), and they have an increased content of cholesterol. Dysbetalipoproteinemia is confirmed by the absence of the E-3 and E-4 isoforms of apo-E when the triglyceride-rich fraction of serum is analyzed by isoelectric focusing.

CLINICAL DESCRIPTIONS OF PRIMARY & SECONDARY DISORDERS OF LIPOPROTEIN METABOLISM

THE HYPERTRIGLYCERIDEMIAS

Atherogenicity

In addition to LDL, certain triglyceride-rich lipoproteins appear to be atherogenic. There is ample clinical evidence that the remnant lipoproteins of dysbetalipoproteinemia are associated with accelerated atherosclerosis in coronary and peripheral vessels. The atherogenicity of other triglyceride-rich lipoproteins is probably dependent upon particle diameter and perhaps on other properties as well. For example, patients with primary chylomicronemia do not appear to have accelerated atherosclerosis despite extremely high levels of triglycerides in serum, whereas there is some clinical evidence in support of the atherogenicity of VLDL of small to moderate particle diameter. Furthermore, VLDL have now been demonstrated in the walls of arteries removed at surgery. Impaired capacity of the VLDL of some individuals to accept cholesteryl esters from the LCAT reaction may also contribute to atherogenesis by impeding centripetal transport of cholesterol.

Cause of Pancreatitis

Very high levels of triglycerides in plasma are associated with risk of acute pancreatitis, probably from the local release of amphipathic free fatty acids and lysolecithin from lipoprotein substrates in the capillary bed of the pancreas. When the concentrations of these lipids exceed the binding capacity of albumin, they could lyse membranes of parenchymal cells, initiating a chemical pancreatitis. Patients who have had previous attacks of pancreatitis appear to be at higher risk.

Many patients with lipemia have intermittent episodes of epigastric pain during which serum amylase does not reach levels commonly considered diagnostic for pancreatitis. This is especially true in patients who have had previous attacks. The observation that these episodes frequently evolve into classic pancreatitis suggests that they represent incipient pancreatic inflammation. The progression of pancreatitis can be prevented by rapid reduction of triglyceride levels in serum, which can usually be accomplished by rigorous restriction of dietary fat and institution of other corrective measures. In more threatening cases, parenteral feeding with glucose may be required for a few days. The clinical course of pancreatitis in patients with lipemia is typical of the general experience with this disease. Fatal hemorrhagic pancreatitis occurs in a few; many develop pseudocysts; and some progress to pancreatic exocrine insufficiency or compromised insulinogenic capacity.

Clinical Signs

When triglyceride levels in serum exceed 3000–4000 mg/dL (34.5–46 mmol/L), light scattering by these particles in the blood lends a whitish cast to the venous vascular bed of the retina, a sign known as **lipemia retinalis.** Markedly elevated levels of VLDL (and perhaps small chylomicrons) in plasma may be associated with the appearance of **eruptive cutaneous xanthomas.** These lesions, filled with foam cells, appear as yellow morbilliform eruptions 2–5 mm in diameter, often with erythematous areolae. They usually occur in clusters on extensor surfaces such as the elbows, knees, and buttocks. They are transient and usually disappear within a few weeks after triglyceride levels are reduced below 2000–3000 mg/dL (23–34.5 mmol/L).

Effects of Hypertriglyceridemia on Laboratory Measurements

Very high levels of triglyceride-rich lipoproteins may introduce important errors in clinical laboratory measurements. Light scattering from these large particles can cause erroneous results in most chemical determinations involving photometric measurements in spite of corrections for blank values. Amylase activity in serum may be inhibited by triglyceride-rich lipoproteins; hence, lipemic specimens should be diluted for measurement of this enzyme. Because the lipoproteins are not permeable to ionic or polar small molecules, their hydrophobic regions constitute a second phase in plasma. When the volume of this phase becomes appreciable, electrolytes (measured by flame photometry) and other hydrophilic species in serum will be underestimated with respect to their true concentration in plasma water. A practical rule for correcting these values is as follows: for each 1000 mg/dL (11.5 mmol/L) of triglyceride in serum, the concentrations of all hydrophilic molecules and ions should be increased by 1%.

1. PRIMARY HYPERTRIGLYCERIDEMIA

Deficiency of Lipoprotein Lipase or Its Cofactor

A. Clinical Findings: Because the clinical expressions of these defects are identical, they will be considered together. Both appear to be transmitted as autosomal recessive traits. On a typical North American diet, lipemia is usually severe (serum triglyceride levels of 2000–25,000 mg/dL) (23–287.5 mmol/L). Hepatomegaly and splenomegaly are frequently present. Foam cells laden with lipid are found in liver, spleen, and bone marrow. Splenic infarct has been described and may be a source of abdominal pain. Hypersplenism with anemia, granulocytopenia, and thrombocytopenia can occur. Recurrent epigastric pain and overt pancreatitis are frequently encountered. Eruptive xanthomas may be present. These disorders are present from birth and may be recognized in early infancy or may go unnoticed until an attack of acute pancreatitis occurs or lipemic serum is noted on blood sampling as late as middle age. Patients with these disorders are classically not obese and have normal carbohydrate metabolism, unless pancreatitis impairs insulinogenic capacity. Estrogens intensify the lipemia by stimulating production of VLDL by liver. Therefore, in pregnancy and lactation or during the administration of estrogenic steroids, the risk of pancreatitis increases.

B. Laboratory Findings: These patients have a preponderance of chylomicrons in serum such that the infranatant layer of serum refrigerated overnight may be nearly clear. Many have a moderate increase in VLDL, however, and in pregnant women or those receiving estrogens, a pattern of mixed lipemia is usually present. Levels of low-density lipoproteins in serum are decreased, probably representing the predominant catabolism of VLDL by pathways that do not involve the production of LDL. Levels of HDL are also decreased. A presumptive diagnosis of these disorders can be made by restricting the oral intake of fat to 10–15 g/d for 3–5 days. The triglyceride level of plasma drops precipitously, usually reaching 200–600 mg/dL (2.3–6.9 mmol/L) within 3–4 days. Confirmation of deficiency of lipoprotein lipase is obtained by measurement in vitro of the lipolytic activity of plasma prepared from blood drawn 10 minutes after heparin, 0.2 mg/kg, is injected intravenously. Analysis of lipolysis is carried out with and without 0.5 M sodium chloride, which inhibits lipoprotein lipase but does not suppress the activity of other plasma lipases, including hepatic lipase. Classically, the lipolytic activity of plasma is very low and is similar in the saline-inhibited and saline-uninhibited incubates. Recent findings suggest that several forms of LPL deficiency can be differentiated by prolonged infusions of heparin. These findings are compatible either with selective deficiencies of the LPL species in different tissues or with the existence of a form of the disorder in which binding to endothelium is abnormal. The latter is supported by heterogeneity in levels of another heparin-releasable enzyme, histaminase, in sera of patients with LPL deficiency. Absence of the cofactor protein of LPL, apo-C-II, is the counterpart of deficiency of LPL and can be demonstrated most readily by electrophoresis or isoelectric focusing of the proteins of VLDL.

C. Treatment: Treatment of primary chylomicronemia is entirely dietary. Intake of fat should be reduced to 10% or less of total calories. In an adult, this represents 15–30 g/d. Because the defect involves lipolysis, both saturated and unsaturated fats must be curtailed. The diet should contain at least 5 g of polyunsaturated fat as a source of essential fatty acids, and an ample supply of fat-soluble vitamins must be provided. Careful adherence to this diet will invariably maintain serum triglyceride levels below 1000 mg/dL (11.5 mmol/L) in the absence of pregnancy, lactation, or the administration of exogenous estrogens. Because this is below the level at which pancreatitis usually occurs, compliant patients with these disorders are at low risk.

Endogenous & Mixed Lipemias

A. Etiology and Pathogenesis: Endogenous lipemia (primary hyperprebetalipoproteinemia) and mixed lipemia probably both result from several genetically determined disorders. The occurrence of multiple cases in a kindred is the basis for considering them primary. Thus, a number of "sporadic cases" may be similar, only lacking evidence of familial occurrence. Because VLDL and chylomicrons are competing substrates in the intravascular lipolytic pathway, saturating levels of VLDL will cause an impedance in the removal of chylomicrons. Therefore, as the severity of endogenous lipemia increases, a pattern of mixed lipemia may supervene. In other cases, the pattern of mixed lipemia appears to be present continuously. Though specific pathophysiologic mechanisms remain obscure, certain familial patterns are known. In all forms, factors that increase the rate of secretion of VLDL from liver aggravate the hypertriglyceridemia—ie, obesity with insulin resistance, or the appearance of fully developed non–insulin-dependent diabetes mellitus (NIDDM); ethanol ingestion; and the use of exogenous estrogens. Studies of VLDL turnover indicate that either increased production or impaired removal of VLDL may be operative in different individuals. It appears that a substantial number of patients with mixed lipemia have partial defects in catabolism of triglyceride-rich lipoproteins. Increases in production rates of VLDL secondary to excess caloric intake, ethanol, or estrogens tend not to be accompanied by increased removal, as in normal individuals, but result in increased levels of circulating triglycerides. Some patients with mixed lipemia have decreased levels of lipoprotein lipase in plasma after a heparin stimulus, which may be of importance in this regard. Most pa-

tients with significant endogenous or mixed lipemia have the hypertrophic form of obesity, in which there is a reduced population of insulin receptors on cell membranes associated with impaired effectiveness of insulin. Mobilization of free fatty acids is maintained at a higher than normal rate, providing an increased flux of fatty acids to the liver, in turn increasing the secretion of triglyceride-rich VLDL. Recent studies also suggest that the removal of triglycerides from circulating chylomicrons is decreased in obesity.

B. Clinical Findings: Clinical features of these forms of hypertriglyceridemia depend upon severity and include eruptive xanthomas, lipemia retinalis, recurrent epigastric pain, and acute pancreatitis (described above). One constellation of clinical features that may be monogenic is endogenous lipemia with obesity, insulin resistance, elevated baseline levels of insulin, hyperlycemia, and hyperuricemia. There is also a tendency toward the development of hypertension in such patients. Some individuals will be more severely affected than others and will have a mixed lipemia, as though they had a double dose of the involved gene or a compound genetic state, including an aggravating trait. Many of the clinical features described above are associated with endogenous lipemia that does not present a clearly monogenic pattern of inheritance, suggesting that several mechanisms may be operative and that endogenous lipemia and mixed lipemia may also be polygenic.

C. Treatment: The primary mode of treatment is dietary. In the short term, severe restriction of total fat intake will usually result in a rapid decline of serum triglyceride levels to 1000–3000 mg/dL (11.5–34.5 mmol/L), averting pancreatitis. The objective of long-term dietary management is reduction to ideal body weight. Because ethanol causes significant augmentation of VLDL production, abstinence is important.

If weight loss is achieved, the serum triglycerides almost always show a marked response, often approaching normal values. When the fall in triglyceride levels is not satisfactory, clofibrate, gemfibrozil, or nicotinic acid will usually produce further reductions. (See Treatment of Hyperlipidemia, below.)

Familial Combined Hyperlipidemia (Multiple Type)

A. Etiology: Epidemiologic studies of the kindreds of survivors of myocardial infarction revealed this common heredofamilial disorder. The underlying process appears to be overproduction of VLDL. Some of the affected individuals have increased levels of both VLDL and LDL in serum (combined hyperlipidemia); some have increased levels of only VLDL or LDL. Without family studies, the latter 2 patterns would not be identified as belonging with this syndrome. Patterns in the serum of an individual patient may change with time. It is known that a mating of an individual having any one of the 3 phenotypic patterns with a normal individual can result in the appearance of one of the other patterns. Children in these kindreds may have hyperlipidemia, but the disorder is usually not fully expressed until adulthood.

B. Clinical Findings: Neither tendinous nor cutaneous xanthomas other than xanthelasma occur. Available data suggest that this disorder is inherited as a mendelian dominant trait. It appears that the factors that increase the severity of hypertriglyceridemia in other disorders aggravate the lipemia in this syndrome as well.

C. Treatment: The risk of coronary vascular disease is significantly increased in these patients, and therefore they should be treated aggressively with diet and drugs. Lipemia responds to clofibrate or gemfibrozil, but these agents may increase LDL levels (beta shift). Hence, niacin may be a better choice. Patients with increased LDL levels respond to bile acid–binding resins but may then have increases in VLDL. Therefore, the combination of a resin and niacin is frequently required. Lovastatin is also useful. (See Treatment of Hyperlipidemia, below.)

Familial Dysbetalipoproteinemia (Broad Beta Disease, Type III Hyperlipoproteinemia)

A. Etiology and Pathogenesis: A permissive genetic constitution for this disease occurs commonly, but expression of hyperlipoproteinemia apparently requires additional genetic or environmental determinants. The molecular basis of this disorder is the presence of mutant forms of apo-E that cannot interact normally with high-affinity receptors. In its fully expressed form, the lipoprotein pattern is dominated by the accumulation of remnants of VLDL and chylomicrons. Two populations of VLDL are usually present: normal prebeta-lipoproteins and remnants with beta-electrophoretic mobility. Remnant particles of intermediate density are also present. Characteristically, levels of LDL in serum are decreased, probably reflecting interruption of the normal transformation of VLDL remnants to LDL. The primary defect appears to involve the uptake of remnants of triglyceride-rich lipoproteins from plasma. Chylomicron remnants are frequently present in serum obtained after a 14-hour fast even when total serum triglycerides are only 300–600 mg/dL (3.45–6.9 mmol/L). All the remnant particles are enriched in cholesteryl esters such that the level of cholesterol in serum is often as high as the level of triglycerides. The "broad beta" electrophoretic pattern of VLDL is highly suggestive of familial dysbetalipoproteinemia. However, this pattern is seen also in hypothyroidism, resolving lipemias of other origins, and certain disorders involving immunoglobulin-lipoprotein complexes. Virtual absence of the E-3 and E-4 isoforms of apo-E, detected on isoelectric focusing of VLDL proteins, confirms the diagnosis of genetic dysbetalipoproteinemia. Hetero-

zygosity for apo-E-2, which may be associated with intensification of hyperlipemia from other causes, occurs in about 15% of the white population. Whereas homozygosity is present in about 1% of the population, the incidence of clinical hyperlipidemia among these patients is much smaller. Additional mutations of apo-E that cannot be distinguished from E-3 by isoelectric focusing are now known to result in dysbetalipoproteinemia.

B. Clinical Findings: Hyperlipidemia and clinical stigmas are not usually evident before age 20. In younger patients with hyperlipidemia, hypothyroidism or obesity is likely to be present. Adults frequently have tuberous or tuberoeruptive xanthomas. Both tend to occur on extensor surfaces, especially elbows and knees. Tuberoeruptive xanthomas are pink or yellowish skin nodules 3–8 mm in diameter that often become confluent. Tuberous xanthomas—reddish or orange, often shiny nodules up to 3 cm in diameter—are usually moveable and nontender. Another type, planar xanthomas of the palmar creases, strongly suggests dysbetalipoproteinemia. The skin creases assume an orange color from deposition of carotenoids and other lipids. They occasionally are raised above the level of adjacent skin and are not tender. (Planar xanthomas are also seen in cholestatic disease.) Xanthelasma—yellowish plaques on the canthus—may occur in dysbetalipoproteinemia.

Some patients have impaired glucose tolerance, which is usually associated with higher levels of blood lipids. Obesity is commonly present and tends to aggravate the lipemia. Patients with the genetic constitution for dysbetalipoproteinemia often develop severe hyperlipidemia if they are hypothyroid.

Atherosclerotic vascular disease of the coronary and peripheral vessels occurs with increased frequency in hyperlipidemic subjects with dysbetalipoproteinemia. The prevalence of atherosclerotic disease of the iliac and femoral vessels appears to be especially high.

C. Treatment: Management should begin with institution of a weight reduction diet providing a reduced intake of cholesterol. The use of alcohol should be minimized. Patients who achieve ideal body weight often do not require drug treatment. When the hyperlipidemia does not respond satisfactorily, clofibrate, gemfibrozil, or niacin in low doses are usually effective. (See Treatment of Hyperlipidemia, below.)

2. SECONDARY HYPERTRIGLYCERIDEMIA

Diabetes Mellitus

In patients with insulin-dependent diabetes mellitus (IDDM), levels of VLDL in plasma are frequently elevated despite the regular use of insulin, reflecting the difficulty of control of carbohydrate metabolism in this disorder.

A. Clinical Findings: Lipemia may be very severe, with elevated levels of both VLDL and chylomicrons when control is poor. Lipemic patients usually have ketoacidosis, but lipemia can occur in its absence. Patients with IDDM who have been chronically undertreated with insulin may have mobilized most of the triglyceride from peripheral adipose tissue, so that they no longer have sufficient substrate for significant ketogenesis. These emaciated individuals may have severe lipemia and striking hepatomegaly.

B. Pathogenesis: The severe lipemia associated with absence or marked insufficiency of insulin is attributable to deficiency of LPL activity, because this enzyme is induced by insulin. The administration of insulin in such cases usually restores triglyceride levels to normal within a few days. However, if massive fatty liver is present, weeks may be required for the VLDL levels to return to normal while the liver secretes its triglyceride into plasma. Conversion of massive amounts of VLDL to LDL, as the impedance of VLDL catabolism is relieved, leads to marked accumulation of LDL that may persist for weeks. This "beta shift" phenomenon may lead to a spurious diagnosis of hypercholesterolemia.

The moderately high levels of VLDL seen in diabetes under average control probably reflect chiefly an increased flux of FFA to liver that stimulates production of triglycerides and their secretion in VLDL. In addition to VLDL, LDL levels are also somewhat increased in insulin-dependent diabetics under poor control, probably accounting in part for their increased risk of coronary heart disease. Mild increases in VLDL and in FFA occur in many individuals with non–insulin-dependent diabetes mellitus (NIDDM). Some have much higher levels of VLDL, suggesting that an additional genetic factor predisposing to lipemia is present. Still another cause of lipemic diabetes is the compromised insulinogenic capacity that can result from acute pancreatitis in individuals with severe primary lipemias. The deficiency may be severe enough to require exogenous insulin, often only in small doses. In diabetics who develop nephrosis as a consequence of their microvascular disease, the secondary lipemia of nephrosis compounds their hypertriglyceridemia.

C. Treatment: The rigid control of blood glucose levels, which can be attained with continuous subcutaneous insulin infusion, is associated with sustained normalization of levels of both LDL and VLDL.

The lipemia of IDDM responds well to control of the underlying disorder of carbohydrate metabolism. In obese, insulin-resistant individuals, weight loss is the key to treatment. Diets containing a large fraction of calories as carbohydrates are actually well tolerated, allowing a decrease in the burden of chylomicron triglycerides in plasma.

Uremia

Uremia is associated with modest isolated increases in VLDL. The most important underlying mechanisms are probably insulin resistance and impairment of cata-

bolism of VLDL. Many uremic patients are also nephrotic. The additional effects of nephrosis upon lipoprotein metabolism may produce a combined hyperlipoproteinemia. Patients who have had renal transplants may be receiving glucorticoids, which also induce a combined hyperlipidemia.

Corticosteroid Excess

In endogenous Cushing's syndrome, there is insulin resistance, and levels of both LDL and VLDL are increased. It appears that the combined hyperlipidemia is primarily due to increased secretion of VLDL, which is then catabolized to LDL. More severe lipemia ensues when steroidogenic diabetes appears, reducing catabolism of triglyceride-rich lipoproteins via the LPL pathway.

Estrogens

When estrogens are administered to normal premenopausal women, triglyceride levels may increase by as much as 15%. This is believed to reflect increased hepatic production of VLDL, though other mechanisms may be operative. Paradoxically, estrogens increase the efficiency of catabolism of triglyceride-rich lipoproteins. Whereas estrogens tend to induce insulin resistance, it is not clear that this is an important mechanism, because certain nortestosterone derivatives decrease plasma triglyceride levels despite the induction of appreciable insulin resistance.

Certain individuals, usually with preexisting mild lipemia, show marked hypertriglyceridemia when receiving estrogens even in relatively small doses. Thus, the triglyceride level of serum should be measured in any woman receiving exogenous estrogens. Contraceptive combinations with predominant progestational effects produce less hypertriglyceridemia than purely estrogenic compounds.

Alcohol Ingestion

Ingestion of appreciable amounts of alcohol may not necessarily result in significantly elevated levels of triglycerides in serum, but many alcoholics are lipemic. Furthermore, alcohol profoundly increases triglyceride levels in patients with primary and secondary hyperlipemias. In Zieve's syndrome, the lipemia is associated with hemolytic anemia and hyperbilirubinemia. Because LCAT originates in liver, severe hepatic parenchymal dysfunction may lead to deficiency in the activity of this enzyme. A resultant accumulation of unesterified cholesterol in erythrocyte membranes may account for the hemolysis seen in Zieve's syndrome.

Ethanol is converted to acetate, exerting a sparing effect on the oxidation of fatty acids. The fatty acids are incorporated into triglyceride in liver, resulting in hepatomegaly due to fatty infiltration and in marked enhancement of secretion of VLDL. In many individuals, there is sufficient adaptive increase in the removal capacity for triglycerides from plasma that triglyceride levels tend to return toward normal if alcohol intake is continued over a period of weeks. In individuals in whom the adaptive response is impaired, marked lipemia may ensue. Increased levels of HDL in plasma associated with ethanol ingestion may be coupled to the increased secretion of VLDL in some individuals.

Nephrosis

The hyperlipidemia of nephrosis is biphasic. Before serum albumin levels fall below 2 g/dL, levels of LDL increase selectively. This is probably a result of increased secretion of albumin by liver to compensate for that lost in the urine. The synthesis of VLDL in the Golgi apparatus of liver appears to be coupled to that of albumin. The increased flux of VLDL from liver would be expected to increase the production of its daughter particles, LDL; however, altered surface properties of LDL, functional hypothyroidism, and even changes in capillary perfusion may contribute to increased levels of LDL. As albumin levels fall below 1–2 g/dL, lipemia ensues. Impaired hydrolysis of triglycerides by LPL may be due in large part to lack of albumin as an FFA receptor. Free fatty acids, which normally circulate complexed to albumin, bind to lipoproteins when albumin levels are low. The ability of these altered lipoproteins to undergo hydrolysis is thus impaired. Lysolecithin and bile acids that normally bind to albumin also associate with lipoproteins. In nephrosis, VLDL contain abundant cholesteryl esters, probably reflecting an increased rate of synthesis of these lipids.

Because coronary vascular disease is quite prevalent in patients with long-standing nephrotic syndrome, treatment of the hyperlipidemia appears to be indicated, though no studies of the effect of treatment have been reported. The hyperlipidemia is relatively resistant to diet. Clofibrate or gemfibrozil may precipitate myopathy even in relatively small doses. Bile acid–binding resins and niacin appear to be the drugs of choice. Lovastatin may prove useful as well. Nephrotic patients may be deficient in tryptophan, and oral administration of this amino acid has been reported to ameliorate the hypertriglyceridemia.

Glycogen Storage Disease

In type I glycogenosis, insulin secretion is decreased, leading to an increased flux of FFA to liver, where a substantial fraction is converted to triglycerides, leading to increased secretion of VLDL. The low levels of insulin in plasma also are the probable cause of reduced activity of LPL, which may cause impaired removal of triglycerides from serum. The fatty liver in these patients tends to progress to cirrhosis.

Frequent small feedings help to maintain blood glucose levels and ameliorate the lipemia. A program of nocturnal nasogastric drip feeding may be of considerable benefit in this disease. In less tractable cases, portacaval shunting may be of use both in maintaining

blood glucose levels and in reducing the hypertriglyceridemia. Other forms of hepatic glycogen storage disease may be associated with elevated levels of VLDL and LDL in serum.

Hypopituitarism & Acromegaly

Part of the hyperlipidemia of hypopituitarism is attributable to secondary hypothyroidism, but hypertriglyceridemia persists in the face of thyroxine replacement therapy. Dwarfism due to isolated deficiency of growth hormone is associated with higher than normal levels of both LDL and VLDL. Decreased insulin levels may be the major underlying defect; however, deficiency of growth hormone may impair the disposal of FFA by oxidation and ketogenesis in liver, favoring synthesis of triglycerides. Mild hypertriglyceridemia is often associated with acromegaly, probably resulting from insulin resistance. Though growth hormone acutely stimulates lipolysis in adipose tissue, FFA levels are normal in acromegaly.

Hypothyroidism

Whereas significant hypothyroidism tends to produce elevated levels of LDL in serum in nearly all individuals, only a fraction will develop hypertriglyceridemia. The increase in LDL levels results at least in part from decreased numbers of B-100:E receptors on cell membranes, although decreased conversion of cholesterol to bile acids may also contribute. Lipemia, when present, is usually mild, though serum triglyceride levels in excess of 3000 mg/dL (34.5 mmol/L) can occur. The underlying mechanisms are not fully understood, though it is probable that impaired removal of triglycerides from blood is involved, perhaps related to decreased activity of hepatic lipase. Increased content of cholesteryl esters and apo-E in the triglyceride-rich lipoproteins suggests that accumulation of remnant particles occurs. Hypothyroidism, even of very mild degree, causes expression of hyperlipidemia in otherwise latent carriers of familial dysbetalipoproteinemia.

Immunoglobulin-Lipoprotein Complex Disorders

Both polyclonal and monoclonal hypergammaglobulinemias may cause hypertriglyceridemia. IgG, IgM, and IgA have each been involved. Of the underlying monoclonal disorders causing hypertriglyceridemia, myeloma and macroglobulinemia are the most important, but lymphomas and lymphocytic leukemias have also been implicated. Lupus erythematosus and other collagen vascular disorders have been associated with the polyclonal type. Binding of heparin by immunoglobulin, with resulting inhibition of LPL, can cause severe mixed lipemia. More commonly, the triglyceride-rich lipoproteins have an abnormally high density, probably as a result of bound immunoglobulin, though some may be remnantlike particles. These complexes, which bind lipophilic stains, usually have gamma mobility on electrophoresis in agarose gel.

Xanthomatosis associated with immunoglobulin complex disease includes tuberous and eruptive xanthomas, xanthelasma, and planar xanthomas of large areas of skin. The latter are otherwise seen only in patients with cholestasis. Deposits of lipid-rich hyaline material can occur in the lamina propria of the intestine, causing malabsorption and protein-losing enteropathy. Circulating immunoglobulin-lipoprotein complexes can fix complement, leading to hypocomplementemia. In such patients, administration of whole blood or plasma can cause anaphylaxis. Hence, washed red cells or albumin are recommended when blood volume replacement is required.

Treatment is directed at the underlying disorder. Because the critical temperature of cryoprecipitation of some of these complexes is close to body temperature, plasmapheresis should be done at a temperature above the critical temperature measured in the serum of individual patients.

THE HYPERCHOLESTEROLEMIAS

1. PRIMARY HYPERCHOLESTEROLEMIA

Familial Hypercholesterolemia

A. Etiology and Pathogenesis: This disorder, which in its heterozygous form occurs in approximately one in 500 individuals in the USA, is transmitted as a mendelian dominant trait with very high penetrance. Because half of first-degree relatives are affected, including children, all members of a proband's family should be screened for this disorder. Hypercholesterolemia, representing a selective increase in LDL, exists from birth. Levels of LDL tend to increase during childhood and adolescence such that average levels of serum cholesterol in adult heterozygotes are usually greater than 350 mg/dL (9.1 mmol/L). VLDL levels are usually normal, though some individuals, especially those in kindreds in which hypertriglyceridemia is present, may have higher than normal levels of both VLDL and LDL. Aside from an increase in content of cholesteryl esters, the LDL are normal in structure.

The underlying defect appears to be a deficiency of normal high-affinity receptor sites for LDL on cell membranes. A number of genetic defects affecting the structure, translation, modification, or transport of the B-100:E receptor protein have been identified. In some of these defects, the gene product either does not appear on the cell surface or completely lacks receptor function. The gene products associated with other defects appear as kinetically impaired receptors.

Some individuals have combined heterozygosity. In cases in which a kinetic mutant is combined with an ablative mutant, the severity of the hypercholesterolemia is greater than that seen in simple heterozygosity, usually in the range of 500–800 mg/dL (13–20.8 mmol/L). Those patients who are homozygous for genes that produce no effective receptors have extremely severe hypercholesterolemia (approaching 1000 mg/dL [26 mmol/L] or greater) and fulminant arteriosclerosis.

Some patients who are heterozygous for receptor defects may have serum levels of LDL that are only mildly elevated or, even less commonly, in the normal range. Mitigating factors, perhaps involving decreased production rates for VLDL and LDL, may exist in such individuals. Production rates for LDL generally appear to be nearly normal in heterozygotes but are increased in the homozygous state, largely owing to increased conversion of VLDL to LDL. In the heterozygote, a greater fraction of LDL is removed by non–receptor-dependent mechanisms than in normal subjects. In homozygotes, all removal of LDL proceeds through such pathways.

B. Clinical Findings: One of the most striking clinical features that may be present is tendinous xanthomatosis. The xanthomas, which usually appear in early adulthood, cause a broadening or fusiform mass in the tendon. They can occur in almost any tendon but are most readily detected in the Achilles and patellar tendons and in the extensor tendons of the hands (Fig 24–5). Patients who are physically active may complain of achillodynia. Arcus corneae (Fig 24–5B) may occur as early as the third decade. Xanthelasma (Fig 24–5A) may also be present. Both arcus and xanthelasma are seen in individuals who do not have hyperlipidemia, however. Coronary atherosclerosis tends to occur prematurely in heterozygotes, commonly in the fifth decade. Eighty-five percent of the men will have had a myocardial infarction before age 60, compared with 15% of unaffected men. Coronary artery disease is particularly prominent in individuals who are relatively deficient in HDL. It is probable that this represents a coincident inheritance of both traits. The homozygous form of familial hypercholesterolemia is catastrophic. Levels of cholesterol in serum may exceed 1000 mg/dL (26 mmol/L), and xanthomatosis progresses rapidly. Patients may have tuberous xanthomas (Fig 24–5C) and elevated plaque-like xanthomas of the extremities, buttocks, and interdigital webs. Many homozygotes have overt coronary disease in the first decade of life.

A serum cholesterol level in excess of 350 mg/dL (9.1 mmol/L) in the absence of significant hypertriglyceridemia makes the diagnosis of heterozygous familial hypercholesterolemia likely. The presence of affected first-degree relatives is supportive of this diagnosis, especially if no other phenotypes of hyperlipidemia are present in the family that would suggest familial combined disease. The finding of tendon xanthomas is nearly pathognomonic—betasitosterolemia and cerebrotendinous xanthomatosis (cholestanolosis) excepted. Although the cholesterol con-

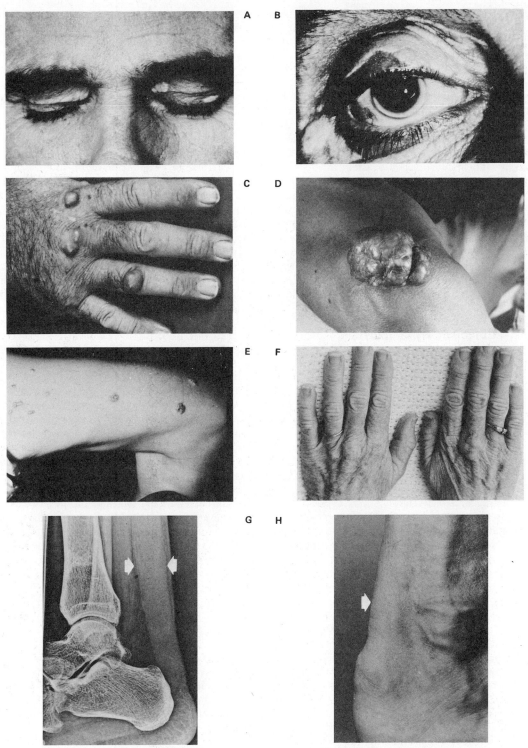

Figure 24–5. Clinical manifestations of hyperlipidemias. A: Xanthelasma involving medial and lateral canthi. B: Severe xanthelasma and arcus corneae. C: Tuberous xanthomas. D: Large tuberous xanthoma of elbow. E: Eruptive xanthomas, singly and in rosettes. F: Xanthomas of extensor tendons of the hands. G: Xeroradiogram of Achilles tendon xanthoma. H: Xanthoma of Achilles tendon (Normal Achilles tendons do not exceed 7 mm in diameter in the region between the calcaneus and the point at which the tendon fibers begin to radiate toward their origins.)

tent of serum from umbilical cord blood is usually elevated in patients with this disorder, the diagnosis is most easily established by measuring serum cholesterol levels after the first year of life.

C. Treatment: Treatment with various single drug regimens is of moderate benefit in decreasing LDL levels in serum. However, complete normalization of LDL levels can be achieved in most compliant heterozygotes with a combination of a bile acid–binding resin and niacin, when they are eating a diet low in saturated fat and cholesterol. Comparable results are achieved with combinations of lovastatin and resin or niacin. Serum cholesterol levels less than 200 mg/dL are often seen with a ternary combination of these drugs. Treatment of homozygotes is extremely difficult. Partial control may be achieved with portacaval shunt or repeated plasmapheresis in conjunction with combined drug regimens. Immunophoresis is of considerable value. Striking reduction of LDL levels is observed after live transplantation, illustrating the important role of hepatic receptors in LDL clearance. (See Treatment of Hyperlipidemia, below.)

Familial Combined Hyperlipidemia (Multiple Type)

In some individuals in kindreds in which this disorder is present (see Primary Hypertriglyceridemia, above), LDL will be the only lipoprotein that is elevated. This pattern may vary in an individual over time, and elevated VLDL alone or combined elevations of LDL and VLDL may be observed in the patient or the patient's relatives. Some affected children express hyperlipidemia. In contrast to most cases of familial hypercholesterolemia, the serum cholesterol level may often be lower than 350 mg/dL, and neither tendinous nor tuberous xanthomas occur. Studies of kindreds suggest a mendelian dominant mechanism of transmission. Coronary atherosclerosis is accelerated in this disorder, which is sufficiently prevalent to be observed in about 10% of survivors of myocardial infarction. The underlying biochemical mechanism appears to involve increased synthesis of apo-B-100.

Treatment of the hypercholesterolemia should begin with diet and niacin. It may be necessary to add resin or lovastatin to normalize levels of LDL.

Lp(a) Hyperlipoproteinemia

A lipoprotein that normally comprises a very minor fraction of circulating lipoproteins, Lp(a), is present in high concentrations in some individuals whose levels of LDL may also be elevated or nearly normal. Upon ultracentrifugation, this lipoprotein ranges on both sides of the density that discriminates LDL from HDL. It contains apo-B-100 and the Lp(a) protein. It is identified in LDL or HDL fractions obtained by ultracentrifugation by its prebeta-electrophoretic mobility. A number of studies implicate it as an independent risk factor for coronary artery disease. Preliminary results

indicate that niacin is the most effective drug used in treatment.

Poorly Defined Types of Hypercholesterolemia

Kindreds have been found in which there are several individuals with higher than normal levels of LDL who respond dramatically to diets low in cholesterol and saturated fats. There are also kindreds in which multiple genetic factors that lead to higher levels of LDL appear to aggregate in individuals (polygenic hypercholesterolemia). The incidence of hyperlipidemia is smaller in the latter kindreds than in those with monogenic disorders, and the LDL increase is not great. There is also a group of recessive types of hypercholesterolemia that show marked responsiveness to dietary restriction of saturated fat and cholesterol. Tuberous or raised planar xanthomas may be present, and in some individuals serum cholesterol levels may reach 600 mg/dL (15.6 mmol/L). Some of these individuals, particularly those with tuberous xanthomas, have primarily phytosterolemia.

2. SECONDARY HYPERCHOLESTEROLEMIA

Hypothyroidism

The typical disorder of lipoproteins associated with hypothyroidism is high LDL and IDL concentrations. Increased content of apo-E in the VLDL and IDL is consistent with an increase in remnant particles in plasma. In addition to elevated LDL, some patients may have lipemia as described in the section on secondary hyperlipemia. The hyperlipidemia of hypothyroidism may occur in individuals with no overt signs or symptoms of decreased thyroid function. Biliary excretion of cholesterol and bile acids is depressed; however, cholesterol biosynthesis is also decreased. Absorption of cholesterol from the intestine is unchanged. Cholesterol stores in tissues appear to be increased, although the number of B-100:E receptors on cells appears to be decreased. Activity of hepatic lipase is also markedly decreased. Atherogenesis is accelerated by myxedema. The hyperlipidemia responds dramatically to treatment with thyroxine.

Nephrosis

As described in the section on secondary hypertriglyceridemias, nephrosis produces a biphasic hyperlipoproteinemia. The earliest alteration of lipoproteins in nephrosis is elevated LDL. The underlying mechanisms are not clearly identified, but increased secretion of VLDL by liver is probably involved. Because the lipids of the lipoprotein surfaces are altered by enrichment with sphingomyelin, lysolecithin, and FFA, the catabolism of LDL could be impaired. Perhaps the low metabolic rate in affected patients introduces metabolic changes similar to those associated with hypothyroidism. The hyperlipidemia may be an important element in the markedly increased risk of atherosclerotic heart disease in these patients. The treatment of choice appears to be bile acid–binding resins with niacin. Lovastatin may also be useful.

Immunoglobulin Disorders

One of the lipoprotein abnormalities that can be associated with monoclonal gammopathy is elevated LDL. A "gamma lipoprotein" that is a stable complex of immunoglobulin and lipoprotein may be observed in agarose gel electrophoretograms of the sera of some patients. Cryoprecipitation, often in the temperature range encountered in peripheral tissues when the environmental temperature is low, may occur. Patients may have symptoms from the vascular effect of complement fixation resulting from complex formation and may have hyperviscosity syndrome from the elevated immunoglobulins per se.

Treatment is directed at the underlying process. Plasmapheresis is often effective. If cryoprecipitation occurs at critical temperatures near or above room temperature, the procedure must be carried out in a special warm environment. Transfusion of whole blood or serum may be dangerous in these patients because of rapid production of anaphylatoxins from complement in the serum, resulting from interaction with circulating antibody-antigen complexes. This risk can be minimized by the use of packed red blood cells and albumin in place of whole blood.

Anorexia Nervosa

About 40% of patients with anorexia nervosa have elevated LDL in serum, and levels of cholesterol in serum may reach 400–600 mg/dL (104.–15.6 mmol/L). The hyperlipidemia, which persists despite correction of hypothyroidism, is probably a result of decreased fecal excretion of bile acids and cholesterol.

Serum lipoproteins return to normal when proper nutrition is restored.

Cholestasis

The hyperlipidemia associated with the obstruction of biliary flow is complex. It occurs either with extrahepatic or intrahepatic obstruction, though it tends to be more severe with the former. Levels of cholesterol in serum exceeding 400 mg/dL (10.4 mmol/L) usually are associated with extrahepatic obstruction or with intrahepatic tumor. At least 3 types of abnormal lipoproteins are present in plasma. The most abundant, termed LP-X, is a bilayer vesicle composed of unesterified cholesterol and lecithin, with associated apolipoproteins but not apo-B. LP-X is apparent on electrophoresis of lipoproteins in agarose gel as a band of zero to gamma mobility which shows metachromatic staining with Sudan black. It is these vesicular particles that cause the serum phospholipid and unesterified cholesterol content to be extremely high. There is another abnormal

species called LP-Y, which contains appreciable amounts of triglycerides and carries apo-B. It may represent a remnant particle derived from chylomicrons. The LDL in cholestasis also contain an unusually large amount of triglycerides.

Patients with cholestasis may have planar xanthomas of the skin, especially at sites of minor trauma, and xanthomas of the palmar creases. Occasionally, eruptive xanthomas are present. Xanthomatous involvement of nerves may lead to symptoms of peripheral neuropathy, and the abnormal lipoproteins may be atherogenic. Whereas bilirubin levels are nearly normal in some patients with chronic cholestasis, all have elevated serum alkaline phosphatase activity.

Neuropathy is the chief indication for treatment of the hyperlipidemia. Bile acid–binding resins are of some value, whereas clofibrate causes an increase in serum cholesterol levels. Plasmapheresis is the most effective treatment.

THE HYPOLIPIDEMIAS

Although the clinician is confronted infrequently by the problem of a striking deficiency in plasma lipids, it is important to recognize the primary and secondary hypolipidemias. A serum cholesterol level less than 110 mg/dL (2.9 mmol/L) in an adult patient is noteworthy. Since levels of triglycerides in normal fasting serum may be as low as 25 mg/dL (0.29 mmol/L), significance is limited to cases in which they are virtually absent.

1. PRIMARY HYPOLIPIDEMIA

DEFICIENCY OF HIGH-DENSITY LIPOPROTEINS

Tangier Disease

A. Etiology and Pathogenesis: Severe deficiency of HDL occurs in the primary disorder known as Tangier disease. Heterozygotes lack clinical signs but have about one-half or less of the normal complement of HDL and apo-A-I in plasma. Homozygotes lack normal plasma HDL, and apo-A-I and apo-A-II are present at extremely low levels. Serum cholesterol levels are usually below 120 mg/dL (3.12 mmol/L) and may be half that value. Mild hypertriglyceridemia is usually present. The genetic defect probably involves alteration of catabolism of HDL.

Several biochemical defects in the metabolism of triglyceride-rich lipoproteins are probably the result of the deficiency of HDL. The chylomicrons and VLDL are deficient in C proteins, which may account for the mild hypertriglyceridemia. Abnormal oblate (oval) lipoproteins in the HDL density interval that contain cholesteryl esters may be remnant particles derived from chylomicrons. The LDL are greatly enriched in triglycerides at the expense of cholesteryl esters.

B. Clinical Findings: The clinical features of this rare autosomal recessive disease include large, orange-colored, lipid-filled tonsils, accumulation of cholesteryl esters in the reticuloendothelial system, and an episodic and recurrent peripheral neuropathy with predominant motor weakness in the later stages. The course of the disease is benign in early childhood, but the neuropathy may appear as early as age 8. Cholesteryl ester accumulates most prominently in peripheral nerve sheaths. Carotenoid coloration may be apparent in pharyngeal and rectal mucous membranes. Splenomegaly and corneal infiltration may also be present.

C. Treatment: Because much of the lamellar lipoprotein material in plasma is believed to originate in chylomicrons, restriction of dietary fats and cholesterol is suggested.

Familial Hypoalphalipoproteinemia

A. Etiology and Pathogenesis: This phenotypic pattern is a partial deficiency of HDL in serum that may involve heterogeneous mechanisms. These presumed constitutional disorders must be differentiated from the condition in which moderately low levels of HDL cholesterol are seen in individuals consuming a diet very low in fat, perhaps reflecting decreased generation of HDL from chylomicrons. For example, white and Asian men on such diets usually have HDL cholesterol levels of 38–44 mg/dL (1–1.1 mmol/L) by ultracentrifugal analysis, in contrast with a median value of 49 mg/dL (1.3 mmol/L) when consuming a typical North American diet. Such levels are commonplace, for example, in Asiatic populations and among vegetarians, where risk of coronary disease is small. The physician must further interpret HDL cholesterol levels in the light of the amount of triglyceride-rich lipoproteins in plasma. Because triglyceride is progressively substituted for cholesteryl esters in the core of HDL as the plasma triglyceride level rises, the HDL cholesterol will decrease as an inverse logarithmic function of the triglyceride level. This decrease causes an apparent decrease in HDL levels, since cholesterol is the component of HDL that is commonly measured. In severe forms of hypertriglyceridemia, there is an additional absolute decrease in levels of the HDL vehicle in the serum of many individuals.

B. Etiologic Factor in Coronary Disease: Clinical experience suggests that familial hypoalphalipoproteinemia is fairly common and is an important risk factor in coronary vascular disease. This abnormality may be the only apparent risk factor in many cases of premature coronary atherosclerosis. Furthermore, it may accelerate the appearance of coronary disease in patients with familial hypercholesterol-

emia or other hyperlipidemias. Hypoalphalipoproteinemia shows a strong familial incidence. Although several mechanisms and modes of transmission may be involved, many kindreds show distributions consistent with mendelian dominance.

C. Treatment: To date, there has been no demonstration that increasing total HDL levels will decrease the risk of progression of arteriosclerotic disease. Furthermore, only limited means of raising HDL levels are at hand. Recent findings that HDL exist in as many as 8 discrete species further complicate this problem. It is not yet known which of these species may be involved in protecting against arteriosclerosis or whether levels of those species can be increased. Thus, though alcohol ingestion can increase total HDL levels in some individuals, it appears that the effect is primarily on the HDL_3 ultracentrifugal fraction, which correlates poorly with decreased risk in epidemiologic studies. Therefore, no recommendation for increased alcohol consumption should be made on this account. Heavy exercise is associated with increases in HDL in some individuals, but exercise must be approached with caution in patients who may have coronary disease. Niacin increases total HDL levels in many subjects, chiefly in the HDL_2 ultracentrifugal fraction. Its effects on individual subspecies of HDL remain to be determined.

Perhaps the most important reason at present for measuring HDL cholesterol levels is to identify patients who are at increased risk. Thus, just as with patients who have premature vascular disease or a family history of early arteriosclerosis, patients with low HDL levels should be treated more aggressively for elevated levels of lipoproteins that appear to be atherogenic (LDL, IDL, and VLDL). Furthermore, vigorous efforts should be directed at the control of other risk factors, such as hypertension and smoking. Because the latter is known to decrease HDL cholesterol levels significantly, smoking should be strongly interdicted. Modest lowering of HDL cholesterol levels by beta-adrenergic blocking agents must be weighed against the need for their cardiovascular effects in individual cases.

Deficiency of LCAT

Another disorder associated with low serum levels of HDL is LCAT deficiency. This rare autosomal recessive disorder is not expressed in clinical or biochemical form in the heterozygote. In the homozygote, clinical characteristics are variable. The diagnosis is usually made in adult life, although corneal opacities may begin in childhood. Proteinuria may be an early sign. Deposits of unesterified cholesterol and phospholipid in the renal microvasculature, leading to progressive loss of nephrons and ultimate renal failure, have been a frequent cause of death. Many patients have mild to moderate normochromic anemia with target cells. Hyperbilirubinemia or peripheral neuropathy may be present. Red blood cell lipid composition is abnormal, with increased content of unesterified cholesterol and lecithin. Most have elevated plasma triglycerides (200–1000 mg/dL [2.3–11.5 mmol/L]), and levels of serum cholesterol vary from low normal to 500 mg/dL (13 mmol/L), only a small fraction of which is esterified. The large triglyceride-rich lipoproteins, presumably derived from VLDL and chylomicrons, are unusually rich in unesterified cholesterol and appear to have abnormal surface monolayers. The LDL are rich in triglycerides, and abnormal vesicular lipoproteins are present in the LDL density interval. Two abnormal HDL species are present: bilayer disks and small spherical particles. Marked restriction of dietary fat and cholesterol results in a decrease of VLDL-like particles and lamellar LDL in plasma and is the recommended treatment.

DEFICIENCY OF APO-B-CONTAINING LIPOPROTEINS

Recessive Abetalipoproteinemia & Familial Hypobetalipoproteinemia

A. Etiology and Pathogenesis: Recessive abetalipoproteinemia and familial hypobetalipoproteinemia probably represent a number of mutations involving the apo-B structural gene, the processing of apo-B, or the secretion of apo-B-containing lipoproteins. Familial hypobetalipoproteinemia is inherited as an autosomal dominant. Affected heterozygotes are usually asymptomatic but have moderately low levels of total plasma cholesterol (55–146 mg/dL [1.4–3.8 mmol/L]), LDL cholesterol levels about 50% of normal (50–90 mg/dL [1.3–2.3 mmol/L]), and normal HDL cholesterol levels. Individuals homozygous for this disorder share features in common with those who have recessive abetalipoproteinemia. In serum of patients homozygous for either disorder, all forms of apo-B are absent. No chylomicrons, VLDL, or LDL are found in plasma, leaving only HDL. Plasma triglyceride levels are usually less than 10 mg/dL (0.12 mmol/L) and fail to rise after a fat load. The plasma cholesterol, essentially all of which is found in HDL, is usually less than 90 mg/dL (2.3 mmol/L). There is a defect in the incorporation of newly synthesized triglycerides into chylomicron particles. However, at low levels of fat intake, about 80% of the ingested triglycerides are absorbed, probably by direct absorption of fatty acids via the portal vein.

B. Clinical Findings: Clinical features include a paucity of adipose tissue, associated with malabsorption of long-chain fatty acids due to failure of the intestine to secrete chylomicrons; red blood cells that may be acanthocytic, with a high cholesterol:phospholipid ratio; progressive degeneration of the central nervous system, including cerebellar degeneration and posterior and lateral spinal tract disease; retinal degeneration that may be severe; and, usually, very low levels of fat-soluble vitamins in plasma. The neurologic defects

may be related to deficiency of vitamin E (normally transported largely in LDL). Patients are apparently normal at birth and develop steatorrhea with impaired growth in infancy. The neuromuscular disorder often appears in late childhood with ataxia, night blindness, decreased visual acuity, and nystagmus. Cardiomyopathy with arrhythmias has been reported and may be a cause of death.

C. Treatment: Treatment includes administration of fat-soluble vitamins. Very large doses of tocopherols (1000–5000 IU/d) appear to limit the progressive central nervous system degeneration. Although vitamin A seems to correct the night blindness, it does not alter the course of the retinitis pigmentosa. Vitamins D and K may also be indicated. Restriction of dietary fat minimizes steatorrhea.

Normotriglyceridemic Abetalipoproteinemia

Normotriglyceridemic abetalipoproteinemia is a group of disorders in which LDL are absent from plasma but fat absorption appears to proceed normally. The underlying defects are mutations that cause truncation of the apo-B-100 protein with sparing of all or most of the B-48 region. Chylomicron secretion is relatively normal. In some cases, VLDL with truncated apo-B-100 appear to be secreted from liver but cannot be converted to LDL. Clinical features may include ataxia, minimal stomatocytosis of erythrocytes, and profound deficiency of tocopherols. Tocopherol levels in plasma can be significantly increased by supplementation with this vitamin.

Chylomicron Retention Disease

This disorder, which presents in the neonate, appears to be based upon the inability of intestinal epithelial cells to secrete chylomicrons. Affected individuals have severe malabsorption of triglycerides with steatorrhea. Levels of LDL and VLDL are about one-half of normal, presumably secondary to malnutrition. Tocopheral levels may be very low and may be associated with neurologic abnormalities. Clinical symptoms diminish somewhat with time if the patient is managed with a low-fat diet and tocopheral supplementation.

2. SECONDARY HYPOLIPIDEMIA

Hypolipidemia may be secondary to a number of diseases characterized by chronic cachexia, eg, advanced cancer. Myeloproliferative disorders can lead to extremely low levels of LDL, probably owing to increased uptake related to rapid proliferation and membrane synthesis. A wide variety of conditions leading to intestinal malabsorption produce hypolipidemia. In these situations, levels of chylomicrons, VLDL, and LDL in serum are low but never absent. Because most of the lipoprotein mass of fasting serum is of hepatic origin, massive parenchymal liver failure can cause severe hypolipidemia. In Reye's syndrome, there appears to be a contravention of the normal production of VLDL by liver, leading to near absence of both VLDL and LDL from serum.

The hypolipidemias associated with immunoglobulin disorders result from diverse mechanisms. Affected patients usually have myeloma or macroglobulinemia but may have lymphomas or lymphocytic leukemia. Any of the major classes of immunoglobulins may be involved. In many cases, the immunoglobulins are cryoprecipitins; thus, the diagnosis may be missed if blood is not drawn and serum prepared at 37 °C and observed for cryoprecipitation. Complexes between immunoglobulins and lipoproteins may circulate in plasma and fix complement, leading to hypocomplementemia and the risk of anaphylaxis on transfusion with whole blood or plasma. The complexes may precipitate in various tissues. When this occurs in the lamina propria of the intestine, a syndrome of malabsorption and protein-losing enteropathy may result. Monoclonal IgA in myeloma may precipitate with lipoproteins, causing xanthomas of the gingiva and cervix. Lesions in the skin are usually planar and xanthomatous and may involve intracutaneous hemorrhage, producing a classic purple xanthoma. Planar xanthomas occurring in cholestasis may be confused with this condition, because the abnormal lipoprotein of cholestasis (LP-X), like the circulating lipoprotein complex of immunoglobulin and lipoprotein, has gamma mobility on electrophoresis.

OTHER DISORDERS OF LIPOPROTEIN METABOLISM

THE LIPODYSTROPHIES

Classification

Current classification of the lipodystrophies is based on their familial or acquired origin and the regional or generalized nature of the fat loss. Among the associated metabolic abnormalities, insulin resistance is the common finding. Two of these disorders are known to be inherited.

Familial generalized lipodystrophy (Seip-Berardinelli syndrome), a rare recessive trait, may be diagnosed at birth and is associated with macrosomia. Genital hypertrophy, hypertrichosis, acanthosis nigricans, hepatomegaly, insulin resistance, hypertriglyceridemia, and glucose intolerance are regularly observed.

Familial lipodystrophy of limbs and trunk (Köberling-Dunningan syndrome) appears to be transmitted as a dominant gene, affects women predominantly, and is not evident until puberty. The face, neck, and upper trunk are usually spared. Growth is normal, but otherwise this syndrome shares features of the generalized form noted above. It is frequently associated with Stein-Leventhal syndrome.

Acquired forms of lipodystrophy, generalized (Lawrence syndrome) and partial (Barraquer-Simmons' syndrome), usually begin in childhood, affect females predominantly, and often follow an acute febrile illness. The generalized type commonly shares the features described above, invariably involving the trunk and extremities but sometimes sparing the face. A sclerosing panniculitis, as seen in Weber-Christian syndrome, may appear at the outset. The partial type usually begins in the face and then involves the neck, upper limbs, and trunk. In this disorder, reduced levels of C3 complement are frequently encountered. Most patients have proteinuria, and some develop overt vascular nephritis.

Associated Disorders

Because a number of patients with disorders resembling both familial and acquired types of lipodystrophy have tumors or other lesions of the hypothalamus, appropriate neurologic evaluation should be obtained. Similarly, the physician should be alert to the association of collagen vascular disorders, including scleroderma and dermatomyositis, with some cases of acquired lipodystrophy.

RARE DISORDERS

Werner's Syndrome, Progeria, Infantile Hypercalcemia, & Sphingolipidoses

These disorders may be associated with hypercholesterolemia, but levels of triglycerides are usually normal. Some patients with Niemann-Pick disease have hypercholesterolemia, but most have hypertriglyceridemia, as do many patients with Gaucher's disease.

Wolman's Disease & Cholesteryl Ester Storage Disease

These recessive lipid storage disorders involve the absence and partial deficiency, respectively, of lysosomal acid lipase, resulting in abnormal cholesteryl ester and triglyceride stores in liver, spleen, adrenal glands, small intestine, and bone marrow. Most patients have elevated levels of both LDL and VLDL in plasma. Wolman's disease is fatal in infancy.

Cerebrotendinous Xanthomatosis

In this recessive disorder, impaired synthesis of bile acids results in increased production of cholesterol and cholestanol, which accumulate in body tissues. Plasma levels of cholesterol and cholestanol are normal or elevated. Cataracts, tendon xanthomas, progressive neurologic dysfunction, and premature coronary atherosclerosis are hallmarks of this disease. Its central nervous system effects include dementia, spasticity, and ataxia. Death usually ensues before age 50 from neurologic degeneration or coronary disease. Treatment with chenodeoxycholic acid appears useful. Resins must be avoided because they aggravate the underlying defect.

Phytosterolemia

This disorder is distinguished by normal or elevated plasma cholesterol levels; high concentrations of plant sterol in serum, adipose tissue, and skin; and prominent xanthomas of both the tendinous and tuberous types. Individuals with this disorder absorb a substantially larger fraction of phytosterols and cholesterol from the intestine than do normal individuals. A more severe form apparently exists in which serum cholesterol levels may be as high as 700 mg/dL (18.2 mmol/L), reflecting an increase in LDL that contain sitosterol esters in addition to cholesteryl esters. Premature coronary arteriosclerosis may be present. Treatment consists of a diet restricted in plant sterols and cholesterol and the use of bile acid-binding resins.

TREATMENT OF HYPERLIPIDEMIA

The first therapeutic measure in all forms of hyperlipidemia is institution of an appropriate diet. In most forms of hyperlipidemia, a single "universal" diet is indicated. In many subjects with lipemia or with hypercholesterolemia of mild to moderate severity, compliance with this diet will be sufficient to control lipoprotein levels. However, many patients with severe hypercholesterolemia or lipemia will require drug therapy. In all of these individuals, the prescribed diet must be continued to achieve the full potential of the medications.

Caution Regarding Drug Therapy

There are insufficient data to evaluate the effects on the fetus of drugs used in treatment of hyperlipoproteinemia. Therefore, women of childbearing age should be advised of the potential risk and should be given these agents only if pregnancy is being actively avoided. If contraceptives are prescribed, estrogens should not be used in patients with hypertriglyceridemia.

In children, hyperlipidemias other than familial hypercholesterolemia rarely require medication. Factors such as the severity and age at onset of symptomatic coronary disease in the child's family and psychologic considerations should be evaluated in deciding when drug treatment should be started. A resin is the drug of choice. Dietary treatment is indicated for all children

with hyperlipidemia and should be started after the first year. The exception is primary chylomicronemia, in which an appropriate diet should be instituted as soon as the disease is detected.

DIETARY FACTORS IN THE MANAGEMENT OF LIPOPROTEIN DISORDERS

Restriction of Caloric Intake

The secretion of VLDL by liver is greatly stimulated by caloric intake in excess of requirements for physical activity and basal metabolism. Therefore, the total caloric content of the diet is of greater importance than its specific composition in treating endogenous hyperlipemia. There is a positive correlation between serum levels of VLDL triglyceride and various measures of obesity, but many obese patients have normal serum lipids. On the other hand, most patients with hypertriglyceridemia are obese. This association is more consistently observed in persons whose weight gain occurred in later childhood or adulthood and who have adipocyte hypertrophy with relative insulin resistance. As obese patients lose weight, plasma VLDL stabilizes at lower levels. In theory, reduction of output of VLDL by the liver should reduce the production rate of its daughter particle, LDL. In fact, there is a modest correlation of LDL levels with body weight in the general population.

Restriction of Fat Intake

In primary chylomicronemia, saturated and polyunsaturated fats both must be restricted rigidly, because the underlying defect is in lipolysis. Similarly, in the acute management of mixed lipemia with impending pancreatitis, elimination of dietary fat leads to a rapid decrease in chylomicron-borne triglycerides in plasma.

The cholesterol-lowering effect of a significant reduction in total fat content of the diet is well known. It has also been shown that a 10–15% fall in serum cholesterol levels is achieved when individuals who have been consuming a typical North American diet restrict their intake of saturated fats to 8% of total calories. The mechanism for these effects remains unclear, but increased bile acid and perhaps also neutral sterol excretion are known to occur at least transiently until a new steady state with lower levels of LDL and VLDL is established. This is accompanied by a decrease in the flux of the apolipoprotein of LDL, suggesting that production of the precursor lipoprotein, VLDL, is decreased. Substitution of polyunsaturated fats for saturates also reduces LDL cholesterol levels. The safety of diets containing large amounts of polyunsaturates has not been established, however. Diets very rich in these fatty acids may lower HDL levels and might lead to increased generation of free radicals as a result of hydroperoxidation. In obese subjects, increased intake of polyunsaturates may induce lithogenicity of bile.

Monounsaturates tend to have a neutral effect on LDL levels.

Recently, it has become apparent that the omega-3 fatty acids found in fish oils have special properties relevant to the treatment of hypertriglyceridemia. Substantial decreases in triglyceride levels can be induced in some patients with severe endogenous or mixed lipemia at doses of 10–15 g/d. Certain members of this class of fatty acids, such as eicosapentaenoic acid, are potent inhibitors of platelet reactivity.

Reduction of Cholesterol Intake

The amount of cholesterol in the diet affects serum cholesterol levels, but individual responses vary. Restriction of dietary cholesterol to less than 200 mg/d (5.2 mmol/L) in normal individuals usually results in a decrease of 10–15% in serum cholesterol. This apparently in part reflects the fact that increased cholesterol intake in humans is not completely balanced by reduced cholesterogenesis in the liver. The ingestion of cholesterol is generally reflected in increased LDL content of serum. Some individuals whose serum levels increase very little with increased dietary intake may have greatly increased tissue stores of cholesterol. Dietary cholesterol and saturated fat content have independent effects on levels of serum cholesterol.

Role of Carbohydrate in Diet

The role of dietary carbohydrate in lipid metabolism is still being investigated, but certain effects seem to have been uniformly observed. There is great individual variation in these responses. When a high-carbohydrate diet is fed, hypertriglyceridemia develops within 48–72 hours, and levels of triglyceride in serum rise to a maximum in 1–5 weeks. Persons with higher basal triglyceride levels and those consuming hypercaloric diets show the greatest effect. After 1–8 months on a high-carbohydrate diet, triglycerides fall to basal levels. An occasional subject shows sustained hypertriglyceridemia. Similar induction of lipemia by carbohydrate is seen in patients with endogenous and mixed lipemia. There is apparently no type of hyperlipemia that is particularly "carbohydrate-sensitive." It must be emphasized, however, that both of these patterns of lipemia are extremely sensitive to excess total caloric intake. Levels of HDL in serum are lower on a high-carbohydrate intake, but the differences are small.

Alcohol Ingestion

Ingestion of alcohol is a common cause of secondary hypertriglyceridemia, owing to overproduction of VLDL. Some individuals with familial hypertriglyceridemia are particularly sensitive to the effects of alcohol, and abstinence may normalize their triglyceride levels. Chronic alcohol intake may also be associated with hypercholesterolemia. Increased cholesterol synthesis and decreased conversion to bile acids have been observed. Alcohol ingestion may account for alimentary lipemia persisting beyond 12–14 hours. This possibility should be excluded by the history or a repeat lipid analysis. A positive correlation has been found between alcohol intake and HDL cholesterol levels; however, increased HDL levels are not observed in all individuals. Because alcohol-induced changes in HDL appear primarily to involve the HDL_3 subfraction, there does not seem to be an indication for the use of alcohol to increase the "protective effect" of HDL against arteriosclerosis.

Fiber in Diet

Although much attention has been devoted to the possible role of fiber in the development of coronary heart disease, there is little evidence that plasma lipids can be significantly affected by intake of most forms of fiber. A modest reduction in LDL cholesterol is associated with the addition of oat bran to the diet, however.

Other Dietary Substances

Several other nutrients have been studied in relation to atherosclerotic heart disease, including calcium, magnesium, trace elements, vitamins D, E, and C, and pyridoxine. The results of these studies are generally equivocal, and the observed effects on serum lipid levels are small. Caffeine and sucrose have negligible effects on serum lipids, and their statistical relationship to coronary heart disease is generally unimpressive when data are corrected for cigarette smoking. Ingestion of large amounts of zinc appears to be associated with decreased levels of HDL.

The "Universal Diet"

Dietary treatment is an important aspect of the management of all forms of lipoprotein disorders and may in some cases be all that is required. Knowledge of the dietary factors reviewed above allows the physician to select appropriate modifications for an individual patient. However, a basic diet is useful in the treatment of most patients. The elements of this diet are as follows:

(1) Ideal body weight should be achieved and maintained.

(2) Fat should provide less than 30% of total calories. Saturated fat should be less than 7% of total calories.

(3) Cholesterol should be reduced to less than 200 mg/d.

(4) Caloric difference should be made up with complex carbohydrate.

(5) Alcohol should be avoided in any patient with hypertriglyceridemia.

This diet is consistent with the Step-Two Diet recommended by the National Cholesterol Education Program Expert Panel.

Caloric restriction and reduction of adipose tissue mass are particularly important for patients with increased levels of VLDL and IDL. Levels of VLDL and LDL tend to be lower during periods of substantial weight loss than can be maintained under isocaloric conditions, even at ideal body weight.

Sources of Dietetic Information

Referral to a local American Heart Association chapter or other source of dietetic consultation is often helpful in ensuring compliance. Several recipe books have been published, and food manufacturers are developing products that add variety and palatability to the restricted diet. Since the prudent diet, as proposed by the American Heart Association and others, is generally recommended, it is helpful to urge the entire family of a hyperlipidemic patient to eat a modified diet, providing greater ease of preparation and an added measure of psychologic support.

DRUGS USED IN TREATMENT OF HYPERLIPOPROTEINEMIA (Table 24–3)

BILE ACID SEQUESTRANTS

Mechanism of Action

Cholestyramine and colestipol are cationic resins that bind bile acids in the intestinal lumen (Fig 24–6). The resin particles are not absorbed by the bowel and

therefore increase the excretion of bile acids in the stool. Normally, 98% of the bile acid secreted in bile is reabsorbed. However, excretion of bile acids can be increased up to 10-fold when bile acid–binding resins are given. There is a large attendant increase in the synthesis of cholesterol by the liver, but the pool of cholesterol in circulating LDL is also tapped for bile acid synthesis by increased expression of high-affinity receptors on cell membranes of the liver. These agents are useful only in disorders involving elevated LDL levels. In fact, patients who have increased levels of VLDL may have further increases in serum triglyceride levels during treatment with resins. Thus, in combined hyperlipidemia, where the resins may be given because of high LDL levels, a second agent such as nicotinic acid may be required to control the hypertriglyceridemia. Levels of LDL will fall 15–30% in compliant patients with heterozygous familial hypercholesterolemia who are receiving maximal doses of the resins. Larger decrements of LDL cholesterol may be seen in patients with other, less severe forms of hypercholesterolemia and in some, levels of LDL will be normalized completely.

Drug Dosage

In disorders involving moderately high levels of LDL, 20 g of cholestyramine (Questran) or colestipol

Table 24–3. The primary hyperlipoproteinemias and their drug treatment.[1]

	Single Drug[2]	Drug Combination
Primary chylomicronemia (familial lipoprotein lipase or cofactor deficiency) Chylomicrons, VLDL increased	Dietary management	
Familial hypertriglyceridemia Severe Chylomicrons, VLDL increased	Niacin, gemfibrozil, clofibrate	Niacin plus gemfibrozil or clofibrate.
Moderate VLDL ± chylomicrons increased	Gemfibrozil, clofibrate, niacin	
Familial combined hyperlipoproteinemia (multiple type hyperlipoproteinemia) VLDL increased	Niacin, gemfibrozil, clofibrate	
LDL increased	Resin, niacin, lovastatin	Niacin plus resin or lovastatin.
VLDL, LDL increased	Niacin	Niacin plus resin or lovastatin; clofibrate plus resin.
Familial dysbetalipoproteinemia VLDL remnants, chylomicron remnants increased	Clofibrate, gemfibrozil, niacin	
Familial hypercholesterolemia Heterozygous LDL increased	Resin, lovastatin, niacin	Two or 3 of the single drugs.
Homozygous LDL increased	Probucol, niacin	Resin plus niacin plus lovastatin; probucol plus agents above.
Lp(a) hyperlipoproteinemia Lp(a) increased	Niacin	Niacin plus lovastatin.
Unclassified hypercholesterolemia	Resin, niacin, lovastatin, clofibrate, gemfibrozil	

[1] Reproduced, with permission, from Katzung BG (editor): *Basic & Clinical Pharmacology*, 4th ed. Appleton & Lange, 1989.
[2] Single-drug therapy should be evaluated before drug combinations are used.

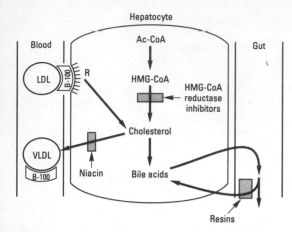

Figure 24–6. Sites of action of HMG-CoA reductase inhibitors, niacin and resins used in treating hyperlipidemias. LDL receptors (R) are increased by treatment with resins and HMG-CoA reductase inhibitors. Reproduced, with permission, from Katzung BG (editor): *Basic & Clinical Pharmacology,* 4th ed. Appleton & Lange, 1989.

(Colestid) daily may lower cholesterol levels effectively. Treatment should commence at one-half of the above dose to minimize gastrointestinal side effects. Maximum doses of 30 g of colestipol or 32 g of cholestyramine daily are required in more severe cases. In familial hypercholesterolemia and combined hyperlipidemia, the resins may be used in combination with niacin (see below).

Side Effects

Because the resins are confined to the lumen of the intestine, few systemic side effects are observed. Patients frequently complain of a bloated sensation and constipation, both of which may be relieved by adding concentrated sources of bran to the diet. Malabsorption of fat or fat-soluble vitamins with a daily dose of resin of up to 30 g occurs only in individuals with preexisting bowel disease or with cholestasis. Hypoprothrombinemia has been observed in patients with malabsorption due to these causes. The resins bind thyroxine, digitalis glycosides, and warfarin and impair the absorption of iron, thiazides, beta-blockers, and other drugs. Absorption of all of these substances is ensured if they are administered 1 hour before the resin. During long-term treatment with the resins, some patients may complain of dry, flaking skin, perhaps reflecting some effect on cutaneous sterols. This minor symptom responds to local application of lanolin. Because they change the composition of bile micelles, bile acid sequestrants theoretically may increase the risk of cholelithiasis, particularly in obese subjects. In practice, this risk appears to be very small. Mild, usually transient, elevations in transaminase and alkaline phosphatase have been reported.

NIACIN
(Nicotinic Acid)

Mechanism of Action

Niacin (but not its amide) is able to effect major reductions in LDL and triglyceride-rich lipoproteins (Fig 24–6). It has been postulated that this is due to decreased flux to liver of free fatty acids, which are normally an important substrate for VLDL production. Niacin is a potent inhibitor of the mobilization of free fatty acids from adipose tissue, at least in the short term; its ability to inhibit intracellular lipolysis chronically has not been established. Niacin appears to inhibit the secretion of VLDL by liver. Incorporation of amino acids into the protein moiety of VLDL is inhibited, and it appears to increase the efficiency of removal of VLDL triglycerides via the LPL pathway. Niacin has several effects on cholesterol metabolism. It increases sterol excretion acutely and mobilizes cholesterol from tissue pools until a new steady state is established. Although it has no effect on the conversion of cholesterol to bile acids, it decreases cholesterol biosynthesis. That it can cause a continued decrease in hepatic cholesterol production even when given with bile acid–binding resins is probably an important feature of the complementary action of these agents. Because niacin does not change the turnover of LDL per se, it appears that the reduction of levels of LDL associated with its use must reflect decreased production of LDL resulting from decreased secretion of its precursor, VLDL. Levels of HDL in plasma, particularly HDL_2, are significantly increased, reflecting a decrease in the fractional catabolic rate of these lipoproteins. Niacin stimulates production of tissue plasminogen activator, an effect that may be of value in preventing thrombotic events.

Drug Dosage

The dose of niacin required for effective treatment varies with the diagnosis. Optimal effect on LDL levels in heterozygous familial hypercholesterolemia is only achieved when a bile acid–binding resin is combined with 4.5–7.5 g of niacin daily (in 3 doses). For other forms of hypercholesterolemia and for hypertriglyceridemia, a dose of 1.5–3.5 g/d often has a dramatic effect. Because niacin causes cutaneous flushing, it is usually started at a dosage of 100 mg 3 times daily and increased slowly. Tachyphylaxis to the flushing often occurs within a few days at any dose, allowing stepwise increases. Many patients have no flushing or only occasional minimal flushing when stabilized on a given dose. Because the flushing is prostaglandin-mediated, 0.3 g of aspirin given 20–30 minutes before each dose may mitigate this symptom. It is important to counsel the patient beforehand that the flushing is a harmless cutaneous vasodilatation. Patients should be advised to take the drug with meals.

Side Effects

Moderate elevations of transaminases are more often observed if the dosage of niacin is increased too rapidly. If a daily dose of 2.5 g is not exceeded by the end of the first month, 5 g after the second month, and 7.5 g after the third month, such abnormalities are uncommon. A daily dose of 7.5 g is the maximum under any circumstances. Some patients have reversible elevations of serum glutamic aminotransferase or alkaline phosphatase activities up to 2.5 times the upper limit of normal that do not appear to be clinically significant. In a group of patients treated continuously for up to 10 years, no significant liver disease developed despite such enzyme abnormalities. About one-fifth of patients have mild hyperuricemia that tends to be asymptomatic unless the patient has had gout. In such cases, a uricosuric agent can be added to the regimen. A few patients will have moderate elevations of blood glucose during treatment. Again, this is reversible except possibly in some patients who have latent maturity-onset diabetes. A more common side effect is gastric irritation, which responds well to antacids. Rarely, patients develop acanthosis nigricans, which clears if the drug is discontinued. Some patients can have cardiac arrhythmias while taking niacin. Reversible macular degeneration has been described rarely.

Niacin should be avoided in patients with peptic ulcer or hepatic parenchymal disease. It should be discontinued in patients who develop markedly elevated levels of transaminases or alkaline phosphatase. Liver function, uric acid, and blood glucose should be evaluated before commencing treatment and periodically thereafter.

CLOFIBRATE
(Ethyl Chlorphenoxyisobutyrate)

Mechanism of Action

Clofibrate appears to act chiefly by increasing the activity of the lipolytic pathway in plasma, specifically increasing levels of LPL activity. It may also increase oxidation of fatty acids by liver and decrease VLDL production modestly. Inhibition of cholesterol biosynthesis in liver may be secondary to changes in VLDL secretion and catabolism. Since decreases in VLDL levels are frequently attended by increased levels of LDL (the so-called beta shift), serum cholesterol levels of some patients may not change despite reductions in triglyceride levels.

Drug Dosage

Clofibrate (Atromid-S) is most useful in treating familial dysbetalipoproteinemia and moderate endogenous hypertriglyceridemia. The usual dose is 1 g twice daily, though patients with dysbetalipoproteinemia may respond well to one-half this dose or less. Clofibrate is of little benefit in familial hyper-

cholesterolemia and has limited effect when severe chylomicronemia is present. In the latter case, niacin may be used with clofibrate or alone.

Side Effects

Side effects include nausea, diarrhea, skin eruptions, leukopenia, and moderate elevations of serum glutamic aminotransferase activity. Impotence has also been reported. Muscle pain or cramps associated with elevated muscle creatine kinase activity have been noted. Because this syndrome is most likely to occur when serum albumin levels are low, clofibrate should not be given to patients with nephrosis. Clofibrate potentiates the activities of coumarin and indanedione anticoagulants, and the hypoglycemic effects of sulfonylureas may be enhanced. It also increases the lithogenicity of bile, particularly in obese patients. Results of a recent multicenter study indicate that clofibrate may have a modest carcinogenic potential for tissues of the gastrointestinal tract.

GEMFIBROZIL

Mechanism of Action

Gemfibrozil, a congener of clofibrate, is bound tightly to plasma proteins and is excreted chiefly by the kidney. It decreases lipolysis in adipose tissue, reduces levels of circulating triglycerides, and causes modest reductions in LDL cholesterol levels. However, in some patients reductions in VLDL levels are attended by increases in LDL levels. It causes moderate increases in levels of HDL, including the protein moiety. In general, the indications are the same as for clofibrate. It is not yet clear whether the increases in HDL with this drug are greater than those resulting from clofibrate.

Drug Dosage

Gemfibrozil (Lopid) is supplied in 300-mg capsules. The usual dose is 600 mg twice daily. Patients with familial dysbetalipoproteinemia may be managed with smaller doses.

Side Effects

Skin eruptions and gastrointestinal and muscular symptoms similar to those associated with clofibrate have been described, as well as blood dyscrasias and elevated plasma levels of transaminases and alkaline phosphatase. It is likely that most of the toxic effects associated with clofibrate will be observed as experience with this drug increases. Like clofibrate, it enhances the effects of the coumarin and indanedione anticoagulants and increases lithogenicity of bile.

NEOMYCIN

Neomycin is of some usefulness in treating hypercholesterolemia, effecting reductions in LDL cholesterol levels of up to 25%. It is not approved by the FDA as a lipid-lowering agent, and its use is considered investigational. It apparently acts by inhibiting absorption of cholesterol and bile acids. The dosage required for this effect is 0.5–2 g/d. Even in this dosage range, some patients develop diarrhea that persists as long as the drug is taken. Patients should be observed for ototoxicity and nephrotoxicity.

DEXTROTHYROXINE
(D-Thyroxine)

Dextrothyroxine is isomeric to the normal thyroid hormone, L-thyroxine. It acts in a fashion similar to L-thyroxine on lipid metabolism, increasing conversion of cholesterol to bile acids. Preparations available in the USA have had hypercalorigenic activity, however, either because of residual L-thyroxine or because of inherent effects of the D-isomer on oxidative phosphorylation. This activity causes increased cardiac work and may induce angina. Dextrothyroxine is no longer indicated, because it has only limited effectiveness in treating hyperlipidemia and because its use may increase the risk of fatal cardiac arrhythmias.

HMG-CoA REDUCTASE INHIBITORS

Mechanism of Action

Several closely related structural analogues of HMG-CoA that have been developed act as competitive inhibitors of HMG-CoA reductase, a key enzyme in the cholesterol biosynthetic pathway. Of these, lovastatin is approved for use in the USA. Inhibition of cholesterol biosynthesis induces an increase in high-affinity LDL receptors in the liver, increasing removal of LDL from plasma and decreasing production of LDL. The latter results from increased uptake of lipoprotein precursors of LDL by hepatic receptors. Modest increases in HDL cholesterol and limited decreases in VLDL levels occur during treatment (Fig 24–6).

Drug Dosage

Lovastatin is the most effective individual agent for treatment of hypercholesterolemia. Its effect is amplified significantly when combined with niacin or resin. Daily doses vary from 20 to 80 mg. A single 20-mg dose, preferably in the evening, may be sufficient to treat moderately elevated LDL levels. Patients with heterozygous familial hypercholesterolemia usually require 20–30 mg twice daily with meals. Because information on long-term safety is lacking, its use in children should be restricted to those with homozygous familial hypercholesterolemia who have some receptor function. Women who are lactating, pregnant, or likely to become pregnant should not be given this drug.

Side Effects

Lovastatin is generally well tolerated. Reported side effects, often transient, include changes in bowel function, nausea, headaches, insomnia, fatigue, and rashes. Myopathy with markedly elevated creatine kinase levels occurs in less than 5% of patients. Rarely, myopathy can progress to rhabdomyolysis with myoglobinuria and renal shutdown. There is an increased incidence of myopathy in patients receiving lovastation with cyclosporine (30%) or fibric acid derivatives (5%). Minor elevations of creatine kinase activity in plasma are noted more frequently, especially with unusual physical activity. Creatine kinase levels should be measured before starting therapy, and monitored at regular intervals.

Moderate, often intermittent, elevations of serum transaminase (up to twice normal) occur in some patients. Therapy may be continued if transaminase levels are measured frequently (at 1- to 2-month intervals). In about 2% of patients, some of whom have underlying liver disease or a history of alcohol abuse, transaminase levels may exceed 3 times the normal limit. This usually occurs after 3–16 months of continuous therapy and may portend more severe hepatic toxicity. Lovastatin should be discontinued in these patients. The drug should be used with caution in patients with a history of liver disease.

Although no effects on the lens have been detected to date, slit lamp examination of the eyes should be done before starting treatment and annually thereafter.

PROBUCOL

Probucol moderately lowers levels of LDL by increasing the fractional clearance of LDL and perhaps by decreasing cholesterol synthesis. It retards atherogenesis in animal models by apparently inhibiting hydroperoxidation of LDL, which in turn reduces uptake of LDL by scavenger cells. HDL cholesterol levels are usually significantly reduced, but emerging data suggest that centripetal transport of cholesterol may be normal. Both atheromas and tendon xanthomas regress in patients with homozygous familial hypercholesterolemia. The use of probucol is indicated in these patients, whose response to bile acid–binding resins and HMG-CoA reductase inhibitors is usually negligible. Other patients with fulminant atheromatous disease might benefit similarly.

Side effects of this agent include nausea, diarrhea, abdominal pain, and increased Q–T intervals. It should be avoided in patients with a predisposition to ventricular arrhythmia or with prolonged Q–T intervals. It should not be given with digitalis, quinidine, erythromycin, or other agents known to prolong Q–T intervals. Elevated levels of transaminases, bilirubin, alkaline phosphatase, creatine kinase, uric acid, and blood glucose have been observed.

Probucol (Lorelco) is available as 250-mg and 500-mg tablets. The usual dose is 500 mg twice daily.

COMBINED DRUG THERAPY
(Table 24–3)

Combinations of drugs are indicated (1) when LDL and VLDL levels are both elevated; (2) in cases of hypercholesterolemia in which significant increases of VLDL occur during treatment with bile acid–binding resins; and (3) where a complementary effect is required to normalize LDL levels, as in familial hypercholesterolemia.

Fibric Acid Derivatives
With Other Agents

Whereas clofibrate or gemfibrozil have some effectiveness in decreasing levels of VLDL in plasma in conjunction with bile acid–binding resins, they usually do not complement the effect of the resins on plasma LDL levels in familial hypercholesterolemia. The effectiveness of these agents is thus generally limited to disorders in which moderate elevations in levels of plasma VLDL occur. Theoretically, they should increase the lithogenicity of bile, which may already be increased by bile acid–binding resins. The combination of clofibrate or gemfibrozil with niacin may be more effective than either drug alone in managing marked hypertriglyceridemia. Gemfibrozil with lovastatin appears to be effective treatment for familial combined hyperlipidemia, but the risk of myopathy is increased.

Niacin & Resins

Niacin usually normalizes the triglyceride levels in individuals who have increased levels of VLDL while taking resins. The combination of niacin and resins is more effective than either agent alone in decreasing LDL levels in familial hypercholesterolemia. The complementarity of action presumably results from additive effects of increased catabolism of LDL due to the resin and decreased production of VLDL induced by niacin. No additional toxicity or side effects have been described with this regimen beyond those encountered when the agents are used individually. The daily dose of niacin required for optimal effect on LDL levels in familial hypercholesterolemia is 6.5 g in conjunction with 24–30 g of resin. On this regimen, levels of HDL cholesterol are significantly elevated, and the diameters of tendon xanthomas are reduced significantly even over a period of only a few months. Patients who have been treated with this combination for 10 years show evidence of a sustained effect on lipoprotein levels and have not developed additional side effects or toxicity. It is also very useful in the treatment of familial combined hyperlipidemia.

The absorption of niacin from the intestine is unimpeded by the presence of resin; the 2 medications may therefore be taken together. Because colestipol has potent acid-neutralizing properties, there is further reason to give the 2 medications together when a patient complains of the gastric irritation that sometimes occurs as an adverse effect of niacin.

Lovastatin With Other Agents

The addition of resin or niacin to lovastatin further decreases plasma levels of LDL in patients with primary hypercholesterolemias. Liver function and plasma creatine kinase activity should be monitored frequently when the combination of lovastatin plus niacin is used. These 3 drugs used together are more effective than any of their binary combinations in reducing plasma LDL levels. Serum cholesterol levels in patients with severe heterozygous familial hypercholesterolemia usually fall below 200 mg/dL. In some patients, a reduction of as much as 80% has been observed. Effects are sustained, and no compound toxicity is observed.

SURGICAL TREATMENT OF HYPERLIPIDEMIA

The operation that has received the most study in the treatment of hyperlipidemia is ileal bypass. This procedure is intended to impede the reabsorption of bile acids and not to cause malabsorption of triglycerides. Evidence supporting impeded absorption of cholesterol is weak. The procedure appears merely to mimic the effect of bile acid–binding resins. Serum cholesterol levels are apparently decreased in a variety of disorders, but, as with bile acid sequestrants, levels of triglycerides in serum may be significantly elevated. Thus, the procedure is not indicated in hypertriglyceridemia. Furthermore, in a series of well-documented cases of heterozygous familial hypercholesterolemia, levels of cholesterol in serum were reduced by only 33%. Clearly, ileal bypass is less effective in that disorder than in drug treatment. A significant number of patients develop diarrhea, which may be difficult to control, and if the procedure is not performed correctly there may be steatorrhea. Absorption of vitamin B_{12} is impaired in all patients, and this necessitates lifelong parenteral administration of the vitamin.

In some patients with homozygous familial hypercholesterolemia, end-to-side portacaval shunts have ameliorated but not normalized LDL levels. Liver transplantation results in dramatic reduction in plasma LDL levels in these patients.

REFERENCES

Relationship of Coronary Heart Disease to Disorders of Lipoprotein Metabolism

Armstrong ML, Warner ED, Connor WE: Regression of coronary atheromatosis in rhesus monkeys. *Circ Res* 1970;**27**:59.

Castelli WP: Epidemiology of coronary heart disease: The Framingham Study. *Am J Med* 1984;**76(Suppl 2A)**:4.

Goldstein JL, Kita T, Brown MS: Defective lipoprotein receptors and atherosclerosis: Lessons from an animal counterpart of familial hypercholesterolemia. *N Engl J Med* 1983;**309**:288.

Gordon T et al: High-density lipoprotein as a protective factor against coronary heart disease: The Framingham Study. *Am J Med* 1977;**62**:707.

Havel RJ: Role of the liver in atherosclerosis. *Arteriosclerosis* 1985;**5**:569.

Kannel WB: High-density lipoproteins: Epidemiologic profile and risks of coronary artery disease. *Am J Cardiol* 1983;**52**:9B.

Kannel WB et al: Overall and coronary heart disease mortality rates in relation to major risk factors in 325,348 men screened for the Multiple Risk Factor Intervention Trial (MRFIT). *Am Heart J* 1986;**112**:825.

Lipid Research Clinics Program: The Lipid Research Clinics coronary primary prevention trial results. (2 parts.) *JAMA* 1984;**251**:351, 365.

Ostrander LD Jr et al: Biochemical precursors of atherosclerosis: Studies in apparently healthy men in a general population, Tecumseh, Mich. *Arch Intern Med* 1974;**134**:224.

Rhoads GG, Gulbrandsen CL, Kagan A: Serum lipoproteins and coronary heart disease in a population study of Hawaii Japanese men. *N Engl J Med* 1976;**294**:293.

Ross R: The pathogenesis of atherosclerosis: An update. *N Engl J Med* 1986;**314**:488.

Lipoprotein Metabolism

Brown MS, Faust JR, Goldstein JL: Role of the low-density lipoprotein receptor in regulating the content of free and esterified cholesterol in human fibroblasts. *J Clin Invest* 1975;**55**:783.

Brunzell JD: Familial lipoprotein lipase deficiency and other causes of the chylomiconemia syndrome. In: *The Metabolic Basis of Inherited Disease*, 6th ed. Scriver CR et al (editors). McGraw-Hill, 1989.

Havel RJ: The formation of LDL: Mechanisms and regulation. *J Lipid Res* 1984;**25**:1570.

Kane JP, Havel RJ: Introduction: Structure and metabolism of plasma lipoproteins. Page 1129 in: *The Metabolic Basis of Inherited Disease*, 6th ed. Scriver CR et al (editors). McGraw-Hill, 1989.

Primary Disorders of Lipoprotein Metabolism

Brown MS, Goldstein JL: Familial hypercholesterolemia. In: *The Metabolic Basis of Inherited Disease*, 6th ed. Scriver CR et al (editors). McGraw-Hill, 1989.

Goldstein JL et al: Hyperlipidemia in coronary heart disease. 2. Genetic analysis of lipid levels in 176 families and delineation of a new inherited disorder, combined hyperlipidemia. *J Clin Invest* 1973;**52**:1544.

Havel RJ, Goldstein JL, Brown MS: Lipoproteins and lipid transport. In: *Metabolic Control Disease*, 8th ed. Bondy PK, Rosenberg LE (editors). Saunders, 1980.

Mahley RW, Rall Jr, SC: Type III hyperlipoproteinemia (dysbetalipoproteinemia: The role of apolipoprotein E in normal and abnormal lipoprotein metabolism. Page 1195 in: *The Metabolic Basis of Inherited Disease*, 6th ed. Scriver CR et al (editors). McGraw-Hill, 1989.

Malloy MJ, Kane JP: Hypolipidemia. *Med Clin North Am* 1982;**66**:469.

Treatment of Hyperlipidemia With Diet

Belfrage P et al: Alterations of lipid metabolism in healthy volunteers during long-term ethanol intake. *Eur J Clin Invest* 1977;**7**:127.

Connor WE, Connor SL: The dietary treatment of hyperlipidemia: Rationale, technique, and efficacy. *Med Clin North Am* 1982;**66**:485.

Keys A: Coronary heart disease, serum cholesterol, and the diet. *Acta Med Scand* 1980;**207**:153.

Nutrition Committee and the Council on Arteriosclerosis of the American Heart Association: Recommendations for the treatment of hyperlipidemia in adults. *Circulation* 1984;**69**:443A.

Treatment of Hyperlipidemia With Drugs

Bernstein MJ: Lowering blood cholesterol to prevent heart disease. *JAMA* 1985;**253**:2080.

Blankenhorn DH et al: Beneficial effects of combined colestipol-niacin therapy on coronary atherosclerosis and coronary venous bypass grafts. *JAMA* 1987;**257**:3233.

Brensike JF et al: Effects of therapy with cholestyramine on progression of coronary arteriosclerosis: Results of the NHLBI Type II Coronary Intervention Study. *Circulation* 1984;**69**:313.

Canner PL et al: Fifteen-year mortality in Coronary Drug Project patients: Long-term benefit with niacin. *J Am Coll Cardiol* 1986;**8**:1245.

Carew TE, Schwenke DC, Steinberg D: Antiatherogenic effect of probucol unrelated to its hypocholesterolemic effect: Evidence that antioxidants in vivo can selectively inhibit low density lipoprotein degradation in macrophage-rich fatty streaks and slow the progression of atherosclerosis in the Wetanabe heritable hyperlipidemic (WHHL) rabbit. *Proc Natl Acad Sci USA* 1987;**84**:7725.

Cleeman JJ: Report of the National Cholesterol Education Program expert panel on detection, evaluation, and treatment of high blood cholesterol in adults. *Arch Intern Med* 1988;**148**:36.

Frick MH et al: Helsinki Heart Study: Primary-prevention trial with gemfibrozil in middle-aged men with dyslipidemia. Safety of treatment, changes in risk factors, and incidence of coronary heart disease. *N Engl J Med* 1987;**317**:1237.

Grundy SM: Hypertriglyceridemia: Mechanisms, clinical significance, and treatment. *Med Clin North Am* 1982;**66**:519.

Grundy SM, Vega GL, Bilheimer DM: Influence of combined therapy with mevinolin and interruption of bile-acid reabsorption on low-density lipoproteins in heterozygous familial hypercholesterolemia. *Ann Intern Med* 1985;**103:**339.

Grundy SM et al: Influence of nicotinic acid on metabolism of cholesterol and triglycerides in man. *J Lipid Res* 1981;**22:**24.

Havel RJ et al: Lovastatin (Mevinolin) in the treatment of heterozygous familial hypercholesterolemia: A multicenter study. *Ann Intern Med* 1987;**107:**609.

Illingworth DR: Mevinolin plus colestipol in therapy for severe heterozygous familial hypercholesterolemia. *Ann Intern Med* 1984;**101:**598.

Kane JP, Havel RJ: Treatment of hypercholesterolemia. *Annu Rev Med* 1986;**37:**427.

Kane JP, Malloy MJ: When to treat hyperlipidemia. *Adv Intern Med* 1988;**33:**143.

Kane JP et al: Normalization of low-density lipoprotein levels in heterozygous familial hypercholesterolemia with a combined drug regimen. *N Engl J Med* 1981;**304:**251.

Levy RI et al: The influence of changes in lipid values induced by cholestyramine and diet on progression of coronary artery disease: Results of the NHLBI Type II Coronary Intervention Study. *Circulation* 1984;**69:**325.

Lipid Research Clinics Program: The Lipid Research Clinics coronary primary prevention trial results. (2 parts.) *JAMA* 1984;**251:**351, 365.

Lovastatin Study Group II: Therapeutic response to lovastatin (Mevinolin) in nonfamilial hypercholesterolemia. A multicenter study. *JAMA* 1986;**256:**2829.

Lovastatin Study Group III: A multicenter comparison of lovastatin and cholestyramine therapy for severe primary hypercholesterolemia. *JAMA* 1988;**260:**359.

Malloy MJ: Disorders of lipoprotein metabolism. In: *Practical Pediatric Therapy,* 2nd ed. Eichenwald HF, Ströder J (editors). Mosby, 1989.

Malloy MJ et al: Complementarity of colestipol, niacin, and lovastatin in treatment of severe familial hypercholesterolemia. *Ann Intern Med* 1987;**107:**616.

Shepherd J et al: Cholestyramine promotes receptor-mediated low-density lipoprotein catabolism. *N Engl J Med* 1980;**302:**1219.

25

Obesity

Mary J. Malloy, MD, & John P. Kane, MD, PhD

Adipose tissue is an organ of metabolism that serves as a capacitor for energy-rich fatty acids. In comparison with glycogen stored in hydrated form in liver and muscle, the unhydrated triglycerides stored in adipose tissue contain over twice the available energy per unit mass. Triglycerides are laid down during times when the supply of circulating energy substrates exceeds the need; in periods of caloric deficit, their constituent fatty acids and glycerol are yielded to the plasma for catabolism at distant tissue sites. Regulation of triglyceride storage involves both neural and endocrine factors but, as would be expected, primarily reflects the net surplus of caloric substrate available to the organism. Obesity, the state of excess storage of triglyceride,* in turn exerts important effects on metabolic processes in adipose tissue and in other organs. The metabolic and pathologic consequences of obesity increase continuously with the extent of deviation above ideal weight.

METABOLISM OF ADIPOSE TISSUE

The preponderant mass of the fatty acids stored in adipose tissue appears to come from circulating triglyceride-rich lipoproteins. The triglycerides of very low density lipoproteins (VLDL) and chylomicrons are hydrolyzed by lipoprotein lipase (LPL) located on the capillary endothelium yielding fatty acids, most of which are transported into adipocytes (Fig 25–1). Insulin, which induces LPL activity, also facilitates the entry of glucose into adipocytes, where it is largely converted to α-glyceryl phosphate. This compound provides the glyceryl moiety for esterification of free fatty acids to triglycerides. Adipose tissue is capable of forming fatty acids from acetate derived from ethanol. Glucose also contributes to the synthesis of fatty acids to a limited extent.

Free fatty acids and glycerol are mobilized from adipose tissue into plasma by the hydrolysis of stored triglycerides, a process mediated by an intracellular

Acronyms Used in This Chapter	
ACTH	Adrenocorticotropic hormone
ATP	Adenosine triphosphate
BMI	Body mass index
cAMP	Cyclic adenosine monophosphate
CCK	Cholecystokinin
FFA	Free fatty acids
LPL	Lipoprotein lipase
SHBG	Sex hormone–binding globulin
VLDL	Very low density lipoprotein(s)

hormone-sensitive lipase system. The first steps of hydrolysis, which are rate-limiting, release 2 mol of fatty acid. The process is rapidly completed by a monoglyceridase. Hormones that stimulate the hydrolysis of triglycerides are epinephrine, norepinephrine, ACTH, glucagon, and growth hormone. Afferent autonomics serving adipose tissue, which also mediate fatty acid mobilization, represent an important pathway by which the central nervous system exerts control over the mobilization of fatty acids. Many of these stimuli increase the activity of adenylate cyclase. The resulting increase in cAMP activates a protein kinase that phosphorylates inactive triglyceridase to its active form. The phosphorylation is reversible via a phosphatase enzyme, allowing tonic control of the lipolytic process. A phosphodiesterase damps the cAMP signal by hydrolysis of the cyclic nucleotide. Inhibition of phosphodiesterase by caffeine and theophylline potentiates the hormonal stimulation of lipolysis. Thyroxine and cortisol have a permissive effect on lipolysis. The hormonal and neural stimuli are opposed by insulin. Thus, when blood glucose and triglyceride levels increase after a meal, insulin promotes storage of fat and inhibits lipolysis, whereas fasting and exercise promote lipolysis relatively unopposed by insulin.

PROLIFERATION OF ADIPOCYTES

In the first few months of life, adipocytes largely increase storage capacity via hypertrophy. In nonobese

---

*The triglycerides are now called triacylglycerols in some current texts.

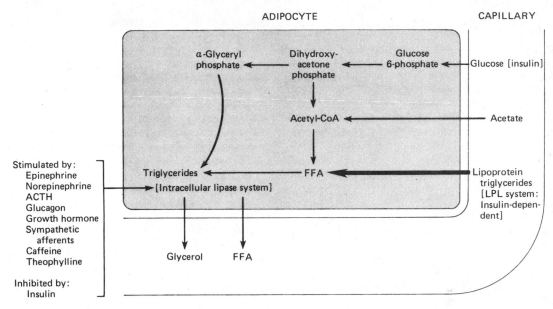

ADIPOCYTE   CAPILLARY

Figure 25–1. Metabolism of adipocytes

children, fat cell size decreases after age 1 year, whereas it remains hypertrophic in obese children. Adipocyte hyperplasia, ie, increase in the number of adipose cells, appears to occur from about 1 year of age through preadolescence, proceeding more rapidly in obese children. Thereafter, increases in adipose tissue mass occur primarily as a result of hypertrophy. However, there is some evidence that there may be increases and decreases in white fat cell numbers in adults. Grossly obese adults generally have increased numbers of adipocytes, whereas moderate obesity is usually hypertrophic. The latter may respond more readily to treatment. The early determination of adipocyte number highlights the importance of obesity in childhood as a predisposing factor in the subsequent development of lifelong obesity. Childhood-onset obesity tends to be distributed both centrally and peripherally, whereas adult-onset obesity is usually centrally distributed. A consequence of hypertrophy of adipocytes is insulin resistance and reduction in the number of cellular insulin receptors. The severity of these consequences generally correlates positively with the degree of cellular hypertrophy. Patients with adipocyte hypertrophy tend to be relatively resistant to the development of ketosis during a fast.

INDICES OF OBESITY

Adipose tissue comprises about 10% of the body mass of normal infants at birth. In early adulthood, nonobese males have about 10–15% of body mass as fat, whereas in normal females, adipose mass is about 15–20%. Because body weight and quantity of fat are continuously distributed in populations, the definition of obesity must be arbitrary. However, some guides are useful in identifying individuals who are significantly obese. A principal problem in defining obesity is the great variation in lean body mass among individuals of the same stature. Persons of mesomorphic body build, with heavy bone structure and musculature, may easily exceed the tabular norms of weight for height without being obese. A number of sophisticated techniques, including measurement of body density, isotopic compartmentation, ultrasonography, and magnetic resonance imaging, have been used to measure body fat. These procedures are generally used only in research.

More practical indices express the relationship of height to weight: weight/height ratio; weight in kilograms divided by the square of height in meters, called the body mass index (BMI or Quetelet index); and height divided by the cube root of weight, called the ponderal index. The BMI correlates best with body composition. The height and weight tables of the Metropolitan Life Insurance Company are divided into 3 arbitrary classes of frame size, permitting a rough accommodation for the effect of lean body mass on total weight. Allowing for frame, patients must be considered obese if their weight exceeds the average by 20% or more.* Another factor that must be considered is that lean body mass decreases somewhat with age. Not only the percent of fat in the body but also its distribu-

---

*A simple rule that does not allow for differences in body frame but is useful as a screening test is as follows: Beginning with a body weight of 100 lb for women and 105 lb for men at 60 inches, an increment of 6 lb per inch for men and 5 lb per inch for women is permissible.

tion differs between the sexes. In men, fat tends to be distributed about the trunk; in women, more adipose mass is present over the limbs and gluteal region. Departures from these patterns are of some importance in differentiating certain disorders associated with obesity. Several studies have established that truncal obesity is associated with an increased risk of acquiring type II diabetes or arteriosclerotic vascular disease. The distribution of adipose mass between the trunk and the gluteal region can be described quantitatively using the ratio of the circumference at the waist to that at the hips. With normal distribution, the ratio falls between 0.7 and 0.85. Skinfold thickness, when measured at the proper sites with constant tension calipers, is also a useful index of fat distribution. In general, adults may be considered obese if skinfolds exceed 19 mm for men and 30 mm for women at the midtriceps level or 22 mm for men and 27 mm for women at the subscapular level. These figures represent the upper 20% in a United States population survey.

ETIOLOGIC FACTORS IN OBESITY

Genetic Factors

Obesity in humans is frequently familial, but separation of genetic from environmental effects is difficult. Some of the observed familial aggregation of obesity may be related to family eating patterns, especially as they affect nutrition in infancy and early childhood. Nevertheless, studies of identical twins reared apart provide convincing evidence for substantial genetic determinacy of adipose mass.

Ultimately, obesity reflects the relative intake and expenditure of energy substrate. Resting metabolism accounts for nearly 70% of total energy expenditure but can differ by as much as 500 kcal per day among individuals of the same body weight. It is highest in infancy and decreases progressively with age after the second decade. The aggregation of similar rates of resting energy expenditure within kindreds may account in large part for the familial distribution of obesity. Resting energy expenditure appears to be lower in a number of obese subjects compared with nonobese individuals and can serve as a predictor of weight gain. It has been observed that the energy expenditure of infants born to obese mothers is lower than that in infants born to nonobese mothers.

Endocrine Factors

There is no established endocrine cause for most cases of obesity. However, several uncommon endocrine disorders do include obesity as one of the clinical features. Cushing's syndrome is characterized by centripetal redistribution of adipose tissue and is readily recognized by other prominent stigmas. Hyperinsulinism associated with insulinoma can lead to obesity, presumably by stimulating hyperphagia as well as by adipotropic metabolic effects. Some individuals with hypothyroidism become obese, probably largely because of diminished catabolic activity, although the permissive role of thyroxine in lipolysis may also be important. It should be remembered, however, that most excess gain with hypothyroidism is due to myxedema. Obesity may also be associated with Klinefelter's and Turner's syndromes, male hypogonadism, and castration.

It is well established that insulin resistance accompanies obesity, often with elevated levels of insulin in plasma and increased rates of insulin secretion. The concentration of insulin receptors in monocytes, fibroblasts, and adipocytes from obese individuals is reduced, probably owing in large part to the hyperinsulinemia per se. This phenomenon is accompanied by decreased insulin-induced glucose transport, glucose oxidation, and lipogenesis by adipocytes. The sensitivity of the inhibition of lipolysis in isolated fat cells from obese subjects appears to be increased. This could result in impaired hydrolysis of stored triglycerides during fasting when insulin levels are relatively low and thus may be significant in the etiology of obesity.

Neurologic Factors

Lesions of the ventromedial hypothalamus in animals regularly produce hyperinsulinism, hyperphagia, and obesity. Rarely, structural or functional lesions of this region in humans, including tumors, trauma, and inflammation, have produced a similar type of hypertrophic obesity. Hypothalamic dysfunction is also postulated in certain rare heredofamilial syndromes of obesity.

Psychologic Factors

Psychologic determinants are of great importance in both the etiology of obesity and its management. Individuals reared in a kindred of obese people tend to regard obesity as the norm. Overeating may represent disturbed family dynamics and involve the whole family. Parents may overfeed children in an attempt to deal with guilt, as an expression of their own unmet emotional needs, or as a distorted expression of love. Such a child often becomes passive, overdependent, and immature in later childhood and as an adult. Overeating and decreased activity leading to obesity may occur as a response to some environmental or emotional stress such as death of a loved one, disruption of a family unit, or school or job pressures or failures. Eating patterns in some obese patients ("night-eating syndrome," "eating binge syndrome") have been associated with periods of psychologic stress. Food may become a substitute for other gratifications or may serve to relieve boredom, loneliness, or anxiety. Eating may help to stave off uncomfortable feelings of anger or depression. Obesity may serve to protect an individual from normal social interaction, sexual conflicts, and exposure to the possibility of failure in such interpersonal relationships.

Habit and environmental factors appear to influence appetite regulation. Thin individuals tend to eat only when hungry, whereas obese people eat in response to such stimuli as time of day, flavor, odors, etc. Another important factor is the Old World cultural view that obesity is a sign of health and prosperity. But in a society such as ours, which favors an image of youthful slimness, obesity can cause serious psychologic problems as well as originate from them.

SYNDROMES ASSOCIATED WITH OBESITY

Prader-Willi Syndrome

This syndrome is not clearly genetic, but several cases have been reported in some kindreds. About half of these patients have a deletion or translocation of chromosome 15. Clinical features include short stature, mental retardation, hypotonia, small hands and feet, and hypogonadism. Generalized obesity begins at age 1–3 years and is progressive into adulthood.

Bardet-Biedl Syndrome (Laurence-Moon-Biedl Syndrome)

Consanguinity is common in this autosomal recessive disorder, which is characterized by mental retardation, polydactyly, and hypogonadism, especially of males, who have small testes and gynecomastia. Generalized obesity begins at age 1–2 years.

Alström-Hallgren Syndrome

The obesity in this syndrome also begins in early childhood and is predominantly truncal. Clinical features include retinal degeneration and nerve deafness. Diabetes frequently occurs, and acanthosis nigricans and male hypogonadism are occasionally present.

Fröhlich's Syndrome (Adiposogenital Dystrophy)

Obesity in this disorder is truncal in distribution. There is hypogenitalism with absence of secondary sex characteristics. Short stature, decreased visual acuity, diabetes insipidus, and mental retardation may be associated findings.

Hyperostosis Frontalis Interna

This syndrome of women may begin as late as the sixth decade. It includes hyperostosis of the frontal bones, with mental obtundation, headache, and occasionally virilism and impaired equilibrium or seizure.

Cohen's Syndrome

In this syndrome, probably transmitted as an autosomal recessive disorder, truncal obesity usually begins in childhood. Patients may have hypogonadism. Associated features include boney abnormalities of the nose and palate and hypotonia.

Carpenter's Syndrome

This autosomal recessive disorder is characterized by central obesity and hypogonadism and by structural abnormalities of the digits and the craniofacial bones.

Multiple Lipomatosis

Several syndromes of lipomatosis are recognized. The lipomas are usually distributed in a bilaterally symmetric fashion. Often they enlarge when the patient is consuming alcohol and may regress with abstinence. One variety, **Madelung's disease,** selectively involves the neck.

PATHOPHYSIOLOGIC CONSEQUENCES OF OBESITY

Truncal Obesity Associated Syndrome

Truncal obesity is frequently associated with a constellation of findings that include insulin resistance with impaired glucose tolerance, hypertension, hypertriglyceridemia, hyperuricemia, and increased risk of coronary arteriosclerosis and stroke. The risk of type II diabetes, coronary vascular disease, and stroke is more positively correlated with truncal obesity than with obesity per se. Whereas it is presumed that the hypertriglyceridemia and hyperglycemia are related to the impaired effectiveness of insulin, the causes of the hypertension and hyperuricemia are unclear.

Hyperlipoproteinemia

Obesity chiefly affects the metabolism of triglyceride-rich lipoproteins and is almost a prerequisite for the appearance of primary hyperprebetalipoproteinemia. Levels of VLDL in plasma fall as soon as body weight begins to decrease and can usually be maintained near normal if ideal body weight can be achieved. Likewise, in primary and secondary mixed lipemias, obesity profoundly amplifies the expression of the underlying defect. In familial dysbetalipoproteinemia, where remnant lipoprotein particles accumulate in blood, obesity is also a major determinant of expression of the metabolic defect. In all forms of lipemia, reduction of adipose mass to normal is an important element of therapy. There is an independent inverse relationship of adipose mass with the levels of plasma high-density lipoproteins.

Diabetes

Obesity associated with adipose cell hypertrophy is an essential element in the development of maturity-onset diabetes, in which insulin resistance, hyperinsulinism, and resistance to ketosis are prominent features. With the exception of those patients who develop severely compromised insulinogenic capacity, reduction of adipose mass to normal is attended by amelioration or even normalization of blood glucose and insulin levels.

Cardiopulmonary Disease

Obesity is associated with a moderate increase in risk of atherosclerotic heart disease, probably mediated at least in part by its effects on circulating lipoproteins and perhaps also by its association with hypertension. Obesity increases cardiac work as a result of the expanded requirement for blood transport, thus increasing the risk of underlying valvular or cariomyopathic disease, where load is important. Cardiac failure is the cause of death in most morbidly obese patients. Hypoventilation with decreased arterial oxygen content, with or without hypercapnia, is encountered in grossly obese persons. The fully developed **pickwickian syndrome** may include somnolence, cyanosis, and muscle twitching.

Complications of Pregnancy, Labor, & Puerperium

Obese women are at significantly increased risk of preeclampsia-eclampsia. Labor tends to be difficult and prolonged, and the incidence of postpartum hemorrhage is increased.

Cholelithiasis

Lithogenic bile, commonly seen in obese patients and largely resulting from increased cholesterol synthesis and excretion, increases the risk of cholelithiasis severalfold, especially in women.

Other Consequences of Obesity

An enlarged, fatty liver is often seen in association with obesity. Nonspecific gastrointestinal symptoms such as bloating and dyspepsia may be reported, and osteoarthritis may appear in its most severe form in obese patients.

A number of effects of obesity on endocrine function are now recognized. The production of cortisol by the adrenal cortex is increased in proportion to body mass. The conversion of androstenedione to estrone is increased up to 5-fold in obese women. In addition, the sex hormone–binding capacity attributable to sex hormone–binding globulin (SHBG) is low in obese individuals, leading to a higher level of unbound estradiol in plasma. Amenorrhea and oligomenorrhea are associated findings in some obese women. However, menarche tends to occur early in obese girls. Plasma levels of progesterone, pregnenolone, androsterone, and dehydroepiandrosterone are elevated in obese prepubertal girls, whereas their levels of 17β-estradiol are much lower than those seen in slender girls. There is a significant association of obesity, impaired glucose tolerance, and endometrial carcinoma.

TREATMENT OF OBESITY

Weight reduction in obese individuals is associated with significantly decreased risk of atherosclerotic cardiovascular disease and decreased rate of mortality.

The metabolic sequelae of weight reduction are also apparent. Data from the Framingham study show that men achieved a mean fall of 11 mg/dL in serum cholesterol levels after a 10% reduction in body weight. Serum levels of glucose and uric acid were also decreased, as was systolic blood pressure.

Efforts to reduce body weight in hyperplastic obesity—ie, in patients with increased adipose cellularity resulting from early proliferation of adipocytes—are frequently unsuccessful. These patients often have no insulin resistance, and the significance of their obesity with respect to carbohydrate and lipid metabolism is therefore probably less than in the case of patients with adult-onset obesity. Especially energetic efforts should be made toward weight reduction in patients with truncal obesity. Management of any obese patient must be individualized and based on information obtained from a complete history of family and environmental factors, eating habits, appetite, and physical activity patterns. The patient's attitude toward and desire for weight loss must be assessed. Causes of secondary obesity that may require specific treatment must be identified by physical examination or appropriate laboratory studies.

The central elements in management are diet and those psychologic interventions that promote adherence to the diet. Exercise, when physical status permits, is a useful adjunct not only because it increases caloric expenditure but also because it has a mood-elevating effect for many people. Infrequently, anorectic drugs may be useful in the short term when a patient has not responded to diet, but they should be used with caution because of their potential for abuse. Even less frequently, in some morbidly obese patients, mechanical interventions may be employed. Patients should be counseled not to expect daily loss of weight, because some water-soluble cell constituents may be retained along with water for brief periods as triglycerides are removed. Ideally, the calories should be distributed over at least 3 meals. Patients should be advised to prepare their food in attractive ways and to eat slowly. Careful dietary counseling should be given to ensure adequate intake of protein, vitamins, and minerals.

Claims have been made for various extreme dietary regimens. One of these, total fasting, leads to substantial ketosis that induces anorexia. A variation of this diet involves severe restriction of carbohydrate; another involves feeding of protein with essentially no carbohydrate or fat. In all these diets, hyperuricemia, hypercholesterolemia, and cholelithiasis may occur. Prolonged metabolic acidosis may lead to demineralization of bone. Certainly, patients with insulin-dependent diabetes, liver disease, renal disease, or gout should not undertake these extreme diet regimens.

A number of cases of sudden death have been reported in patients ingesting only collagen-based liquid formulas. These deaths are attributed to ventricular arrhythmias resulting from electrolyte disturbances. Supplementation with potassium is not sufficient to prevent arrhythmias, however, and other micronutrients appear to be involved. Because of their intermittence, there is no way of anticipating the appearance of the arrhythmias, which can occur as early as 10 days after commencement of the diet. However, use of a balanced fixed-composition liquid formula as a substitute for one ordinary meal a day may facilitate successful initiation of weight loss.

Experience with very low calorie diets indicates that they may be safe in most patients if they supply necessary minerals, vitamins, and enough protein of high biologic value to meet the amino acid requirements of the body. Only patients in good general health should be given these diets, and regular medical supervision, with visits at least every 2 weeks, is important. Very low calorie diets are contraindicated in children and in pregnant or lactating women. Numerous side effects include diarrhea, orthostatic hypotension, muscle cramps, amenorrhea, a sense of coldness, thinning of the skin, and hair loss. Because nearly 50% of patients experience some side effects, these diets should be reserved for those patients in whom weight loss is medically imperative and for whom conventional diets have failed in the face of appropriate behavior modification.

In general, consistent application of a nutritionally balanced reducing diet appears to be the most judicious course. In patients with severe chylomicronemia, fat should be restricted specifically to achieve the greatest reduction in plasma triglycerides. Alcohol should be avoided by patients with hypertriglyceridemia. Patients must be seen frequently for nutritional monitoring and psychologic support if success is to be achieved.

Psychologic Interventions

In patients who prove refractory to the initial dietary intervention, it is important to evaluate underlying psychologic mechanisms more thoroughly. Psychotherapy, group therapy, and behavior modification are all of potential benefit. The latter technique, particularly when used in a group format, appears to effect a modest reduction in weight that is generally better maintained than that produced by other nonsurgical methods. In morbidly obese patients, the weight loss will not be sufficient, but behavior modification may be of some help in avoiding relapse. The most successful weight loss and long-term weight maintenance programs employ behavior modification, general nutritional education, dietary counseling, and an individualized exercise program.

In a seriously disturbed patient, rapid weight reduction may lead to severe depression or even psychosis. Goals for weight loss in any patient must be individualized. Reduction to ideal body weight is not realistic for the patient with the lifelong type of obesity. Supportive therapy, building on the patient's strengths, should be the goal in such cases rather than persistent striving for the unattainable. Physicians must be aware of the importance of their relationship with the obese patient and the patient's need for help in achieving a sense of personal worth.

Drug Therapy

Drugs that will increase thermogenesis safely or direct fatty acids toward oxidation rather than storage eventually may be introduced. Currently available agents are directed at appetite suppression. A group of these appears to act through adrenergic mechanisms; some are associated with effects on blood pressure and heart rate, making them undesirable in patients with cardiovascular disease, and others appear to have significant abuse potential. Among those with the least apparent abuse potential and cardiovascular effects are diethylpropion, mazindol, and phentermine. The use of these drugs, however, has been associated with cardiovascular and neurologic adrenergic effects and, in the case of diethylpropion, with bone marrow suppression. None of these agents should be given to women who are or may become pregnant.

Other currently available agents have a mechanism of action that appears to involve the appetite-suppressing effects of increased levels of serotonin in blood. This is presumed to be the mechanism of action of fenfluramine. This agent also has many side effects. Its cardiovascular side effects may include systemic hypertension or hypotension and pulmonary hypertension. A variety of central nervous system effects have been described; this agent should not be given to persons with psychiatric disorders or to those consuming alcohol.

Surgical Treatment

Jejunoileal bypass was formerly employed to induce intestinal malabsorption in patients with morbid obesity. However, the morbidity and mortality rates were unacceptable. Gastric procedures have replaced intestinal surgery, and a number of techniques of bypass and gastroplasty have been tried. The American Society for Clinical Nutrition has developed guidelines for selection of patients for surgery. Because of serious and potentially lethal complications, surgery should be considered only for individuals with extreme, life-threatening obesity. Close, long-term follow-up is essential.

Other Mechanical Treatments

Jaw wiring is being performed very infrequently, because although weight is usually lost, it is almost always regained. Balloon bezoars endoscopically inserted into the stomach have caused gastric erosion and intestinal obstruction and produce no differences in weight loss when compared to sham-operated controls. Weight is regained promptly. A recent national conference recommended that gastric balloons be used only in approved clinical trials.

REFERENCES

Alpers DH: Surgical therapy for obesity. *N Engl J Med* 1983;**308:**1026.

Amer P et al: Influence of obesity on the antilipolytic effect of insulin in isolated human fat cells obtained before and after glucose ingestion. *J Clin Invest* 1984;**73:**873.

Bray GA, Gray DS: Obesity. 1. Pathogenesis. 2. Treatment. *West J Med* 1988;**149:**429, 555.

Bogardus C et al: Familial dependence of the resting metabolic rate. *N Engl J Med* 1986;**315:**96.

Donahue RP et al: Central obesity and coronary heart disease in men. *Lancet* 1987;**1:**821.

Edman CD, MacDonald PC: Effect of obesity on conversion of plasma androstenedione to estrone in ovulatory and anovulatory young women. *Am J Obstet Gynecol* 1978;**130:**456.

Flier JS: Insulin receptors and insulin resistance. *Annu Rev Med* 1983;**34:**145.

Foster WR, Burton BT (editors): Health implications of obesity. (National Institutes of Health Consensus Development Conference.) *Ann Intern Med* 1985;**103(6–Part 2 Suppl):**981. [Entire issue.]

Garrison RJ et al: Obesity and lipoprotein cholesterol in the Framingham offspring study. *Metabolism* 1980;**29:**1053.

Kannel WB, Gordon T: Page 125 in: *Physiological and Medical Concomitants of Obesity: The Framingham Study.*

Publication No. (NIH) 79-359. Bray GA (editor). US Department of Health, Education, and Welfare, 1975.

Keill N (editor): *Psychology of Obesity.* Thomas, 1973.

Knittle JL et al: The growth of adipose tissue in children and adolescents: Cross-sectional and longitudinal studies of adipose cell number and size. *J Clin Invest* 1979;**63:**239.

Mott DM et al: Altered insulin binding to monocytes and diploid fibroblasts from obese donors. *J Clin Endocrinol Metab* 1983;**57:**1.

Pedersen O, Hjollund E, Sorensen NS: Insulin receptor binding and insulin action in human fat cells: Effects of obesity and fasting. *Metabolism* 1982;**31:**884.

Ravussin E et al: Reduced rate of energy expenditure as a risk factor for body-weight gain. *N Engl J Med* 1988;**318:**467.

Roberts SB et al: Energy expenditure and intake in infants born to lean and overweight mothers. *N Engl J Med* 1988;**318:**461.

Siiteri PK: Extraglandular estrogen formation and serum binding of estradiol: Relationship to cancer. *J Endocrinol* 1981;**89:**119.

Sjöström L, William-Olsson T: Prospective studies on adipose tissue development in man. *Int J Obes* 1981;**5:**597.

Stunkard AJ et al: An adoption study of human obesity. *N Engl J Med* 1986;**314:**193.

Hormones & Cancer

26

Christopher C. Benz, MD, & Brian J. Lewis, MD

HORMONAL EFFECTS ON TUMORS

GROWTH PROMOTION & MALIGNANT TRANSFORMATION

It would be logical to suppose that hormones which support normal growth might also promote tumorigenesis. However, although a great deal is known about endocrine factors regulating normal pre- and postnatal growth, very little from that body of information can be applied to our current understanding of tumorigenesis. Growth hormone (GH), thyroid hormone, insulin, and sex and adrenal steroids have permissive roles in prenatal growth (see Chapter 8). Of these hormones, only the sex steroids directly stimulate tissue growth during the postnatal period; genetic rather than endocrine factors play the major role in determining body stature. Gigantism, for example, results from excessive secretion of GH by a pituitary tumor; however, the end-organ tropic responses to GH as well as the responses to thyroxine and insulin are mediated by mitogenic growth factors that have also been called somatomedins (see Chapter 7). Specifically, somatomedins C and A (also known as insulinlike growth factors, IGF-I and IGF-II) are polypeptides with structural homology to proinsulin, and their serum concentrations are regulated by hormones. Acting via membrane receptors, these somatomedins and other more recently identified growth factors directly stimulate growth and proliferation of both normal and neoplastic cells. Several of the better characterized growth factors of nonhematopoietic and nonlymphoid tissue origin are shown in Table 26–1; recent reviews on cellular growth factors and their relation to cellular oncogenes are also provided in the reference list that accompanies this chapter.

In brief, many human tumors appear to produce, perhaps constitutively, mitogenic polypeptides that are called cellular or transforming growth factors (TGF). In addition, tumor cells synthesize membrane-binding proteins for these same growth factors, and these growth factor receptors commonly possess protein

Acronyms Used in This Chapter	
ACTH	Adrenocorticotropic hormone
APUD	Amine precursor uptake and decarboxylation
CCK	Cholecystokinin
CMF	Cyclophosphamide, methotrexate, fluorouracil
DES	Diethylstilbestrol
DNA	Deoxyribonucleic acid
EGF	Epidermal growth factor
ER	Estrogen receptor(s)
FGF	Fibroblast growth factor
FSH	Follicle-stimulating hormone
GH	Growth hormone
GnRH	Gonadotropin-releasing hormone
hCG	Human chorionic gonadotropin
IGF-I	Insulinlike growth factor-I (somatomedin C)
IGF-II	Insulinlike growth factor-II (somatomedin A)
LH	Luteinizing hormone
LTR	Long terminal repeat (segments)
MMTV	Murine mammary tumor virus
NGF	Nerve growth factor
PDGF	Platelet-derived growth factor
PgR	Progesterone receptor(s)
PRL	Prolactin
PSA	Prostate-specific antigen
SIADH	Syndrome of inappropriate secretion of vasopressin (antidiuretic hormone)
TGFα, TGFβ	Transforming growth factors
TSH	Thyroid-stimulating hormone (thyrotropin)
VIP	Vasoactive intestinal polypeptide

kinase activity that transduces the mitogenic signal from cytoplasm to nucleus. Many of these growth factors and receptors are encoded by DNA sequences that are homologous or identical to normal proto-oncogene sequences (eg, c-*sis* and PDGF beta chain, c-*int*-2 and basic FGF; also, c-*erb* B-1 and EGF receptor, c-*src* and IGF-I receptor), indicating that a structural relationship exists between cellular growth-promoting mechanisms and oncogene products (Table 26–1).

Proto-oncogenes are cellular genes believed to have been captured and recombined into the transform-

Table 26–1. Growth factors and receptors potentially involved in the autocrine and paracrine regulation of human tumor growth.

Growth Factor (Homologous Oncogene)	Tissue Source of Factor	Receptor (Homologous Oncogene) Expressed by Normal Target
EGF	Submaxillary gland, Brunner's glands	170 kD tyrosine kinase (c-*erb* B-1) on epithelial and mesenchymal cells.
TGF-α	Transformed cells, placenta, embryos	Cross-reacts with EGF receptor on same cells.
TGF-β	Platelets, kidney, placenta	615 kD tyrosine kinase on epithelial, epidermal, and mesenchymal cells.
PDGF (c-*sis* with beta chain)	Platelets, endothelial cells, placenta	185 kD tyrosine kinase on smooth muscle, mesenchymal cells, and placenta.
IGF-I/ Somatomedin C	Liver, smooth muscle, other cells	450 kD tyrosine kinase (c-*ros* and c-*src* with beta chain) on epithelial and mesenchymal cells.
IGF-II/ Somatomedin A	Fetal liver, placenta	250 kD glycoprotein on epithelial and mesenchymal cells.
FGF (*int*-2 with basic form)	Brain, pituitary, kidney, cartilage	Possible intracellular receptor in endothelial and mesenchymal cells.
NGF	Submaxillary gland, keratinocytes	130 kD protein kinase on sympathetic and sensory neurons, melanocytes.

ing genes found in certain oncogenic retroviruses. Although yet unproved, the intracellular activation of these proto-oncogenes is thought to account for the development and progression of a variety of human cancers. Carcinogenic mutation, chromosomal rearrangement, and gene amplification are several of the known genetic mechanisms that can activate normal proto-oncogenes.

Specific studies have addressed the development of tumors occurring in hormonally regulated tissues. It is known that both chemical carcinogens (including steroidal and nonsteroidal estrogens) and the genomic integration of viral DNA can potentially induce tumorigenesis. Long-term or in utero exposure to exogenous estrogens is epidemiologically associated with an increased incidence of human uterine and breast carcinomas. It is also known that murine mammary cancers are commonly induced by the murine mammary tumor virus (MMTV), which is a weakly oncogenic type B retrovirus. The regional insertion of MMTV DNA activates genomic c-*int*-1 or c-*int*-2 proto-oncogenes, which are then constitutively expressed in mammary epithelium, leading to pre-malignant hyperplastic lesions and, finally, to infiltrating adenocarcinomas. Since there are closely linked steroid receptor-binding sequences within the integrated MMTV long terminal repeat (LTR) segment, this process of malignant transformation can be promoted by exposure to steroids. In transgenic animal experiments, fusion of the MMTV LTR promoter region to various oncogenes (including c-*myc*, v-Ha-*ras*, c-*int*-1, and activated c-*neu*/*erb* B-2), and introduction of these fused constructs into viable eggs of female mice leads to breast tumors in otherwise normal mouse offspring. Despite widespread genomic incorporation of the transgene in all mouse tissues, only breast, salivary gland, and epididymal tissues express the incorporated oncogene, and essentially only breast adenocarcinomas occur over a time course and with an increased incidence that depends on the particular oncogene. To date, the most effective breast cancer-inducing construct is the MMTV/c-*neu* transgene, which encodes an activated EGF receptorlike molecule that has potent tyrosine kinase activity. Although preliminary, these basic studies have also provided important insights into the molecular mechanisms underlying hormone-dependent tumor promotion in humans. One notable finding is an apparent correlation between clinically aggressive disease and amplification of c-*int*-2 and overexpression of c-*neu*/*erb* B-2 in a significant percentage of human breast tumors.

TUMOR GROWTH MEDIATED BY AUTOCRINE & PARACRINE FACTORS

During human growth and development, as well as during normal tissue response to injury, proliferation and invasion of diploid cells is regulated by exogenous and endogenous cellular growth factors. In the absence of these mitogenic factors, normal cells will become reversibly arrested in G1/G0 phase, permitting normal expression of the differentiated phenotype. In the process of tumorigenesis, these growth factors become inappropriately and constitutively activated, leading to the invasive and autonomous growth that characterizes malignancy. Ectopic expression of these growth factors may also account for a host of other tumor-related complications. Specific factors such as nerve growth factor (NGF), which are important for the maintenance and differentiation of some normal cells (eg, sensory and sympathetic neurons), may exert mitogenic effects on other related cells (eg, adrenal chromaffin cells). These effects may explain the selective expression of specific factors in certain types of malignant tumors (eg, pheochromocytomas, melanomas, and small-cell carcinomas). The concept that autonomous tumor growth can be driven by unregulated expression of locally produced and locally acting growth factors is exemplified by the mitogenic effect of NGF on cells derived from neural crest. Normal keratinocytes express mitogenic concentrations of NGF, which can stimulate local melanocytes or melanoma cells that possess NGF receptors to overexpress the growth-related oncogenes c-*myc* and c-*fos*. This potential model of tumorigenesis illustrates the functional relationship between growth factors and oncogenes that may exist in addition to the structural relationship described earlier.

There are now abundant in vitro and in vivo models showing growth factor production by a tumor that also possesses receptors for the same autostimulating factor (autocrine loop). Autocrine factors synthesized by some activated oncogenes (eg, c-*sis*) may not even be secreted extracellularly; rather, they may be simply bound to internally sequestered receptors that, when stimulated, result in malignant transformation. Possibly as important in tumorigenesis as the autocrine loop is a more indirect process of autostimulation in which transformed cells recruit local normal cells of stromal or epithelial origin to secrete growth factors that stimulate the receptor-bearing malignant cells (paracrine loop). This paracrine interdependence between adjacent normal and malignant tissues may also explain a variety of commonly observed neoplastic phenomena, including site-specific metastases, fibroblast and endothelial chemotaxis and proliferation (leading to stromal reactivity and tumor neovascularity), local bone resorption or malignant hypercalcemia, and suppression of normal immune reactions seen with advancing malignancy.

Hormonal influences on tumor-promoting autocrine and paracrine loops have been well described in studies using cultured human breast cancer cell lines. For example, estrogen-induced growth stimulation of receptor-positive tumor cells actually occurs via rapid modulation of autocrine and paracrine growth factor release by estradiol. Estradiol enhances breast cancer cell production of autostimulating mitogens, such as TGF-α, EGF, IGF-I, and IGF-II, and of paracrine factors, such as PDGF. Additionally, estradiol can depress synthesis of the bifunctional growth factor, TGF-β, which normally inhibits proliferation of breast cancer epithelial cells while paradoxically stimulating growth of mesenchymal cells. The net paracrine effect from PDGF, IGF-II, and TGF-β causes a rapid increase in fibroblast expression of several oncogenes (eg, c-*myc*, c-*fos*, c-*jun*) and the release of additional growth factors that can mitogenically stimulate breast cancer cells. Besides inducing a stromal proliferative response, these paracrine influences also stimulate fibroblasts to enzymatically alter the local composition of basement membrane and extracellular matrix, facilitating further invasion and growth by the malignant mammary epithelial cells.

STEROID-DEPENDENT TUMORS

The early studies of Bittner, Huggins, Furth, and others established the concept that sex steroids can cause or at least promote tumor growth. Until recently, the only cancers believed to be promoted by sex steroids included the common tumors arising from breast (male and female), endometrial, and prostatic tissue (Table 26–2).

It may be generally true that endocrine dependency can develop as an associated trait of tumors derived from any tissue whose normal growth is stimulated by a hormone. Studies in fact have demonstrated associations between sex steroids (especially estrogens) and vaginal, ovarian, and laryngeal carcinomas as well as hepatomas. It has been suggested that sex steroids alone may play a pathogenic role in almost 30% of all cancer cases in the USA. Thyroid, testicular, and ovarian tumors occur in glands under the tropic influences of TSH, FSH, and LH and may also be putatively included in the list of endocrine-dependent cancers. With increasing epidemiologic data, it is likely that

Table 26–2. Endocrine-responsive tumors.

Primary treatment involves endocrine therapy
  Breast carcinoma
  Endometrial carcinoma
  Prostatic carcinoma
  Leukemia
  Lymphoma
Tumor treatment may include endocrine therapy
  Renal cell carcinoma
  Thyroid carcinoma
  Ovarian carcinoma
  Pituitary adenoma
Tumor subsets may be endocrine-dependent
  Vaginal carcinoma
  Meningioma
  Melanoma and apudoma
  Gastrointestinal carcinoma
  Sarcoma

this list will increase. For example, the incidence of osteosarcoma closely parallels the different age-specific growth patterns of men and women, implicating pubertal hormonal changes in the etiology of this tumor. Meningiomas and thyroid and renal cell carcinomas show a marked discrepancy in male-female incidence (and prognosis), also suggesting trophic sex hormone influences on tumor growth.

In contrast to the tropic sex steroids, glucocorticoids are capable of cytolytic responses mediated by steroid-induced enzymatic pathways. Since the realization several decades ago that glucocorticoids could lyse human lymphoblasts, these steroids have been extensively employed in the treatment of leukemia and lymphoma.

TUMORS AFFECTING ENDOCRINE STATUS

Tumors that are not hormone-responsive (or amenable to endocrine therapy) may still affect endocrine status, and these tumor-induced endocrine effects are important for clinical diagnosis and management.

NONSECRETORY TUMORS

Nonsecretory primary or metastatic tumors may invade and replace normal glandular tissue and thereby cause loss of endocrine function. The most common syndrome in this category is hypopituitarism due to pressure necrosis that occurs gradually during tumor growth or that occurs abruptly from tumor infarction and bleeding. Tumors such as breast cancer, leukemia, or lymphoma may be metastatic to the sella; may directly invade, as with a craniopharyngioma or hypothalamic glioma; or may originate from a primary adenoma in the anterior pituitary. Rarely, infarction of the posterior pituitary and the clinical development of diabetes insipidus may be the presenting sign of metastatic cancer. Adrenal insufficiency can also occur with metastatic infiltration of both glands by a variety of epithelial cancers (eg, lung cancer, breast cancer, melanoma). However, clinical evidence of adrenal insufficiency produced by metastatic infiltration is unusual relative to the high overall incidence of adrenal metastases found at autopsy. Although extensive pancreatic or ovarian replacement can occur with metastatic retroperitoneal tumor spread, diabetes mellitus or ovarian failure virtually never results. Ovarian failure may develop in association with a primary ovarian carcinoma that secretes steroid precursors which in turn inhibit pituitary gonadotropin production.

SECRETORY TUMORS

Several types of benign and malignant tumors secrete hormones or hormonelike substances. When these chemicals are produced ectopically or "inappropriately" (by a tumor arising in a tissue not normally associated with the hormone), the resulting paraneoplastic syndrome may provide a diagnostic clue or may signify recurrence of an otherwise undetectable lesion (see Chapter 27). For example, gynecomastia associated with an elevated titer of human chorionic gonadotropin (hCG) strongly suggests an underlying testicular carcinoma that can be cured with chemotherapy. "Appropriate" hormone production by secretory tumors arising within endocrine tissue may also produce symptoms leading to early tumor detection and cure, as is occasionally observed with insulinomas. On the other hand, endocrine symptoms from secretory tumors may develop in association with advanced disease and result in life-threatening or debilitating clinical complications. Palliation of symptoms of carcinoid or one of the other apudomas (see Chapter 27) can actually become of greater clinical concern than controlling the tumor itself, and symptomatic control of these unresectable lesions can only be achieved with chemotherapeutic agents. These secretory tumors are usually well differentiated and may occur in genetic patterns (eg, Klinefelter's syndrome associated with a breast or pituitary tumor) or in familial patterns involving multiple endocrine glands (eg, multiple endocrine neoplasia type I, IIa, or IIb; see Chapter 28). Table 26–3 lists the

Table 26–3. Secretory tumors of endocrine glands.

Tumor Origin	Secretory Product(s)
Anterior pituitary	GH, PRL, ACTH, TSH, FSH, LH
Adrenal	
Cortex	Aldosterone, glucocorticoids, androgens, estrogens (rare)
Medulla	Catecholamines
Kidney	Erythropoietin
Gonads	
Germ cell, trophoblast	hCG
Stroma	Estrogens, androgens, progestins
Pancreas and gut (APUD cells)	Serotonin, kallikrein, prostaglandins, somatostatin, gastrin, glucagon, insulin, VIP, CCK, vasopressin, ACTH, neurotensin
Parathyroids	Parathyroid hormone
Thyroid	
Parafollicular (medullary) cells	Calcitonin
Follicular cells	Thyroglobulin, T_3 and T_4 (rare)

origin of commonly occurring secretory tumors and their associated secretory products.

TREATMENT-INDUCED ENDOCRINOPATHY

With the improved prognosis of patients with leukemia, lymphoma, stage II breast cancer, and germ cell neoplasms treated with irradiation and chemotherapy, there is a growing awareness of the long-term endocrine complications of treatment. The glands associated with treatment-induced endocrinopathy include the hypothalamus, pituitary, thyroid, parathyroids, and gonads. As shown in Table 26–4, local or regional effects from radiation therapy and the systemic effects of radiomimetic drugs (alkylating agents) produce the greatest clinical problems.

Brain & Pituitary

Children receiving cranial irradiation either to prevent leukemia of the central nervous system or to treat a curable brain tumor have blunted GH responses, impaired growth rates, and some impairment of intellectual function. Less commonly, they may have reduced secretion of TSH, ACTH, FSH, and LH. In adults, apart from the use of hormonal agents, antitumor therapy results in very few abnormalities in the hypothalamic-pituitary-neuroendocrine axis. Adjuvant chemotherapy for breast cancer has been reported to lower serum PRL levels, but the underlying mechanism is unclear. Vincristine and cyclophosphamide have both been associated with a syndrome of inappropriate secretion of vasopressin (antidiuretic hormone), or SIADH. While a direct effect on renal tubules is be-

lieved to be the cause of the antidiuresis that occurs with cyclophosphamide, vincristine may increase vasopressin release by disrupting microtubules within the neurohypophysis.

Thyroid

One-third of patients with cervical lymphomas or carcinomas of the pharynx or larynx treated with curative doses of radiation (which includes the thyroid) develop increased TSH levels, and most of these also develop decreased thyroxine levels. A few become clinically hypothyroid. Both low-dose and (less frequently) high-dose irradiation increase the incidence of thyroid carcinomas occurring 10 or more years after treatment (see Chapter 10).

Adrenals

Adrenal gland function appears resistant to the toxic effects of conventional doses of radiation or chemotherapy. However, prolonged busulfan administration for chronic granulocytic leukemia results in a clinical syndrome resembling adrenocortical insufficiency. Some investigators believe that pituitary secretion of ACTH—rather than adrenocortical function—is damaged by the drug. This mechanism could be similar to that resulting in impaired PRL secretion, mentioned above.

Gonads

Perhaps the most frequently encountered endocrinopathy resulting from antitumor therapy is gonadal failure. Radiation therapy and chemotherapy can cause infertility in both men and women. In women, amenorrhea (or oligomenorrhea), dyspareunia, decreased libido, and hot flushes may follow either form

Table 26–4. Treatment-induced endocrinopathy.

	Hormone Abnormality	Clinical Abnormality
Radiation therapy Brain	↓ GH; less commonly, ↓ TSH, ACTH, FSH, LH	Growth retardation.
Head and neck Low-dose (≤ 750 rads)	↑ Parathyroid hormone	Hyperparathyroidism, thyroid cancer.
High-dose (≥ 1400 rads)	↓ Thyroxine; ↑ TSH	Hypothyroidism, thyroid cancer.
Abdomen and pelvis (including gonads)	↓ Estrogen; ↑ FSH, LH	Sterility, menopause, azoospermia.
Chemotherapy Alkylating agents, vinblastine, others	↓ Estrogen; ↑ FSH, LH (normal testosterone, adrenal steroids)	Sterility, menopause, azoospermia.
Vincristine	↑ Vasopressin	SIADH[1]
Cyclophosphamide	(Normal vasopressin)	SIADH[1]
Mitotane	↓ Adrenal steroids	Primary adrenal insufficiency.
Aminoglutethimide	↓ Estrogens, adrenal steroids	Primary adrenal insufficiency.
	↓ Thyroxine; ↑ TSH	Hypothyroidism.

[1]Syndrome of inappropriate secretion of vasopressin (antidiuretic hormone).

of therapy. These symptoms are associated with reduced plasma estradiol and increased levels of FSH and LH. In fact, ovarian failure occurs so frequently after adjuvant chemotherapy for breast cancer that some have suggested that the effectiveness of adjuvant therapy results from "chemical oophorectomy." In younger women, there is a greater probability that gonadal function will return to normal. In men, azoospermia (or oligospermia) occurs in association with reduced testicular size, increased FSH, and (occasionally) gynecomastia. Leydig cells are much more resistant to toxic therapy, and serum testosterone levels therefore usually remain normal, although there may be evidence for partial Leydig cell failure compensated for by higher levels of LH. Depending on radiation or drug dosage, male gonadal function and fertility may recover. With the aggressive drug combinations used to cure lymphomas, however, gonadal recovery is unlikely, and men should be offered the opportunity for sperm storage before chemotherapy begins. Recent successes with in vitro fertilization and cryopreservation have provided a similar option for women. GnRH analogues, which decrease serum gonadotropin levels, are currently being investigated for their ability to protect the gonads during cytotoxic therapy. The use of birth control pills to reversibly suppress gonadotropins and suspend ovarian function has reportedly been successful in sparing women from gonadal toxicity during chemotherapy. It should be recognized that gonadal toxicity varies with the type of chemotherapy being used; alkylating agents and procarbazine are the most potent toxins. Certain combinations of drugs used to treat lymphomas may, in fact, cause little permanent gonadal damage.

ENDOCRINE THERAPY FOR CANCER

STEROID RECEPTORS & TREATMENT

At present, endocrine treatment is of major therapeutic value in breast, endometrial, and prostatic cancers. The specific applications of endocrine therapy in these diseases will be discussed later. However, the measurement of steroid receptors has added a further refinement to the technology of determining which tumors are endocrine-sensitive. Estrogen receptors (ER) and progesterone receptors (PgR), useful for predicting the clinical responsiveness of breast cancer, are now being detected in a variety of other human tumors, including ovarian and endometrial carcinomas, hepatomas, sarcomas, meningiomas, renal cell carcinomas, as well as melanomas and colorectal and pancreatic carcinomas. On average, however, most of these tumors have a very low frequency of receptor positivity and a much lower receptor content than that found in breast cancer. Thus, with the exception of endometrial cancer, clinical studies have failed to detect a significant role for endocrine therapy in the management of these other tumors.

The mere presence of a steroid receptor does not ensure either a functioning receptor mechanism or a cytostatic or cytolytic response when endocrine treatment is employed. For example, glucocorticoids are known to alter liver metabolism, but they do not produce the cytolytic effects on hepatocytes that are observed with lymphocytes, although both cell types contain high levels of glucocorticoid receptor. Additionally, ER-positive tumors capable of making PgR are the breast tumors most responsive to endocrine treatment. While most endocrine agents do not exert their antitumor effects by binding to PgR, the mere presence of PgR identifies those tumor subsets with a well-functioning ER mechanism. In short, the therapeutic importance of receptors depends on both a functioning receptor mechanism and a growth-regulating receptor response.

Additional comments should be made in reference to the potential clinical significance of the different available means of assaying for tumor ER and PgR content. Biochemical assays have traditionally involved the competitive binding of a radioligand to a cell-free receptor extract prepared by homogenizing fresh tumor specimens. The calculated receptor content (fmol/mg protein cytosol) is very sensitive to procedural conditions, provides no measure of receptor heterogeneity within the tumor specimen, and can be falsely depressed by endogenous or exogenously administered receptor-binding agents. For instance, it has been shown that exogenously administered nonsteroidal antiestrogens can depress receptor levels to about 25% of their pretreatment values; thus, it is recommended that at least 2 months elapse after treatment cessation before assaying the tumor if the assay technique utilizes competitive ligand binding. Treatment with radiation therapy or chemotherapy may result in a true reduction in receptor levels, independent of the assay procedure, and this may persist for 12–24 months following cessation of therapy. New assays utilizing monoclonal antibodies to measure ER and PgR content are easier to perform, and they avoid the problems related to receptor occupation by competing ligands. Monoclonal antibody assays provide an immunohistochemical means of assessing receptor heterogeneity within tumor tissue and permit the detection of receptor-positive cells in small cytologic samples, eg, fine needle aspiration biopsies of tumors. Furthermore, immunohistochemical assay enables the unequivocal detection of receptor-positive malignant cells within receptor-positive normal tissue, such as occurs with uterine cancers. Table 26–5 relates the incidence of ER positivity (assayed by monoclonal antibody) of newly diagnosed breast, endometrial, and

Table 26–5. Response to endocrine therapy of tumors known to contain estrogen receptor (ER).

Tumor Type	Percentage Positive for ER	Rate of Response to Endocrine Therapy[1]
Breast carcinoma	50–60%	30%
Endometrial carcinoma	40–50%	30%
Ovarian carcinoma	30–40%	<20%

[1]Objective clinical response after antiestrogen or progestin therapy in advanced cases unselected with regard to ER status.

ovarian cancer samples with the clinical response rates observed when treating unselected advanced cases with endocrine therapy (antiestrogen or progestins). Clinical response rates for selected ER-positive tumor patients are only available for breast cancer, and these will be reviewed in a later section.

RECEPTOR AGONISTS & ANTAGONISTS

Surgeons in the late 19th century first observed the regression of breast cancer following bilateral oophorectomy, thus marking the beginning of endocrine therapy and the awareness of endocrine-dependent tumors. Surgical ablation has only recently been challenged by drugs that can chemically ablate selected endocrine organs. Unfortunately, the long-standing empiricism surrounding endocrine therapy has not yet been totally supplanted by scientific rationale. Although the biology and biochemistry of ER and PgR are of primary importance in predicting breast cancer treatment response and prognosis, at present there is insufficient experience on which to base any recommendations about using receptor data in deciding upon the clinical management of prostatic cancer, leukemia, or lymphoma.

The empiricism of endocrine therapy is also evident from studies showing little difference in response rates when receptor agonists or antagonists are compared with surgical ablative therapy. For example, premenopausal breast cancer patients respond to either oophorectomy, tamoxifen, or medroxyprogesterone acetate. Similarly, patients with prostatic carcinoma respond equally well to orchiectomy, diethylstilbestrol (DES) or GnRH analogues. These generalities seem puzzling only because of our limited understanding of receptor function and the mechanisms resulting in either cytostatic or cytolytic tumor control and of the effect of treatment on hypothalamic and pituitary factors that also modify tumor growth. How do we explain that when hormone agonists bind to cellular receptors in tumors, they can trigger either a complete or a partial response? Prolonged agonist binding may exhaust the cellular response or down-regulate the receptor (tachyphylaxis). We also know with certainty that individual tumors are heterogeneous—they may contain subpopulations of cells with and without receptor proteins and with quantitative and qualitative variations in receptor function.

Apart from the commonly administered steroid agonists (estrogens, androgens, progestins, and glucocorticoids), there are also analogues of nonsteroid hormones currently being tested for antitumor potential. For example, bromocriptine and other tight-binding dopamine agonists are capable of shrinking pituitary adenomas. Agonists and antagonists of GnRH that reduce serum PRL and gonadotropin levels can produce clinical responses in breast and prostatic cancers.

The classic concept has been that hormone antagonists bind to receptors and block the subsequent steps to hormonal response, including the signals to undergo cell division and synthesize proteins. However, clinically effective steroid antagonists such as tamoxifen, clomiphene, cyproterone, and flutamide may or may not share the steroid ring structure of the hormones they antagonize and may bind with high affinity to nonreceptor sites within the cytoplasm. Some, in addition to blocking hormonal response, also induce synthesis of bifunctional growth factors and unique proteins with as yet unknown functions. Flow cytometric studies comparing the cell cycle responses of tumors to either antiestrogen administration or estrogen deprivation have shown different points of cell cycle arrest, again suggesting dissimilar mechanisms of antitumor activity. Equally disconcerting to investigators is the therapeutic significance of "spillover" among steroid hormones: the potential cross-reactivity of androgens for ER, progestins for ER and glucocorticoid receptors, and glucocorticoids for androgen receptors.

ENZYME INHIBITORS

Within the subcellular microsome system of endocrine-responsive cells are enzymes necessary for interconverting steroids to more active hormonal derivatives. These enzymes have become the targets of a growing family of synthetic agents used to treat breast and prostatic cancers. Aminoglutethimide was the first of such agents released for use; it was initially introduced as an anticonvulsant in 1960 but then was found to inhibit adrenal steroidogenesis, resulting in "medical adrenalectomy." This drug is now used to treat breast cancer in postmenopausal women and has subsequently been found to be a potent inhibitor of aromatase activity. Aromatase is actually a complex of enzymes found in many extra-adrenal tissues, including breast cancers, that converts circulating androgens to estrogens (see Fig 17–4). The estrogen products (estrone and estradiol) can then bind to intracellular ER and produce estrogen-specific responses.

The predominant circulating estrogen in postmenopausal women is estrone sulfate, which is derived from adrenal steroid synthesis, peripheral aromatization, and hepatic conjugation. To be reutilized in ER-positive tissues, estrone sulfate must first be reactivated by another microsomal enzyme, sulfatase. Active investigation is under way to develop inhibitors of sulfatase that could be used clinically in ovariectomized or postmenopausal women with breast cancer.

Estrogen responsiveness is also related to the activity of a catabolic enzyme, estradiol 17β-dehydrogenase. High-dose medroxyprogesterone acetate exerts part of its antitumor effect by increasing 17β-dehydrogenase levels and internally depriving the breast tumor cells of active estrogens.

COMBINATION ENDOCRINE THERAPY

Medroxyprogesterone acetate and other steroid agonists and antagonists are now being combined with enzyme inhibitors to try to increase endocrine response rates. There can be multiple mechanisms at work when such combinations are employed; for instance, besides increasing 17β-dehydrogenase activity, medroxyprogesterone acetate is also known to suppress adrenal production of androstenedione and thereby deplete cells of their androgenic substrate for aromatase and reduce conversion to estrogen. Thus, combining medroxyprogesterone acetate with aminoglutethimide brings into play at least 2 mechanisms of interaction that could result in enhanced inhibition of ER-positive tumors. Furthermore, higher doses of medroxyprogesterone acetate can bind (spill over) to glucocorticoid receptors, obviating the need for administering replacement doses of cortisol to patients receiving aminoglutethimide.

In benign and malignant prostatic tissues, it is believed that ER-positive stromal cells provide the tropic androgens required by the androgen receptor-containing epithelial cells. In the stromal cells, 5 α-reductase converts testosterone to the most active androgen, dihydrotestosterone. Strategy for the endocrine treatment of prostatic cancers has focused on androgen ablation, by either surgical or medical means. Because of the hormonal interdependence between epithelial and stromal cells and the overall dependence of prostatic tissue on pituitary factors (FSH, LH, and PRL), medical ablation can be accomplished using estrogen agonists and antagonists, GnRH analogues, or inhibitors of 5 α-reductase. All of these nonsurgical modalities are under clinical investigation, and preliminary studies suggest that combining some of these agents may vastly improve response rates in prostatic carcinoma.

CHEMO-ENDOCRINE THERAPY

Combining chemotherapy and endocrine therapy is emerging as a popular treatment approach for endocrine-sensitive tumors (especially breast cancer) de-spite a lack of biochemical or cytokinetic rationale. Estramustine and prednimustine are 2 chemically similar steroid alkylating agents designed to be selectively toxic against receptor-positive cells. At present, it appears that these derivatives are little more effective than their parent compounds, suggesting that impaired receptor binding or systemic drug metabolism is limiting their cytotoxic potential. Simultaneous administration of tamoxifen with drug combinations such as CMF (cyclophosphamide, methotrexate, fluorouracil) may indeed increase response rates in selected groups of breast cancer patients; however, such additive effectiveness has not generally been observed in all patients, in all endocrine-sensitive tumors, or with other drug-hormone combinations. In fact, the potential for adverse therapeutic effects with chemo-endocrine combinations has also been pointed out, and this form of treatment must still be considered investigational. Specifically, by suppressing tumor cell growth, hormonal therapy may protect the tumor from chemotherapeutic agents that are most effective against replicating cells.

In summary, endocrine therapy has a long and established history of empiric usefulness; because the mechanism of its antitumor activity is predominantly cytostatic, the duration of endocrine therapy is necessarily longer than that required for cytotoxic chemotherapy. With the recent emergence of some biochemical understanding of the mechanisms underlying endocrine response and hormonal growth promotion, we are now witnessing the advent of more scientifically based applications. The hope is that this new understanding will lead to better tumor control.

CLINICAL PROBLEMS

BREAST CANCER IN WOMEN

Epidemiology

Breast cancer is a common tumor in the USA. There are over 120,000 new cases annually, and a woman in the USA has roughly a 7–8% lifetime risk of developing the disease. The cause of breast cancer is unknown. Associated risk factors are listed in Table 26–6.

A. Family History: It is well established that the daughters of women with breast cancer are at higher risk of developing the disease than other women in the general population. The highest lifetime risk, 50%, is borne by women whose mothers had bilateral breast cancer with onset before menopause.

B. Menstrual History: Early age at menarche and late age at menopause increase the risk of breast cancer. Conversely, late age at menarche or early menopause (natural or surgical) reduces the risk.

C. Parity: Younger age of the mother at the time of her first pregnancy and history of full-term pregnancy lower the subsequent risk of breast cancer.

D. Population Differences: There are striking variations across cultures in the incidence of breast cancer. Asian women have a much lower risk than women in Western countries. Women of Japanese descent who grow up in the USA have a higher incidence of breast cancer than those who grow up in Japan. Within the USA, the probability of developing breast cancer by age 75 shows significant ethnic variation: 8.2% for whites, 7% for blacks, 4.8% for Hispanics, 2.5% for Native Americans, 5.4% for Japanese Americans, and 6.1% for Chinese Americans.

E. Endogenous Hormones: The data on menstrual function and parity in women—and experimental work in animals, where estrogen is clearly permissive or even carcinogenic in the induction of breast cancer—strongly implicate estrogen exposure as an important factor in the development of breast cancer. Many case control studies have examined estrogen profiles as well as PRL levels, but no clear pattern or association has emerged. There is also no linkage with androgens or thyroid hormone levels. An inherent flaw in these studies is that the induction of breast cancer is a long-term process, and if the estrogen profile of a patient or a control were to be related to cancer, it is probable that a short-term analysis of hormones—a snapshot, as it were—when the cancer was detected would not tell enough of the story. One would need instead a longitudinal, integrated profile starting at least at the menarche in a large cohort of women in order to reliably detect differences in endocrine physiology and relate them to the development of cancer.

F. Exogenous Hormones: Retrospective analyses of users of birth control pills or of postmenopausal women who take estrogen are contradictory. There is, however, some suggestion that increased duration of estrogen exposure may increase the risk of breast cancer. Prospective studies of birth control pill usage do not indicate an increased risk, and there might even be a slight reduction in risk in some studies; but because of the considerable latent period for induction of breast cancer—presumably decades—further observation will be necessary to resolve the issue. The data certainly do not justify withholding birth control pills, but it would be prudent to limit the overall period of use as much as possible. The administration of estrogen to postmenopausal patients is a hotly debated issue, especially because estrogen use is associated with endometrial cancer. The possibility that prolonged use or high doses can increase the risk of breast cancer warrants further caution. One should keep the dose and duration of exposure to exogenous estrogen to a minimum (see Chapter 17).

G. Benign Breast Disease: "Fibrocystic disease" is not a very specific term and usually refers to painful breast nodules that may wax and wane during the menstrual cycle. This commonly diagnosed condition occurs in up to 50% of women and reflects variability in end-organ response to fluctuations in endogenous hormone levels. The condition is less frequent in users of birth control pills and may also respond to the elimination of caffeine from the diet. Histologically, one can see macrocysts, microcysts, adenosis, apocrine change, fibrosis, fibroadenomas, or ductal hyperplasias. These conditions are not found with higher frequency in patients who develop breast cancer, but it has been noted that having had a previous biopsy for benign breast disease increases the relative risk (from 1.86 to 2.13) of developing breast cancer compared to the general population.

Retrospective analysis of a large group of patients was performed to better define who within the benign breast disease category had an increased relative risk for subsequent breast cancer. The presence of a proliferative lesion without atypical hyperplasia (atypia) increased the risk to 1.9 relative to the presence of a nonproliferative lesion without atypia. Atypia increased the risk to 5.3, and patients with atypia plus a family history of breast cancer had a relative risk of 11. It should be noted that the majority of patients (70%) who underwent biopsy for benign breast disease did not have lesions associated with an increased risk of breast cancer.

H. Other Factors: Obese habitus may correlate positively with an increased risk of breast cancer. Ionizing radiation is an established carcinogen. Atomic bomb survivors, patients who received therapeutic radiation for mastitis, and those who had repeated chest fluoroscopy for tuberculosis show increased rates of breast cancer. Cancer in one breast is associated with a 10–20% lifetime chance of developing primary cancer in the opposite breast. A history of endometrial or ovarian cancer also increases the chances for developing breast cancer.

It appears from the above data that the hormonal milieu is a critical element in the development of breast cancer. Estrogen seems to be the most important factor. There may be a dose-response effect, as suggested by the correlation with an increased duration of ovulatory cycling or with obesity. In the latter instance, there may be added estrogen contribution by peripheral conversion of sex steroids in adipose tissue. Early pregnancy may cause subtle changes in the set points for estrogen and PRL levels, or it may induce a protective change at a critical time in the breast tissue itself. In women with a strong family history of breast cancer, endogenous estrogen may enhance some inherent genetic susceptibility to breast carcinogenesis. Radiation is clearly a carcinogen for the breast, but other exogenous factors (eg, diet) that might account for population differences in the attack rate of breast cancer are less easy to document. Diet could be influential through specific elements such as fat or fiber content, or it could have a more complex interaction. The overall calorie content and balance of foodstuffs could produce variations in growth, hormone profiles (anterior pituitary hormones such as GH as well as sex steroids), age at menarche, and the like, and these could influence susceptibility to breast cancer later in life.

Treatment of Metastatic Breast Cancer

A. Steroid Receptors and Other Considerations: Hormonal therapy is a main feature in the treatment of advanced breast cancer. A fairly straightforward algorithm to guide the selection of treatment utilizes the patient's menopausal status and the ER and PgR profile of the tumor (Fig 26–1). The chance of responding to endocrine therapy increases directly with tumor concentrations of ER and PgR. Table 26–7 shows how breast cancer response rates vary with receptor status. These data also indicate that postmenopausal patients are more apt to have receptor-positive tumors than premenopausal patients and, by implication, to respond more frequently to endocrine therapy.

Important ancillary data include the performance status of the patient, the tempo of tumor growth, the extent of visceral involvement, and the prior treatment history. The better the general condition of the patient and the lower the tumor burden, the more likely that an appropriately chosen hormonal treatment will be effective. Since the response to hormonal treatment is often not evident for several weeks and it can take several months for maximum response to occur, patients who are critically ill from breast cancer and require an im-

Table 26–6. Associated risk factors for breast cancer in women.

Family history
Menstrual history
Parity
Population differences
Endogenous hormones
Exogenous hormones
Benign breast disease
Obesity
Ionizing radiation
Prior breast cancer
Prior endometrial or ovarian cancer

mediate antitumor effect should receive chemotherapy. Likewise, patients with explosive tumor growth or with a short interval between mastectomy and the development of metastases are less likely to benefit from hormonal therapy than those with more indolent tumor growth. Skin, soft tissue, lymph nodes, and bone are the metastatic sites most responsive to endocrine maneuvers. Significant lung or liver involvement and brain metastases require chemotherapy and radiation therapy, respectively. Limited lung or liver infiltration may well respond to hormone treatment. The patient who has responded favorably to a prior hormonal maneuver has some likelihood of responding to subsequent endocrine treatment. Conversely, if a patient's tumor is refractory to one form of endocrine therapy, subsequent hormone treatments are usually of

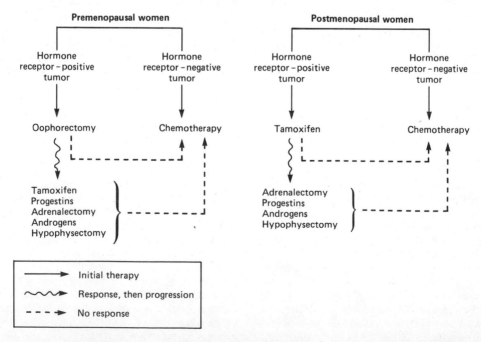

ADVANCED BREAST CANCER

Figure 26–1. Treatment algorithm for advanced breast cancer in women.

Table 26–7. Rates of response to endocrine therapy according to estrogen and progesterone receptors (ER, PgR) in women with breast cancer.[1]

Tumor Receptor Status	Frequency Distribution		Rate of Response to Endocrine Therapy
	Premeno-pausal Women	Postmeno-pausal Women	
ER−, PgR−	30%	19%	11%
ER−, PgR+	9%	3%	46%
ER+, PgR−	12%	23%	27%
ER+, PgR+	49%	55%	77%

[1]Modified and reproduced, with permission, from McGuire WL: Steroid hormone receptors in breast cancer treatment strategy. *Recent Prog Horm Res* 1980;**36**:135.

little value, and it is better to consider starting chemotherapy.

B. Premenopausal Endocrine Therapy: For premenopausal patients with ER-positive tumors, ablative treatment with oophorectomy is one first-line hormonal maneuver, although the antiestrogen tamoxifen appears to be equally effective in this role. However, because it can lead to increased circulating estrogens and gonadotropins—and because (by mass action effect) it may not adequately block the higher endogenous estrogen level—some clinicians believe that tamoxifen may not be entirely equivalent to oophorectomy as first-line treatment in premenopausal patients. Studies also suggest that women who respond favorably to tamoxifen have some chance of responding to oophorectomy, but the converse is not true. In general, the response rate to either oophorectomy or tamoxifen as initial treatment ranges from 30 to 60%, depending upon the level of ER protein and the sites of metastatic disease. Responses average 12–15 months in duration.

In premenopausal patients who respond to oophorectomy or tamoxifen but whose tumors progress, several options are available. They can next receive a trial of progestational agents or androgens. Progestational agents have few side effects, can increase appetite and sense of well-being, and produce clinical response in 15–30% of patients when used as second-line treatment. Androgens are effective in 10–20% of patients but have masculinizing effects. Attempts to develop less virilizing analogues of testosterone have been only moderately successful, and it is argued that the frequency of virilization may not be all that different between various congeners at equipotent antitumor doses. Another ablative maneuver, adrenalectomy—either surgical or medical (using aminoglutethimide)—can be employed as either second- or third-line treatment, with a response rate in the range of 15–30%. Medical adrenalectomy appears equal to surgical ablation in antitumor effect, but its effects are reversible once the drug is stopped. However, like surgical adrenalectomy, it also requires the administration of replacement hydrocortisone. In ad-

dition to maintaining vital functions, this replacement therapy also prevents increased pituitary ACTH production and overriding of the adrenal blockade. Since dexamethasone metabolism is augmented by aminoglutethimide, it should not be used as the replacement steroid during treatment. Up to 30% of patients receiving aminoglutethimide will initially experience somnolence or rash, side effects that usually subside with continued treatment and which can be minimized by gradually working up to full doses over several weeks.

Finally, the development of transsphenoidal surgery has made hypophysectomy a more feasible ablative maneuver. Before the advent of receptor analyses, hypophysectomy was used as palliative treatment in end-stage patients, especially those with extensive and painful bone metastases. Patients who were responders would often awaken from anesthesia with dramatic pain relief. That it occasionally benefits hormone-refractory cases suggests that its palliative effects are not mediated via sex steroid mechanisms. When compared to adrenalectomy in ER-positive tumors as second- or third-line treatment, hypophysectomy is equally effective and may have a slightly longer duration of action. However, the availability of aminoglutethimide, the operative risk, and the requirement for permanent adrenal replacement make hypophysectomy a less desirable option.

Premenopausal patients with ER-negative tumors would bypass endocrine therapy and be placed on a chemotherapy protocol.

C. Postmenopausal Endocrine Therapy: The initial endocrine maneuver in postmenopausal patients with ER-positive tumors is the administration of the antiestrogen tamoxifen. In the recent past, additive therapy with diethylstilbestrol (DES) was used. However, this agent is associated with many more side effects than tamoxifen and has now largely been abandoned. Response rates to tamoxifen or DES range from 30 to 60%, again in proportion to the disease-free interval, metastatic sites, and the ER content of the tumor. Response durations are similar to those for oophorectomy. Once the breast cancer of a patient who has responded to tamoxifen progresses, second-line endocrine therapy is either medical adrenalectomy or administration of progestins, with response rates ranging from 15 to 40%. It should be noted that 10–20% of patients initially failing to respond to tamoxifen may have a clinical response to adrenalectomy. Thus, if the tempo of the disease and the clinical status of the patient permit, one can offer a trial of adrenalectomy before proceeding to chemotherapy.

When DES was in wider use, induction of therapy in patients with skeletal metastases would occasionally be accompanied by a "flare" with exacerbation of bone pain and hypercalcemia. This phenomenon usually heralded a clinical response and did not necessarily require prolonged interruption of treatment. When the cancer of patients who had responded to

DES progressed, drug withdrawal was frequently followed by another clinical remission in up to 30% of patients, and this could last for several months. The flare phenomenon and the response to withdrawal are less frequently seen with tamoxifen; these effects have also been noted to occur with androgen therapy. Postmenopausal patients with ER-negative tumors would bypass hormonal treatment and begin chemotherapy.

Current investigational endocrine agents include cogeners of tamoxifen and a variety of GnRH agonists and antagonists.

BREAST CANCER IN MEN

Cancer of the male breast is extremely rare, occurring with a frequency of about 1% of that of cancer of the female breast. There is an association with Klinefelter's syndrome and with exogenous estrogen exposure (eg, in transsexuals), emphasizing the importance of hormonal factors, especially estrogen.

Up to 80% of tumors in men are ER-positive. Sixty to 70% of patients with metastatic tumors will respond to orchiectomy, and adrenalectomy and hypophysectomy are effective as second-line hormonal treatments. More recently, tamoxifen has shown activity as primary treatment and may eventually supplant orchiectomy. As in female patients with breast cancer, male patients whose tumors become refractory to hormone therapy go on to receive chemotherapy. Androgens are contraindicated because of their potential for facilitating tumor growth.

ENDOMETRIAL CANCER

Epidemiology

There are approximately 30,000 new cases of endometrial cancer annually in the USA. In contrast to the somewhat equivocal role of estrogen in the induction of breast cancer, its place in the causation of endometrial cancer appears more certain.

At the clinical level, as shown in Table 26–8, a variety of conditions have been associated with an increased risk of developing endometrial cancer. Their common denominator is unopposed or increased estrogen stimulation of the endometrium. This produces endometrial hyperplasia, a condition that can in turn

Table 26–8. Conditions associated with an increased risk of developing endometrial cancer.

Prolonged or unopposed estrogen effect on the uterus
Exogenous estrogen administration
Late menopause
Obesity (increased peripheral conversion of precursors to estrogen)
Polycystic ovary syndrome
Ovarian cortical stromal hyperplasia
Estrogen-secreting ovarian tumors

progress to frank cancer. Progesterone antagonizes this effect of estrogen and induces the endometrium to mature or differentiate to a secretory state. Its action may be mediated by augmentation of enzymes in endometrial cells that metabolize estrogen and by decreasing levels of ER in this same tissue. There is a more frequent history of irregular menses in patients who develop endometrial cancer, and while combination birth control pills may have no influence on or may even decrease the risk of uterine cancer, sequential birth control pills may impart an increased risk, possibly because of the days of therapy where only estrogen is being administered.

At the population level, an upsurge in the incidence of endometrial cancer was noted in the USA in the early 1970s. This followed and paralleled an increase in the number of prescriptions written over the preceding years for replacement estrogen therapy in postmenopausal women. Case control studies of this phenomenon have clearly shown that exogenous estrogen use imparts a 3- to 8-fold increase in the risk of developing uterine cancer. The higher the dose and the longer the duration of estrogen use, the greater the risk. One follow-up study from the late 1970s reported that a decline in the number of estrogen prescriptions (after the initial recognition of their association with endometrial cancer) was accompanied by a decline in the incidence of endometrial cancer in the same population base.

Taken together, the above observations strongly support a conservative approach to the use of exogenous estrogens. They should be given in the smallest possible dose, for the shortest duration feasible, and on an intermittent schedule, with consideration given to adding a progestin to the treatment regimen. (See also Chapters 11 and 17 for further discussion of estrogen therapy.)

Treatment of Metastatic Endometrial Cancer

A. Steroid Receptors: As is true in breast cancer, hormonal therapy is a primary therapeutic modality for advanced endometrial cancer. Unlike the situation in breast cancer, receptor profiles are not used to guide treatment selection in cases of endometrial cancer, although it was from uterine tissue that Jensen first isolated and characterized estrogen receptors in the 1960s. Uterine estrogen receptors increase during the proliferative phase of the menstrual cycle and fall in the presence of exogenous progesterone or with the rise of endogenous progesterone during the luteal phase. Progesterone receptors are induced by estrogen, and their level peaks coincident with the estradiol peak in the menstrual cycle. Most endometrial carcinomas contain ER, and, in contrast to breast cancer, levels are higher and inversely proportionate to the degree of histologic differentiation of the tumor. Progesterone receptors are also present in endometrial cancer, and their presence correlates directly with the degree of differentiation. As yet, ER and PgR have no practical application in the management of patients, probably because of the difficulty in distinguishing tumor from receptor-positive normal tissue.

B. Endocrine Therapy: Approximately one-third of metastatic tumors will respond to progestins. The probability of response is highest in patients with the most differentiated tumors and in those with the longest interval between primary treatment and the appearance of metastases. Responders live an average of 2 years after treatment is started, while nonresponding patients survive only about 6 months. Until recently, parenteral preparations such as hydroxyprogesterone and medroxyprogesterone were used. An orally effective compound, megestrol, has simplified treatment and appears to be as potent as the earlier parenteral formulations. Potential side effects of these compounds include salt retention and an increased predisposition to thrombophlebitis.

In patients who progress on progestational therapy or who do not respond initially, disease may be palliated with chemotherapy. However, in many patients, advanced disease stage, poor general health, and a history of pelvic irradiation limit tolerance to the most effective agents, ie, doxorubicin, cyclophosphamide, fluorouracil, and cisplatin.

PROSTATIC CANCER

Epidemiology

There are approximately 55,000 new cases annually of prostatic cancer in the USA. Prostatic cancer is essentially a disease of men in their 60s and 70s, and autopsy series have shown occult carcinoma in over one-third of men over age 70.

Several lines of evidence support the idea that testosterone plays a role in the development of prostatic cancer. Testosterone can induce adenocarcinoma of the prostate in rats; castrated men do not develop prostatic cancer; and the disease is less frequent in patients with cirrhosis. Cirrhotic patients tend to be in a stage of relative estrogen excess from decreased hepatic estrogen metabolism, and they frequently exhibit testicular atrophy and gynecomastia.

Less clearly understood are racial and geographic differences. American blacks have a much higher incidence of prostatic cancer than Nigerian blacks, and Japanese-Americans who live in Hawaii have an attack rate intermediate between the low rate seen in Japan and the higher rates seen in whites in the USA. There are inconclusive data suggesting that patients may have higher testosterone production than controls; that viruses with oncogenic potential may play a permissive role; and that the number of sexual partners and a history of sexually transmitted disease also influence the incidence of prostatic cancer.

Treatment of Metastatic Prostatic Cancer

A. Steroid Receptors: Cytosol receptors for androgen have been isolated from prostatic cancers, and

while they may predict for response, they are not used as a basis for selecting therapy because (1) initial response rates to standard endocrine therapy are high, and alternative choices are far less promising (ie, second-line hormonal manuevers or chemotherapy); (2) androgen receptor assays are still technically difficult and often unreliable; and (3) the volume of tumor specimens from primary sites or metastatic sites (eg, bone) is not usually adequate for biochemical determination of tumor receptor content. When assays using monoclonal antibodies to detect androgen receptors on histologic sections become available, they may prove useful in selecting patients unlikely to respond to endocrine therapy.

B. Endocrine Therapy: It is difficult to compare the response data and therapies from different treatment centers. Typically, a patient with metastatic disease will complain of bone pain and manifest abnormalities on bone scan or plain x-ray. The acid phosphatase level may be specifically elevated in prostatic cancer, along with increased levels of the relatively nonspecific enzyme, alkaline phosphatase. Response to therapy is hard to quantitate, since subjective complaints are difficult to measure, bone lesions resolve slowly, and the acid phosphatase does not always correlate reliably with variation in tumor volume. Only in less common instances of discrete lung, lymph node, or liver metastases is it possible to objectively and directly measure antitumor response. The advent of an assay for prostate-specific antigen (PSA) may improve the monitoring of therapeutic response, since its serum level and change in titer appear to correlate well with tumor bulk and therapeutic response.

Within these limitations, it appears that one-half to three-fourths of patients will benefit from treatment. Initial therapy is hormonal and is based upon the pioneering work of Huggins, showing that prostatic cancer is a testosterone-dependent tissue. Therapy consists of lowering testosterone levels either by orchiectomy or by the administration of DES. Since DES may have direct suppressive effects on the tumor and may inhibit pituitary gonadotropin secretion, some advocate the use of both DES and orchiectomy. However, the response rates with all 3 maneuvers—DES, orchiectomy, or DES plus orchiectomy—are essentially the same. Disease that progresses after initially responding to orchiectomy or to DES rarely responds to crossover treatment with the other maneuver.

A large Veterans Administration study established that 1 mg of DES daily orally was as effective as 5 mg but imposed less risk of cardiovascular complications. Since a 1-mg dose may lead to submaximal reduction in testosterone levels, a 3-mg does is frequently employed. Patients who take DES may be troubled by painful gynecomastia; this can be prevented by low-dose breast irradiation prior to initiation of treatment. The average response duration to orchiectomy or DES is 15 months.

The presence of low levels of circulating androgens after orchiectomy has led to trials of adrenalectomy or hypophysectomy in patients with progressive disease. However, subsequent response rates to these ablative therapies are quite low, and responses are short-lived. More recently, alternative methods of depriving prostatic cancer of the tropic stimulus of testosterone have been tested. Androgen antagonists such as cyproterone or flutamide appear to be potent agents in previously untreated patients, but they are much less effective in patients who have been treated by orchiectomy. Most recently, GnRH analogues have been quite effective in reducing testosterone to castrate levels and producing response rates equivalent to those achieved with DES or orchiectomy. The side effects from these analogues are virtually nil. GnRH analogues alone—or in combination with antiandrogens—have now become frontline agents for treatment of prostatic cancer. Limitations in their use include cost, and, in the case of some GnRH analogues, the requirement for daily parenteral administrations.

MISCELLANEOUS TUMORS

Steroid hormone receptors have been isolated from tumors arising from organs not usually considered to be under primary endocrine control. Corticosteroid receptor protein is present in leukemia and lymphoma cells. It shows some correlation with response to steroid therapy, but levels are not used prospectively to guide treatment.

As mentioned earlier, there are reports of low but reproducible levels of ER or ER-like proteins in some human renal, ovarian, hepatic, bone and pancreatic tumors and in melanomas. Progestational agents produce regression in 10% of hypernephromas; there are case reports that tamoxifen and progestins have caused regressions in ovarian cancer; and there are also reports that tamoxifen can cause regressions in melanomas that contain ER. Hepatomas have responded to progestational agents on occasion, and trials are in progress to determine whether hormonal agents can produce regressions in pancreatic cancer.

In summary, it can be said that endocrine treatments for these tumor types do not appear promising at present. This reservation relates to the observation that traditional targets of endocrine therapy (eg, breast cancer) arise from a physiologic "target" issue, and the probability of response appears to increase with increasing concentration of steroid receptor protein. The miscellaneous tumors just mentioned are not from obvious physiologic target tissues and contain low levels of steroid receptors; it is not surprising that they have shown no more than a glimmer of response to the endocrine modalities tested to date.

REFERENCES

Bittner JJ: The causes of mammary cancer in mice. *Harvey Lect* 1947;**42**:221.

Bresciani F et al (editors): *Hormones and Cancer 2*. Vol 31 of: *Progress in Cancer Research and Therapy*. Raven Press, 1984.

Burck KB, Liu ET, Larrick JW: Growth factors and receptors. Pages 156–181 in: *Oncogenes*. Springer-Verlag, 1988.

Dickson RB, Lippman ME: Estrogenic regulation of growth and polypeptide growth factor secretion in human breast carcinoma. *Endocr Rev* 1987;**8**:29.

Dupont WD, Page DL: Risk factors for breast cancer in women with proliferative breast disease. *N Engl J Med* 1985;**312**:146.

Furth J: Hormones as etiological agents in neoplasia. Pages 75–120 in: *Cancer: A Comprehensive Treatise*. Vol 1. Becker FF (editor). Plenum Press, 1975.

Goustin AS et al: Growth factors and cancer. *Cancer Res* 1986;**46**:1015.

Henderson BE et al: Endogenous hormones as a major factor in human cancer. *Cancer Res* 1982;**42**:3232.

Huggins C: Endocrine-induced regression of cancers. *Science* 1967;**156**:1050.

King RJ: Oestrogen and progestin receptors as markers for the behavior of human breast tumors. Pages 357–370 in: *Biochemical and Biological Markers of Neoplastic Transformations* Chandra PP (editor). Plenum Press, 1983.

Lane MA, Sainten A, Cooper GM: Activation of related transforming genes in mouse and human mammary carcinomas. *Proc Natl Acad Sci USA* 1981;**78**:5185.

Leclercq G et al (editors): *Clinical Interest of Steroid Hormone Receptors in Breast Cancer*. Vol 91 of: *Recent Results in Cancer Research*. Springer-Verlag, 1984.

Lippman ME: Endocrine responsive cancers of man. In: *Williams Textbook of Endocrinology*, 7th ed. Wilson JB, Foster DW (editors). Saunders, 1985.

May FE et al: Mouse mammary tumour virus-related sequences are present in human DNA. *Nucleic Acids Res* 1983;**11**:4127.

Muller WJ et al: Single-step induction of mammary adenocarcinoma in transgenic mice bearing the activated c-*neu* oncogene. *Cell* 1988;**54**:105.

Salomon DS et al: Presence of transforming growth factors in human breast cancer cells. *Cancer Res* 1984;**44**:4069.

Shalet SM: Disorders of the endocrine system due to radiation and cytotoxic chemotherapy. *Clin Endocrinol* 1983; **19**:637.

Spona J, Gitsch E, Kubista E, Salzer H, Kohler B: Enzyme immunoassay and Scatchard plot estimation of estrogen receptor in gynecological tumors. *Cancer Res* 1986;**46(8 Suppl)**:4310s.

Sporn MB, Roberts AB: Autocrine growth factors and cancer. *Nature* 1985;**313**:745.

Sporn MB, Roberts AB: Peptide growth factors are multifunctional. *Nature* 1988;**332**:217.

Humoral Manifestations of Malignancy   27

Gordon J. Strewler, MD

GENERAL CONCEPT OF ECTOPIC HORMONE SECRETION

The idea that tumors can cause endocrine syndromes by secreting hormones inappropriately was first proposed by Fuller Albright. In 1941 he suggested that the cause of hypercalcemia and hypophosphatemia in a patient with renal carcinoma might be production of parathyroid hormone (PTH) by the tumor. The term "ectopic hormonal syndrome" was subsequently coined by Liddle to describe such situations. By now the idea of "ectopic hormone production" is widely held, and some humoral syndromes induced by nonendocrine tumors are recognized as being among the commonest of endocrine disorders. However, the term "ectopic" is probably a poor descriptor of most of these syndromes. Ectopic means "out of place," implying abnormal secretion of a hormone by tissues that do not normally do so. Yet, tumors that produce hormones most often arise from cells that are normally committed to producing the same hormone. For example, adrenocorticotropic hormone (ACTH) is produced by lung carcinomas that develop from ACTH-producing lung cells. Many other examples will be encountered in this chapter. Although truly ectopic secretion of hormones is probably a rarity, the term ectopic is firmly ingrained and will not soon be abandoned.

Of all the paraneoplastic syndromes, the ectopic production of hormones is probably the commonest. Virtually all the peptide hormones are produced by nonendocrine tumors (Table 27–1), and a wide variety of neoplasms are associated with syndromes of hormone excess. However, strong associations exist between specific hormones and specific tumors. For example, the PTH-like protein associated with hypercalcemia (see below) is most commonly produced by squamous carcinomas, while ACTH, vasopressin, and calcitonin are most commonly produced by small-cell lung carcinoma and other neuroendocrine tumors. It should be noted that nearly all the peptide hormones are represented in Table 27–1, but none of the steroid or thyroid hormones are listed; it is presumed that steroid hormones are not produced by tumors because their synthesis requires expression of a whole series of enzymes, while synthesis of a peptide requires ex-

Acronyms Used in This Chapter	
ACTH	Adrenocorticotropic hormone
ADH	Antidiuretic hormone (vasopressin)
APUD	Amine precursor uptake and decarboxylation
cAMP	Cyclic adenosine monophosphate
CRH	Corticotropin-releasing hormone
EGF	Epidermal growth factor
FSH	Follicle-stimulating hormone
GRH	Growth hormone–releasing hormone
GRP	Gastrin-releasing peptide
hCG	Human chorionic gonadotropin
hPLP	Human PTH-like protein
IGF-I	Insulinlike growth factor-I (somatomedin C)
IGF-II	Insulinlike growth factor-II (somatomedin A)
LH	Luteinizing hormone
mRNA	Messenger ribonucleic acid
PDGF	Platelet-derived growth factor
PTH	Parathyroid hormone
SIADH	Syndrome of inappropriate secretion of vasopressin (antidiuretic hormone)
TRH	Thyrotropin-releasing hormone
TSH	Thyroid-stimulating hormone (thyrotropin)
VIP	Vasoactive intestinal peptide

pression of only a single gene. The exception—secretion of the sterol hormone $1,25(OH)_2D_3$ by certain lymphomas—occurs because its synthesis from the circulating precursor $25OHD_3$ requires only a single step.

Secretion of hormones by tumors often differs qualitatively from glandular secretion of hormones. First, secretion by tumors is rarely suppressible. Second, tumors often lack the ability to process peptide hormones normally, and they secrete larger precursor forms whose biologic activity is reduced. Third, tumor-associated syndromes may involve physiologically different forms of the same peptides. For example, in hyperparathyroidism hypercalcemia is caused by PTH excess, but in malignant disease hypercalcemia may be caused by excess of other physiologi-

Table 27–1. Hormones produced by tumors.

Hypercalcemia factors
  PTH-like protein
  Tumor necrosis factor-α
  $1,25(OH)_2D_3$
  Prostaglandins
Vasopressin
ACTH
Calcitonin
Human chorionic gonadotropin (hCG)
Placental lactogen
Growth hormone–releasing hormone
Corticotropin-releasing hormone
Somatostatin
Erythropoietin
Oncogenous osteomalacia factor
Hypoglycemia factor
Renin
Other gut hormones (gastrin-releasing peptide, somatostatin, pancreatic polypeptide, vasoactive intestinal peptide, substance P, motilin)

cally similar peptides, one of which is closely related to PTH.

Criteria for deciding whether a nonendocrine tumor is responsible for producing hormone excess are listed in Table 27–2. Not every one of the criteria has been fulfilled for every hormone listed, but for most of these hormones there is evidence of production by tumor cells in vitro or of mRNA expression.

Cellular Basis of Ectopic Hormone Secretion

It was once held that "derepression" of tumor genes was responsible for ectopic hormone secretion, ie, that tumor cells express a random assortment of genes that are normally repressed, including genes that encode hormones. This hypothesis cannot readily explain the nonrandom association of certain hormonal syndromes (eg, ACTH and vasopressin excess) with specific cancers (eg, small-cell lung carcinoma). Moreover, the derepression hypothesis is obviated by the aforementioned finding that tumors typically express the same hormones as their cell of origin. The "dedifferentiation" hypothesis posits a retrograde movement of tumor cells along the pathway of differentiation, leading to the expression of fetal proteins (eg, alpha-fetoprotein, carcinoembryonic antigen) or hormones normally present in immature cells (eg, human chorionic gonadotropin [hCG]). While this hypothesis would account for the nonrandom nature of hormone expression and the presence of low-level expression in mature normal cells, there is no supporting evidence for the occurrence of dedifferentiation. A more sophisticated model is the "dysdifferentiation" hypothesis of Baylin and Mendelsohn, which holds that epithelial malignancy is the result of clonal expansion of a particular cell type along a complex pathway of epithelial differentiation. This is viewed as giving rise to overexpression of hormones, as by clonal expansion of a normally rare population of cells committed to expression of the hormone, or to expression of hormones not present in the mature epithelium, as by clonal expansion of a primitive cell.

Hormone Secretion by APUD Cells

The most celebrated attempt to explain the nonrandom patterns of hormone secretion by tumors is the APUD hypothesis of Pearse. A characteristic shared by many endocrine cells and some tumor cells that secrete hormones is the capacity to synthesize and store biogenic amines (*Amine Precursor Uptake and Decarboxylation*). The APUD hypothesis suggests that APUD cells, although widely scattered in many tissues, have a common origin in neural crest and are specialized for production of peptide hormones. Histologic analysis shows that APUD cells do contain typical neurosecretory granules associated with secretion of peptides and biogenic amines. Besides such endocrine cells as thyroid C cells, pituitary corticotrophs, and adrenal medullary cells, APUD cells are scattered in the bronchial and gastrointestinal mucosa, and hormone-producing neoplasms (carcinoids, small-cell lung carcinoma) are frequently composed of APUD cells. Pearse proposed that APUD cells were a "diffuse neuroendocrine system," a third branch of the nervous system.

The APUD theory probably requires modification in 2 respects. First, it has been clearly shown that not all APUD cells are of neural crest origin—some arise from primitive endoderm. Thus, hormone-producing APUD cells do not necessarily have a common origin. Second, hormones are produced not only by APUD cells but by a variety of non-APUD tumor cells. However, the APUD cell is the type most likely to be associated with the secretion of biologically active hormones that leads to a clinical syndrome of hormone excess. The best example is ACTH in Cushing's syndrome. Although the biologically inactive ACTH precursor pro-opiomelanocortin is produced by many tumors, Cushing's syndrome is typically associated with APUD tumors containing neurosecretory granules, presumably because these are capable of processing and secreting ACTH. Thus, the rubric APUD identifies cytochemical or ultrastructural features associated not so much with production of hormones as with se-

Table 27–2. Criteria for determining whether a nonendocrine tumor is a source of hormone.[1]

Association of clinical syndrome or inappropriate hormone level with presence of tumor.
Reversal of syndrome with tumor-specific therapy.
Presence of hormone in tumor tissue.
Demonstration of arteriovenous gradient for hormone across tumor.
Synthesis or release of hormone by tumor tissue in vitro.
Expression of hormone mRNA by tumor.

[1]Criteria are listed in order of their rigor; the first 2 are clinical and the rest are primarily investigational.

cretion of active hormones. However, it is preferable to refer to APUD cells as **neuroendocrine cells,** a term that denotes the presence of neurosecretory granules that are involved in hormone secretion.

Oncogenes & Growth Factors

The transformation of cells from normal to malignant is thought to involve activation of oncogenes. Oncogenes are aberrant forms of normal genes (proto-oncogenes) that control growth and differentiation, encoding growth factors (*sis* encodes platelet-derived growth factor [PDGF]), growth factor receptors (*erb*-B encodes a portion of the epidermal growth factor [EGF] receptor) or cellular effector systems coupled to growth factor receptors (*sarc* encodes a tyrosine kinase). The process of transformation thus involves the inappropriate activation of a variety of normal cellular pathways. In many instances, the production of hormones by malignant cells will probably be the consequence of activation of a specific oncogene.

Why should hormone secretion be linked to proto-oncogenes controlling normal growth and differentiation? One possible answer is that production of hormones may have survival value, both for cancer cells and for their normal cells of origin. Among the characteristic tumor products of small-cell lung carcinoma is gastrin-releasing peptide (GRP), the mammalian counterpart of the amphibian hormone bombesin. GRP/bombesin fulfills most criteria as an autocrine growth factor in small-cell carcinoma: it is secreted, it can stimulate replication of the cells via specific receptors, and blockade of its action by specific antibodies to GRP inhibits cell replication and tumor formation in vivo. Studies may eventually show whether other hormonal products of small-cell lung carcinoma (ACTH, vasopressin, calcitonin) also serve as growth factors.

MALIGNANCY-ASSOCIATED HYPERCALCEMIA

Hypercalcemia is the commonest paraneoplastic endocrine syndrome. The incidence is 15 cases per 100,000 person-years, about half the incidence of primary hyperparathyroidism. Hypercalcemia develops as a complication in up to 10% of patients with advanced malignant disease. In hospitalized patients, malignant disease is the commonest cause of hypercalcemia. Table 27–3 shows the frequency with which various tumors cause hypercalcemia. Lung carcinoma, breast carcinoma, and multiple myeloma together account for more than 50%. Among lung carcinomas, hypercalcemia is seen most commonly in squamous carcinoma and is also associated with large-cell carcinoma and adenocarcinoma. Small-cell lung carcinoma rarely causes hypercalcemia, despite its propensity for other endocrinopathies. Squamous carcinomas of the head, neck, esophagus, and other organs are also strongly associated with hypercal-

Table 27–3. Tumors that cause hypercalcemia.[1]

Primary Site	No. (%) of Cases		Known Metastatic Disease (%)
Lung	111	(25)	62
Breast	87	(19.6)	92
Multiple myeloma	43	(9.7)	100
Head and neck	36	(8.1)	73
Kidney and urinary tract	35	(7.9)	36
Esophagus	25	(5.6)	53
Female genitalia	24	(5.2)	81
Unknown primary	23	(5.2)	--
Lymphoma	14	(3.2)	91
Colon	8	(1.8)	--
Liver and biliary	7	(1.6)	--
Skin	6	(1.4)	--
Other	25	(5.6)	--
Total	444	(100.0)	

[1]Modified and reproduced, with permission, from Stollerman GH et al (editors): *Advances in Internal Medicine*. Vol. 32. Year Book, 1987.

cemia, as is renal cell carcinoma. In contrast, hypercalcemia is rarely seen in gastrointestinal adenocarcinoma or in sarcomas, even lytic sarcomas of bone. The offending neoplasm is apparent in 98% of cases when hypercalcemia is first detected. Except in patients with multiple myeloma and breast cancer, the course of which can be punctuated by self-limited episodes of hypercalcemia, the prognosis of the cancer patient with hypercalcemia is grim, with a 3-month survival rate of less than 50%.

Differential Diagnosis

The principal entity in the differential diagnosis of hypercalcemia associated with malignancy is primary hyperparathyroidism, which may present as an intercurrent illness in a patient with a malignant tumor. The presence of primary hyperparathyroidism may be indicated by an elevated PTH value. In commonly used mid region assays, the immunoreactive PTH levels in cancer patients are usually normal. However, PTH levels may be slightly high in some patients with mild hypercalcemia. In assays that measure intact PTH by immunoradiometric techniques, PTH levels are suppressed, greatly facilitating the differential diagnosis of hypercalcemia in malignancy-associated hypercalcemia. The use of the PTH assay in the differential diagnosis of hypercalcemia is discussed in Chapter 11.

Chronic, long-standing hypercalcemia preceding the diagnosis of cancer or radiographic changes of subperiosteal bone resorption may also indicate the presence of primary hyperparathyroidism.

Etiology & Pathogenesis

In patients with cancer, excessive bone resorption is the most important cause of hypercalcemia. The most important stimulus to bone resorption is local or systemic release of tumor-derived mediators, the nature of which is currently under investigation (see below). Direct bone resorption by lytic metastases is less important as a pathogenetic mechanism, as most patients with widespread lytic metastases are not hypercalcemic. Decreased renal calcium excretion may contribute to the pathogenesis of hypercalcemia in many patients. Tumors can secrete hypocalciuric substances, such as the PTH-like protein associated with solid tumors (see below), and the effects of hypercalcemia itself, eg, reduction of the glomerular filtration rate, also contribute to defective renal calcium excretion. The relative roles of excess bone resorption and excess renal reabsorption of calcium are difficult to define, but calcium absorption from the gut probably plays no role in the development of malignancy-associated hypercalcemia, except in rare patients with lymphoma and elevated levels of $1,25(OH)_2D_3$.

The molecular basis of hypercalcemia associated with cancer involves the production of at least 3 different hypercalcemic factors, giving rise to several distinct clinical syndromes. In addition, a variety of other mediators have been suggested, eg, prostaglandins. Prostaglandins of the E series are potent bone-resorbing substances. It is clear that prostaglandins are secreted by some tumors, and elevated levels of their metabolites are found in blood and urine in some cancer patients. However, only rare patients with hypercalcemia respond to inhibition of prostaglandin synthesis with nonsteroidal anti-inflammatory agents.

A. Solid Tumors: Solid tumors other than breast cancer, especially squamous carcinoma and renal cell carcinoma, produce a characteristic syndrome of hypercalcemia. This syndrome often occurs in the absence of bone metastases (Table 27–3) and is characterized by hypophosphatemia and elevated nephrogenous cyclic adenosine monophosphate (cAMP) excretion, both of which occur in hyperparathyroidism. As nephrogenous cAMP is a specific indicator of PTH action, these findings have been thought to implicate a PTH-like substance in the pathogenesis of hypercalcemia. Recently, a unique protein has been isolated from both squamous and renal carcinomas (Fig 27–1). This 141-amino-acid protein possesses an amino-terminal domain that is strongly homologous with PTH, binds to PTH receptors

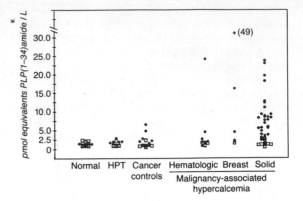

Figure 27–2. Serum levels of the PTH-like protein in normal subjects and in patients with hyperparathyroidism or malignant disease. Cancer controls are normocalcemic. Levels of PLP are increased in 3 of 9 patients with multiple myeloma and normal in the remaining patients with hematologic cancers (lymphoma or leukemia). Of patients with solid tumors, 70% have increased levels of PLP. (Modified and reproduced, with permission, from Budayr A et al: Increased serum levels of a parathyroid hormone–like protein in malignancy-associated hypercalcemia. *Ann Intern Med* 1989;**111:**807.)

in both bone and kidney with the same affinity as PTH, and mimics all the classic effects of PTH (eg, excess bone resorption, hypercalcemia, increased renal calcium reabsorption, decreased renal phosphate reabsorption, and increased renal synthesis of $1,25(OH)_2D_3$). The tumor-derived protein, which has been called human **PTH-like protein** (hPLP) or **PTH-related protein,** is the probable cause of humoral hypercalcemia in solid tumors other than breast cancer. It has recently been shown by immunoassay techniques that the protein is actually present in the circulation in hypercalcemic cancer patients (Fig 27–2). Even in patients with bone metastases, hypercalcemia may well have a humoral basis; this is supported by evidence that bone metastasis correlates poorly with hypercalcemia. Despite its limited sequence homology with PTH (Fig

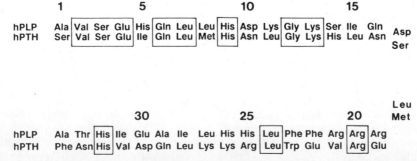

Figure 27–1. Comparison of the amino acid sequences of human PTH and the human PTH-like protein of malignancy.

27–1), hPLP does not cross-react with PTH antisera and is probably not the cause of the PTH-like immunoreactivity often detectable in patients with malignancy-associated hypercalcemia.

Despite the ability of hPLP to stimulate production of $1,25(OH)_2D_3$, plasma levels of $1,25(OH)_2D_3$ are often normal or even suppressed in patients with cancer, in contrast to the high levels seen in hyperparathyroidism. The reason for this is unclear, but it is known that production of $1,25(OH)_2D_3$ is suppressed by hypercalcemia per se, and it is likely that $1,25(OH)_2D_3$ production is more sensitive to hypercalcemia in cancer patients than in patients with primary hyperparathyroidism.

HPLP is present in the normal human genome and is expressed in normal cells, notably keratinocytes, from which squamous carcinomas arise. This is another example of hormone production by the cells from which a tumor originates. Presumably, hPLP subserves a physiologic role in tissues such as skin and lactating breast that express the protein.

HPLP is unusual among mediators of paraneoplastic syndromes because it causes a well-defined clinical syndrome by mimicking another hormone that is a distinct gene product. Other as yet unidentified tumor products, such as the mediator of tumor-induced hypoglycemia, may well fit the same pattern.

B. Breast Carcinoma: In breast cancer, hypercalcemia occurs almost invariably in patients with extensive bone metastases (Table 27–3). In one study, 35% of patients with advanced breast cancer had hypercalciuria, and 14% developed severe hypercalcemia requiring therapy. Episodes of hypercalcemia are often triggered by estrogen, androgen, or antiestrogen therapy and are often self-limited if hormonal therapy is stopped. These characteristics define a different syndrome from that associated with other solid tumors.

The strong association of hypercalcemia with bone metastases suggests an unidentified local osteolytic factor as the etiologic agent. Although breast carcinoma cells sometimes secrete prostaglandins, hypercalcemia in these patients rarely responds to treatment with inhibitors of prostaglandin synthesis. The local factor in breast cancer could be the same PTH-like protein that probably causes humoral hypercalcemia in other solid tumors; the protein has been isolated from a breast tumor, and findings in a minority of patients showed increased levels of nephrogenous cAMP and of hPLP (Fig 27–2).

C. Multiple Myeloma: Patients with myeloma are the most likely of all cancer patients to develop hypercalcemia. Hypercalciuria is even more common than hypercalcemia in this group, and hypercalcemia is probably precipitated in many cases by declining renal function with reduced clearance of calcium. As in patients with breast cancer, hypercalcemic episodes in patients with multiple myeloma are sometimes circumscribed, with prolonged subsequent survival. Hypercalcemia in patients with myeloma may respond to glucocorticoids.

The etiologic factor is probably a cytokine produced locally by myeloma cells, and current evidence favors lymphotoxin (tumor necrosis factor-β) as the most important of these. The term "osteoclast-activating factor," which was introduced as a rubric for a bone-resorbing factor secreted by normal and malignant leukocytes, should be abandoned. It is now clear that leukocytes secrete a variety of cytokines with bone-resorbing activity (eg, interleukin-1, tumor necrosis factor-α, granulocyte-macrophage colony-stimulating factor [GM-CSF], granulocyte colony-stimulating factor [G-CSF]); for example, normal monocytes predominantly secrete interleukin-1β, a bone-resorbing substance that is not secreted by myeloma cells.

D. Lymphoma: Hypercalcemia occurs in 2–3% of patients with lymphoma, usually in patients with bone involvement. It is seen in all varieties of lymphoma, but a strong predisposition to hypercalcemia is seen in only one—the adult T-cell leukemia/lymphoma syndrome, in which hypercalcemia occurs in two-thirds of cases. The disorder runs an aggressive course, and the associated hypercalcemia responds poorly to steroids and other measures. The causative agent of the syndrome is a retrovirus, the human T-cell leukemia/lymphoma virus (HTLV). The mediator of hypercalcemia has not been identified with certainty, but available evidence suggests a role for hPLP.

The etiology of hypercalcemia in lymphoma is variable. In the majority of patients, hypercalcemia is probably caused by secretion of a cytokine. In some patients, $1,25(OH)_2D_3$ appears to be the mediator of hypercalcemia. The latter patients probably have increased intestinal calcium absorption, as well as increased bone resorption, and they respond to glucocorticoid therapy. It is recognized that human monocytes in sarcoid granulomas can produce $1,25(OH)_2D_3$, and it is likely that lymphoma cells are similarly capable of synthesis of this metabolite. The histology of the tumor in patients with high levels of $1,25(OH)_2D_3$ is diverse; histiocytic, lymphocytic, Hodgkins', and HTLV-positive T-cell lymphomas are seen. That a single pathogenetic mechanism would cut across histologic lines of classification in this manner is surprising.

Treatment

The treatment of hypercalcemia is discussed in Chapter 11.

THE SYNDROME OF INAPPROPRIATE ADH SECRETION

The syndrome of inappropriate secretion of antidiuretic hormone (SIADH) is probably the second most common endocrine complication seen in cancer patients. The syndrome is seen in 7–8% of patients with small-cell carcinoma of the lung, the tumor that most commonly produces vasopressin excess. Other causative tumors, many of which are neuroendocrine tumors, include adenocarcinoma and large-cell carcinoma of the lung, bronchial carcinoids, carcinoma of the duodenum, small-cell carcinoma of the prostate, thymoma, and adrenocortical carcinoma.

Etiology & Pathogenesis

SIADH is now recognized as the most common cause of hyponatremia in hospitalized patients, but most cases result from central or eutopic secretion of vasopressin, with only 16–50% of cases in different series resulting from ectopic secretion of vasopressin by tumors. The differential diagnosis of hyponatremia is discussed in Chapter 9.

In the presence of vasopressin, excretion of free water is impaired. If the intake of free water exceeds the limited excretion of free water, water intoxication and hyponatremia ensue, with the appearance of symptoms as the serum sodium falls below 125 meq/L. However, if the thirst mechanism is intact and the patient appropriately reduces water intake, a moderate excess of vasopressin may be well tolerated. Thus, the severity of the syndrome depends on water intake as well as on the vasopressin level.

Lung cancer cells have been shown to synthesize a molecule closely resembling propressophysin, the vasopressin precursor, and to secrete immunoreactive vasopressin together with a neurophysin, the other product of its precursor. (Ectopic secretion of the sister octapeptide hormone oxytocin is very rare, if it occurs at all.) The levels of both vasopressin and neurophysin are inappropriately high for the level of plasma osmolality, not only in symptomatic patients, but also in 17–65% of asymptomatic patients with small-cell lung carcinoma. Many of the latter patients may in fact have asymptomatic, compensated ectopic secretion of vasopressin. However, some cancer patients with hyponatremia and elevated plasma vasopressin levels probably have central or eutopic, rather than ectopic, hypersecretion of vasopressin. For example, in some patients the vasopressin level increases as the plasma osmolality is increased by infusion of hypertonic saline; ie, secretion is under osmotic control. As tumors have not been shown to express an osmoreceptor, these patients probably have a pituitary source of vasopressin. Pituitary secretion of vasopressin could result from stimulation of baroreceptors by tumor or by hypovolemia.

Clinical Features

Progressive weakness, lethargy, somnolence, and confusion often appear when the serum sodium is less than 125 meq/L; coma, seizures, and death usually occur when the serum sodium is less than 110 meq/L. Patients experience weight gain but no edema, as the retained water is distributed among both intracellular and extracellular spaces. By definition, the urinary osmolality is inappropriately high for the systemic hypo-osmolality. Blood urea nitrogen is often relatively low and the urinary excretion of sodium relatively high, reflecting the expansion of body fluid spaces by retained water. Hypouricemia is often seen. The diagnosis of SIADH is established by excluding other causes of hyponatremia, such as hypovolemia, edematous states, hypothyroidism, and adrenal insufficiency. The presence of inappropriately elevated vasopressin levels can be confirmed by radioimmunoassay, but this step is often unnecessary. The treatment is restriction of water intake. In patients who cannot tolerate a reduction of water intake to correct hypo-osmolality, therapy with hypertonic saline, diuretics, or demeclocycline should be started (see Chapter 9).

CUSHING'S SYNDROME

The ectopic ACTH syndrome (Cushing's syndrome) is strongly associated with neuroendocrine (APUD) tumors. Small-cell lung carcinoma accounts for 50% of all cases; 20% are caused by bronchial or thymic carcinoid tumors (epithelial thymomas), 5% by abdominal carcinoid tumors, 5% by pancreatic islet cell tumors, and 5% by medullary carcinoma of the thyroid. There is also a strong association of neuroendocrine tumors with secretion of calcitonin and GRP. Neuroendocrine cells are scattered throughout the normal bronchial mucosa, indicating that neuroendocrine cells may represent the cell of origin of small-cell carcinomas.

Many, perhaps most, lung tumors contain immunoreactive pro-opiomelanocortin, the ACTH precursor. However, processing of pro-opiomelanocortin by nonpituitary tumors is frequently abnormal. It is primarily tumors of the neuroendocrine type that process and secrete enough ACTH to cause the clinical manifestations of Cushing's syndrome. It is likely that the ability of neuroendocrine tumors to process and secrete ACTH is related to the dense secretory granules that characterize neuroendocrine cells. However, processing of ACTH is probably abnormal even in a majority of neuroendocrine tumors; it is secreted in a large form that results from incomplete processing of its precursor, and it has reduced biologic activity. At least 25% of patients with small-cell lung carcinoma show elevated immunoreactive ACTH levels, but most of these patients have no evidence of cortisol excess.

Clinical Features

The classic somatic features of Cushing's syndrome are not present in most patients with Cushing's syndrome associated with nonendocrine tumors. Although cortisol levels are often very high, moon facies, truncal obesity, and cutaneous striae, which reflect the effect of cortisol on protein and fat metabolism, probably do not have time to develop. The syndrome usually develops rapidly and presents with weight loss, wasting, hypokalemia, and muscle weakness.

The treatment of Cushing's syndrome is discussed in Chapter 12.

Diagnosis

The differential diagnosis of glucocorticoid excess is presented in Chapter 12. The ectopic ACTH syndrome can usually be distinguished from other forms of Cushing's syndrome by its clinical presentation and by the failure of glucocorticoids to suppress the secretion of ACTH. There is typically no response to administration of corticotropin-releasing hormone (CRH). However, certain slow-growing tumors are associated with chronic secretion of ACTH and produce classic Cushing's syndrome. These tumors are often bronchial or thymic carcinoid tumors, about half of which may be suppressed by administration of dexamethasone in high doses. These tumors are a diagnostic challenge, because they are sometimes too small to be detected radiologically and because they may mimic perfectly the secretory dynamics of pituitary Cushing's disease. Their suppressibility is rare among ectopic hormone syndromes and may be due to their expression of both the glucocorticoid receptor and a glucocorticoid-responsive element in the pro-opiomelanocortin gene.

An alternative explanation for the suppressibility of bronchial and thymic carcinoids is that they may produce CRH, whose effect on pituitary corticotrophs is suppressed by glucocorticoids. Several tumors have been reported to secrete both ACTH and CRH; the role of CRH in the pathogenesis of hypercortisolism in patients with such tumors is not clear in all cases. In a small number of these patients it seems clear that ectopic secretion of CRH was the basis for the development of Cushing's syndrome. Unexpectedly, in several of these patients ACTH was not suppressible by dexamethasone. The reason for this finding is unknown.

NON-ISLET-CELL TUMORS & HYPOGLYCEMIA

Fasting hypoglycemia has been associated with a variety of non-islet-cell tumors. Bulky mesenchymal tumors arising in the retroperitoneum, abdomen, or chest (eg, fibrosarcomas, rhabdomyosarcomas, mesotheliomas, and hemangiopericytomas) account for half of all cases. Hepatocellular carcinomas (hepatomas), gastrointestinal carcinomas, carcinoids, and adrenocortical carcinomas together account for about 25%. A wide variety of carcinomas make up the remaining 25%.

The clinical presentation and differential diagnosis of fasting hypoglycemia are discussed in Chapter 23. A distinctive feature of hypoglycemia associated with nonpancreatic tumors is that insulin levels are suppressed. What then is the cause of hypoglycemia? High rates of glucose utilization have been observed in some patients. It has been suggested that excessive utilization of glucose by extremely large tumors could outstrip hepatic glucose output, but hepatic production

of glucose can normally be increased severalfold. These findings could be accounted for by elaboration of an insulinlike factor that increases glucose utilization while suppressing glucose output. An IGF-II-like substance has been detected by radioreceptor assay in the serum of some patients with hypoglycemia associated with cancer, and IGF-II in mRNA has been found in some tumors. However, in other patients neither IGF-I nor IGF-II was detectable using both radioimmunoassay and radioreceptor assay. It is likely that production of IGF-II (but not IGF-I) is sometimes involved in hypoglycemia, but other factors may be contributive. Besides increased glucose utilization by the tumor, such factors include deficiency of the glucose counterregulatory hormones and inanition, with decreased amino acid flux to the liver as substrate for hepatic gluconeogenesis.

OTHER HORMONES SECRETED BY TUMORS

Gonadotropins & Other Glycoprotein Hormones

hCG is produced eutopically by trophoblastic and other germ cell tumors, including testicular embryonal carcinoma and extragonadal germ cell tumors such as ectopic pinealoma, and in these cases it is highly useful as a tumor marker. hCG is secreted "ectopically" by many tumors. Elevated serum levels are found in 10–30% of patients with lung, breast, gastrointestinal, and ovarian tumors, and in some patients with melanoma. hCG has also been detected in low levels in a variety of normal tissues. In one study elevated levels were found in 9% of patients with various benign diseases, including inflammatory bowel disease, duodenal ulcer disease, and cirrhosis.

Some tumors do not process hCG normally; they secrete free subunits. hCG is a heterodimeric glycoprotein hormone composed of an alpha subunit, which is shared with the other glycoprotein hormones, and a unique beta subunit. Secretion of free alpha subunits is much more common than secretion of free βhCG. One instance in which measurement of subunits is indicated is in patients with pancreatic islet-cell tumors. Secretion of intact hCG is rare in islet-cell tumors, but about half of malignant functional islet-cell tumors secrete alpha subunit while benign islet-cell tumors rarely do.

hCG is the only ectopically secreted hormone composed of multiple subunits, thus requiring the expression of 2 different genes. The other glycoprotein hormones, follicle-stimulating hormone (FSH), luteinizing hormone (LH), and thyroid-stimulating hormone (TSH) are rarely, if ever, produced by extrapituitary tumors. Presumably, the propensity of tumors to secrete hCG is related to its expression at low levels in many of their cells of origin in normal tissues.

The clinical syndromes associated with tumor production of hCG are isosexual precocious pseudopuberty in children and bilateral gynecomastia in adult males. Isosexual precocity occurs in boys with hepatoblastoma. Gynecomastia in adult males probably results from increased estrogen levels resulting from conversion of circulating androgens, rather than a direct effect of hCG on the breast. Ectopic secretion of hCG is a relatively uncommon cause of gynecomastia (see Chapter 16).

Growth Hormone–Releasing Hormone, Growth Hormone, & Placental Lactogen

Since 1980, 30 cases of acromegaly have been associated with extrapituitary production of growth hormone–releasing hormone (GRH). In fact, GRH was first isolated from pancreatic tumors associated with acromegaly. The tumors involved have all been neuroendocrine tumors of the pancreas, lung, or gut (85% involved pancreas or lung). The clinical features of acromegaly induced by GRH do not differ from the common form induced by growth hormone (GH) except for the symptoms and signs of the extrapituitary tumor. The response to provocative testing is also unhelpful in detecting GRH-induced acromegaly, but elevated levels of plasma GRH on radioimmunoassay are diagnostic, and this determination should be performed in patients with acromegaly and extrapituitary malignant disease.

Ectopic secretion of GH itself is very rare. A single well-documented case exists, in which secretion from a pancreatic islet-cell tumor was confirmed by measurement of an arteriovenous gradient for GH across the tumor and a high tumor content of both GH and GH mRNA. In contrast to growth hormone, human placental lactogen (chorionic somatomammotropin) is frequently secreted by tumors. In a large series, placental lactogen was detectable in plasma in 9% of patients with malignant disease. Lung carcinoma was the commonest source. Galactorrhea was not present in these patients. The pituitary lactotrophic hormone prolactin is rarely secreted ectopically.

Calcitonin

Like ACTH, vasopressin, and GRP, calcitonin is present in neuroendocrine cells of the normal bronchial epithelium. Calcitonin is frequently secreted by tumors of the neuroendocrine type, including 60% of small-cell lung carcinomas. Calcitonin is also secreted by other lung carcinomas (15% of large-cell lung carcinomas), breast cancer, leukemia, and a broad spectrum of other cancers. Secretion of calcitonin is not associated with a distinctive clinical syndrome. In part, this may result from incomplete processing of large forms of ectopic calcitonin with reduced biologic activity. However, hypercalcitoninemia is also asymptomatic in medullary thyroid carcinoma, where levels of monomeric calcitonin are sometimes greatly elevated. Secretion of calcitonin by extrathyroid tumors may respond to secretagogues such as pentagastrin, but the response is smaller than in medullary thyroid carcinoma.

Oncogenous Osteomalacia Factor

Osteomalacia, or rickets, accompanied by hypophosphatemia occurs in association with tumors of mesenchymal origin, usually small benign tumors of the extremities. Over 50 cases have been reported, making this the commonest cause of late-onset hypophosphatemic rickets. The tumors associated with this syndrome are often highly vascular (hemangiomas, hemangiopericytomas) and frequently include giant cells. The presentation is of osteomalacia with renal phosphate wasting and low levels of $1,25(OH)_2D_3$. The syndrome is rapidly and completely reversed by resection of the tumor, clearly establishing its humoral basis. However, the humor involved has not been identified. The only type of epithelial malignancy strongly associated with this syndrome is prostate carcinoma, in which 20% of patients may be hypophosphatemic and a smaller percentage develop osteomalacia.

Hypothalamic-Pituitary Hormones

Ectopic secretion of CRH and GRH was discussed above. Beta-endorphin, β-lipotropin, and other products of pro-opiomelanocortin are associated with the ectopic ACTH syndrome, but they do not produce clinical syndromes other than hyperpigmentation (see Chapter 6). Thyrotropin-releasing hormone (TRH) and somatostatin are detectable in a variety of tumors, mostly of the neuroendocrine type, but clinical disorders that are due to their ectopic secretion have not been reported.

Gut Hormones

Vasoactive intestinal peptide (VIP) secretion has produced the watery diarrhea-hypokalemia-achlorhydria syndrome in patients with squamous lung carcinoma, ganglioneuroma, and ganglioneuroblastoma. Somatostatin, VIP, GRP (bombesin), motilin, pancreatic polypeptide, and substance P have repeatedly been found in tumors, often of the neuroendocrine type, but have not clearly produced symptoms.

Erythropoietin

One to three percent of renal carcinomas, 5% of hepatocellular carcinomas, and 10% of cerebellar hemangioblastomas are associated with erythrocytosis, probably resulting from secretion of erythropoietin. In some cases production of erythropoietinlike activity or expression of erythropoietin mRNA by tumor cells has been demonstrated. However, serum erythropoietin levels on radioimmunoassay reportedly correlate poorly with the presence of erythrocytosis in patients with hepatocellular carcinoma.

Renin

See Chapter 15.

REFERENCES

General
Baylin, SB, Mendelsohn G: Ectopic (inappropriate) hormone production by tumors: Mechanisms involved and the biological and clinical implications. *Endocr Rev* 1980;**1**:45.

Hansen M, Pedersen AG: Tumor markers in patients with lung cancer. *Chest* 1986;**89(4 Suppl)**:219S.

LeDouarin NM: On the origin of pancreatic endocrine cells. *Cell* 1988;**53**:169.

Orth DN: Ectopic hormone production. In: *Endocrinology and Metabolism,* 2nd ed. Felig P. et al (editors). McGraw-Hill, 1987.

Hypercalcemia of Cancer
Breslau NA et al: Hypercalcemia associated with increased serum calcitriol levels in three patients with lymphoma. *Ann Intern Med* 1984;**100**:1.

Broadus AE et al: Humoral hypercalcemia of cancer: Identification of a novel parathyroid hormonelike peptide. *N Engl J Med* 1988;**319**:556.

Budayr A et al: Increased serum levels of a parathyroid hormone-like protein in malignancy-associated hypercalcemia. *Ann Intern Med* 1989;**111**:807.

Bunn PA Jr et al: Clinical course of retrovirus-associated adult T-cell lymphoma in the United States. *N Engl J Med* 1983;**309**:257.

Fisken RA, Heath DA, Bold AM: Hypercalcemia: A hospital survey. *Q J Med* 1980;**49**:405.

Fukumoto S et al: Clinical evaluation of calcium metabolism in adult T-cell leukemia/lymphoma. *Arch Intern Med* 1988;**148**:921.

Galasko CS, Burn JI: Hypercalcaemia in patients with advanced mammary cancer. *Br Med J* 1971;**3**:573.

Garrett IR et al: Production of lymphotoxin, a bone-resorbing cytokine, by cultured human myeloma cells. *N Engl J Med* 1987;**317**:526.

Rosenthal N et al: Elevations in circulating 1,25-dihydroxyvitamin D in three patients with lymphoma-associated hypercalcemia. *J Clin Endocrinol Metab* 1985;**60**:29.

Stewart AF et al: Biochemical evaluation of patients with cancer-associated hypercalcemia: Evidence for humoral and nonhumoral groups. *N Engl J Med* 1980; **303**:1377.

Strewler GJ et al: Parathyroid hormone-like protein from human renal carcinoma cells: Structural and functional homology with parathyroid hormone. *J Clin Invest* 1987;**80**:1803.

Suva LJ et al: A parathyroid hormone-related protein implicated in malignant hypercalcemia: Cloning and expression. *Science* 1987;**237**:893.

Syndrome of Inappropriate Secretion of ADH
Anderson RJ et al: Hyponatremia: A prospective analysis of its epidemiology and the pathogenetic role of vasopressin. *Ann Intern Med* 1985;**102**:164.

Forrest JN Jr et al: Superiority of demeclocycline over lithium in the treatment of chronic syndrome of inappropriate secretion of antidiuretic hormone. *N Engl J Med* 1978;**298**:173.

Zerbe R, Stropes L, Robertson G: Vasopressin function in the syndrome of inappropriate antidiuresis. *Annu Rev Med* 1980;**31**:315.

Cushing's Syndrome
Cagliero E, Lorenzi M: The corticotropin-releasing factor test in the diagnosis of ectopic ACTH secretion. *West J Med* 1987;**146**:614.

Carey RM et al: Ectopic secretion of corticotropin-releasing factor as a cause of Cushing's syndrome: A clinical, morphologic, and biochemical study. *N Engl J Med* 1984;**311**:13.

de Keyzer Y et al: Altered propiomelanocortin gene expression in adrenocorticotropin-producing nonpituitary tumors: Comparative studies with corticotropic adenomas and normal pituitaries. *J Clin Invest* 1985; **76**:1892.

Findling JW, Tyrrell JB: Occult ectopic secretion of corticotropin. *Arch Intern Med* 1986;**146**:929.

Hypoglycemia
Daughaday WH et al: Synthesis and secretion of insulin-like growth factor II by a leiomyosarcoma with associated hypoglycemia. *N Engl J Med* 1988;**319**:1434.

Gorden P et al: Hypoglycemia associated with non-islet-cell tumor and insulinlike growth factors. *N Engl J Med* 1981;**305**:1452.

Widmer U et al: Is extrapancreatic tumor hypoglycemia associated with elevated levels of insulin-like growth factor III? *J Clin Endocrinol Metab* 1982;**55**:833.

Gonadotropins
Bates SE, Longo DL: Use of serum tumor markers in cancer diagnosis and management. *Semin Oncol* 1987;**14**:102.

Kahn CR et al: Ectopic production of chorionic gonadotropin and its subunits by islet-cell tumors: A specific marker for malignancy. *N Engl J Med* 1977; **297**:565.

GRH, Growth Hormone & Placental Lactogen
Melmed S et al: Acromegaly due to secretion of growth hormone by an ectopic pancreatic islet-cell tumor. *N Engl J Med* 1985;**312**:9.

Sano T, Asa SL, Kovacs K: Growth hormone-releasing hormone-producing tumors: Clinical, biochemical, and morphological manifestations. *Endocr Rev* 1988; **9**:357.

Weintraub BD, Rosen SW: Ectopic production of human chorionic somatomammotropin by nontrophoblastic cancers. *J Clin Endocrinol Metab* 1971;**32**:94.

Calcitonin
Roos BA et al: Plasma immunoreactive calcitonin in lung cancer. *J Clin Endocrinol Metab* 1980;**50**:659.

Samaan NA et al: Serum calcitonin after pentagastrin stimulation in patients with bronchogenic and breast cancer compared to that in patients with medullary thyroid carcinoma. *J Clin Endocrinol Metab* 1980; **51**:237.

Zajac JD et al: Biosynthesis of calcitonin by human lung cancer cells. *Endocrinology* 1985;**116**:749.

Oncogenous Osteomalacia Factor

Lyles KW et al: Hypophosphatemic osteomalacia: Association with prostatic carcinoma. *Ann Intern Med* 1980;**93**:275.

Ryan EA, Reiss E: Oncogenous osteomalacia: Review of the world literature of 42 cases and report of two new cases. *Am J Med* 1984;**77**:501.

Weidner N et al: Neoplastic pathology of oncogenic osteomalacia/rickets. *Cancer* 1985;**55**:1691.

Hypothalamic-Pituitary Hormones

Melmed S, Rushakoff RJ: Ectopic pituitary and hypothalamic hormone syndromes. *Endocrinol Metab Clin North Am* 1987;**16**:805.

Gut Hormones

Noseda A et al: Increased plasma motilin concentrations in small cell carcinoma of the lung. *Thorax* 1987; **42**:784.

Erythropoietin

Kew MC, Fisher JW: Serum erythropoietin concentrations in patients with hepatocellular carcinoma. *Cancer* 1986;**58**:2485.

Syndromes Involving Multiple Endocrine Glands

28

Leonard J. Deftos, MD, & Bayard D. Catherwood, MD

MULTIPLE ENDOCRINE NEOPLASIA

Astute clinical observation has resulted in the identification of neoplastic syndromes involving multiple endocrine glands. The glands most commonly involved in such syndromes are the parathyroid, pituitary, pancreas, thyroid, and adrenal. The cell types involved in these tumors are postulated to have a common embryologic precursor in the neuroectoderm. This embryologic feature may be accompanied by the presence of the metabolic pathway for *amine precursor uptake and decarboxylation*—thus the appellation APUD cells. Oncogenic mutational factors may also influence expression of these tumors. The multiple endocrine neoplasia syndromes are usually transmitted in an autosomal dominant inheritance pattern, but there may be considerable variability in penetrance and in specific tumor incidences among kindreds. The gene or genes associated with multiple endocrine disorders have recently been mapped, and new syndromes are being recognized. The availability of genetic markers may revolutionize the diagnosis of inherited endocrine tumors.

There are 3 well-defined types of multiple endocrine neoplasia (MEN) syndromes (Table 28–1): **MEN type I** (also called Wermer's syndrome), **MEN type IIa** (also called Sipple's syndrome and MEN type II), and **MEN type IIb** (also called MEN type III). The clinical descriptions and terminology for these syndromes have evolved from 1954 to the present. The first MEN syndrome was clearly described by Wermer in 1954 and was characterized by tumors of the parathyroids, pituitary, and pancreas. Shortly thereafter, Zollinger and Ellison described a syndrome that consisted of gastric hypersecretion and severe peptic disease associated with a non–insulin-producing islet cell tumor of the pancreas. This syndrome, the Zollinger-Ellison syndrome, is found in association with MEN type I in some cases but more commonly occurs by itself. In 1961, Sipple reported the association between thyroid

Acronyms Used in This Chapter

ACTH	Adrenocorticotropic hormone
APUD	Amine precursor uptake and decarboxylation
CGRP	Calcitonin gene–related peptide
CT	Calcitonin
GH	Growth hormone
HLA	Human leukocyte antigen
LH	Luteinizing hormone
MEN	Multiple endocrine neoplasia
MSH	Melanocyte-stimulating hormone
POEMS	Polyneuropathy, organomegaly, endocrinopathy, M protein, and skin changes
PP	Pancreatic polypeptide
PRL	Prolactin
PTH	Parathyroid hormone
TSH	Thyroid-stimulating hormone (thyrotropin)
VIP	Vasoactive intestinal polypeptide

cancer and pheochromocytoma. Through the subsequent studies of Williams and Hazard, a distinct thyroid tumor of the calcitonin-producing cells (C cells) of the thyroid—ie, medullary thyroid carcinoma—was defined. Characterization of the second MEN syndrome, consisting of medullary thyroid carcinoma, parathyroid tumors, and pheochromocytoma, evolved from these observations. The additional observation that there were 2 accompanying somatotypic features—ie, a marfanoid habitus and multiple mucosal neuromas—in some patients with this second type of MEN syndrome has led to the classification of a third type of MEN syndrome. In summary, the **major components** of the 3 syndromes are as follows: **MEN type I**—tumors of the parathyroids, pituitary, and pancreas, and, in some cases, components of the Zollinger-Ellison syndrome; **MEN type IIa**—medullary thyroid carcinoma, hyperparathyroidism, and pheochromocytoma; and **MEN type IIb**—medullary thyroid carcinoma, pheochromocytoma, marfanoid habitus, and multiple mucosal neuromas.

In general, the clinical and biochemical characteristics of component tumors of MEN syndromes do

Table 28–1. Components of the multiple endocrine neoplasias (MEN).

MEN Type I
  Parathyroid tumors
  Pituitary tumors
  Pancreatic tumors
MEN Type IIa
  Medullary thyroid carcinoma
  Pheochromocytoma
  Hyperparathyroidism
MEN Type IIb
  Medullary thyroid carcinoma
  Pheochromocytoma
  Mucosal neuromas

not differ markedly from characteristics of each tumor when it occurs by itself; therefore, those aspects are only briefly described in this chapter. For example, primary hyperparathyroidism as part of a MEN syndrome has most of the characteristics of primary hyperparathyroidism occurring alone, and the reader should consult Chapter 11 for a more detailed description of the features of primary hyperparathyroidism. However, the presence of multiple endocrinopathies presents a unique clinical picture (Table 28–2), and the presence of multiple endocrine tumors does have specific implications for therapy.

MULTIPLE ENDOCRINE NEOPLASIA TYPE I

MEN type I is characterized by tumors of the parathyroids, pituitary, and pancreas. The most common pituitary tumor is benign chromophobe adenoma; the

most common pancreatic tumor is gastrinoma; and the most common parathyroid lesion is multiglandular primary hyperparathyroidism. Table 28–3 shows the approximate frequency of occurrence of the components of MEN type I. The actual pattern may vary among kindreds. Tumors other than the 3 principal components of the syndrome (Table 28–3) are rare, and their relationship to the genetic disorder is unclear. This disorder has been mapped to chromosome 11.

Primary Hyperparathyroidism

Primary hyperparathyroidism is the most common endocrine neoplasia of MEN type I. Thus, upon identifying a patient with primary hyperparathyroidism, it is important to determine whether other components of the syndrome are present. The pathologic characteristics of the parathyroid glands can be best understood by recognizing the multiglandular nature of the disorder. The glands have been described in various terms ranging from adenomatous to hyperplastic. The histologic features necessary to make these classifications are not always apparent. Although chief cells are usually dominant, clear cells or a mixed picture may also be seen. The most important practical point to be derived from pathologic descriptions is the potential for all parathyroid glands to be involved in the neoplastic process, even ectopic glands. This means that aggressive surgical therapy directed toward subtotal parathyroidectomy may be necessary for effective treatment.

Pituitary Tumors

The most common pituitary tumor of MEN type I is chromophobe adenoma. This nonfunctioning tumor is usually benign by histologic criteria but can cause en-

Table 28–2. Abnormal hormone production by endocrine tumors of MEN syndromes. Measurement of these substances or their metabolites in blood and urine can serve as diagnostic tests.

	Pituitary	Pancreas	Parathyroid	Thyroid	Adrenal
PTH			+		
CT		+		+	
ACTH	+			+	
GH	+				
Somatostatin	+	+			
PRL	+				
VIP		+			
PP		+			
Gastrin		+			
Insulin		+			
Glucagon		+			
Catecholamines				+	+
Chromogranin A	+	+	+	+	+

Table 28–3. Components of MEN type I and their approximate frequency of occurrence in patients with MEN type I.

Component	Frequency
Hyperparathyroidism	80%
Pancreatic tumors	75%
Gastrinomas	
Benign	20%
Malignant	30%
Insulinomas	
Benign	20%
Malignant	5%
Nonfunctioning tumors	
Benign	< 5%
Malignant	< 5%
Pituitary tumors	65%
Chromophobe or nonfunctioning adenomas	
Benign	40%
Malignant	< 5%
Eosinophilic tumors or acromegaly (benign)	15%
Cushing's disease, basophilic	5%
Mixed and other types (benign)	< 5%
Prolactin-secreting tumors	< 5%
Other tumors	
Carcinoid and bronchial adenomas	< 5%
Lipomas and liposarcomas	5%
Adrenocortical adenomas	10%

docrine abnormalities by the effect of its mass on adjacent endocrine cells. Tumors producing growth hormone (GH), adrenocorticotropic hormone (ACTH), prolactin (PRL), and somatostatin have also been described in this syndrome, and their manifestations are classically related to their location and hormonal products. The incidence of pituitary microadenomas is not well defined.

Pancreatic Tumors

Gastrin-producing islet cell tumors are the most common pancreatic neoplasias of MEN type I, accounting for at least 50% of all pancreatic tumors. Gastrinomas can also occur at other sites such as the duodenal wall and stomach. Insulinomas are the next most common neoplasias. In addition, there are case reports of tumors producing vasoactive intestinal polypeptide (VIP), glucagon, pancreatic polypeptide (PP), somatostatin, and calcitonin (CT). Measurement by radioimmunoassay of these hormones in serum is an important diagnostic procedure. The "tumors" are usually composed of hyperplastic islet cells or multiple small tumors. The secretory products of these tumors can explain some of the associated findings. Examples are the peptic ulcer diathesis with gastrin, hypoglycemia with insulin, and secretory diarrhea with VIP and perhaps with PP. Glucagonomas can be associated with bullous dermatitis, but the pathogenesis of this lesion is obscure.

The production of excess gastrin leading to peptic ulceration by a pancreatic islet cell tumor is called **Zollinger-Ellison syndrome.** Zollinger-Ellison syn-

drome more commonly occurs by itself, but it can also be part of MEN type I. The ulcer diathesis of Zollinger-Ellison syndrome makes gastrointestinal symptoms a dominant clinical feature. Gastrointestinal symptoms may also be dominant in a patient with a VIP-producing islet cell tumor (VIPoma).

Other Tumors

The other tumors indicated in Table 28–3 are also found in patients with MEN type I, but their link to this disorder is not clearly established. Carcinoid tumors associated with MEN type I are more likely to be found in foregut-derived structures such as the thymus and bronchial tree than in midgut-derived structures, where sporadic carcinoid tumors usually occur. Bronchial carcinoid can produce its vasoactive symptoms without metastasizing. Adrenal and thyroid adenomas occurring in MEN type I represent predominantly the results of autopsy findings and are usually nonfunctioning. Lipomas may be present in some kindreds in MEN type I, and when cutaneous they may provide a useful sign of the syndrome.

MULTIPLE ENDOCRINE NEOPLASIA TYPES IIa & IIb

In the early reports of medullary thyroid carcinoma as part of a multiple endocrine disorder, the associated lesions were pheochromocytoma, hyperparathyroidism, and a syndrome consisting of multiple mucosal neuromas and marfanoid habitus (mucosal neuroma syndrome). It is now appreciated that 2 distinct clinical syndromes can be defined by these associated endocrinopathies: MEN type IIa (Table 28–4) and MEN type IIb (Table 28–5). MEN type IIa consists of medullary thyroid carcinoma, pheochromocytoma, and hyperparathyroidism; MEN type IIb consists of medullary thyroid carcinoma, pheochromocytoma, multiple mucosal neuromas, and marfanoid habitus. The component tumors of MEN type IIa and MEN type IIb vary in their incidence and prevalence. Since medullary thyroid carcinoma is the central tumor, it will be discussed first. MEN type IIa has been mapped to chromosome 10.

Medullary Thyroid Carcinoma

Medullary thyroid carcinoma, a tumor of the calcitonin-producing cells (C cells) of the thyroid gland, is a component of MEN type IIa and IIb. The thyroidal

Table 28–4. Components of MEN type IIa and their approximate frequency of occurrence in patients with MEN type IIa.

Component	Frequency
Medullary thyroid carcinoma	97%
Hyperparathyroidism	50%
Pheochromocytoma	30%

Table 28–5. Components of MEN type IIb and their approximate frequency of occurrence in patients with MEN type IIb.

Component	Frequency
Multiple mucosal neuromas	100%
Medullary thyroid carcinoma	90%
Marfanoid habitus	65%
Pheochromocytoma	45%

C cells are now generally accepted to be of neural crest origin. These cells migrate to the ultimobranchial bodies from the neural crest. In submammals, the cells form a distinct organ, the ultimobranchial organ, which harbors C cells and their secretory product, calcitonin. In mammals, C cells become incorporated into the thyroid gland and perhaps other sites. The neural crest origin of C cells offers an explanation for the association of medullary thyroid carcinoma with other tumors of neural crest origin and also appears to explain the production by these tumors of a wide variety of bioactive substances.

Medullary thyroid carcinoma is usually a firm, rounded tumor located in the middle or upper lobes of the thyroid gland. The cells usually are polyhedral or polygonal and are arranged in a variety of patterns. Calcification is commonly found in the tumor, and a characteristic calcification may be visible on x-ray. Although the presence of amyloid has long been considered to be important in the diagnosis of medullary thyroid carcinoma, the diagnosis is best established by the use of specific immunohistochemical procedures for calcitonin that demonstrate the abnormal C cells. The frank malignancy of medullary thyroid carcinoma, at least in familial cases, is preceded by a progressive hyperplasia of C cells referred to as **C cell hyperplasia.** This predecessor of medullary thyroid carcinoma can become manifest in early childhood or as late as the second decade. There may be corresponding changes in the parathyroid and adrenal glands. Several instances of **C cell adenoma** have also been reported. The natural history of medullary thyroid carcinoma can vary greatly, and this may make decisions regarding therapy difficult. The tumor is generally regarded as intermediate between the aggressive behavior of anaplastic thyroid carcinoma and the more indolent behavior of papillary and follicular thyroid carcinoma. The most common presentation is a thyroid nodule, and the most common symptom is diarrhea.

There are 2 general groups of factors that can contribute to the diarrhea commonly seen in patients with medullary thyroid carcinoma—humoral factors and anatomic ones. Many of the various bioactive substances produced by medullary thyroid carcinoma have been implicated in the pathogenesis of the diarrhea seen with this tumor. These peptide hormones include (1) calcitonin, (2) ACTH and melanocyte-stimulating hormone (MSH), (3) neurotensin, (4) somatostatin, (5) β-endorphin, and (6) nerve growth factor. The various anatomic abnormalities discussed subsequently that can be found in the gastrointestinal tract of patients with medullary thyroid carcinoma may also account for the diarrhea. These anatomic lesions may reflect and perhaps even produce fundamental abnormalities in gastrointestinal innervation that can produce abnormal motility.

A. Calcitonin and Related Peptides and Proteins: Since medullary thyroid carcinoma is a neoplastic disorder of the C cells of the thyroid gland, the tumor produces abnormally high amounts of calcitonin. As a result, patients with this tumor have elevated concentrations of calcitonin in peripheral blood and urine. In many patients, basal concentrations of the hormone are sufficiently elevated to be diagnostic of the presence of medullary thyroid carcinoma. However, in an increasing percentage of patients with this tumor, basal levels of calcitonin are indistinguishable from normal. Thus, **provocative tests** with calcium and pentagastrin have been developed for the diagnosis of medullary thyroid carcinoma and its histologic antecedents. These tests are based on the observation that calcium and pentagastrin are potent calcitonin secretagogues.

Opinion differs regarding the relative clinical value of pentagastrin and calcium infusion in the diagnosis of medullary thyroid carcinoma. One must remember that most tumors respond to either agent and that both infusion procedures sometimes give false-negative results. Therefore, either procedure can be recommended, and if one procedure gives negative results in a patient suspected of having medullary thyroid carcinoma, the alternative procedure should be considered before the diagnosis is excluded. In general, both the sensitivity and the specificity of the calcitonin immunoassay are probably just as important as the choice between calcium and pentagastrin in provocative testing of a patient suspected of having medullary thyroid carcinoma. Selective venous catheterization with measurements of calcitonin can also be useful, but its greatest value is probably not in primary diagnosis but in the location of tumor metastases (or sources of ectopic calcitonin production), since knowledge of the presence of metastatic (or ectopic) disease can greatly influence therapy. The effectiveness of therapy in patients with calcitonin-producing tumors can be monitored by serial measurements of plasma calcitonin. In addition to determining the relatively acute effects of a given treatment regimen, periodic surveillance with appropriate provocative testing can be conducted for recurrence of tumor.

The calcitonin gene encodes other peptides, among them a 37-amino-acid peptide termed CGRP (calcitonin gene–related peptide) (Table 28–6). Although the function of these peptides is unknown, they are secreted by medullary thyroid carcinoma and may thus serve as tumor markers. C cells also secrete chromogranin A, a high-molecular-weight protein origi-

Table 28–6. Calcitonin gene-related peptides and other products secreted by medullary thyroid carcinoma.

Catecholamines	Adrenocorticotropic hormone	Amyloid
Dopa decarboxylase	Melanocyte-stimulating hormone	Carcinoembryonic antigen
Histaminase	Somatostatin	Melanin
Serotonin	β-Endorphin	Neuron-specific enolase
Prostaglandins	Substance P	Chromogranin A
Kallikrein and kinins	Vasoactive intestinal polypeptide	
	Corticotropin-releasing hormone	
	Prolactin-releasing hormone	
	Nerve growth factor	

nally discovered in the secretory granules of pheochromocytomas and now known to be present in other endocrine tissues, among them the parathyroid, pancreas, and pituitary (Table 28–2). This protein could thus be a marker for each of the endocrine neoplasias encountered in any of the multiple endocrine neoplasias (Table 28–7).

B. Other Secretory Products: In addition to calcitonin, medullary thyroid carcinoma produces other substances, nonpeptides as well as peptides (Table 28–6). Their measurement in blood, eg, chromogranin A, may also be useful in diagnosis and management. This unusual biosynthetic capacity of medullary thyroid carcinoma may be related to the neural crest origin of C cells.

Pheochromocytoma

Pheochromocytoma is a component of MEN type IIa and IIb. Pheochromocytomas occurring in association with medullary thyroid carcinoma have several distinct features. Bilateral and multifocal pheochromocytomas are very common in this clinical setting, with an incidence of over 70%. This contrasts with a bilateral incidence of usually less than 10% for sporadic pheochromocytomas and only 20–50% with familial pheochromocytomas. Pheochromocytomas are much more likely to occur in patients with familial rather than sporadic medullary thyroid carcinoma. The thyroid tumor may antedate the pheochromocytoma by as much as 2 decades. Furthermore, a second pheochromocytoma may become manifest after removal of the first. Thus, there is a greater incidence of pheochromocytomas in older patients with medullary thyroid carcinoma. If hyperparathyroidism also exists, it too is likely to be diagnosed before the pheochromocytoma. **Adrenal medullary hyperplasia** may be a predecessor of the pheochromocytomas seen with medullary thyroid carcinoma, just as C cell hyperplasia may be a predecessor of medullary thyroid carcinoma and chief cell hyperplasia a predecessor of primary hyperparathyroidism in these patients. The increase in adrenal medullary mass results from diffuse or multifocal proliferation of adrenal medullary cells, primarily those found within the head and body of the glands. Diagnostic tests for pheochromocytoma should be pursued vigorously, because the biochemical as well as clinical manifestations of this tumor may be subtle. A high ratio of epinephrine to norepinephrine—rather than absolute levels—is considered an important diagnostic criterion (see Chapter 14).

Hyperparathyroidism

The exact incidence of hyperparathyroidism in patients with medullary thyroid carcinoma is difficult to establish. Hyperparathyroidism is much more common in MEN type IIa than in MEN type IIb. Recent research suggests that hyperplasia is more common than adenoma. Despite these uncertainties, the concurrence of hyperparathyroidism and medullary thyroid carcinoma in MEN syndromes is well established, and although it cannot be quantitated, the presence of one tumor should always make one suspect the presence of the other. Hyperparathyroidism does not easily fit into a unitary concept of embryogenesis, since parathyroid cells are not classically considered to be of neural crest origin. However, some authorities have suggested a neural crest origin for the parathyroid gland. An alternative explanation for the hyperparathyroidism is a functional relationship between it and medullary thyroid carcinoma. According to this hypothesis, the abnormal concentrations of calcitonin induce hyperparathyroidism, which is secondary to the hypocalcemic actions of the calcitonin. This type of functional relationship between the neoplasias is unlikely; the most convincing evidence supports a genetic relationship between medullary thyroid carcinoma and hyperparathyroidism.

Table 28–7. Plasma calcitonin and chromogranin A concentrations (mean ± SE) in patients with endocrine tumors.

Group	Chromogranin A (ng/mL)	Calcitonin (pg/mL)
Normal controls (n = 16)	82 ± 16	60 ± 15
Pheochromocytoma (n = 11)	1614 ± 408[1]	. . .
Medullary thyroid carcinoma (n = 6)	789 ± 333[1]	7485 ± 3009[1]
Parathyroid adenoma (n = 7)	218 ± 13[1]	. . .

[1]$p \leq .01$ compared to control.

Mucosal Neuromas

The presence of neuromas with a centrofacial distribution is the most consistent component of MEN type IIb. The most common location of neuromas is the oral cavity (tongue, lips, buccal mucosa), but other sites may be involved (Table 28–8). The oral lesions (Fig 28–1) are almost invariably present by the first decade and in some cases even at birth. The most prominent microscopic feature of neuromas is an increase in the size and number of nerves.

Mucosal neuromas can be present in the eyelids, conjunctiva, and cornea. The thickened medullated corneal nerves traverse the cornea and anastomose in the pupillary area. These hypertrophied nerve fibers are readily seen with a slit lamp but occasionally may be evident even on direct ophthalmoscopic examination.

Gastrointestinal tract abnormalities are part of the multiple mucosal neuroma syndrome. The most common of these is **gastrointestinal ganglioneuromatosis.** Ganglioneuromatosis is best observed in the small and large intestine but has also been noted in the esophagus and stomach. The anatomic lesions are sometimes associated with functional difficulties in swallowing, megacolon, diarrhea, and constipation. Similar lesions may be present on other mucosal surfaces.

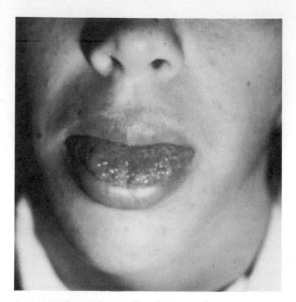

Figure 28–1. Mucosal neuromas on the tongue of a 12-year-old child with MEN type IIb.

Marfanoid Habitus

The term "marfanoid habitus" denotes a tall, slender body with long arms and legs, an abnormal ratio of upper to lower body segment, and poor muscle development. It is seen commonly in multiple mucosal neuroma syndrome. The extremities are thin, and there may be lax joints and hypotonic muscles. Other features associated with the marfanoid habitus may include dorsal kyphosis, pectus excavatum or pectus carinatum, pes cavus, and high-arched palate. In contrast to patients with true Marfan's syndrome, no patients with multiple mucosal neuromas have been reported to have aortic abnormalities, ectopia lentis, homocystinuria, or, notably, mucopolysaccharide abnormalities.

OTHER MULTIPLE ENDOCRINE NEOPLASIAS

Several additional syndromes exist that are characterized by the autosomal dominant inheritance of multiple endocrine tumors. The **von Hippel-Lindau syndrome** consists of cerebelloretinal hemangioblastomas occurring with pheochromocytomas and pancreatic islet cell tumors along with renal cell carcinoma. It has been linked to a deletion on chromosome 3. In addition to Schwann-cell tumors, patients with neurofibromatosis (**Recklinghausen's disease**) have pheochromocytomas and duodenal carcinoid tumors. This disorder has been mapped to chromosome 17, the location of the nerve growth factor receptor.

As with some other tumors, such as retinoblastoma

Table 28–8. Summary of clinical features in 41 patients with MEN type IIb.

	Number of Patients With Findings[1]		
	Positive	Probable	Negative
Family history of MEN type IIb	14	2	15
Neuroma (any type) Oral type	41 37		4
Ocular type	24		16
Other type	4		36
"Bumpy" lips	35	2	
Pheochromocytoma	19[2]	4	18
Medullary thyroid carcinoma	38		2
Marfanoid habitus	26	5	
Hypertrophied corneal nerves	23		
Skeletal defects	24		4
Gastrointestinal tract abnormalities	23		10

[1]In some cases, the status of some of the clinical features was not known.
[2]Unilateral in 7 patients; bilateral in 12 patients.
Modified from Khairi et al.

and small-cell lung carcinoma, the presence of chromosomal deletions in endocrine tumors has led to the hypothesis that the deleted gene encodes an anti-oncogene whose absence allows oncogenesis to occur. Studies with the tools of molecular biology (see Chapter 2) will provide important insights into the pathogenesis of inherited endocrine tumors.

MANAGEMENT OF PATIENTS WITH MULTIPLE ENDOCRINE NEOPLASIA (MEN) SYNDROMES

The individual endocrine components of MEN syndromes have, in general, the same clinical and biochemical manifestations as when they occur as individual entities. The unique clinical aspect of the patient with MEN is the way in which the individual presents to the physician. The patient may be part of a kindred with well-established MEN, and the physician must then evaluate the patient for each potential component of the kindred's syndrome. Or the physician may search for the presence of MEN when a patient presents with one of the endocrine components; in this latter circumstance, the yield will not be great, but when one patient with MEN is discovered, it leads to the identification of other patients.

Surgery is the treatment of choice for the 3 neoplasias in MEN type IIa. All are potentially lethal—especially medullary thyroid carcinoma and pheochromocytoma—but all can be cured by early diagnosis followed by operation. Aggressive therapy is thus warranted, and special consideration should be given to certain aspects of the treatment, since one is dealing with a patient with 3 potential endocrine tumors.

Management of the individual components of MEN syndromes generally follows the accepted procedures for each of the neoplasias, and these are discussed in detail elsewhere in this book. Thus, the management of pituitary tumors is guided by the availability of transsphenoidal hypophysectomy and the management of mucosal neuromas by cosmetic factors. However, the clinical setting does influence the sequence and extent of surgical therapy. The sequence of treatment is guided by the presence of multiple endocrine tumors. Pheochromocytomas, which are commonly bilateral, especially in MEN type IIb, should be treated first, medically or surgically, in order to obviate their cardiovascular effects on surgical procedures. Thyroid and parathyroid surgery must be aggressive, because all glandular tissue may be involved.

An essential feature of appropriate clinical management is evaluation of family members, since MEN syndromes are transmitted in an autosomal dominant pattern. Family members must be reevaluated periodically because of the varying penetrance of the component tumors.

FAILURE OF MULTIPLE ENDOCRINE GLANDS

This section deals mainly with the syndromes involving autoimmune destruction of multiple endocrine and specific other tissues. Historically, the first of these associations was Schmidt's syndrome of nontuberculous Addison's disease and lymphocytic thyroiditis. In a 1964 review of Schmidt's syndrome, Carpenter et al found coexisting diabetes mellitus in 10 out of 15 patients with Addison's disease and thyroiditis. They broadened the definition of the syndrome to include diabetes mellitus associated with nontuberculous Addison's disease. However, multiglandular failure may also involve the parathyroids, ovaries, testes, and possibly adenohypophysis. Schmidt's syndrome (the Carpenter definition will be used in this chapter) is thus but one subset of these disorders. In addition, these endocrinopathies are frequently associated with other disorders of tissue-specific autoimmunity, notably pernicious anemia and vitiligo. This discussion will emphasize the evidence for clinical, immunologic, and possibly genetic heterogeneity among groups of patients with these disorders.

Six mechanisms of immunologic tissue injury have been described (Table 28–9). The primary effectors in autoimmune reactions are immunoglobulins, T cells (thymus-dependent lymphocytes that become sensitized to specific antigens and release soluble nonimmunoglobulin mediators), and monocytes (which possess receptors for the Fc region of immunoglobulins and cytotoxic capabilities in the presence of tissue-specific antibody). The role of these mechanisms in autoimmune endocrine disease has been most extensively studied in Hashimoto's thyroiditis and Graves' disease. Although immune complexes are present in the sera of some patients with autoimmune thyroid disease, T cell-mediated immunity and antibody-dependent cell-mediated cytotoxicity have received the greatest attention as mechanisms of target organ destruction in Hashimoto's thyroiditis. Evidence for specifically sensitized T cells has been found in other

Table 28–9. Types of immunologic tissue injury.[1]

IgE-mediated immediate hypersensitivity
Complement-dependent direct humoral cytotoxicity
Antigen-antibody complex deposition
T cell–mediated immunity
Receptor autoantibody binding (blocking or stimulating)
Antibody-dependent cell-mediated cytotoxicity

[1]Modified and reproduced, with permission, from Deftos LJ, Catherwood BD, Bone HG: Multiple endocrine disorders. Chapter 28 in: *Endocrinology and Metabolism.* Felig P et al (editors). McGraw-Hill, 1981.

autoimmune endocrinopathies as well. To explain this apparent break in the immunologically privileged status of autologous tissues, Volpe has proposed a unifying theory of pathogenesis of autoimmune thyroid disease based on a defect in immuno-regulation by suppressor T cells (thymus-dependent lymphocytes that suppress immune responses, possibly including recognition of autoantigens). In vitro reconstitution experiments have shown that normal suppressor T cells can depress the production of migration-inhibiting lymphokines by leukocyte cultures from Hashimoto's thyroiditis patients and can also inhibit the differentiation of antithyroid antibody-secreting cells. Patients with autoimmune thyroid disease, but not other autoimmune diseases, appear to lack suppressor T cells capable of these functions.

The events that initiate immune sensitization to antigens of the endocrine system remain unclear. Class II histocompatibility molecules, normally borne only by macrophages and a few other cells, can be expressed on endocrine cells (as manifest by the Ia+ determinant of HLA-DR). This observation has suggested the theory that some environmental event (such as a viral infection) might first cause antigens that are otherwise sequestered to be displayed in conjunction with these essential antigen-presenting molecules. However, Ia antigen expression is also seen in localized areas of lymphocytic reaction in other thyroid diseases such multinodular goiter and thyroid carcinoma. Additional factors must therefore be necessary for progression to established autoimmunity. It remains to be determined for each endocrine cell whether all 3 factors (display of otherwise sequestered antigens, expression of antigen-presenting molecules, and antigen-specific suppressor cell defect) are necessary and sufficient for the development of autoimmunity.

A number of methods have been used for assessment of tissue-specific immunity in the autoimmune endocrinopathies (Table 28–10). Immunoprecipitation, latex or tanned red cell agglutination, and radioimmunoassay have been used to detect thyroglobulin autoantibodies, the last being the most sensitive method. The indirect immunofluorescence test for autoantibodies to endocrine cells in frozen tissue sections is a versatile technique that has demonstrated autoan-

Table 28–10. Methods for assessment of tissue-specific immunity.

Methods Reflecting T Lymphocyte Function
  T cell help (for B cell differentiation)
  Direct lymphocytotoxicity
  Induced lymphocyte proliferation
  Induced lymphokine production
  Lymphocyte activation (Ia+)
Methods Reflecting B Lymphocyte Function
  Precipitin reaction
  Complement fixation
  Indirect immunofluorescence
  Direct serum cytotoxicity
  Enablement of cell-mediated cytotoxicity

tibodies to adrenal, thyroid, islet cell, parathyroid, and gonadal "cytoplasmic" antigens. Thyroperoxidase is now recognized as a major component of the thyroid cytoplasmic antigen, which has been localized to microsomal fractions and titered by complement fixation. With the exception of these principal antithyroid antibody tests, the immunofluorescence tests are performed only in specialized laboratories.

PROTOTYPICAL AUTOIMMUNE ENDOCRINOPATHY: ADDISON'S DISEASE

Addison's disease plays a central role in several groups of patients with failure of multiple endocrine glands, and there is strong evidence that idiopathic Addison's disease is the end result of autoimmune adrenalitis in most cases. Addison's disease has also provided a good focus for investigation of endocrine autoimmunity (1) because few of these patients should escape medical attention and (2) because tuberculous Addison's disease has provided a natural control group for clinical and immunologic comparison.

Autoimmune Addison's disease is diagnosed when there is no evidence of tuberculosis or any other reasonable explanation for adrenal failure. Pulmonary tuberculosis and adrenal calcification justify a presumptive diagnosis of tuberculous Addison's disease; however, in patients with granulomatous disease on chest film but without adrenal calcification, the cause of adrenal failure is indeterminate. Autoantibodies to adrenal tissue can be detected by indirect immunofluorescence in a high percentage (48–74%) of patients with presumed autoimmune Addison's disease, while the incidence of adrenal autoantibodies is essentially zero in patients with unequivocal tuberculous Addison's disease. Although comparable data are not available for patients with Addison's disease due to other causes such as histoplasmosis, this information suggests that adrenal autoantibodies are not an epiphenomenon due to tissue destruction. In vitro evidence of T cell activation (increased Ia+ number) and of cell-mediated immunity to adrenal antigen is also present in many patients with autoimmune Addison's disease but not in patients with tuberculous Addison's disease. The autoimmune nature of idiopathic Addison's disease is further substantiated by its specific association with a wide variety of second endocrinopathies with in vitro evidence for tissue-specific autoimmunity. Table 28–11 shows the strikingly higher frequency of second diseases in autoimmune compared with tuberculous Addison's disease. The diseases found with tuberculous Addison's disease have generally been diabetes mellitus and thyroid disease. These results support the conclusion that idiopathic Addison's disease is part of a larger autoimmune endocrine syndrome.

The presence of adrenal autoantibodies in the blood

Table 28–11. Incidence of other autoimmune disorders in patients with Addison's disease.

	Autoimmune Addison's Disease (n = 419)	Tuberculous Addison's Disease (n = 114)
Diabetes mellitus	10%	. . .
Hyperthyroidism	8%	. . .
Thyroiditis and primary myxedema	9%	. . .
Pernicious anemia	4%	. . .
Hypogonadism	16%	. . .
Hypoparathyroidism	5%	. . .
One or more disorders	39%	8%

may be a marker for activity of the autoimmune diathesis. Adrenal autoantibodies tend to have disappeared in patients studied later than 1–5 years after the onset of Addison's disease. Table 28–12 shows the relationship of adrenal autoantibody to the sex of the patient, the age at onset of adrenal insufficiency, and the presence of a second autoimmune disorder. The higher prevalence of autoantibodies in Addison's disease associated with other disorders is particularly striking. Patients with autoimmune Addison's disease with adrenal autoantibodies have a 2- to 3-fold greater incidence of other clinically manifest endocrinopathies compared with patients without adrenal autoantibodies. Several investigators have found a higher prevalence of adrenal autoantibodies in women, although this has not been uniformly reported. The frequency of autoantibodies is much less in patients with Addison's disease alone who are male or whose onset of adrenal insufficiency was before age 20 years. Adrenal autoantibodies have been found in 13% of patients with idiopathic hypoparathyroidism alone. They are found rarely in first-degree relatives of patients with autoimmune Addison's disease, in patients with Cushing's

Table 28–12. Incidence of adrenal autoantibodies in patients with autoimmune Addison's disease according to sex, age at onset of adrenal insufficiency, and presence of other disease.[1]

	Sex		Age at Onset		
	Female	Male	<20	>20	Total
Addison's disease alone	14/27 (52%)	7/40 (18%)	4/26 (15%)	16/36 (44%)	21/67 (31%)
Addison's disease plus other disease	23/30 (77%)	13/21 (62%)	15/21 (71%)	20/28 (71%)	36/51 (71%)
					57/118 (48%)

[1]Source of data: Blizzard RM, Chee D, Davis W: *Clin Exp Immunol* 1967;**2**:19. Modified and reproduced, with permission, from Deftos LJ, Catherwood BD, Bone HG: Multiple endocrine disorders. Chapter 28 in: *Endocrinology and Metabolism.* Felig P et al (editors). McGraw-Hill, 1981.

disease, and in patients with Hashimoto's thyroiditis or diabetes mellitus alone. The prevalence of adrenal autoantibodies in apparently normal individuals is less than one per 1000 population.

Many investigators have found an increased prevalence of subclinical autoimmunity to other tissues in patients with autoantibody-positive Addison's disease, as evidenced by autoantibodies to parathyroid, islet cell, thyroid, and gastric mucosa. Nerup found a 6-fold higher frequency of thyroid autoantibodies and a 10-fold increase in parietal cell autoantibodies in patients with adrenal autoantibody-positive Addison's disease, but patients with Addison's disease without adrenal autoantibodies showed no difference from age- and sex-matched controls. When a panel of in vitro immunologic tests was used along with clinical data, 84% of patients with Addison's disease and adrenal autoantibodies were found to have evidence of extra-adrenal autoimmune involvement.

CLINICAL & IMMUNOLOGIC HETEROGENEITY

From what has been said, it can be inferred that autoimmune Addison's disease is not a homogeneous disorder with a random coincidence of other autoimmune endocrine disease and that patients with failure of additional glands might also be heterogeneous. Fig 28–2 supports this thesis, showing the distribution of the age at onset in 3 clinical subsets of patients with Addison's disease studied in the USA and the UK. It is clear that Addison's disease associated with hypoparathyroidism has a much earlier age at onset than Addison's disease associated with Schmidt's syndrome or without other endocrinopathy. Analyzing 182 patients from 140 families with autoimmune Addison's disease, idiopathic hypoparathyroidism, or both disorders, Spinner et al found evidence for genetic as well as clinical heterogeneity among these patients and divided their patients into 4 groups: Addison's disease with hypoparathyroidism, isolated hypoparathyroidism, isolated Addison's disease, and Schmidt's syndrome. Immunologic differences also distinguish groups of patients with autoimmune endocrine disease. Patients with Addison's disease in adulthood are predominantly female and frequently have thyroid autoantibodies. They therefore resemble the group with complete Schmidt's syndrome. However, patients with childhood-onset Addison's disease without other endocrinopathy tend to be male and have predominantly autoantibodies to parathyroid tissue, resembling more closely the patients with Addison's disease associated with clinical hypoparathyroidism. Some of these patients may represent a forme fruste of pluriglandular endocrine insufficiency. Several types of study have thus led to the concept that multiglandular autoimmune endocrinopathy is not a uniform syndrome nor the random coincidence of a number of individual diseases but

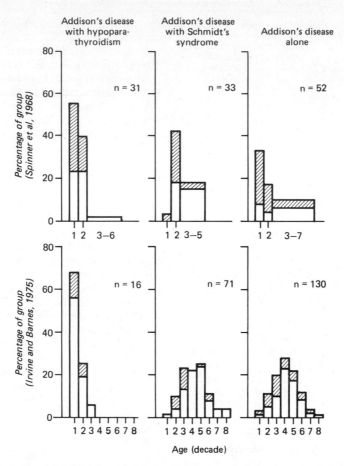

Figure 28–2. Clinical heterogeneity of Addison's disease. Distribution of age at onset (upper) or of diagnosis (lower) of Addison's disease with hypoparathyroidism, Addison's disease with Schmidt's syndrome, and Addison's disease alone. The open area represents females; the closed area represents males. Note that age is measured in decades. (Reproduced, with permission, from Deftos LJ, Catherwood BD, Bone HG: Multiple endocrine disorders. Chapter 28 in: *Endocrinology and Metabolism,* 2nd ed. Felig P et al [editors]. McGraw-Hill, 1985.)

that there are at least 2 distinct patterns of glandular involvement. These ideas are summarized as major types and variations in Figure 28–3. Besides the groups of patients with Addison's disease outlined above, there are groups in which a direct association of thyroiditis and diabetes mellitus is found in the absence of Addison's disease. In addition, other endocrine and some nonendocrine disorders occur with increased frequency in these patients.

Addison's Disease With Hypoparathyroidism

In the set of patients with Addison's disease and hypoparathyroidism, male and female patients are usually affected in childhood (Fig 28–2). Chronic mucocutaneous candidiasis frequently precedes both endocrinopathies; conversely, 84% of patients with this infection and an associated endocrinopathy have hypoparathyroidism. The typical sequence of events is shown in Figure 28–4: Hypoparathyroidism develops

in the first decade in 88% of patients. Addison's disease follows in about 2 years, and in 75% of patients it occurs within 9 years of the onset of the syndrome. These patients may be affected by a third endocrinopathy, including thyroid disease, diabetes mellitus, pernicious anemia, and ovarian failure. The probability that the sibling of an affected person will have Addison's disease or hypoparathyroidism or any one of the above-mentioned secondary disorders has been estimated to be 0.35.

Patients with idiopathic hypoparathyroidism frequently have circulating autoantibodies to parathyroid tissue; patients with Addison's disease and hypoparathyroidism also have an increased frequency of thyroid and parietal cell autoantibodies. A number of defective immune responses have been reported in patients with chronic mucocutaneous candidiasis with or without endocrinopathies. These include defective blast transformation, macrophage migration inhibition, and lymphocytotoxicity. The role of these abnor-

PLURIGLANDULAR ENDOCRINE FUNCTION

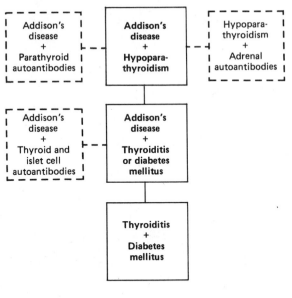

OTHER ENDOCRINE
DISORDERS

Graves' disease
Ovarian failure
Testicular failure
? Hypophysitis

NONENDOCRINE
DISORDERS

Mucocutaneous candidiasis
Pernicious anemia
Vitiligo
Alopecia
Chronic active hepatitis
Malabsorption

Figure 28–3. The 3 major clinical categories of pluriglandular autoimmune endocrinopathy (center column), with forme fruste variants (dashed boxes) and less frequently associated endocrine disorders and nonendocrine disorders. Graves' disease may substitute for thyroiditis. Gonadal failure is associated with a pan–steroid cell autoantibody in Addison's disease, and candidiasis is strongly associated with hypoparathyroidism. (Modified and reproduced, with permission, from Deftos LJ, Catherwood BD, Bone HG: Multiple endocrine disorders. Chapter 28 in: *Endocrinology and Metabolism,* 2nd ed. Felig P et al [editors]. McGraw-Hill, 1985.)

malities in the pathogenesis of immune sensitization to endocrine tissue is unclear.

Isolated Hypoparathyroidism

Patients with isolated hypoparathyroidism are similar to those with Addison's disease plus hypoparathyroidism in having an early onset of disease (73% in the first decade) and associated candidiasis. The frequency of parathyroid autoantibodies in this group is similar to that in the group with Addison's disease. Immunofluorescent adrenal autoantibodies are detected in 7% of patients with hypoparathyroidism, whereas in hypoparathyroidism with candidiasis, most patients have subclinical adrenal autoimmunity. The occurrence of adrenal autoantibodies and candidiasis thus indicates that this subset may represent a forme fruste of pluriglandular endocrine insufficiency.

Isolated Addison's Disease

As noted above, patients with isolated autoimmune Addison's disease still have an increased prevalence of thyroid, parathyroid, and islet cell autoantibodies when compared with control populations. These immunologic findings suggest that despite the absence of clinically evident involvement of other glands, isolated Addison's disease should be considered part of the spectrum of multiple endocrine autoimmunity, since some patients with this disorder may ultimately develop an associated endocrinopathy.

Schmidt's Syndrome

As shown in Figure 28–2, Schmidt's syndrome (defined in the introduction) is more frequent in females, and all of the components including the Addison's disease commonly have their onset in the age range from 20 to 50 years. Table 28–11 shows that the occurrence of diabetes mellitus in autoimmune Addison's disease is 10% and that of Hashimoto's thyroiditis and primary myxedema 9% overall. Although many of these patients may have onset of diabetes in young adulthood, most of them have been treated with insulin. Hashimoto's thyroiditis or diabetes develops an average of 7 years after adrenal insufficiency. Schmidt's syndrome is frequently accompanied by additional autoimmune diseases, including ovarian failure and pernicious anemia (see below).

Patients with Schmidt's syndrome have the highest rate of thyroid autoantibodies of any group with Addison's disease, which suggests that thyroid autoantibodies in Addison's disease may be predictive of thyroid failure. Activation of cell-mediated immunity is evidenced in Hashimoto's thyroiditis by an increased circulating number of Ia+ T cells.

Islet cell autoantibodies may also be important in Schmidt's syndrome. These autoantibodies circulate in the majority of patients at the time of diagnosis of insulin-dependent diabetes mellitus, even in the absence of any other tissue-specific autoimmune disease. The incidence is substantially lower in patients not requiring insulin therapy at the time of diagnosis. In most patients, islet cell autoantibodies disappear with time; their persistence in the blood is associated with the presence of other autoimmune disorders (19%) or autoantibodies to thyroid or gastric tissue (65%). In patients without insulin dependence at the time of diagnosis of their diabetes, the presence of islet cell autoantibodies appears to predict future insulin requirement and failure of oral hypoglycemic agent therapy.

For about half of index individuals, one or more other family members can be found with autoimmune endocrinopathies. These relatives frequently have only thyroiditis and diabetes without adrenal disease. Such family members may be assigned to this syndrome on the basis of their relative with Addison's disease.

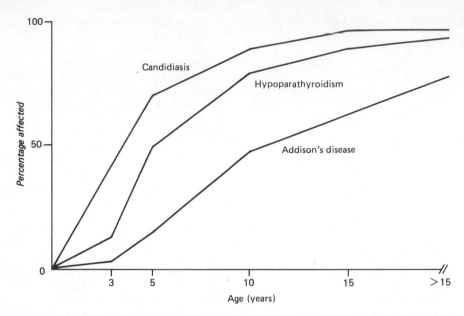

Figure 28–4. Typical sequence for childhood onset of chronic mucocutaneous candidiasis, autoimmune hypoparathyroidism, and Addison's disease. Patients with hypoparathyroidism may not develop Addison's disease, but frequent adrenal autoantibodies suggest that the polyendocrine diathesis is still present. (Source of data: Neufeld et al: *Medicine* 1981;**60**:355. Reproduced, with permission, from Deftos LJ, Catherwood BD, Bone HG: Multiple endocrine disorders. Chapter 28 in: *Endocrinology and Metabolism,* 2nd ed. Felig P et al [editors]. McGraw-Hill, 1985.)

Many more family members have been found to have thyroid autoantibodies in the blood.

Other Endocrinopathies Associated with Addison's Disease

Ovarian failure is common in women with autoimmune Addison's disease. In one large series, the prevalence of amenorrhea was 24%, and another 6% had oligomenorrhea. Abnormal reproductive function persists after adrenal replacement therapy and is uncommon in tuberculous Addison's disease, which leads to the conclusion that it is not related to deficiency of adrenal corticosteroids. The presumed autoimmune oophoritis is closely correlated with the onset of the patient's adrenal failure. In girls with Addison's disease and hypoparathyroidism occurring before the age of menarche, the presentation of oophoritis is that of primary amenorrhea, and in some cases streak gonads have been found at laparoscopy.

Ovarian failure in Addison's disease is closely related to a distinctive type of autoantibody against common antigens present in multiple steroid-producing cells, including theca interna, corpus luteum, Leydig cells, placenta, and adrenal cortex. These autoantibodies are cytotoxic for granulosa cells in monolayer cell culture. The presence of such autoantibodies is not only a risk factor for ovarian failure but may also be an independent risk factor for other extra-adrenal endocrinopathies. Steroid cell autoantibodies are uncommon in men with Addison's disease, but several instances of testicular failure associated with Addison's disease have been reported.

Although decreased function or failure is the most common consequence of attack on the endocrine glands, Graves' disease is intimately associated with these disorders; thyrotoxicosis occurs in about 8% of patients with Addison's disease. In patients with autoimmune Addison's disease, clinical atrophic gastritis may occur with or without diabetes, thyroid disease, hypoparathyroidism, or ovarian failure. Pernicious anemia is found in approximately 4% of patients with Addison's disease (Table 28–11).

Direct Association of Thyroid Disease & Diabetes Mellitus

The general frequency of diabetes mellitus and thyroid disease makes the study of a link between these disorders difficult. Nevertheless, an increased frequency of autoimmune thyroid disease in diabetics has been reported by many authors; pernicious anemia is also associated. Comparison of the frequency of tissue-specific autoantibodies in unselected diabetics versus age- and sex-matched controls provides additional support for this association. Table 28–13 provides a representative summary of the interrelationships of autoimmunity against islet, parietal, and thyroid cells.

Table 28–13. Interrelationships of autoimmunity against islet, parietal, and thyroid cells: Representative frequencies of occurrence.[1]

Index Disease	Associated Finding	Frequency
Diabetes mellitus	Thyroid autoantibodies	16%
	↑ TSH (males)	6%
	↑ TSH (females)	17%
	Parietal cell autoantibodies	17%
Thyroiditis	Islet cell autoantibodies	9%
	Intrinsic factor autoantibodies	2%
	Pernicious anemia	9%
Hyperthyroid- ism	Islet cell autoantibodies	3%
	Intrinsic factor autoantibodies	3%
	Pernicious anemia	3%
Pernicious anemia	Islet cell autoantibodies	11%
	Thyroid autoantibodies	38%
	Hypothyroidism	12%
	Hyperthyroidism	9%

[1]Modified and reproduced, with permission, from Deftos LJ, Catherwood BD, Bone HG: Multiple endocrine disorders. Chapter 28 in: *Endocrinology and Metabolism,* 2nd ed. Felig P et al (editors). McGraw-Hill, 1985.

Other Disorders

A dozen cases of presumed "autoimmune hypophysitis" have been reported, and half were associated with autoimmune diseases, especially lymphocytic thyroiditis and atrophic gastritis. All of these cases have been temporally related to pregnancy and have presented as sellar masses or sudden collapse. A diagnosis of hypopituitarism has been made in life in at least one of these patients. Diabetes insipidus has been associated with autoimmune adrenalitis and hypoparathyroidism in one instance, but the pathogenesis of this defect is unclear.

Vitiligo may occur with any autoimmune endocrinopathy. This disorder probably represents tissue-specific autoimmunity to melanin-producing cells.

MANAGEMENT OF PATIENTS WITH FAILURE OF MULTIPLE ENDOCRINE GLANDS

The history, physical examination, laboratory findings, and treatment of the hormonal disorders discussed in this section are similar to those of the disorders as they occur individually and are discussed in other chapters in this book.

The most serious pitfall in diagnosis of multiple autoimmune endocrinopathy would be to confuse adrenal, thyroid, and ovarian failure with hypopituitarism. In every such case, the integrity of pituitary function should be proved by showing elevated blood levels of TSH, LH, or ACTH. Failure of other glands not dependent on pituitary function (hypoparathyroidism or diabetes mellitus) should be an indicator of autoimmune endocrinopathy.

Patients with Addison's disease should receive particular attention in surveillance for failure of previously uninvolved glands, as these individuals are at greater risk. The physician should be alert for signs of the insidious onset of hypothyroidism and pernicious anemia. Elevation of serum TSH may be seen in untreated Addison's disease because of a lack of the normal regulatory effects of the steroid hormone on thyrotroph function and does not necessarily indicate thyroid disease unless it persists on glucocorticoid replacement. In a random population, slight elevation of serum TSH does not necessarily indicate future clinical hypothyroidism, but simultaneous observation of thyroid autoantibodies predicts an incidence of clinical hypothyroidism estimated to be 4% per year, and when autoantibody titers are markedly elevated, the incidence may be as high as 26% per year. These rates may be higher in patients with Addison's disease. First-degree relatives of patients with Addison's disease should also be observed carefully and evaluated with an ACTH stimulation test if they develop any autoimmune disorder. Cases have been reported in which secondary amenorrhea remitted following glucocorticoid replacement therapy of associated Addison's disease. It may thus be important to consider this association in any case of unexplained premature ovarian failure.

The implications of multiglandular endocrine failure for treatment are not well characterized. Since cortisol antagonizes the intestinal calcium transport effects of vitamin D, including vitamin D metabolites used to treat hypoparathyroidism, the development of adrenal failure can result in sudden vitamin D intoxication in affected patients.

GENETIC ASPECTS OF AUTOIMMUNE DISORDERS

Early genetic studies of autoimmune disorders have estimated probabilities of clinical involvement of 0.25–0.35 for siblings of probands with Schmidt's syndrome and Addison's disease with hypoparathyroidism.

Typing of antigens coded by the major histocompatibility (HLA) complex on chromosome 6 has provided genetic correlations with the clinical and immunopathologic findings in the individual autoimmune endocrinopathies. At least 3 classes of HLA glycoproteins are displayed by human cells. Class I molecules (antigens of the A and B loci) are expressed on all nucleated cells. They are quantitively regulated by lymphokines and may play a secondary role in autoimmune disorders. HLA-A and -B typing is useful, primarily because these molecules serve as markers closely linked to the HLA-D locus. Class II HLA molecules (HLA-DR, HLA-DQ, and others) are normally displayed only on a few antigen-presenting cells, such as the macrophage, but can be induced on many other cell types. The presence of HLA-DR on cell surfaces can be detected by the reaction of antibodies to common determinants such as Ia. Individuals can be classified into phenotypic groups using panels of antisera to class II antigens; further polymorphism can be detected functionally by the presence or absence of the mixed lymphocyte culture reaction against homozygous allogeneic lymphocytes. The immunologic defect in immune regulation resulting in autosensitization to endocrine tissue may be a gene in the HLA region genetically linked to certain HLA antigens. HLA-D antigens are most closely associated with the endocrine disorders (Table 28–14). Common haplotypes such as HLA-A1-B8-D3- and HLA-A2-B15-D4 occur because of linkage disequilibrium. HLA studies in type I diabetes mellitus have suggested that only the HLA-(B8)-D3-linked diabetogenic gene is associated with persistent islet cell autoantibodies and with other autoimmune disease and that homozygosity for this haplotype confers no increased risk of development of diabetes.

HLA typing of a number of kindreds with pluriglandular autoimmune endocrinopathy has been reported. In most families, this type of analysis has suggested dominant inheritance linked to either HLA-D3 or -D4. Data on the interaction of D3 and D4-linked genes are not available for Addison's disease. In a few kindreds the predictive value of HLA typing appeared questionable, and lack of HLA association has been reported for Addison's disease with hypoparathyroidism.

NONAUTOIMMUNE ENDOCRINE FAILURE

Bardwick et al have recently reviewed a syndrome, previously reported mostly from Japan, to which they give the acronym POEMS (polyneuropathy, organomegaly, endocrinopathy, M protein, and skin changes) (Table 28–15). Gonadal failure, gynecomastia, and glucose intolerance are frequent endocrine disorders,

Table 28–14. HLA antigen associations with autoimmune diseases (Caucasians).

Addison's disease	HLA-DR3 or -DR4
Atrophic thyroiditis	HLA-DR3
Graves' disease	HLA-B8 and -DR3
Diabetes mellitus	HLA-DR3 and -DR4
Hashimoto's thyroiditis	HLA-DR3 and -DR5
Hypoparathyroidism	?

Table 28–15. Incidence of abnormalities in patients with "POEMS" syndrome.[1]

Polyneuropathy	
Peripheral neuropathy	100%
Papilledema	68%
Increased cerebrospinal fluid	94%
Organomegaly	
Hepatomegaly	67%
Splenomegaly	37%
Lymphadenopathy	64%
Endocrinopathy	
Gynecomastia	70%
Impotence	67%
Amenorrhea	100%
Glucose intolerance	48%
Hypothyroidism	10%
M protein	61%
IgG	41%
IgA	20%
Marrow plasma cells	48%
Sclerotic bone lesions	71%
Skin changes	
Hyperpigmentation	98%
Thickening	85%
Hirsutism	78%
Hyperhidrosis	66%
Other	
Peripheral edema	92%
Ascites	68%
Pleural effusions	24%
Fever	48%

[1]Reproduced, with permission, from Bardwick PA et al: Plasma cell dyscrasia with polyneuropathy, organomegaly, endocrinopathy, M protein, and skin changes. *Medicine* 1980;59:311.

while adrenal failure is uncommon. Seventy-five percent of affected patients are male, and they have plasma cell dyscrasias with onset in the fourth or fifth decade, usually sclerotic plasmacytomas. In one of the cases reported by Bardwick et al, insulin-dependent diabetes mellitus remitted with irradiation of the patient's plasmacytoma, returned 3 years later with the appearance of a new tumor, and disappeared again with another course of radiation treatment. Neither the polyneuropathy nor the endocrinopathy appears to be due to amyloidosis. In contrast to findings in autoimmune endocrinopathies, Bardwick et al did not find tissue-specific endocrine autoantibodies. The mechanism of this interesting syndrome needs to be elucidated.

Pseudohypoparathyroidism type Ia is due to hereditary deficiency of the guanine nucleotide–binding regulatory protein of the cell membrane–adenylate cyclase complex and is characterized by resistance to multiple hormones besides parathyroid hormone. This disorder is discussed in Chapter 11.

REFERENCES

Multiple Endocrine Neoplasia

Austin LA, Heath H III: Calcitonin: Physiology and pathophysiology. *N Engl J Med* 1981;**304:**269.

Carney JA, Sizemore GW, Tyce GM: Bilateral adrenal medullary hyperplasia in MEN, type 2. *Mayo Clin Proc* 1975;**50:**3.

Chong GC et: Medullary carcinoma of the thyroid gland. *Cancer* 1975;**35:**695.

Copp DH, Crockroft DW, Kueh Y: Calcitonin from ultimobranchial glands of dogfish and chickens. *Science* 1967;**158:**924.

Cushman P Jr: Familial endocrine tumors: Report of two unrelated kindred affected with pheochromocytomas, one also with multiple thyroid carcinomas. *Am J Med* 1962;**32:**352.

Deftos LJ: *Medullary Thyroid Carcinoma.* Karger, 1983.

Deftos LJ: Radioimmunoassay for calcitonin in medullary thyroid carcinoma. *JAMA* 1974;**227:**403.

Deftos LJ, Bone HG, Parthemore JG: Immunohistological studies of medullary thyroid carcinoma and C-cell hyperplasia. *J Clin Endocrinol Metab* 1980;**51:**857.

Fung Y-K T et al: Structural evidence for the authenticity of the human retinoblastoma gene. *Science* 1987;**236:**1657.

Gagel FR et al: Natural history of the familial medullary thyroid carcinoma–pheochromocytoma syndrome and the identification of preneoplastic stages by screening studies: A five-year report. *Trans Assoc Am Physicians* 1975;**88:**177.

Gagel RF et al: The clinical outcome of prospective screening for multiple endocrine neoplasia type 2a. *N Engl J Med* 1988;**318:**478.

Genetic markers in multiple endocrine neoplasia type 2. (Editorial.) *Lancet* 1988;**1:**396.

Griffiths DFR, Williams GT, Williams ED: Duodenal carcinoid tumors, phaeochromocytoma and neurofibromatosis: Islet cell tumor, phaeochromocytoma and the Von Hippel-Lindau complex: Two distinctive neuroendocrine syndromes. *Q J Med* 1987;**245:**769.

Hazard JB: The C cells (parafollicular cells) of the thyroid gland and medullary thyroid carcinoma: A review. *Am J Pathol* 1977;**88:**213.

Hennessey JF et al: A comparison of pentagastrin injection and calcium infusion as provocative agents for the detection of medullary thyroid carcinoma. *J Clin Endocrinol Metab* 1974;**39:**487.

Jackson CE et al: The two-mutational-event theory in medullary thyroid carcinoma. *Am J Hum Genet* 1979;**31:**704.

Khairi MRA et al: Mucosal neuroma, pheochromocytoma and medullary thyroid carcinoma: MEN, type III. *Medicine* 1975;**54:**89.

Melvin KE, Tashjian AH Jr, Miller HH: Studies in familial (medullary) thyroid carcinoma. *Recent Prog Horm Res* 1972;**28:**399.

Naylor SL et al: Loss of heterozygosity of chromosome 3p markers in small-cell lung cancer. *Nature* 1987;**329:**451.

O'Connor DT, Burton D, Deftos LJ: Immunoreactive human chromogranin A in diverse polypeptide hormone–producing human tumors and normal endocrine tissues. *Clin Endocrinol Metab* 1983;**57:**1084.

Pearse AGE, Ewen SEB, Polak JM: The genesis of APUD amyloid in endocrine polypeptide tumors: Histochemical distinction from immunamyloid. *Virchows Arch [Cell Pathol]* 1972;**10:**93.

Parthemore JG et al: A short calcium infusion in the diagnosis of medullary thyroid carcinoma. *J Clin Endocrinol Metab* 1974;**39:**108.

Ponder BAJ et al: Risk estimation and screening in families of patients with medullary thyroid carcinoma. *Lancet* 1988;**1:**397.

Rouleau GA, Wertelecki W, Haines JL et al: Genetic linkage of bilateral acoustic neurofibromatosis to a DNA marker on chromosome 22. *Nature* 1987;**329:**246–248.

Schimke RN, Hartman WH: Familial amyloid-producing medullary thyroid carcinoma and pheochromocytoma: A distinct genetic entity. *Ann Intern Med* 1965; **63:** 1027.

Seizinger BR, Martuza RL, Gusella JF: Loss of genes on chromosome 22 in tumorigenesis of human acoustic neuroma. *Nature* 1986;**322:**644.

Seizinger BR et al: Genetic linkage of von Recklinghausen neurofibromatosis to nerve growth factor receptor gene. *Cell* 1987;**49:**589.

Seizinger BR et al: Von Hippel-Lindau disease maps to the region of chromosome 3 associated with renal cell carcinoma. *Nature* 1988;**332:**268.

Sipple JH: The association of pheochromocytoma with carcinoma of the thyroid gland. *Am J Med* 1961; **31:**163.

Steiner AL, Goodman AD, Powers SR: Study of a kindred with pheochromocytoma, medullary thyroid carcinoma, hyperparathyroidism, and Cushing's disease: MEN, type II. *Medicine* 1968;**47:**371.

Takai S et al: Loss of genes on chromosomes 22 in medullary thyroid carcinoma and pheochromocytoma. *Jpn J Cancer Res* 1987;**78:**894.

Wermer P: Genetic aspects of adenomatosis of endocrine glands. *Am J Med* 1954;**16:**363.

Williams ED: A review of 17 cases of carcinoma of the thyroid and phaeochromocytoma. *J Clin Pathol* 1965; **18:**288.

Wolfe HJ et al: C-cell hyperplasia preceding medullary thyroid carcinoma. *N Engl J Med* 1973;**289:**437.

Zollinger RM, Ellison EH: Primary peptic ulceration of the jejunum associated with the islet cell tumors of the pancreas. *Ann Surg* 1955;**142:**709.

Failure of Multiple Endocrine Glands

Ahmann AJ, Burman KD: The role of T lymphocytes in autoimmune thyroid disease. *Endocrinol Metab Clin North Am* 1987;**16:**287.

Asa SL et al: Lymphocytic hypophysitis of pregnancy resulting in hypopituitarism: A distinct clinicopathologic entity. *Ann Intern Med* 1981;**95:**166.

Bardwick PA et al: Plasma cell dyscrasia with polyneuropathy, organomegaly, endocrinopathy, M protein, and skin changes: The POEMS syndrome. *Medicine* 1980;**59:**311.

Betterle C et al: Complement-fixing adrenal autoantibodies as a marker for predicting onset of idiopathic Addison's disease. *Lancet* 1983;**1:**1238.

Blizzard RM, Chee D, Davis W: The incidence of adrenal and other antibodies in the sera of patients with idiopathic adrenal insufficiency (Addison's disease). *Clin Exp Immunol* 1967;**2**:19.

Blizzard RM, Chee D, Davis W: The incidence of parathyroid and other antibodies in the sera of patients with idiopathic hypoparathyroidism. *Clin Exp Immunol* 1966;**2**:19.

Bottazzo GF et al: Autoimmunity in juvenile diabetics and their families. *Br Med J* 1978;**2**:165.

Carpenter CCJ et al: Schmidt's syndrome (thyroid and adrenal insufficiency): A review of the literature and a report of fifteen new cases including ten instances of coexistent diabetes mellitus. *Medicine* 1964;**43**:153.

Chan JY, Walfish PG: Activated (Ia+) T-lymphocytes and their subsets in autoimmune thyroid diseases: Analysis by microfluorocytometry. *J Clin Endocrinol Metab* 1986;**62**:403.

Deftos LJ, Catherwood BD, Bone HG: Multiple endocrine disorders. Chapter 28 in: *Endocrinology and Metabolism*, 2nd ed. Felig P et al (editors). McGraw-Hill, 1985.

Dwyer JM: Chronic mucocutaneous candidiasis. *Annu Rev Med* 1981;**32**:491.

Eisenbarth GS et al: The polyglandular failure syndrome: Disease inheritance, HLA type, and immune function. *Ann Intern Med* 1979;**91**:528.

Foulis AK: Class II major histocompatibility complex and organ specific autoimmunity in man. *J Pathol* 1986; **150**:5.

Gordin A, Lamberg BA: Spontaneous hypothyroidism in symptomless autoimmune thyroiditis: A long-term follow-up study. *Clin Endocrinol* 1981;**15**:537.

Iitaka M et al: Studies of the effect of suppressor T lymphocytes on the induction of antithyroid microsomal antibody-secreting cells in autoimmune thyroid disease. *J Clin Endocrinol Metab* 1988;**66**:708.

Irvine WJ, Barnes EW: Addison's disease, ovarian failure and hypoparathyroidism. *Clin Endocrinol Metab* 1975;**4**:379.

Irvine WJ et al: Immunological aspects of premature ovarian failure associated with idiopathic Addison's disease. *Lancet* 1968;**2**:883.

Irvine WJ et al: Pancreatic islet cell antibodies in diabetes mellitus correlated with the duration and type of diabetes, coexistent autoimmune disease, and HLA type. *Diabetes* 1977;**26**:138.

Irvine WJ et al: Thyroid and gastric autoimmunity in patients with diabetes mellitus. *Lancet* 1970;**2**:164.

Maclaren NK, Riley WJ: Inherited susceptibility to autoimmune Addison's disease is linked to human leukocyte antigens -DR3 and/or -DR4, except when associated with type I autoimmune polyglandular syndrome. *J Clin Endocrinol Metab* 1986;**62**:455.

McCarthy-Young S, Lessof MH, Maisey MN: Serum TSH and thyroid antibody studies in Addison's disease. *Clin Endocrinol* 1972;**1**:45.

Nerup J: Addison's disease. *Acta Endocrinol* 1974; **76**:127.

Okita N, Row VV, Volpe R: Suppressor T-lymphocyte deficiency in Graves' disease and Hashimoto's thyroiditis. *J Clin Endocrinol Metab* 1981;**52**:528.

Pujol-Borrell R et al: Inappropriate major histocompatibility complex class II expression by thyroid follicular cells in thyroid autoimmune disease and by pancreatic beta cells in type I diabetes. *Mol Biol Med* 1986;**3**:159.

Rabinowe SL et al: Ia-positive T lymphocytes in recently diagnosed idiopathic Addison's disease. *Am J Med* 1984;**77**:597.

Rabinowe SL et al: Lymphocyte dysfunction in autoimmune oophoritis: Resumption of menses with corticosteroids. *Am J Med* 1986;**81**:347.

Rapoport B: Recombinant DNA technology in the study of autoimmune thyroid disease. *Endocrinol Metab Clin North Am* 1987;**16**:445.

Spinner MW, Blizzard RM, Childs B: Clinical and genetic heterogeneity in idiopathic Addison's disease and hypoparathyroidism. *J Clin Endocrinol* 1968;**28**:795.

Spinner MW et al: Familial distribution of organ-specific antibodies in the blood of patients with Addison's disease and hypoparathyroidism and their relatives. *Clin Exp Immunol* 1969;**5**:461.

Sridama V, Pacini F, Degroot L: Decreased suppressor T-lymphocytes in autoimmune thyroid diseases detected by monoclonal antibodies. *J Clin Endocrinol Metab* 1982;**54**:316.

Volpe R: Autoimmune thyroid disease—A perspective. *Mol Biol Med* 1986;**3**:25.

Weetman AP: Regulation and role of thyroid cell class II antigen expression. *Immunol Res* 1986;**5**:81.

Wuepper KD, Wegienka LC, Fudenberg HH: Immunologic aspects of adrenocortical insufficiency. *Am J Med* 1969;**45**:206.

Geriatric Endocrinology

29

Susan L. Greenspan, MD, & Neil M. Resnick, MD

Individuals over age 65 comprise the fastest growing segment of the United States population; each day this group increases by over 1000 people. This increase has led to a remarkable situation—of all the people who have ever lived to the age of 65, more than two-thirds are still alive. Thus, it is becoming increasingly important for the endocrinologist to understand how endocrine physiology and disease may differ in the elderly.

Before considering specific conditions, however, it is worthwhile to review some general principles that account for many of the age-related changes in disease presentation in the elderly. First, aging itself—in the absence of disease—is associated with only a gradual and linear decline in the physiologic reserve of each organ system (Fig 29–1). Since the reserve capacity of each system is substantial, age-related declines have little effect on baseline function and do not significantly interfere with the individual's response to stress until the eighth or ninth decade. Second, because each organ system's function declines at a different physiologic rate, and because 75% of the elderly have at least one disease, endocrine dysfunction in the elderly often presents disparately, with initial symptoms derived from the most compromised organ system. For example, hyperthyroidism in an elderly patient with preexisting coronary and conduction system disease may present with atrial fibrillation and a slow ventricular response, while in another, equally hyperthyroid patient with a prior stroke, it may present with confusion or depression; neither patient may tolerate hyperthyroidism long enough for the classic thyroid-related manifestations (eg, goiter) to become apparent. Third, elderly patients often have multiple diseases and take many medications that may mimic or mask the usual presentation of endocrine disease.

THYROID FUNCTION & DISEASE

The prevalence of thyroid disease in the elderly is approximately twice that in younger individuals; hy-

Acronyms Used in This Chapter

ACTH	Adrenocorticotropic hormone
AVP	Argine vasopressin
BMD	Bone mineral density
cAMP	Cyclic adenosine monophosphate
CRH	Corticotropin-releasing hormone
DHEA	Dehydroepiandrosterone
FSH	Follicle-stimulating hormone
hCG	Human chorionic gonadotropin
HPA	Hypothalamic-pituitary-adrenal
LH	Luteinizing hormone
LHRH	Luteinizing hormone–releasing hormone
NPH	Neutral protamine Hagedorn
PTH	Parathyroid hormone
SIADH	Syndrome of inappropriate secretion of antidiuretic hormone
TRH	Thyrotropin-releasing hormone
TSH	Thyroid-stimulating hormone (thyrotropin)

pothyroidism and hyperthyroidism each affect roughly 3–4% of older individuals. In addition, some studies suggest that up to 9% of hospitalized elderly patients have overt thyroid disease. Finally, "subclinical hypothyroidism"—normal serum levels of thyroid hormones (thyroxine, T_4; triiodothyronine, T_3) but an elevated level of thyrotropin (TSH)—is more prevalent, with estimates of 4–14% in the elderly.

There are no major age-related changes in the physiology of the hypothalamic-pituitary-thyroid axis (see Chapter 10). TSH release remains pulsatile (Fig 29–2), although the nocturnal rise in serum TSH appears to be blunted with age. Balanced decreases in T_4 secretion and clearance result in no change in serum T_4; T_3 resin uptake, free T_4, and the free T_4 index are also unchanged. There is a slight age-related decline in serum T_3, but values usually remain within normal limits. Serum TSH increases slightly with age, but this too remains within normal limits. The effect of age on the release of TSH by thyrotropin-releasing hormone (TRH) is less clear, but most recent studies show little change in either sex. The 24-hour radioiodine uptake is also unchanged. Thyroid antibodies occur more commonly in the elderly (15% compared to 2.5% in younger

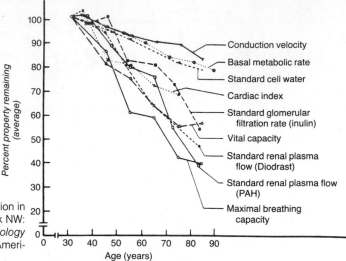

Figure 29–1. Influence of age on physiologic function in humans. (Reproduced, with permission, from Shock NW: Discussion on mortality and measurement. In: *The Biology of Aging: A Symposium*. Strehler BL et al [editors]. American Institute of Biological Sciences, 1960.)

counterparts), but their presence does not serve as a specific screening test for thyroid disease.

DISORDERS OF THE THYROID GLAND

1. HYPERTHYROIDISM

Clinical Findings

With age, the prevalence of Graves' disease decreases (although it remains the most common cause of hyperthyroidism) and the prevalence of multinodular goiter and toxic nodules increases. Elderly hyperthyroid patients tend to present with symptoms or complications related to the most vulnerable organ system, usually the cardiovascular system (atrial fibrillation, congestive heart failure, angina, and acute myocardial infarction) or the central nervous system (apathy, depression, confusion, or lassitude). Occasionally, they present with gastrointestinal symptoms, but these differ from those seen in younger patients because they include constipation, failure to thrive, and anorexia and weight loss. Because of degeneration of the sinus node and fibrotic changes in the cardiac conduction system, older patients are less likely than younger patients to present with palpitations (Table 29–1).

The physical signs of hyperthyroidism also differ in the elderly (Table 29–1). Resting tachycardia is less frequent, the thyroid feels normal in size or is not palpable in two-thirds of patients, and lid lag is uncommon. Ophthalmopathy is less common, not only because Graves' disease occurs less often, but also because even with Graves' disease ophthalmopathy occurs less frequently in the elderly. However, although they are less common in the elderly, some findings appear to be highly suggestive of hyperthyroid-

ism. These include increased frequency of bowel movements, weight loss despite increased appetite, fine finger tremor, eyelid retraction, and increased perspiration.

Diagnosis

As in younger patients (see Chapter 10), the diagnosis is usually confirmed by standard thyroid function tests. A TRH test is rarely required. There are potential pitfalls, however. T_3 toxicosis may be more difficult to diagnose because concomitant nonthyroid illness is common and can depress serum T_3. Euthyroid hyperthyroxinemia (due to nonthyroid illness) may also cause confusion. Elderly patients may also be taking medications such as propranolol, which may elevate levels of serum T_4. Finally, iodide-induced hyperthyroidism, known also as the jodbasedow effect, is becoming more common in elderly patients with multinodular goiter because of increased exposure to radiocontrast studies; the resultant hyperthyroidism is generally transient.

Treatment

Beta-blocking agents are useful in alleviating symptoms, but radioactive iodine is the therapy of choice in elderly patients because it is efficient, uncomplicated, and inexpensive. Antithyroid drugs can be used prior to radioactive iodine treatment to render the patient euthyroid and to avoid radiation-induced thyroiditis, but they are not definitive treatment and are more toxic in this age group. Surgery has a more limited role because of its increased morbidity.

Following radioactive iodine treatment, patients become euthyroid over a period of 6–8 weeks. They should receive careful follow-up, because hypothyroidism develops in 80% or more of those patients who have been adequately treated. Once hyperthyroidism has abated, the metabolic clearance rate of other medi-

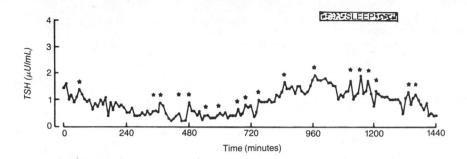

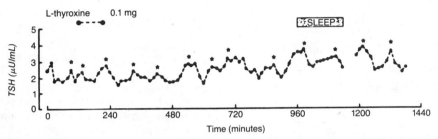

Figure 29–2. Twenty-four-hour serum TSH pulsation profiles in a healthy 34-year-old (●———●) and 67-year-old (●--------●) receiving levothyroxine (0.1 mg/d). Pulses are identified with stars. (Reproduced, with permission, from Greenspan SL et al: Pulsatile secretion of thyrotropin in man. *J Clin Endocrinol Metab* 1986;**63**:661.)

cations may decrease and doses may require readjustment.

2. HYPOTHYROIDISM

Hypothyroidism in the elderly is most often due to Hashimoto's thyroiditis or radioactive iodine ablative therapy.

Clinical Findings

It is easy to overlook hypothyroidism in an older person because many euthyroid elderly patients have the same symptoms. Moreover, elderly patients with hypothyroidism are more likely than younger patients with hypothyroidism to present with cardiovascular symptoms (eg, congestive heart failure or angina), or neurologic findings (eg, cognitive impairment, confusion, depression, paresthesias, deafness, psychosis, or coma). Finally, in the older hypothyroid patient, the physical findings are frequently nonspecific, although puffy face, delayed deep tendon reflexes, and myoedema support the diagnosis.

Diagnosis

The diagnosis can be established by a low serum T_4, T_3 resin uptake, and free T_4 index, in conjunction with an elevated TSH. Measurement of serum T_3 is unnecessary and potentially misleading, because T_3 is the

form of thyroid hormone most likely to decrease in nonthyroid illness. Although an increased serum TSH is the most sensitive indicator of decreased thyroid function, it should not be used alone to diagnose hypothyroidism because it will not always differentiate symptomatic from "subclinical" hypothyroidism. Furthermore, in hypothyroid patients, serum TSH levels can be reduced to within the normal range by treatment with dopaminergic drugs and corticosteroids. In such patients, determination of free T_4 and reverse T_3 may help to differentiate those with true hypothyroidism from those with nonthyroid illness.

Treatment

The doses of thyroid hormone required for adequate replacement decrease with age (Table 29–2). Elderly patients should be started on approximately 25–50 μg of levothyroxine, and the dose should be increased by approximately 25 μg every 3–4 weeks. In patients with cardiovascular disease, even lower initial doses can be used and increased at a slower rate. Dessicated thyroid hormone and preparations containing T_3 should be avoided because T_3 is rapidly absorbed and cleared. The metabolic clearance of other drugs will change as hypothyroidism is corrected, and their doses may require readjustment.

It is still not known whether treating "subclinical hypothyroidism" is beneficial in older patients. However, two-thirds of these patients will remain chem-

Table 29–1. Percentages of patients with symptoms and clinical findings attributable to thyrotoxicosis.[1]

	Old[1]	Old[2]	Young
Symptoms			
Number	25	85	247
Mean age	81.5	68.6	40[2]
Range	75–95	60–82	5–73
Symptoms			
Weight loss	44	35	85
Palpitations	36	42	89
Weakness	32	28	70
Dizziness, syncope	20	—	—
Nervousness	20	38	99
No symptoms	8	—	—
Memory loss	8	—	—
Tremor	8	—	—
Local symptoms[3]	8	11	—
Pruritus	4	4	—
Heat intolerance	4	63	89
Clinical Findings			
Pulse > 100	28[4]	58	100
Atrial fibrillation	32	39	10
New-onset atrial fibrillation	20[5]	—	—
Lid lag	12	35	71
Exophthalmos	8	8	—
Fine skin	40	81	97
Tremor	36	89	97
Myopathy	8	39	—
Hyperactive reflexes	24	26	—
Gynecomastia	(1 male)	1	10
None	8	—	—
Thyroid			
Impalpable or normal	68	37	—
Diffusely enlarged	12	22	100
Multinodular goiter	12	20	—
Isolated nodule	8	21	—

[1]Modified and reproduced, with permission, from Tibaldi JM et al: Thyrotoxicosis in the very old. *Am J Med* 1986;**81**:619.
[2]Approximated from graph of patients' ages.
[3]Dysphagia, enlarging neck mass, etc.
[4]Includes 5 patients with normal sinus rhythm as well as 2 who had atrial fibrillation.
[5]This was transient in 4 of 5 patients with conversion to normal sinus rhythm. Old[1] = Tibaldi JM et al: Thyrotoxicosis in the very old. *Am J Med* 1986;**81**:619. Old[2] = Davis PJ, Davis FB: Hyperthyroidism in patients over the age of 60 years. *Medicine* 1974;**53**:161. Young = Ingbar SH et al: The thyroid gland. In: *Williams' Textbook of Endocrinology.* Williams RH (editor). Saunders, 1981.

ically euthyroid for at least 4 years, and low titers of antimicrosomal antibodies may identify patients at lowest risk for progression. At present, careful annual follow-up is recommended.

3. MULTINODULAR GOITER

The prevalence of multinodular goiter increases with age. However, if swallowing and breathing are not compromised and thyroid function tests are normal, the goiter can be observed without treatment. Levothyroxine therapy rarely shrinks the gland, and although it may prevent further enlargement, the risk of inducing hyperthyroidism is significant because multinodular goiters may develop areas of autonomous function.

4. THYROID NODULES & CANCER

Thyroid nodules are more common in the elderly. Ninety percent of these nodules are benign, but the prognosis for elderly patients with malignant nodules may be worse than that for younger patients with malignant nodules. The prognosis also correlates with the size of the tumor. The outcome in elderly patients may therefore be substantially improved by early evaluation of nodules in patients who are surgical candidates.

Papillary carcinoma is more common in young and middle-aged patients. However, it has a poorer prognosis in the elderly, possibly because it is detected at a more advanced stage. Follicular carcinoma accounts for 15% of thyroid cancers and usually occurs in middle-aged and older patients. Anaplastic thyroid carcinoma is almost exclusively found in middle-aged and older patients. It presents as a rapidly growing hard mass, which is locally invasive, often has metastatic lesions, and has a very poor prognosis.

Table 29–2. Daily dose of thyroxine in hypothyroid patients.[1,2]

	Daily Dose of Thyroxine (μg/day)		
	<40 Years	40–60 Years	>60 Years
All patients	167 ± 62[4] (20)	135 ± 37 (34)	109 ± 42[3] (40)
Men	185 ± 82[5] (5)	149 ± 36 (19)	116 ± 48[4] (16)
Women	148 ± 33[5] (5)	116 ± 15 (15)	105 ± 37[5] (24)

[1]Reproduced, with permission, from Sawin CT et al: Aging and the thyroid. *Am J Med* 1983;**75**:206.
[2]Values are mean ± 1 standard deviation (SD); numbers of patients are indicated in parentheses.
[3]$p < 0.01$ (all p values are compared to ages 40–60).
[4]$p < 0.05$.
[5]NS.

CARBOHYDRATE INTOLERANCE & DIABETES MELLITUS

AGING & THE PHYSIOLOGY OF CARBOHYDRATE INTOLERANCE

Even healthy elderly individuals demonstrate an age-related increase in fasting blood glucose (1 mg/dL [0.6 mmol/L] per decade) and a more significant increase in blood glucose (5 mg/dL [0.28 mmol/L] per decade) in response to a standard glucose tolerance test. According to the criteria of the National Diabetes Data Group, nearly 10% of the elderly have glucose intolerance. The possible causes of this intolerance include changes in body composition, diet, physical activity, insulin secretion, and insulin action.

With aging, lean body mass decreases and body fat increases. The percentage of body fat correlates positively with fasting levels of serum glucose, insulin, and glucagon. However, when obesity (or the percentage of body fat) is taken into account, the basal levels of glucose, insulin or glucagon are not influenced by age.

Insulin release appears to be unaffected by age. Decreased physical activity and a low-carbohydrate diet also impair glucose tolerance, but the major contribution to glucose intolerance in healthy, active elderly individuals appears to be a decrease in insulin-mediated uptake of glucose in peripheral tissues (Fig 29–3). This is probably due to a postreceptor defect that has not yet been characterized. However, recent findings suggest that much of the carbohydrate intolerance found in average elderly individuals is caused by diet, drugs, lack of exercise, or environmental factors.

DIABETES MELLITUS

Clinical Findings

The prevalence of diabetes mellitus increases with age, affecting 17% of persons over age 65. Most diabetes in the elderly is type II, or non-insulin-dependent, diabetes. Diabetes may be difficult to diagnose in the elderly because of its often atypical and asymptomatic presentation. For example, polyuria or polydipsia are not present in many elderly patients, because the glomerular filtration rate and thirst threshold decline with age while the renal threshold for glycosuria increases. Instead, symptoms in these individuals are usually nonspecific (eg, weakness, fatigue, weight loss, or minor infection). These patients may also present with neurologic findings such as cognitive impairment, acute confusion, or depression.

The diagnosis is established by obtaining a fasting blood glucose above 140 mg/dL (7.8 mmol/L) on 2 separate occasions (in the absence of acute illness); a 2-hour oral glucose tolerance test is needed rarely, if

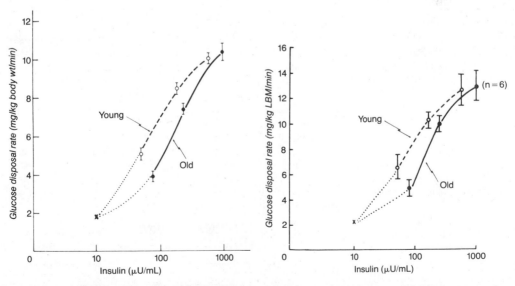

Figure 29–3. Dose-response curves for insulin-mediated disposal in young (O-----O) and old (●——●) subjects. In the left panel, glucose disposal is expressed as milligrams per kilogram of body weight. In the right panel, glucose disposal rates are normalized for lean body mass. (Reproduced, with permission, from Rowe JW et al: Characterization of the insulin resistance of aging. *J Clin Invest* 1983;**71**:1581.)

ever. Because the renal threshold for glycosuria increases in the elderly, the diagnosis should not be based on the presence of glycosuria. Increased blood levels of glycosylated hemoglobin support the diagnosis, but this test is more useful in monitoring treatment.

Since the complications of diabetes mellitus are related to the duration of disease, elderly patients who live long enough will suffer the same complications of nephropathy, neuropathy, and ophthalmopathy as their younger counterparts.

Treatment

A reasonable treatment goal in the elderly patient with diabetes mellitus is to maintain the fasting blood glucose below 150 mg/dL (8.3 mmol/L) and the postprandial blood glucose below 220 mg/dL (12.2 mmol/L). Achieving this goal is often difficult and complicated by other medications commonly prescribed for the elderly, eg, thiazide diuretics, phenytoin, and glucocorticoids, which have hyperglycemic effects.

Similar to the strategy used in younger patients (see Chapter 22), initial therapy should include dietary manipulation, weight reduction, and an exercise program tailored to the individual's capabilities. If mild to moderate hyperglycemia persists (fasting blood glucose < 300 mg/dL [16.7 mmol/L]), an oral hypoglycemic agent should be tried. Chlorpropramide should be avoided because of its long half-life and its propensity to induce both hyponatremia and hypoglycemia. Because of their convenience and potency, second-generation agents such as glipizide and glyburide are often used, but no data yet support their superiority to older agents such as tolazamide or tolbutamide.

If the fasting blood sugar remains above 300 mg/dL (16.7 mmol/L), insulin therapy should be started. The usual initial dose is 15–30 units of NPH (neutral protamine Hagedorn, or isophane) or another intermediate-acting insulin. One daily injection is usually sufficient. Since elderly patients often lack symptoms of hypoglycemia, the fasting, postprandial, and bedtime blood glucose levels must be checked initially even if symptoms are absent. Finally, as in younger patients, it is important to control other adverse factors such as hypertension and smoking, which can contribute to vascular complications associated with diabetes.

Diabetic ketoacidosis is rarely seen in the elderly. It should be treated cautiously, following a strategy similar to one used in younger patients (see Chapter 22), with particular attention to the correction of electrolytes and water balance.

NONKETOTIC HYPEROSMOLAR COMA

Clinical Findings

Nonketotic hyperosmolar coma occurs almost exclusively in the elderly. Predisposing factors include inadequate insulin secretion in response to hyper-

glycemia and a reduction in the peripheral effectiveness of insulin. Both factors lead to a progressive increase in serum glucose concentrations. The age-related increased renal threshold prevents osmotic diuresis until significant hyperglycemia is present, while an age-related decline in thirst predisposes to dehydration. Blood glucose concentrations often exceed 1000 mg/dL (55.5 mmol/L) and are coupled with marked elevation of plasma osmolality without ketosis.

This syndrome is frequently seen in elderly patients with type II diabetes who are in nursing homes. However, one-third of such patients have no previous history of diabetes, and nonketotic hyperosmolar coma can be precipitated by medications (eg, thiazide, furosemide, phenytoin, glucocorticoids) or an acute medical illness. Patients present with an acute confusional state, lethargy, weakness, and, occasionally, coma. Neurologic findings can be generalized or focal and can mimic an acute cerebrovascular event. Marked volume depletion, orthostatic hypotension, and prerenal azotemia are also usually present.

Treatment

The average extracellular fluid volume deficit is 9 L. It should be replaced initially with normal saline, especially when significant orthostatic hypotension is present. After 1–3 L of isotonic saline have been administered, fluids can be changed to half-normal (0.45%) saline. Half of the fluid and ion deficits should be replaced in the first 24 hours and the remainder over the next 48 hours.

Intravenous insulin in small doses (10–15 units) should be given initially, followed by a drip infusion of 3–5 units/h. Insulin therapy should not be used in lieu of fluids because it will exacerbate intravascular fluid depletion and further compromise renal function as it shifts glucose intracellularly. Potassium deficits should be corrected when the patient is producing urine. Possible precipitating events—such as an acute myocardial infarction, pneumonia, or administration of a medication—must be investigated and treated. Although metabolic abnormalities may improve in 1–2 days, mental status deterioration and confusion may persist for one week or more. Over one-third of patients can be discharged without insulin treatment, but they are at significant risk for recurrence and should be monitored carefully.

OSTEOPOROSIS & CALCIUM HOMEOSTASIS

OSTEOPOROSIS

Despite the considerable prevalence, morbidity, and expense of osteoporosis, most of our knowledge is derived from studies of perimenopausal women. Yet it is the older woman who typically experiences the ravages of the disease. Twenty-five percent of women have vertebral fractures by age 70; by age 80, the figure is closer to 50%. Over 90% of hip fractures occur in women over age 70, and by age 90, one woman in 3 will have sustained such a fracture. Hip fractures are associated with significant morbidity, an increased risk of institutionalization, and up to a 20% increase in mortality rates. Despite the significant differences between perimenopausal and older women, diagnostic and therapeutic approaches for older women are derived largely from studies of perimenopausal women. The relevance of such studies for older women has only recently been questioned.

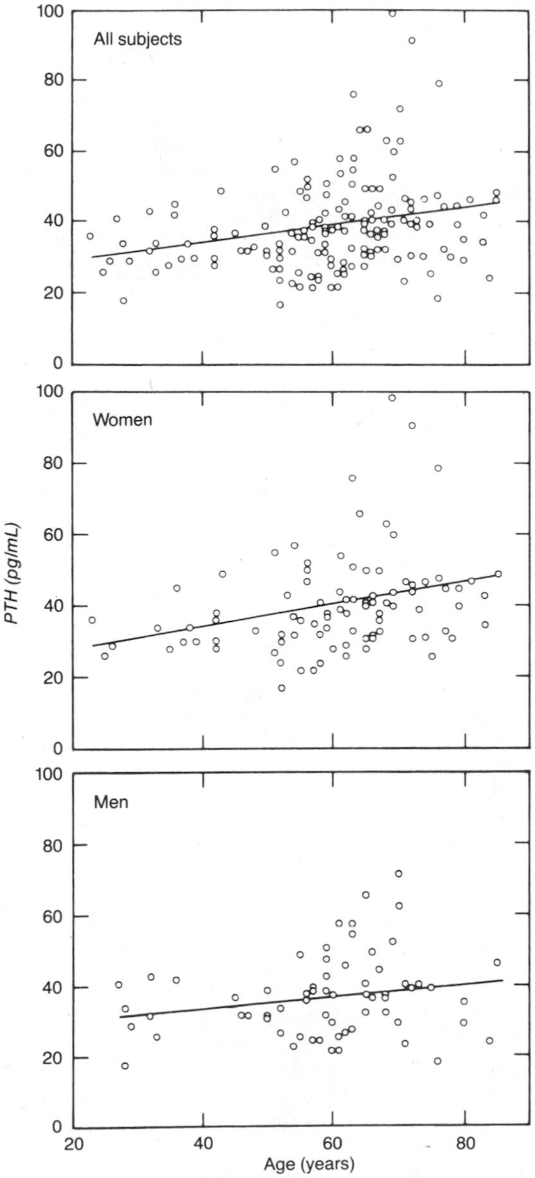

Factors Affecting Bone Physiology

There are significant physiologic differences between perimenopausal and older women with respect to maintenance of skeletal integrity. While calcium intake is inadequate in both age groups, calcium absorption declines with age, despite an age-related increase in serum levels of parathyroid hormone (PTH) (Fig 29–4); this increase is not due solely to a decrease in renal clearance, and it is associated with other biochemical evidence of increased PTH activity, including elevated levels of bone GLA protein (osteocalcin) and nephrogenous cyclic adenosine monophosphate (cAMP).

A. Vitamin D: Vitamin D metabolism also changes with age. The ability to convert vitamin D to its active moiety (calcitriol) is impaired with age, as is the skin's ability to form vitamin D precursors. Elderly individuals also experience decreased sun exposure and have a decreased dietary intake of vitamin D. As a result, vitamin D deficiency is common in the elderly. Up to 15% of healthy, elderly residents of communities in the sunny southwestern USA have frank vitamin D deficiency; still more have subclinical vitamin D deficiency; and up to 50% of elderly nursing home residents are deficient in vitamin D. Finally, bone formation also appears to decrease with age. These factors are summarized in Figure 29–5.

B. Bone Loss and Architectural Changes: The rate of bone loss also differs between perimenopausal and older women. Cortical and (possibly) trabecular bone are lost rapidly at menopause, but in older women,

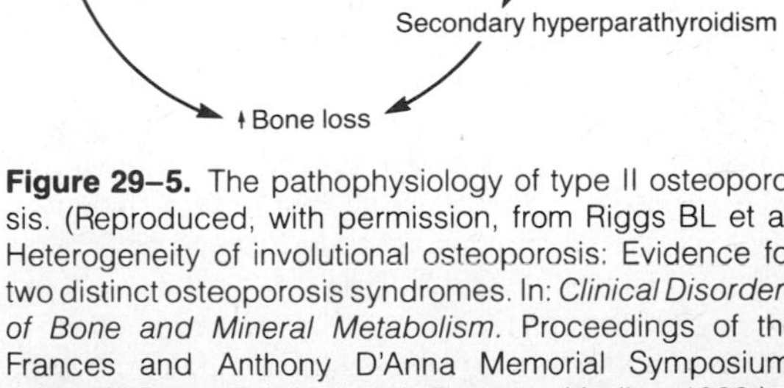

Figure 29–4. The effect of age on serum PTH. Upper panel, entire study group (p = 0.27, p < 0.001); middle panel, women (r = 0.31, p < 0.001); lower panel, men (r = 0.21; p < 0.05). (Reproduced, with permission, from Marcus R et al: Age-related changes in parathyroid hormone and parathyroid action in normal humans. *J Clin Endocrinol Metab* 1984;**58**:223.)

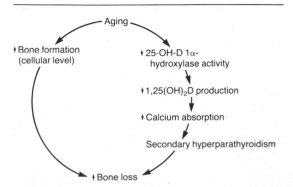

Figure 29–5. The pathophysiology of type II osteoporosis. (Reproduced, with permission, from Riggs BL et al: Heterogeneity of involutional osteoporosis: Evidence for two distinct osteoporosis syndromes. In: *Clinical Disorders of Bone and Mineral Metabolism.* Proceedings of the Frances and Anthony D'Anna Memorial Symposium. Frame B, Potts JT Jr [editors]. *Excerpta Medica,* 1983.)

Panel 1

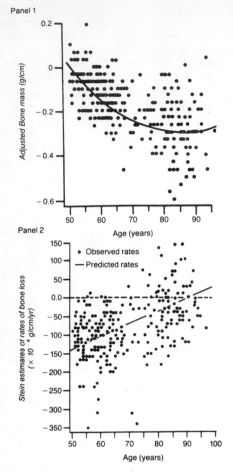

Panel 2

Panel 3

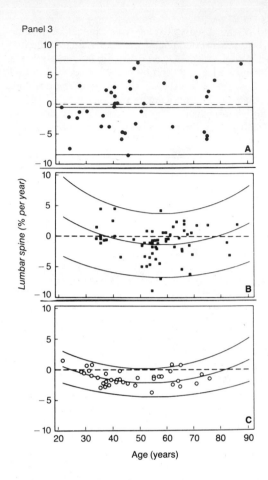

Figure 29–6. Rate of bone loss in perimenopausal and older women. *Panel 1:* Cross-sectional data showing the average bone mass at the midshaft site of the radius measured by single-photon absorptiometry for each subject adjusted for body size plotted against mean age during the time of measurement. *Panel 2:* Longitudinal data for subjects followed for a mean of 7 years, showing the linear rate of bone loss plotted against age for each subject. The rate of bone loss declines with age. (Modified, with permission, from Hui SL et al: A prospective study of change in bone mass with age in postmenopausal women. *J Chronic Dis* 1982;**35**:715.) *Panel 3:* Longitudinal rates of *trabecular* bone loss in 139 normal women measured by dual photon absorptiometry. The rate of change in bone mineral density (BMD) of the lumbar spine is plotted against age at time of the first BMD measurement. Subjects are identified by time on study: A ~ 1 year; B ~ 2 years; ~ 3 years. When all data were analyzed, mean bone loss occurred across life. When only subjects in the groups having mean scan intervals of ~ 2 years or ~ 3 years were analyzed, however, age regression was best fitted with a parabolic equation. Center line denotes age regression and upper and lower line denotes 95% confidence limits for the equation. Broken line shows zero rate of change in BMD. (Modified, and reproduced, with permission, from Riggs BL et al: Rates of bone loss in the appendicular and axial skeletons of women. *J Clin Invest* 1986;**77**:1487.)

cortical bone loss (at least in the forearm) may slow and in some cases cease; the data on trabecular bone loss are still inconclusive (Fig 29–6).

In addition, there are changes in bone geometry; cortical bone remodeling in older women is insufficient to compensate for the loss of bone mineral content (Fig 29–7). There are also qualitative changes in trabecular bone, since an age-related reduction in trabecular bone jeopardizes plate integrity or "connectivity"; trabecular plates not only become perforated and disconnected, but with aging they continue to thin, causing further loss of bone strength and compromising the bone's ability to regain structural integrity with conventional therapy (Fig 29–8).

C. Risk Factors: Fracture risk factors differ in perimenopausal and older women. While a "fracture threshold" is helpful in determining which perimenopausal women are at risk for fracture, by age 70 most women have bone density measurements below this threshold (Fig 29–9), yet less than one-fourth of them will ever suffer a hip fracture. Falling is often cited as major risk factor for hip fracture in the older woman. Although more than one-third of elderly women fall annually, however, less than 5% of falls result in a fracture and those falls that do still cannot be predicted. Weakened muscles, decreased proprioception, and reduced soft tissue padding may contribute to the risk but have not yet been well evaluated. Moreover,

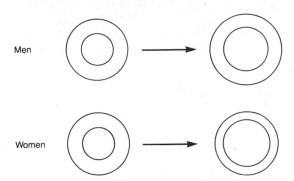

Figure 29–7. Schematic representation of cortical bone remodeling with age in males and females. Note that with age-related bone loss, bone is remodeled in men to increase its diameter and partially offset the loss of strength. In women, bone diameter changes little with age so that bone strength decreases proportionately more than in men. (Reproduced, with permission, from Ruff CB, Hayes WC: Sex differences in age-related remodeling of the femur and tibia. *J Orthop Res* 1988;**6**:886.

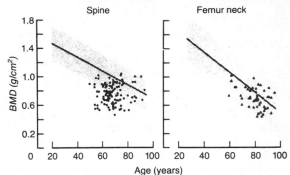

Figure 29–9. Bone mineral density (BMD) levels for spine and femur neck, plotted as a function of age for 111 patients with vertebral fractures (·) and 49 patients with hip fractures (△). The line represents the regression with age; the cross-hatched area shows the 90% confidence limits for 166 normal women. Note that the fracture threshold (90th percentile of the measurements for patients with fractures) is about 1 g/c² and is independent of age. (Reproduced, with permission, from Riggs BL et al: Involutional osteoporosis. *N Engl J Med* 1986;**314**:1676).

the factors that protect the older woman from fractures in over 95% of falls are still unknown. Finally, although not considered a risk factor for fractures in perimenopausal women, medications that affect the sensorium or postural blood pressure (eg, psychotropic and sedative agents) are associated with fractures in older women.

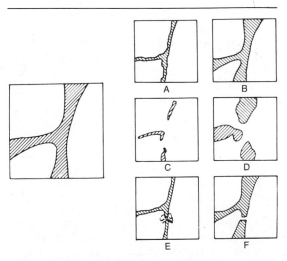

Figure 29–8. Possible effects of osteoporotic treatment regimens on trabecular bone. *Left panel:* Normal trabecular bone mass and architecture. Treatment resulting in anabolic effects on bone volume may restore normal bone volume and architecture in thin trabeculae (*A,B*). If trabecular integrity is disrupted before treatment, similar effects on bone volume may not reverse architectural abnormalities (*C,D*), particularly if treatment impairs the repair of microfractures (*E,F*). (Modified and reproduced, with permission, from Kanis JA: Treatment of osteoporotic fracture. *Lancet* 1984:**1**:27.)

Treatment

Because the factors that affect bone physiology—the rate of bone loss, the structure of remaining bone, and the risk of fracture—are substantially different in perimenopausal and elderly women, interventions appropriate for perimenopausal women may be inappropriate for older women. Unfortunately, few therapeutic studies include older individuals, and the studies that do generally use bone density (rather than bone fracture) as an endpoint. Bone density as an endpoint may be less relevant for the elderly woman whose bone density is already depleted, because even if further bone loss could be slowed, it is not clear that fracture risk would be reduced, especially if the structure of the remaining bone is still impaired. Since all but one of the currently accepted modalities only slow further bone loss, it is still difficult to estimate their efficacy in preventing hip fractures in the elderly.

A. Calcium: Considerable controversy surrounds the use of calcium supplementation in perimenopausal women, and few data are available regarding its use in older women. Theoretically, calcium supplementation seems appropriate because calcium intake in the elderly is low and the ability to adapt to a low-calcium diet declines with age. However, there are potential problems with prescribing high doses of calcium in the elderly. First, calcium induces or exacerbates constipation. Second, when given with vitamin D to patients who are also taking a diuretic, calcium supplementation may provoke hypercalcemia, especially if dehydration occurs. Third, since compliance with other drug regimens decreases as the number of drugs increases, calcium therapy may supplant more important medications.

B. Vitamin D: There are few data to support the use of vitamin D or its metabolites. In fact, one study demonstrated a small but significantly harmful effect of calcitriol on vertebral fractures. Additionally, there is a small therapeutic ratio for vitamin D; toxicity from hypercalcemia can occur with doses as low as 50 μg (2000 IU), especially in individuals who are also taking a thiazide diuretic and calcium supplementation.

C. Estrogen: Estrogen therapy slows bone loss and prevents osteoporotic fractures in perimenopausal women, but there is little evidence supporting its use for the first time in women over age 65. Of 4 available studies, 2 are positive and 2 show no effect, and each had significant design limitations. The most recent report is a longitudinal analysis from the Framingham study. Although estrogen was reported to have a positive effect, it was not significant in women over age 65, only half of the elderly women had been given estrogen for the first time, and all of the fracture protection occurred in just a few months. The last point cannot be readily explained by current concepts of estrogen's mode of action.

Estrogen's protective effect against cardiovascular disease is another benefit frequently cited to support its use. However, there are few data to support the suggestion that such a benefit will accrue when estrogen is newly prescribed to elderly women in whom the prevalence of heart disease is already high. Since estrogen, like calcium, only slows bone loss in women who already have insufficient and inadequate bone, and since estrogen may provoke menses and the need for gynecologic surveillance and endometrial sampling to prevent cervical cancer, it is difficult at present to advocate prophylactic use of estrogen in the elderly woman.

D. Exercise: Although the rationale for exercise therapy is sound, there is little evidence that it will benefit the elderly woman. One study prescribed exercise for older women and found that forearm bone mineral content increased in those who continued exercising during a 3-year trial. However, it is unclear whether the benefit extends to other more important sites, such as the hip. In addition, exercise is potentially dangerous because sedentary older women who newly engage in exercise may increase their exposure to accidents and subsequent fractures.

In summary, there is ample reason to question the validity of extrapolating data from studies of perimenopausal women when formulating a treatment plan for older women. However, given the prevalence of the problem and the current lack of alternatives, it is reasonable to recommend an adequate daily intake of vitamin D (10–20 μg contained in 1–2 multivitamin tablets), an adequate daily intake of calcium (totaling 800–1500 mg), and judicious participation in an individually tailored exercise program.

Perhaps more importantly, the risk of falls should be addressed. This can be accomplished by reviewing medications (including nonprescription agents) and discontinuing (when possible) those with adverse effects on cognition, balance, or blood pressure. It is also important to correct reversible sensory losses and medical conditions and to educate patients about hazards in their environment, such as throw rugs, extension cords, and poorly lit stairways, that could lead to falls and fractures.

HYPERPARATHYROIDISM

Clinical Findings

Hyperparathyroidism becomes increasingly prevalent with age. While its incidence is less than 10 per 100,000 in women under age 40, the incidence increases to 190 per 100,000 in women over age 60. As a result, over half of all cases of hyperparathyroidism occur in individuals over the age of 65. Most cases are mild. Detection is by routine screening of serum calcium, and few, if any, symptoms are present. However, with relatively minor elevations of serum calcium (up to 11–12 mg/dL [2.8–3 mmol/L]), some elderly subjects may experience weakness, fatigue, depression, and confusion. Failure to thrive and constipation are commonly seen; renal, gastrointestinal, and skeletal complications occur less often. Other causes of hypercalcemia in the elderly—especially multiple myeloma, malignancy, vitamin D intoxication, and thiazide diuretics—must be considered in the differential diagnosis.

Treatment

For symptomatic patients with serum calcium levels above 12 mg/dL (3 mmol/L), parathyroidectomy is well tolerated and is the treatment of choice. For those with more modest elevations, treatment decisions are less certain because it is difficult to differentiate symptoms and signs due to the disease from those seen in older individuals without hyperparathyroidism. Moreover, asymptomatic individuals—especially those with levels of serum calcium under 11 mg/dL (2.8 mmol/L)—have been observed to remain asymptomatic for over a decade. Until more data become available, the decision to treat asymptomatic individuals surgically should be made on an individual basis.

In patients whose symptoms may be due to hyperparathyroidism, it is worthwhile to observe the response to medical therapy before considering surgery. In women, a course of estrogen may be effective. Ethinyl estradiol (30–50 μg/d) or conjugated estrogens (1.25–2.5 mg/d) reduce serum calcium by an average of 0.8 mg/dL, diminish urinary calcium excretion, and antagonize the skeletal effect of PTH. In men and in women with higher elevations of serum calcium, oral phosphates can be used, but they are less well tolerated in the elderly because of their gastrointestinal side effects. Furosemide is a less satisfactory alternative in frail elderly patients because it increases the risk of dehydration with resultant hypercalcemia.

CHANGES IN WATER BALANCE

With age, major changes in renal function and homeostatic mechanisms result in significant changes in water balance. Renal blood flow, cortical mass, glomerular number, and tubular function all decline with age, although medullary mass is preserved. Clinically, however, the most relevant change is the age-related decline in creatinine clearance (Fig 29–10), which is largely due to relative hypertension in the elderly. Because of the decrease in muscle mass associated with aging, however, serum creatinine levels are unchanged and may not accurately reflect the extent of renal functional impairment.

Extrarenal modulators of water balance also change significantly with age. Although there are no changes in the basal level, half-life, volume of distribution, or metabolic clearance of vasopressin, the stimulated responses of vasopressin are significantly altered. Hyperosmolar stimuli increase serum vasopressin levels in older subjects to 5 times those achieved in younger subjects (Fig 29–11). On the other hand, the normal vasopressin increase observed in response to overnight dehydration and postural change is impaired in the elderly. Additionally, basal and stimulated levels of serum renin and aldosterone decline with age. In contrast, basal levels of atrial natriuretic factor are 3-fold higher in healthy elderly individuals than in young controls. Finally, the thirst sensation appears to be somewhat impaired in healthy elderly individuals and is more impaired in those who are frail.

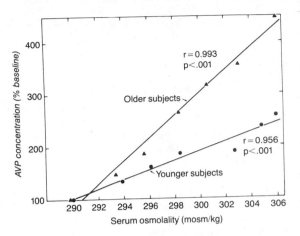

Figure 29–11. Relationship between serum osmolality and arginine vasopressin (AVP) concentration in young (mean age 35 years) and old (mean age 67 years) subjects who received 3% saline, 0.1 mL/kg/min intravenously for 2 hours. The relationship, ΔAVP : Δosmolality, defines osmoreceptor sensitivity; hence, the differences in slopes shown here indicate heightened osmoreceptor sensitivity in elderly subjects. (Reproduced, with permission, from Helderman JH et al: The response of arginine vasopressin to intravenous ethanol and hypertonic saline in man: The impact of aging. *J Gerontol* 1978;**33**:39.)

DISORDERS OF WATER BALANCE

In addition to physiologic changes, many diseases and drugs further increase the vulnerability of the elderly to changes in water balance. These include kidney disease, hypertension, and congestive heart failure, as well as medications that alter water balance (eg, narcotics, diuretics, lithium, chlorpropamide, carbamazepine, amphotericin-B, intravenous hypotonic fluids, and hypertonic contrast agents).

1. HYPERNATREMIA

Clinical Findings

The incidence of hypernatremia in elderly patients admitted to the hospital is approximately 1% and is higher in institutionalized elderly patients. Signs and symptoms are usually nonspecific, eg, lethargy, weakness, confusion, depression, and failure to thrive. The cause is usually multifactorial, including impaired thirst, renal disease, sedative-induced confusion, use of restraints, impaired access to free water, excess water loss due to fever, and decreased response to vasopressin.

Treatment

As in younger patients, initial therapy involves correcting the volume deficit with isotonic saline and then correcting the water deficit with half-normal (0.45%)

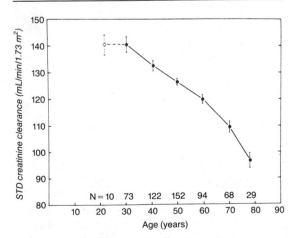

Figure 29–10. Cross-sectional differences in standard creatinine clearance with age. The number of subjects in each age group is indicated above the abscissa. Values plotted indicate mean ± standard error of mean (SEM). (Reproduced, with permission, from Rowe JW et al: The effect of age on creatinine clearance in man: A cross-sectional and longitudinal study. *J Gerontol* 1976;**31**:155.)

saline. Roughly 30% of the deficit should be corrected within 24 hours and the remainder within the next 24–48 hours.

2. HYPONATREMIA

Clinical Findings

The prevalence of hyponatremia is approximately 2.5% in the general hospital setting, is higher in geriatric units, and rises to 20% in the nursing home setting. Presenting symptoms and signs are often nonspecific and include lethargy, weakness, and confusion. The mechanisms predisposing to hyponatremia include the exuberant response of vasopressin to osmolar stimuli, a decreased ability to excrete a water load, and the sodium-wasting tendency of the older kidney. Additionally, elderly patients often use medications and have diseases that impair free water excretion. Common hyponatremic syndromes in the elderly include the syndrome of inappropriate antidiuretic hormone secretion (SIADH) and thiazide-induced hyponatremia.

Treatment

The treatment of hyponatremia in the elderly does not differ from that in younger patients (see Chapter 9).

3. HYPORENINEMIC HYPOALDOSTERONISM

Hyporeninemic hypoaldosteronism usually occurs in elderly patients with diabetes and mild renal insufficiency. Patients are usually asymptomatic, and hyperkalemia and acidosis are found on routine screening. On the other hand, symptoms of hyperkalemia (eg, heart block) may be provoked by administration of a beta-adrenergic blocking agent, which further compromises extrarenal regulation of potassium homeostasis. After other causes of persistent hyperkalemia are ruled out, patients respond well to administration of small doses of fludrocortisone (0.05 mg/dL) or furosemide combined with restriction of potassium.

GLUCOCORTICOIDS & STRESS

Because of equivalent decreases in secretion and clearance, serum cortisol and corticosteroid-binding globulin change little with age. However, the morning peak of cortisol secretion occurs several hours earlier in the elderly (Fig 29–12).

In healthy elderly individuals, dynamic testing of the hypothalamic-pituitary-adrenal axis (HPA) is normal; expected responses to insulin-induced hypo-

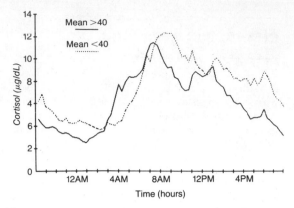

Figure 29–12. Mean 24-hour plasma cortisol concentration derived from 20-minute sampling for 12 subjects more than 40 years of age and for 22 subjects less than 40 years of age. (Reproduced, with permission, from Sherman B et al: Age-related changes in the circadian rhythm of plasma cortisol in man. *J Clin Endocrinol Metab* 1985;**61**:439.)

glycemia, metyrapone, dexamethasone, ACTH and to CRH are preserved (Fig 29–13).

DISORDERS OF THE HYPOTHALAMIC-PITUITARY-ADRENAL AXIS

1. ABNORMAL RESPONSE TO STRESS

In contrast to the normal responses of the HPA in the elderly to dynamic testing, increased stress elicits abnormal responses. For example, although serum cortisol levels increase to the same extent in young and old patients undergoing elective surgery, the increase is protracted in the elderly (Fig 29–14). It is not known whether other, more commonly encountered types of stress provoke persistent elevations of cortisol, but if so, these elevated levels may contribute to the increased hypertension, glucose intolerance, muscle atrophy, osteoporosis, and impaired immune function observed in the elderly.

2. ADRENAL HYPERSECRETION

While adrenal hypersecretion (Cushing's syndrome) is uncommon in the elderly, it is easily overlooked because it mimics normal aging processes. Signs such as hypertension, glucose intolerance, weight gain, and osteoporosis are less specific in elderly than in younger patients, but as in younger patients the diagnosis is established or excluded using the usual criteria (see Chapter 12).

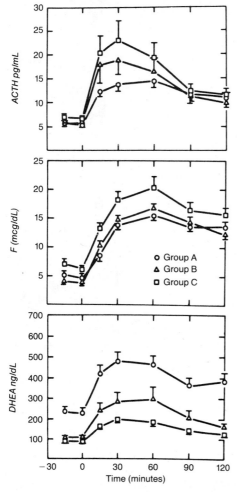

Figure 29–13. Mean values for groups A, B and C of plasma ACTH (*upper panel*), F or cortisol (*middle panel*), and DHEA (*lower panel*) before, and up to 120 min after, bolus intravenous injection of ovine CRH (1 μg/kg). Group A, 21–49 yr, mean age 35.2 yr, n = 19. Group B, 50–69 yr, mean age 60.7 yr, n = 15. Group C, 70–86 yr, mean age 77.1 yr, n = 15. (Reproduced, with permission, from Pavlov EP et al: Responses of plasma adenocorticotropin, cortisol, and dehydroepiandrosterone to ovine corticotropin-releasing hormone in healthy aging men. *J Clin Endocrinol Metab* 1986;**62**:767.)

3. ADRENAL INSUFFICIENCY

Symptoms of adrenal insufficiency in younger patients, eg, failure to thrive, weakness, weight loss, confusion, and arthralgias, are common complaints in adrenally intact elderly patients; the most specific sign of adrenal insufficiency in the elderly is hyperpigmentation. The laboratory findings of adrenal insufficiency are similar to those found in younger patients and in-

clude azotemia, hypoglycemia, hyponatremia, hyperkalemia, and eosinophilia. Because the metabolic clearance rate of cortisol decreases with age, older patients generally require lower replacement doses of cortisol.

CHANGES IN REPRODUCTIVE FUNCTION IN MEN

Overall, while sexual activity decreases with age, there are only minor physiologic changes in the hypothalamic-pituitary-testicular axis. There is no consensus on the effect of age on the production or metabolism of dihydrotestosterone, estrone, and estradiol. Studies of testosterone economy show that serum testosterone (Fig 29–15), sex hormone-binding globulin, and free testosterone change little, if at all, while testosterone clearance decreases. A decrease in the number or responsiveness of testicular Leydig cells is likely because serum FSH and LH increase with age, and the testosterone response to human chorionic gonadotropin (hCG) decreases. On the other hand, with age there is probably a decrease in the ratio of circulating bioactive to immunoreactive LH. Finally, minor pituitary changes are suggested by a decreased gonadotropic response to luteinizing hormone-releasing hormone (LHRH) stimulation (Fig 29–16).

The clinical relevance of these changes is questionable. The correlation between sexual activity and the minor age-related changes described is weak, and although early studies found decreased spermatozoa concentrations in the ejaculate of older men, the difference disappeared after corrections were made for frequency of ejaculation. Sperm motility and the volume of ejaculate do decrease with age, and the proportion of abnormal spermatozoa also increases.

Impotence becomes more prevalent with age and is more likely to have several possible causes. The incidence in men under age 45 is 5%; the incidence in men over age 75 is 50%. Unfortunately, there are few studies of this problem in the elderly. However, one study of men over age 50 found that 90% had coexistent medical conditions or were taking medications that contributed to their impotence. Often there were multiple overlapping causes of impotence—psychosocial, neurovascular, and arteriolar—in the same individual.

The evaluation of impotence in the elderly is similar to that in younger individuals (see Chapter 16), although more emphasis must be placed on the effects of drugs (both prescribed and nonprescribed), and a search for multiple causative factors should be undertaken.

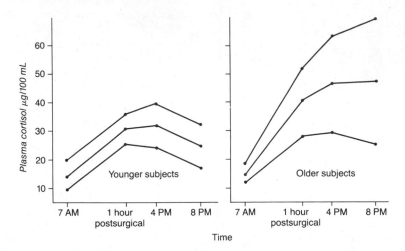

Figure 29–14. Plasma cortisol response to surgery in 20 young and 15 elderly patients. The average values are calculated, the dotted area indicating ± standard deviation (SD). (Reproduced, with permission, from Blichert-Toft M et al: Secretion of corticotropin and somatotropin by the senescent adenohypophysis in man. *Acta Endocrinol (Copenh)* [Suppl 195] 1975;**78:**1.)

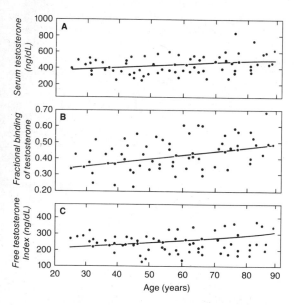

Figure 29–15. Total and free serum testosterone in men in relation to age. *A:* Serum testosterone concentration in men of various ages. The solid line in this and subsequent figures is drawn from least squares linear regression. *B:* Fractional binding of testosterone by column chromatography determined in sera from men of different ages. *C:* Free testosterone index determined from serum testosterone and fractional binders in sera from men of different ages. (Reproduced, with permission, from Harman SM et al: Reproductive hormones in aging men. 1. Measurement of sex steroids, basal luteinizing hormone, and Leydig cell response to human chorionic gonadotropin. *J Clin Endocrinol Metab* 1980;**51:**35.)

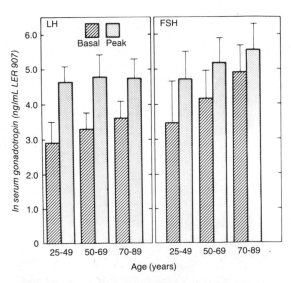

Figure 29–16. Log-transformed mean basal and peak serum LH and FSH levels obtained for each group of men before and after LHRH stimulation. (Error bars indicate one SD.) Reproduced, with permission, from Harman SM et al: Reproductive hormones in aging men. 2. Basal pituitary gonadotropins and gonadotropin responses to luteinizing hormone–releasing hormone. *J Clin Endocrinol Metab* 1982;**54:**547.

REFERENCES

Thyroid Function & Disease

Davis PJ, Davis FB: Hyperthyroidism in patients over the age of 60 years. *Medicine* 1974;**53**:161.

Greenspan SL et al: Pulsatile secretion of thyrotropin in man. *J Clin Endocrinol Metab* 1986;**63**:661.

Harman SM, Wehman RE, Blackman MR: Pituitary-thyroid hormone economy in healthy aging men: Basal indices of thyroid function and thyrotropin responses to constant infusions of thyrotropin releasing hormone. *J Clin Endocrinol Metab* 1984;**58**:320.

Livingston EH et al: Prevalence of thyroid disease and abnormal thyroid tests in older hospitalized and ambulatory persons. *J Am Geriatr Soc* 1987;**35**:109.

Meneilly GS et al: Endocrine systems. In: *Geriatric Medicine,* 2nd ed. Rowe JW, Besdine R (editors). Little, Brown, 1988.

Nordyke RA, Gilbert FI, Harada ASM. Graves' disease: Influence of age on clinical findings. *Arch Intern Med* 1988;**148**:626.

Robuschi G et al: Hypothyroidism in the elderly. *Endocr Rev* 1987;**8**:142.

Rosenthal MJ et al: Thyroid failure in the elderly: Microsomal antibodies as discriminant for therapy. *JAMA* 1987;**258**:209.

Sawin CT et al: Aging and the thyroid. *Am J Med* 1983;**75**:206.

Sawin CT et al: The aging thyroid: Relationship between elevated serum thyrotropin level and thyroid antibodies in elderly patients. *Am J Med* 1985;**79**:591.

Sawin CT et al: The aging thyroid: Thyroid deficiency in the Framingham study. *Arch Intern Med* 1985; **145**:1386.

Tibaldi JM et al: Thyrotoxicosis in the very old. *Am J Med* 1986;**81**:619.

Carbohydrate Intolerance & Diabetes Mellitus

Cahill GF: Hyperglycemic hyperosmolar coma: A syndrome almost unique in the elderly. *J Am Geriatr Soc* 1983;**31**:103.

Chen M, Halter JB, Porte D: The role of dietary carbohydrate in the decreased glucose tolerance of the elderly. *J Am Geriatr Soc* 1987;**35**:417.

Davidson MB: The effect of aging on carbohydrate metabolism: A review of the English literature and a practical approach to the diagnosis of diabetes mellitus in the elderly. *Metabolism* 1979;**28**:688.

Elahi D et al: Effect of age and obesity on fasting levels of glucose, insulin, growth hormone and glucagon in man. *J Gerontol* 1982;**37**:385.

Harris MI et al: Prevalence of diabetes and impaired glucose tolerance and plasma glucose levels in US population aged 20–74 years. *Diabetes* 1987;**36**:523.

Hollenbeck CB et al: Effect of habitual physical activity on regulation of insulin-stimulated glucose disposal in older males. *J Am Geriatr Soc* 1985;**33**:273.

Kannel WB: Lipid diabetes in coronary heart disease: Insights from the Framingham Study. *Am Heart J* 1985;**110**:1100.

Kannel WB, McGee DL: Diabetes and glucose tolerance as risk factors for cardiovascular disease: The Framingham Study. *Diabetes Care* 1979;**2**:210.

Minaker KL et al: Clearance of insulin: Influence of steady state insulin levels and age. *Diabetes* 1982; **31**:851.

Reaven GM, Reaven EP: Age, glucose tolerance, and non-insulin-dependent diabetes mellitus. *J Am Geriatr Soc* 1985;**33**:286.

Rowe JW, Minaker KL, Pallotta JA: Characterization of the insulin resistance of aging. *J Clin Invest* 1983; **71**:1581.

Zavaroni I et al: Effect of age and environmental factors on glucose tolerance and insulin secretion in a worker population. *J Am Geriatr Soc* 1986;**34**:271.

Osteoporosis & Calcium Homeostasis

Cummings SR et al: Epidemiology of osteoporosis and osteoporotic fractures. *Epidemiol Rev* 1985;**7**:178.

Heath DA et al: Surgical treatment of primary hyperparathyroidism in the elderly. *Br Med J* 1980; **280**:1406.

Heath H III et al: Primary hyperparathyroidism. *N Engl J Med* 1980;**302**:189.

Holick MF: Vitamin D requirements for the elderly. *Am J Clin Nutr* 1986;**5**:121.

Hui SL et al: A prospective study of change in bone mass with age in postmenopausal women. *J Chronic Dis* 1982;**35**:715.

Jensen GF, Christiansen C, Transbol I: Treatment of post menopausal osteoporosis: A controlled therapeutic trial comparing oestrogen/gestagen, 1,25-dihydroxy-vitamin D_3 and calcium. *Clin Endocrinol* 1982;**16**:515.

Kiel DP et al: Hip fracture and the use of estrogens in postmenopausal women: The Framingham Study. *N Engl J Med* 1987;**317**:1169.

Mannix H Jr et al: Hyperparathyroidism in the elderly. *Am J Surg* 1980;**139**:581.

Marcus R, Madvig P, Young G: Age-related changes in parathyroid hormone and parathyroid hormone action in normal humans. *J Clin Endocrinol Metab* 1984; **58**:223.

Marcus R et al: Conjugated estrogens in the treatment of post-menopausal women with hyperparathyroidism. *Ann Intern Med* 1984;**100**:633.

Melton LJ III, Riggs, BL: Risk factors for injury after a fall. *Clin Geriatr Med* 1985;**1**:525.

Omdahl JL et al: Nutritional status in a healthy elderly population: Vitamin D. *Am J Clin Nutr* 1982;**36**:1225.

Parfitt AM: Trabecular bone architecture in the pathogenesis and prevention of fracture. *Am J Med* 1987;**82** **(Suppl 1B)**:68.

Parfitt AM et al: Vitamin D and bone health in the elderly. *Am J Clin Nutr* 1982;**36**:1014.

Quigley MET et al: Estrogen therapy arrests bone loss in elderly women. *Am J Obstet Gynecol* 1987;**156**:1516.

Ray WA et al: Psychotropic drug use and the risk of hip fracture. *N Engl J Med* 1987;**316**:363.

Resnick NM, Greenspan SL. Senile Osteoporosis reconsidered. *JANA* 1989;**261**:1025.

Riggs BL, Melton LJ III: Involutional osteoporosis. *N Engl J Med* 1986;**314**:1676.

Riggs BL et al: Rates of bone loss in the appendicular and axial skeletons of women. *J Clin Invest* 1986;**77**:1487.

Ruff CB, Hayes WC: Sex differences in age-related remodeling of the femur and tibia. *J Orthop Res* 1988; **6**:886.

Selby PL et al: Ethinyl estradiol and norethindrone in the treatment of primary hyperparathyroidism in postmenopausal women. *N Engl J Med* 1986; **314**:1481.

Smith EL Jr, Reddan W, Smith PE: Physical activity and calcium modalities for bone mineral increase in aged women. *Med Sci Sports Exerc* 1981;**13**:60.

Tibblin S et al: Hyperparathyroidism in the elderly. *Ann Surg* 1983;**197**:135.

Wilson PWF, Garrison RJ, Castelli WP: Postmenopausal estrogen use, cigarette smoking, and cardiovascular morbidity in women over 50. *N Engl J Med* 1985; **313**:1038.

Changes in Water Balance

Anderson RJ et al: Hyponatremia: A prospective analysis of its epidemiology and the pathogenetic role of vasopressin. *Ann Intern Med* 1985;**102**:164.

Cyus JC, Krothapalli RK, Arieff AL: Treatment of symptomatic hyponatremia and its relation to brain damage. *N Engl J Med* 1987;**317**:1190.

Helderman JH et al: The response of arginine vasopressin to intravenous ethanol and hypertonic saline: The impact of aging. *J Gerontol* 1978;**33**:39.

Philips PA et al: Reduced thirst after water deprivation in healthy elderly men. *J Clin Endocrinol Metab* 1987; **64**:81.

Rowe JW et al: The effect of age on creatinine clearance in man: a cross-sectional and longitudinal study. *J Gerontol* 1976;**31**:155.

Shannon RP, Minaker KL, Rowe JW: Aging and water balance in humans. *Semin Nephrol* 1984;**4**:346.

Snyder NA, Feigal DW, Arieff AL: Hypernatremia in elderly patients: A heterogenous, morbid, and iatrogenic entity. *Ann Intern Med* 1987;**107**:309.

Glucocorticoids & Stress

Blichert-Toft M, Blichert-Toft B, Jensen HK: Pituitary-adrenocortical stimulation in the aged as reflected in levels of plasma cortisol and compound. *Acta Chir Scand* 1970;**136**:665.

Blichert-Toft M, Hippe E, Jensen HK: Adrenal cortical function as reflected by the plasma hydrocortisone and urinary 17-ketogenic steroids in relation to surgery in elderly patients. *Acta Chir Scand* 1967;**133**:591.

Blichert-Toft M, Hummer L: Serum immunoreactive corticotropin and response to metyrapone in old age in man. *Gerontology* 1977;**23**:236.

Blichert-Toft M et al: Secretion of corticotropin and somatotropin by the senescent adenohypophysis in man. *Acta Endocrinol (Copenh)* [Suppl 195] 1975; **78**:1.

Muggeo M et al: Human growth hormone and cortisol response to insulin stimulation in aging. *J Gerontol* 1975;**30**:546.

Pavlov EP et al: Response of plasma adrenocorticotropin, cortisol and dehydro-epiandrosterone to ovine corticotropin-releasing hormone in healthy aging men. *J Clin Endocrinol Metab* 1986;**62**:767.

Sapolsky RM, McEwen B: Why dexamethasone resistance? Two possible neuroendocrine mechanisms. In: *HPA Physiology and Pathophysiology*. Schatzberg A, Nemeroff C (editors). Raven Press, 1987.

Sherman B, Wysham C, Pfohl B: Age-related changes in the circadian rhythm of plasma cortisol in man. *J Clin Endocrinol Metab* 1985;**61**:439.

West CD et al: Adrenocortical function and cortisol metabolism in old age. *J Clin Endocrinol Metab* 1961; **21**:1197.

Reproductive Function in Men

Davis SS et al: Evaluation of impotence in older men. *West J Med* 1985;**142**:499.

Harman SM, Tsitouras PD: Reproductive hormones in aging men. 1. Measurement of sex steroids, basal luteinizing hormone, and Leydig cell response to human chorionic gonadotropin. *J Clin Endocrinol Metab* 1980;**51**:35.

Harman SM et al: Reproductive hormones in aging men. 2. Basal pituitary gonadotropins and gonadotropin responses to luteinizing hormone-releasing hormone. *J Clin Endocrinol Metab* 1982;**54**:547.

Pearlman CK: Frequency of intercourse in males at different ages. *Med Aspects Hum Sex* 1972;**6**:92.

Sparrow D, Bosser, Rowe JW: The influence of age, alcohol consumption and body build on gonadal function in men. *J Clin Endocrinol Metab* 1980;**51**:508.

Tsitouras PD, Martin CE, Harman SM: Relationship of serum testosterone to sexual activity in healthy elderly men. *J Gerontol* 1982;**37**:288.

Appendix

Appendix. Table of normal hormone test results[1]

Test	Source	Value: Per ML or DL		Value: SI Units[2]
Adrenocorticotropic Hormone, ACTH	Plasma	20–100 pg/mL		4.4–22.2 pmol/L

(Collect in plastic syringe with 100 U heparin/5 mL blood; keep iced, centrifuge in plastic tube under refrigeration; store frozen at −60 °C.)

Test	Source	Value: Per ML or DL		Value: SI Units[2]
Antidiuretic Hormone ADH (Vasopressin)	Plasma	If serum osmolarity > 290 mosm/kg, 2–12 pg/mL		1.85–11.1 pmol/L
		If serum osmolarity < 290 mosm/kg, < 2 pg/mL		<1.85 pmol/L

(Collect in EDTA tubes, keep iced, centrifuge refrigerated, store at −70 °C within 2 hr.)

Test	Source	Value: Per ML or DL		Value: SI Units[2]
Aldosterone	Serum, fasting	Sodium intake 100–200 meq/d:	ng/dL	pmol/L
		0700 hr, recumbent	3–9	83–250
		0900 hr, upright	4–30	111–832
		adrenal vein	200–400	5548–11096
		Sodium intake 10 meq/d:		
		0700 fasting, recumbent	12–36	333–999
		0900 hr, upright	17–137	472–3800
	Urine	On normal diet (100–200 meq Na/d), 2–19 μl/24 h		5.5–52.7 nmol/24 h
		On low-sodium diet (<20 meq Na/d), 10–40 μg/24 h		28–112 nmol/24 h

Test	Source	Value: Per ML or DL		Value: SI Units[2]
Androstanediol Glucuronide	Serum	ng/ml Male: 2.6–16		nmol/L 5.7–35.2
		Female: 0.6–8.1		1.3–17.8

(Freeze serum and store at −20 °C.)

Test	Source	Value: Per ML or DL		Value: SI Units[2]
Androstenedione	Serum	0.4–2.3 ng/mL (adults)		1.4–7.9 nmol/L

Test	Source	Value: Per ML or DL		Value: SI Units[2]
			ng/mL	μg/L
C Peptide of Insulin	Serum	Fasting:	0.5–3	0.5–3
		Stimulated:	1.5–9	1.5–9

(Freeze serum at −20 °C within 8 hrs of collection.)

Test	Source	Value: Per ML or DL		Value: SI Units[2]
			pg/mL	pmol/L
Calcitonin	Plasma	Male:	<91	<24.5
		Female:	<71	<19.2

(Refrigerate, spin down immediately, store at −20 °C.)

Calcitonin Stimulation Test: Pentagastrin, 0.5 μg/kg administered intravenously; plasma specimens obtained at 0, 1.5, 5, 10, and 15 min. A positive response is a 1.5-minute level of >190 pg/mL (51.4 pmol/L) in a male, or >80 pg/mL (21.6 pmol/L) in a female.

Test	Source	Value: Per ML or DL		Value: SI Units[2]
			pg/mL	nmol/L
Catecholamines	Plasma	Norepinephrine	110–410	0.7–2.4
		Epinephrine	<50	<.27
		Dopamine	<30	<.19

(Collect and centrifuge under refrigeration. Freeze in plastic at −60 °C.)

			μcg/24 h	nmol/24 h
	Urine	Norepinephrine	15–56	88.6–331
		Epinephrine	<15	<82
		Dopamine	100–440	625–2750

(24-hr urine preservative: 25 mL 6N HCl)

(continued)

Test	Source	Value: Per ML or DL			Value: SI Units[2]	
Cortisol	Plasma	µg/dL AM: 5–20 PM: 2.5–10			µmol/L 0.14–0.55 0.07–0.28	
(Collect and process under refrigeration; spin down immediately.)						
	Urine (free)	25–95 ng/mg creatinine			78–297 nmol/mmol creatine	
Dehydroepiandros-terone (DHEA)	Serum	Age <6 yr 6–8 yr 8–10 yr 10–12 yr 12–14 yr >14 yr Postmenopause	Male ng/dL 26–72 29–66 53–135 183–383 240–520 307–835	Female ng/dL 19–42 73–165 74–180 234–529 224–611 282–771 30–450	Male nmol/L 0.9–2.5 1–2.3 1.8–4.7 6.3–12.3 8.3–18 10.6–29	Female nmol/L 0.7–1.5 2.5–5.7 2.6–6.2 8.1–18.3 7.8–21.2 9.8–26.7 1–15.6
Dehydroepiandros-terone Sulfate (DHEAS)	Serum	Age 1–8 yr 8–10 yr 10–12 yr 12–14 yr 14–16 yr >16 yr Postmenopause Pregnancy (term)	Male µg/dL 6–15 34–54 25–43 76–138 138–234 199–334	Female µg/dL 6–15 34–54 53–136 70–169 138–234 82–338 17–77 23–117	Male µmol/L 0.16–0.4 0.9–1.4 0.7–1.1 2.0–3.6 3.6–6.1 5.2–8.7	Female µmol/L 0.16–0.4 0.9–1.4 1.4–3.5 1.8–4.4 3.6–6.1 2.1–8.8 0.4–2 0.6–3
Dihydrotestosterone	Serum	Age Prepubertal Adult	Male ng/dL <3–13 30–300	Female ng/dL <3–10 6–33	Male nmol/L <0.1–0.4 1–10.4	Female nmol/L <0.1–0.3 0.2–1.1
Erythropoietin	Serum	4–26 mIU/mL			4–26 IU/L	
Estradiol	Serum	Age Prepubertal 8–12 yr 12–14 yr 14–16 yr Adult Early follicular Preovulatory Luteal Postmenopause	Male pg/mL < 10 16.8–23.2 20–50	Female pg/mL < 7 8.2–17.8 16–34 20–68 20–100 100–500 100–500 10–301	Male pmol/L < 37 62–85 62–184	Female pmol/L < 26 30–65 59–125 73–250 73–367 367–1836 367–1836 37–110
Estriol (Pregnancy)	Serum	Week of Gestation 30–32 33–35 36–38 39–40	ng/mL 2–12 3–19 5–27 10–30	nmol/L 7–42 10–66 17–94 35–104		
	Male and nonpregnant female: <2 ng/mL		<7 nmol/L			
Estrone	Serum	Male pg/mL 10–50	Female pg/mL Follicular 30–100 Ovulatory >150 Luteal 90–160 Postmenopausal 20–40		Male pmol/L 37–185	Female pmol/L 111–370 >555 333–592 74–148
Follicle-Stimulating Hormone (FSH)	Serum	Male 2–17 mIU/mL	Female 4–20 mIU/mL		Male 2–17 IU/L	Female 4–20 IU/L
Gastrin (No heparin, store at −20 °C.)	Serum	<200 pg/mL			<52 pmol/L	

(*continued*)

Test	Source	Value: Per ML or DL	Value: SI Units[2]
Glucagon (Centrifuge immediately under refrigeration, store in plastic vial at −20 °C.)	Plasma	50–200 pg/mL	14–57 pmol/L
Growth Hormone (Store at −20 °C.)	Serum (fasting)	Children <10 ng/mL Adults <5 ng/mL	<465 pmol/L <232 pmol/L
17-Hydroxycorticoids (Preservative: 10 mL 6N HCl)	Urine	Male: 3–15 mg/24 h Female: 2–12 mg/24 h (or 3–7 mg/g creatinine)	8.3–41.4 μmol/24 h 5.5–33 μmol/24 h (or 0.9–2.2 mmol/mol creatinine)

17-Hydroxypregnenolone — Serum

	ng/dL	nmol/L
Prepubertal child:	<100	<3.2
Adult male:	40–250	1.3–8
Adult female:	20–400	0.6–13

Test	Source	Value: Per ML or DL	Value: SI Units[2]
17-Hydroxyprogesterone	Serum	10–300 ng/dL	0.3–9.5 nmol/L
Hydroxyproline (Preservative: 25 mL 6N HCl)	Urine	Total: 25–77 mg/d Free: <2 mg/24 h	191–588 nmol/24h <15 nmol/24h

Insulin (fasting) — Serum (Cold centrifuge, freeze at −20 °C.)

	μU/mL	ng/mL	pmol/L
Newborn:	3–20	0.12–.8	21–138
Adult:	5–25	0.2–1	34–172

Insulin (with oral glucose tolerance test) — Serum

	μU/mL	ng/mL	pmol/L
0 min:	7–24	0.28–.96	48–165
30 min:	25–231	0.96–9.4	165–1618
1 hr:	18–276	0.72–11	124–1893
2 hr:	16–166	0.64–6.6	110–1136
3 hr:	4–38	0.16–1.5	28–258

17-Ketosteroids — Urine (Preservative: 10 mL 6N HCl)

Age	mg/24h	nmol/24h
0–8 yr:	0–1	0–3.5
8 yr-puberty:	1–10	3.5–35
Adult male:	9–22	31–76
Adult female:	5–15	17–52

Luteinizing Hormone — Serum (hCG will interfere with the measurement of LH in most assays. Freeze specimen at −20 °C.)

	mIU/mL	IU/L
Male:	4–18	4–18
Female:		
Premenopause	5–25	5–25
Postmenopause	30–200	30–200

Test	Source	Value: Per ML or DL	Value: SI Units[2]
Metanephrine (total) (Preservative: 30 mL 6N HCl)	Urine	0.3–0.9 mg/24 h	1.5–4.5 nmol/24 h
Osmolality	Serum Urine	285–293 mosm/kg 300–900 mosm/kg	
Pancreatic Polypeptide (Process immediately and freeze plasma at −60 °C.)	Plasma	<350 pg/mL	<86 pmol/L
Parathyroid Hormone (Intact hormone assay: Freeze serum at −20 °C.)	Serum	11–54 pg/mL	1.2–5.6 pmol/L

Pregnenetriol — 24-hr urine

Age	mg/24 h	μmol/24 h
0–3 yr:	<0.2	<.06
3–12 yr:	<1	<2.8
>12 yr:	<2	<5.5

(*continued*)

Test	Source	Value: Per ML or DL			Value: SI Units[2]	

Progesterone
 	
(Freeze at −20 °C.)
	Serum	Female:
		  Follicular phase:
		  Luteal phase:
		Male:
			ng/mL
			0.3–0.8
			4–20
			0.12–0.3
					pmol/L
					0.9–2.3
					11.6–58
					0.3–0.9	

Prolactin (Freeze serum at −20 °C.)	Serum	 Newborn 1–5 mo Childhood Adult	Female ng/mL 141–189 6–14 4–8 <20	Male ng/mL 141–189 6–14 4–8 <15	Female nmol/L 6.4–8.6 0.27–0.64 0.18–0.36 <0.9	Male nmol/L 6.4–8.6 0.27–0.64 0.18–0.36 <0.7
Renin	Plasma	8 AM recumbent: 3.4 ± 0.7 ng/mL/h 12 N upright: 8.8 ± 1.7 ng/mL/h			0.97 ± 0.19 ng/(L/s) 2.44 ± 0.47 ng/(L/s)	
(Draw in cold tube, separate plasma, and freeze in plastic within 15 min of collection.)						
Semen Analysis (See Table 16–3.)						
Somatomedin C **(SM-C, IGF-I)** (Freeze at −20 °C. Results with plasma are 10–15% higher.)	Serum or Plasma	Age 0–3 yr 3–6 yr 6–10 yr 10–13 yr 13–16 yr 16–18 yr >18 yr	Male ng/mL 14–56 13–81 29–108 102–182 98–319 136–293 43–178	Female ng/mL 14–60 18–97 34–137 104–374 192–347 132–305 24–153	Male U/mL 0.1–0.4 0.1–0.6 0.2–0.8 0.7–1.3 0.7–2.3 1.0–2.1 0.3–1.3	Female U/mL 0.1–0.4 0.1–0.7 0.2–1 0.7–2.7 1.4–2.5 0.9–2.2 0.2–1.1
Testosterone, total (Freeze at −20 °C.)	Serum	 ng/dL Prepubertal Pubertal Adult	Male 8–14 84–180 300–1000	Female 5–13 9–24 30–70	nmol/L Male 0.28–0.49 2.91–6.24 10.4–34.7	Female 0.17–0.45 0.31–0.83 1.04–2.43
Testosterone, free (Freeze at −20 °C.)	Serum	 Adult Male Adult Female	pg/mL 80–280 3–13		pmol/L 69.3–970.9 10.4–45.1	

Thyroglobulin
 	
	Serum	Normal: <40 ng/mL
		After Total Thyroidectomy:
		  on T_4: <5 ng/mL
		  off T_4: <10 ng/mL
					<40 µg/L
					
					<5 µg/L
					<10 µg/L	

(Freeze at −20 °C. The presence of thyroglobulin autoantibodies in the patient's serum may falsely lower the result.)						
Thyroid Auto- **antibodies** (Freeze at −20 °C.)	Serum	Microsomal antibodies: titer <100 Thyroglobulin antibodies: titer <10				
Thyroxine-Binding **Globulin**	Serum	16–34 µg/mL			16–34 mg/L	
Thyroid-Stimulating **Hormone (TSH)**	Serum	0.4–4.8 µU/mL			0–4.8 mU/L	
(Neonatal and cord blood levels are 2–4 times higher.)						
Thyroid-Stimulating **Immunoglobulin** **(TSI)** (Freeze at −20 °C.)	Serum	Negative = <2 µU TSH equivalent/mL. 2–3 µU TSH/mL = equivocal. Based on cAMP generation in thyroid cell tissue culture.				

Thyroid Uptake of
Radioactive Iodine
(RAIU)
	Activity over
	  thyroid gland
		Fractional uptake: 2 hr: 4–12%
		                  6 hr: 6–15%
		                 24 hr: 8–30%				

(Ingestion or administration of iodide will decrease thyroid uptake of RAI.)						

(*continued*)

Test	Source	Value: Per ML or DL		Value: SI Units[2]
Thyroxine (T$_4$)	Serum	Age	μg/dL	nmol/L
		Cord Blood	4.6–13	59.2–167
		1–3 d	11.8–23.2	151.9–298.6
		3–10 d	9.9–21.9	127.4–281.9
		10–45d	8.2–16.2	105.5–208.5
		45–90 d	6.4–14	82.4–180.2
		3–12 mo	7.8–16.5	100.4–212.4
		1–5 yr	7.3–15	94–193.1
		5–10 yr	6.4–13.3	82.4–171.2
		10–15 yr	5.6–11.7	72.1–150.5
		15–20 yr	4.2–11.8	54.1–151.9
		>20 yr	5–12	64.4–154.4
(Refrigerate serum. Fasting preferred. Elevated levels in pregnancy due to increased TBG.)				
Thyroxine, free (F T$_4$)	Serum	0.9–1.7 ng/dL		11.5–21.8 pmol/L
Resin T$_3$ Uptake (RT3U)	Serum	25–35%		0.25–0.35
Free Thyroxine Index	Serum	(Product of T$_4$ × RT3U) = 1.3–4.2 arbitrary units		
		(Expressed as T$_4$ adjusted for TBG-binding) = 5–12 arbitrary units		
Thyroxine: TBG Ratio	Serum	T$_4$ (μg/dL)/TBG (μg/mL) = 0.2–0.5		T$_4$ (nmol/L)/TBG (mg/L) = 2.7–6.4
Triiodothyronine (T$_3$)	Serum	Age	ng/dL	nmol/L
		Cord blood	15–75	0.23–1.2
		1–3 d	32–216	0.49–3.3
		3–30 d	50–250	0.77–3.8
		1–12 mo	105–280	1.6–4.3
		1–5 yr	105–269	1.6–4.1
		5–10 yr	94–241	1.4–3.7
		10–15 yr	83–213	1.3–3.3
		15–20 yr	80–210	1.2–3.2
		>20 yr	95–190	1.5–2.9
(Refrigerate serum. Elevated levels in pregnancy due to increased TBG.)				
Free T$_3$ Index (F T$_3$ I)	Serum	(Expressed as product of T$_3$ × RT3U) = 24–67 (arbitrary units)		
Free T$_3$ (F T$_3$)	Serum	0.2–0.52 ng/dL		3–8 pmol/L
Reverse T$_3$ (RT$_3$)	Serum	25–75 ng/dL		0.39–1.15 nmol/L
Vanillylmandelic Acid (VMA)	Urine (24 hr)	Age	mg/d	nmol/d
		Newborn	<1	<5.8
		Infant	<2	<11.7
		Child	1–3	5.8–17.6
		Adolescent	1–5	5.8–29.4
		Adult	2–7	11.8–41.2
	Urine (24 hr or "spot")		μVMA/mg creatinine	nmol VMA/nmol creatinine
		1–12 mo	<36	<24
		1–2 yr	<31	<20.5
		2–5 yr	<17	<11.3
		5–10 yr	<15	<10
		>10 yr	<11	<7.4
Vasoactive Intestinal Peptide (Freeze at −60 °C.)	Plasma	<70 pg/mL		<21 pmol/L
Vitamin D (25 Hydroxy)	Serum	10–50 ng/mL		25–126 nmol/L
(Measures both D2 and D3. Freeze serum in plastic tube at −20 °C.)				
Vitamin D (1,25 Di-Hydroxy)	Serum	20–76 pg/mL		48–184 pmol/L
(Measures both D2 and D3. Freeze serum at −60 °C in plastic tube.)				

[1]These normal values are taken from the *Clinical Laboratories Manual* of the University of California Hospitals and Clinics, San Francisco, California, August 10, 1988. The factors used in converting conventional units to Système International d'Unites (SI units) were derived, in part, from the *CRC Handbook of Chemistry and Physics.* It is important to emphasize that normal ranges vary among different laboratories; it is essential for the clinician to know the normal range for the test of interest in the laboratory performing the test.

[2]SI units = Système International Units (*JAMA* 1985;**253:**2553–2554).

Index

Fructose, diabetic patient and, 617
FSH. *See* Follicle-stimulating
hormone
Furosemide
for hypercalcemia, 281–82
for SIADH, 186

GABA. *See* Gamma-aminobutyric
acid
Galactopoiesis, 556
Galactorrhea
amenorrhea with, 467
prolactinomas and, 114
Galactorrhea-amenorrhea syndromes,
113
Gallbladder disease, oral contraceptives and, 486
Gamma-aminobutyric acid (GABA),
prolactin secretion and, 89
Ganglioneuromatosis, gastrointestinal, 730
Gangrene of feet, diabetic patients
and, 645
Gastrectomy, alimentary hypoglycemia due to, 661
Gastric inhibitory polypeptide (GIP),
577
distribution of, 573
duodenal ulcer and, 583
major action of, 570
Gastric outlet obstruction, basal hypergastrinemia and, 582–83
Gastrin, 573–75
distribution of, 573
major action of, 570
normal test results for, 758
serum, measurement of, 585
Gastrinoma, 584–86
basal hypergastrinemia and, 582
clinical findings in, 584–85
diagnosis of, 585
treatment of, 585–86
Gastrin-releasing peptide (GRP), 581
distribution of, 573
duodenal ulcer and, 583
major action of, 570
Gastrointestinal ganglioneuromatosis,
730
Gastrointestinal tract
disorders of
hormonal abnormalities in, 582–
88
motility, 583–84
oral contraceptives and, 486
eicosanoids and, 60
hormones of, 569–88
delivery of, 569–70
distribution of, 572, 573
mechanisms of action of, 570–
71
structure of, 571
ulcers of, eicosanoids and, 64
Gastroparesis, diabetic, 644, 656
Gemfibrozil, for hyperlipoproteinemia, 689

Genes
chromosomal, molecular cloning
and, 31
cloned, transfer into mammalian
cells, 31–32
evolution of, 25–26
expression of, 20–24
initial steps in, 23
regulation of, 24–25
families of, 25–26
structure of, 22–24
therapy with, 36
Genetic disease
diagnosis using DNA, 34–35
mechanisms of, 26
Genetic markers, 35
Genetic polymorphisms, 34–35
Genital ducts, differentiation of, 495–
97
Genitalia
ambiguous
degenerative renal disease and,
515
management of patients with,
516–18
external, differentiation of, 497,
498
male
normal, androgen resistance in
men with, 513–14
stages of development of, 522
Genitourinary system
female, menopause and, 479
infections of, male infertility and,
434
Geriatric endocrinology, 741–54
Germ cell tumors, 437–38
Germinal epithelium, 443
Germinoma, 465
Gestational diabetes, 562
diagnosis of, 562
management of, 563
GIF. *See* Glucocorticoid-increasing
factor
Gigantism, 118–24, 143–44
cerebral, 173
clinical findings in, 119–21
diagnosis of, 122
differential diagnosis of, 122–23
etiology and pathogenesis of, 118
pathology of, 118
pathophysiology of, 118–19
pituitary, 174
treatment of, 123–24
GIP. *See* Gastric inhibitory
polypeptide
Glibenclamide (DiaBeta, Micronase),
for diabetes mellitus, 619
Glipizide (Glucotrol)
for diabetes mellitus, 619
hypoglycemia due to, 656
Glucagon, 598–99
action of, 599
amino acid sequence of, 598
biochemistry of, 598–99
enzymes induced/repressed by, 604

fuel metabolism and, 601–5
hypoglycemia and, 651–52
normal test results for, 758
secretion of, 599
Glucagonoma, 586–87
Glucagon stimulation test
insulinoma and, 658
pheochromocytoma and, 394
Glucocorticoid-increasing factor
(GIF), hypothalamic-
pituitary-adrenal-thymic
axis and, 50
Glucocorticoid regulatory element
(GRE), 24
Glucocorticoids, 323–59
action of, regulatory structure mediating, 25
adrenal adenomas secreting, 349
agonists of, 332
antagonists of, 332
biologic effects of, 331–34
brain function and, 77
deficiency of, familial, adrenal insufficiency in, 341–42
effects on tissues, 333–34
for hirsutism in women, 473
for hypercalcemia, 281
immune response and, 45
intermediary metabolism and, 332–
33
osteoporosis and, 307
postnatal growth and, 152
pregnancy and, 551–52
receptors for, 331–32
stress and, 752–53
Glucocorticoid suppression test, primary hyperparathyroidism
and, 278–79
Glucose
blood, testing of, 612–13
cellular uptake of, hormones and,
15
metabolism of, glucocorticoids
and, 332
Glucose-dependent insulin-releasing
polypeptide, 577
Glucose-growth hormone suppression
test, hypothalamic-pituitary
function and, 99
Glucose suppression test, acromegaly
and, 122
Glucose tolerance test
intravenous, 615
oral, 614–15
insulinoma and, 658
Glucotrol. *See* Glipizide
γ-Glutamyltranspeptidase, 57
Glutathione-S-transferase, 57
Glyburide (DiaBeta, Micronase)
for diabetes mellitus, 619
hypoglycemia due to, 656
Glycemic index, 616–17
Glycogen
phosphorylation-dephosphorylation
of, 601, 603
synthesis and breakdown of, 17